Lecture Notes in Computer Science 7946

Commenced Publication in 1973
Founding and Former Series Editors:
Gerhard Goos, Juris Hartmanis, and Jan van Leeuwen

Andreas Holzinger   Martina Ziefle
Martin Hitz   Matjaž Debevc (Eds.)

Human Factors
in Computing
and Informatics

First International Conference, SouthCHI 2013
Maribor, Slovenia, July 1-3, 2013
Proceedings

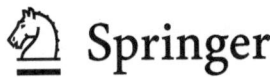 Springer

Volume Editors

Andreas Holzinger
Medical University of Graz (MUG)
Institute for Medical Informatics, Statistics and Documentation (IMI)
Auenbruggerplatz 2/V, 8036, Graz, Austria
E-mail: andreas.holzinger@medunigraz.at

Martina Ziefle
RWTH Aachen University, Human-Computer Interaction Center
Theaterplatz 14, 52056 Aachen, Germany
E-mail: ziefle@comm.rwth-aachen.de

Martin Hitz
Alpen-Adria-Universität Klagenfurt, Institute of Informatics Systems
Universitätsstrasse 65-67, 9020, Klagenfurt, Austria
E-mail: martin.hitz@aau.at

Matjaž Debevc
University of Maribor, Faculty of Electrical Engineering and Computer Science
Smetanova 17, 2000 Maribor, Slovenia
E-mail: matjaz.debevc@um.si

ISSN 0302-9743   e-ISSN 1611-3349
ISBN 978-3-642-39061-6   e-ISBN 978-3-642-39062-3
DOI 10.1007/978-3-642-39062-3
Springer Heidelberg Dordrecht London New York

Library of Congress Control Number: 2013940616

CR Subject Classification (1998): H.4-5, D.2, C.2, I.2, J.3, K.4.2

LNCS Sublibrary: SL 2 – Programming and Software Engineering

Typesetting: Camera-ready by author, data conversion by Scientific Publishing Services, Chennai, India

Printed on acid-free paper

Springer is part of Springer Science+Business Media (www.springer.com)

Preface

The field of Human–Computer Interaction (HCI) has been extremely successful for the last 30 years, especially when it comes to changing computing to the benefit of end users. Advanced mobile, ubiquitous, and pervasive computing have dramatically changed the way we *interact with information,* which turns "human factors" into an essential part of computer science and informatics in all areas of our daily life. SouthCHI – the International Conference on Human Factors in Computing & Informatics (formerly USAB), is dedicated to this field and particularly wants to build a bridge between experts from Southern Europe with the world.

SouthCHI is the successor of the well-established USAB Conference series, which was born in 2005 at Vienna University of Technology, Austria, when it took place as the "First USABility Symposium" with Ben Shneiderman as the first keynote speaker. Whereas the USAB series always focused on a certain topic, e.g., on Information Quality in e-Health in 2011, the SouthCHI conference series promotes all aspects of HCI and usability engineering – which was a big wish from the participants of the USAB series and took shape during USAB 2010 at the Alpen-Adria-Universität Klagenfurt, where the idea arose of organizing such a conference particularly to connect experts from the southern countries of Europe with the whole world.

This first event was organized in Maribor, Slovenia, the European Capital of Culture 2012. The conference was organized by the University of Maribor and supported by the world's largest computing organizations: IEEE and ACM.

HCI is important in all application domains, including medical and life sciences, automotive industry, social media, Web 2.0 etc., which are rapidly increasing in popularity and importance, particularly in South and South-Eastern European countries and thus are bringing about fundamental changes in the area of user-friendly computer-supported tools. With their multi- and interdisciplinary approach and research, solutions are becoming essential in modern human work and life.

HCI is an interdisciplinary profession/field and requires the ability to communicate with professionals from other disciplines and the willingness to accept and incorporate also their points of view. Consequently, SouthCHI 2013 was organized so as to promote a close collaboration between scientists, engineers, industrial and business representatives, and experts from the regions of Alpe-Adria, South and South-East Europe as well as Mediterranean countries with the "rest of the world." This was a unique opportunity to meet experts from around the world for networking and discussing business opportunities, in order to gain new connections, knowledge, and possibilities of exchanging expertise. The main mission of this conference, therefore, is to build this bridge between people from Central and Southern Europe and other countries.

SouthCHI 2013 received a total of 169 submissions. We followed a careful and rigorous two-level, double-blind review scheme, assigning each paper to a minimum of three and maximum of six reviewers from our international scientific board. On the basis of the reviews, only 38 full papers were accepted (resulting in an acceptance rate of approx. 22 %). Additionally, 12 short papers, four posters, and three doctoral thesis papers were accepted; i.e. 57 regular papers plus 2 keynote lectures from 30 countries: Austria, Belgium, Canada, China, Croatia, Cyprus, Czech Republic, Denmark, Finland, Germany, Greece, India, Ireland, Italy, Japan, The Netherlands, Norway, Poland, Portugal, Romania, Saudi Arabia, Slovenia, Spain, Sweden, Switzerland, Taiwan, Tunisia, Turkey, UK, and USA.

The organizers see SouthCHI as a bridge within the scientific community, between various technological disciplines as well as social sciences that meets end users' needs and brings them benefits and values. The people who gathered together to work for this conference showed great enthusiasm and dedication.

We cordially thank each and every person who contributed toward making SouthCHI 2013 a success, for their participation and commitment: the authors, reviewers, partners, organizations, supporters, the team of the Institute of Media Communication from University of Maribor, Slovenia, the team from the Research Unit Human–Computer Interaction for Medicine and Health Care (HCI4MED) of the Institute of Medical Informatics, Statistics and Documentation of the Medical University Graz, Austria, the team at the Alpen-Adria-Universität Klagenfurt, Austria and all the volunteers; without their help, this bridge would never have been built.

July 2013

Andreas Holzinger
Martina Ziefle
Martin Hitz
Matjaž Debevc

Organization

General Chairs

Matjaž Debevc   University of Maribor, Slovenia
Martin Hitz   Alpen-Adria-Universität Klagenfurt,
Austria

Program Chairs

Andreas Holzinger   Medical University of Graz, Austria
Martina Ziefle   RWTH Aachen University, Germany
Vlado Glavinić   Zagreb University, Croatia

Program Committee

Julio Abascal   University of the Basque Country, Spain
Sheikh Iqbal Ahamed   Marquette University, USA
David Ahlström   Alpe-Adria-Universität Klagenfurt,
Austria
Henning Andersen   Technical University Denmark,
Denmark
Russell Beale   Birmingham University, UK
Marilyn Sue Bogner   Institute of Study of Human Error, LLC
Bethesda, USA
John N. A Brown   EMJD ICE, Austria
John M. Carroll   Pennsylvania State University, USA
Tiziana Catarci   Università di Roma La Sapienza, Italy
Luca Chittaro   University of Udine, Italy
Remy Choquet   Université Paris, France
Andy Cockburn   University of Canterbury, New Zealand
Alireza Darvishy   ZHAW, Zürich, Switzerland
Matjaz Debevc   University of Maribor, Slovenia
Paloma Diaz   University Carlos III Madrid, Spain
Alan Dix   Lancaster University, UK
Pier Luigi Emiliani   National Research Council, Italy
Jan Engelen   Katholieke Universiteit Leuven, Belguim
Kapetanios Epaminondas   University of Westminster, London, UK
Paolo Federico   Vienna University of Technology,
Austria

Alexandru Floares   Oncological Institute Cluj-Napoca,
                                         Romania
Jonathan Freeman   Goldsmiths University of London, UK
Adinda Freudenthal   Technical University Delft,
                                         The Netherlands
Qiang Gao   Beihang University, China
Vlado Glavinic   University of Zagreb, Croatia
Sabine Graf   Athabasca University, Canada
Andrina Granic   University of Split, Croatia
Eduard Groeller   Vienna University of Technology,
                                         Austria
Lisa Gualtieri   Tufts University School of Medicine
                                         Boston, USA
Sissel Guttormsen Schaer   University Bern, Switzerland
Martin Hitz   Alpen-Adria-Universität Klagenfurt,
                                         Austria
Timo Honkela   Helsinki University of Technology,
                                         Finland
Bin Hu   Birmingham City University, UK
Bo Hu   SAP Research Belfast, UK
Ebba P. Hvannberg   University of Iceland, Reykjavik,
                                         Republic of Iceland
Homa Javahery   IBM Centers for Solution Innovation,
                                         Canada
Chris Johnson   University of Glasgow, UK
Gregor Jošt   University of Maribor, Slovenia
Kinshuk   Athabasca University, Canada
Jiří Klema   Czech Technical University, Prague,
                                         Czech Republic
Katja Kous   University of Maribor, Slovenia
Mihael Kukec   Polytechnic of Varazdin, Croatia
Effie Lai-Chong Law   University of Leicester, UK
Denise Leahy   Trinity College Dublin, Ireland
Gerhard Leitner   Alpen-Adria-Universität Klagenfurt,
                                         Austria
ZongKai Lin   Chinese Academy of Science Peking,
                                         China
Sandi Ljubić   University of Rijeka, Croatia
Luca Longo   Trinity College Dublin, Ireland
Suzana Loshkovska   University of Skopje, The former
                                         Yugoslav Republic of Macedonia
András Lukacs   Hungarian Academy of Sciences, University
                                         Budapest, Hungary
Ljiljana Majnaric-Trtica   Josip Juraj Strossmayer University,
                                         Osijek, Croatia
Flora Malamateniou   University of Pireaus, Greece

Marino Menozzi	ETH Zürich, Switzerland
Silvia Miksch	Vienna University of Technology, Vienna, Austria
Małgorzata Moleda	Warsaw School of Economics, Poland
Antonio Moreno-Ribas	Universitat Rovira i Virgili, Tarragona, Spain
Danijela Milošević	University of Kragujevac, Serbia
Shogo Nishida	Osaka University, Japan
Hiromu Nishitani	University of Tokushima, Japan
Nuno J.Nunes	University of Madeira, Portugal
Anne-Sophie Nyssen	Université de Liege, Belgium
Patricia Ordonez-Rozo	University of Maryland, Baltimore County, Baltimore, USA
Ant Ozok	UMBC Baltimore, USA
Jan Paralic	Technical University of Kosice, Slovakia
Gabriella Pasi	Università di Milano Bicocca, Milan, Italy
Vimla Patel	Arizona State University, USA
Helen Petrie	University of York, UK
Armando J.,Pinho	Universidade the Aveiro, Portugal
Maja Pivec	University of Applied Sciences, Graz, Austria
Margit Pohl	Vienna University of Technology, Austria
Gregor Polančič	University of Maribor, Slovenia
Robert W. Proctor	Purdue University, USA
Heri Ramampiaro	Norwegian University of Science and Technology, Norway
Harald Reiterer	University of Konstanz, Germany
Yvonne Rogers	University College Londen (UCL), UK
Demetrios Sampson	University of Piraeus, Greece
Giuseppe Santucci	La Sapienza, University of Rome, Italy
Anthony Savidis	ICS FORTH, Heraklion, Greece
Albrecht Schmidt	Fraunhofer IAIS/B-IT, University of Bonn, Germany
Gig Searle	Medical University Graz, Austria
Paola Sebastiani	Boston University, USA
Ahmed Seffah	Troyes University of Technology, France
Klaus-Martin Simonic	Medical University Graz, Austria
Andrzej Skowron	University of Warsaw, Poland
Neil R. Smalheiser	University of Illinois at Chicago, USA
Snežana Šćepanović	University Mediterranean, Montenegro
Hironomu Takagi	Tokyo Research Laboratory, IBM, Japan
Harold Thimbleby	University of Swansea, UK

Geoff Underwood   Nottingham University, UK
William Wong   Middlesex University, London, UK
Pinar Yildirim   Okan University, Istanbul, Turkey
Panayiotis Zaphiris   University of Cyprus, Cyprus
Jiajie Zhang   University of Texas Health Science
                         Center, USA
Ping Zhang   Syracuse University, USA
Minlu Zhang   University of Cincinnati, USA
Xuezhong Zhou   Beijing Jiaotong University, China
Martina Ziefle   RWTH Aachen University, Germany

External Reviewers

Richard Coshott   Gamercize, USA
George Demiris   Washington University, USA
Joost van Hoof   Fontys University of Applied Sciences,
                         The Netherlands
Sheryl Flynn   Blue Marble Game Company, USA
Lynne Coventry   University of Northumbria, UK
Ralf Klamma   RWTH Aachen University, Germany
Ulrik Schroeder   RWTH Aachen University, Germany
Tom Langhorst   Fontys University of Applied Sciences,
                         The Netherlands
Hannah Marston   German Sport University Cologne,
                         Germany
Philippe Brauner   RWTH Aachen University, Germany
Martina Ziefle   RWTH Aachen University, Germany
André Calero-Valdez   RWTH Aachen University, Germany
Anne Kathrin Schaar   RWTH Aachen University, Germany
Beul Shirley   RWTH Aachen University, Germany
Felix Heidrich   RWTH Aachen University, Germany
Bob de Schutter   Group T e-Media lab, Belgium
Zijlstra Wiebren   German Sport University Cologne,
                         Germany
Barbara Chamberlin   New Mexico State University, USA
Stuart Smith   Neuroscience Research Australia,
                         Australia

Organizing Committee

Matjaž Debevc   University of Maribor, Slovenia
Simon Hauptman   University of Maribor, Slovenia
Ines Kožuh   University of Maribor, Slovenia

David Podgorelec   University of Maribor, Slovenia
Borut Žalik   University of Maribor, Slovenia
Suzana Žilič Fišer   University of Maribor, Slovenia

Special Session on Design Culture for Ageing Well: Designing for »Situated Elderliness«(DCAW)

Chairs

Özge Subasi   HCI Group, Vienna University of
                         Technology, Vienna, Austria
Geraldine Fitzpatrick   HCI Group, Vienna University of
                         Technology, Vienna, Austria
Lone Malmborg   The IT University of Copenhagen,
                         Denmark
Britt Östlund   Rehabiliation Engineering, Design
                         Sciences, Lund University, Sweden

International Scientific Committee

Marie Ertner   IT University of Copenhagen, Denmark
Geraldine Fitzpatrick   Vienna University of Technology,
                        Austria
Jean Hallewell   Fachhochschule Wels, Austria
Dave Harley   University of Brighton, UK
Michael Leitner   Northumbria University, UK
Charlotte Magnusson   Lund University, Sweden
Lone Malmborg   IT University of Copenhagen, Denmark
Francisco Nunes   Vienna University of Technology,
                        Austria
Kirsten Rassmu-Gröhn   Lund University, Sweden
Marjo Rauhala   Vienna University of Technology,
                        Austria
Tomas Sokoler   IT University of Copenhagen, Denmark
Özge Subasi   Vienna University of Technology,
                        Austria
Britt Östlund   Lund University, Sweden
John Vines   Northumbria University, UK

Workshop for Assessing the State of HCI Research and Practice in South-Eastern Europe (WS-HCI-SEE)

Chair

Bojan Blažica   Xlab, Slovenia

International Scientific Committee

Bojan Blažica	Xlab, Slovenia
Ciril Bohak	University of Ljubljana, Slovenia
Luka Čehovin	University of Ljubljana, Slovenia
Jože Guna	University of Ljubljana, Slovenia
Gerhard Leitner	Alpen-Adria-Universität Klagenfurt, Austria
Matevž Pesek	University of Ljubljana, Slovenia
Domen Tabernik	University of Ljubljana, Slovenia

Partners

We are grateful to the following companies and institutions for their support in our aims to bridge science and industry. Their logos are displayed on our conference website: http://southchi.org/sponsors

Keynote Speaker 1: Prof. Dr. Helwig Hauser

Biographical Note

Helwig Hauser is professor at the University of Bergen in Norway, where he leads a research group on visualization in the Department of Informatics since 2007. Before that, he was the scientific director of the VRVis Research Center in Vienna, Austria, where he cared about many projects in collaboration of science and industry. Helwig Hauser graduated in 1998 from Vienna University of Technology, Austria, with a PhD thesis on the visualization of dynamical systems. He then worked at the Institute of Computer Graphics and Algorithms (TU Wien) as assistant, first, and then as assistant professor, before he changed to the newly founded VRVis Research Center in 2000. In 2004, he finished his habilitation at TU Wien with a thesis entitled "Generalizing Focus+Context Visualization" – in 2006 this work was awarded with the Heinz-Zemanek Preis from OCG (given every two years for exceptional works in computer science or a related area). Prof. Hauser is a visualization researcher and teacher since the mid-1990s with a focus on scientific visualization, information visualization, visual analytics, etc., and he enjoys exercising his research in the context of several different application domains (including medicine, geosciences, engineering, biology, climatology, etc.). He was/is member of the Editorial Boards of the major visualization journals, including IEEE Transactions on Visualization and Computer Graphics and Computer Graphics Forum by Eurographics. Prof. Hauser is also member of several Steering Boards, including the EuroVis Steering Committee. Frequently, he is invited to talk about his research (in particular about interactive visual analysis), repeatedly also as keynote speaker. Regularly, Helwig Hauser chaired/chairs central visualization events, e.g., TopoInVis 2011, EuroVis 2011, PacificVis 2012, and IEEE InfoVis 2013, more recently.

Lecture: Integrating Interactive and Computational Analysis in Visualization

In our emerging information age it becomes important that we can exploit the wealth of available data for the sake of learning, decision making and other tasks. A promising approach – not at the least targeted by the new concept of visual analytics in visualization research – is to cleverly integrate the strengths of computers (fast computation, efficient handling of large datasets, comparably low costs, etc.) with the strengths of the users (outstanding perceptual and cognitive capabilities, domain knowledge, etc.). In this talk, we look at one possible solution, originating in visualization research within computer science, i.e., the concept of interactive visual analysis, and describe it as an iterative process, enabling the integration of computational and interactive means for data exploration and analysis. Thinking of interactive visual analysis as an iterative process enables that each step is performed on the basis of a toolbox with computational and interactive visual solutions. In order to substantiate the conceptual aspects of this solution, we also look at several examples that document the successful application of interactive visual analysis.

Keynote Speaker 2: Dr. rer. nat. Dr. phil. Norbert A. Streitz

Biographical Note

Dr. Dr. Norbert Streitz (Ph.D. in physics, Ph.D. in psychology) is a Senior Scientist and Strategic Advisor with more than 30 years of experience in information and communication technology. He is the founder and scientific director of the Smart Future Initiative (SFI) which was launched in January 2009. From 1987 - 2008, he was at the Fraunhofer Institute IPSI in Darmstadt, Germany, where he held different positions as Division Manager and Deputy Director. Prominent examples of his activities are the user-centered design and development of cooperative hypermedia systems, local and distributed electronic meeting rooms, ubiquitous computing, ambient intelligence, and smart environments. Roomware ® - the integration of furniture, walls, doors, etc. with information technology became much cited pioneering work in these areas. He also taught at the Department of Computer Science of the Technical University Darmstadt for more than 15 years. Before joining IPSI in Darmstadt, he was an Assistant Professor at the Technical University Aachen (RWTH), Germany, teaching and doing research in cognitive science and human-computer interaction and founding the ACCEPT-Group (AaChen Cognitive Ergonomics ProjecT). This was preceded by his work in elementary particle physics and general relativity theory at the University of Kiel, Germany. Furthermore, he was a post-doc research fellow at the University of California, Berkeley, USA, a visiting scholar at Xerox PARC, USA, and at the Intelligent Systems Lab of MITI, Tsukuba Science City, Japan. He is regularly asked to present keynote speeches and tutorials at scientific as well as commercial events in Europe, USA, South America, Middle East (Qatar), Malaysia, Singapore, Hongkong, China, Korea and Japan.

Lecture: Smart Cities as New Challenges for Human-Centered Design

Having entered what is being called the Urban Age, where more than half of the world population is living in cities, economic prosperity and quality of life will largely depend on the abilities of cities to reach their full potential. One important dimension is the information technology perspective deploying appropriate infrastructures and providing ambient intelligence-based support for smart urban living. Real urban spaces become increasingly interactive spaces reflecting social networks created in the virtual world now also again in the real world. Since the origin and initial meaning of social networks derive from real world encounters one could label this "a return trip to the real world". At the same time, it shows the importance of real human beings living in a real world. Combining these information and experience spaces with ubiquitous and ambient computing in urban contexts constitutes what we are calling a "smart hybrid city".

This keynote talk addresses issues and challenges for designing ambient intelligence environments in urban contexts, especially from a human-environment interaction perspective. This includes the shift from information design to experience design, spreading social communication behavior from virtual worlds back into real spaces, and the relevance of hybrid symmetric interaction. We are arguing for a people-oriented, empowering smartness where smart spaces make people smarter by keeping the human in the loop. The implications of sensor-enriched – one could also call them "sensor-polluted" - smart environments will be discussed (e.g., availability and use of location-based services), because they reach a new dimension, especially with respect to privacy. Privacy is endangered to become a commodity people have to pay for and thus a privilege. Privacy issues constitute an important part of a new research agenda that will be presented. It consists of 12 research lines that were developed on the basis of an umbrella scenario on "Urban life management". Needing a vision for reconciling humans and technology in the Urban Age, we argue for a human-centered design approach resulting in a Humane Smart Hybrid City where people can exploit their creative potential and lead a self-determined life.

Table of Contents

Measurement and Usability Evaluation

Usability Evaluation - Medical Environments

Accessibility Methodologies

Game-Based Methodologies

Web-Based Systems and Attribution Research

Virtual Environments

Special Session on Design Culture for Ageing Well: Designing for Situated Elderliness (DCAW)

Input Devices

Adaptive Systems and Intelligent Agents

Workshop for Assessing the State of HCI Research and Practice in South-Eastern Europe (WS-HCI-SEE)

Doctoral Consortium

Poster Presentations

Design and Development Methodology for the Emotional State Estimation of Verbs

Georgios Kouroupetroglou, Nikolaos Papatheodorou, and Dimitrios Tsonos

National and Kapodistrian University of Athens,
Department of Informatics and Telecommunications, Athens, Greece
koupe@di.uoa.gr

Abstract. The use of words and particularly the verbs in Human-Human Interaction reveals significant aspects of both human's social and mental state. This work presents a novel methodology towards the emotional assessment of verbs by users. Essentially we would like to study whether the emotions that user experience are comparable with the corresponding results obtained through a mixture of natural language and statistical classifiers in SentiWordNet. Following the paper and pencil guidelines of the International Affective Picture System (IAPS) we have developed a web-based unsupervised version of the Self Assessment Manikin (SAM) test, designed for the emotional assessment of verbs in English and Greek language. Thirty five men and seventeen women participated in an internet survey version of the experiment. In the first part of the process, the participants had to assess their induced emotional state while reading a verb (totally 75 Greek verbs), on 5-point scales of "Pleasure", "Arousal" and "Dominance". The results comprise coherence and consistency. As a rule, all verbs obtained low to mid range scores on Arousal and Dominance axis and only on the Pleasure dimension scores are close to the edge.

Keywords: verbs, emotional state, SentiWordNet, Self-Assessment Manikin test.

1 Introduction

Emotions are considered as an integral part of human existence and thus of our daily activity. The scientific domain of emotions, as an expression of human behavior, constitutes a multidisciplinary effort, with Human-Computer Interaction (HCI) to be one of its aspects. Similarly, it is not the first research area that investigates the way to make emotions experimentally available and conceptually compatible with existing research models. The definition of the word "emotion" is open to several interpretations. According to Scherer [1] emotion is defined as: "An episode of interconnected, synchronized changes in circumstances of all or most of the five organic subsystems in response to the evaluation of an external or internal stimulus on the key concerns of the organism". An alternative and also simpler definition given by Brave and Nass [2]: "The emotion is the reaction to events associated with the needs, goals or concerns of a person and includes the ingredients of physiology, influence, behavior and

A. Holzinger et al. (Eds.): SouthCHI 2013, LNCS 7946, pp. 1–15, 2013.

cognitive". Therefore, emotional behavior in HCI shows that expressiveness incorporates a significant amount of individual variability. This point out that people signifies their emotions with a variety of styles and in a rather wide range of intensity.

This work aims to design, implement and test an online web-based tool for self-assessment of the induced emotional state of the participant when reading certain verbs. Existing similar studies have been conducted using semi-automated methods and algorithms (SentiWordNet) without being so far confirmed by users for their validity. The present study introduces a systematic way to study the emotional response of the reader by using a standard experimental procedure. The results can be incorporated to augment the users' experience during Human-Computer Interaction (details presented in section 6).

The basic requirement was that the methodology could be accessed by a large statistical sample of participants in different languages and cultures. For this reason, the focus was on developing a web application so that the research could be easily accessible by users with diverse interests, educational background or occupation, covering a wide range of ages.

In this work, we first describe a SentiWordNet based methodological approach for the proper selection of the verbs. In section 3 we present an interactive web-based Self Assessment Manikin (SAM) Test we have developed for the emotional assessment of verbs along with the experimental setup. Last, the results of the study are presented and discussed, along with their possible uses in Human-Computer Interaction, focusing on augmenting acoustic interaction through Expressive Speech Synthesis.

2   Methodology for the Selection of Verbs

2.1   WordNet

The ontology based English WordNet of Princeton University [3] contains information about the conceptual meaning of verbs and much more. It incorporates a classification of the main parts of speech (i.e. nouns, verbs, adjectives and adverbs) into *synsets, i.e.* sets of semantically or conceptually equivalent words that express an individual concept. WordNet interconnects words not only morphologically, but also with the specific meanings of words. As a result, words that are in close proximity with others in the lexical base are not semantically ambiguous. In addition, WordNet characterizes the semantic relationships between words, in contrast to a dictionary which does not follow a clear pattern, except the concept of similarity. Relations among synsets create an interconnected network. Different senses of polysemous words are members of distinct synsets that are related to different synsets (i.e., occupy different locations in the network). For example, {stock. broth} has superordinate synset {dish} and {stock, breed} has superordinate synset {variety}. These different synsets are also linked to different parts/whole synsets.

2.2   SentiWordNet

Every synset in the SentiWordNet [4] lexical resource is correlated with three scores: Obj(s), Pos(s) and Neg(s), that indicate how much Objective, Positive, and Negative are the terms included in the specific synset [5], [6]. These scores take a numerical value between 0 to 1 and the sum of the three scores for each synset must be always 1. It is possible different senses of the same term to have different opinion-related properties. This supports the transition for terms to synsets. It is obvious that a synset may have all of its three scores with nonzero values. In that case, according to the sense indicated by the synset, the respective term has the three opinion-related properties only to a certain degree. Fig. 1 shows the graphical model representation of the three scores for each synset.

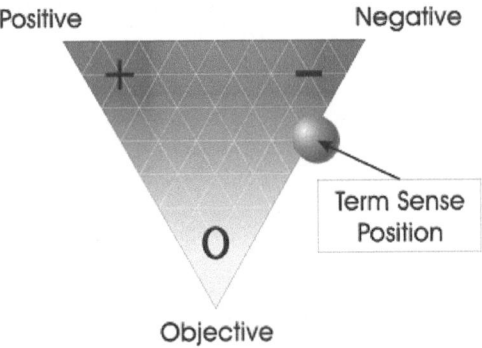

Fig. 1. Graphical model representation of the three scores for each synset

SentiWordNet provides scores for all the different meanings that a verb can have in a synset. For example, the verb "teach" under SentiWordNet corresponds to two different concepts: a) *impart skills or knowledge of* and b) *accustom gradually to some action or attitude*. For this reason, our study focused on the score of the first concept of each verb which is also the most common. Fig. 2 shows the two meanings of the verb "teach" and the respective ratings in the graphical model representation.

2.3   Selection of Verbs

The following methodology was applied for the selection of the appropriate verbs for the experiments. From the lexical database of the Corpus of Contemporary American English [7] a list of the 5.000 most frequently used words in the English language was originally determined. From this list we choose the most commonly occurring verbs in English. After comparing the lexical database of verbs in SentiWordNet to the corresponding database of the Corpus of Contemporary American English we selected the 1.000 most commonly occurring verbs in English along with their emotional annotation.

Studying the emotion rating of these verbs, we noticed that a very large proportion of them were similarly rated in more than one axis (grade <0.6 per axis), resulting in the characterization on the three axes being ambiguous. Then, we separated the 1.000 verbs in three different groups according to their emotional value (positive, negative, neutral) preserving in each group those verbs with the highest score in one of the three emotional axes (grade> 0.8). As a result we got a list with the 25 verbs that have the highest scores in each group. Thus, we selected 75 verbs for the evaluation which were then translated into Greek. The translation was done in accordance with the widely known online dictionary Babylon English - Greek [8].

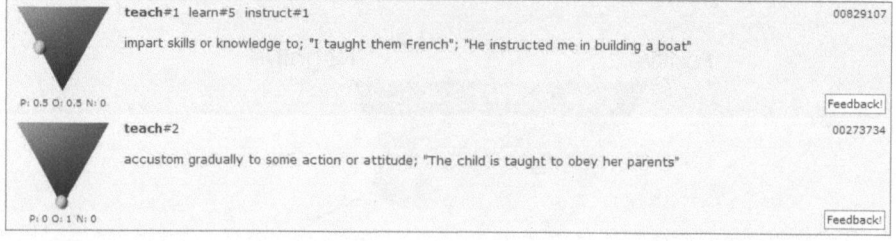

VERB

Fig. 2. The two different meanings of verb "teach" and their corresponding rating in the graphical model representation

Tables 1, 2 and 3 present the three classes (Positive, Neutral and Negative) respectively of the 75 verbs finally selected. The ranking of each verb in the list of the 5.000 most frequently English words is shown in the second column of the three tables.

3   Emotional Assessment of Verbs

To investigate the emotion that elicited each verb to the reader, we used the Self-Assessment Manikin (SAM) Test [9] [10]. The SAM method measures the emotional response, based on the dimensional approach of emotions [1] [11], giving the user the ability to avoid the verbal expression of emotions in the assessment. It implies a quick and easy procedure (Fig. 3). The tool has been designed to follow a visual, rather than verbal, self-assessment course of the emotions. This makes it easy to use and therefor fast in the application. One of its major advantages can be seen in its reproducibility which allows a comparison of studies from different laboratories or statistical samples. In addition it has been shown to be independent from cultural and linguistic characteristics, suitable for use in different countries and cultural groups [10] [12].

By applying the SAM Test, one can measure emotions in three axis:

- "Pleasure" (also used as "evaluation", "valence").
- "Arousal" (also used as "activation", "activity").
- "Dominance" (also used as "power", "potency").

Participants in the SAM test can choose one from at least five figures (manikins). In the present study we used a 5-point scale (Fig. 4). To assess the emotional state of "Pleasure", the extreme values are a smiling and a sad figure. In case of "Arousal" one pole is represented by a figure of great vigor and the opposite with a calm manikin, with eyes closed. Similarly, "Dominance" dimension is represented as controlled by a small manikin and non-controlled by a large one. When evaluating the results, users' answers can be easily converted from scale points to a group of values which ranges in the interval [-1, 1] or [-100%, 100%]. The value "0" represents the neutral state in each of the three dimensions, whereas the middle values represent an intermediate state.

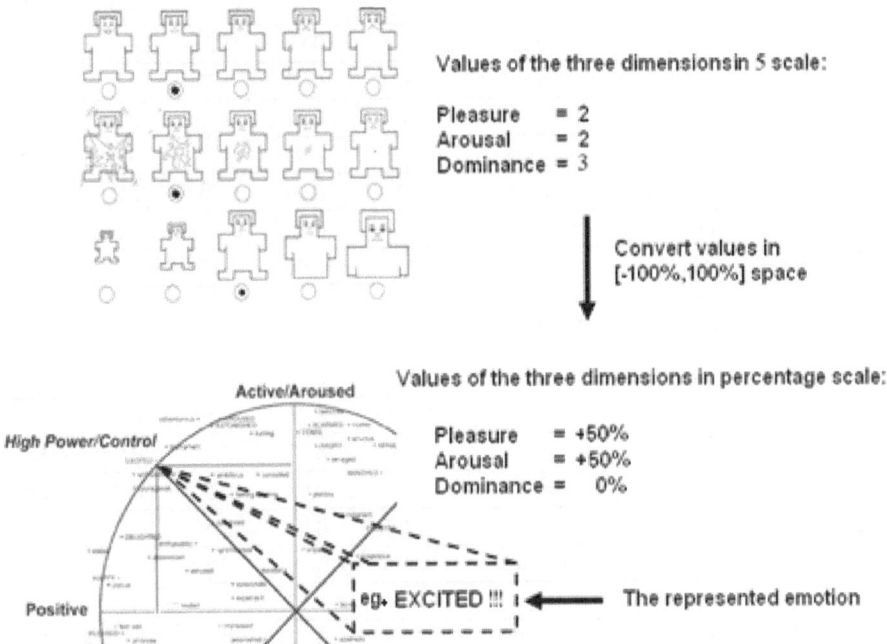

Values of the three dimensions in 5 scale:

Pleasure   = 2
Arousal   = 2
Dominance = 3

Convert values in
[-100%,100%] space

Values of the three dimensions in percentage scale:

Pleasure   = +50%
Arousal   = +50%
Dominance =   0%

The represented emotion

Fig. 3. Extracting the emotion under the SAM Test. Participants assess their emotional state using the manikins. The 5-point scale values are converted into a percentage scale and then mapped on to the emotion wheel for the verbal-semantic representation of the emotion.

By applying the SAM test on specific projected stimuli we can have two different results that are closely related: the dimensional perspective / modeling of both the emotional states and the emotions of the participants.

An application system for the automated estimation of emotion primitives (the dimensional approach) from speech using acoustic features has been proposed recently [13], [14], [15]. Moreover, a study [16] on the automated detection of pleasant and unpleasant emotions in spoken dialogs derived from a call center has been presented.

The SAM test has been used also by Busso et al. [17] in order to evaluate the modelling of the head motion sequences in an experiment of expressive facial animations analyzed in terms of their naturalness and emotional salience during perception.

Table 1. The 25 positively classified verbs in English with their rank number according to Corpus of Contemporary American English and the corresponding Greek translation

				Positive Verbs				
ID	Rank	Word	Greek Translation	Frequ-ency	Dispe-rsion	Posi-tive	Nega-tive	Obje-ctive
1	1728	prefer	προτιμώ	20946	0.96	0.875	0.0	0.125
2	1356	fit	ταιριάζω	27875	0.96	0.75	0.0	0.25
3	1964	question	ερωτώ	17924	0.97	0.75	0.0	0.25
4	2244	deserve	αξίζω	14944	0.97	0.75	0.125	0.125
5	3197	suit	αρμόζω	9477	0.95	0.75	0.0	0.25
6	3753	accommodate	διευκολύνω	7571	0.94	0.75	0.0	0.25
7	3075	qualify	δικαιούμαι	10090	0.95	0.625	0.0	0.375
8	3305	admire	θαυμάζω	9016	0.96	0.625	0.125	0.25
9	4125	please	ευχαριστώ	6565	0.95	0.625	0.0	0.375
10	4134	donate	δωρίζω	6606	0.94	0.625	0.0	0.375
11	391	love	αγαπώ	103681	0.95	0.5	0.0	0.5
12	546	teach	διδάσκω	72668	0.95	0.5	0.0	0.5
13	735	save	σώζω	52067	0.97	0.5	0.0	0.5
14	857	check	ελέγχω	45760	0.95	0.5	0.0	0.5
15	1043	tend	τείνω	38295	0.94	0.5	0.125	0.375
16	1214	define	ορίζω	33958	0.90	0.5	0.125	0.375
17	1319	contribute	συνεισφέρω	30090	0.92	0.5	0.25	0.25
18	2836	respect	σέβομαι	11083	0.97	0.5	0.0	0.5
19	2864	possess	κατέχω	11474	0.93	0.5	0.0	0.5
20	3026	satisfy	ικανοποιώ	10194	0.96	0.5	0.0	0.5
21	3066	rid	απαλλάσω	10104	0.95	0.5	0.0	0.5
22	3583	lend	δανείζω	7961	0.96	0.5	0.25	0.25
23	3852	rescue	διασώζω	7187	0.96	0.5	0.0	0.5
24	3868	diagnose	διαγιγνώσκω	7255	0.94	0.5	0.0	0.5
25	4286	instruct	καθοδηγώ	6117	0.95	0.5	0.0	0.5

Following the paper and pencil IAPS Guidelines [18] we have developed a web-based unsupervised version of the SAM test, designed for the emotional assessment of verbs in English and Greek language. This automated SAM test helps to create an easy to use experiment and the rapid collection and process of the results.

Table 2. The 25 neutrally classified verbs in English with their rank number according to Corpus of Contemporary American English and the corresponding Greek translation

				Neutral Verbs				
ID	Rank	Word	Greek Translation	Frequency	Dispersion	Positive	Negative	Objective
1	18	do	κάνω	2573587	0.95	0.0	0.0	1,0
2	19	say	λέγω	1915138	0.95	0.0	0.0	1.0
3	35	go	πηγαίνω	1151045	0.93	0.0	0.0	1.0
4	37	can	μπορώ	1022775	0.98	0.0	0.0	1.0
5	45	make	κατασκευάζω	857168	0.98	0.0	0.0	1.0
6	47	know	γνωρίζω	892535	0.93	0.0	0.0	1.0
7	48	will	διαθέτω	824568	0.97	0.0	0.0	1.0
8	56	think	σκέφτομαι	772787	0.91	0.0	0.0	1.0
9	63	take	λαμβάνω	670745	0.97	0.0	0.0	1.0
10	67	see	βλέπω	663645	0.96	0.0	0.0	1.0
11	70	come	έρχομαι	628254	0.95	0.0	0.0	1.0
12	85	look	κοιτάζω	491707	0.93	0.0	0.0	1.0
13	92	use	χρησιμοποιώ	420781	0.96	0.0	0.0	1.0
14	95	find	βρίσκω	395203	0.98	0.0	0.0	1.0
15	103	tell	διηγούμαι	388155	0.94	0.0	0.0	1.0
16	117	work	εργάζομαι	318210	0.98	0.0	0.0	1.0
17	127	try	προσπαθώ	294023	0.96	0.0	0.0	1.0
18	131	ask	ζητώ	284632	0.96	0.0	0.0	1.0
19	139	become	γίνομαι	259102	0.97	0.0	0.0	1.0
20	150	leave	φεύγω	240482	0.96	0.0	0.0	1.0
21	151	put	θέτω	237480	0.96	0.0	0.0	1.0
22	154	mean	εννοώ	242198	0.93	0.0	0.0	1.0
23	156	keep	κρατώ	231760	0.96	0.0	0.0	1.0
24	159	let	αφήνω	240300	0.93	0.0	0.0	1.0
25	164	begin	αρχίζω	218617	0.98	0.0	0.0	1.0

For the development of the application, PHP [19] was used on an Apache Web Server and MySQL [20]. PHP allowed us to develop dynamic web pages, for the presentation of the stimuli, and to automate the registration of the participants' answers. The answers are stored in a database (MySQL). Moreover, technologies like HTML (Hyper Text Markup Language) [21], JavaScript [22] and CSS [23] were used in order to enhance the usability, administration and visual characteristics of the tool (e.g. to accurately control the projection time of the verb).

Table 3. The 25 negatively classified verbs in English with their rank number according to Corpus of Contemporary American English and the corresponding Greek translation

			Negative Verbs					
ID	**Rank**	**Word**	**Greek Translation**	**Frequency**	**Dispersion**	**Positive**	**Negative**	**Objective**
1	1413	deny	αρνούμαι	26675	0.96	0.0	0.875	0.125
2	750	protect	προστατεύω	50649	0.97	0.0	0.75	0.25
3	1535	hate	μισώ	24921	0.93	0.0	0.75	0.25
4	1874	complain	παραπονούμαι	19102	0.97	0.0	0.75	0.25
5	3024	damage	ζημιώνω	10163	0.96	0.0	0.75	0.25
6	3778	abuse	καταχρώμαι	7554	0.94	0.0	0.75	0.25
7	1670	fear	φοβούμαι	21333	0.98	0.125	0.625	0.25
8	3508	murder	δολοφονώ	8462	0.93	0.0	0.625	0.375
9	3679	average	υπολογίζω	8106	0.91	0.0	0.625	0.375
10	3782	apologize	απολογούμαι	7485	0.94	0.0	0.625	0.375
11	4639	spare	εξοικονομώ	5492	0.95	0.0	0.625	0.375
12	284	lose	χάνω	134102	0.97	0.0	0.5	0.5
13	554	face	αντικρίζω	69493	0.98	0.0	0.5	0.5
14	912	imagine	φαντάζομαι	43487	0.95	0.0	0.5	0.5
15	973	worry	ανησυχώ	40210	0.96	0.25	0.5	0.25
16	1186	replace	αντικαθιστώ	32688	0.96	0.0	0.5	0.5
17	1382	ignore	αγνοώ	27023	0.97	0.0	0.5	0.5
18	1587	disappear	χάνομαι	23389	0.94	0.0	0.5	0.5
19	1786	warn	προειδοποιώ	19996	0.97	0.0	0.5	0.5
20	1798	steal	κλέβω	20296	0.95	0.0	0.5	0.5
21	2083	mind	νοιάζομαι	17378	0.93	0.0	0.5	0.5
22	2437	confront	αντιμετωπίζω	13757	0.96	0.0	0.5	0.5
23	3685	endure	αντέχω	7586	0.97	0.0	0.5	0.5
24	3755	injure	τραυματίζω	7574	0.94	0.0	0.5	0.5
25	3982	vanish	εξαφανίζομαι	7154	0.91	0.0	0.5	0.5

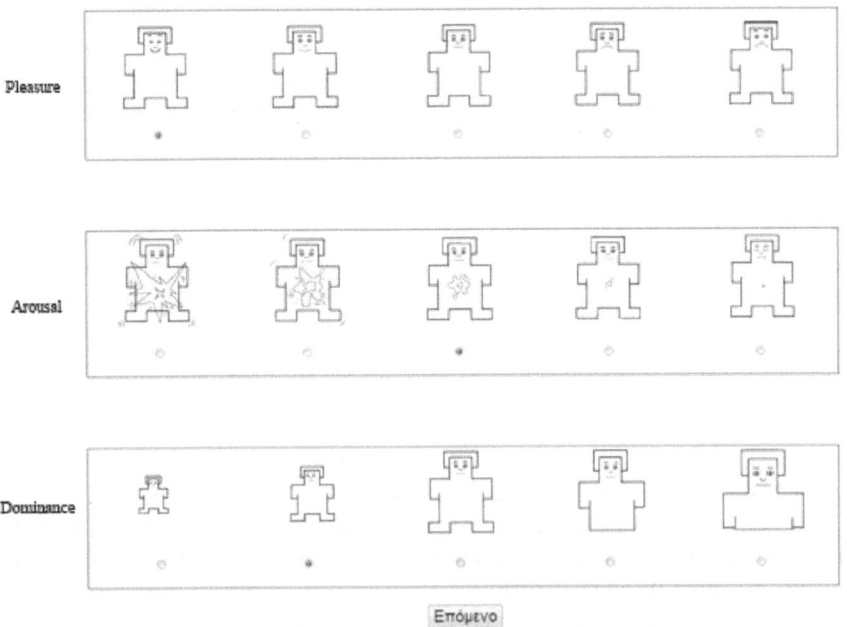

Fig. 4. The manikins of the 5-point scale SAM Test as presented during the test. The verbal expressions of "Pleasure", "Arousal" and "Dominance" do not appear during the test.

Just before the tests, all the participants have to read a brief text explain the purpose of this research study as well as a short simplified introduction on the emotional states theory. Standard guidelines are followed for all participants during the experimental process [18]. Also, they have to fill in an electronic form with demographic information, for example about their age, education level, for any visual problems, and also if she/he agrees to participate in the test.

The participants are familiarized with the SAM test before the measurements. Each stimulus is presented for a few seconds and then they are asked to select the manikins as presented in Fig. 4. By pressing the "continue" button, the next stimulus is presented to the user. Stimuli are given in a random sequence to all the participants. To avoid possible biased results, we have designed the manikins' presentation layout on the screen in such a way to eliminate any interruption of the participants during the test.

In order to evaluate the mental condition of the participants they have to fill in two questionnaires: a) the Symptom Check List-90-Revised (SCL-90-R) [24] to investigate the relationship between psychosomatic disorders and emotional verbal assessment and b) the Eysenck Personality Questionnaire (EPQ) [25].

4   Experimental Setup

Fifty two native Greek speakers, 35 men and 17 women, university students (mean age = 21.7 years, SD = 3.5 years) participated in the experiment. The stimuli were 75 Greek verbs, 25 positively, 25 negatively and 25 objectively characterized (Tables 1, 2 and 3) selected with the methodology described in section 3. Each participant had to fill her/his demographic information and complete a consent form that she/he agrees to participate in the test. Then, they were familiarized with the experiment, through a demo of the SAM test (three stimuli). Certain guidelines were followed for all participants during the experimental process [18]. After the completion of the SAM test, they completed the SCL-90-R and EPQ questionnaires both standardized to the Greek population [26] [27].

5   Results

Figures 5, 6 and 7 present the average values of participants' responses for each verb, on each scale, namely "Pleasure", "Arousal" and "Dominance", respectively. Each verb is represented by an integer ID number in the interval [1, 25] (Tables 1, 2 and 3 show the matching ID number-verb).

The results of the study comprise coherence and consistency. Specifically, observing Fig. 5, 6 and 7, we can assume that the verb "save" (Table 1, verbID=13 - "σώζω" in

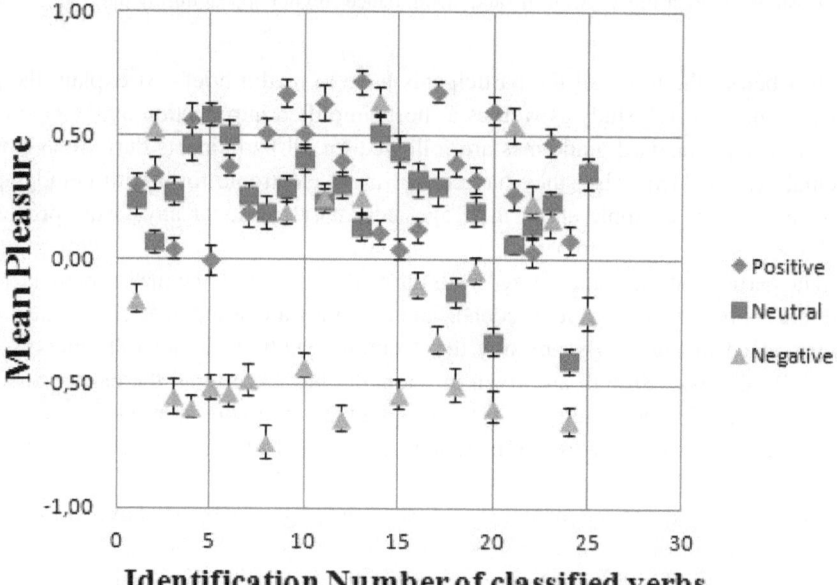

Fig. 5. The graphical representation of the average rating (with the corresponding standard error of mean) of the 75 classified verbs on "Pleasure" dimension in [-1,1] scale. Positive values correspond to positively assessed emotions, while negative values correspond to negatively assessed emotions.

Greek) obtained the highest value on "Pleasure" and "Arousal" dimensions whereas the verb "murder" (Table 3, verbID=8 - "δολοφωνώ" in Greek) has the lowest value. Additionally, it is noticeable that among the negatively classified verbs, the verb "spare" (Table 3, verbID=11 - "εξοικονομώ" in Greek) show a very low score on the Arousal field in contrast to the verb "worry" (Table 3, verbID=15 - "ανησυχώ" in Greek) which held the lead in its classification. Finally, regarding Dominance it is obvious that the verb with the highest score is "apologize" (Table 3, verbID=10 - "απολογούμαι" in Greek) suggesting a submissive emotion unlike the verb "know" (Table 2, verbID=6 - "γνωρίζω" in Greek) which shows a strong dominant emotion (Fig. 7).

We observe that all the 25 positively classified verbs recorded a positive score with only two verbs being at the very middle of the "Pleasure" axis (Fig. 5), namely "suit" (Table 1. verbID=5 - "αρμόζω" in Greek) and "lend" (Table 1, verbID=22 - "δανείζω" in Greek). Regarding the 25 neutrally classified verbs, it is worth noting that the majority's score is concentrated above the middle of the Pleasure axis (22 verbs) and below the middle of the Dominance axis (23 verbs). Furthermore, we observe that the 25 negatively classified verbs are spread out on all three axis. In general, we notice that the neutrally classified verbs show a significant approach towards the positively classified rather than the negative classified ones. As a rule, all verbs obtained low to mid range scores on Arousal and Dominance axis and only on the Pleasure dimension scores are close to the edge.

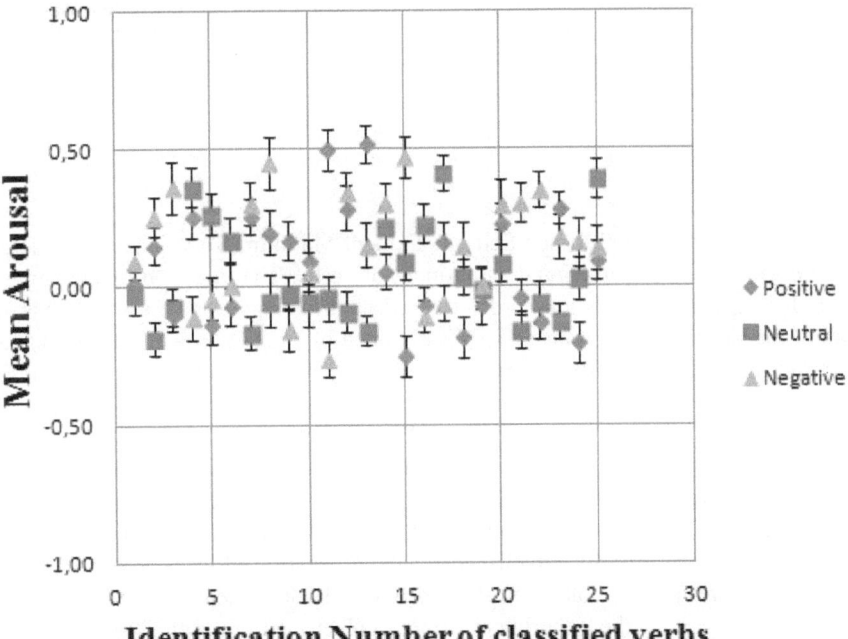

Fig. 6. The graphical representation of the average rating (with the corresponding standard error of mean) of the 75 classified verbs on "Arousal" dimension in [-1,1] scale. Positive values indicate higher intensity.

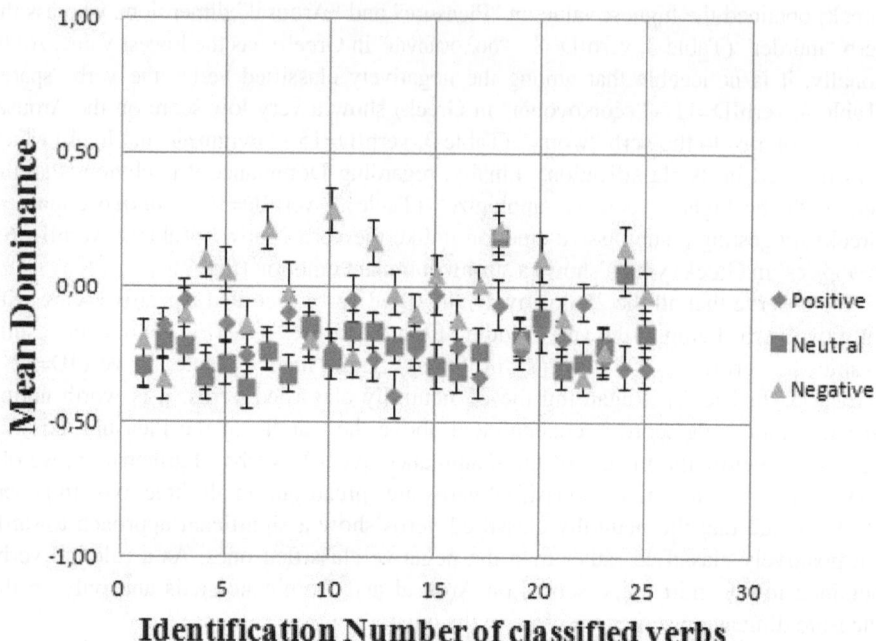

Identification Number of classified verbs

Fig. 7. The graphical representation of the average rating (with the corresponding standard error of mean) of the 75 classified verbs on "Dominance" dimension in [-1,1] scale. Positive values correspond to submissive emotions, while negative values correspond to dominant emotions.

6   Conclusions

We have described a web-based Self-Assessment Manikin (SAM) Test [18] designed and developed for the emotional assessment of verbs. The selection of the verbs has been done according to SentiWordNet based methodology. Apart from the verification of the validity of the relative results obtained by SentiWordNet, our study makes a further step regarding the formalism and the correlation of the exported results. Obviously, the format (as shown in Fig. 1) that SentiWordNet has established in order to present the measured sentiment for each verb is very simple and lacks additional information, such as other factors that influence the final score (e.g. mental and psychological state, educational background), as well as supplementary scales which could highlight different interesting aspects of each verb. For instance, due to the alternative way we initially established for the evaluation of each verb, we managed to export the results in relation to three different scales (Pleasure, Arousal, Dominance). Consequently, the experiment offered enhanced information and showed the different influences that contributed to the final result, in comparison with SentiWordNet which characterizes each verb as positive, objective or negative.

With regard to the issues we faced during the development of the whole experiment, the application's background response time tracking system which was implemented from the beginning, showed that some users showed lack of concentration after the first half of the experiment which suggests that the large number of verbs could be potentially decreased [31]. In addition, while this study was held we noticed that almost 50% of the users who started the test quit it after some minutes which emphasizes the assumption above. All these cases were excluded from the participants' set.

During the experiment, users were evaluated with regard to their emotional and psychological state (EPQ & SCL-90-R) at the very moment after the completion of the verbs evaluation. The addition of the above tests to our methodology, can lead to further statistical analysis of the exported results. For example, it is possible to identify users with certain emotional and psychological disorders, so as to distinguish them from the rest examined sample and determine whether the emotional and psychological state of a user has an impact on the sentiment evaluation or not and to what extent after a deeper analysis of that particular sample [31].

It should be noticed that the presented experimental procedure has the advantage of being developed and designed for a significant number of users as it is widely open to the public as opposed to SentiWordNet which started by a very small group of experts and maintained by semi-automatic algorithms later on. As a result, we have the capability to investigate a statistically significant population sample, depending on the experimental design and needs.

An interesting future study would be to investigate whether emotion/emotional state semantics of the verbs are cross-cultural and/or language independent. Due to "manikin description" of emotional states during the experimental procedure, instead of using their verbal description, we can easily conduct a multilingual and/or multicultural research. There is a growing interest for the results of such kind of studies as they can be merged into software systems for the automated emotional annotation of text documents, e.g. using EmotionML [28]. This kind of information would very useful for systems that can automatically emotionally rank a document by its content in order to accomplish users' information retrieval needs. Also, this kind of annotation can be used to augment expressions during Human-Computer Interaction. For example, combining the results of the current study with Expressive Speech Synthesis [29], we can augment the user experience during multimodal interaction, focusing on acoustic, as proposed in [30].

The experience obtained from the implementation of this particular study could probably set new standards regarding the sentiment evaluation of verbs and even expand relative research for the analysis of nouns, adjectives as well as adverbs. Consequently, the implemented methodology we used to analyze the available data from the web based application with the help of users' interaction, can be proven valuable regarding its effectiveness in the opinion mining field of interest [32].

Moreover, the current design of the web application does not support interaction with blind users which leads to improve the user interface-interaction adding support for the acoustic and/or haptic modality. Finally, the support of touch sensitive controls is in our plans as it would make the experimental process easier and more directly straight forward.

Acknowledgements. This research has been co-financed by the European Union (European Social Fund – ESF) and Greek national funds through the Operational Program "Education and Lifelong Learning" of the National Strategic Reference Framework (NSRF) under the Research Funding Project: "THALIS-University of Macedonia- KAIKOS: Audio and Tactile Access to Knowledge for Individuals with Visual Impairments", MIS 380442.

References

1. Scherer, K.R.: What are emotions? And how can they be measured? Social Science Information 44(4), 695–729 (2005)
2. Brave, S., Nass, C.: Emotion in human-computer interaction. In: Sears, A., Jacko, J.A. (eds.) The Human-Computer Interaction Handbook: Fundamentals, Evolving Technologies and Emerging Applications, pp. 77–92. Taylor and Francis Group (2007)
3. WordNet, Lexical database of English, http://wordnet.princeton.edu/
4. SentiWordNet, http://sentiwordnet.isti.cnr.it/
5. Esuli, A., Sebastiani, F.: SENTIWORDNET: A Publicly Available Lexical Resource for Opinion Mining. In: 5th Conference on Language Resources and Evaluation (LREC 2006), Genoa, Italy, pp. 417–422 (2006)
6. Esuli, A., Baccianella, S., Sebastiani, F.: SentiWordNet 3.0: An Enhanced Lexical Resource for Sentiment Analysis and Opinion Mining. In: 7th Conference on International Language Resources and Evaluation (LREC 2010), Malta (2010)
7. Word frequency lists and dictionary from the Corpus of Contemporary American English, http://www.wordfrequency.info/intro.asp
8. Babylon 9 translation Software and Dictionary Tool, http://www.babylon.com
9. Lang, P.J., Bradley, M.M., Cuthbert, B. N.: International affective picture system (IAPS): Affective retings of pictures and instruction manual. Technical report A-8, University of Florida, Gainesville, FL (2005)
10. Bradley, M.M., Lang, P.J.: Measuring emotion: The self-assessment manikin and the semantic differential. Journal of Behavior Therapy and Experimental Psychiatry 25(1), 49–59 (1994)
11. Russell, J.A., Mehrabian, A.: Evidence for a three-factor theory of emotions. Journal of Research in Personality 11(3), 273–294 (1977)
12. Morris, J.D.: Observations SAM: The Self-Assessment Manikin - An Efficient Cross-Cultural Measurement of Emotional Response. Journal of Advertising Research 35(8), 63–68 (1995)
13. Grimm, M., Mower, E., Narayanan, S., Kroschel, K.: Combining categorical and primitives-based emotion recognition. In: Proceedings of 14th European Signal Processing Conference (EUSIPCO), Florence, Italy (September 2006)
14. Grimm, M., Kroschel, K., Mower, E., Narayanan, S.: Primitives-based evaluation and estimation of emotions in speech. Speech Communication 49(10-11), 787–800 (2007) ISSN: 0167-6393
15. Grimm, M., Kroschel, K., Narayanan, S.: Support Vector Regression for Automatic Recognition of Spontaneous Emotions in Speech. In: IEEE International Conference on Acoustics, Speech and Signal Processing 2007 (ICASSP 2007), Hawaii, USA, April 15-20, vol. 4, pp. IV-1085-IV–1088 (2007) ISBN: 1-4244-0728-1
16. Chul, M.L., Narayanan, S.S.: Toward detecting emotions in spoken dialogs. Transactions on Speech and Audio Processing 13(2), 293–303 (2005) ISSN: 1063-6676

17. Busso, C., Deng, Z., Grimm, M., Neumann, U., Narayanan, S.: Rigid Head Motion in Expressive Speech Animation: Analysis and Synthesis. IEEE Transactions on Audio, Speech, and Language Processing 15(3), 1075–1086 (2007) ISSN: 1558-7916
18. Lang, P.J., Bradley, M.M., Culthbert, B.N.: International Affective Picture System (IAPS): Instruction Manual and Affective Ratings. Technical Report A-6, The Center for Research in Psychophysiology, University of Florida, U.S.A. (2005)
19. PHP Hypertext Preprocessor, http://www.php.net/
20. Welling, L., Thomson, L.: PHP and MySQL Web Development, 4th edn. Addison-Wesley Professional (2008)
21. HTML Tutorial, http://www.w3schools.com/html/default.asp
22. JavaScript Tutorial, http://www.w3schools.com/js/default.asp
23. CSS Reference, http://www.w3schools.com/cssref/default.asp
24. Derogatis, L.R.: The Symptom Checklist-90-revised. NCS Assessments, Minneapolis (1992)
25. Corulia, W.J.: A psychometric investigation of the Eysenck Personality Questionnaire (revised) and its relationship to the I7 Impulsiveness Questionnaire. Personality and Individual Differences 8, 651–658 (1987)
26. Donias, S., Karastergiou, A., Manos, N.: Standardization of the symptom checklist-90-R rating scale in a Greek population. Psychiatriki (1), 42–48 (1991)
27. Demetriou, E.X.: The Eysenck Personality Questionnaire: Standardization to the Greek population, Adult and Junior. Engefalos 23, 41–54 (1986)
28. Emotion Markup Language (EmotionML) 1.0,
    http://www.w3.org/TR/emotionml/
29. Campbell, N., Hamza, W., Hoge, H., Tao, J., Bailly, G.: Editorial Special Section on Expressive Speech Synthesis. IEEE Trans. Audio, Speech, and Language Processing 14(4), 1097–1098 (2006)
30. Kouroupetroglou, G., Tsonos, D.: Multimodal Accessibility of Documents. In: Pinder, S. (ed.) Advances in Human-Computer Interaction, pp. 451–470. I-Tech Education and Publishing, Vienna (2008)
31. Stickel, C., Ebner, M., Steinbach-Nordmann, S., Searle, G., Holzinger, A.: Emotion Detection: Application of the Valence Arousal Space for Rapid Biological Usability Testing to Enhance Universal Access. In: Stephanidis, C. (ed.) Universal Access in HCI, Part I, HCII 2009. LNCS, vol. 5614, pp. 615–624. Springer, Heidelberg (2009)
32. Petz, G., Karpowicz, M., Fürschuß, H., Auinger, A., Winkler, S.M., Schaller, S., Holzinger, A.: On Text Preprocessing for Opinion Mining Outside of Laboratory Environments. In: Huang, R., Ghorbani, A.A., Pasi, G., Yamaguchi, T., Yen, N.Y., Jin, B. (eds.) AMT 2012. LNCS, vol. 7669, pp. 618–629. Springer, Heidelberg (2012)

Automatic Recognition of the Unconscious Reactions from Physiological Signals

Leonid Ivonin, Huang-Ming Chang, Wei Chen, and Matthias Rauterberg

Eindhoven University of Technology, Eindhoven, The Netherlands
{l.ivonin,h.m.chang,w.chen,g.w.m.rauterberg}@tue.nl

Abstract. While the research in affective computing has been exclusively dealing with the recognition of explicit affective and cognitive states, carefully designed psychological and neuroimaging studies indicated that a considerable part of human experiences is tied to a deeper level of a psyche and not available for conscious awareness. Nevertheless, the unconscious processes of the mind greatly influence individuals' feelings and shape their behaviors. This paper presents an approach for automatic recognition of the unconscious experiences from physiological data. In our study we focused on primary or archetypal unconscious experiences. The subjects were stimulated with the film clips corresponding to 8 archetypal experiences. Their physiological signals including cardiovascular, electrodermal, respiratory activities, and skin temperature were monitored. The statistical analysis indicated that the induced experiences could be differentiated based on the physiological activations. Finally, a prediction model, which recognized the induced states with an accuracy of 79.5%, was constructed.

Keywords: Affective computing, archetypes, the collective unconscious.

1 Introduction

Since the beginning of the last decade affective computing has become a prominent research direction and attracted attention of researches who work on new generations of human-computer interfaces. Originally, Rosalind Picard defined affective computing as a computing that "relates to, arises from, or deliberately influences emotions" [1]. However, later affective computing gave an impulse to a more generic research area of physiological computing. The latter was introduced by Fairclough [2] and extended the scope of investigation from emotions to general psychological states of users. Physiological computing is seen as a novel mode of human-computer interaction (HCI) that enables development of computer systems, which are aware of the users' emotional and cognitive states and, thus, can dynamically adapt to their needs without the requirement of purposeful and overt communication from the users.

The research in physiological computing has built upon and confirmed many findings from psychophysiology, the field that extensively studies the physiological bases of psychological processes. In particular, it has become clear that responses of the autonomic nervous system have a good potential of being applied in computing

A. Holzinger et al. (Eds.): SouthCHI 2013, LNCS 7946, pp. 16–35, 2013.

applications because they are capable of predicting changes in psychological states of individuals and can be measured with relatively cheap, quick and unobtrusive methods [3]. The possible applications of physiological computing cover a range of domains and can be roughly divided into two branches: cognitive and affective. Cognitive physiological computing is directed at monitoring and improvement of the users' performance. For instance, in adaptive automation scenarios where an operator needs to control an aircraft or a vehicle, it is important to identify the states of boredom and low vigilance because they are likely to increase the risk of accidents [4, 5]. On the other hand, affective physiological computing is aimed at increase of pleasure in interaction with computer systems and is well suited for domains such as entertainment or computer-based learning [6]. Naturally, there is an overlap between these two branches of physiological computing [3] due to the fact that cognition and affect are interrelated in the human psyche.

One course of investigation in physiological computing involves study of the psychological states that have been identified in psychology but have not yet been considered with regard to HCI. It is of little surprise that research in psychology and neuroscience has collected more knowledge about human cognition, affect and behavior than any other disciplines. For this reason, physiological computing is largely based on original experiments in psychophysiology [2] and adoption of new insights from these fields seems rational. An emerging trend in psychological science over the past 30 years is understanding and acceptance of the fact that human experience is extensively tied to a deeper level of psyche, which is not directly available to conscious awareness and, thus, defined as the unconscious. Although it may sound controversial and surprising, often people are not very well aware of and not able to accurately report on their higher order cognitive processes [7]. The absence of introspective awareness about the unconscious mental processes does not mean that they have no influence or effect on behaviors, experiences and memories. On the contrary, carefully designed experiments with both healthy volunteers and brain-damaged patients have indicated that a large part of people's everyday behaviors is conducted without any conscious control [8]. As the phenomenon of the unconscious is still to be fully understood by the scientific community, there has not been developed an established definition for it yet. However, in order to avoid ambiguity and confusion, the unconscious processes have been operationally defined by Bargh "in terms of a lack of awareness of the influences or effects of a triggering stimulus and not of the triggering stimulus itself" [9]. This definition emphasizes the important distinction between *unconscious* and *subliminal* by resolving the common confusion about these two phenomena. People outside of psychological science often equate the unconscious with processing of stimuli, which are too weak or short to enter the conscious awareness and, therefore, are referred to as subliminal. In fact, the unconscious information processing is not necessarily associated with presentations of subliminal stimuli and runs continuously as a parallel background process in human mind [10].

Carl Jung, a Swiss psychiatrist, developed his concept of the unconscious in the beginning of the previous century. According to Jung, the unconscious consists of two components: the *personal unconscious* and the *collective unconscious*. The personal unconscious is a repository for all of one's feelings, memories, knowledge and thoughts that are not conscious at a given moment of time [11]. They may be retrieved from the personal unconscious with a varying degree of difficulty that depends on how actively they are being repressed. On the other hand, the collective component of the unconscious is universal and has contents and modes of behavior that are uniform in all individuals [12]. The collective unconscious represents the deepest level of the psyche and does not arise individually but is inherited and contains innate behavior patterns for survival and reproduction developed over evolutionary time. The content of the collective unconscious was conceptualized by Jung as archetypes or pre-existent forms. Archetypes are very close analogies to instincts because the latter are impersonal, inherited traits that present and motivate human behavior long before any consciousness develops [13]. Furthermore, feelings and ideas emerged from archetypes continue to influence people despite any degree of consciousness later on. Archetypes define the patterns of instinctual behaviors and are conceptualized as images or representations of the instincts.

The unconscious side of the human psyche is a profoundly intriguing phenomenon guiding smart and adaptive processes that shape behaviors and experiences of people and yet remain hidden from their conscious awareness. While research in physiological computing has made a considerable progress in recognition of cognitive and affective states of the users, the investigation has been primary focused on conscious psychological states. Thus, sensing a deeper level of human experiences defined by the unconscious processes remains a largely unexplored area. Interestingly, there is some initial evidence from psychophysiology [14] that the unconscious experiences of people can be indirectly assessed with their physiological signals. This fact implies that although the unconscious processes are hidden from the conscious mind, traces of the unconscious can be observed from bodily activations. However, a further investigation is required in order to evaluate the feasibility of sensing the users' unconscious mental processes in HCI scenarios by means of physiological computing.

In this study our primary goal was the evaluation of the possibility to sense the unconscious experiences of the users in an automatic and unobtrusive manner. However, as the unconscious is a complex phenomenon, the scope of our study was limited to the collective unconscious. Unlike the personal unconscious that is highly diverse and individual, the collective unconscious consists of the universal archetypes. For this reason, it is better suited for computing applications where a range of common archetypal experiences could be employed for system adaptation to psychological states of the users. More specifically, this study was aimed at investigating the feasibility of sensing and distinguishing various archetypal experiences of the users based on the analysis of physiological signals such as heart rate or skin conductance.

In accordance with our research objectives an experiment was designed where explicit emotional feelings, such as fear or joy, and a range of common archetypal experiences were elicited in individuals. The explicit emotions were included in this study to serve as a benchmark that can be used to compare our results with other affect recognition studies. Simultaneously with the presentation of emotional and archetypal stimuli physiological signals of the participants were unobtrusively measured with a number of wireless sensors. Subsequently, signal processing methods were applied to the collected physiological data and a set of appropriate features was extracted with advanced data mining techniques. In order to explore the obtained dataset several statistical tests were utilized. Finally, predictive models that allow for a meaningful classification of the subjects' psychological states were constructed based on the vector of features extracted earlier.

2 Methods

2.1 Experimental Design

Stimuli. An appropriate set of stimuli was required for the elicitation of the explicit emotions and the archetypal experiences in the experiment. Past research in affect elicitation have applied different media types for emotion induction in laboratory conditions, including images and sounds [15, 16], music [17], and films [18]. These media types differ from one another in many aspects. For instance, still images and sounds are commonly presented to subjects for very short periods of time and have a high temporal resolution. On the other hand, music and film clips accommodate a lower degree of temporal resolution lasting for several minutes and deliver heterogeneous cognitive and affective activations. In comparison with the other types of media, film clips are powerful in capture of attention because of their dynamic display that includes both visual and auditory modalities [18]. Another characteristic of film clips is the ability to elicit intensive emotional responses that lead to activations in cognitive, experiential, central physiological, peripheral physiological and behavioral systems [19]. Taking into account the pros and cons of each media type film clips were chosen for this study because they effectively elicit emotions and last for several minutes. The latter fact was important for calculation of heart rate variability parameters that require at least 5 minutes of data [20]. With regard to the archetypal stimuli we assumed that the media with a high affective impact would also have a large influence on the collective unconscious. For this reason, film clips were utilized for the induction of both the explicit emotions and the archetypal experiences.

Emotions or feelings are commonly represented in affective computing with the dimensional model [21]. This model projects emotions in the affective space with two or three dimensions. In case of two dimensions an emotional state in the affective space is characterized by values of arousal and valence. The dimension of arousal ranges from calm to aroused states while the dimension of valence ranges from negative to positive states [22]. For this study five explicit emotions, amusement, fear, joy, sadness and neutral state, were selected. They uniformly cover the two-dimensional affective space. According to the previous work in this field [23], the neutral state is located close to the origin of the affective space and each one of the other four emotions is situated in a separate quadrant of the space. The film clips for elicitation of each chosen explicit emotional state were identified based on the previous studies in affect induction and recognition. The seminal work of Gross [18] and Pantic [24] provides guidance with regard to application of video in emotion research and even proposes sets of film clips that can be readily used as emotional stimuli. However, we could not always use the recommended clips for the two following reasons. First, some of the film clips were considerably shorter than 5 minutes. Second, from the pilot study we learnt that some of the clips taken from old movies do not emotionally engage people because they are perceived as old-fashioned. Thus, we introduced five film clips that were selected according to the requirements of this study and presented them in Table 1.

Having prepared stimuli for the explicit emotions, it was next necessary to obtain film clips for the archetypal experiences. Jung discovered that symbolic representations of archetypes had been present across cultures for thousands of years. Archetypal symbols are commonly found in artwork, myths, storytelling, and continue to be actively employed in modern mass media [25]. This fact led us to the idea that the set of stimuli could be constructed by extracting typical archetypal appearances from a variety of rich media sources. However, beforehand we had to determine which archetypes would be included in the experiment.

Table 1. Information about sources of the film clips

Film clip	Movie	Film clip	Movie
Stimuli for Explicit Emotions			
Neutral	Coral Sea Dreaming: Awaken [26]	Fear	The Silence of The Lambs [27]
Amusement	Mr. Bean [28]	Joy	The Lion King [29]
Sadness	Forrest Gump [30]		
Archetypal stimuli			
Anima	American Beauty [31]	Hero Return	Braveheart [32]
Animus	Black Swan [33]	Mentor	The King's Speech [34]
Hero Departure	Braveheart [32]	Mother	All About My Mother [35]
Hero Initiation	Braveheart [32]	Shadow	Fight Club [36]

For this study eight archetypes (anima, animus, hero-departure, hero-initiation, hero-return, mentor, mother and shadow) were selected based on their importance and representativeness. Therefore, only films depicting the most common archetypes [12] formed our set of stimuli. The archetypes of anima, animus and shadow were chosen based on their appearance in the manuscripts of Jung [13]. Three archetypes of a hero exemplify important stages in the hero's journey described by Joseph Campbell [37]. He identified that a prototypic journey, which a hero undertakes in a generic narrative, includes stages of departure, initiation, and return. The archetype of mentor is found in the research of Campbell as well and signifies a character that supports the hero in acquiring knowledge and power. Finally, mother is yet another major archetype [38] that was picked for this study.

Next, film clips embodying these eight archetypes were needed. Similar to the stimuli for the explicit emotions and to the previous studies that employed films [19] we obtained our clips by editing fragments of full-length commercial movies. However, unlike the explicit emotions, there was no guidance from the past research with regard to the selection of the stimuli. Thus, our choices had to be evaluated and, if necessary, corrected by experts in the area of archetypal research. Therefore, we pursued collaboration with The Archive for Research in Archetypal Symbolism (ARAS), which is an organization that since the early 1930s has been collecting and annotating mythological, ritualistic, and symbolic images from all over the world [39]. Thanks to the cooperation with ARAS and their feedback, our set of archetypal stimuli was constructed from the clips, which were obtained from the movies listed in Table 1.

Unfortunately, copies of the film clips employed in the study cannot be shared due to the fact that they were extracted from commercial movies. However, all of the movies are freely available on the market and we will provide the editing instructions to produce exactly the same clips upon request.

Participants. Thirty-six healthy volunteers were recruited for this study. Many of them were undergraduate or graduate students. Eventually, 10 participants had to be excluded from the data analysis due to technical problems with Shimmer wireless physiological sensors. One more participant was excluded because he did not comply with the procedure of the experiment and the validity of his data was questionable. For this reason, only data from 25 subjects, consisting of 12 women and 13 men, was utilized in this study. Of these, 11 participants were from Europe, 10 participants originally came from Asia, 3 participants were from Middle East and one participant was from South America. The average age for the women was 23.0 years (SD = 1.9) and for the men 25.4 years (SD = 4.5). Participants had normal or corrected to normal vision and hearing. Prior to the experiment each subject signed an informed consent form and was later financially compensated for participation in the laboratory session that took approximately 2 hours.

Apparatus. The laboratory was equipped with a high definition beamer that in a cinema like settings projected the film clips on a white wall with dimensions 592 x 222 cm. The couch that accommodated participants during the study was situated at a viewing distance of approximately 4 meters in front of the white wall. Additionally to the beamer, a computer screen and a mouse were located near the couch. After watching a film clip subjects were required to use the mouse for providing a self-report about their feelings by rating them against a number of scales, which were displayed on the screen. The procedure of the experiment including presentation of the clips, collection of the feedback, and time tracking was synchronized and automated with a website. Heart activities and skin conductance of participants were monitored with Shimmer wearable wireless sensors that streamed physiological data to a computer via Bluetooth connection. The three-lead Shimmer electrocardiogram sensor was connected with four disposable pregelled Ag/AgCl spot electrodes. Two of the electrodes were placed below the left and right collarbones and the other two were attached to the left and right sides of the belly. The electrode placed on the right side of the belly served as a reference. The same type of electrodes was used to connect the Shimmer GSR sensor to thenar and hypothenar eminences of the participant's palm on a non-dominant hand for measurement of the skin conductance. Regrettably, due to the malfunctioning of the Shimmer ECG sensor, physiological data of 10 participants was partly missing and had to be excluded from the analysis. A Refa amplifier from TMSI BV in combination with an inductive respiration belt and a temperature sensor was used for the measurement of the respiration and skin temperature. A respiration belt with an appropriate size was strapped around the participant's chest and the temperature sensor was fixed on the subject's belly with a sticky tape.

Procedure. Each participant went through a session of the experiment individually. Upon arrival to the laboratory, a participant was invited to sit upright on the couch. Then, the participant was asked to read and sign the provided informed consent form. Next, the experimenter demonstrated the required positioning of the physiological sensors on a body, assisted the participant to attach them, and ensured that the sensors streamed signals of good quality. After placement of the sensors the experimenter allowed a time interval of approximately five minutes to pass before presentation of the first film clip. This interval was necessary for the electrode gel to soak into the participant's skin and thereby establish a stable electrical connection [40]. Meanwhile, an overview of the study was given to the subject. The overview further clarified the procedure of the study explaining that several film clips would be played, and the participant's physiological signals would be continuously recorded during the film's demonstration. However, the actual goal of the experiment remained undisclosed and, for this reason, the participant was not aware of any emotions or archetypes pictured in the clips. Following the overview, the subject was asked to make her comfortable on the couch and refrain from unnecessary movements during the session. The light in the laboratory was dimmed so that the viewing experience became similar to the one in a movie theater. The demonstration of the film clips always started with the neutral film (Coral Sea Dreaming: Awaken [26]) because the participants had to be brought to the same psychophysiological baselines. Piferi et al. [41] argued that a relaxing aquatic video could be used for establishing the baseline. Then, the other film clips were shown in random order. A short video demonstrating a breathing pattern preceded presentation of each film clip (including the neutral one). This video lasted for 40 seconds and its purpose was to dismiss psychological and physiological effects of the previous stimuli. During this video the participant was required to follow the breathing pattern and thereby adjust her respiration rate to the common baseline. Upon completion of viewing a film clip, the participant provided a retrospective self-report by rating her feelings along a number of dimensions using the computer screen and the mouse located near the participant's dominant hand. The discussion of the data collected in self-reports is out of the scope of this manuscript and will be presented elsewhere. As soon as the participant submitted the self-report for the last film clip, the light in the room was turned on and the experimenter helped the subject with detaching the physiological sensors from her body. Finally, the participant was debriefed and reimbursed.

Physiological Signals. A number of physiological signals were monitored in this study. The decision regarding inclusion of a particular signal in the experiment was made based on the background literature in psychophysiology and will be further discussed in this section.

Electrocardiogram (ECG) is a measurement of the heart's electrical activity conducted with electrodes attached to the skin surface and recorded over a period of time. ECG was monitored at 512 Hz and then cleaned with low-pass, high-pass, and notch filters. ECG contains plenty of information about the cardiovascular activity, and in the psychophysiological domain it is commonly used for the calculation of the heart rate (HR) and heart rate variability (HRV). The heart rate is a simple measurement that characterizes the heart's activity in terms of the number of heart beats per minute [42]. The HR was obtained from the ECG signal by identifying beats with an algorithm provided in [43] and computing the average heart rate over a moving window of 10 seconds. We expected to see a relation between the psychological states of the subjects and their HR because this measure had been widely applied in physiological computing and, according to Kreibig [44], the HR is the most often reported cardiovascular measure in psychophysiological studies of emotion. Next, several HRV parameters from time and frequency domains were calculated based on the heart beats data with an HRVAS software package [45]. Time domain parameters included the standard deviation of the beat to beat intervals (SDNN), the square root of the mean of the sum of the squares of differences between adjacent beat to beat intervals (RMSSD), and the standard deviation of differences between adjacent beat to beat intervals (SDSD) [20]. A pool of frequency domain parameters consisted of a total power, a power in a very low frequency range (VLF, 0-0.04 Hz), a power in a low frequency range (LF, 0.04-0.15 Hz), a power in a high frequency range (HF, 0.15-0.4 Hz), and a ratio of the power in a low frequency range to the power in a high frequency range (LF/HF) [20].

Skin conductance describes variations in the electrodermal activity of skin and is associated with processes of eccrine sweating, which are controlled by the sympathetic branch of the autonomic nervous system [40]. According to [23], skin conductance is closely related to psychological processes and particularly to the level of arousal. Skin conductance has tonic and phasic components. The tonic component reflects relatively slow changes in skin conductance over longer periods of time lasting from tens of seconds to tens of minutes. Thus, it is indicative of a general level of arousal and is known as the skin conductance level (SCL). A different perspective is given by the phasic component of skin conductance, which is called the skin conductance response (SCR), because it reflects high frequency variations of the conductance and is directly associated with observable stimuli [40]. The skin conductance signal was recorded at 512 Hz. Although such a high sampling rate is not imperative for measurement of the skin conductance signal, complex analysis approaches and smoothing procedures can benefit from higher resolution data [40]. The SCL was obtained from the raw skin conductance signal by applying a low pass filter at 1 Hz. An additional high pass filter was set at 0.5 Hz for the SCR.

Respiration is yet another physiological signal that has been often studied in psychophysiology [46]. This signal is correlated with processes in the sympathetic nervous system and is indicative of psychological states of individuals [47]. The raw respiration signal was monitored at 512 Hz and treated with low pass and high pass filters. Then, the respiration rate (RR) was obtained from the signal based on the guidelines provided by the manufacturer of the respiration sensor (*TMSI BV*). Afterwards, the RR was averaged with a moving window of 10 seconds.

Skin temperature (ST) fluctuates due to localized variations in the blood flow characterized by vascular resistance or arterial blood pressure that are in turn modulated by the sympathetic nervous system [48]. It has been previously reported in literature [49] that affective stimuli can cause variations in ST of individuals. The ST signal was monitored at 512 Hz. However, the raw data was later harmlessly resampled to 64 Hz because it is a slow changing signal. High frequency noise was eliminated with a low pass filter of 10 Hz that was applied to the resampled signal. Finally, the signal was smoothed with a moving window of 10 seconds.

Keeping in mind practical HCI applications, we preferred not to include electroencephalography (EEG) measures in this study due to concerns about the robustness of the EEG signal.

2.2   Statistical Analysis

As stated in the introduction, one of the motivations for this study was the question whether the patterns of physiological responses to various archetypal experiences are different and, furthermore, if the difference is statistically significant. We were also interested how physiological activations modulated by the explicit emotions of the participants are different comparing to their responses elicited by the archetypal stimuli. A number of statistical tests had to be conducted in order to answer these questions.

Each subject watched all the film clips that formed our sets of stimuli for the explicit emotions and the archetypal experiences. Thus, the study had repeated-measures design where physiological measurements were made on the same individual under changing experimental conditions. An appropriate statistical test for this type of design would be multivariate analysis of variance (MANOVA) for repeated measures [50]. However, certain assumptions of this test were violated for some of the physiological signals' features in our study. Namely MANOVA does not allow inclusion of time-varying covariates in the model and an unequal number of repeated observations per an experimental condition. The former requirement could not be fulfilled because the physiological baselines that were introduced to the statistical model as covariates consisted of multiple data points. Although this assumption could easily be satisfied by transforming a number of data points into a single feature, we preferred to preserve the richness of our dataset and refrained from, for instance, averaging the baseline record. The latter prerequisite of MANOVA demands an equal number of repeated measurements per experimental condition. It could not be met due to the fact that the film clips presented during the experiment had slightly different length and, consequently, the size of vectors with physiological data varied. While all the clips lasted for approximately 5 minutes, there was a considerable difference between some of the stimuli. The shortest film clip had duration of 4 minutes and 46 seconds whereas the longest one was 6 minutes and 35 seconds.

The limitations of MANOVA can be overcome if the statistical analysis is performed with linear mixed models (LMM). LMMs are parametrical statistical models for clustered, longitudinal or repeated-measures data that characterize the relationships between continues dependent variables and predictor factors [51]. LLMs have another advantage over MANOVA – they allow participants with missing data points to be included in the analysis. In contrast, MANOVA drops the entire dataset of a subject even if just one data point is absent. The general specification of an LMM for a given participant i can be defined as follows:

$$Y_i = X_i\beta + Z_iu_i + \varepsilon_i \tag{1}$$

In this equation Y_i is a vector of continues responses for the i-th subject and X_i is a design matrix that contains values of the covariates associated with the vector of fixed-effect parameters β. The Z_i matrix is comprised of covariates that are associated with random effects for the i-th subject. The vector or random effects is assumed to follow a multivariate normal distribution and is denoted with u_i. Finally, the ε_i vector represents residuals. A more elaborate introduction into LMMs can be found in, for instance, [51] or [52].

A software implementation of statistical procedures included in SPSS Version 19 (SPSS, Inc.) was utilized to answer the research questions pointed out earlier. Physiological responses of the subjects were treated as dependent variables (continuous responses), the film clips represented fixed variables and the physiological baselines measured during the presentation of the video with a breathing pattern before each stimulus were used as covariates. The LMMs main effect tests whether the patterns of the participants' physiological responses are different between various stimuli. The HRV features were analyzed with MANOVA as they met the requirements of this method. All statistical tests used a 0.05 significance level.

2.3   Data Mining Techniques

The statistical analysis can enable us to determine whether or not it is possible to distinguish the archetypal experiences of people based on the patterns of their physiological activations corresponding to each of the archetypes. However, a statistically significant difference between the physiological responses associated with various archetypes does not allow evaluation of the practical feasibility to accurately predict psychological states of the participants. On the other hand, a prediction model that maps physiological signals and the unconscious states of the users is what will be appreciated by HCI practitioners. Thus, besides the statistical analysis, data mining techniques were applied to the dataset in order to obtain a predictive model that would facilitate evaluation of the classification accuracy among the archetypal experiences. In order to make physiological data from different individuals comparable, the baseline values were subtracted from the data corresponding to stimuli presentations. The result of the subtraction was then normalized to a range from 0 to 1 for each subject separately.

Classification Methods. As demonstrated film clips had a duration of approximately 5 minutes, the physiological data that was recorded for each stimulus formed temporal sequences. The time sequences classification is different from the recognition of static information due to the increased complexity of the classification task. In general three main kinds of sequence classification algorithms can be distinguished [53] as shown below. However, there are also alternative approaches (see, for instance, [54]).

- Feature based classification essentially transforms a sequence classification problem to a representation amenable for conventional classification methods such as decision trees and neural networks.
- Sequence distance based classification relies on a distance measure that defines the similarity between a pair of time sequences. Similar to the feature based classification the idea of this method is to translate a sequence classification task into a domain where some existing classification algorithm can be used.
- Model based classification makes an assumption that time series are generated by an underlying model. This method requires a statistical model that given a class of data sequences defines the probability distribution of the sequences in the class [53].

In physiological computing, the feature based method of time sequence classification currently dominates [3]. From our point of view, this approach was also well tailored to this study. It has several advantages comparing to the other classification methods. First, this method provides a convenient way to include non-temporal attributes, such as some of the HRV features or the gender of subjects, into the analysis, which sequence distance or model approaches do not [55]. Second, contrary to HMM, this method does not require a considerable amount of training data in order to demonstrate a satisfying performance [55]. Taking into consideration the fact that the physiological data of 10 participants had to be discarded from the analysis, the quantity of data was clearly not enough to achieve competitive classification accuracy with HMM. Third, the identification of model streams representing typical time series that correspond to various psychological states is not trivial in the sequence distance method.

After the selection of attributes, several classifiers were used to construct predictive models for classification. In our analysis 5 classification methods frequently used in physiological computing [3] were evaluated. K-nearest neighbor (kNN) is a simple algorithm that performs instance-based learning classifying an object based on the classes of its neighbors. The second classifier was support vector machine (SVM) that constructs a set of hyperplanes for classification purposes. The third classification method relied on a probabilistic model built with the naïve Bayes algorithm. The fourth approach was linear discriminant analysis (LDA) that is well suited for small data samples and is easy in implementation [3]. Finally, the fifth classification method was the C4.5 algorithm for generation of decision trees. The decision trees were used in conjunction with Adaptive Boosting (AdaBoost) [56] in order to achieve higher accuracy. It was important to guarantee that the classification algorithms are not trained and tested on the same dataset because we wanted to obtain subject independent results. Therefore a leave-one-out cross-validation technique was employed for assessments of the classification performance.

Selection of Features. An essential prerequisite of the classification is the extraction of feature vectors from data sequences. The main goal pursued by the extraction of features is a compression of data sequences to smaller sets of static features. The sliding window, the Discrete Wavelet Transform (DWT) and the Discrete Fourier Transform (DFT) [57–59] are three methods for conversion of time series to static data. The sliding window method performs best with low frequency and relatively short time sequences because an increase of the signal's frequency and length leads to generation of high dimensional feature vector. For long and high frequency data series the DWT and DFT approaches have been introduced. The idea behind these methods is the transformation of a sequence from the time domain to the time-frequency plane (DWT) or to the frequency domain respectively (DFT). Taking into consideration the aspects of our setup, the sliding window method for extraction of feature vectors was an appropriate way to prepare the dataset for the classification. Another name of this approach is segmentation since it first involves partition of a time axis into multiple segments with equal length and then averaging of temporal data along the segments [59].

Our next step was to use the segmentation method with the collected physiological data. The ECG signal provided 38 features in total: 30 features were obtained from the HR temporal data by averaging values of the HR along the segments of 10 seconds; 8 features of the HRV signal (SDNN, RMSSD, SDSD, total power, VLF, LF, HF, and LF/HF). A total of 60 features were extracted from the skin conductance signal. The first 30 features belonged to the SCL signal that was averaged over 30 segments of 10 seconds each. The remaining 30 features were generated in a similar manner from the SCR signal. Then, the respiration signal was converted to 30 features representing the average RR calculated on each of the segments. Another 30 features were obtained from the ST signal by calculating average values over the 30 segments. Finally, we had 158 features ready for the classification.

Dimension Reduction. Reduction of dimensionality is a recommended step in the data mining process. There are various techniques for the reduction of features including principal component analysis (PCA) and LDA. For the purposes of our study LDA was chosen over PCA because in general PCA has the weakness of only capitalizing on between-class information, while LDA uses both within- and between-class information for better performance [60]. Two aspects of LDA should be mentioned here. First, strictly speaking, LDA is not a feature selection but a feature extraction method that obtains the new attributes by a linear combination of the original dimensions. The reduction of dimensionality is achieved by keeping the components with highest variance. Second, LDA can be used for both the identification of important features and classification [3]. Dimension reduction with LDA reduced 158 features into 7 components. For illustration of the importance of each physiological signal in the extracted components, coefficients of determination (R^2) were calculated and put in Table 2. The coefficients of determination specify the amount of variance in one of the 7 discriminant functions that can be described by all the features of a certain physiological signal. The data in Table 2 suggests that electrocardiography and skin conductivity were two measurements which contributions to the discriminant functions were the strongest.

Table 2. Coefficients of determination (R^2) for the seven discriminant functions

	1	2	3	4	5	6	7	Average
ECG	0.553	0.228	0.607	0.971	0.742	0.905	0.184	0.599
SC	0.098	0.060	0.151	0.098	0.164	0.299	0.507	0.197
RR	0.003	0.000	0.003	0.005	0.006	0.001	0.000	0.003
ST	0.004	0.030	0.004	0.000	0.006	0.056	0.002	0.015

3 Results

3.1 Statistical Analysis

The initial motivation of this study was to explore the relationships between the archetypal experiences and their physiological correlations. The statistical analysis was to answer the question whether the archetypal experiences of the participants elicited with the film clips have a significant effect on their physiological signals. The features extracted from ECG, skin conductance, respiration and skin temperature recordings were arranged to form three types of datasets: one with the data for the explicit emotions, another with the data for the archetypal experiences and the unified dataset.

LMMs were fit to each of the datasets with the HR features. The analysis, which the HR entered as a dependent variable, demonstrated a significant interaction effect between the film clips and the HR baselines for all the datasets: the explicit emotions dataset, [$F_{(4, 541.443)} = 2.513$, $p = 0.041$], the archetypal experiences dataset [$F_{(7, 1028.618)} = 3.503$, $p = 0.001$] and the unified dataset, [$F_{(12, 1521.573)} = 3.929$, $p <= 0.001$].

As the HRV features were calculated over the whole duration of every stimulus and were represented with a single data point, they could be easily analyzed with MANOVA for repeated measures. This test showed a significant main effect of the film clips on the HRV parameters of the participants' physiological responses for two of the datasets: the explicit emotions dataset, [$F_{(32, 329.811)} = 2548$, $p <= 0.001$ (Wilks' lambda)] and the unified dataset, [$F_{(96, 1903.193)} = 1987$, $p <= 0.001$ (Wilks' lambda)]. However, the same test for the archetypal experiences dataset was not significant, [$F_{(56, 872.323)} = 1281$, $p = 0.085$ (Wilks' lambda)].

The relationship between the SCL features and the presentations of the stimuli was investigated with LMMs. The statistical tests indicated a significant interaction effect between the film clips and the SCL baselines for the explicit emotions dataset [$F_{(4, 2884,487)} = 42.130$, $p <= 0.001$], the archetypal experiences dataset [$F_{(7, 5880.869)} = 38.795$, $p <= 0.001$] and the unified dataset [$F_{(12, 9868.854)} = 27.615$, $p <= 0.001$]. Next, we ran analysis for the SCR features in a similar manner. A significant interaction effect between the film clips and the baseline covariates was discovered for the explicit emotions dataset, [F(4, 707.582) = 13.473, p <= 0.001], the archetypal experiences dataset, [F(7, 1391.923) = 11.401, p <= 0.001] and the unified dataset, [F(12, 2109.957) = 10.667, p <= 0.001].

Then, we looked at the respiration data and performed tests with LMMs that were fit to the RR measurements. The interaction between the film clips and the baseline RR did not demonstrated significance for the archetypal experiences dataset, [F(7, 1071.446) = 1.070, p = 0.380] and the unified dataset [F(12,1686.540) = 1.667, p = 0.068]. Nevertheless, the same test was significant for the explicit emotions dataset, [F(4, 611.304) = 2.931, p = 0.020].

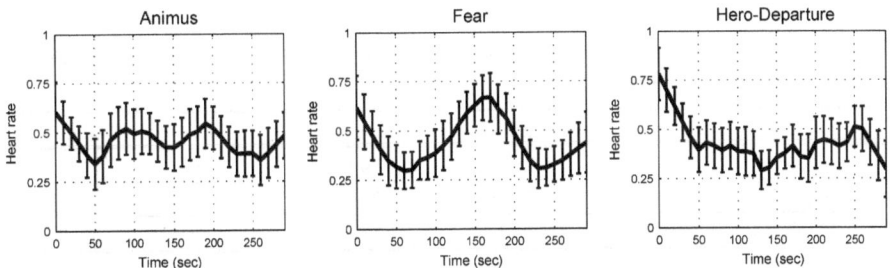

Fig. 1. Heart rate responses of the subjects to the film clips. The mean values and 95% confidence intervals of the HR are represented with the bold lines and the vertical bars.

Finally, the features of the skin temperature recordings were analyzed. Again, LMMs built on the ST data were used for the statistical testing. However, we could not complete the analysis because the statistical software did not achieve a convergence within 100 of iterations.

For illustrative purposes, the data of HR signal that contributed to the discriminant functions the most is presented on Fig. 1. The mean values and 95% confidence intervals of the HR are indicated for several of the stimuli.

3.2   Classification

After the statistical analysis an evaluation of several predictive models was conducted. This evaluation was aimed at answering the question of how accurate the archetypal experiences can be predicted and classified by computational intelligence algorithms from physiological data.

Similar to the statistical analysis the classification was performed on three collections of data records: the explicit emotions dataset, the archetypal dataset and the unified dataset that integrated all the available data. Every selected classification method (kNN, SVM, naïve Bayes, LDA and AdaBoost with decision trees) was applied to each of the datasets.

For the archetypal dataset the model constructed with the kNN method was able to correctly classify 74% of the instances. However, the same classification approach resulted in the recognition rate of 72% for the explicit emotions dataset and of 49.8% for the unified dataset. The number of nearest neighbors equal to 20 ($k = 20$) lead to the optimal performance in all the cases. The SVM algorithm provided better classification accuracy than kNN for the archetypal dataset (75.5%) and for the unified dataset (68.3%). On the other hand it demonstrated slightly lower recognition rate on the explicit emotions dataset (71.2%). The naïve Bayes and LDA approaches enabled us to achieve similar performance on the archetypal dataset (79.5%) and the explicit emotions dataset (74.4%). The recognition rate on the unified dataset was higher with the LDA method (61.2%) comparing to the naïve Bayes classifier (57.2%). Finally, decision trees in conjunction with AdaBoost led to the poorest classification results: 67% for the archetypal dataset, 68.8% for the explicit emotions dataset and 47.1% for the unified dataset. A summary of the classification results is provided in Table 3.

Table 3. Classification performance achieved with different methods for the archetypal, the explicit and the unified datasets

Dataset	kNN	SVM	Naïve Bayes	LDA	AdaBoost
Archetypal	74%	75.5%	79.5%	79.5%	67%
Explicit	72%	71.2%	74.4%	74.4%	68.8%
Unified	49.8%	68.3%	57.2%	61.2%	47.1%

4   Discussion

4.1   Statistical Analysis

A number of statistical tests were run on the collected data. Their outcomes gave evidence of a significant relationship between some of the physiological signals and the psychological conditions of the subjects. Whereas the patterns in three out of the four measurements reflected the induced explicit emotions, no association could be inferred from the skin temperature signal. These findings were anticipated and go along with the state of the art of physiological computing. Unfortunately, the skin temperature signal did not justify our expectations and, from our point of view, its variations are too slow to successfully contribute to the differentiation of emotions. The archetypal states of the participants demonstrated statistically significant relationship with the HR, SCL and SCR features extracted from the ECG and skin conductance signals. In comparison with the explicit emotions, the archetypal experiences lead to observable activations in a smaller number of the physiological features. Nevertheless, our results show that the patterns of physiological responses to various archetypal experiences are different and the difference is statistically significant. Furthermore, the analysis performed with the unified dataset, which integrated the explicit emotions and the archetypal experiences, supported the hypothesis of possibility to distinguish between these two types of stimuli.

4.2   Classification Accuracy

Having conducted the statistical analysis we were curious how accurately computational intelligence methods can classify the archetypal experiences. The findings of our study indicate that prediction models built with data mining techniques and trained on the physiological data of the subjects achieved reasonably high precision. Five different classification methods were used to obtain the models that demonstrated classification rates from 67% to 79.5%. These results are not subject-depended and characterize the ability of the models to predict the correct archetypal conditions from the physiological recordings of an unknown user. While it is easy to check the classification accuracy of the explicit emotions against other studies in affect recognition, the same comparison for the archetypal experiences is challenging. We are aware of only one study [61] where the responses of people to brief presentations of *mandala* symbols, which are considered to express the archetype of the self, were measured with physiological sensors. The reported classification rate of 23.3% is considerably lower than the results obtained in this study. This fact can be explained with the differences in the design of the experiments. In particular, the duration of stimuli presentation and the type of stimuli seem to be important. Indeed, the film clips extracted from blockbuster movies are likely to be more powerful than the images of mandala presented for several seconds. Our findings for the archetypal experiences can also be set against previous studies in affect recognition just to have a relative benchmark. Judging by the review provided in [3], the classification accuracy of our models is on par with the ones demonstrated in those studies. Although in some cases higher recognition rates have been reported, for instance in [62–64] researchers achieved classification precision of up to 97.4%, two types of limitations, which seem to exist in these studies, have to be taken into account. First, in some cases the classification is subject-dependent, meaning that recognition algorithms are adjusted to perform well only with the data belonging to a particular individual and cannot be generalized. Second, the number of the psychological conditions that are being predicted is important because the more classes to be classified, the more difficult the problem becomes. This can be illustrated with a simple example – in a case of two classes problem, accuracy of 50% is attained simply by chance, while in a situation with 8 classes the chance level drops to 12.5%. In our experiment we had 8 conditions to be differentiated, but the best recognition rates were obtained in the studies that considered only 2 or 3 affective states.

Looking at the obtained results it seems clear that the Naïve Bayes and LDA classification methods generally outperformed other approaches. A particularly interesting finding is that higher prediction accuracy was obtained for the archetypal dataset comparing to the explicit emotions dataset. The better recognition rate was achieved despite of the fact that the archetypal dataset contained 8 classes while the explicit emotion dataset only 5. From our point of view, the archetypes were classified more accurately than the explicit emotions because by definition they elicit cognitive and affective activations that are universal across the population. On the other hand, the explicit emotions are more subject-dependent and considerably vary due to an individual's personality.

In the future work it will be necessary to improve the classification accuracy. From our point of view, an increase of the recognition rate can be achieved by taking into account additional parameters of physiological signals and performing subject-dependent classification.

4.3   Archetypal Stimuli

The stimuli for induction of the archetypal experiences were a crucial component of the study. However, as it was the first experiment where the archetypal experiences were elicited with film clips, we did not have an empirical evidence that the stimuli we identified with the help of ARAS [39] would successfully express the 8 targeted archetypes. Another concern was related to the length of the film clips. Due to the fact that they each lasted approximately five minutes, it was reasonable to expect highly heterogeneous affective and cognitive responses of the participants that would complicate the recognition problem. Judging by our findings, the selection of the film clips was satisfactory and the universal unconscious reactions in subjects from various regions of the world were elicited successfully. This conclusion can be made based on the accurate recognition rate that otherwise would not be possible to attain.

4.4   Limitations

Several limitations of this study should be highlighted. First, a relatively small number of participants can be considered as a limitation. Next, during the presentation of the film clips the subjects generally sit still and the amount of movements was small. For this reason, we did not have to implement any dedicated signal processing methods for combating the movement artifacts that would likely be necessary in many HCI scenarios. The third limitation is the generalizability of the results. Only a single example of each archetype was presented to the participants. This fact limits the generalizability of our findings and demands new studies with more representations for every archetype to be carried out. Finally, it is necessary to perform comparison of the physiological data and the self-reports provided by the subjects. Such a comparison will indicate to which extent the participants were able to consciously perceive the archetypal appearances in the film clips.

4.5   Conclusion

To a large extent people are driven by the collective unconscious in their decisions, motivations, and behaviors. So far, the unconscious experiences of the users have received little attention in physiological computing because it has been primary dealing with cognition and affect. In this study the feasibility of recognizing the archetypal experiences of users, which constitute the collective unconscious, with wireless sensors and without human interventions, was evaluated. The experiment that featured 8 archetypes visualized with the film clips was executed in order to collect physiological data. We then applied data mining methods to the obtained dataset, performed statistical analysis and built several prediction models that demonstrated prediction accuracy of up to 79.5%. Thus, physiological sensors coupled with computational intelligence algorithms can facilitate development of HCI interfaces that sense archetypal experiences of the users and use this information for system adaptation.

Acknowledgements. The authors thank The Archive for Research in Archetypal Symbolism (ARAS) and in particular John Beebe, Baruch Gould, Iden Goodman, Allison Tuzo and Tom Singer for the help with identification and selection of the archetypal stimuli. We also thank the anonymous reviewers for their helpful comments. This work was supported in part by the Erasmus Mundus Joint Doctorate (EMJD) in Interactive and Cognitive Environments (ICE), which is funded by Erasmus Mundus under the FPA no. 2010-2012.

References

1. Picard, R.W.: Affective computing, MIT Media Laboratory Perceptual Computing Section Technical Report No. 321 (1995)
2. Fairclough, S.H.: Fundamentals of physiological computing. Interacting with Computers 21, 133–145 (2009)
3. Novak, D., Mihelj, M., Munih, M.: A survey of methods for data fusion and system adaptation using autonomic nervous system responses in physiological computing. Interacting with Computers 24, 154–172 (2012)
4. Zhou, F., Qu, X., Helander, M.G., Jiao, J.(R.): Affect prediction from physiological measures via visual stimuli. International Journal of Human-Computer Studies 69, 801–819 (2011)
5. Wu, D., Courtney, C.G., Lance, B.J., Narayanan, S.S., Dawson, M.E., Oie, K.S., Parsons, T.D.: Optimal arousal identification and classification for affective computing using physiological signals: virtual reality stroop task. IEEE Transactions on Affective Computing 1, 109–118 (2010)
6. Stickel, C., Ebner, M., Steinbach-Nordmann, S., Searle, G., Holzinger, A.: Emotion detection: application of the valence arousal space for rapid biological usability testing to enhance universal access. In: Stephanidis, C. (ed.) Universal Access in HCI, Part I, HCII 2009. LNCS, vol. 5614, pp. 615–624. Springer, Heidelberg (2009)
7. Nisbett, R.E., Wilson, T.D.: Telling more than we can know: verbal reports on mental processes. Psychological Review 84, 231–259 (1977)
8. Van Gaal, S., Lamme, V.A.F.: Unconscious high-level information processing: implication for neurobiological theories of consciousness. The Neuroscientist 18, 287–301 (2012)
9. Bargh, J.A., Morsella, E.: The unconscious mind. Perspectives on Psychological Science 3, 73–79 (2008)
10. Rauterberg, M.: Emotions: The voice of the unconscious. In: Yang, H.S., Malaka, R., Hoshino, J., Han, J.H. (eds.) ICEC 2010. LNCS, vol. 6243, pp. 205–215. Springer, Heidelberg (2010)
11. Sally, W.: Algorithms and archetypes: evolutionary psychology and Carl Jung's theory of the collective unconscious. Journal of Social and Evolutionary Systems 17, 287–306 (1994)
12. Jung, C.G.: The archetypes and the collective unconscious. Princeton University Press, Princeton (1981)
13. Jung, C.G.: Man and his symbols. Doubleday, Garden City (1964)
14. Miller, N.E.: Some examples of psychophysiology and the unconscious. Applied Psychophysiology and Biofeedback 17, 3–16 (1992)
15. Lang, P.J., Bradley, M.M., Cuthbert, B.N.: International affective picture system (IAPS): affective ratings of pictures and instruction manual. Technical Report A-8, Gainesville, FL, USA (2008)
16. Bradley, M.M., Lang, P.J.: International affective digitized sounds (IADS): stimuli, instruction manual and affective ratings (Tech. Rep. No. B-2), Gainesville, FL, USA (1999)
17. Eich, E., Ng, J.T.W., Macaulay, D., Percy, A.D., Grebneva, I.: Combining music with thought to change mood. In: Coan, J.A., Allen, J.J.B. (eds.) The Handbook of Emotion Elicitation and Assessment, pp. 124–136. Oxford University Press, New York (2007)

18. Gross, J.J., Levenson, R.W.: Emotion elicitation using films. Cognition & Emotion 9, 87–108 (1995)
19. Rottenberg, J., Ray, R.D., Gross, J.J.: Emotion elicitation using films. In: Coan, J.A., Allen, J.J.B. (eds.) Handbook of Emotion Elicitation and Assessment, pp. 9–28. Oxford University Press, New York (2007)
20. Task Force of the European Society of Cardiology and the North American Society of Pacing and Electrophysiology: Heart rate variability: standards of measurement, physiological interpretation, and clinical use. Circulation 93, 1043–1065 (1996)
21. Russell, J.A.: A circumplex model of affect. Journal of Personality and Social Psychology 39, 1161–1178 (1980)
22. Ivonin, L., Chang, H.-M., Chen, W., Rauterberg, M.: A new representation of emotion in affective computing. In: Proceeding of 2012 International Conference on Affective Computing and Intelligent Interaction (ICACII 2012), Taipei, Taiwan. Lecture Notes in Information Technology, pp. 337–343 (2012)
23. Lang, P.J., Greenwald, M.K., Bradley, M.M., Hamm, A.O.: Looking at pictures: affective, facial, visceral, and behavioral reactions. Psychophysiology 30, 261–273 (1993)
24. Soleymani, M., Pantic, M., Pun, T.: Multimodal emotion recognition in response to videos. IEEE Transactions on Affective Computing 3, 211–223 (2011)
25. Faber, M.A., Mayer, J.D.: Resonance to archetypes in media: there is some accounting for taste. Journal of Research in Personality 43, 307–322 (2009)
26. Hannan, D.: Coral sea dreaming: awaken. Roadshow Entertainment (2010)
27. Demme, J.: The silence of the lambs. Orion Pictures (1991)
28. Atkinson, R., Curtis, R.: Mr. Bean (season 1, episode 1). Pearson Television International (1990)
29. Allers, R., Minkoff, R.: The Lion King. Walt Disney Pictures (1994)
30. Zemeckis, R.: Forrest Gump. Paramount Pictures (1994)
31. Mendes, S.: American beauty. DreamWorks Pictures (1999)
32. Gibson, M.: Braveheart. 20th Century Fox (1995)
33. Aronofsky, D.: Black swan. Fox Searchlight Pictures (2010)
34. Hooper, T.: The king's speech. The Weinstein Company (2010)
35. Almodóvar, P.: All about my mother. Warner Sogefilms (1999)
36. Fincher, D.: Fight club. 20th Century Fox (1999)
37. Campbell, J.: The hero with a thousand faces. New World Library, Novato (2008)
38. Maloney, A.: Preference ratings of images representing archetypal themes: an empirical study of the concept of archetypes. Journal of Analytical Psychology 44, 101–116 (2002)
39. Gronning, T., Sohl, P., Singer, T.: ARAS: archetypal symbolism and images. Visual Resources 23, 245–267 (2007)
40. Figner, B., Murphy, R.O.: Using skin conductance in judgment and decision making research. In: Schulte-Mecklenbeck, M., Kuehberger, A., Ranyard, R. (eds.) A Handbook of Process Tracking Methods for Decision Research, pp. 163–184. Psychology Press, New York (2011)
41. Piferi, R.L., Kline, K.A., Younger, J., Lawler, K.A.: An alternative approach for achieving cardiovascular baseline: viewing an aquatic video. International Journal of Psychophysiology 37, 207–217 (2000)
42. Neuman, M.R.: Vital signs: heart rate. IEEE Pulse 1, 51–55 (2010)
43. Afonso, V.X., Tompkins, W.J., Nguyen, T.Q.: ECG beat detection using filter banks. IEEE Transactions on Biomedical Engineering 46, 192–202 (1999)
44. Kreibig, S.D.: Autonomic nervous system activity in emotion: a review. Biological Psychology 84, 394–421 (2010)

45. Ramshur, J.T.: Design, evaluation, and application of heart rate variability software (HRVAS). Master's thesis, The University of Memphis, Memphis, TN (2010)
46. Fairclough, S.H., Venables, L.: Prediction of subjective states from psychophysiology: a multivariate approach. Biological Psychology 71, 100–110 (2006)
47. Boiten, F.A.: The effects of emotional behaviour on components of the respiratory cycle. Biological Psychology 49, 29–51 (1998)
48. Kim, K.H., Bang, S.W., Kim, S.R.: Emotion recognition system using short-term monitoring of physiological signals. Medical & Biological Engineering & Computing 42, 419–427 (2004)
49. Ekman, P., Levenson, R., Friesen, W.: Autonomic nervous system activity distinguishes among emotions. Science 221, 1208–1210 (1983)
50. O'Brien, R.G., Kaiser, M.K.: MANOVA method for analyzing repeated measures designs: an extensive primer. Psychological Bulletin 97, 316–333 (1985)
51. West, B.T., Welch, K.B., Galecki, A.T.: Linear mixed models: a practical guide using statistical software. Chapman and Hall/CRC, Boca Raton (2006)
52. Cnaan, A., Laird, N.M., Slasor, P.: Using the general linear mixed model to analyse unbalanced repeated measures and longitudinal data. Statistics in Medicine 16, 2349–2380 (1997)
53. Xing, Z., Pei, J., Keogh, E.: A brief survey on sequence classification. ACM SIGKDD Explorations Newsletter 12, 40 (2010)
54. Holzinger, A., Stocker, C., Bruschi, M., Auinger, A., Silva, H., Gamboa, H., Fred, A.: On applying approximate entropy to ECG signals for knowledge discovery on the example of big sensor data. In: Huang, R., Ghorbani, A.A., Pasi, G., Yamaguchi, T., Yen, N.Y., Jin, B. (eds.) AMT 2012. LNCS, vol. 7669, pp. 646–657. Springer, Heidelberg (2012)
55. Kadous, M.W., Sammut, C.: Classification of multivariate time series and structured data using constructive induction. Machine Learning 58, 179–216 (2005)
56. Freund, Y., Schapire, R.E.: A decision-theoretic generalization of on-line learning and an application to boosting. Journal of Computer and System Sciences 55, 119–139 (1997)
57. Agrawal, R., Faloutsos, C., Swami, A.: Efficient similarity search in sequence databases. In: Lomet, D.B. (ed.) FODO 1993. LNCS, vol. 730, pp. 69–84. Springer, Heidelberg (1993)
58. Chan, F.K.: Haar wavelets for efficient similarity search of time-series: with and without time warping. IEEE Transactions on Knowledge and Data Engineering 15, 686–705 (2003)
59. Geurts, P.: Pattern extraction for time series classification. In: Siebes, A., De Raedt, L. (eds.) PKDD 2001. LNCS (LNAI), vol. 2168, pp. 115–127. Springer, Heidelberg (2001)
60. Martinez, A.M., Kak, A.C.: PCA versus LDA. IEEE Transactions on Pattern Analysis and Machine Intelligence 23, 228–233 (2001)
61. Ivonin, L., Chang, H.-M., Chen, W., Rauterberg, M.: Unconscious emotions: quantifying and logging something we are not aware of. Personal and Ubiquitous Computing 17, 663–673 (2013)
62. Healey, J.A., Picard, R.W.: Detecting stress during real-world driving tasks using physiological sensors. IEEE Transactions on Intelligent Transportation Systems 6, 156–166 (2005)
63. Picard, R.W., Vyzas, E., Healey, J.: Toward machine emotional intelligence: analysis of affective physiological state. IEEE Transactions on Pattern Analysis and Machine Intelligence 23, 1175–1191 (2001)
64. Sakr, G.E., Elhajj, I.H., Huijer, H.A.-S.: Support vector machines to define and detect agitation transition. IEEE Transactions on Affective Computing 1, 98–108 (2010)

Technique for Evaluating Photo Sharing Interfaces with the Early Prototypes - Group Simulation

Jarno Aulis Olavi Ojala[1], Dhaval Vyas[2], and Arto Juhani Lehtiniemi[3]

[1] Tampere University of Technology, Human-Centered Technology,
P.O. Box 589, 33101 Tampere, Finland
[2] Industrial Software Systems, ABB Corporate Research, Bangalore, India
[3] Nokia Research Center, Visiokatu 3, FIN-33270, Tampere, Finland
`jarno.ojala@tut.fi`, `dhaval.vyas@yahoo.com`,
`arto.lehtiniemi@nokia.com`

Abstract. User evaluations using paper prototypes commonly lack social context. The *Group simulation technique* described in this paper offers a solution to this problem. The study introduces an early-phase participatory design technique targeted for small groups. The proposed technique is used for evaluating an interface, which enables group work in photo collection creation. Three groups of four users, 12 in total, took part in a simulation session where they tested a low-fidelity design concept that included their own personal photo content from an event that their group attended together. The users' own content was used to evoke natural experiences. Our results indicate that the technique helped users to naturally engage with the prototype in the session. The technique is suggested to be suitable for evaluating other early-phase concepts and to guide design solutions, especially with the concepts that include users' personal content and enable content sharing.

Keywords: User studies, participatory design, mobile interfaces, personal content management, content sharing, social interaction, user experience, design.

1 Introduction

The number of social networking services (SNS) [1], content management and sharing services hand in hand with the devices for capturing and storing content has exploded in recent years. Digital content sharing has grown rapidly hand in hand with the development of capturing devices, social networking and file sharing services. Social media and social networking services are growingly relying on personal content that is shared or published in these services. Since capturing images and editing them has become easier and applications available and usable to everyone, the new focus is designing experience of photo enjoyment [2]. While producing the photos has become easier, practices for enjoying the digital photos together as when people gathered to watch the freshly developed set of printed photos some years ago has changed [3]. Users capture personal content with multiple devices such as mobile phones, digital cameras and video

A. Holzinger et al. (Eds.): SouthCHI 2013, LNCS 7946, pp. 36–53, 2013.

capturing devices. Organizing and managing the massive collections on hard disks and online has become a burden for the users.

Users are not only dealing with the photos taken by themselves, but also those taken by others. Managing and maintaining the growing personal inventories [4, 5] of photos and other personal media [6, 7] and sharing the meaningful content with others [8, 9, 10, 11] has become an interesting area for research and development. Novel solutions and design methods for creating pleasurable user experiences are needed.

The first objective of the simulations in this research was to create real interaction within the group using their own personal content. As previous studies show, collectively created and shared content can develop into highly emotional objects and work as a central motivator for the interaction in a group [12, 13]. The research contribution of this work is two-folded. Firstly, it evaluates the concept and, secondly, it contributes to the field of participatory design with a group simulation technique that involving users' actual personally created content.

Goals of this study are:

- To evaluate the technique of using participants' own content in early phase prototype simulation.
- To identify habits of collaboration in the photo organization and sharing by observing users' interactions with the prototype in the simulation sessions.
- To evaluate the concept by using the early prototype in the simulation sessions
- To contribute to design recommendations and implications for photo-sharing systems we aim to identify the weak signals that users give in their group working and learn how social context can actualized in the prototype.

This work contributes to Human-Computer interaction research field firstly, by introducing a concept for small group photo sharing and, secondly, by introducing a technique for designing and evaluating similar content sharing applications in an early phase of development.

2   Related Work

New photographing devices support users in taking the photos, but all the effort that is made after photographing offers more interesting areas for development. Kirk et al. [14] have identified and named the process that happens after the photo capturing as *"photowork"* and the authors have identified and categorized the activities that people perform on their digital photos. In the study [14] photowork was categorized in to actions of finding, sharing and receiving. Similarly, Lehikoinen and others [15] introduce "get, enjoy, maintain and share" –model for the personal content, which describes the process of the content experiencing. The work identifies patterns that occur before sharing and publishing PC use of digital photographs and paper prints have been extensively studied in the past [16]. Frohlich et al. introduce four categories of photo-sharing activities: co-present and remote sharing, archiving and sending.

Current solutions of *photoware* [16] should enable all of these activities within a single system and remove the boundaries between these practices.

In a study by Miller and Edwards [17], users described a habit of downloading pictures of others as a part of their own photo collection. Most of the users added photos of others to their collection in the study and did not see any particular problems in that. The study describes two cultures of photo sharing "snaprs" and "Kodak-culture". The Snaprs had shifted their photowork and sharing almost entirely to SNS, where Kodak-culture shared digital photos through mail very limitedly [17]. Due to the different channels these groups had different socialization styles related to photos.

2.1   Designing Photo Sharing Technology for Small Groups

Previous studies of photo sharing and photowork have identified problems in archiving the photos. Some of these problems are still not answered with technology. Photos are identified in many studies as highly personal content. For this reason, people are very sensitive with sharing photos and videos of their close-ones and the groups they belong to. The people are more eager to share personal content within the private circles such as family and close friends, as previous studies show [18]. Sharing photos to small groups, such as relatives, close friends or private groups has different motivations and needs than sharing to bigger audiences. Olsson [10] introduces three-fold motivations for photo collecting and sharing. The main motivator for storing personal photos and making private collection is claimed to be personal growth and identity building. Sharing to small groups mostly includes documenting everyday life, sharing memories and telling stories of meaningful events or extraordinary occasions

In the study by Petrelli and Whittaker [19] meaningful objects for family memories were studied and results show that 16% of the meaningful objects that participants chose from their homes were physical photos. Functions of the memorial objects that were identified in the study were: important event, relationship, activities, personal reminiscence, identity and personal achievements.

When people share photos with relatives and friends, the main motivator is be strengthening the existing social ties [10]. The most public level of sharing, where photos are put out to whole community or service, includes motivational factors of self-expression and getting attention from others [19, 20 21]. Self-expressional needs and presenting oneself through the photographs come up in both sharing photos regardless of the size of the target audience [20, 21]. Adjustments of privacy levels become an issue, when photos are shared through online systems. For some users personal photos are the most sensitive objects of their personal content. Frohlich and others [16] introduce taxonomy of sharing usage, where time and presence are the most important factors. Sharing of photos includes personal archiving as a starting point ("sharing to self"), sending and remote sharing with others online and co-present sharing that can include co-present sharing with online-services or other devices.

Cloud computing technology allows new solutions for archiving the photos outside the hard disks and drives. Databases and storages that are accessible everywhere and through different devices have been introduced [22]. MyLifeBits is a personal collection, which aims for managing all the other digital content. Other services and concepts such as Dropbox [23] for all the digital content and Picasa for photos only have been introduced lately for full content management and sharing. Idea of these collections is to create a personal inventory that is accessible anywhere and with many devices. The fragmentation of the personal content also means that content is accessible from many locations and devices, also across the platforms [24].

Co-present or collocated [25, 26] sharing of photos with mobile phones has been studied widely earlier. These studies introduce new concepts that support novel interaction models with many mobile devices. Sharing can happen collaboratively by synchronous and shared screens. "pass-them-around" prototype introduces way of using multiple mobile phones to view the photo collection of the group [18].

New technologies to share and present photos for selected and limited group have been developed recently. Most of these technologies use mobile phones as photographing device but as a device for group formation and photo presentation and viewing. Feed me–system supports "directed sharing" [7] that recognizes users close contacts and their interests and aims to more effective and targeted sharing of content. Nunes et al. [27] introduced "Souvenirs" prototype that enables users to link photos with physical memorabilia in the home environment. In the study, it was seen that photo collections only on the hard disk of the computer can prevent users from spontaneous presenting and experiencing the photos together. Digitalization of the photo collections [28] can evoke feeling of inability to access digital photos freely, which can be a source of frustration, as a study by Petrelli and Whittaker [19] suggests.

Battarbee suggests that designing for co-experience should always include the social context and that "more than one person is involved in a unit of study, to create the conditions for co-experience in a manner that is appropriate for the design context." [29]. Battarbee suggests that designers should take part as the co-experiencers. Group simulation aims to support participation of users in a design process in a novel and light-weight way.

2.2   Participatory Design in an Early Phase Development

Social features in interfaces introduce a new area for early evaluation of the services and devices. Systems and software that enable social interaction and are targeted for sharing personal content can only be fully understood by using the users' actual content instead of generated content that is normally used in paper prototypes or even in more functional prototypes.

The problem with classical paper prototypes is the generic nature of the content, which mostly is added or created by the researchers, designers or developers. The interaction with content created by the researchers can vary from the interaction with personal content. Same problem may occur in the implemented interactive prototypes, as the critical mass of users to produce the content is hard to reach. In the systems, applications and services that enable management and sharing personal content the privacy aspects as well as the motivations to use the solutions are revealed only when the actual content is available. By investing time and resources to collect actual personal content that is created by the users themselves, the work aims to make the prototype more personal and thereby more meaningful to users. User interviews and focus groups are suitable methods for collecting feedback for developing new concepts and collecting ideas from current needs and practices, but early evaluation of concepts needs other kinds of study designs.

The use of early stage prototypes in a participatory design has been studied before. Hagen and others [30] describe characteristics of a *simulation* study in mobile research. Simulations aim to "reflect or recreate a mobile use situation" [30]. However, traditional simulations are criticized of not including the social context or "social environment" [31] to the early-stage evaluations. The *Group simulation* described in this paper aims to solve this problem by adding the social context of a group and users' personally created content to the prototype. Prototype is evaluated by participatory design sessions by using the technique of simulation [30].

Participatory design workshops have used mock-ups and physical, but non-functional prototypes to create hands-on experiences [32] as well as imaginary "make tools" [33] to give users free hands to imagine the features they need but are not yet present. Using tangible and physical mock-ups and real objects that may have "magical" or imagined features is a powerful way to generate ideas. Through the use of make tools users are able to express the needs they have for new technology that may not yet exist. Another participatory design direction is "bodystorming" [34] in a sense to arrange workshops in real contexts. This paper uses these ideas to generate real social context and facilitate the interaction in the session through tangible prototype that is a real world "photo book" object with added functionality that is facilitated by the researchers acting as the service intelligence in the sessions. "Wizard of Oz"-technique in participatory design as well as in usability testing is a technique where user interacts with a prototype that is actually manipulated by a researcher [32, 35]. In these settings, users are sometimes aware of the setting, but sometimes left uninformed that actually the device intelligence is not artificial.

3   Prototype Design

The idea of a system that enables instant photo sharing and uploading was crafted in the project. Earlier studies have shown that users had a need for instant sharing of photos especially within their close contacts [15, 27, 5, 10]. In order to evaluate the created concept idea and to validate the actual features to be implemented the concept was introduced to the participants with a paper prototype in the group simulation sessions. As a paper prototype, we used dedicated *photo books*. The construction and content collection of these photo books are described later in the methods part. All of the functions in the system were introduced to the participants by using "Wizard of Oz"-technique. The researchers worked as the "intelligence" of the system in the simulations sessions. They performed as facilitators of the social interaction functionality and the features in the system, so the users could get idea of the complete functionality prototype offers. The private group setting and instant sharing are the key differentiators from conventional photo sharing tools such as Facebook [36] or Flickr [37]. In our current setup, user's photos are directly uploaded to a shared album, which is accessible to relevant users [38].

The prototype implementation included special features that were introduced to the users in the sessions. In the start of the session, users were introduced with two novel ways to interact with the system: *FingerPrints* and *MoodPhotos*. Additionally the prototype also included *My Picture Everywhere* function.

MoodPhotos gathers users' facial expression during the use of system. When user browses through photos in the album, system captures certain expressions by front camera of the mobile for example. These expression photos can then be shared to other watchers browsing the same photo. User can add her mood photos from a sequence of photos that the device has automatically taken while you were viewing the image. User can either select from the captured mood photos or pose and take a new one to share. The concept uses front camera of mobile phones or laptops to detect the face of the viewer. When a user browses a photo from a shared album for a prolonged time, a counter indicates mood photos and fingerprints that other people have left on the image. Mood Photos feature aims for target experience of instantly sharing emotional reactions to photos [38] and thus give users feel of relatedness through the technology [2].

The FingerPrint concept uses the metaphor of physical photo sharing where viewers unintentionally leave their fingerprints on photos. Idea is to use the metaphor in more positive sense in order to disclose other users the activities of watchers of the photo. Users are able to view consumption patterns of their photos. The fingerprints are shown in different colours, sizes and intensity to represent type of friends (e.g. colleague, family), frequency, recent activity and the length of viewing [38].

My Picture Everywhere concept gives users information of the photos in which they appear. My Picture Everywhere uses face recognition algorithms to detect the photos that user appears in and provides then option to contact the author of the photo.

4   Research Method

Simulation sessions were held with each group. In the session participants were introduced with a concept that enables instant photo sharing within their small group.

Each session with groups started with an introductory session, where users were given instructions for their co-creation event in which they took part together. After the event they were invited to the simulation sessions. Sessions included introduction to the concept prototype service and feature concepts, individual browsing sessions and in the end group interview.

During the introductory session each user was guided to take at least 20 photographs in an event that they arranged. This event was planned in a way it would be optimal for being a *co-creation event* where users would spend time together and take as many photos of the event, each other and the whole group.

After their co-creation event together users shared the photos with the researchers. They were ordered not to show the photos to each other before the simulation sessions, so they would see the photos taken by others first time in the event. Simulation sessions were organized 1-2 weeks after their *content co-creation event*. Researchers analyzed the photos and created dedicated *photo books* for the simulation sessions from the event photos.

4.1   Background of the Participating Groups

Participant groups were recruited from the mailing lists, social media services, forums and researchers' contacts. Study included three groups of potential users of the studied system. Each group consisted of four members. The participant groups were recruited through multiple mailing lists for students of Tampere Universities and through forums of photographers.

Background data of the participants was collected by using a web form before the interviews. The participants were screened for the study by their answers in the web form. The selection was made on basis of their equipment usage, age and activity of photographing and sharing habits in social networking services. The aim was to have four groups with different backgrounds. The participant groups include both non-technical photographers who do not use professional equipment and more advanced photographers with semi-pro or pro equipment.

All the participant groups had organized an event together, where they captured the photos for the simulation (Fig. 1).

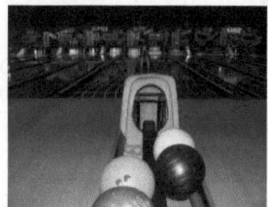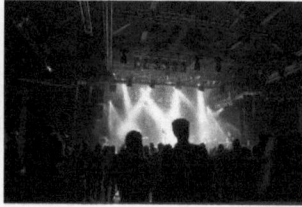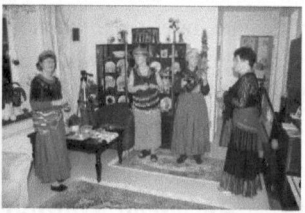

Fig. 1. Users photos from their events. Photo on the left is from Group 1 and their bowling event, photo on the center shows Group 2 in a music concert, photo on the right shows Group 3 and their social event at one of the members' home.

The participant groups were informed to select events where they would normally take photos. Selections of photos to describe the nature of the main events the groups participated in is given in Fig. 1. Bowling group consisted of students (2 males, 2 females, ages 27-30). The group went bowling and had a dinner together. Music festival group consisted of students (3 males, 1 female, ages 22-26) and they took part in "Lost in Music 2011" indoor festival in Tampere. Senior photographers consisted of four pensioners (all females, ages 67-72). They arranged a party together at one of the group members' home in Tampere. Participants were instructed to take at least 20 photos in their co-creation sessions. The activity of participants was surprising, and they took totally 782 photos for the photo books in their events (Table 1).

Table 1. Number of photos captured in the co-creation events

Participant	Number of photos added by participant	Group (total number of photos)
U1	112	Bowling (273)
U2	23	Bowling (273)
U3	66	Bowling (273)
U4	22	Bowling (273)
U5	160	Music (378)
U6	48	Music (378)
U7	56	Music (378)
U8	114	Music (378)
U9	35	Camera club (181)
U10	47	Camera club (181)
U11	55	Camera club (181)
U12	44	Camera club (181)
Total	**782**	**All groups (782)**

Music group was the most active in the photo taking, and partial reason may be the event that they attended. All the groups kept their photos in privacy and did not show them to others before the simulations, so the simulations could really represent the first browsing session of the folders (Table 1).

4.2   Simulating the Prototype Functionality with the Photo Books as Prototype

For demonstrating the functionality and the features in a tangible and physical approach, the *photo books* were created (Figure 1). For every session three different photo books were created from the photos that users had captured. Each photo book consisted of 15-20 photos totally. The photos selected from collection that they had created during the co-creation events. The photos were added to the book in a random sequence. The photos were added on the background graphic layer of photo book prototype service. A transparency that showed the graphic user interface and the features was added in top of each picture.

Paper prototypes were selected for the study instead of using actual interactive implementations at the early phase in order to test the validity and suitability of the concept as early in the development process as possible. Using the real life objects such as photo books can reveal ways of interaction that may not occur with the implementations. This study aims to exploit physical world and real interactions in order to duplicate similar interaction in the actual implementation later on.

Photo books (Fig. 2) were used as a paper prototype of the photo sharing service where people are able to easily share their photos within the small group. Photo books included Moods and FingerPrints functionality as represented earlier.

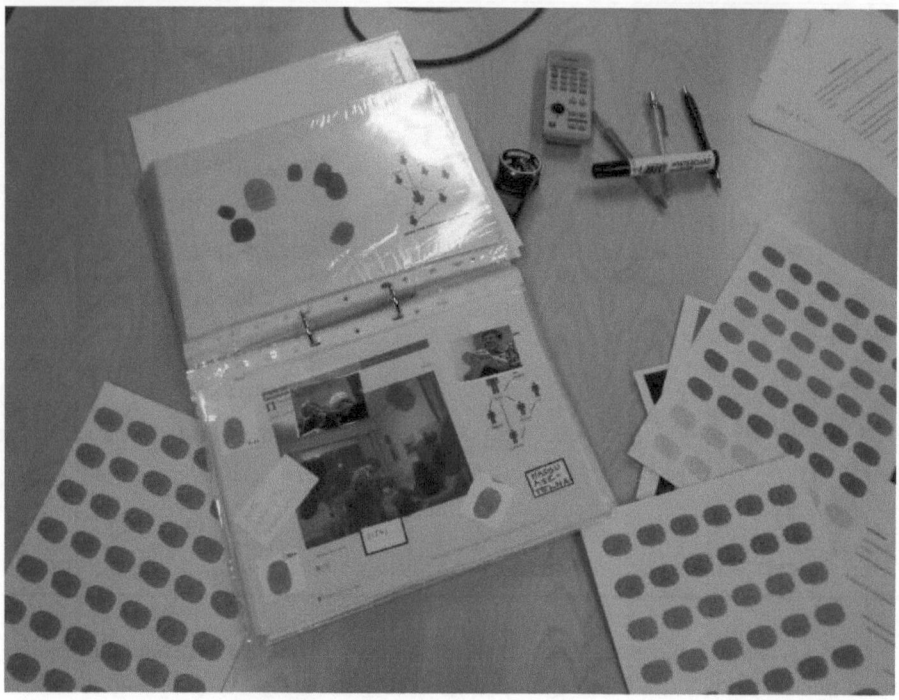

Fig. 2. Photo book was created of the photos users had taken together in their co-creation events. Functionalities are added on a transparency layer on the top of the pages.

Users were given brief description of the photo book at the start of the simulation. It represents a shared group folder on the cloud where all the group photos they have taken in the event have automatically appeared. In the simulation sessions they were able to see the photos taken by others for the first time. As the Fig. 2 describes, functionalities in the service were shown to the users in transparencies that were added on top of the photo book pages. So users were able to browse folders with the functional layer, or remove it and watch only the photos by turning the transparency pages.

Mood Photos functionality was demonstrated to the users by using web cameras and printers in order to give users option to add pictures of their reactions to other users' photos. They were able to add them by their own will.

Photo book functionality was intentionally explained in a rather low detail and instead users were instructed to interact and add comments in the way they felt natural and their actions were observed and recorded. These observations were analyzed in order to identify natural interaction habits for design ideas to the concept.

4.3   Setup of the Simulation Sessions

Simulation sessions were organized in a way that participants had time to get to know to the interviewing group and the surroundings. This created relaxed and open atmosphere to the session, which helped participants to express their ideas and set them to right mood of creativity.

In order to simulate usage sessions of the photo sharing service four users were divided into three stations. Each member was observed individually at 4 sessions where they browsed the photo books. Each session lasted for 30 minutes.

The 3 user Stations were organized in the session as follows: the Station A with two users, B and C with single user. In the station A the system use was simulated together with two participants. Researchers started from the decided stations, circulated all the stations carrying the same photo book all the time. During the individual sessions users added comments and thus communicated with each other through the photo book (Fig. 3).

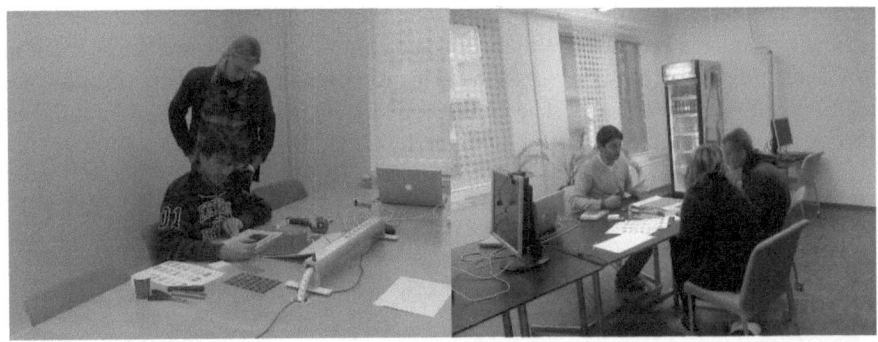

Fig. 3. On the left, individual photo browsing session in the group simulations on the station B. On the right, station A with two participants browsing and commenting the content in a joint session. Web camera is monitoring the interaction on the left.

The photo books circulated through each station collecting the comments and content from each participant (Fig. 3). After the photo books had circulated each station, a summative group interview was held. Each researcher completed thus totally four sessions with users, including the ending session where they returned to the station where they started from. At the end of the circulation session the participants were shown photo book they started working with, with additions made by others (Figure 4 and 5). This technique allowed researcher to become familiar with all the users and to gain deep knowledge of their own photo book and its contents. As mentioned before, simulations used modified technique of "Wizard of Oz" [32]. Researchers worked as the intelligence and functionality of the service in the simulation supporting and facilitating the interaction. Users were aware of the role of the researchers all the time.

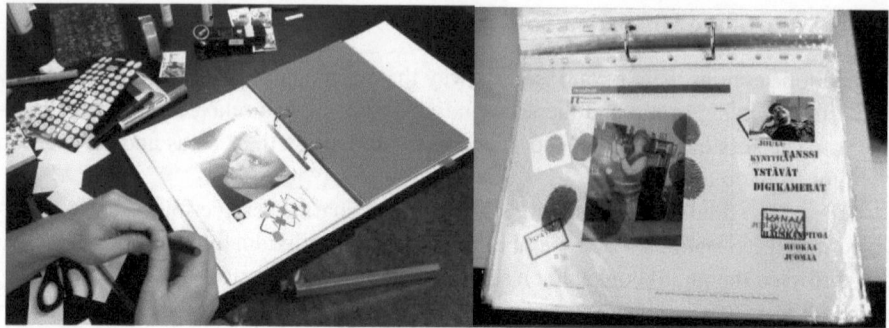

Fig. 4. Social interaction cues added to the transparency layer of the photobooks. Picture on the left, during the session. Picture on the right, after the session with all the interaction cues added.

The circulation was arranged to represent photo application browsing sessions of the shared folder of photos in the system. In the individual session the users created collaborative collection together. Their collaboratively created album was represented in the group interview at the end of the session (Fig. 4). The pictures that appeared in the final collection were the ones that collected comments, or the ones users spent the most time with in the browsing sessions. This represents the detection of most meaningful pictures in the concept. The collaboratively commented album was in the end of the sessions represented in the group interview (Fig. 5).

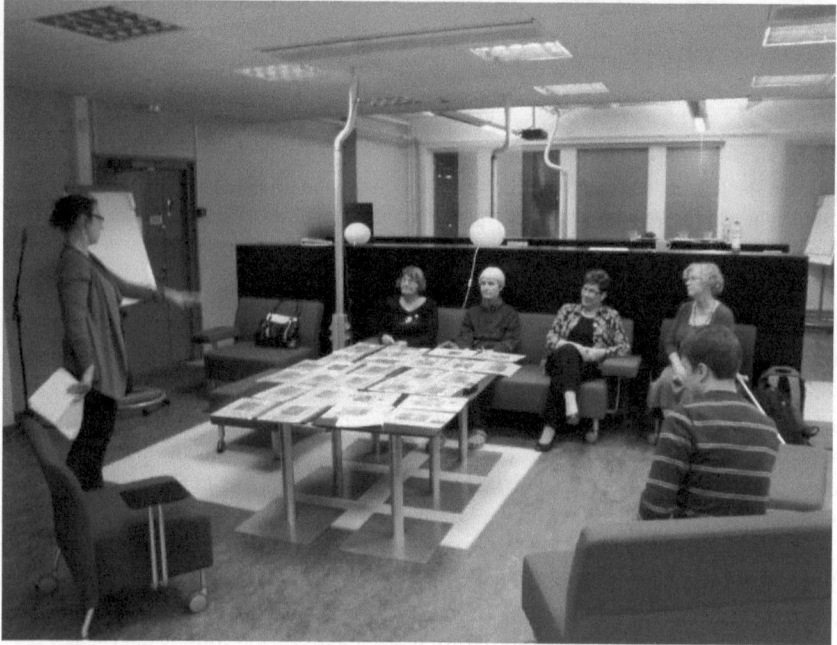

Fig. 5. Group interview session. The users are gathered around the table full of photos they have commented and browsed in the simulation.

The pictures that appeared in the final collection, which was presented in the group interview session, were the ones that evoked emotions, comments or which users spent most time with in the browsing sessions. This phase of the session represents the automatic detection of most meaningful pictures that have gained the most interest in the concept (Fig. 5). In the end of the simulation sessions, users were gathered together around the table where the most commented photos were scattered (Fig. 4) and the actual group interview was completed in the vicinity of the groups' photo content. Users were able to see the collection they had created together in the events, by additional content and comments from the simulation sessions (Fig. 4) to fully understand the interaction possible through the concept.

5   Results

Users were given three detailed concepts in the simulation sessions for interacting with other people in the simulation sessions by using the prototype. Two of these features are designed for social interaction and one to notify the user when her photos appear in the service. Usage of these concepts was observed. From the observations, conclusions were made on the interaction between the members of a group through their shared album.

All of the concepts were seen suitable for working with personal, emotional photos that are shared within a close group. There were differences especially regarding to the openness of sharing and commenting. Some of these concerns are related to the age and experience of SNS use. However, habits of commenting and collaborating repeated regardless of the age and experience. All of the participants commented and created collaborative content to the book in a rather similar fashion.

The idea of collecting all the photos from every photographer into a same album was highly appreciated. The users appreciated seeing the different viewpoints and styles of photographing, to get pictures of themselves in the events and to get an idea of how others experienced the event.

5.1   Design Implications and Considerations Related to Small-Group Sharing

Creating a shared photo book together was stated to be a peak experience. Even using Dropbox for photo sharing was a new and pleasant experience for many. The concept of shared or collaboratively created and maintained folder was also much appreciated. The concept was described by the participants as shared folder or a pool of photos by many authors that the members could join and contribute to.

The first round of the analysis of the results concentrated on the groups as study cases [39]. The group session records were observed and analysed individually utilizing a qualitative and descriptive approach. This phase was completed by three researchers individually. In the second round, the analysis followed "grounded theory" methodology [40]. In this analysis phase, all the groups where studied and analyzed together, using the affinity diagram method. In this phase, all the researchers collaborated in the analysis. Findings from the second round of analysis were organized under the themes and statements that are presented in the following.

Users appreciate simplicity in the system design; they want to be able to concentrate on the content. If there are too many different features in the system the overview may become messy. Nonetheless, commenting and leaving marks for other users was much appreciated and evoke emotions, all users demonstrated the willingness to concentrate on the content of the photos only. They wanted features of removing all of the additional data, so that the photo could rise to the top, and they could really enjoy watching the photos.

To have a sense of control over the content is important even in small group setting. Users wanted to remove pictures that they did not like or wanted to give a suggestion for removal to the author. Viewers of the shared folder need to be visible, so everyone knows how publicly the photos are shared. Authorship, in a sense, poses a difficult question, since users want to be able to remove the photos where they are presented. On the other hand, others removing the photos from the author can lower the sense of control over one's own content.

Recognition and feedback from others adds value to pictures. Users expected others to react and comment on their pictures if they are shared between the closed group. However, if the photos are automatically transferred to a shared folder, users need automatic notifications that others have seen them. One of the concepts had solution of informing the members of the visits of others.

Users want to know about actions of others: who have seen their photos. Others' consumption activities can work as social navigation cues. Photos became more meaningful for the participants when the circulations were done, and others had commented on them. Even the photos they did not see interesting at the start tend to become interesting when there was content from others. They wanted to see which photos gathered others attention.

Users appreciated neutral way to notify others that they have seen the photos. On the other hand, participants were interested in seeing the popularity and activity in their photos even in limited small group setting. Following popularity is identified as a motivator for content creation in other contexts as well [9, 10].

Identity of others and contextual cues are important. Users wanted to know who saw and commented their photos. Anonymous comments were frustrating. If persons who do not belong to the group see their photos, or appear in their photos, they want a clarification about how they relate to their group or networks of friends. Comments are only made on the most interesting or special pictures. Some wanted to browse through all the pictures before giving comments or other messages. Some gave comment or reaction right after seeing a photo that got their attention. The pictures that had collected attention and comment from others had a tendency to collect more comments from the viewer as well. The Mood photos worked reciprocally: users wanted to respond to others' reactions with their own.

Shared ownership of the photos divides opinions. Some of the photographers wanted to get credit of the photos they had taken and shared even inside the closed group. They were willing to add the photos to the shared pool for commenting, but they wanted to maintain the info who has taken the picture. Some were concerned about the authorship and editing rights of the photos in shared pool: who can remove the photos and who can publish them outside the group, and is the permission needed from the object in the picture. *Group formation and sharing outside the group are essential.* Since one of the concepts introduced idea of getting notifications and photos outside the closed group, and for sharing the photos outside the group, users started to consider the privacy issues of this shared collection. Seeing the pictures where they appear was seen as a nice feature, but informing others of their photos that include people outside the group was more problematic.

5.2   Evaluation of the Group Simulation Technique

As the study shows, the group simulation technique with the paper prototypes and users' own content is an effective tool for evaluating the social concepts in an early phase. It is efficient in testing the basic design of the concept as well as to get an idea whether the target experiences are reached with the concept. In the simulation, users were able to understand the features that the concept will offer when it is fully implemented.

The technique of circulating the photo books to simulate the browsing sessions in the photo sharing service was seen as an effective approach to demonstrate the functionality of the concepts and observe users in the sessions. Leaving some functionalities and features of the concepts open for discussion and ideas worked for the most creative users, but some were confused and wanted more concrete ideas and instructions how the functionalities really work in the prototype.

Users personally created content, which was utilized in the prototype, was highly motivating for the user groups to work with. Especially in a concept that is related to actual personal content of users, the demonstration or prototype with content generated by the researchers or demo content will leave the experience superficial, and users may not understand the system in a way that they would actually use it with their own content included. This study shows users own content really motivates them to react and comment in the simulation. Users were actually interested in the content, because they saw the photos of others in the group for the first time in the session, which evoked emotional responses to a certain photos. The simulation added to the amount of commenting, and most said that they would not comment that much in real use of the services. Results and feedback concerning the actual features of the prototype are introduced in details in another publication [38].

6   Discussion

The technique was suitable for collecting information about the social use of the photographs in a small group. The paper prototype was effective in collecting information how participants would naturally comment and interact with the shared photos they have captured as a group. Giving users free hands in the commenting and creating content together gave valuable information on interaction methods to add to the collaborative implementation. The ideology of "make tools" [33] and using the real world object such as photo book gave users freedom to be creative and take part in the design process. The technique is suggested to be a tool for design as well as collecting data of the content sharing habits and interactions within the group.

Researchers acting as the "intelligent features" of the system and facilitators of the interaction through the system offered a method of demonstrating and evaluating the sophisticated features in the early phase prototype. At certain points of the sessions participants had problems interacting in a natural manner when the researchers facilitated the interaction, but with only a couple of exceptions users accepted that researchers facilitate and simulate the interaction. Using several researchers in the session saves implementation time and allows the concepts to be tested in an early phase of the implementation – before actual software is completed. Using the group simulation session with more complete implementations or "demo features" could add one level to the simulation. Demo functionality presented by videos or partly functional prototypes could be compensated with the researchers circulating and delivering the messages and interaction.

The technique can be utilized in a design process of many kinds of applications that aim for content sharing. Other media content formats may require implementation of prototype software instead of paper prototypes. Nevertheless, investing time on the content collection can give more realistic evaluation results for the prototype.

In the future the group simulation method could be studied in a more controlled setting by comparing it to the test group using generated content in a similar simulation. Comparing the technique to classical paper prototypes should be completed to validate the efficiency of the technique.

7   Conclusions

This study contributes to the HCI and participatory design field by introducing technique for arranging simulation sessions with paper prototypes to small groups, involving the aspect of social context that previously has been missing from the prototype evaluation sessions. The research contribution of this work is two-folded. Firstly, it evaluates the concept and, secondly, it contributes to the field of participatory design with group simulation technique that uses users' actual personal content. As the study results describe, users saw simulation sessions with the content they had previously created together highly motivating and fun.

The technique is suitable for evaluating concepts that include personal content such as photos and enable sharing with small groups. It poses problems in finding the actual usability and design flaws that can be found in an actual usability test but it offers possibility to evaluate the concepts in an early stage of the process. In spite of the before mentioned problems, it was proven to be a effective tool for evaluating the designs in an early phase. It is suggested for the design cases, where implementing the interactive prototype will take time and populating the service with the users and the user-generated content even more time and effort. This study concentrated on the development of a photo sharing application, but by slight modifications the simulation technique can be applied to cover different kinds of solutions for group working as well. From the findings of the sessions a functional prototype was implemented. Testing of the functional prototype with the group of users will continue the work presented in this paper.

Acknowledgements. Authors would like to thank the participating groups for their valuable feedback and Kaisa Väänänen-Vainio Mattila, Guido Grassel, Sanna Malinen, Yanqing Cui and Rod Walsh for their valuable contributions to the work.

References

1. Iriberri, A., Leroy, G.: A life-cycle perspective on online community success. In: ACM Computing Surveys (CSUR). ACM Press, New York (2009)
2. Hassenzahl, M.: Experience Design; Technology for all the right reasons. Morgan & Claypool Publishers (2010)
3. Whittaker, S., Bergman, O., Clough, P.: Easy on that trigger dad: a study of long term family photo retrieval. Personal Ubiquitous Computing 14, 31–43 (2008)
4. Odom, W., Pierce, J., Stolterman, E., Blevis, E.: Understanding why we preserve some things and discard others in the context of interaction design. In: CHI 2009, pp. 1053–1062. ACM Press, New York (2009)
5. Odom, W., Zimmerman, J., Forlizzi, J.: Teenagers and their virtual possessions. In: CHI 2011, pp. 1491–1500. ACM Press, New York (2011)
6. Bentley, F., Metcalf, C., Harboe, G.: Personal vs. commercial content: the similarities between consumer use of photos and music. In: CHI 2006 Conference on Human Factors in Computing Systems, pp. 667–676. ACM Press, New York (2006)
7. Bernstein, M., Marcus, A., Karger, D., Miller, R.C.: Enhancing Directed Content Sharing on the Web. In: CHI 2010, pp. 971–980. ACM Press, New York (2010)
8. Ojala, J., Malinen, S.: Photo sharing in small groups: identifying design drivers for desired user experiences. In: International Academic MindTrek Conference, pp. 69–76. ACM Press, New York (2012)
9. Ojala, J.: Personal content in online sports communities: motivations to capture and share personal exercise data. International Journal of Social and Humanistic Computing 2(1/2), 68–85 (2013) doi:10.1504/IJSHC.2013.053267
10. Lehtiniemi, A., Ojala, J.: MyTerritory: evaluation of outdoor gaming prototype for music discovery. In: International Conference on Mobile and Ubiquitous Multimedia, MUM 2012, article 35. ACM Press, New York (2012)
11. Olsson, T.: Understanding Collective Content: Purposes, Characteristics and Collaborative Practises. In: Communities and Technologies, C&T 2009, pp. 21–30. ACM, New York (2009)
12. Patel, N., Clawson, J., Voida, A., Lyons, K.: Mobiphos: A study of user engagement with mobile collocated-synchronous photo sharing application. International Journal of Human-Computer Studies, IJHCS 67(12), 1048–1059 (2009)
13. Malinen, S., Ojala, J.: Maintaining the instant connection - Social media practices of smartphone users. In: Proceedings of the 10th International Conference on the Design of Cooperative Systems, pp. 197–211 (2012), doi:197-211.10.1007/978-1-4471-4093-1_14
14. Kirk, D., Sellen, A., Rother, C., Wood, K.: Understanding photowork. In: CHI 2006, pp. 761–770. ACM Press, New York (2006)

15. Lehikoinen, J., Aaltonen, A., Huuskonen, P., Salminen, I.: Personal Content Experience. Wiley (2007)
16. Frohlich, D., Kuchinsky, A., Pering, C., Don, A., Ariss, S.: Requirements for photoware. In: CSCW 2002, pp. 166–175. ACM Press, New York (2002)
17. Miller, A., Edwards, W.K.: Give and take: a study of consumer photo sharing culture and practice. In: CHI 2007, pp. 347–356. ACM Press, New York (2007)
18. Kairam, S., Brzozowski, M.J., Huffaker, D., Chi, E.H.: Talking in circles: selective sharing in Google+. In: Proc. CHI 2012, pp. 1065–1974. ACM Press, New York (2012)
19. Petrelli, D., Whittaker, S.: Family memories in the home: contrasting physical and digital mementos. Personal Ubiquitous Computing 14(2), 153–169 (2010)
20. Malinen, S.: Strategies for gaining visibility on Flickr. In: HICSS 2011: Proceedings of the 2011 44th Hawaii International Conference on System Sciences, pp. 1–9. IEEE (2011)
21. Malinen, S.: ICI Photo Exhibition or Online Community? The Role of Social Interaction in Flickr. In: ICIW 2010 Proceedings of the 2010 Fifth International Conference on Internet and Web Applications and Services, pp. 380–385. IEEE (2010)
22. Gemmell, J., Bell, G., Lueder, R.: MyLifeBits: a personal database for everything. In: Communications of the ACM, pp. 88–95. ACM Press, New York (2004)
23. Dropbox, http://www.dropbox.com (accessed September 1, 2012)
24. Wäljas, M., Segerståhl, K., Väänänen-Vainio-Mattila, K., Oinas-Kukkonen, H.: Cross-Platform Service User Experience: A Field Study and an Initial Framework. In: MobileH-CI 2010, pp. 219–228. ACM Press, New York (2010)
25. Van House, N.: Collocated photo sharing, story-telling and the performance of self. International Journal of Human-Computer Studies, IJHCS 67(12), 1073–1086 (2009)
26. Lucero, A., Holopainen, J., Jokela, T.: Pass-them-around: collaborative use of mobile phones for photo sharing. In: CHI 2011, pp. 1783–1793. ACM Press, New York (2011)
27. Nunes, M., Greenberg, S., Neudstaedter, C.: Sharing digital photographs in the home through physical mementos, souvenirs and keepsakes. In: ACM Conference on Designing Interactive Systems, DIS 2008, pp. 250–260. ACM Press, New York (2008)
28. Rodden, K., Wood, K.R.: How do people manage their digital photographs? In: CHI 2003, pp. 409–416. ACM Press, New York (2003)
29. Battarbee, K.: Co-experience, Understanding User Experiences in Social Interaction. Doctoral dissertation in UIAH (2004)
30. Hagen, P., Robertson, T., Kan, M., Sadler, K.: Emerging research methods for understanding mobile technology use. In: Australia Conference on Computer-Human Interaction, OZCHI 2005, Australia, pp. 1–10 (2005)
31. Sa, M., Carrico, L.: Lessons from early stages design of mobile applications. In: Mobile-HCI 2008, pp. 127–136. ACM Press, New York (2008)
32. Ehn, P., Kyng, M.: Cardboard Computers: Mocking-it-up or Hands-on the Future. In: Greenbaum, J., Kyng, M. (eds.) Design at Work: Cooperative Design of Computer Systems, pp. 169–195. Lawrence Erlbaum Associates, Hillsdale (1991)
33. Vaajakallio, K., Mattelmäki, T.: Collaborative Design Exploration: Envisioning future practices with make tools. In: Designing Pleasurable Products and Interfaces, DPPI 2007. ACM Press, New York (2007)
34. Oulasvirta, A., Kurvinen, E., Kankainen, T.: Understanding contexts by being there: case studies in bodystorming. Personal and Ubiquitous Computing 7(2), 125–134 (2003)
35. Kelley, J.F.: An iterative design methodology for user-friendly natural language office information applications. ACM Transactions of Office Information Systems 2(1), 26–41 (1984)

36. Facebook, http://www.facebook.com (accessed September 1, 2012)
37. Flickr, http://www.flickr.com (accessed September 1, 2012)
38. Vyas, D., Cui, Y., Ojala, J., Grassel, G.: *Producing while consuming*: social interaction around photos shared within private group. In: Nijholt, A., Romão, T., Reidsma, D. (eds.) ACE 2012. LNCS, vol. 7624, pp. 133–150. Springer, Heidelberg (2012)
39. Yin, R.: Case study research, design and methods. Sage Publications Inc. (2003)
40. Strauss, A., Corbin, J.: Grounded theory methodology. An Overview Handbook of Qualitative Research, 273-285 (1994)

Usability Evaluation of Configuration-Based API Design Concepts

Thomas Scheller and Eva Kühn

Institute of Computer Languages
Vienna University of Technology
1040 Wien, Austria
{ts,eva}@complang.tuwien.ac.at

Abstract. Usability is an important quality attribute for designing APIs, but usability-related decision factors are often unknown. This is also the case when looking at APIs for configuration tasks, like for dependency injection or object-relational mapping. In these areas three different API design concepts can be found, which are annotations, fluent interfaces, and XML. There exists no research concerning usability-related characteristics and differences between these concepts.

In this paper, we present a usability study that identifies such characteristics and differences between the three concepts, by comparing three different variants of an API for dependency injection. From the study results we evaluate advantages and disadvantages in different use cases, and show how to build more usable configuration-based APIs.

Keywords: API Usability, API Design, Fluent Interfaces, Annotations, XML.

1 Introduction

There are many areas in programming where APIs (application programming interfaces) are used for some kind of configuration. Examples are APIs for object-relational mapping like Hibernate[1], APIs for dependency injection like Unity[2], or APIs for communication like the Windows Communication Foundation[3] (see Table 1). Next to logging and unit testing, these are the most prominent areas where external APIs are used. When looking at such "APIs for configuration", many of them share the same basic design concepts, independent from the area of usage. We identified three design concepts that are used for such APIs: The first is *XML*, where the whole configuration is not written in code, but stored in a separate XML file. The second is *annotations*, where the configuration is done by annotating code elements with additional information. The third is *fluent interface* [1], which has only recently become popular, and tries to make use of the natural language by defining methods that are concatenated to form a readable sentence.

---

[1] http://www.hibernate.org

[2] http://unity.codeplex.com

[3] http://msdn.microsoft.com/en-us/library/dd456779.aspx

A. Holzinger et al. (Eds.): SouthCHI 2013, LNCS 7946, pp. 54–73, 2013.

Table 1. Examples for configuration-based APIs

API for	Configures	Then does
Dependency Injection	bindings and injections	create instances
Serialization	which fields are serialized	serialize/deserialize objects
Object-Relational Mapping	mappings from code to db	insert, update and read data to/from the db
Communication	which messages are sent, which transport layer is used	send/receive messages

When evaluating the usability of such an API, it is therefore important to understand the usability implications of the used design concept(s). There is not yet any research concerning the usability of XMLs, annotations, or fluent interfaces in this context. Some existing papers deal with the usability evaluation of APIs [2,3,4,5]. They analyze the impact of parameters in objects' constructors, compare the usability of constructors and static factory methods, check the implications of method placement on API learnability, and evaluate the usability implications when using classes and methods in different scenarios. These papers cover well the usage of basic elements of object oriented APIs, but do not take higher level design concepts into account like the ones mentioned above. In the context of XML there are a few papers dealing with usability [6,7], but they are either too problem specific or not applicable in the context of programming. Further, there is a number of API design guidelines like [8] and [9], which give a good overview how to build usable APIs. While such guidelines show how to build APIs with each of the mentioned design concepts, there are none comparing them and/or saying when it is best to use which one. Further, they don't have a scientific basis. Today, when a programmer e.g. wants to choose a dependency injection framework, he/she has a large selection of different APIs with different design concepts. It has often been shown that usability is an important factor [10,11,12], both for API developers who need to know how to design an API, as well as for API users who want to choose the best usable API. But usability can only be taken into account if the according differences between design concepts are known.

Therefore, in this paper we want to evaluate the usability of the three API design concepts *XML*, *annotations* and *fluent interface*, and compare them to each other. We therefore conducted a usability study with three different APIs, each implementing one of these design concepts. As a result of the study, we want to show which designs perform better or worse in which situations, and which factors influence usability for each design concept.

In section 2 we present the design of the study, including the used APIs and details about the test execution and data analysis. Section 3 presents the study results, with statistical evaluations for each measured performance detail. An interpretation of the results is shown in section 4, where we present advantages, disadvantages and measurable properties for each design concept.

2   Design of the Study

To compare the three design concepts XML, annotations and fluent interface, we implemented an API for each one, all providing the same functionality. From the areas shown in Table 1 we chose dependency injection [13], because it is widely known, tests are easy to setup because there are no external dependencies (e.g. for testing an object-relational mapping API, a database would be needed) and there are many different APIs available for all three design concepts. To identify which tasks are most often done with a dependency injection (further in short: DI) API, as well as to see how the three design concepts are used in this context, we looked at a number of existing APIs. We examined Spring, Java EE, Google Guice and PicoContainer on the Java side, as well as Unity, Ninject, Castle Windsor, StructureMap, AutoFac and the Managed Extensibility Framework (MEF) on the .Net side. We concentrate our research on Java and C# because they are two of the most widely used object oriented programming languages.

2.1   Design of the APIs

Concerning the tasks the users should solve during the study, we chose the ones that were most common with existing DI APIs and ordered them so that users can use their knowledge from previous tasks, allowing us to monitor the learning effect. The following 6 tasks had to be solved in the given order:

1. creating a simple binding from an interface type to an implementation type
2. creating named bindings
3. defining for a class which constructor is used (constructor injection)
4. defining for a class which constructor parameters are injected, when it is instantiated using the DI API (constructor injection)
5. creating a binding with a singleton scope (so only a single instance is created)
6. applying all of the functions used in previous tasks on a more complex class structure, with three different bindings and two constructor injections

For each task, we evaluated the cognitive steps for solving it, e.g. for the first task this would be (1) choosing the interface type for the binding, (2) choosing the implementation type. The three APIs were then implemented following these cognitive steps as closely as possible, also using the same terms (e.g. "bind/binding", "inject", "instantiate") wherever possible, so that there is no impact on the study results from such differences. We also closely followed the domain language dictated by existing APIs. Figure 1 shows for two examples how functionality was implemented in the three different APIs. To be able to test a more diverse range of programmers we implemented our APIs both in Java and C#.

Concerning the XML-based API, we observed that a majority of the available APIs do not directly provide an XML schema. Even if a schema is provided, it needs to be added manually to the IDE in a separate step from referencing the API (e.g. in Visual Studio this feature is rather hidden). We therefore decided that it would be more representative for existing APIs to not provide an XML schema for the study participants.

Class for binding:	Class for constructor injection:
| ```
public class ConsoleLogger
    : ILogger {}
``` | ```
public class Service {
    public Service() {...}
    public Service(ILogger logger)
        {...}
}
``` |
| Annotations:<br>```
[BindingFor(typeof(ILogger))]
public class ConsoleLogger...
``` | Annotations:<br>```
[Inject]
public Service(ILogger logger)
    ...
``` |
| Fluent Interface:<br>```
container.Bind<ILogger>()
    .To<ConsoleLogger>();
``` | Fluent Interface:<br>```
container
    .WhenInstantiating<Service>()
    .UseConstructorWithTypes<
        ILogger>();
``` |
| XML:<br>```
<DIContainer>
<Bindings>
<Binding type="Classes.ILogger"
bindTo="Classes.ConsoleLogger"/>
</Bindings>
</DIContainer>
``` | XML:<br>```
<DIContainer>
  <Instantiations>
   <Instantiation
    type="Classes.Service">
     <Constructor>
        <Param name ="logger" />
     </Constructor>
   </Instantiation>
  </Instantiations>
</DIContainer>
``` |

Fig. 1. Code examples in C# for (a) creating a binding and (b) defining an injection constructor for all three APIs

In addition to the API itself, a short tutorial document was created for each API. Again attention has been paid to make the three tutorials as similar as possible, to minimize influence of the documentation structure on the study.

2.2   Participants and Measurement

Our study included 27 programmers (9 per API). 17 were Java programmers using Eclipse as IDE, 10 were .Net programmers using Visual Studio. The study involved both programmers with academic and industrial background, which had experience with a variety of different APIs. The participants were between 22 and 46 years old and had between 2 and 20 years of programming experience. All programmers were recorded using a screen capturing software, and a supervisor was sitting next to the programmer to explain each task. The tests were designed as unittests, so users could evaluate the code at any time (a successful test run marks the end of each task). Additionally, an eye tracker was used to capture the participants' eye movements, allowing us to add gaze replays to the screen capture data. A between-subjects design was used for the study, meaning each participant was only tested with one of the three APIs, to prevent a falsification of the data from cross-API learning effects.

Overall 180 values were measured per participant. From the captured video data, we extracted times for specific steps that programmers had to do in each task, in the same way as we did in [3]. These steps include instantiating the DI container, creating a certain binding, defining the constructor injection for a certain class, reading a certain part of the tutorial, running a test and searching for errors. This way of fine grained evaluation removes unnecessary noise and by that allows a more accurate statistical evaluation.

When participants used the tutorial, we focused on identifying how long they took to understand certain parts of it, and how long they spent on reading either the running text or the included code examples. In this case the eye tracking data was especially helpful, because participants would sometimes put code and tutorial side-by-side on the screen, which would have made it impossible to detect what the user was looking at without this data.

In addition to performance times some other values were evaluated, like the number of switches between tutorial and code, the number of switches between classes in the IDE, and the number of needed test runs. At the end of the study participants had to fill out a short questionnaire concerning their experience with other DI frameworks, their satisfaction with the used API, and what they thought were advantages and disadvantages of each of the three design concepts.

3   Study Results

We evaluated all our results with statistical data analysis methods. If not mentionend otherwise, a *t-test* was used, which is a parametric statistical hypothesis test for assessing whether one of two samples of independent observations tends to have larger values than the other. For each applied test the p-value is given below, which represents the probability that there are significant differences between the two samples (a significant difference is present when $p<0.05$).

In the following sections, the letters A, F and X are used as short forms for the three API variants (annotations, fluent interface, XML).

3.1   Performing Simple Tasks (Creating a Binding)

The action of creating a binding represents a simple task which can be solved using a single annotation, or only very few methods or xml elements. The basic code for this task is shown in Figure 1(a). In the first task, users had to write exactly this code, in successive tasks they had to additionally define a binding name, with one additional value/method/xml attribute needed in the code.

Figure 2(a) compares the times for all tasks that were needed for first reading the tutorial section about bindings and then creating the binding. The median times are 42s for A, 34s for F and 65s for X. A check for statistical significance shows that the times for both A and F are significantly smaller than X (t-test: $p<0.001$). When removing one extreme outlier of F, the times for F are also significantly smaller than A ($p=0.042$). So, for simple tasks users performed best with the fluent interface, closely followed by the annotations API. The large gap from X to the other two APIs is not unexpected, as users of the XML API spent much time writing the XML configuration without auto completion features available.

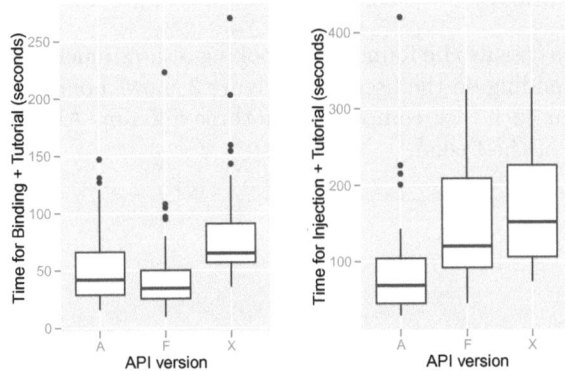

Fig. 2. Boxplots: (a) Time needed for creating a binding incl. reading tutorial, (b) time needed for constructor injection incl. reading tutorial.

3.2   Performing Complex Tasks (Constructor Injection)

Performing constructor injection represents a more complex task. Users had to use multiple annotations, chain a higher number of methods in the fluent interface, and use more xml elements and attributes. The basic code for this task is shown in Figure 1(b). Users first had to use constructor injection in task 3, and later in tasks 4 and 6. In tasks 4 and 6 users additionally had to specify which bindings are used for the injection of the constructor parameters, resulting in additional complexity.

Figure 2(b) compares the times for all tasks that were needed for reading the tutorial section about constructor injection and configuring the injection. The median times are 69s for A, 120s for F and 152s for X. A check for statistical significance shows that the times for A are significantly smaller than both F and X (t-test: p=0.017 for A<F and 0.002 for A<X). The times for F are not significantly smaller than X (p=0.195). The result of the annotations API being the best was expected because in this case much work is done implicitly just by choosing on which code element the annotation is placed. E.g. when the injection for constructor parameters needed to be defined, an annotation needed to be placed directly on the constructor parameter. With the other two APIs, users first needed to explicitly define the class and the constructor before they could even start with defining the injection of the parameters. This leads to the conclusion that the deeper within a hierarchy something needs to be configured, the greater the advantage of annotations against the other API variants will be.

What is surprising is that compared to simple tasks (see above) users with the fluent API were now much slower. This may indicate that a more complex method chain with a higher number of chaining options imposes a significant difficulty on the users.

3.3   Overall Times

Interesting details can also be found when looking at how much time users needed for each task depending on the used API. Figure 3 shows boxplots for the overall times per task, for each task comparing the three different APIs (see section 2.1 for a description of the tasks).

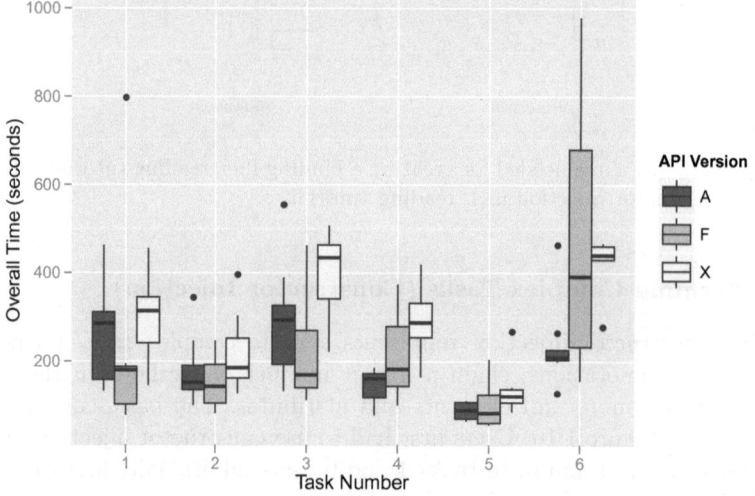

Fig. 3. Boxplot: Overall times per task and API version

The first thing that can be noticed is the learning effect. This can best be observed when comparing tasks 1 and 2 (users needed to create a binding), as well as when comparing tasks 3 and 4 (users needed to use constructor injection). While both the annotations and the XML API show a clear speedup, there is hardly one to see for the fluent interface. This implies that the fluent interface has a more flat learning curve than the other two.

A second thing that confirms this suspicion are the times for task 6. For this task, users had to use everything they had previously learned, and we asked them to try to do it without looking into the tutorial if possible. Only for the XML API 5 of the 9 users had to look into the tutorial to solve the task, which was simply because they did not remember all needed XML elements and attributes any more, and were not able to use auto completion for this. When looking at the times for task 6, it can be noticed that while the spread is very small for A and X, it is very large for F. From this we interpret that users of A and X all had at this point gained a complete understanding of the APIs and knew exactly how to use them – so solving a task of this complexity takes about 200-230 seconds with the annotations API, and about 420-470 seconds with the XML API. On the other hand, with the fluent interface some users were very fast (about 200 seconds), but others were extremely slow (up to 15 minutes), which means that many users still did not understand the API well enough to use it in a fast and efficient way. This could also be observed during the test, where users that had a good understanding of the API were very focused on the task and used API functions intuitively, while others needed to stop and think about how something is done with the API and also needed much more time searching for errors that were related to wrong API usage.

3.4 Information Sources

For each action the users needed to take during the test we analyzed where he/she acquired the information needed for that action. We distinguished between three different sources of information: The first was that users needed to look into the tutorial, the second that they used the auto completion mechanisms of the IDE, and the third was that they already had all the information they needed and therefore didn't need to look anywhere. For auto completion we expected that it would be most useful for the fluent interface, since it always presents the methods that can be chained next.

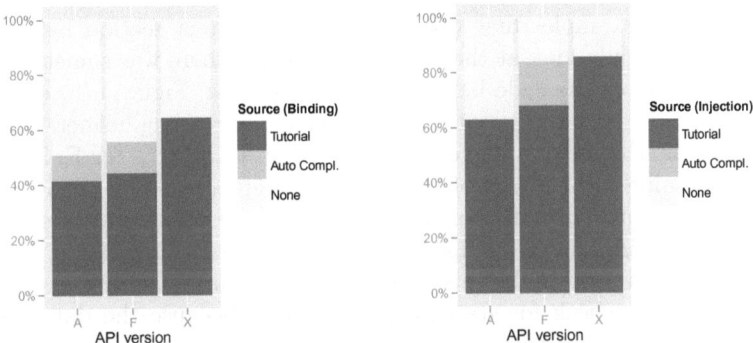

Fig. 4. Which information source was used how often, compared by Task, for the action of (a) creating a binding, (b) constructor injection

Figure 4 shows the evaluation of information sources for the actions of creating a binding (the simple task as explained in section 3.1) and constructor injection (the complex task, see section 3.2). Unsurprisingly the tutorial was used most often with the XML API (65% of the time for creating a binding, 85% for constructor injection), which is partly because of the missing auto completion. The users of the annotations API needed the tutorial the least often (40% and 60%), especially for the task of injection, where 20% more of the tasks were solved without using any information source than with the other APIs. Auto completion was most used with the fluent interface as expected (most clearly visible in Figure 4(b)), but an advantage due to using auto completion can only be seen compared to XML.

Generally, the main advantage of using auto completion was actually not that users could search for a method within the IDE, but simply that they didn't need to remember the whole class or method name. If the users only remembered the first few letters, they could still easily use a method by just auto-completing it. So, although it may appear in Figure 4 that auto completion was rarely used, it was actually used very often, but only in 10-20% of the cases it was really used for searching. For simple completion of class, method and property names it was used in about 80% of all cases.

3.5   Time Spent in Tutorial

We analyzed how much time users spent in the tutorial and what they were reading there. The result can be found in Figure 5(a). It shows that users spent about 30 to 35 seconds per task in the tutorial, with no significant differences between the three APIs.

The eye tracking data additionally allowed us to evaluate how much time user spent reading the running text, and how much reading only the headers and code examples (in all tutorials about 50% was running text, and the other 50% code examples). By doing that we intend to gain evidence on the self-explainability of each API. We observed that users almost always tended to look at the code examples first (after finding the correct section by scanning the headers), and only look at the running text when there was something they didn't understand or the code behaved not as expected. Figure 5(b) shows the percentage of time that was spent in the tutorial only reading headers and code examples. While the median percentage is 81% for A and 63% for F, it is 100% for XML, meaning in over half of the cases users spent no time at all reading the text in the tutorial. This can also be seen when looking at Figure 5(c), which shows the time spent reading running text. The median values are 9s for A, 21s for F and 0s for X. In this case we used the non-parametric *Wilcoxon Rank Sum Test* to check for statistical significance because the data shows a strong floor effect and is therefore not normally distributed. X is significantly lower than F ($p=0.010$), but not significantly lower than A ($p=0.155$), and A is very close to being significantly lower than F ($p=0.052$). This leads us to the conclusion that the XML code has the highest self-explainability because most of the time users didn't need to read any additional text to understand it. On the other hand, users of the fluent interface did not get enough understanding from just the code examples and therefore needed to read the whole tutorial more thoroughly.

The question may arise why the overall tutorial time for XML was not lower than the others. One reason is that due to the missing auto completion users often needed to switch into the tutorial just for looking how XML elements and attributes are written or how the exact structure looks like. Users of the XML API also switched into the tutorial much more often because of that.

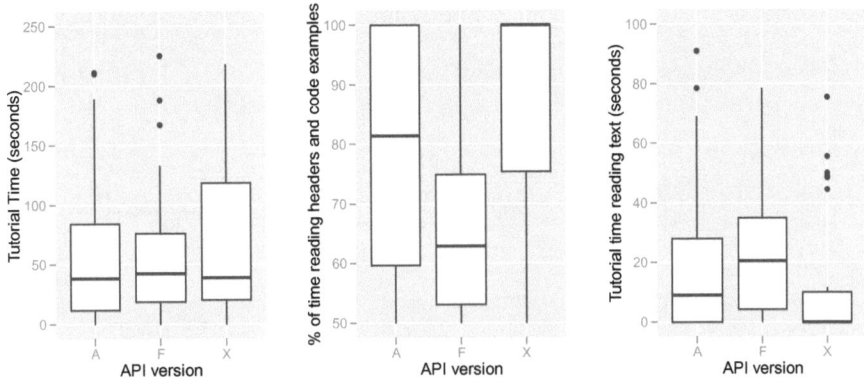

Fig. 5. Boxplots: (a) Overall tutorial times per API, (b) Percentage of time spent reading only headers and code examples, (c) Time spent reading running text

3.6 Switches between Classes

We observed that the three APIs differed in the number of times that users needed to switch between different classes in the IDE. Figure 6(a/b) compares how often users switched between classes, for the tasks of creating a binding (a) and constructor injection (b). While A and X show only a slight difference between the two different tasks, there is a large one with F. This is because with the fluent interface, users only switched between classes when they wanted to take a look at the class contents. This was mostly when doing constructor injection, to look at the available constructors and their parameters, but hardly ever happened for creating a binding. When looking at the large time differences between simple and complex tasks for the fluent interface (see Figure 2), it is highly probable that this is also due to an impact from the number of class switches. While the switching itself doesn't take much time, it is the act of looking up information in the configured class (e.g. parameter types and names of the constructor) that is time-consuming.

A check for statistical significance shows that for creating a binding (Figure 6(a)), the number of switches with F is significantly lower than for A and X (t-test: both $p<0.001$). In the other hand, for constructor injection (Figure 6(b)) the number of switches for A is the lowest ($p=0.062$ for A<F and 0.002 for A <X). The result that X has equal or more switches than A was unexpected, since with the annotations API users needed to switch a lot because annotations need to be applied directly to the targeted classes. The reason for the XML API needing so many switches was that most users opened every class to copy-paste the class name and often a second time to copy-paste the package/namespace name, because there is no auto completion of class names in the XML. Especially when doing constructor injection, users of F and X needed to switch back and forth multiple times, while with A switching to the class once was often enough.

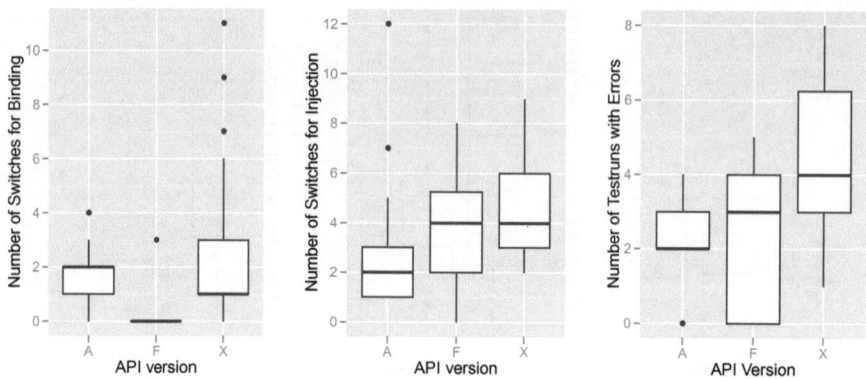

Fig. 6. Boxplots: (a) Number of switches between classes in IDE for creating a binding, (b) Number of switches for constructor injection, (c) Number of test runs with errors

3.7 Error Rate

To check if more errors were made with one API than with another, we compared the number of test runs that were needed to finish all tasks, as shown in Figure 6(c). All tasks were designed as unit tests, and to show that a task was finished correctly (or to check for runtime errors), users had to run the tests. The median number of test runs with errors was 2 for A, 3 for F and 4 for X. So with the XML API an error happened twice as often as with the annotations API. The number of errors with XML is significantly higher than with the other two (t-test: p=0.019 for X>A, p=0.043 for X >F). There is no significant difference between A and F (p=0.485 for A<F).

The main reason for this is of course the missing auto completion in the XML configuration, and that errors are therefore also not discovered at compile time. Errors happened especially often for longer and more complex words like "Instantiation". Another typical error was that the package/namespace of a class was incorrect, because the classes were sometimes placed in a different namespace/package than the one that was normally used (which was actually prepared exactly to show that this can lead to errors in the XML configuration, while not affecting the other two API variants).

3.8 Programmer Satisfaction

After the test we asked each programmer to rate 3 aspects of the used API on a 5 point differential scale as suggested in [14]. The measured aspects were simplicity (Simple ... Complicated), satisfaction (Pleasing ... Irritating/Frustrating) and speed (Fast to use ... Slow to use).

The results are shown in Figure 7. For *Simplicity*, both A and X were rated with a median value of 5 (the highest rating). F achieved a median value of 4, which is significantly lower than the other two (t-test: p=0.016 for F<A and

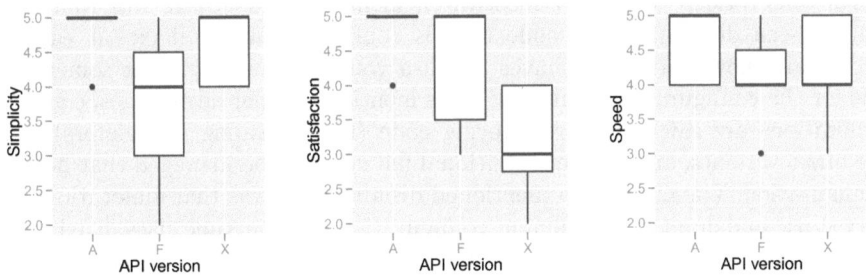

Fig. 7. Boxplots displaying the results of the post-test questionnaire (1-5, 5=highest): (a) Simplicity, (b) Satisfaction, (c) Speed

0.041 for F<X). On the first look it may be unexpected that the XML API was rated significantly higher in simplicity than the fluent interface. But this result also supports the assumptions made in section 3.5, that XML has an especially high self-explainability and can be easily understood. With the fluent interface users had difficulties in this area – often users stated that they were unsure which methods can be chained or which must be used consecutively, especially when using more complex functions.

For *Satisfaction*, A and F were rated with a median value of 5, while X was rated significantly lower with a median of 3 ($p<0.001$ for X<A and 0.014 for X<F). The reason for XML being rated worst is clearly the missing auto completion, both for typing XML element and attribute names, and for typing class names in the XML. Although working with the fluent interface was less simple, it was still more satisfying because nothing needed to be typed in manually.

The smallest differences are shown for *Speed* with a median value of 5 for A and 4 for F and X. There are no significant differences in the speed values, with F<A being the one closest to significance ($p=0.060$). Especially the fluent interface and XML APIs were rated very equally, although when looking at the performance the fluent interface actually was almost always significantly faster.

When combining the results for all three rated aspects, the annotations API was rated significantly higher than the fluent interface and XML APIs, which were both rated equally.

3.9 Programmer Preferences

In addition to the questionnaire, we asked users about their general opinions on the used API and, in case they had used the other two design patterns, which one they preferred and why. From the 27 test users, 10 users had never used a DI API before, 5 had worked with an annotations-based API, 9 had used an API with a combination of XML and annotations, and 3 a fluent interface. When asked which kind of API they preferred, 9 users had no preferences because of insufficient experience, 12 preferred an annotations-based API, and 6 and API with a fluent interface. None of the users gave a preference for XML.

For annotations the by far most often mentioned advantage was that they can be seen directly in the code that is configured, which makes it easy to understand how the code behaves because you don't need to look somewhere else for the configuration. Only few users mentioned other advantages, e.g. that annotations are safer when refactoring code (like renaming parameters) than the other variants, and that no additional file needs to be managed that holds a configuration. The most often mentioned disadvantage was that annotations are very static and don't allow different configurations for the same class, like having one configuration for unittesting and another for the production environment. Further, some mentioned it was a disadvantage that you have to look into every file separately to see the configuration, so it can be difficult to gain an overview.

Some advantages were mentioned for both the fluent interface and XML, which is not surprising because they are similar in certain points. These advantages were that the whole configuration is in one place and is therefore easier to overview (which is interestingly the opposite of the most popular advantage of annotations), and that the configuration is independent from the configured code, also allowing different configurations if needed.

For the fluent interface, other mentioned advantages were that the chaining of methods is very comfortable and easy to use once you are familiar with it, and that you can do almost everything with auto completion (unlike with XML). Especially for users that mentioned the former it could often be observed that they were mumbling to themselves in sentences similar to the method chains. For example, when users needed to write the code for constructor injection, which starts like `container.WhenInstantiating<Service>().UseConstructorWith Types<...`, they mumbled something like "when I am instantiating the class Service, then I want to use the constructor with the types ...". We also see this as a confirmation that once the structure of a fluent interface is understood, it allows coding by building such sentences very intuitively. The main mentioned disadvantage of the fluent interface was that as soon as you need to configure something that cannot be accessed with methods and generics, like constructor parameters, you need to use strings which feels very unpleasant and is not safe to refactoring (unlike annotations, which don't have this problem). All other disadvantages were centered around the concept of chaining methods, and displayed well the problems we observed during the tests. Users said that it was unclear in the beginning which methods could be chained with which others, that they were unsure if a method chain was complete or if they had forgotten anything, and that longer method chains (4+ methods) were increasingly complex.

For XML, a mentioned advantage was that the configuration can be changed without recompiling, though on the other hand favourers of the fluent interface mentioned that this was completely unnecessary in most cases. Further, the actual API that is needed in the code is very small and simple: For the DI API it only needed one function, which was creating instances. The main disadvantage was unsurprisingly the missing auto completion, and that due to this there is also no compile-time error checking. A few users noted that this would not have been as much a problem if a schema file had been provided. Some additionally mentioned the problem of refactoring, that most of the time the configuration file is not included in the refactoring process, so refactorings can easily destroy the configuration without directly being noticed.

3.10   Impact of Programmer Experience

An important question is if the study results can be applied to both experienced and inexperienced users. In [3] we analyzed if the years of programming experience and/or the domain knowledge had any impact on performance, with the result that there was none. We did the same tests for this study, with the same results. Additionally we asked users if they were using any DI framework frequently. A performance comparison shows that users that were using a DI framework regularly were not significantly faster while writing code (all needed about 16 minutes overall). But they spent significantly less time in the tutorial (t-test: p<0.001): The median times are 338s for non-regular DI users and 201s for regular ones. It should be noted though that the significance of these results is limited since only 4 of the 27 users were regular DI framework users.

4   Interpretation of Results

Based on the study results we can now present an overview of advantages and disadvantages of the three design concepts, as well as an analysis which one should be used in which cases. Further we analyze the possibilities for automatically measuring usability and/or making suggestions on the usage of these concepts, which would be necessary for integration into an automated measurement method as we proposed in [15].

4.1   Advantages and Disadvantages

Annotations. The annotations API performed either best for almost all measured results. Users were fastest especially when performing more complex tasks, the API was well understood from the tutorial, the learning curve was high, the error rate low, and it was also rated overall best for simplicity, satisfaction and speed. As the main reason for this we see the fact that considerable amount of information is given simply by the fact where the annotation is placed. So, while with the other APIs the users needed to explicitly say "I want to configure the class Service, and use the constructor with the following parameters...", this was naturally defined with annotations just by the fact that the annotation was placed at this constructor. Therefore also much fewer code elements were needed, e.g. only a single parameterless annotation for defining the injection constructor, compared to two different methods with multiple parameters with the fluent interface. This advantage was stronger, the deeper in a hierarchy the annotation was placed. It was strongest when it needed to be placed at a constructor parameter, which is in the third hierarchical level (class>constructor>parameter). An additional reason for the performance advantage was found in the number of class switches. For complex tasks users needed to look into the classes to create the configuration, which made it necessary for users of the fluent interface and XML to switch back and forth between class and configuration. For annotations this was not an issue, since the class and configuration were at the same place. Only for very simple tasks (operating on the first hierarchical level) the fluent interface had a small performance advantage against annotations (as shown in section 3.1), in which case the users could solve the task without ever switching into the configured class.

The simpleness of annotations was also well expressed by the opinions of the users, since a majority of them gave a preference to annotations. What users like most about annotations, and what was also the most often made statement concerning preferences, is that they are applied directly to the code that is configured. By having the configuration and the element that is being configured at the same place, the code is especially easy to understand, and there is no need to look somewhere else.

There are only few mentioned disadvantages, one being that it gets complicated to get an overview in larger projects because the configuration is spread out across a large number of classes. This was out of the scope of this study, but would be interesting to evaluate in future studies. In general it can be said that from a usability viewpoint, if the use case allows it, an annotations based API should be preferred to fluent interfaces and XML.

Fluent Interface. The fluent interface showed its main advantages in type safety (especially when compared to XML), as well as in the intuitive way that a method chain can be formed like a sentence in natural language. This enabled users to program in the same way they were thinking, e.g. when thinking "I want to bind ILogger to ConsoleLogger", the code they needed to write was `container.Bind<ILogger>().To<ConsoleLogger>()`.

On the other hand, the chaining of methods was also the main source for complications. While there was no problem chaining only two or three methods, users got confused when more methods were needed, and were wondering whether there was a needed order or if a certain method needed to be used or not. Most users seemingly thought that it was not ensured by the API itself that methods can only be called in a valid order (which the API of course did), and that they needed to do that themselves. To illustrate that, Figure 8 shows the chaining tree for the methods that were available in the study. The arrows show which methods can be called in succession, e.g. to define a named binding with singleton scope, the methods `Bind>To>Named>InSingletonScope` can be chained. In this case, either of the methods `Named` and `InSingletonScope` could be called first, or only one of them could be used alone if the other was not needed. Most often this problem occurred with the more complex chaining tree starting with `WhenInstantiating`. Users were often unsure if `UseConstructorWithTypes` was needed before defining injections for the parameters with `ForConstructorParam`, although the tutorial even contained examples where one was used without the other.

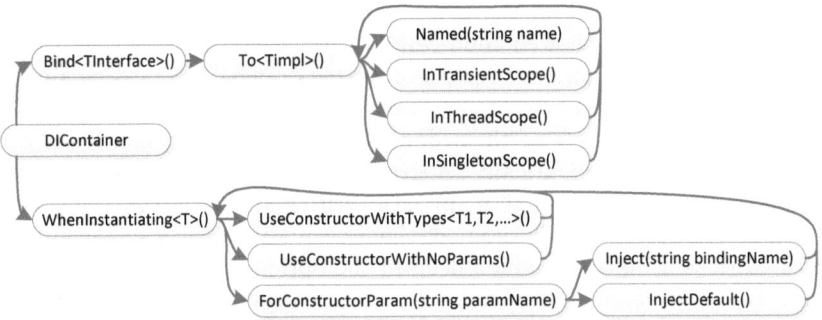

Fig. 8. Method chaining tree of the fluent interface API

In addition to not knowing if the order is correct or a certain method was needed, users had problems because they were missing some kind of visible ending to a method chain. This is certainly a problem with fluent interfaces, because you can of course just stop writing after any method without the compiler marking any errors. So, an error because of an incomplete method chain would only be found at runtime. In some fluent interfaces we evaluated, an ending method was used to mark the ending of a configuration (like "Start" or "Do'"), but with such an ending the chain unfortunately looses readability, since a natural sentence would never end with such a word.

It is to be expected that many of these problems occurred because most of the users had never used a fluent interface before. But rather than that being a threat to the validity of the study, we think that this just shows that fluent interfaces are not widely known, which makes them harder to learn and use.

When looking at these results and the statements of the users, there are some things that can be done to maximize the usability of fluent interfaces: First, users performed much better with short chains (up to 3-4 methods), so if some use cases would require the users to build especially long chains, this could be improved by changing the methods so that the chain is shortened. Second, to minimize the insecurity of users concerning the order and selection of chained methods, the API should whenever possible prevent the user to chain methods that would build an invalid chain. This can be a very difficult task, especially when the API has a large number of chainable methods, but can prevent many potential usability problems.

XML. As a main advantage of XML we identified its understandability and self-explainability. This can be seen when looking at the times spent in the tutorial, where most of the time the code examples alone were sufficient for understanding how to create the XML configuration. We see the reasons for that in the simpleness of the XML language itself (there are just two components that need to be understood, namely elements and attributes, which is far less than in a programming language like Java or C#), as well as the fact that nearly every programmer has already used XML in some way. This makes the users comfortable with XML from the start, which is also shown in the ratings for simplicity, where XML showed good results.

Unfortunately, this cannot compensate the big drawback of missing auto completion. Again it needs to be said that a result of the evaluation of various XML based APIs was that most of them don't offer an XML schema. Even if they offered one, it is not automatically integrated into the IDE, and manual integration is often not done. Although many users criticised that an XML schema was missing, e.g. for Visual Studio none of them even knew how a schema could be integrated (it is a function hidden deep in the options menu). Since we wanted to show the most common use case, we therefore decided that the study should also not contain an XML schema.

If a schema is present, this would definitely improve the performance of XML since it makes creating the configuration faster and prevents typing errors. But it doesn't remove all disadvantages, because there is still no checking of package, class and parameter names. Especially when creating a larger configuration, users rely strongly on copy-pasting the XML elements (this was also observed in the study), which minimizes the problem of typing errors for XML elements, but doesn't change anything about the problems with package/class/parameter names. To prevent this problem, users in the study often copy-pasted the class and package names, which was a significant slowdown. These problems are also displayed in the ratings for satisfaction, where the XML API was rated lowest.

From the performance results it can be said that in general one of the other two design concepts should be preferred to XML, as long as the use case allows it. In all performance ratings except for the tutorial, XML performed worst of the three, sometimes even taking twice as much time, because of the mentioned disadvantages (Figure 3 makes this especially obvious). If XML needs to be used, the study has shown that especially an intuitive and simple XML structure with short and easy to memorize element and attribute names can improve working with the API and prevent unnecessary errors. Further, an XML schema should always be made available.

4.2   Suitability Per Use Case

The design concept that has been identified as easiest to use is annotations, so it should be the first choice when deciding for a configuration-based API to use. An annotations API can be used whenever the targets of the configuration are classes (e.g. for the areas shown in Table 1), and when it is possible to statically apply the configuration directly to the classes (which can only be done when the source code of the classes is accessible and can be changed). A fluent interface can be considered alternatively, if the configuration is not too complex (if the configuration of constructors, methods and parameters is not involved). The fluent interface is not limited to only a single configuration, so for simple configurations it could be preferred to annotations.

The only reason to use XML would be a case where it is absolutely necessary that the configuration can be changed without recompiling. Such a case would for example be logging. To be able to switch logging on and off (or change the log level), it would make no sense to compile the configuration into the program. In all other cases, where Annotations cannot be used, fluent interfaces should be the first choice, since despite being harder to learn the study showed that they provide significantly better usability than XML. Examples where a fluent interface can be the best choice are APIs for unit testing and mocking.

Many existing APIs show that also a combination of multiple design concepts can make sense, e.g. to have a fluent interface and combine it with annotations for more complex class configurations.

4.3   Automated Measurement

One of our goals is to find properties that could be integrated into an automated measurement method as described in [15]. Usability is evaluated by analyzing the structure of an API as well as usage examples.

Automatic recognition of the three design concepts can easily be done: Annotations and XML can both be recognized by the presence of the corresponding elements. A fluent interface can be recognized in the code examples by two or more methods of the API being chained together. In case of the presence of XML, a recommendation could be given to use either annotations or a fluent interface instead. In case of a fluent interface, if longer method chains are present annotations could be recommended as an alternative, if the configuration involves classes (this could be recognized by checking if one of the fluent methods takes a class as parameter type).

For XML, the understandability of the structure is very important. One measurable parameter can be the number of elements and attributes necessary to solve a certain task. Especially when compared to a fluent interface, elements and attributes are mostly equivalent to methods and parameters, not only in their structure but also in the necessary numbers for solving a task. Overall, the usage the XML took about 50% more time than the fluent interface, and should be rated accordingly more complex. Additionally, the fact that more complicated element names were especially hard to memorize could be considered by checking the length of the names. In the study, names with more than 11 letters were perceived especially difficult.

For the fluent interface, an important parameter is the number of chained methods. The complexity showed more an exponential than a linear increase, especially for 4+ methods. Other than that, the number of chaining possibilities (size of the chaining tree) could be an indicator for a hard to understand fluent interface.

The study shows that while the number of code elements increases with more complex tasks when using XML or fluent interfaces, it stays mostly the same for annotations, because they are simply placed deeper in the hierarchy. So, this advantage could be measured by the number of needed code elements. While applying an annotation needs more effort than calling a single method, the advantage is simply achieved by the small number of code elements. According to the study results, using one annotation with a single parameter is about equal to two methods with a single parameter each in the fluent interface.

4.4 Validity and Applicability of the Study Results

The general validity of the study has been ensured by the usage of common statistical data analysis methods, as well as by having a sufficient number of participants with different backgrounds and different levels of experience.

To ensure that our study is not only applicable to APIs for dependency injection, we evaluated a much wider range of APIs, for the areas that were shown in Table 1. For all of these areas, there are implementations available using the three presented design concepts. The evaluation showed that the general structure, as well as the usability-specific differences between the different design concepts are basically the same for all of these areas. We therefore conclude that our study results are also applicable to at least these areas.

Of course there are also limits to what can be checked with such a study, like how efficient users can work with an API after they having used it for several hours, days or weeks of experience. Especially for the fluent interface, it can be expected that users would have been able to improve further (see section 3.3), although it is unlikely that it would perform better for complex tasks than annotations, so there would be little change to the overall results.

While the study focused on evaluating how programmers work with an API, an additional interesting fact to research in the future would be reading and understanding existing code. This could further strengthen the study results and/or show additional interesting usability aspects. Also a usability evaluation in the context of large projects could bring additional valuable results. Especially the missing support for refactoring in an XML could become a serious problem in this case, and with Annotations the scattering of the configuration over a large number of classes could make it difficult to maintain.

5   Conclusions

In this paper, we presented a study for evaluating three configuration-based API design concepts: annotations, fluent interfaces and XML. Users performed best and were most satisfied with annotations, while they performed worst with XML. Annotations proved especially useful when configuring elements deeper in a hierarchy, but can in general only be used when the targets of a configuration are classes. For most other cases, the best choice is a fluent interface, where users performed very well with small method chains, but had often problems when four or more methods needed to be chained. Also, the fluent interface paradigm proved hardest to understand, partly because of the fact that it is the least common one. XML showed its strengths by being very easy to understand and self-explainable, but proved the most cumbersome to use because of its missing auto completion, which was an issue both for XML elements and attributes, as well as for class and package names. Based on these results, we gave suggestions how usability could be improved, and extracted several properties that could be integrated into an automated measurement method. The paper hereby presents an important step towards a better understanding of API usability.

For future work, we plan to conduct further studies to gain more understanding of API usability. In the area of configuration-based APIs, a study on the understandability of existing code and suitability for larger projects would be especially interesting.

Acknowledgments. The work is funded by the Austrian Government under the program BRIDGE (Brückenschlagprogramm der FFG), project 827571 Agi-Log – Middleware technologies to reduce complexity for agile logistics. Special thanks go to our project partner pcsysteme.at, all study participants and the Interactive Media Systems Group at TU Vienna for lending us their eye tracker.

References

1. Fowler, M.: Domain-Specific Languages. In: The Addison-Wesley Signature Series. Addison-Wesley (2010)
2. Ellis, B., Stylos, J., Myers, B.: The factory pattern in API design: A usability evaluation. In: Proc. of the 29th International Conference on Software Engineering, ICSE 2007, pp. 302–312. IEEE Computer Society, Washington, DC (2007)
3. Scheller, T., Kühn, E.: Influencing factors on the usability of api classes and methods. In: 19th Annual IEEE International Conference and Workshops on the Engineering of Computer Based Systems, ECBS 2012, Novi Sad, Serbia, pp. 232–241. IEEE Computer Society (2012)
4. Stylos, J., Clarke, S.: Usability implications of requiring parameters in objects' constructors. In: Proc. of the 29th International Conference on Software Engineering, ICSE 2007, pp. 529–539. IEEE Computer Society, Washington, DC (2007)
5. Stylos, J., Myers, B.A.: The implications of method placement on API learnability. In: Proc. of the 16th ACM SIGSOFT International Symposium on Foundations of Software Engineering, SIGSOFT 2008/FSE-16, pp. 105–112. ACM, New York (2008)
6. Graaumans, J.: A qualitative study to the usability of three xml query languages. In: Proc. of the Conference on Dutch Directions in HCI, Dutch HCI 2004, pp. 6–9. ACM, New York (2004)
7. Sapienza, F.: Usability, structured content, and single sourcing with xml. Technical Communication 51(3), 399–408 (2004)
8. Cwalina, K., Abrams, B.: Framework design guidelines: conventions, idioms, and patterns for reusable. net libraries, 1st edn. Addison-Wesley Prof. (2005)
9. Tulach, J.: Practical API Design: Confessions of a Java Framework Architect, 1st edn. Apress, Berkely (2008)
10. Clarke, S.: Measuring API usability. Dr. Dobb's Journal 29, S6–S9 (2004)
11. Henning, M.: API design matters. Queue 5, 24–36 (2007)
12. Robillard, M.P.: What makes APIs hard to learn? answers from developers. IEEE Software 26, 27–34 (2009)
13. Fowler, M.: Inversion of Control Containers and the Dependency Injection pattern (January 2004), http://martinfowler.com/articles/injection.html
14. Nielsen, J.: Usability Engineering. Morgan Kaufmann, San Francisco (1994)
15. Scheller, T., Kühn, E.: Measurable concepts for the usability of software components. In: Proc. of the 37th EUROMICRO Conference on Software Engineering and Advanced Applications, SEAA 2011, pp. 129–133. IEEE Computer Society, Oulu (2011)

Monitoring Learning Activities in PLE Using Semantic Modelling of Learner Behaviour

Selver Softic[1], Benham Taraghi[1], Martin Ebner[1],
Laurens De Vocht[2], Erik Mannens[2], and Rik Van de Walle[2]

[1] Graz University of Technology - Department for Social Learning
Muenzgrabenstr. 35A, 8010 Graz, Austria
{selver.softic,b.taraghi,martin.ebner}@tugraz.at
http://www.tugraz.at
[2] Ghent University - iMinds - Multimedia Lab
Gaston Crommelaan 8, 9000 Ghent, Belgium
{laurens.devocht,erik.mannens,rik.vandewalle}@ugent.be
http://www.ugent.be

Abstract. We report on the reflection of learning activities and revealing hidden information based on tracked user behaviour in our widget based PLE (Personal Learning Environment) at Graz University of Technology. Our reference data set includes information of more then 4000 active learners for a period of around two years. We have modelled activity and usage traces using domain specific ontologies like Activity Ontology and Learning Context Ontology from the IntelLEO[1] EU project. Generally we distinguish three different metrics: user centric, learning object (widget) centric and activity centric. We have used Semantic Web query languages like SPARQL and representation formats like RDF to implement a human and machine readable web service along with a learning analytics dashboard for metrics visualization. The results offer a quick overview of learning habits, preferred set-ups of learning objects (widgets) and overall reflection of usages and activity dynamics in the PLE platform over time. The architecture delivers insights for intervening and recommending as closure of a learning analytics cycle[1] to optimize confidence in the PLE.

Keywords: PLE, Semantic Web, Learning Analytics, Reflection, RDF, SPARQL.

1 Introduction

The Web 2.0 introduced intensive and wide-spread participation in online activities: the Social Web became a reality and derivate of such circumstances are visible nowadays in form of social networks (e.g. Facebook, Twitter), resource sharing platforms or interactive collaborative environments for problem solving [2,3]. The transformation of internet from consuming into interacting medium

---

[1] http://intelleo.eu

A. Holzinger et al. (Eds.): SouthCHI 2013, LNCS 7946, pp. 74–90, 2013.
© Springer-Verlag Berlin Heidelberg 2013

along with the corresponding web technologies determinates more and more how we think, inform ourselves, organize our every day activities but also how we learn. This evolution is bringing new approaches to education. Massive Open On-line Courses (MOOCs) for example aim for large-scale worldwide participation. This became possible on the one hand thanks to advances in the technology and on the other hand by challenges resulted by organising the education in general in order to provide to the needs of modern learners adequate time contemporary environments. The idea about open knowledge and open access also contributed to the developments in this direction. E-Learning platforms turned to be more efficient for tackling the problem of organisational and cost-effective matter[2]. Since the Web became not only consuming but also a producing medium evolving problem of Big Data is one of the next challenges for E-Learning to tackle in the near future. Limited availability of resources along with a time efficiency focus forces the designers and decision makers of learning platforms to revise their methodologies and techniques in order to respond the challenges of time and the needs of their targeted groups. On the other side learners are expecting a focused and simple way to organize their learning process, without losing time on information and actions which could disturb or prolong their learning, which also has a strong impact on acceptance of such platform [4].

Therefore todays learning process became more individual, multi faceted and activity driven with the tendency to ad-hoc initiated collaboration and infor-mation exchange. These circumstances imply the need for a scalable, adaptive learning environment enriched with multimedia supportive materials, communi-cation channels, personalized search and interfaces to external platforms from Social Web like e.g. Slideshare, Youtube channels etc. All these parameters in-crease the complexity of online learning platform design and organization. Dy-namics involved in this process require nowadays shorter optimization cycles in adaptation process of Learning Management Systems and Personal Learn-ing Environments. In order to provide the learners an attractive surrounding and to tackle the named problems use of learning analytics for optimization of learning process and design of learning surrounding emerges as the time passes by. Personalized Learning Dashboards with focus to the learning objectives are necessary. Additionally learning platforms need a more focused view on overall learning management system performance and activities. Growth of data pro-duced as monitoring material to the common state of the art learning platforms reveals a new dimension of optimization possibility to monitor the usage of learn-ing artefacts and learning activities of users individually and overall aiming at the analysis of emotion and affective data in learning environments. Such data contributes to the personalization and adaptation of the learning process and deliver out of the results new interfaces for learning analytics.

Our widget based Personal Learning Environment (PLE)[3] was developed for the needs of Graz University of Technology. The PLE serves currently more then

---

[2] http://www.insidehighered.com/news/2012/10/16/u-texas-aims-use-moocs-reduce-costs-increase-completion

[3] http://ple.tugraz.at

4000 users. We tracked the usage, activities and the use of the learning Widgets. Widget-based interfaces have been considered by Reinhardt et al. to cope with learner awareness requirements as they allow dynamic addition of functionalities [5]. We used data collected over 2 years in order to generate learning analytics services with visualization support, which reflects the overall usage and process view on our environment following the research trends of previous years [6,7]. We want to gain insights [8] to optimize our PLE and adapt the PLE to the learners by using more personalized methods of learning possibilities e.g. through recommendations[9]. In the following section we introduce our findings and concepts based upon semantic modelling for visual data exploration to improve learning management systems with respect to social and semantic analysis of the determining parameters on a user, widget and activity centred level [10]. A PLE does not intend to substitute a Learning Management Systems (LMS), but it is an additional learning environment to support self regulated learning. So our model and analysis does not actually improve LMS, but it may have a role to improve the quality of learning by supporting students in their personal learning process. We model the learning context using domain specific ontologies and describe them semantically. We realize as such accessible interfacing and extendibility on machine and human level while offering advantages such as the possibility to enrich the analysis results with Linked Data[4]

2   Related Work

The current learning analytics research community defines [11] learning analytics as the analysis of communication logs [10,12], learning resources [13], learning management system logs as well existing learning designs [14,15] and the activity outside of the learning management systems [7,16]. The result of this analysis improves the creation of predictive models [17,18], recommendations [19,9] and refection [20].

Learning Analytics resides on algorithms, formulas, methods, and concepts that translate data into meaningful information. Modelling, structuring and processing the collected data derived from e.g. user behaviour tracking plays a decisive role for the evaluation. Different works outlined the importance of tracking activity data in Learning Management Systems [11,21]; none of them addressed the issue of intelligently structuring learner data in context and processing it to provide a flexible interface that ensures maximum benefit from collected information. Emerging technologies like the Semantic Web along with RDF[5] and SPARQL[6] where data is structured and queried as graphs and projected on specific knowledge domain using adequate ontologies. Linked Data has been fairly successful used to generate correct interpretation of webtables [22] and the DEPTHS environment demonstrates how a synergistic combination of

---

[4] http://linkeddata.org/
[5] http://www.w3.org/RDF/
[6] http://www.w3.org/TR/rdf-sparql-query/

social and semantic technologies and Linked Data advances the learning process in software engineering [23]. Additionally the Semantic Web introduces a retrieval standard: SPARQL, which enables easily querying of semantically enriched data. This potential is partly the topic of current research in the EU project *Intelligent Learning Extended Organisation (IntellLEO)* which produced in the published ontology framework: Activities Ontology [7] to model learning activities and events related to them along with the surrounding environment and Learning Context Ontology[8] which offers formalization of learning context as general learning situation. Due to their accuracy to the problem that is addressed by this work these ontologies have been used to model the context of analytic data collected used in following observations.

Our work focuses on tracking learner's widget activity in a PLE system. Further the reflection of different views on the trackers is tended to be presented using our learning analytics dashboard. Our method is based on a tracking model as a knowledge domain related context using Semantic Web ontologies and query languages like SPARQL similar to current research in the area of Self-regulated Learners(SRL)[24]. Exploratory graphics show that the sum of (web) user data on the access paths and the linkage of the resources within an environment (site) at a particular time window gives sufficient insight at what constitutes relevance; important properties and linkages between data resources[25]. The overall goal of is summarization of visualizations and evaluation of statistic data that enable the PLE optimization and present the research community used generic techniques and metrics for problems in design and adaptation of learning environments.

3   Use Case

In a PLE by definition there are no teachers and learners, producers and consumers like in Learning Management Systems (LMS). PLE lies in the category of self regulated learning where students have the whole control over the services and resources they may need and would like to use. Teachers may recommend their students to use some widgets or resources in PLE as they may recommend them to read some books, but they provide nothing in PLE.

3.1   Modelling Statistics of Learners Logs

Concept Modelling statistics in dimensions for the PLE: reflection (by tracking users), prediction (tracking activities) and unveiling hidden information (tracking widgets - LOs). All three dimension are directly in relation to each other which implies that reflection influences prediction and vice versa. The hidden information regarding the learning objects (widgets) is derived from these bidirectional bounds. This implication relies on modelling and the native concept of widget as learning object as it will be shown in following sections.

---

[7] http://www.intelleo.eu/ontologies/activities/spec/

[8] http://www.intelleo.eu/ontologies/activities/spec/

Revealing hidden information enables to find out how the learning process is going on in general and individually for each student in respect of what learners are learning: how often are they learning and whether it is continuously or not. This shows which learning objects are mostly used and hence is a possible indicator for usefulness.

Prediction: following the activities of learners, assumed that we can extract some patterns within activities (what they do and also what goals and to which extent they achieve a goal) teachers can predict the overall performance of their learners according to their activities.

Plotting the overall activities of learners reflects their learning process within PLE: this is reflection.

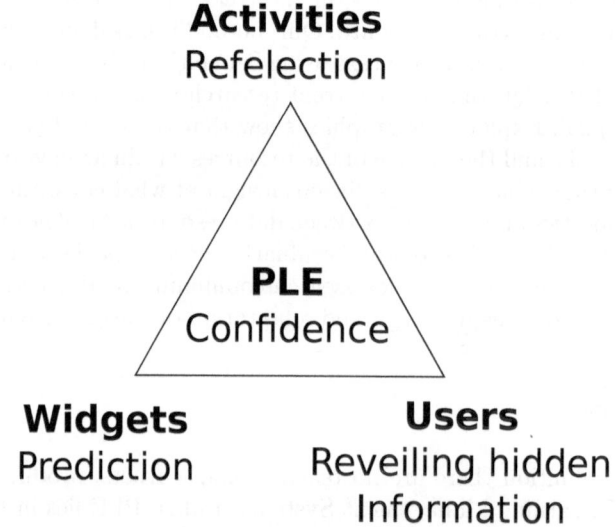

Fig. 1. Dimensions of PLE Measuring confidence by monitoring widgets, activities and users

Purpose. All statistics combined establish confidence in modules/widgets as interface between teacher (knowledge provision) and learner (knowledge consumer). The context of widgets is important to achieve reliable outcomes of the analysis of learner's activities. Figure 1 depicts the analysis of learner's activities ensures the optimization of the PLE focus to cover three modelling dimensions maximally by constructing a coherent view to support a call to action with high confidence.

Application. Specific use cases based on statistics learned on the modeled learners logs should: contribute to better understanding of PLE usage, and reveal favored designs of widget. Further intention that should be covered with this investigation is to orchestrate the insights into a recycling feedback loop to increase the overall acceptance of PLE as useful learning environment. Last targeted but not less important appliance of lesson learned should deliver initial information for improvements in our recommender system for widgets already integrated in PLE.

3.2   Dashboard for Analytics

Concept To get an overview, PLE administrators have access to a 'Dashboard' facilitating browsing the learning analytics from the PLE as shown in Figure 2. The dashboard contains views containing a graph visualization on the modelled information. The view is split in a summary which displays several graphs of measures derived from the raw statistics data to monitor the confidence and the balance of the learning environment.

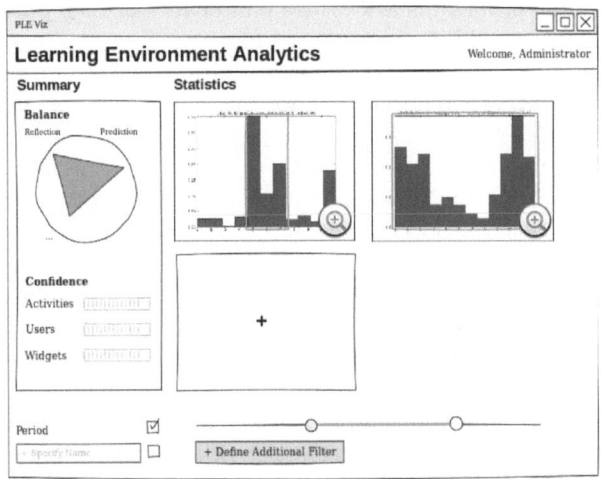

Fig. 2. `PLE Analytics Dashboard` Overview of the available statistics and measures of the PLE

Purpose. The dashboard is a collection of indicators for administrators to get to-the-point feedback. Administrators can deduct new views, broader or narrower; based on actions in the existing views because we allow intelligently adding new views on the statistics data to the dashboard. The combination of different views and visualizations of analytics based learner's log data encourages administrators to take action and further optimize the learning environment.

Application. The widget based interface for the dashboard guides users in constructing complex queries and revealing hidden correlations among the datasets. It is an excellent way for putting analytics into context using categories, assumptions, and reason towards relating perspectives in a broader context trough the addition and linking of multiple data resources.

4   Semantics for Learning Analytics

4.1   Modelling

In current work we are aiming at visualisation of three different kind of monitoring aspects interesting for optimisation of PLE: User centric view where relations between the learner and the learning surrounding along with aligned activities should be outlined. Activity centric view where activities bound to the widgets that a learner is using are tracked. Finally widget centric where the whole perspective is reflected out of the sight of learning widgets. With this purpose the data that was collected was tracked out of the PLE using simple log files which included information about a user (in anonymous way), about widget and activities related to the learning widget with additional time stamp when this logging event happened. Simple logging of data is unstructured and not easy queryable, the same problem is also with maintenance of such data. Generating specific visualization would in unstructured form imply formatting data into the form of visualisation interfaces and requires additional efforts for each new visualization framework that would be used for implementation of such monitoring dashboard.

In order to provide flexible data model that also delivers all wide accepted formats as e.g. XML or JSON as final output since those formats are very wide spread as input in visualization libraries our consideration lead us towards more operable and flexible data modelling framework and standards, for maintenance of tracking data. We wanted also to make the data model extensible and scalable, and to additionally enrich the data with the context reflection in which such data was collected. Since Semantic Web offers flexible and scalable approach to modelling, formatting data in this way was the next logical step. SPARQL as retrieval technology driven by the efforts of W3C community reached mature level comparable to common occurrences. Output of SPARQL frameworks support XML, JSON or comma separated values.

The challenge is to choose an adequate modelling vocabulary (in our case Ontology) since RDF offers only the framework how the data is aligned and organized in such constructions. Fortunately current research in *IntellLEO* EU project resolved our dilemmas. One of the main goals of this project is building an *innovative ontological framework for learning representation which includes learners, context and collaboration models, serving to achieve the targeted synergy*[9]. In the realm of the *IntellLEO* project inside the provided ontology framework two special ontologies are eminent. The first is the Activity Ontology which offers a vocabulary to represent different activities and events related to them inside of a learning environment with possibility to describe and reference the environment (in this case PLE) where these activities occur. The second contribution from current Ontology research work in *IntellLEO* project is the Learning Context Ontology which describes the context of a learning situation.

Our logs include the events about learners who use a PLE while performing different learning activities in a certain period of time. Their activities comply

---

[9] http://intelleo.eu/index.php?id=5

Listing 1.1. `LearningContext` in N3 RDF notation.

```
@prefix ao: <http://intelleo.eu/ontologies/activities/ns/> .
@prefix foaf: <http://xmlns.com/foaf/0.1/> .
@prefix lc: <http://www.intelleo.eu/ontologies/learning−context/ns/> .
@prefix rdfs: <http://www.w3.org/2000/01/rdf−schema#> .
@prefix um: <http://intelleo.eu/ontologies/user−model/ns/> .


<https://ple.tugraz.at/ns/activity/#Viewing> a ao:Viewing .

<https://ple.tugraz.at/ns/users/#FSKSN> a um:User;
    foaf:name "FSKSN" .

<http://ple.tugraz.at/ns/events/log/#7912> a ao:Logging;
    ao:performedBy <https://ple.tugraz.at/ns/users/#FSKSN>;
    ao:timestamp "2012−10−04T07:52:52" .

<https://ple.tugraz.at/ns/widgets/#LatexFormulaToPngWidget>
    a ao:Enivironment;
    rdfs:label "LaTeXFormulaPNG Converter" .

<http://ple.tugraz.at/ns/learningcontext/#7912> a lc:LearningContext;
    lc:activityRef <https://ple.tugraz.at/ns/activity/#Viewing>;
    lc:environmentRef
    <https://ple.tugraz.at/ns/widgets/#LatexFormulaToPngWidget>;
    lc:eventRef <http://ple.tugraz.at/ns/events/log/#7912>;
    lc:userRef <https://ple.tugraz.at/ns/users/#FSKSN> .
```

to our use cases very well, which implicitly solved our modelling vocabulary dilemma stated before. Representation of log entries from PLE as instance of a learning context concept can be seen in N3 RDF Notation in Listing 1.1.

As stated in listing 1.1 depicted instance of `lc:LearningContext` class descibes in compact N3 RDF Notation that a `ao:Logging` event occured which tracked the learning activity of `ao:Viewing` by certain `um:User` inside the learning widget named *LatexFormulaToPngWidget* as `ao:Enviroment` at certain time.

4.2 Querying

Beside the scalability and flexibility of data models Semantic Web also includes the advantage of traceability of such models using SPARQL. Common storage and retrieval systems for semantic data instances support the exposure of so-called SPARQL endpoints, where the data from the storages (RDF triple stores) can be easily retrieved by simple SQL like queries defined by SPARQL standard. Additional advantage of such endpoints is that most of them deliver result data in common formats like XML,JSON or comma separated values. This functionality is essential for processing the retrieved results for visualisation dashboard

Listing 1.2. SPARQL query filtering Viewing action on LatexFormulaPNG widget.

```
PREFIX ao: <http://intelleo.eu/ontologies/activities/ns/> .
PREFIX foaf: <http://xmlns.com/foaf/0.1/> .
PREFIX lc: <http://www.intelleo.eu/ontologies/learning−context/ns/> .
PREFIX rdfs: <http://www.w3.org/2000/01/rdf−schema#> .
PREFIX um: <http://intelleo.eu/ontologies/user−model/ns/> .

SELECT ?user WHERE
{
 ?x a lc:LearningContext;
        lc:activityRef <https://ple.tugraz.at/ns/activity/#Viewing>;
        lc:environmentRef
        <https://ple.tugraz.at/ns/widgets/#LatexFormulaToPngWidget>;
        lc:eventRef ?e;
        lc:userRef ?u.

 ?e a ao:Logging;
        ao:timestamp ?date.

 ?u a um:User;
        foaf:name ?user.

 FILTER ( ?date > "2011−01−01T00:00:00Z"^^xsd:dateTime )
}
```

(PLE-Viz). Also very important function is that the endpoints offer implicitly standardized interfaces based upon RDF for data exchange to other platforms. Operability over the data is much easier then in the case if the log data would be stored in specific structure without standardization. In this way humans and machines readable, reusable activity knowledge artefacts has been produced with broader appliance field then a simple tracking log entry.

Listing 1.2 depicts in the best way how easily a question like: "Which users performed viewing in *LaTeXFormulaPNG Converter* widget after the first of January 2011?" can be answered by simple SPARQL query. This approach obviously enables easy preprocessing and thanks to SPARQL endpoints output configuration, the desired inputs for visualizations can be delivered in the same step. Semantic Web uses a "closed world" representation which means if there are no results when there is no answer possible in the system. The advantages of Semantic Web technologies combined with adequate vocabularies and ontologies do not only support easy and flexible analysis, it extends the repositories to the outside world while implementing implicitly many interoperability options for external analytic systems.

5   Results

5.1   Visualization of Statistics

In this section we intend to describe some possible statistics that can be generated by the first prototype of PLE Analytics Dashboard. According to the PLE
measuring confidence triangle described before, the statistics has been modeled
into three dimensions. These dimensions are illustrated through some examples
in the following sections. The dataset used to generate the following statistics
contains the user log data of about last two years in PLE.

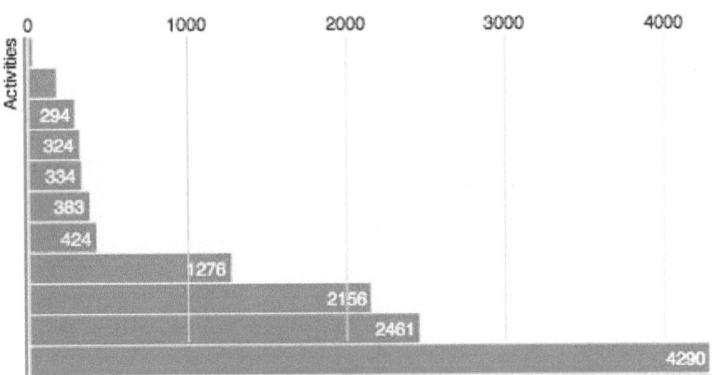

Fig. 3. PLE statistics Distribution of users over activities in PLE

User Centered. Each widget in PLE is associated to one or more activities depending on the functionality that is provided by the widget. To give an example,
Twitter widget is associated to the activities *Reading, ContentSharing, Discus-
sAsynchronouly, Viewing* and *Search*. The other defined activities in PLE are
Authoring, Learning, Game, Quizzing, Computing and *Listening*. Figure 3 depicts the distribution of users over all activities in PLE. The diagram illustrates
that most of all users are engaged in the activities *Reading* (4290 users) followed
by *Authoring* (2461 users) and *Search* (2156 users). In contrast *Listening* (33
users), *Computing* (181 users) and *Quizzing* (294 users) are rarely popular for
users.

Widget Centered. Figure 4 demonstrates an example for widget centered
statistics. It shows how often each widget is used in each period of time in PLE.
The widgets *ZID News* (representing the actual news related to the Central Infor-
matic Service), *TUGraz online* (Administration System), *TUGraz Newsgroups*
(News groups), *TUGMail* (E-Mail service) and *TeachCenter Courses* (LMS platform) are listed on the top as the most frequent used widgets in the last two

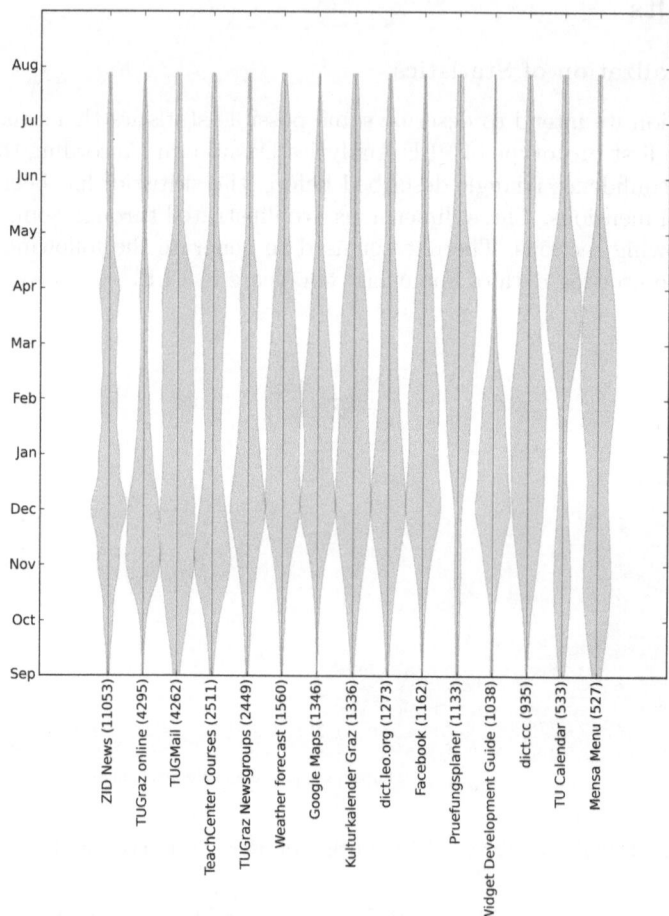

Fig. 4. PLE statistics Distribution of usage of the 15 most popular widgets each month in PLE

years. All these widgets represent university services that students daily use. According to the visualized statistics the highest range of user activity can be monitored from October (begin of the winter semester) until July (end of the summer semester). On the first week of January as well as in summer holidays no active usage cam be seen in PLE that is actually expected. The visualisation helps to detect widgets that are not popular at all or have been rarely used over the whole monitored period. Interestingly we can observe no significant change on this behaviour considering differnt period of times and different users. Widgets *Google Search, Address Book, Plane-Sweep Algorithmus* and *laengste gemeinsame Teilfolge* (a learning object to support learning the algorithm) are such examples that must be revised in a further development process. The other observations can be taken from this visualisation is the development of ple usage

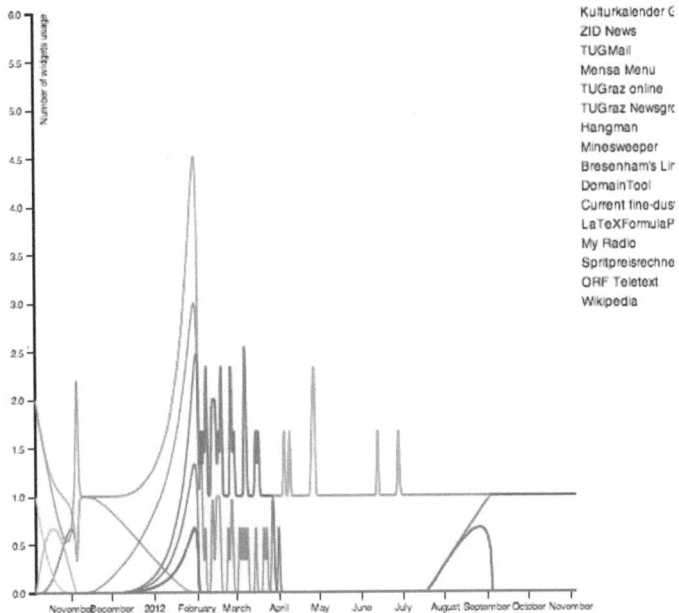

Fig. 5. PLE statistics Distribution of usage of widgets by a sample active user over time in PLE

in general during the time. It is obvious that the frequency and quantity of used widgets have been increased in year 2012 in comparison with 2011.

Figure 5 demonstrates an example that can be of high interest. It demonstrates the activities of a specific user during a time period (in this example over the whole monitored time). The sorted list of widgets that the user have been actively using can be seen on the diagram. It shows that the user has been constantly using some widgets (*KulturKalender Graz, ZID News* and *TUGMail*) since February 2012. *TUGMail* widget is an exception. The user has stopped using it from April to August 2012. Figure 6 demonstrates the activity of another user who uses only two widgets: *ZID News* and *TUGraz Newsgroup*. It is obvious that she has been using *ZID News* continuously.

Activity Centered. Figure 7 depicts the distribution of user activity over all activities in PLE. This diagram resembles figure 3 which depicts the distribution of users over all activities in PLE. The diagram shows that the activities *Reading* (28406 times) followed by *Search* (10588 times) and *Authoring* (9437 times) are most top popular ones. In contrast *Listening* (194 times), *Computing* (295 times) and again *Quizzing* (530 times) are rarely popular for users.

Figure 7 depicts the same situation over the whole monitored time period: an overall picture of the activity usage intensity. Again our observations from previous statistics can be confirmed. The list of activities on figure 7 are sorted

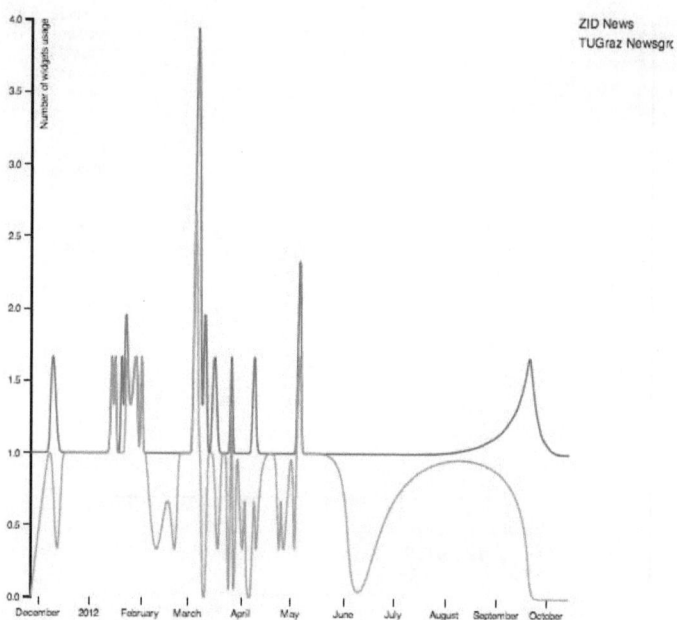

Fig. 6. PLE statistics Distribution of usage of widgets by a sample active user over time in PLE. Widgets: ZID News and TUGraz News

according to the popularity and dominance during the whole monitoring period. The same results can be achieved here. *Reading, Authoring* and *Search* are dominant activities, clearly seen in the year 2012 compared with 2011.

5.2 Discussion

The overview over distribution of activities can reflect the overall interest of the learners within PLE. It can be concluded that in case of our PLE users are more consumers that contributers. Visualisation of statistics can help to improve the PLE in general. Activities such as *Quizzing* and *Learning* (supported by some learning object widgets) are not quite popular. Our investigation showed that the corresponding widgets that support those activities must be revised in regard to some usability issues.

We can obtain a kind of rating/quality measure for the widgets that can be used as an indicator of likely future activity in the PLE. Distribution of usage of widgets over time in PLE showed exactly which widgets have been popular in certain period of time.

Widget centered statitics for a specific user reflect user oriented statistics on which widgets are favoured by a single user: We can observe if this trend is trackable over time or not. It delivers fast overview of affinities of single user

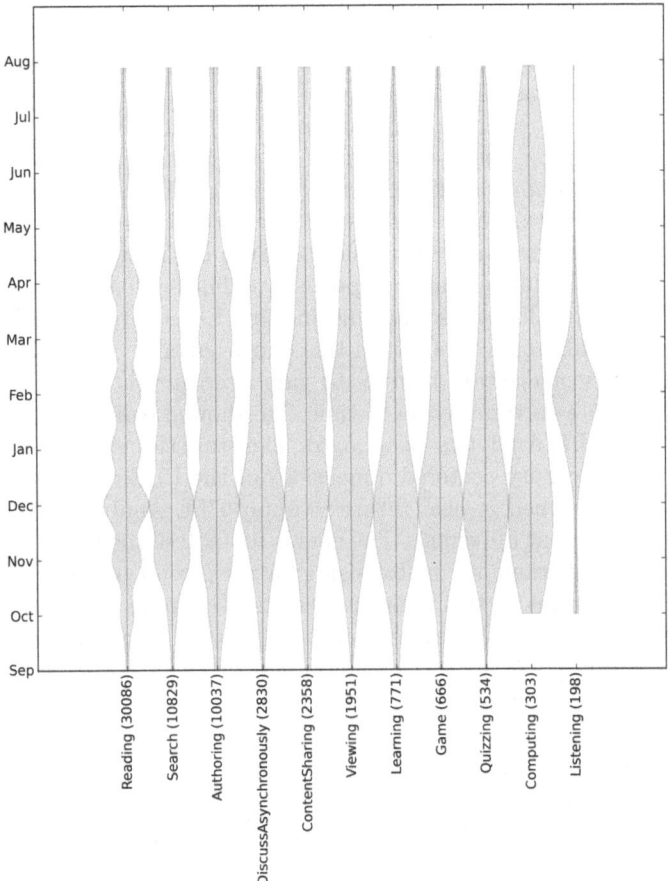

Fig. 7. PLE statistics Distribution of activities occurrence each month in PLE

considering the usage of special widgets. It can also be used e.g. as a basis for recommendation of new widgets in the widget store within PLE.

Through activity centered statistics we gain a better insight in the activities done in the PLE and their use. We can get insight about dominant activities, activity dissemination over time and activity peak usage periods.

6 Conclusions

The interactivity and relations between teachers and students has changed since the introduction of online technology such as the Web with environments such as PLE or LMS. The teacher is no longer the provider of knowledge but rather a middleman between information and student. Instead of being a passive knowledge consumer, the student has now become active in procuring, organizing and managing information. Further development of this technology helps students to understand concepts better and improve their skills.

We demonstrated that using semantic technologies enables the extensibility of learning analytics dashboards. Our approach generates uniform interfaces for information exchange, enables flexibility for visual analytics, and also includes the flexibility regarding the enrichment of learning analytics data with Linked Data. The spread of applicability covers wide range of analytics methodologies like prediction, reflection and as result of these the intervention field. Future efforts regarding improvement semantic structure data layer, besides the mentioned Linked Data could also include precisely defined categorisation of learning widgets, since PLE includes also this information. Especially the learning widget store as part of PLE could profit from this improvement.

The statistics visualisation help us to gain deep insight into the behaviour of a single user in a certain period of time .We showed examples what we have achieved with a PLE Analytics Dashboard. The statistics examples covered the user, widget and activity centered dimensions of the PLE confidence model we introduced. It is planned in near future to apply PLE Analytics Dashboard for some specific courses at university. The goal is to analyse the learner's behaviour in detail, the widgets they use or stop using for the given learning goals and map their monitored actions to their learning results. The main question will be how or if the PLE Analytics Dashboard must be further improved to meet these goals. The examples demonstrated for now show that it would be possible. We will do this survey as the next step in the near future.

Acknowledgements. The research activities that have been described in this paper were funded by Graz University of Technology, Ghent University, iMinds (an independent research institute founded by the Flemish government to stimulate ICT innovation), the Institute for the Promotion of Innovation by Science and Technology in Flanders (IWT), the Fund for Scientific Research-Flanders (FWO-Flanders), and the European Union.

References

1. Clow, D.: The learning analytics cycle: closing the loop effectively. In: Proceedings of the 2nd International Conference on Learning Analytics and Knowledge, LAK 2012, pp. 134–138. ACM, New York (2012)
2. Ebner, M., Holzinger, A., Maurer, H.A.: Web 2.0 technology: Future interfaces for technology enhanced learning? In: Stephanidis, C. (ed.) HCI 2007. LNCS, vol. 4556, pp. 559–568. Springer, Heidelberg (2007)
3. Pohl, M., Holzinger, A., Rester, M., Motschnig, R., Ebner, M., Leitner, G.: Gestaltung von innovativen technologiegesttzten lernsystemen am beispiel von web 2.0-anwendungen. eine herausforderung fr hci. OCG Journal (33), 20–23 (2008)
4. Holzinger, A., Searle, G., Wernbacher, M.: The effect of previous exposure to technology on acceptance and its importance in usability and accessibility engineering. Universal Access in the Information Society 10, 245–260 (2011)

5. Reinhardt, W., Mletzko, C., Drachsler, H., Sloep, P.: Awesome: A widget-based dashboard for awareness-support in research networks. In: Learning, PLE Conference, pp. 1–15 (2011)

6. Santos Odriozola, J.L., Verbert, K., Govaerts, S., Duval, E.: Visualizing PLE usage. In: Proceedings of EFEPLE 2011 1st Workshop on Exploring the Fitness and Evolvability of Personal Learning Environments, CEUR WS, pp. 34–38 (August 2011)

7. Pardo, A., Kloos, C.D.: Stepping out of the box: towards analytics outside the learning management system. In: Proceedings of the 1st International Conference on Learning Analytics and Knowledge, LAK 2011, pp. 163–167. ACM, New York (2011)

8. Mazza, R., Milani, C.: Exploring usage analysis in learning systems: Gaining insights from visualisations. In: Workshop on Usage Analysis in Learning Systems, Proceedings of Artificial Intelligence in Education, Amsterdam (2005)

9. Drachsler, H., Bogers, T., Vuorikari, R., Verbert, K., Duval, E., Manouselis, N., Beham, G., Lindstaedt, S., Stern, H., Friedrich, M., Wolpers, M.: Issues and considerations regarding sharable data sets for recommender systems in technology enhanced learning. Procedia Computer Science 1(2), 2849–2858 (2010); Proceedings of the 1st Workshop on Recommender Systems for Technology Enhanced Learnin (RecSysTEL 2010)

10. Rosen, D., Miagkikh, V., Suthers, D.: Social and semantic network analysis of chat logs. In: Proceedings of the 1st International Conference on Learning Analytics and Knowledge, LAK 2011, pp. 134–139. ACM, New York (2011)

11. Santos, J.L., Govaerts, S., Verbert, K., Duval, E.: Goal-oriented visualizations of activity tracking: a case study with engineering students. In: Proceedings of the 2nd International Conference on Learning Analytics and Knowledge, LAK 2012, pp. 143–152. ACM, New York (2012)

12. Bakharia, A., Dawson, S.: Snapp: a bird's-eye view of temporal participant interaction. In: Proceedings of the 1st International Conference on Learning Analytics and Knowledge, LAK 2011, pp. 168–173. ACM, New York (2011)

13. Niemann, K., Schmitz, H.C., Scheffel, M., Wolpers, M.: Usage contexts for object similarity: exploratory investigations. In: Proceedings of the 1st International Conference on Learning Analytics and Knowledge, LAK 2011, pp. 81–85. ACM, New York (2011)

14. Lockyer, L., Dawson, S.: Learning designs and learning analytics. In: Proceedings of the 1st International Conference on Learning Analytics and Knowledge, LAK 2011, pp. 153–156. ACM, New York (2011)

15. Richards, G., DeVries, I.: Revisiting formative evaluation: dynamic monitoring for the improvement of learning activity design and delivery. In: Proceedings of the 1st International Conference on Learning Analytics and Knowledge, LAK 2011, pp. 157–162. ACM, New York (2011)

16. Blikstein, P.: Using learning analytics to assess students' behavior in open-ended programming tasks. In: Proceedings of the 1st International Conference on Learning Analytics and Knowledge, LAK 2011, pp. 110–116. ACM, New York (2011)

17. Sharkey, M.: Academic analytics landscape at the university of phoenix. In: Proceedings of the 1st International Conference on Learning Analytics and Knowledge, LAK 2011, pp. 122–126. ACM, New York (2011)

18. Fancsali, S.E.: Variable construction for predictive and causal modeling of online education data. In: Proceedings of the 1st International Conference on Learning Analytics and Knowledge, LAK 2011, pp. 54–63. ACM, New York (2011)

19. Verbert, K., Drachsler, H., Manouselis, N., Wolpers, M., Vuorikari, R., Duval, E.: Dataset-driven research for improving recommender systems for learning. In: Proceedings of the 1st International Conference on Learning Analytics and Knowledge, LAK 2011, pp. 44–53. ACM, New York (2011)
20. Verbert, K., Manouselis, N., Drachsler, H., Duval, E.: Dataset-driven research to support learning and knowledge analytics. Educational Technology & Society 15(3), 133–148 (2012)
21. Prinsloo, P., Slade, S., Galpin, F.: Learning analytics: challenges, paradoxes and opportunities for mega open distance learning institutions. In: Proceedings of the 2nd International Conference on Learning Analytics and Knowledge, LAK 2012, pp. 130–133. ACM, New York (2012)
22. Mulwad, V., Finin, T., Syed, Z., Joshi, A.: Using linked data to interpret tables. In: Hartig, O., Harth, A., Sequeda, J. (eds.) COLD. CEUR Workshop Proceedings, vol. 665. CEUR-WS.org (2010)
23. Jeremic, Z., Jovanovic, J., Gasevic, D.: Personal learning environments on the social semantic web. Semantic Web 4(1), 23–51 (2013)
24. Siadaty, M., Jovanovic, J., Pata, K., Holocher-Ertl, T., Gasevic, D., Milikic, N.: A semantic web-enabled tool for self-regulated learning in the workplace. In: ICALT, pp. 66–70. IEEE Computer Society (2011)
25. Kirchberg, M., Ko, R.K.L., Lee, B.S.: From linked data to relevant data – time is the essence. CoRR abs/1103.5046 (2011)

Back to User-Centered Usability Testing

Kimmo Tarkkanen[1], Pekka Reijonen[1], Franck Tétard[2], and Ville Harkke[1]

[1] Information Systems Science,
University of Turku, Turku, Finland
{kimmo.tarkkanen,pekka.reijonen,ville.harkke}@utu.fi
[2] Department of Informatics and Media,
Uppsala University, Uppsala, Sweden
franck.tetard@im.uu.se

Abstract. Usability testing is a widely used evaluation method for product design during and after the development. Conventional usability testing applies short and discrete test tasks and task scenarios that are based on the tasks the product is designed to support. Thus, conventional test task design relies heavily on the representations of the specified context of use and the specified user requirements of the proposed design solution. However, a premature commitment to the specified context, requirements and proposed solutions may limit the scope of usability testing in a manner that hinders its capability to elicit and validate new user requirements, which is one of the objectives of the evaluation phase in the iterative user-centered design process. In this paper, we introduce a user-centered task design approach, which allows test participants to follow their natural work flow and freely express their needs during a test session. The main idea of this open-ended task approach is to break the tight link between the produced design solutions and the tasks used in the usability test and in this way increase the probability that novel user needs can emerge during a test session. Empirical results from a case study are used to depict the approach and its prerequisites, strengths, and limitations are discussed.

Keywords: Usability testing, task design, usability evaluation, user-centered design, requirements elicitation.

1 Introduction

In user-centered product development iterations the designs are routinely evaluated for usability. Usability testing is one of the most discussed usability evaluation techniques in academic usability journals [1] and the most widely applied method among the user-centered design (UCD) practitioners [2]. The method is included in the UCD techniques in the human-centered design process to evaluate if a design meets the specified user requirements. An evaluation using the usability testing method deploys potential users, i.e. subjects who are asked to perform tasks that should be real, meaningful and represent user activity [3].

A. Holzinger et al. (Eds.): SouthCHI 2013, LNCS 7946, pp. 91–106, 2013.

In conventional usability testing test tasks are created by a test designer, in order to direct the evaluation to specific goals and concerns and to get comparable results between the subjects [4]. Creation of tasks is typically based on earlier experience and knowledge of the context of use and the product features. While usage domain knowledge is of the utmost importance for both the developers [5] and the usability evaluators [6], many products, product versions and upgrades are launched in isolation from the actual users [4]. Involving users in the product development requires expertise and experience from its conductors. A careful execution of the UCD and requirements engineering processes acknowledge that the product requirements do not freeze but immediately begin to evolve after the product has been built and actual usage begins [7-8]. The design and redesign of many systems inevitably involves some vagueness of exactly how the users or the intended users will perform their actions in order to fulfill their work goals. Therefore, the requirements elicitation is a constant discovery process that can and should continue also during the product evaluation with usability testing. Regarding usability testing as an inherent part of the requirements process could be of great value for trawling the requirements and the true nature of the work.

However, conventional designer-created usability test tasks with correct answers and clear endings [9] that are always doable [10] are weak in answering usability questions concerning user needs and situated work practices. Usability testing carried out with conventional test task design misses users' point of view and thus can discontinue the user-centeredness of the whole development life cycle. In other words, the tasks may contain implicit premature commitment to a design detail [11] that actually hinders the emergence of new user needs.

In this paper, we propose an approach to early usability testing that is a modified version of the user-defined task approach [10] and applies an open-ended test task that is not based on product functions but is a broad work task from the context of use. The open-ended task allows the users to act freely and therefore improves requirements elicitation and validation and enhances the maintenance of the user-centeredness of the evaluation phase. Next we enlighten the role of usability testing and task design in user-centered design process and then introduce an example of the application of the open-ended task approach. Last, the empirical results and their relation to previous research as well as the prerequisites, strengths, and limitations of the approach are discussed.

2   User-Centeredness and Usability Test Tasks

The ISO (9241-11) standard defines usability as the "extent to which a system, product or service can be used by specified users to achieve specified goals with effectiveness, efficiency and satisfaction in a specified context of use" [12]. The method umbrella for usability creation, development and evaluation is commonly referred to as the user-centered design (UCD) approach. In the UCD, methods adapted from anthropology and sociology such as interviews, focus groups, and direct observations are applied in answering the basic questions of design: who the users are, what they need to accomplish and what user goals the product should support [13]. The general process of UCD follows the four steps of human-centered design for interactive systems (ISO 9241-210) [14]: The product designers need to 1) understand and specify the context of use, 2) specify the user requirements, 3) produce design solutions to meet user requirements, and 4) evaluate the designs against requirements. The design process is iterative; if the proposed product does not satisfy the specified requirements after the evaluation phase, the process continues to specify context, requirements and improved solutions (the phase depends on the type of problems found in the evaluation phase). Thus, usability creation and usability evaluation alternate throughout the life-cycle of product development.

The methods for user-centered design have been developed since its introduction in the late 1980's [15]. The methods vary from holistic development life-cycle methods with a step-by-step guidance, such as contextual design [16] and interaction design [17] to a mix of independent techniques, such as task analysis [18], scenarios [19] and focus groups [4]. The common denominator in the HCI discipline and the UCD approach is that they both favor user studies in the field. For example, in the contextual inquiry the designer interviews, observes and interprets users' activities in the field in order to construct a shared understanding of the goals of the users [16]. The specified goals of the potential users manifest themselves in the representations produced with the UCD methods. The representations of the reality and users' goals can be presented in different ways, for example, as user stories and work models [20], personas [21], iterative requirements specification documents, mock-ups, prototypes and scenarios [19], [22].

In usability evaluation, the users' goals or the user requirements specified during the design process are typically taken as given. In other words, the tasks used in the usability test are created from the representations created in the earlier phases of the development process, possibly without involvement of the users. There has lately been a small change in the design standards: In the ISO 13407 standard from 1999 the focus of the evaluation was "the designs" [23] whereas in the ISO 9241-210 standard from 2010 the focus is "designs against user requirements" [14]. The ISO 9241-210 standard specifically suggests to "collect new information about user needs" in the evaluation phase [14]. The focus shift has, however, rather marginal effect on the actual testing procedure and its outcomes if the user requirements are still the same ones that form the basis for the design. This may easily happen if user needs are not deliberately attended in usability task creation, i.e. the UCD principles are not rigorously followed. In this situation, the usability test reveals if the design matches the requirements but it cannot reveal if the requirements match users' needs.

If existing user requirements are applied anyway, it should be remembered that the user requirements are representations of users' reality and these representations have proved to be more or less incomplete [24] and change over time [7]. Incomplete representations lead to incomplete specifications and inadequate implementations of information system products. Many products fail due to inadequate understanding of the requirements that the products should fulfill. Products may not support the work processes they are designed for and later these practices need to be refuted and amended locally [25]. After the implementation, users must sometimes create workarounds [26], the product usage may become drifted [27], or users' work practices become incoherent [28]. Usability of the product may significantly deteriorate due to non-uniform work practices in all kinds of information systems mediated work [28]. Therefore, usability test tasks should be based on recent user requirements and current work practices.

Just as any interview and observation session for knowledge creation, a usability testing method can provide information only about what has been asked, observed and previously planned to focus on in a test session. The focus of usability testing is realized in test tasks (or task scenarios) that form the core of the data collection method. According to the literature, test scenarios should be real and meaningful [3]. Test scenarios are typically brief prose stories about the use [19] and can comprise several individual test tasks [29]. In the task creation, emphasis is in the tasks that users can do with the product, tasks that an evaluator assumes to relate to potential usability problems, concerns, and goals [4], tasks that will be performed during the course of using the product [29], tasks that are critical or frequent, appear in several UIs, involve new features or make first impression of the product [30] and tasks that include five most important functions of the product [31]. It is obvious from the above that there exists a lot of advice for creation and selection of test tasks that are based on the existing design solutions and representations. The effects of different task types on the test results are, however, scarcely discussed in the research literature [32-33].

If the test tasks in a usability test are selected from a set of tasks that the product is designed to support, the usability test becomes a validation method of the designed users' goals and needs – not a method that would reveal the potential premature commitments to the defined requirements (see [11]). Conventional test tasks include clear endings and correct answers that do not emerge in every work setting [9]. For example, too simple questions for too complex systems may provide misleading usability evaluation results due to the disconnection between the design assumptions and the holistic view of the work [34]. Complex systems introduce usually much higher level goals than applied in typical usability testing tasks, which may be hard to specify beforehand while lower level usability testing may result in an easy-to-use solution for the wrong set of requirements [9]. If usability testing is used to validate and gather requirements, the usefulness (and effectiveness) of the tested product becomes an important unit of analysis (see [35]). We claim, however, that practical evaluation methods, especially the widely applied usability testing, have not evolved towards this direction.

In recent years, a lot of attention has been paid, for example, to determine the appropriate number of participants for usability tests, but task coverage is more or less overlooked. Task coverage is, however, an important issue, as for example the reanalysis [36] of the CUE-4 study [37] revealed that more tasks provided more found usability problems. There are also a few attempts to pinpoint the importance of task design in usability testing and its effects on test results [38], [10], [30].

When the results of two different types of tasks were compared [38], it was found that structured tasks, which are the conventional usability testing tasks, help to detect minor and superficial usability problems while problem solving tasks seemed to uncover usability disasters.

In order to include at least some of the actual users' needs into the evaluation, it has been suggested [10] that the potential user brings some own tasks to the test session. This way users' perspective can be taken into consideration instead of evaluating usability only from the perspective of the design solutions. This approach is depicted in Fig. 1. Usability test tasks are typically based on product functions, i.e. potential tasks are situated inside the boundaries of produced design solutions (the numbered tasks in the Fig. 1). The user-defined tasks can, in principle, be situated anywhere in the sphere of the context of use (the unnumbered shaded tasks in the Fig. 1). Some of the tasks fall inside the produced design solutions, i.e. product functions support their execution while some fall outside, i.e. these users' needs have not been implemented into the design solution.

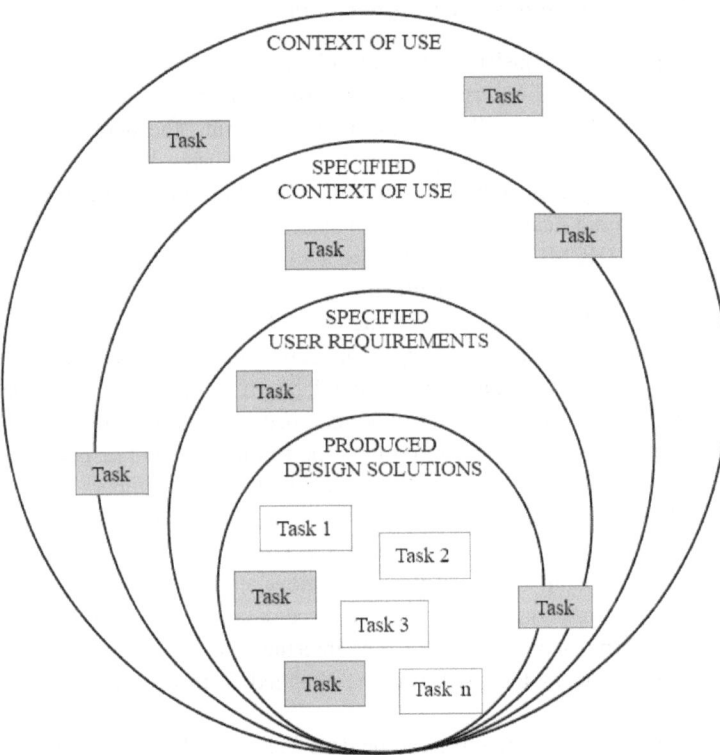

Fig. 1. The phases of the UCD process as nested circles. The tasks refer to the evaluation phase: the numbered tasks are based on design solutions and the unnumbered (shaded) tasks are user-defined and may hence fall anywhere in the context of use.

We have developed a modified version of the user-defined task approach (see [10]) in order to ensure that users' needs have better possibility to emerge in a usability test. The basic idea is that the subject (the test user) is given an open-ended task that does not point to any product function but to a whole work process inside the sphere of the context of use. This procedure allows the subjects to follow their natural work process and to show how they conceptualize their work and what kind of information and actions are needed in real work situations. As the tasks that a subject will carry out during a test session can be situated anywhere in the sphere of the context of use, some of them may fall outside the scope of the design solution (see Fig. 1). These tasks can be, however, the most interesting ones as they highlight user requirements that have not been included into the design solution. Exactly this was the case in the application example that is presented in the next chapter.

3   Application Example

3.1   Work Practices and Studied Application

Homecare nurses' work consists of visits to clients living in their homes where they carry out the planned and emerging care activities. In order to do this a home care nurse must know where the client lives, how to get into the department and what treatment and service the client is planned to receive during this particular visit. Information concerning client's health situation, care plan, and care contracts are managed in an electronic health record (EHR) system. An application called the Home Care Mobile Unit (HCMU) is planned to be a supportive tool in this field work and hence built on the tablet computer platform.

The design of the HCMU is based on the larger EHR system that covers the whole area of municipal health care, including home care. This system has been used in the target organization for about ten years and the deployment of the system in daily work has become routine for all actors. When actions become routine they are usually carried out quickly and, what is more important, the routines are not disputed. If the routines are not disputed by the users, it is obvious that the IS developers do not question the functionality of the system either. In this case this means that the HCMU application was based on the original requirements and specifications of the earlier system, the only difference being the mobility of the new application. In short, the tablet-based application (HCMU) had access to the same data and had the same functions as the stationary system used at the office. The interface, i.e. the access to the functions, was naturally different as the platform was changed from a desktop computer to a tablet computer.

Home care nurses' work practice can be described as a flow of actions as depicted in Table 1. The description was created by the authors prior to the usability testing and it is based on the documents of use cases, requirements, and specifications and the "use" of the paper prototype of the application. The latter was rather intensive as it comprised of a heuristic evaluation of the application by two usability experts.

Table 1. The work practices of a home care nurse while deploying the old EHR system at the office and the new HCMU on the field

Work process (flow of actions)	Software functions		Use location	
	EHR system	HCMU	EHR	HCMU
Prepare today's home care visits	Print today's visit schedule from EHR to a paper	Browse 'daily tasks' –list if needed	office	field
Check the purpose of the next visit	View client's info in the paper schedule	View client's info field in the daily tasks list	office	field
Orientate to client's current health situation	View client's health record in EHR and handwrite significant remarks on the paper schedule	Browse client's earlier care entries	office	field
Travel and access client's home	Check access information from the paper schedule	View client's basic data	field	field
Perform care actions	View the paper schedule and handwrite plan realizations on the schedule	View the care plan and record plan realizations	field	field
Document the visit	Copy realization data from the paper schedule and record visit in the statistics	Record the visit in the statistics	office	field

The heuristic evaluation focused on the conformance of the user interface with solid UI design principles, the work flow of the application and how it supports the nurses in their work and takes patient safety into account. In the heuristic evaluation, 53 problems were observed, but they were not so severe that they would hinder the use of the application in the usability test without changes. However, heuristic evaluation provided a detailed understanding of the application functionality and designed work practices, which greatly helped in planning and carrying out the usability test.

In short, before a visit the home care nurse gets acquainted in the client's health situation and care plan, performs the care actions at the client's home, and documents the visit after it has been completed. Even though the old and the new applications have the same functions, the HCMU application changes the daily routines of the home care nurses. While using a tablet-based mobile application nurses can access updated EHR information during visits whenever needed whereas the desktop computer based application can be used only at the office before and after the daily visit round. This means that all the information needed during the day must be printed out in the morning, the documentation must be handwritten during the day, and in the end of the day copied into the system. With the HCMU application some of these actions can be omitted and some carried out at the client's home or field.

3.2   Usability Testing Procedure

The usability test took place in an early phase of the HCMU application development and a functioning prototype was not available; hence a paper prototype of the application was created for testing purposes. The aim of the test was to locate possible usability problems of the design solution and to gain knowledge of its suitability in home care nurses' work practices. Other prominent issues and stakeholders like security, dependability and effects on patients were consciously excluded from the test. The user interface of the paper prototype was as realistic and detailed as possible and over the 170 printed screens and buttons covered the main functions of the application. The paper prototype was used by pointing with fingers on the print outs of the screens and thus simulated well the real use of a tablet computer. In a sense, the paper prototype was a high-fidelity prototype even though it lacked all computer-based functionality.

Test sessions were carried out in a room that situated at the home care nurses' workplace. During the test, the subject was sitting at a table between two test leaders. The "screens" of the paper prototype were placed in front of the subject by one of the test leaders and the other test leader had a role of a facilitator. A small video camera was placed in front of the subject towards the table so that the use area of the prototype and the sounds were recorded. The recordings of the session were later transcribed for analysis purposes. The recording computer was placed so that the third test leader, a developer representative, was able to monitor the recording and follow the flow of events from the computer screen. The main role of the third test leader was to confirm that the "computer", i.e. the test leader reacting to subject's use maneuvers, performed according to the designed manner.

Four female home care nurses served as subjects. They had been working in municipal home care for 6-15 years as either nurses or attendants and were accustomed to the use of the office-based EHR-system in their daily work. None had used a tablet computer but all had used a touch screen mobile phone. Each individual test session started with a short presentation of the use of a tablet computer and lasted about two hours. The subjects were encouraged to think-out-loud during the application use and occasionally test sessions turned to longer discussions and informal interview about the details of work practices.

The aim of the usability test was to gain knowledge and understanding about the home care nurses' work practices and to evaluate the usability of the supporting HCMU application. The situation was, however, new for the subjects as they did not have any experience of a mobile application use in their field work, so they must improvise and try to apply the practices familiar from the old EHR. Under these circumstances we decided to use somewhat different approach than in conventional usability testing: instead of giving to the subjects product-feature focused, short and answerable test tasks one by one, they were given only one broad task to act on. The task was simple: *"Your name is N.N and you are going to the third scheduled home visit of the day. The name of the client is Y.Y. Perform your work and use this new HCMU application for support when needed."* This approach gave the subjects the autonomy to exhibit their own conceptualization of the work flow, i.e. they could decide what actions are carried out and in which order, what information is needed or must be written down.

It is obvious that while executing the broad task they would need to use different functions of the application and do several subtasks. This was anticipated by creating a set of conventional usability test tasks. These tasks were used as a hint in case users confronted a problem in their main task or halted for some reason. This way the test leader was able to return the session focus on some specific work situation or product function by suggesting one of the supporting tasks to be performed. If a supporting task was used, the participant was asked to validate its meaningfulness and correct placement within the current state of the main task performance. The approach was tested in a pilot test where a member of the development team served as the subject. The pilot test showed that the approach is feasible but rather laborious. It became also obvious that the presence of a developer representative in the test situation is necessary in order to guarantee a proper interpretation of the application functionalities and intended ways of use.

3.3   Results

The test results of the tests indicate that the activities in home care visits have become rather standardized and that significant work flow variations between the four subjects were not observed. In other words, the flow of actions presented in the first column of Table 1 is valid, although minor variations in the sequence between checking the visit purpose and access information were identified. Due to the broad test task approach, three participants were able to start their home care visit by looking for the purpose of the visit while one participant tried to search the home address of the client first. The reason for variation is that the data are visible simultaneously in the EHR but the HCMU application represents the data in separate but following views.

Already in the beginning of the first test session it became clear that there is a major flaw in the second column of Table 1: home care nurses do not base their daily activities on care plan but on a detailed list of tasks that is maintained by them, unofficially, in the EHR. The subjects could easily find from the HCMU who they should visit and where, but they had unexpected difficulties in finding the information about the purpose of the visit. In turn, the test team was puzzled why the participants were not carrying out the care plan and its scheduled activities for the visit that were easily found and recognized by the subjects. The following conversation illustrates the information needs and difficulties of the subjects:

— [Researcher] What information are you looking for?
— [Participant] Well, the purpose of the visit… that what you do in a visit.
— There you can see some information? [Researcher points the approved care plan in the screen]
— Yes, but that is too general information.

— Hmmm... What are you looking for if not this generic?
— Just the information for today. Those can be different care actions that you need to do today than written in the care plan...
— So it's not these actions that you need to perform in today's visit [Researcher points again the actions in the care plan]?
— That's right. These are broader issues [in the care plan], like "weight once a month"... how should I know if it should be done today or does every nurse weight that patient on every visit? I need just the information what should I do right now!

It was immediately apparent that the detailed, daily task information is the most critical piece of data for nurses to even start working. In the EHR system the daily task information is entered as free text, printed on paper, carried along trough the daily visits, and used in making notes for next visit. This way a nurse can inform other nurses about client's current health situation and list to-do care tasks for the near future. Nurses comprehend a client's health situation as these daily events, actions and separate to-do tasks and notes on the paper. Orientation to client's health situation occurs mainly through this daily information and not trough reading care plan or earlier entries of health records.

The field for the daily task information was actually present in the opening view of the HCMU paper prototype (see table 1 View client's info field in the task list), but the field was filled with dummy text (Lorem ipsum). This means that the designers knew about this field but did not know about its importance. In the session interviews, it was found that the practice of this daily task information usage is not something that has been designed into the EHR system but has evolved among the users. When users had noted that the care plans created and maintained in the EHR must be written on somewhat general level they began to use a field intended for additional information to make detailed notes on tasks that must be carried out on the next visit. Currently, three different fields in the EHR system are used to input daily task information, which can be printed along with the patient address information and taken with to the daily round. The HCMU paper prototype implemented only one of these fields.

The daily tasks list does not have, however, a direct relation to the accepted care plan with identified care needs, objectives and planned care activities. The overall health situation of a client is fragmented to a detailed visit task list, outdated care plan, unutilized care realization entries and evaluations. According to the subjects the information in the care plan as well as its realization (as entries of earlier care actions) are hardly read and exploited during the visits.

- "We don't necessarily read or very few read [earlier care actions]."
- " I have no time to read... if you have not seen the client for a long time then yes, then I check."
- "We don't browse them much unless you know that something special has happened"

The HCMU prototype had been designed in the faith that the care plan is the central means in managing the home care activities, as it actually should be according to legislation and local recommendations. In other words, every client must have a care plan and every performed care activity must be categorized for statistical purposes. Unfortunately, compilation of statistics is separated from the care plan into an own function. This way the care plan and its activities may become somewhat outdated as they are rarely updated. The general problem is that the care plan supports only static and permanent data instead of communicative data useful for daily visits. If nurses read the client's care plan, the current practice is to read them before the first visit of the day due to health record availability only at the office. The HCMU design may change this work practice as it allows browsing the care plan and its realization also during a visit. However, the subjects in the test sessions were not spontaneously exploiting these features.

HCMU emphasizes the care plan and its realization by bringing those into perception and manageable on every visit, which may result into more updated care plan information in the future. For example, home care workers are recommended to frequently evaluate the effectiveness of their care acts, but *"there are not enough resources to do evaluations and we don't do much that"*. The implementation into HCMU is, however, promising: *"[...] this seems very simple. I don't even remember how this was done with the current system...this is easy. You can do it right away [not at office]."*

The test approach with only one broad task turned out a success as the subjects were able to conceptualize their work with the new tool and bring forth their needs. It must be, however, kept in mind that one broad task might not bring forth all the needs of the users nor cover all the necessary functions. For this purpose conventional usability test tasks must be used during the test. For example, as the subjects did not spontaneously change clients' medicines a preplanned supportive task was used: *"A doctor called you and said that sleeping medicine Zopinox needs to put on a break. Do this entry."* This task was validated as meaningful and possible scenario by the subjects. The HCMU is designed to nurses and attendants instead of doctors and thus it supports only the documentation of instructions coming from a doctor, i.e. documentation of the delivery of medicine instead of prescription. However, the test participants were used to modify the list of medicines by themselves in the EHR and therefore searched for this possibility also in the HCMU prototype. Several different places for documenting a break in medicine delivery were observed. One would write the break information under the "dosing need" and other the "written instructions of medicines needed" of the care plan. The correct place for the entry is to add new care action and to select the medicine the break is applied to. After selecting the medicine two participants shared their concern and uncertainty about whether the change was derived to the list of medicines, which is followed on daily basis for dosing the clients (the care actions are not read during the visit as presented above). Possibility to misunderstand the effect is obvious. This poses a safety issue that needs to be solved by giving home care workers access to modify the list of medicines or confirm its changes made by the doctor.

4   Discussion

Conventional test tasks in usability testing require careful planning of task formulation and representation order. Special attention must be paid for what is to be "asked" as the answers will be limited by the question as is the case in normal structured interviews. Conventional test tasks as strict, narrow, and structured questions about users' low-level work tasks will provide answers to specific usability questions. Conventional structured tasks are relevant in testing usability of specific product features, functions, representations, terminology etc. of the design and allow adjusting the number of tasks so that they cover all the necessary product features.

The test approach with the open-ended task, however, provides different types of results than the conventional tasks. As our empirical results show the open-ended task allows the subjects to follow their natural work flow, to express their needs freely, and to change their course of action during a test session. For example, the non-uniformity of home care nurses performing two work tasks in different order was revealed by the open-ended task approach, which would not have happened if these tasks were presented as separate conventional test tasks. Most importantly, the open-ended task provided information about how nurses exploit home care plans in their current work practices. The designers' assumption that the care plan has a central role and is the principal source of information during the home care visits was clearly refuted by the subjects. Thanks to the subjects' freedom to integrate the care plan use into the work process the test showed that a low usage of the care plan is also an organizational issue to be solved and to some degree outside the power of the HCMU designers. It is also worthwhile to note that this state of affairs was not observed neither in the heuristic evaluation nor in the pilot test carried out before the usability test as they were both based on the implemented design solution.

Even though the open-ended task approach turned out to a success, due to its permissive nature it seems to require complementary conventional tasks in order to cover all the necessary product features that are planned to be tested. A broad coverage of user tasks implies also more usability problems found [36]. Therefore, to guarantee a good coverage of tasks and features of the product one should not forget to design also low-level tasks, and apply those when the open-ended task does not bring any new information about certain product features. Fig. 2 describes the relation between conventional, structured tasks and open-ended tasks against users' freedom to act and express their needs (i.e. test session's user-centeredness) and the amount of features included in the test (i.e. task coverage from the product point of view). The latter is dependent on the task design as the likelihood of the occurrence of a certain task diminishes when open-ended tasks are applied.

Some prerequisites and limitations for applying the open-ended task can be identified. To begin with, the approach requires a careful control of time during the test session as usually a test session has a limited time and a good feature coverage must be achieved. In our experience a top-down approach is favorable, i.e. the moderator begins with the open-ended task and allocates the end of the session for conventional

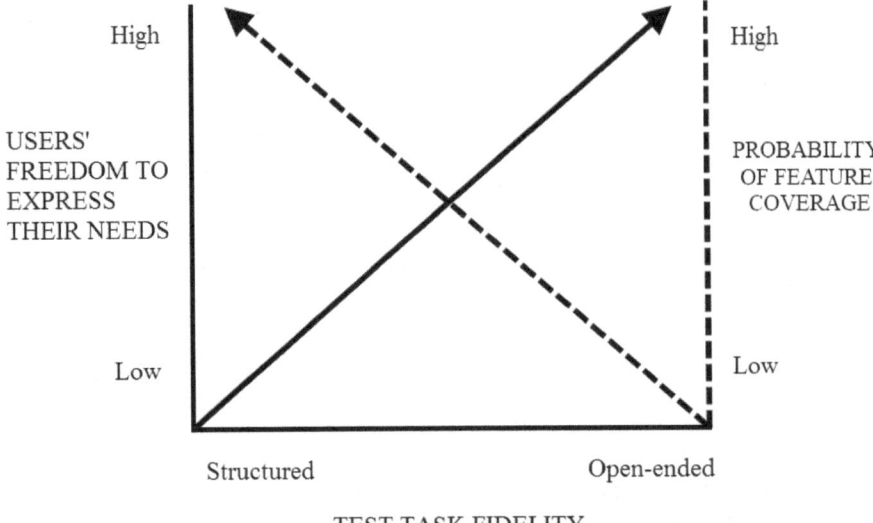

Fig. 2. Effect of test task fidelity on users' freedom to express their needs (arrow on the left) and feature inclusiveness (arrow on the right) during a test session

tasks in order to cover all the necessary features. Another and even a more important prerequisite for applying the open-ended task is good domain knowledge of the test moderator. Poor domain knowledge is a significant hindrance in any usability evaluation [6], but the role of domain knowledge is emphasized with the open-ended approach. That is due to the constant need of the moderator to interpret and react to subjects' unexpected courses of action. With the conventional tasks the moderator can concentrate on how the subjects perform the predefined tasks, and even rehearse and simulate a possible performance beforehand, while with the open-ended task the moderator must acknowledge on-the-fly what the subjects do and why. In this regard the moderator needs similar skills and plans with the open-ended task approach as with any unstructured interview.

A limitation in the open-ended task approach is that it does not necessarily provide data that is comparable, because the subjects are allowed to take actions of their own and thus may perform different set of tasks. That is, however, a minor limitation in a formative and qualitative usability testing, which does not pursue results based on statistical analysis. In our experience the advantages of revealing situated work practices and eliciting new requirements override the downside of incomparableness. Lastly, the approach is beneficial only if the subjects know what they need to accomplish without a moderator giving them an exact task. Therefore, the approach fits well to situations and contexts in which there are definable goals, which is not always the case, for example, with all web pages. One possible solution for testing such products is to co-construct the open-ended task together with the participant in a short interview session and concurrently examine the participant's eligibility to act as a subject in the test. The authors have successfully applied the co-construction approach in another evaluation case.

Our study contributes to the discussion of the importance of tasks in usability testing, i.e. how testing simultaneously fulfills its objective as a method for uncovering new user needs and validating the produced design solutions. The approach certainly needs further validation in different use contexts and with different applications. We acknowledge also that even though our paper prototypes and low fidelity task structures used in this case helped to capture some fundamental misinterpretations of the user requirements in the design process, the fidelity of the prototype itself may have had effect on the type of results achieved. A low-fidelity prototype typically makes users to comment more about work practices and outputs of the tasks whereas with high-fidelity prototype users comment more about ease of use and usefulness of the product [39], [40]. On the other hand, it has been found that a high fidelity prototype provides richer and more useful information for design due to greater number of needs expressed by the users [41].

The main point in this paper is, however, to emphasize the existing links between context of use, user requirements and evaluation premises. Even though usability and product development standards emphasize the evaluation of early prototypes as a means to define the requirements for the product we claim that practical evaluation methods, especially the widely applied usability testing, have not evolved towards this direction. Rather, there has been a tendency to develop usability testing to a method that is more easily conducted, cheaper and therefore even remote, asynchronous and unmoderated by using test settings through different automated web services. The open-ended task approach is a step towards the realization of the HCI standards that maintain user-centeredness along the whole product development life cycle. It can be characterized as a top-down approach, which begins to test our own understanding about the context of use, our abstractions of work and users and the specified requirements for the product, and finally proceeds to a more conventional bottom-level tasks that sufficiently cover the product features and also uncover potential usability problems.

Acknowledgements. The corresponding author would like to thank The Foundation for Economic Education for the grant number 31209.

References

1. Dumas, J., Saparova, D.: The First Seven Years of the JUS. Journal of Usability Studies 8, 1–10 (2012)
2. Vredenburg, K., Mao, J.-Y., Smith, P.W., Carey, T.: A Survey of User-Centered Design Practice. In: CHI 2002, pp. 471–478. ACM (2002)
3. Barnum, C.M.: Usability testing essentials: ready, set...test!. Morgan Kaufmann, Burlington (2011)
4. Dumas, J., Redish, J.: A practical guide to usability testing, revised edn. Intellect Ltd., Exeter (1999)

5. Curtis, B., Krasner, H., Iscoe, N.: A field study of the software design process for large systems. Communications of the ACM 31, 1268–1287 (1988)
6. Chilana, P.K., Wobbrock, J.O., Ko, A.J.: Understanding usability practices in complex domains. In: Proceedings of the 28th International Conference on Human Factors in Computing Systems CHI 2010, pp. 2337–2346. ACM, New York (2010)
7. Robertson, S., Robertson, J.: Mastering the Requirements Process. ACM Press (1999)
8. Jarke, M., Loucopoulos, P., Lyytinen, K., Mylopoulos, J., Robinson, W.: The brave new world of design requirements. Information Systems 36, 992–1008 (2011)
9. Redish, J.: Expanding Usability Testing to Evaluate Complex Systems. Journal of Usability Studies 2, 102–111 (2007)
10. Cordes, R.E.: Task-Selection Bias: A Case for User Defined Tasks. Int. J. of Human Computer Interaction 13(4), 411–419 (2001)
11. Diaper, D.: Scenarios and task analysis. Interacting with Computers 14, 379–395 (2002)
12. International Organization for Standardization: ISO 9241-11:1998 Guidance on usability (1998), http://www.iso.org
13. Ferré, X., Juristo, N., Windl, H., Constantine, L.: Usability Basics for Software Developers. IEEE Software 18, 22–29 (2001)
14. International Organization for Standardization: ISO 9241-210:2010 Human-centred design for interactive system (2010), http://www.iso.org
15. Abras, C., Maloney-Krichmar, D., Preece, J.: User-centered design. In: Bainbridge, W. (ed.) Encyclopedia of Human-Computer Interaction. Sage Publications, Thousand Oaks (2004)
16. Beyer, H., Holtzblatt, K.: Contextual design: defining customer-centered systems. Morgan Kaufmann, San Francisco (1998)
17. Preece, J., Rogers, Y., Sharp, H.: Interaction design: Beyond human-computer interaction. John Wiley & Sons Inc., New York (2002)
18. Diaper, D., Stanton, N.A.: The Handbook of Task Analysis for Human-Computer Interaction. Lawrence Erlbaum Associates Inc. Publishers, Mahwah (2004)
19. Rosson, M.B., Carroll, J.M.: Usability engineering: scenario-based development of human-computer interaction. Academic Press, San Diego (2002)
20. Beyer, H., Holtzblatt, K., Baker, L.: An Agile Customer-Centered Method: Rapid Contextual Design. In: Zannier, C., Erdogmus, H., Lindstrom, L. (eds.) XP/Agile Universe 2004. LNCS, vol. 3134, pp. 50–59. Springer, Heidelberg (2004)
21. Cooper, A.: The inmates are running the asylum: Why high-tech products drive us crazy and how to restore the sanity. SAMS, Indianapolis (1999)
22. Bødker, S.: Scenarios in user-centred design—setting the stage for reflection and action. Interacting with Computers 13, 61–75 (2000)
23. International Organization for Standardization.: ISO 13407:1999 Human-centred design processes for interactive systems (1999), http://www.iso.org
24. Suchman, L.: Plans and situated actions: the problem of human-machine interaction. Cambridge University Press, New York (1987)
25. Wagner, E.L., Scott, S.V., Galliers, R.D.: The creation of 'best practice' software: myth, reality and ethics. Information and Organization 16, 251–275 (2006)
26. Gasser, L.: The integration of computing and routine work. ACM Transactions on Office Information Systems 3, 205–225 (1986)
27. Ciborra, C.U.: From control to drift: the dynamics of corporate information infrastructures. Oxford University Press, UK (2000)

28. Tarkkanen, K.: Business process modeling for non-uniform work. In: Filipe, J., Cordeiro, J. (eds.) Enterprise Information Systems. LNBIP, vol. 19, pp. 188–200. Springer, Heidelberg (2009)

29. Rubin, J., Chisnell, D.: Handbook of usability testing: How to plan, design and conduct effective tests, 2nd edn. Wiley Publishing Inc., Indianapolis (2008)

30. Wilson, C.: Taking usability practitioners to task. Interactions 14, 48–49 (2007)

31. Kuniavsky, M.: Observing the user experience: a practioner's guide to user research. Morgan Kaufmann, San Francisco (2003)

32. van Waes, L.: Thinking Aloud as a Method for Testing the Usability of Websites: The Influence of Task Variation on the Evaluation of Hypertext. IEEE Transactions on Professional Communication 43, 279–291 (2000)

33. van den Haak, M.J., de Jong, M.D.T., Schellens, P.J.: Evaluating Municipal Websites: A Methodological Comparison of Three Think Aloud Variants. Government Information Quarterly 26, 193–202 (2009)

34. Albers, M.J.: Design and Usability: Beginner Interactions with Complex Software. Journal of Technical Writing and Communication 41, 271–287 (2011)

35. Mirel, B.: Dynamic usability: designing usefulness into systems for complex tasks. In: Albers, M.J., Mazur, B. (eds.) Content and complexity: Information Design in Technical Communication, Lawrence Erlbaum Associates, Mahwah (2003)

36. Lindgaard, G., Chattratichart, J.: Usability testing: What have we overlooked? In: Proceedings of CHI 2007, pp. 1415–1424. ACM Press (2008)

37. Molich, R., Dumas, J.S.: Comparative usability evaluation (CUE-4). Behaviour & Information Technology 27, 263–281 (2008)

38. Alshamari, M., Mayhew, P.: Task design: Its impact on usability testing. In: The Third International Conference on Internet and Web Applications and Services, pp. 583–589. IEEE Press (2008)

39. Atladottir, G., Hvannberg, E.T., Gunnarsdottir, S.: Comparing task practicing and prototype fidelities when applying scenario acting to elicit requirements. Requirements Engineering 17, 157–170 (2011)

40. Lindgaard, G., Dillon, R., Trbovich, P., White, R., Fernandes, G., Lundahl, S., Pinnamaneni, A.: User Needs Analysis and Requirements Engineering: Theory and Practice. Int. Comp. 18, 47–70 (2006)

41. Anastassova, M., Mégard, C., Burkhardt, J.-M.: Prototype evaluation and user-needs analysis in the early design of emerging technologies. In: Jacko, J.A. (ed.) HCI 2007. LNCS, vol. 4550, pp. 383–392. Springer, Heidelberg (2007)

Comparing the Levels of Frustration between an Eye-Tracker and a Mouse: A Pilot Study

Hildegardo Noronha, Ricardo Sol, and Athanasios Vourvopoulos

Madeira Interactive Technologies Institute,
University of Madeira 9000-390 Madeira, Portugal
hildegardo.noronha@m-iti.org, rsol@alummni.carnegiemellon.edu,
athanasios.vourvopoulos@m-iti.org
http://m-iti.org

Abstract. This paper tries to identify increases in user frustration when using Eye-Tracking devices as compared to common interfacing devices like a standard mouse. For this, we used an electroencephalograph (EEG) to measure frustration levels while users navigated within a maze using each of the referred devices. Results from the analysis performed on the EEG data indicate that Eye-tracking has the same amount of frustration as a standard mouse for common mouse tracking tasks. In addition, a correlation between the users reported frustration and the extracted EEG data could not be found rendering the above result virtually invalid. The users' self-reported frustration lends support to our hypothesis but it still is not statistically significant and hence does not confirm the hypothesis.

Keywords: Human Computer Interaction, Natural User Interfaces, Eye-Tracker, Mouse, Electroencephalography.

1 Introduction

Computer interface devices are continuously improving towards a more natural user interaction. Natural User Interfaces (NUI) unlike the traditional devices like keyboard and mouse do not require training and familiarization. Devices like Microsoft Kinect (Microsoft Co.) and Nintendo Wii (Nintendo Co., Ltd.) are examples of this transition into a more compelling experience without the use of any mediatory device that users have to learn to use and operate. Going a step further, eye-tracking interfaces using eye position and eye movement for pointing and selecting can act as Natural User Interfaces. Using an eye-tracker as a pointing device is a self-evident way of using eye-gaze as input in a computerized device. Studies conducted over the past three decades have shown that the performance of the eye-tracking devices has steadily improved in the recent years [1]. A major improvement in video-based eye-trackers systems is the range of freedom given to the users head movements. Since these systems are essentially composed of video cameras and software, a substantial decrease in price is soon to be expected. Thus these systems can potentially become part of future computers without major additional costs.

A. Holzinger et al. (Eds.): SouthCHI 2013, LNCS 7946, pp. 107–121, 2013.

Nevertheless current eye-tracking technology still fails to achieve fulfilling interaction with targets of recent applications or websites.

The lack of overall performance might translate into frustration from the user's point of view. This frustration can be quantified for further analysis and performance assessment. Relating these two quantities (low performance triggering high frustration) a tool can be built for assessing future interactive systems that require speed and precision (intrinsic to user interfaces). Understanding the levels of frustration that the users are exposed to can also give us an indication of the potential success of such devices.

The evaluation of such a system can capture the effects on the user experience, quantitatively and qualitatively, by collecting extensive synchronized brain activity and behavioral data on users performance during the testing process. Additionally, such a system can provide us with extremely valuable data that can be used to propose a generalization of it for future systems that can eventually be used by all users, either for entertainment, education or general use.

Technological advances with the synchronization of eye tracking gaze data and electrophysiological data like electroencephalographic (EEG) signals can be combined for scientific research purposes, market research, and a wide range of other application areas. EEG is already a multi-purpose scientific tool used for diseases diagnosis, biofeedback, medical applications and general scientific research. This technology and the data captured from it, can leverage the knowledge of where the users attention is focused (through the eyes) when an event is taking place.

The hypothesis, H1, that we try to verify, is that user frustration is higher when using eye-tracking as the input device instead of a standard mouse for common mouse tracking tasks.

Our research reported in this paper uses a questionnaire and electroencephalographic (EEG) data to analyze the levels of frustration in a sample of 10 users while they try to navigate through several labyrinths with a cursor controlled by eye-gaze or mouse system.

2   Background and State of the Art

Each area of the human brain is responsible for different functions including problem solving, emotion, complex thought, movement, visual stimuli and auditory information [2]. Through the use of electroencephalography (EEG), there are different wave patterns or rhythms that are distinguished and associated to different cognitive or motor actions [3]. This kind of knowledge has been used with Brain-Computer Interfaces (BCIs) based on the pattern recognition approaches for communication and control of computers [4] ranging from Brain-controlled robots, modern computer games [5], prosthetics, control systems [6] through to medical diagnostics. The mental tasks are chosen in such a way that they activate different parts of the brain. In the last few years commercial low cost EEG equipment has been introduced as an alternative game controller by various companies such as Emotiv [7], setting a milestone in user experience with brain-controlled computer games and virtual worlds [5].

Recent evaluations of the detection accuracy of such devices indicate an acceptable level of accuracy for performing mental actions [8] although for the Emotivs Affectiv Suite that is used also for this experiment, similar tests suggest that further examination is needed to verify Emotivs' ability to accurately track cognitive state [9].

The merge of eye-tracking technology with EEG has only been implemented quite recently with the SMI RED-m eye tracker (SensoMotoric Instruments Co.) and the Emotiv EEG Neuro-headset for market research purposes [10]. This online analysis of emotional responses can give an insight into consumers subconscious behavior by merging visual perception and brain response introducing a new type of marketing, neuromarketing [11].

In 2005, Ashmore, Duchowsky and Shoemaker specified and defined four reasons why eye pointing has more problems than manual pointing [13]. The four reasons are: Eye tracker accuracy, Sensor lag, Fixation jitter, and Midas touch.

Eye tracker accuracy depends on the visual angle. The visual angle is associated with the reflection of the eye and not the actual position of the eyes when facing the screen that should be around 90o. In less recent literature, it is possible to find references to visual angles of 3o, however a visual angle around 0.5-1o is commonly accepted. This means that when looking at our 23" computer monitor with a resolution display of 1980x1080 at a viewing distance of 65 cm, the eye pointing will be limited in accuracy to around 22-44 pixels.

Sensor lag is a delay in processing the gaze position. In our system this delay is typical 0.005 seconds (200 Hz frame rates).

Fixation jitter occurs with the dwell time (or fixation time, i.e. time spent selecting through fixation) associated with eye pointing. Three types of these involuntary eye movements (microsaccades) disturb fixation: flicks, drifts, and tremors. The biggest of these movements has a visual angle that is less than 1o.

Midas touch is a problem defined by Jacob in 1991 that occurs because the eyes are always active making the selection task indistinct from the search task [14].

Researchers worldwide have been dealing with the above problems and trying to find ways to improve the interaction.

Mouse and Gaze Input Cascaded (MAGIC) that uses gaze to dynamically redefine the position of the cursor is one of those improvements [15]. In MAGIC after the eye redefines the cursor position the user will makes a small manual input action to select the target. MAGIC has two approaches. In the first approach, referred to as the liberal approach, the cursor moves to the top of the new target that the user looks at. The second approach, the conservative approach that, leaves the cursor at the boundaries of the target.

Salvucci and Anderson presented their intelligent gaze-added interfaces [16]. They addressed accuracy problems that we also face. In their work any target positioned where the users' eye gaze is, is a highlighted target. Then a gaze key gives the user the chance to trigger the action. The system uses a probabilistic algorithm to guess the targets the user is going to look at.

McGuffin and Balakrishnan showed that expanding targets facilitates the pointing task [17]. Their results show that working with expanding targets can be accurately modeled by Fitts' law. They have also shown that targets that expand just as the user is about to reach them can be acquired approximately as fast as targets that are always in an expanded state. They specifically found strong evidence that user performance is consistently aided by target expansion. Miniotas and Spakov used an expansion of targets visible to the users [18]. To facilitate pointing they used dynamic target expansion for fixing the calibration of the eye tracker, basing the correction on the relative change in the gaze position after the expansion.

Ashmore and Duchowsky refined a fisheye lens to support eye pointing [13]. They hid the lens during visual search and obtained improvements in speed and accuracy. Fisheye interaction was evaluated by Fitts pointing and, a visual search. In contrast to MAGIC pointing, where the cursor was quickly moved to the vicinity of one's gaze prior to mouse movement, they directly slaved the lens to the gaze position.

EyePoint used expansions of interactive targets, and used a key for input [19]. When the key is pressed the gaze area is enlarged. When the key is released the selections are made according to where the eye gaze is.

All of the above mentioned work reflect the idea that simple eye gaze interaction is not promising [15]. Quantifying this dissatisfaction by looking into frustrations levels is the goal of this work.

3   Materials and Methods

3.1   Hardware

EEG headset. The Emotiv EPOC Headset is a neuro-signal acquisition and processing wireless neuro-headset with 14 wet (using a common contact lens liquid) sensors and 2 reference sensors being able to detect brain signals and facial expressions. An integrated gyroscope generates positional information, connected wirelessly through a USB dongle and comes with a lithium battery providing 12 hours of continuous use [7]. Detailed specifications are illustrated in Table 1. The sixteen (14 plus 2 reference) sensors are placed on the international 10-20 system [11], an internationally recognized method which describes the electrode placement on the scalp for EEG tests or experiments.

Eye-Tracker. The Tobii TX300 is an eye tracker that uses infrared diodes to illuminate the users eye [20]. The back part of the eye called fovea, reflects when illuminated, and this refection is then collected by the image sensor. Using this reflection, the eye tracker uses complex image processing to determine where in screen is the user looking. Detailed specifications are illustrated in Table 2.

Table 1. Headset specification

Characteristic	Definition
Number of channels	14 (plus CMS/DRL references)
Channel name (10-20 locations)	AF3/4, F3/4/7/8, FC5/6, P3/4/7/8, T7/8, O1/2
Sampling method	Sequential sampling, Single ADC
Sampling rate	~128Hz (2048Hz internal)
Resolution	16 bits (14 bits effective) 1 LSB = 0.51 μV
Bandwidth	0.2 - 45Hz, d. notch filters at 50Hz and 60Hz
Dynamic range (input referred)	$256mV_{pp}$

Table 2. Eye-Tracker specification

Characteristic	Definition
Sampling rate (binocular/variability)	300 Hz / 0.3%
Latency	$\leq 10ms$
Freedom of head mov. (65 cm) (w x h)	37 x 17 cm (15 x 7)
Max gaze angle	35○
Screen size	23$^{"}$ TFT
Screen resolution (Max)	1920 x 1080 pixel
Bandwidth	0.2 - 45Hz, d. notch f. at 50Hz and 60Hz
Response time	~5ms

3.2 Software

EEG Headset. For acquiring the frustration levels, we used the Emotiv SDK. Emotiv uses a black box algorithm for the detection of cognitive characteristics in a suite called Affectiv.

The Affectiv Suite reports real time changes in the subjective emotions experienced by the user. Emotiv currently offers three distinct Affectiv detections: Engagement, Instantaneous Excitement, and Long-Term Excitement.

The Affectiv detections look for brainwave characteristics that are universal in nature and dont require an explicit training or signature-building step on the part of the user.

Eye-Tracker. The Tobii TX300 comes with several software programs. One of them is worth mentioning, the Tobii Software Development Kit that enables the development of software to control the eye tracker.

Custom Made Software. Since no current software was adequate for our research we developed our own custom software. It is composed of four main components: The Emotiv EEG interaction, the Tobbi Eye-Tracker interaction, the test and a log.

Both the Emotiv and Tobbi interaction components use their respective and commercially available SDK as a base to communicate with the hardware. The logging component logs the data enumerated on the section D-Data Description that is gathered from the EEG and the input method (either the mouse or the Eye-Tracker). Finally, the test component is responsible for merging all the components, drawing the mazes and the user interfaces and implementing all the test logic. Fig. 1 shows the visualization created by the software. It corresponds to the last maze of the least thickness. It illustrates an example of what the user has to traverse during the test.

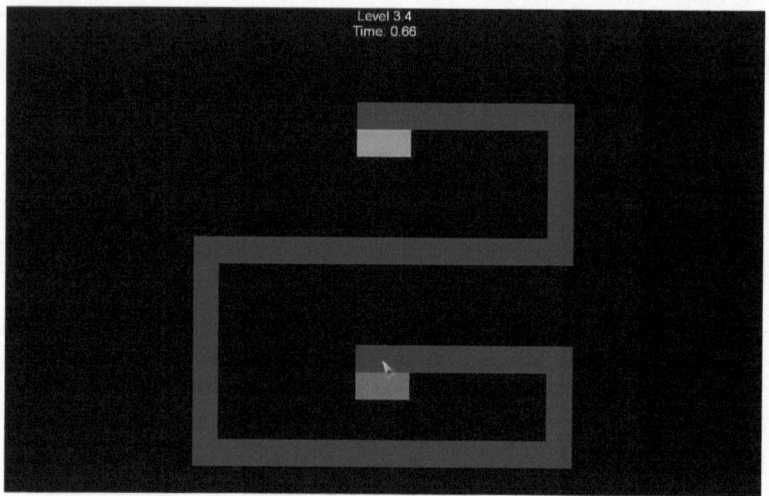

Fig. 1. Example of a maze presented to the user

3.3 Experimental Procedure

The tests are composed of a sequence of simple mazes in which the user navigates from the starting point to the end within the maze borders. If the user moves outside this area, the cursor position is reset back to the starting point. The mazes vary in thickness and in complexity (amount of curves/length of the maze). Every user navigates through a fixed number of different levels of varying thickness and increasing complexity. The first level of thickness is for training purposes. The participant using the eye-tracker, even with poor calibration, can easily control it. The second level is of a comfortable thickness that the user can easily navigate but where he/she has to exercise carein order not to move outside the maze limits. The last thickness is purposely thin to a degree that the failure rate increases significantly, again, with the eye-tracker (some users were not even able to complete a single maze on this difficulty) in the hope of noticing an effect in the frustration levels between the devices. Still, it is easily traversed with a mouse, making the test less artificial. Since there is repetition the user can always come back to the mouse version to compare his performance with the eye tracker.

The users have to complete the whole set four mazes times the tree thickness once for each condition (mouse Vs eye tracker) and repeat it three times. The first condition is selected randomly and from then on the user alternates between conditions.

For every maze, if a user fails 5 times in a row he/she is be sent to the next maze. This number was chosen as a compromise between getting enough data and not taking too long to get it, and to avoid user fatigue.

3.4   Data Description

The raw data was automatically logged by custom-made software that was used for the user tests. The data was split in two files both using a standard comma-separated-values (csv) format. The first file logs the onscreen cursor position along with frustration and engagement levels, sampled every frame. The second file is an event log that logs data when special events happen. The events are Level Mouse and Level Eye, indicating the start of a level for mouse and eye respectively, Failed, indicating that the user moved the cursor outside the maze area, GaveUp, indicating that the user failed too many times and the experiment had just advanced, and finally, Complete, indicating that the user reached his/her goal.

The first file logs the following:

Timestamp in milliseconds, starting from the system initialization;
Cursor Position (either by using the mouse or by using the eye-tracker), in pixels;
Frustration Levels values between 0 and 1;
Engagement Levels values between 0 and 1;

The second file logs the following:

Timestamp in milliseconds, starting from the system initialization;
Type of Event string (single or double word) describing the event;
Event Data string with extra data when needed, 0 if not.

3.5   Conditions

The test is very sensitive to the mental state of the user and external stimulation. This makes this experiment difficult to condition and control. The room where the hardware was located was not dedicated exclusively for the experiment. However, the participants did not face any interruption or disturbance during the tests.

3.6   The Questionnaire

A modified version of the NASA TLX questionnaire was used for the users to fill up after completing the assessment. NASA-TLX is a workload assessment tool with six sub-scales including Mental Demands, Physical Demands, Temporal Demands, Own Performance, Effort and Frustration [12]. This is used to corroborate the accuracy of the headsets frustration data. The whole questionnaire set was used, even if some questions did not seem relevant to the experiment, since some of the standard analyses require the whole data set.

In Fig. 8 and Fig. 9 it is possible to analyze the questionnaire answers.

3.7   Sample

Since we chose Convenience Sampling as our sampling method, users were selected from friends and colleagues, as they were easily accessible to the researchers.

The experiment was performed with 10 participants, 5 males and 5 females, with normal or corrected-to-normal vision. The participants were between 20 and 33 years old. All participants were regular computer and mouse users.

3.8   Statistical Analysis

Central Tendency and Dispersion. There are two input devices (Mouse and Eye-tracker), each one representing a condition and also two data sets that represent the same variable (the EEG data and the questionnaire answers).

Fig. 2 and Fig. 3 demonstrates a large overlapping of the frustration results. This overlap is bigger for the EEG than it is for the Questionnaire.

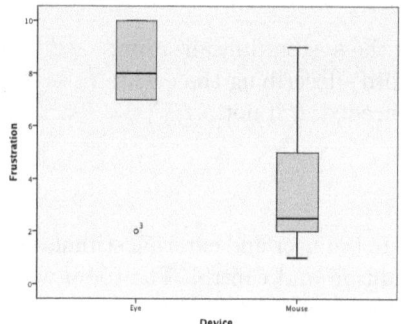

Fig. 2. Whiskers plots Questionnaire

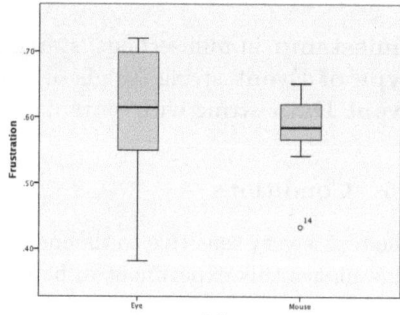

Fig. 3. Whiskers plots for the EEG

Data Normality. Before deciding which statistical test is appropriate for testing the hypothesis of this project, it is important to check the normality of the acquired data as a necessary statistical procedure to avoid incorrect usage of tests that require normality. The distribution of the data will help us choose between parametric or non-parametric tests.

We did several tests, including Histograms (Fig. 4 and Fig. 5), QQ-Plots and several quantitative tests. These tests indicate Normality, but this was not confirmable with the current sample size.

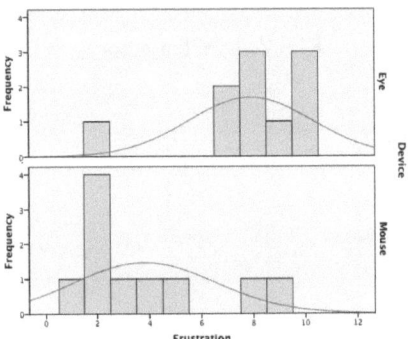

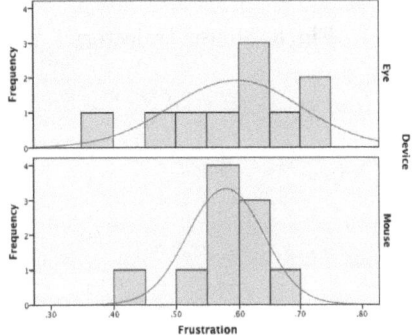

Fig. 4. Histograms and Normality curve for the Questionnaire

Fig. 5. Histograms and Normality curve for the EEG

4   Results

4.1   Central Tendency and Dispersion

For the EEG Headset, the range of the ratio data is from 0.0 to 1.0. The Eye has a Mean of 0.5965, a Median of 0.6149 and a Standard Deviation of 0.10461 and the Mouse has a Mean of 0.5790, a Median of 0.5850 and a Standard Deviation of 0.06003.

The Interquartile Range is 0.34 for the Eye-Tracker and 0.06 for the Mouse. This indicates a fairly larger variability in the Eye-Tracker data than in the Mouse data. Also, this value of 0.34 represents a third of the whole range, suggesting that the data might not be very good.

For the Questionnaire, the data range is from 1 to 10, ordinal. The Eye has a Median of 8 and a Standard Deviation of 2.378 and the Mouse has a Median of 2.5 and a Standard Deviation of 2.741.

The Interquartile Range is 3 for the Eye-Tracker and 4 for the Mouse. This represents from 33% to 44% of the data range, making it an even worse data than that of the EEG.

Fig. 6 and Fig. 7 show the result of the visualization of the cursor trajectory when users navigated through the maze. One can notice higher loss of intended

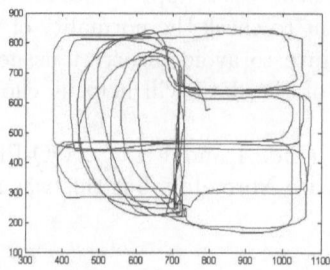

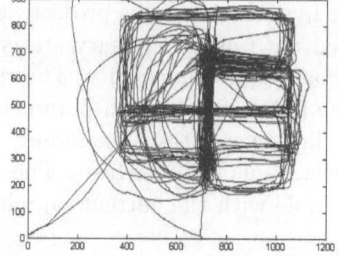

Fig. 6. Mouse Trajectory   **Fig. 7.** Eye Trajectory

Participant No.	Gender	Mental Demand	Physical Demand	Temporal Demand	Performance	Effort	Frustration
1	M	3	1	7	2	3	2
2	M	2	1	1	2	2	2
3	M	3	2	3	9	3	9
4	F	3	1	1	1	1	1
5	F	4	6	5	8	7	8
6	F	3	3	4	3	4	2
7	F	2	2	3	7	3	3
8	F	5	5	5	5	5	5
9	M	3	4	6	2	4	4
10	M	2	2	2	2	2	2

Fig. 8. Mouse questionnaire results

Participant No.	Gender	Mental Demand	Physical Demand	Temporal Demand	Performance	Effort	Frustration
1	M	9	1	8	5	9	8
2	M	8	1	9	6	8	9
3	M	8	6	4	3	5	2
4	F	3	1	6	3	10	10
5	F	5	5	5	8	6	7
6	F	7	8	6	10	8	8
7	F	7	3	5	3	8	8
8	F	10	7	6	8	5	7
9	M	1	10	7	9	8	10
10	M	6	9	9	9	9	10

Fig. 9. Eye-gaze questionnaire results

control while using an Eye-Tracker as compared to a Mouse for normal pointing tasks. The eye-gaze control (Fig. 7) is less accurate.

The tables in Fig. 8 and Fig. 9 show the questionnaire results for the Mouse and the Eye respectively.

Table 3 and Table 4 show the EEG log results for events an data respectively, it demonstrates what happens when a user fails 5 times in a row: it is considered a give up and the user goes on to the next maze.

Table 3. Event Log

Time	X Y	Frustration Engagement
121249441	801 578	0.584 0.879

Table 4. Data Log

Time	Type Data
12149424	Level Mouse 1
12196613	Level Eye 1
12221551	Failed 0
12226329	Failed 0
12232051	Failed 0
12233392	Failed 0
12238636	GaveUp 0

4.2   Effect: EEG

Wilcoxon Signed Ranks Test. The data was found not to have a normal distribution. Due to this, a non- parametric test had to be used to verify our hypothesis. The experiment was within-subjects with two conditions (Mouse and Eye- Tracker). For these reasons, a Wilcoxon Signed Ranks test was conducted. The results of the test follow:

We can infer that, from the 10 users that participated in the experiment, 4 found the Mouse more frustrating to use as compared to the Eye-Tracker, while the other 6 users felt the other way around.

The T value is 22 with a $\rho = 0.575$, higher than the standard $\rho \leq 0.05$. The $T_{critical}$ for a two-tail test with $\alpha = 0.05$ is 8. Hence $22 \geq 8$ then $T \geq T_{critical}$. We can now conclude that we should keep the null hypothesis H0 - Eye-tracking has the same amount of frustration as a standard mouse for common mouse tracking tasks.

The Power. There is a chance that we are making a Type II error, especially due to the small sample size. In order to address this, we did a test of power to check the probability of such error. We found a power of 0.8000817, indicating a high probability of mistakenly not finding an effect that was there. Another interesting value is the amount of tests we would need to perform in order to see an effect. This value is 380 tests.

4.3   Effect: Questionnaire

Wilcoxon Signed Ranks Test. To check the accuracy of the EEG headset data, we provided a questionnaire at the end of the tests for the users to indicate their frustration for each of the conditions (Mouse and Eye-Tracker). We then checked the correlation between the two.

4.4   EEG: Questionnaire Correlation

We first did a Spearmans ρ test to obtain the correlation coefficient. We got a result of ρ = -0.131. The $\rho_{critical}$ is 0.45 for Spearmans ρ test with α = 0.05, for N = 20. Since $|$-0.131$| \leq$ 0.45, $\rho \leq \rho_{critical}$ and so the correlation is not significant.

To complement this result we plotted the linear regression plot (Fig. 10). While we expected a linear relationship close to y = x , we got an almost horizontal line.

Looking into those results, we conclude that there is no evidence of correlation.

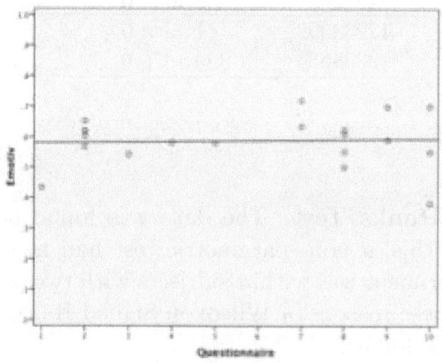

Fig. 10. Linear regression between the Questionnaire and the EEGs Frustration

5   Discussion and Conclusion

5.1   Main Hypothesis Rejection

According to the EEG data, 4 out of 10 users had higher frustration levels using the Mouse whole the remaining 6 users had higher frustration levels with the Eye-Tracker and not the Mouse. The performed Wilcoxon T showed a value of T = 22, with a ρ = 0.575 resulting in a non-significant result. Also, the T value is higher than the $T_{critical}$ = 8. The sum of ranks for a less frustrating Eye-Tracker is 33 and 22 for the Mouse. However, a Type II error could be present. To investigate this, we tested the power of the test. A value of 0.8 was found, indicating a high probability of an undetected effect.

As there is no clear relation between the users reported frustration levels and the frustration levels registered by the EEGs, we did a statistical analysis of the questionnaire results.

We then found a T value is of 8.5 with a ρ = 0.52, which is still higher than the standard $\rho \leq$ 0.05. The $T_{critical}$ for a two-tail test with α = 0.05 is 8. This time 8.5 $\geq$ 8 so T $\geq T_{critical}$. This value is close to the critical value but the significance is still low.

Taking this subsequent statistical analysis into account, we now arrive at a different result from the one we got with the EEG. These subsequent results suggest that 8 users felt more frustrated using the Eye-Tracker as compared to using the Mouse, while the other 2 users felt the other way around. One of the users has extreme values (very frustrated using the mouse and very not frustrated using the Eye-tracker) going against both the expected results and the gathered results. Another result that is not consistent with the expected results is from a user that answered very closely for both devices (7 for Eye-Tracker, 8 for the Mouse).

The lack of agreement in the data may be a due to a combination of two technical issues:

First, the users tended to use the scale relatively, gathering around one of the extremes of the scale: they feel they are either very frustrated or not at all. On the other hand, EEG headsets measures absolute frustration;

Second, the EEG Headset may not be accurate or sensitive enough to output good enough data for scientific usage.

The amount of noise that is generated during the task performance on the headset electrodes can lead to false classification of the frustration, as it is output from the Emotiv algorithm. In addition, the sense of frustration is subjective.

The lack of agreement in the data can also be due to the small sample size or the conditions of the environment under which the experiment was conducted. Another explanation could be that the EEGs algorithm cannot really extract true frustration.

5.2   Conclusion

The data from our experiment was not found to be normally distributed, although it shows some tendency towards normality. Yet, given the small sample, we treated the data as not normal and performed non-parametric tests. We performed a Wilcoxon Signed Ranks test on the frustration data which led us to conclude that we cannot reject the null hypothesis - H0 - Eye-tracking has the same amount of frustration as a standard mouse for common mouse tracking tasks.

Since we suspected that the EEG data might not be accurate, supported by the strong effect power, we ran a questionnaire to gauge how frustrated the user felt while using each of the devices and then compared this data with the EEGs. A correlation was not found, suggesting that the EEG might not be accurate or that the users might be answering incorrectly.

We then further analyzed the questionnaire results and found out that there was a bigger effect, even if it was still not statistically significant.

Thus, we draw two conclusions:

First, the frustration data from the EEGs might be inaccurate - further research is required to prove or refute this.

Second, no effect was found but both the power of the frustration data from the EEGs as well as the data from the questionnaire seem to indicate a possible missed effect.

5.3 Future Work

A better frustration measurement method should be found. After a sufficiently reliable method is found, a bigger sample should be acquired to gather enough information for a significant result to be achieved. Future work can also compare different kinds of input devices in order to arrive at a more complete understanding of users frustration levels with these devices.

Acknowledgments. We would like to thank our friends and colleagues that were kind enough to serve as users in our experiment. We would like to thank Professors Mónica Cameirão and Mon-Chu Chen, for giving us valuable comments.

References

1. Zuchowski, A.: Eye Tracking Methodology: Theory and Practice. Springer, Berlin (2003)
2. Carew, T.J.: Behavioral Neurobiology: The Cellular Organization of Natural Behavior. Sinauer Associates Inc. (2004)
3. Gevins, A., Zeitlin, G., Yingling, C., Doyle, J., Dedon, M., Schaffer, R., Roumasset, J., Yeager, C.: EEG patterns during cognitive tasks. I. Methodology and analysis of complex behaviors. Electroencephalography and Clinical Neurophysiology 47(6), 693–703 (1979)
4. Wolpaw, J.R., Birbaumer, N., McFarland, D.J., Pfurtscheller, G., Vaughan, T.M.: Braincomputer interfaces for communication and control, Clinical neurophysiology? Official Journal of the International Federation of Clinical Neurophysiology 113, 767–791 (2002)
5. Lecuyer, A., Lotte, F., Reilly, R.B., Leeb, R., Hirose, M., Slater, M.: Brain-Computer Interfaces, Virtual Reality, and Videogames. Computer 41, 66–72 (2008)
6. Loudin, J.D., Simanovskii, D.M., Vijayraghavan, K., Sramek, C.K., Butterwick, A.F., Huie, P., McLean, G.Y., Palanker, D.V.: Optoelectronic retinal prosthesis: system design and performance. J. Neural Eng. 4(1), S72–S84 (2007)
7. Emotiv — EEG System — Electroencephalography,
   http://emotiv.com/ (accessed: December 16, 2012)
8. Taylor, G.S., Schmidt, C.: Empirical Evaluation of the Emotiv EPOC BCI Headset for the Detection of Mental Actions. In: Proceedings of the Human Factors and Ergonomics Society Annual Meeting, vol. 56(1), pp. 193–197 (September 2012)
9. Goldberg, B., Brawner, K.W., Holden, H.K.: Efficacy of Measuring Engagement during Computer-Based Training with Low-Cost Electroencephalogram (EEG) Sensor Outputs. In: Proceedings of the Human Factors and Ergonomics Society Annual Meeting, vol. 56(1), pp. 198–202 (September 2012)

10. SensoMotoric Instruments GmbH Gaze and Eye Tracking Systems Applications Neuromarketing,
    `http://www.smivision.com/en/`
    `gaze-and-eye-tracking-systems/applications/neuromarketing.html`
    (accessed: December 16, 2012)
11. Klem, G.H., Lders, H.O., Jasper, H.H., Elger, C.: The ten-twenty electrode system of the International Federation. The International Federation of Clinical Neurophysiology, Electroencephalogr. Clin. Neurophysiol. Suppl. 52, 3–6 (1999)
12. Hart, S.G.: NASA-Task Load Index (NASA-TLX); 20 Years Later. In: Proceedings of the Human Factors and Ergonomics Society 50th Annual Meeting, pp. 904–908. HFES, Santa Monica (2006)
13. Ashmore, M., Duchowski, A.T., Shoemaker, G.: Efficient Eye Pointing with a Fisheye Lens. In: Proceedings of Graphics interface 2005, ACM International Conference Proceeding Series, vol. 112, pp. 203–210 (2005)
14. Jacob, R.J.K.: What You Look at is What You Get: Eye Movement-Based Interaction Techniques. In: Proc. CHI 1990, pp. 11–18. ACM Press (1990)
15. Zhai, S., Morimoto, C., Ihde, S.: Manual and gaze input cascaded (MAGIC) pointing. In: Proc. of CHI 1999, pp. 246–253. ACM (1999)
16. Salvucci, D.D., Anderson, J.R.: Intelligent Gaze-Added Interfaces. In: Proceedings of the SIGCHI Conference on Human Factors in Computing Systems, CHI 2000, pp. 273–280. ACM Press (2000)
17. McGuffin, M., Balakrishnan, R.: Acquisition of Expanding Targets. In: Proceedings of the SIGCHI Conference on Human Factors in Computing Systems CHI 2002, pp. 57–64. ACM Press (2002)
18. Miniotas, D., Špakov, O., MacKenzie, I.S.: Eye Gaze Interaction with Expanding Targets. In: CHI 2004 Extended Abstracts on Human Factors in Computing Systems, pp. 1255–1258. ACM Press (2005)
19. Kumar, M., Paepcke, A., Winograd, T.: EyePoint: Practical Pointing and Selection Using Gaze and Keyboard. In: Proceedings of the SIGCHI Conference on Human Factors in Computing Systems CHI 2007, pp. 421–430. ACM Press (2007)
20. Tobii Technology, Tobii TX300 Eye Tracker Users Manual (2011)

Study of the Influence of Prototype Aesthetic Fidelity (A Realism Factor) in Usability Tests

Diana Rueda, René Hoto, and Andrés Conejero[*]

Universitat Politècnica de València
ancoro@idf.upv.es

Abstract. Tools (virtual and physical) currently available for product interactive design are becoming better and more affordable. Thus, it is now easier for designers to apply high degrees of appearance refinement to a prototype at early stages of design. This paper presents the findings of a study investigating the effect of aesthetic fidelity of digital and physical prototypes of a musical metronome device on user's perception of usability, in a series of experimental trials. The study examined user behavior and subjective user evaluation and emotion. Four groups of users were created and assigned different kind of prototypes (physical or digital with low and high aesthetic fidelity). This paper presents results indicating that there is an effect of aesthetic fidelity on user's perception of attractiveness and usability in both digital and physical prototypes and that user's assessment becomes more critical as the prototype gets closer to the real product.

Keywords: Design process, Usability test, Prototype fidelity, Aesthetics.

1 Introduction

Usability testing is one of the most important and most widely applied methods in usability practice [1], [2]. Furthermore, usability tests can be a vehicle for improving the co-operation between users and product designers [3] and to teach product designers about usability [4]. According to the user centered design approach, the usability of a product should be tested very early in its development process. Hence a not yet developed and functional product needs to be simulated for testing. Due to constraints of the design process such as time pressure and budgetary limitations, this is usually done by means of a prototype. Prototypes can be very basic (low-fidelity prototypes) such as drawn images and handwritten features on a piece of paper, or more advanced (medium-fidelity prototypes) such as interactive computer simulations [5], [6]. Low-fidelity prototypes are often used in usability practice since they are easy, fast and inexpensive to deploy [7]. Similar to that, also medium-fidelity prototypes are very common in usability practice [5] which may be due to the availability of software tools for prototype development that are easy to learn and to use (e.g. Dreamweaver, Powerpoint, DENIM, SILK or PatchWork). However,

---

[*] Corresponding author.

A. Holzinger et al. (Eds.): SouthCHI 2013, LNCS 7946, pp. 122–136, 2013.

prototypes might differ considerably from the final product (e.g.: with regard to aesthetic design, level of functionality, way of interaction etc.) which might have an influence on the results of usability tests [8].

1.1   Prototype Aesthetic Fidelity

The fidelity of a prototype is usually considered to be the resolution (the refinement and detail) of the model. Tullis [9] contends that the fidelity of a prototype is judged by how it appears to the person viewing it, and not by its similarity to the actual application. A number of publications have been focused on the effect of fidelity and the advantages and disadvantages of different prototyping techniques. Sefelin et al. [10] looked at the user's willingness to criticize paper prototypes versus computer based models. Virzi et al. [11] found that there was little difference in usability data for high and low fidelity models of standard two dimensional graphical interfaces and an interactive voice response system. McCurdy et al. [12] argued for a mixed approach that allowed various aspects of a prototype to be built at different fidelity levels according to the design component being prototyped. They go on to suggest that there are five 'dimensions' or fidelity aspects that can be defined as somewhere between high and low within the same prototype, namely, aesthetics, depth of functionality, breadth of functionality, richness of data and richness of interactivity. Other studies have analyzed the influence of the fidelity of prototypes in perceived usability in terms of functionality and interactivity, comparing paper-based and computer-based prototypes with real products [13]. Also, the influence of design aesthetics in usability evaluations has been studied and been proposed that it might be a determining factor in the perceived usability [8] [14]. However, we had not found any specific study considering the prototype aesthetic fidelity as a key factor, this being the central subject of this study.

1.2   Present Study

The present research aims to contribute elucidation of the influence of prototype aesthetic fidelity as a factor of realism in usability tests. With this purpose we have taken advantage of the improvement that have experienced product design tools as Graphic Design and 3D Modelling Softwares and Rapid Prototyping Technologies. Thanks to them, the cost in terms of time and money, in both virtual and physical prototyping, is becoming lower making them more affordable for the designer in the early stages of design. Thus, it is of particular interest the comparison between different degrees of aesthetic fidelity applied to a prototype, in our case: a sketch versus a digital render or a foam model versus a 3D printing prototype.

This investigation presents the comparative analysis of the influence of aesthetic fidelity in prototypes with different levels of interactivity: "medium" in the case of digital prototypes and "low" in physical prototypes. The study aims to analyze whether there is a correlation between these two factors (aesthetic fidelity and interactivity) and the perceived usability, attractiveness, and emotional state.

2   Experimental Design

Forty participants (60% men, 40% women), aged between 11 and 49 years (M = 27.5 years) were involved this study. They all had musical knowledge or notions. A selection criterion was that the participants were regular users of metronome.

The study employed a factorial (2 x 2) design. The main independent variable was the level of interaction of the prototype, which was divided into two levels: physical prototype (low interaction, through cards) and digital prototype (medium interaction, using a computer mouse). A second independent variable was the prototype aesthetic fidelity that was manipulated at two levels: high fidelity vs. low-fidelity. Each participant was assigned one of four experimental conditions (10 participants per prototype). To avoid possible learning effect across the different conditions that could affect the overall assessment each participant was allowed to participate in only one test.

The statistical study has been carried out through analysis of variance using SPSS Software.

2.1   User Performance

Three measures of user performance were made:

- The completion time of the tasks (s) that refers to the time required to perform each task.
- The efficiency of the interaction, a composite parameter that was found by dividing the optimal number of entries required in the task by the actual number of user entries.
- The number of errors made by the user, which appear when the user selects an erroneous navigation option.

2.2   Subjective Usability Evaluation

As user performance, measuring user satisfaction represents a standard procedure in usability tests, often in the form of perceived usability [15]. It is of special relevance the collection of both subjective and objective data, since both types of data do not always coincide [15], [16].

There is a wide range of standardized instruments that can be used to measure the perceived usability and all its facets [2]. The criteria for selecting one of the instruments were: the degree of specificity (generic vs. very specific for a particular product), size (ranging from 10-item to 71-item SUS QUIS) and type of facets covered (for e.g.: ISO standard). Most instruments have acceptable psychometric properties, so they could be applied from a methodological point of view.

In the first part of the usability perception measurement was chosen the ITS method with 10 questions, rated on a 5-point Likert scale (agree, partly agree, neither agree nor disagree, partly disagree, disagree) [17]. The SUS questionnaire (System Usability Scale) was:

- I think I would use this metronome frequently.
- I found the metronome unnecessarily complex.

- I think the metronome is easy to use.
- I think I would need assistance to use this metronome.
- I found the various functions of this metronome were well integrated.
- I thought there was too much inconsistency in this metronome.
- I would imagine that most people would learn to use this metronome very quickly.
- I found the metronome very cumbersome to use.
- I felt very confident using this metronome.
- I needed to learn a lot of things before I could get going with this metronome.

For the other part it was used the Multimetrix questionnaire [18]. This instrument is based on design principles suggested by the ISO (ISO 9241-11). The questionnaire was modified slightly by the removal of items that were irrelevant to the intended application area. The statements had to be rated on a 5-point Likert scale. The subscales of the instrument were:

- Suitability for the task ("The system forces me to carry out unnecessary actions").
- Conformity with user expectations ("Messages of the software always appear at the same place").
- Information and information structure ("The software contains all relevant information").
- Suitability for learning ("The functions of the software can be easily learnt").
- Self-descriptiveness ("I can use the software straight away without the help from others").

2.3   Emotions and Attractiveness

Learning Affect Monitor (LAM). This is a 32-item questionnaire developed by Reicherts et al. [19] to capture emotions experienced in daily life. It was slightly adapted to make it suitable for the purpose of the present study. Only a subset of 10 items were employed and analysed, excluding those items that were considered less relevant for user–product interaction. The items had a 9-point Likert scale.

2.4   Attractiveness

The attractiveness of the product was measured on a one-item 5-point Likert scale, with the item being phrased: "The design of the metronome is appealing" (agree, partly agree, neither agree nor disagree, partly disagree, disagree).

3   Materials

The proposed study was conducted to evaluate a proposed design of an interactive device by users, namely a digital musical metronome. The metronome is a device used to indicate beat and tempo of musical compositions. This digital metronome includes an uncommon feature, which is the ability to create composite compasses, also called amalgam. There were four prototypes to which we applied different ranges of interactivity and aesthetic fidelity. Each prototype allows users to interact with the metronome and carry out a designed task, as if it was a real product.

3.1   Digital Prototypes (Medium Interactivity)

Two digital prototypes with high or low aesthetic fidelity were made. The interaction was considered as medium fidelity because it uses a peripheral device: the mouse. In this case, the representation of the metronome was made by a picture of a frontal view of it, to simulate both housing and screen. The navigation was developed using Dreamweaver (software for web page design). The test was performed by a computer. The interaction was simulated by a web page showing the digital prototype. Depending on which button was pressed in the prototype, the web page was refreshed and changed automatically. When the user made a mistake, a warning message appeared on the screen. The screens were made in animated gif format to achieve a simulation of symbols and flashing LEDs.

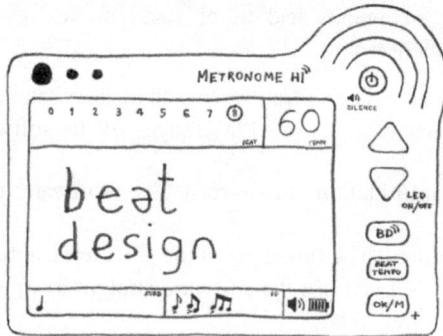

Fig. 1. The low aesthetic fidelity digital prototype was developed with low cost materials and fast processing. Images displayed on this website were previously drawn with a black marker and then scanned and processed in Photoshop (software for image processing). Time spent in the graphics was 2 days. In total it is estimated that the realization of the prototype took one week and a half, with the web programming.

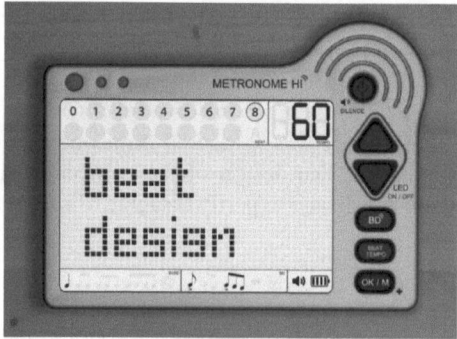

Fig. 2. In contrast, the high aesthetic fidelity digital prototype involves simulating aesthetics in a greater degree of appearance of the different physical elements, such as shape, color and texture both in the housing and screen. The screen images shown on this website were made in Illustrator (software for vector image creation) and then processed in Photoshop. In addition, the body of the metronome was simulated by a render (by using 3D Studio Max Software) of a CAD model (by using Unigraphics Software). The final images were then processed in Photoshop.

3.2   Physical Prototypes (Low Interactivity)

Two physical prototypes were made, respectively with low and high aesthetic fidelity. The interaction was considered as low-fidelity because the simulation was performed with cards [7]. Depending on which button was pressed in the prototype, the examiner returned a card in response to the result of the action. The user performed the task pointing the finger at one of the buttons on the prototype. When the user made a mistake, the examiner informed the user about his decision. Being static images, the simulation of the blinking was done with red stripes covering the flashing. 44 cards were used for this simulation (size 62 mm 44 mm).

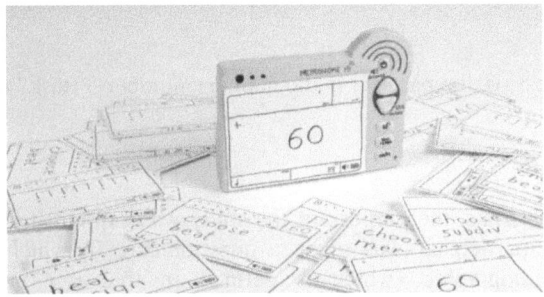

Fig. 3. The low aesthetic fidelity physical prototype was made entirely by hand. Housing and buttons were made of extruded polystyrene foam. The inscriptions and cards were made with a black marker. In total it is estimated that the realization of the prototype took 2 days.

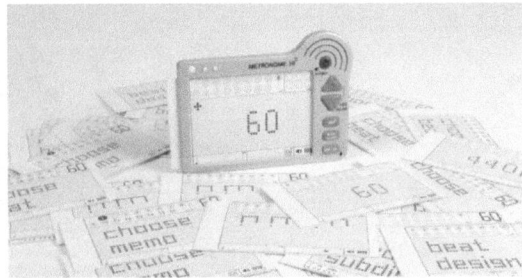

Fig. 4. The high aesthetic fidelity physical prototype housing was previously modelled in Unigraphics design software and. manufactured in ABS by 3D printing in two parts. Keypad was done by pouring elastomeric polyurethane and inscriptions with adhesive vinyl. The graphic design of the cards was made in Illustrator software and then printed. In total it is estimated that the realization of the prototype took three weeks and a half.

3.3   User Tasks

Participants were divided into two separate groups according to the degree of interactivity of the prototype. Each of these groups was separated into two groups, according to the aesthetic fidelity of the prototype (high or low) with a total of four different categories. Each participant was given a series of four tasks:

- Task 1:
  Start the metronome: Press the appropriate button to turn on the metronome (task "on").
- Task 2:
  Change the beat (pulse): Create a rhythm of 8 pulses subdivided into triplets, keeping the tempo to 60 bpm (task "beat/tempo").
- Task 3:
  Design an amalgam compass (Beat Design): Choose the menu "Beat Design" and create a compass composed of 8 pulses by a 2/4, ¾ and another ¾ ((strong-weak)+(semistrong-weak-weak)+(semistrong-weak-weak)) and store (task "beat design").
- Task 4:
  Save memory: Save the pace set in the memory number 3 (task "memorize").

4   Procedure

Before starting the trials, the purpose of the study was explained to the participants. Afterwards, each participant was given a questionnaire in which four parts were differentiated: demographic (which is defined in the user profile), perceived attractiveness (relation with aesthetic fidelity), emotional perception (LAM questionnaire) and the perception of usability (Multimetrix and SUS questionnaire).

Participants were assigned one of the experimental conditions. Throughout the test procedure, notes about the users´ performances and their reactions were taken.

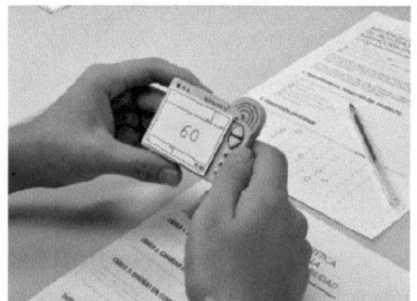 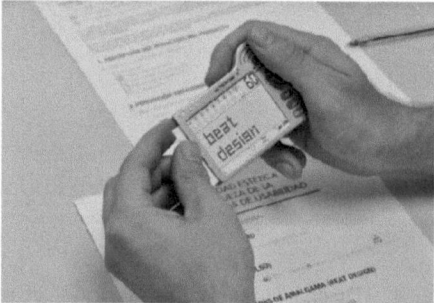

Fig. 5. User test with physical prototypes. Left: low aesthetic fidelity; right: high aesthetic fidelity.

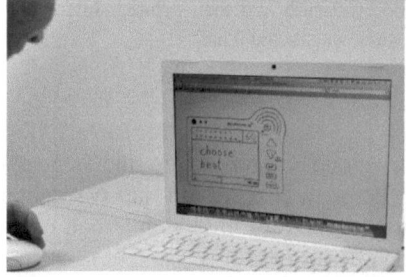 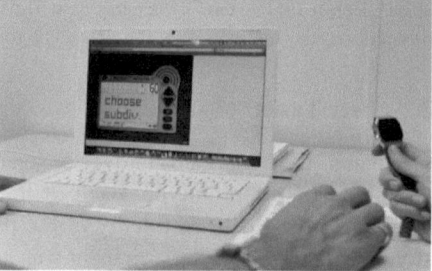

Fig. 6. User test with digital prototypes. Left: low aesthetic fidelity; right: high aesthetic fidelity.

5   Results

5.1   User Behaviour

Task Completion Time. The data obtained show a strong variation among participants regarding the measure of performance (e.g.: timing of the completion of tasks ranging from 145-851 s). The analysis revealed a main effect of the fidelity of the prototype (see Fig. 7), users require more time when they use the physical prototype (F=14,712, df=3, p< 0.001). There was also a significant difference between the physical prototypes due to prototype design, since in the high aesthetic fidelity physical prototype cards were inserted into a slot, so the screen appearance was more real, but causing an increase of time to complete the test. In contrast, in the low aesthetic fidelity physical prototype cards were adhered with adhesive to the foam. Analysing each task separately, a significant effect was found in each of the tasks (p<0.005) except for the first one (F<1). We found no significant effect of the aesthetics of the device (F<1).

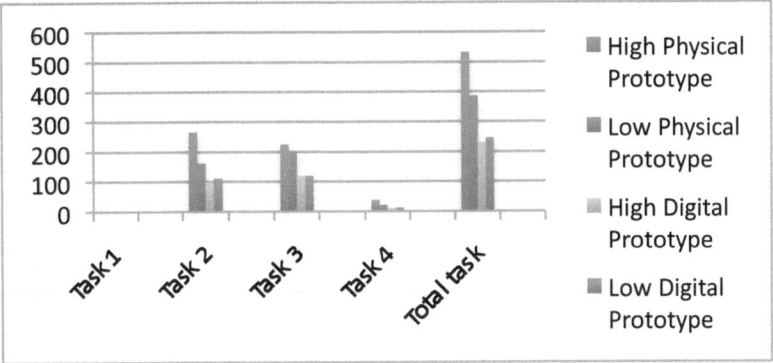

Fig. 7. Average times (s) required to complete the tasks in the indicated type of interaction and aesthetics fidelity prototypes

5.2   Interaction Efficiency

The results o the efficiency of the user-product interaction (i.e.: optimal number of user commands divided by the actual number of commands executed by users) are presented in table 1. There are significant differences between the prototypes in task 2 (F=4.152, df=3; p<0.05) and 3 (F=5.503, df=3; p<0.005). Analyzing in detail, it is shown that the fidelity of the prototypes is related to this difference, the values of the two physical prototypes are similar to each other, like the two digital ones. However, it showed no effect of aesthetic fidelity (F<1). An interesting observation is that in the usability testing of digital prototypes, users thought the screen-touch-metronome was presented and clicked several times directly on the screen instead of using the mouse until they realized or instructors warned them about it. This type of error related to the interactivity of the prototype was not observed on physical prototypes. Regarding the

Table 1. Average ratings of the efficiency of user–prototype interaction

Index	Physical Prototype		Digital Prototype	
	High A. F.	Low A. F.	High A. F.	Low A. F.
Task 1	1.000 (0.000)	0.950 (0.158)	1.000 (0.000)	1.000 (0.000)
Task 2	0.787 (0.181)	0.854 (0.209)	0.602 (0.195)	0.610 (0.202)
Task 3	0.741 (0.264)	0.756 (0.218)	0.481 (0.184)	0.486 (0.139)
Task 4	0.975 (0.079)	1.000 (0.000)	0.975 (0.079)	0.975 (0.079)

Table 2. Averages ratings of the number of errors of user–prototype interaction

Errors	Physical Prototype		Digital Prototype	
	High A. F.	Low A. F.	High A. F.	Low A. F.
Task 1	0.000 (0.000)	0.010 (0.316)	0.000 (0.000)	0.000 (0.000)
Task 2	0.800 (0.632)	0.010 (0.316)	1.600 (1.265)	1.300 (0.823)
Task 3	0.700 (1.160)	0.500 (0.972)	0.800 (1.317)	0.400 (0.516)
Task 4	0.000 (0.000)	0.000 (0.000)	0.300 (0.483)	0.100 (0.316)
Total	1.500 (1.269)	0.700 (0.949)	2.700 (1.418)	1.800 (0.919)

errors in the interaction (table 2), only noticed a significant difference in task 2 ($F=6.192$, $df=3$, $p<0.005$), showing a greater number of errors in digital than in physical prototypes, especially in the high aesthetic fidelity ones.

5.3   Subjective Usability Evaluation

For both the questionnaire Multimetrix as SUS, a multivariate analysis of the variance was performed (MANOVA) to test the overall effects of the independent variables in the different rating scales.

The Multimetrix analysis did not detect any effect on 8 items ($F = 1743$, $df = 8$, $p> 0.05$). Although this indicates no correlation, when examining carefully the table values more pronounced changes were found between the two low aesthetics fidelity prototypes in the following items: "Information", "learning" and "management", ... to be better assessed the physical than the digital (table 3). In "error tolerance" was better rated the physical prototype of high aesthetic fidelity than the digital one. In the case of "intuitive" it is perceived a difference between aesthetic fidelity prototypes, achieving higher scores on physical prototypes. Analyzing the effects that might

Table 3. Average ratings (with deviation) of user–prototype interaction on a global scale and for each subscale (1-5) of Multimetrix

	Physical Prototype		Digital Prototype	
	High A. F.	Low A. F.	High A. F.	Low A. F.
Suitable	4.60 (0.699)	4.80 (0.632)	4.60 (0.516)	4.20 (0.789)
Expectations	4.40 (0.699)	4.40 (1.075)	4.70 (0.483)	4.20 (0.632)
Information	4.30 (0.823)	4.50 (0.707)	4.00 (1.054)	3.50 (0.972)
Learning	4.00 (1.054)	4.60 (0.516)	4.10 (0.994)	3.70 (1.059)
Intuitive	4.00 (1.054)	4.10 (0.994)	3.60 (0.516)	3.70 (0.823)
Handling	4.30 (0.823)	4.60 (0.516)	3.80 (0.919)	3.50 (0.850)
Error Tolerance	4.10 (0.738)	3.90 (1.370)	3.40 (1.174)	3.70 (0.675)
Acceptance	4.50 (0.707)	4.60 (1.265)	4.30 (0.823)	4.30 (0.675)
Overall	4.275 (0.824)	35.5 (0.844)	32.5 (0.809)	3.85 (0.809)

Table 4. Average ratings (with deviation) of user–prototype interaction on a global scale and for each subscale (1-5) of SUS

	Physical Prototype		Digital Prototype	
	High A. F.	Low A. F.	High A. F.	Low A. F.
Answer 1	4.40 (0.966)	4.60 (0.699)	4.00 (1.247)	4.10 (0.876)
Answer 2	2.10 (1.197)	1.50 (0.972)	1.60 (1.075)	2.70 (1.059)
Answer 3	4.00 (1.247)	4.60 (0.966)	4.30 (0.949)	3.90 (0.738)
Answer 4	1.40 (0.516)	1.40 (0.966)	1.60 (0.966)	1.40 (0.966)
Answer 5	4.50 (0.707)	5.00 (0.000)	4.50 (0.972)	4.50 (0.707)
Answer 6	1.30 (0.675)	1.10 (0.316)	1.70 (1.059)	1.90 (0.876)
Answer 7	4.20 (1.033)	4.20 (0.789)	4.30 (0.949)	3.80 (1.135)
Answer 8	1.40 (0.966)	1.10 (0.316)	1.70 (0.949)	1.70 (0.823)
Answer 9	3.80 (0.919)	4.60 (0.516)	3.80 (1.135)	3.20 (0.919)
Answer 10	1.70 (1.059)	1.10 (0.316)	1.40 (0.699)	1.50 (0.527)
Overall	2.88 (0.928)	2.92 (0.585)	2.90 (1.00)	2.87 (0.862)

result from the different prototypes, an interaction was found with the item "management" (F = 3352, df = 3, P <0.05), with the evaluations of digital prototypes lower than physical ones.

The analysis of the questionnaire SUS showed no overall effects in any of the 10 questions (F = 1.998, df = 10, p> 0.05). By looking at table 4, one sees that the most significant values are found in question 2 (The system was needlessly complex I), 3 (I think the system is easy to use), 6 (I think there is not much consistency in the system) and 9 (I felt very confident using the system). The questions are affected by the difference in the valuation between low aesthetic fidelity prototypes (physical vs. digital). Furthermore, in question 2 there is a difference between digital prototypes and in question 3 between physical prototypes. In question 9 there is an interaction between all prototypes (F = 4068, df = 3, p <0.02).

5.4   Emotions and Attractiveness

Emotions. We performed a MANOVA in the 9 items of LAM. The analysis shows no interaction between prototypes (F <1 or p> 0.05). Table 5 and 6 shows the mean scores of the participants at the initial time t_0 (i.e.: before the usability test) and the end time t_1 (i.e., after usability test) as a function of aesthetics fidelity and type of interaction. The strongest effect was found in "disappointed", followed by "down", "bored", "interested", "surprised" and "impotent". Note that the initial valuation time is guided by the prototype perceived attractiveness of the user: however, in the final time emotions are influenced by the outcome of the usability test rather than the perceived attractiveness.

Table 5. Average ratings of emotions at t_0 (before the usability test) and t_1 (after the usability test) on a Likert scale of 9-points. Physical prototoypes.

	High A. F. Physical prototype			Low A. H. Physical prototype		
	t_0 (SD)	t_1(SD)	Difference (t_1-t_0)	t_0 (SD)	t_1(SD)	Difference (t_1-t_0)
Irritated	1.40 (0.966)	2.30 (1.337)	0.90	1.10 (0.316)	1.80 (2.201)	0.70
Bored	1.80 (1.317)	1.60 (1.075)	- 0.20	2.40 (1.647)	2.70 (3.093)	0.30
Disappointed	1.30 (0.949)	1.70 (1.059)	0.40	1.60 (1.897)	1.60 (1.578)	0
Helpless	1.30 (0.949)	2.70 (2.058)	1.40	1.70 (1.494)	1.70 (1.889)	0
Enthusiastic	4.50(1.581)	5.00 (2.261)	0.50	5.80 (1.687)	6.00 (1.491)	0.20
Satisfied	4.90 (1.912)	5.40 (1.713)	0.50	7.00 (1.414)	7.10 (1.287)	0.10
Surprised	5.30 (2.452)	6.20 (1.549)	0.90	6.00 (2.309)	6.80 (2.348)	0.80
Interested	5.60(2.271)	6.60 (1.174)	1.00	6.40 (2.221)	6.80 (2.348)	0.40

Table 6. Average ratings of emotions at t_0 (before the usability test) and t_1 (after the usability test) on a Likert scale of 9-points. Digital protototypes.

	High A. F. Digital Prototype			Low A. H. Digital Prototype		
	t_0 (SD)	t_1(SD)	Difference $(t_1\text{-}t_0)$	t_0 (SD)	t_1(SD)	Difference $(t_1\text{-}t_0)$
Irritated	1.10 (0.316)	1.70 (1.567)	0.60	2.00 (1.944)	2.20 (1.619)	0.20
Bored	1.50 (0.707)	1.10 (0.316)	- 0.40	2.50 (1.269)	1.60 (1.265)	- 0.90
Disappointed	1.40 (0.966)	1.50 (0.972)	0.10	2.50 (1.958)	1.70 (0.949)	- 0.80
Helpless	2.40 (2.227)	3.00 (1.826)	0.60	2.30 (2.163)	3.00 (1.886)	0.70
Enthusiatic	5.80 (1.549)	5.90 (1.729)	0.10	3.90 (1.729)	4.70 (1.337)	0.80
Satisfied	6.70 (1.494)	7.00 (1.563)	0.30	5.10 (2.183)	5.80 (1.687)	0.70
Surprised	6.30 (0.823)	7.60 (1.578)	1.30	6.10 (2.132)	6.20 (1.989)	0.10
Interested	7.20 (1.033)	7.10 (1.663)	-0.10	6.90 (1.101)	7.00 (1.563)	0.10

5.5   Attractiveness

The MANOVA analysis determined that there was no effect of the perception of attractiveness ($F < 1$). No interactions were found between groups of prototypes ($F = 2.42$, $df = 3$, $P > 0.05$), however, a significant difference was detected between digital prototypes ($p < 0.05$). This is because the low fidelity digital prototype was worse assessed (table 7). The most interesting is that the perception of attractiveness on physical prototypes reaches a higher value in the case of reduced fidelity.

Table 7. Average ratings of atracttiveness on a Likert scale of 5-points

	Physical Prototype		Digital Prototype	
	High A. F.	Low A. F.	High A. F.	Low A. F.
Attractiveness	4.200 (1.229)	4.500 (0.850)	4.500 (0.707)	3.500 (0.972)

6   Conclusions

The tools currently available in the product and services design process allow to reach higher levels of fidelity and to increasingly reduce the time to obtain the prototypes. But the design of interactive applications poses a dilemma and a challenge to the design community due to the wide range of elements of different nature that have to be taken in to account, not only physical (size, shape, buttons, etc.) but also, electronic or digital (screens with information and navigation menus). Although recent research and commercial systems have demonstrated the capacity of providing software abstractions to physical devices [20], [21], [22] the expertise threshold and time investment required, make them inappropriate for designers, particularly at the early stages. So, we intentionally selected the computer-based and paper prototypes to carry out this study, because they are the cheapest approaches currently available for designers in the initial stage of the design process.

What we have learnt from the present research, in the first place, is that even though physical prototyping of the device presents obvious advantages over the degree of tangibility experienced by the user, there is a significant loss in the degree of interaction, mainly due to the fact that the response of the screen navigation is simulated by using exchanging paper cards. By contrast, in the digital prototyping of these devices it is possible to achieve a high degree of interactivity through multimedia programmes, obtaining an immediate response in the simulated screen navigation. However, in this case there is a significant loss of physical manipulation.

Even if we found a dilemma: physicality vs. interactivity, the main question was how prototype aesthetic fidelity (degree of aesthetic realism) could affect user perception in both physical and digital prototypes.

Our results about the attractiveness assessment, first factor rated by users, showed that this factor was positively influenced by aesthetic fidelity only in the case of digital prototypes. On the contrary, this influence was negative in the case of physical ones. The explanation for this could be that user attractiveness assessment becomes more critical as the prototype gets closer to the real product in terms of appearance (physical shape, colour and material characteristics). I.e.: The greater the degree of fidelity, the stronger the critical perception of the users. We could also see this effect in the usability assessment of digital prototypes which obtained the lowest ratings. Users expected more from the digital prototype because the level of interaction response is higher. In contrast, as Sonderegger and Sauer [14] has suggested, under reduced fidelity conditions, users created a mental model of the real appliance presenting a much more attractive design. This may suggest a kind of "deficiency compensation" effect. Thus, confirming this assumption, our work shows that the low aesthetic fidelity physical prototype was the best rated in both usability and attractiveness perception. Users seem to project an idealized image of the final product into the prototype because it is unfinished and hence, more perfectible, this being in accordance with Sonderegger and Sauer [14].

Another key result is that there is a positive correlation between the perceived attractiveness and the perceived usability (Multimetrix). This is in agreement with previous studies on the influence of design aesthetics in usability tests [23], [24] and supports the contention that perceived usability may be more strongly associated with attractiveness ratings than with objectively measured usability parameters. Also, with the findings of Tractinsky [25] who proposed that the beauty of design would positively affect the perceived usability. In this respect it has to be pointed out that this study provides evidences on that attractiveness assessment is not only influenced by the aesthetics of the design; it is also determined by the prototype aesthetic fidelity (degree of aesthetic realism). These results also clarify why in other studies [14] user attractiveness assessment of moderate aesthetic design real appliances were given lowest ratings as compared to with their paper prototype versions.

From these results, it seems that it is important to get a degree of refinement of the prototype aesthetics fidelity in order to reach more reliable conclusions in user evaluations. As we have seen in this study, aesthetic fidelity could be an influencing factor. In this sense, realistic virtual images can be helpful in digital prototyping. Nevertheless, to get a really critical assessment of the attractiveness of an interactive device design, is necessary to have a physical prototype with a high aesthetic refinement, as close as it could be to the future real product.

References

1. Holzinger, A.: Usability Engineering for Software Developers. Communications of the ACM 48(1), 71–74 (2005)
2. Lewis, J.R.: Usability testing. In: Salvendy, G. (ed.) Handbook of Human Factors and Ergonomics, pp. 1275–1316. John Wiley, New York (2006)
3. Buur, J., Bagger, K.: Replacing Usability Testing with User Dialogue. Communications of the ACM 42(5), 63–66 (1999)
4. Nielsen, J.: Usability engineering. Morgan Kaufmann, Amsterdam (1993)
5. Engelberg, D., Seffah, A.: A Framework for Rapid Mid-Fidelity Prototyping of Web Sites. In: IFIP World Computer Congress 2002. Kluwer Academic Publishers, Montréal (2002)
6. Vu, K., Proctor, R.W.: Web site design and evaluation. In: Salvendy, G. (ed.) Handbook of Human Factors and Ergonomics, pp. 1317–1343. John Wiley, New York (2006)
7. Snyder, C.: Paper Prototyping: The Fast and Easy Way to Define and Refine User Interfaces. Morgan Kaufmann Publishers, San Francisco (2003)
8. Sauer, J., Sonderegger, A.: The Influence of Prototype Fidelity and Aesthetics of Design in Usability Tests: Effects on User Behaviour, Subjective Evaluation and Emotion. Applied Ergonomics 40, 670–677 (2009)
9. Tullis, T.S.: High-Fidelity Prototyping Throughout the Design Process. In: Proceedings of the Human Factors Society 34th Annual Meeting, p. 266. Human Factors Society, Santa Monica (1990)
10. Sefelin, R., Tscheligi, M., Giller, V.: Paper Prototyping - What is it Good For?: A Comparison of Paper- and Computer-Based Low-Fidelity Prototyping. In: CHI 2003 Extended Abstracts on Human Factors in Computing Systems. ACM, Ft. Lauderdale (2003)
11. Virzi, R.A., Sokolov, J.L., Karis, D.: Usability Problem Identification Using Both Low- and High-Fidelity Prototypes. In: Proceedings of the SIGCHI Conference on Human Factors in Computing Systems: Common Ground, pp. 236–243. ACM Press, Vancouver (1996)
12. McCurdy, M., Connors, C., Pyrzak, G., Kanefsky, B., Vera, A.: Breaking the Fidelity Barrier: An Examination of our Current Characterization of Prototypes and an Example of a Mixed-Fidelity Success. In: Proceedings of the SIGCHI Conference on Human Factors in Computing Systems, pp. 1233–1242. ACM, New York (2006)
13. Youn-kyung, L., Apurva, P., Subashini, P., Shweta, A.: Comparative Analysis of High and Low-Fidelity Prototypes for More Valid Usability Evaluations of Mobile Devices. In: NordiCHI 2006, Oslo, Norway, pp. 14–18 (2006)

14. Sonderegger, A., Sauer, J.: The Influence of Design Aesthetics in Usability Testing: Effects on User Performance and Perceived Usability. Applied Ergonomics 41, 403–410 (2010)
15. Jordan, P.W.: An Introduction to Usability. Tylor & Francis, Lodon (1998)
16. Wickens, C.D., Hollands, J.G.: Engineering Psychology and Human Performance. Prentice-Hall, Upper Saddle River (2000)
17. Brooke, J.: SUS: A Quick and Dirty Usability Scale. In: Jordan, P.W., Thomas, B., Weerdmeester, B.A., McClelland, I.L. (eds.) Usability Evaluation in Industry, pp. 189–194. Taylor & Francis, London (1996)
18. Ollermann, F.: Evaluation von Hypermedia-Anwendungen: Entwicklung und Validierung eines Instruments. Unpublished Diploma thesis. Institute of Work and Organisational Psychology, University of Osnabrück, Germany (2001)
19. Reicherts, M., Salamin, V., Maggiori, C., Pauls, K.: Psychometric characteristics of a computer-based monitoring system for emotion processing and affective states. In: Proceedings of the 10th Spanish Conference on Biometrics, Oviedo, May 25-27 (2005)
20. Greenberg, S., Fitchett, C.: Phidgets: Easy Development of Physical Interfaces through Physical Widgets. In: UIST: ACM Symposium on User Interface Software and Technology, pp. 209–218. ACM, New York (2001)
21. Ballagas, R., Ringel, M., Stone, M., Borchers, J.: iStuff: a Physical User Interface Toolkit for Ubiquitous Computing Environments. In: SIGCHI Conference on Human Factors in Computing Systems, Ft Lauderdale, Florida, pp. 537–544 (2003)
22. Klemmer, S.R., Li, L., Lin, J., Landay, J.A.: Papier-Mâché: Toolkit Support for Tangible Input. In: CHI 2004: Proceedings SIGCHI Conference on Human Factors in Computing Systems, pp. 399–406. ACM Press, New York (2004)
23. Nakarada-Kordich, I., Lobb, B.: Effect of Perceived Attractiveness of Web Interface Design on Visual Search of Web Sites. In: Proceedings CHINZ 2005, Auckland, July 6-8, pp. 25–27 (2005)
24. Brady, L., Phillips, C.: Aesthetics and usability: A look at color and balance. Usability News 5, 1–4 (2003)
25. Tractinsky, N.: Aesthetics and Apparent Usability: Empirically Assessing Cultural and Methodological Issues. In: Proceedings of the CHI, pp. 115–122. ACM, New York (1997)

Exploiting Classical Bibliometrics of CSCW: Classification, Evaluation, Limitations, and the Odds of Semantic Analytics

António Correia[1], Benjamim Fonseca[2],
and Hugo Paredes[2]

[1] UTAD – University of Trás-os-Montes e Alto Douro,
Quinta de Prados, Apartado 1013, Vila Real, Portugal
ajcorreia1987@gmail.com
[2] INESC TEC/UTAD,
Quinta de Prados, Apartado 1013, Vila Real, Portugal
{benjaf,hparedes}@utad.pt

Abstract. The purpose of this study is to conduct a bibliometric and taxonomy-based analysis of the field of CSCW to map its recent evolution at a quantitative and qualitative level. A model for semantic analytics and social evaluation is also discussed with emphasis on the hypothesis of putting crowds into the loop of bibliography classification process to improve the current labor-intensive, time-consuming, unrepeatable and sometimes subjective task of scientometricians. A total of 1,480 publications were carefully reviewed and subjected to scientometric data analysis methods and techniques. Analyzed parameters included document orientation, deviation from trend in the total number of citations, and publication activity by author's affiliation country. A semantic classification of 541 publications allows identifying growing trends and lacking research indicators. At a human-centered perspective, limitations are unfilled in the limitative analytical spectrum, laborious and time-consuming processes of data seeking, gathering, cataloguing and analysis, subjective results at a taxonomic level, lack of more bibliographic data analytics perspectives, and absence of human-centered results concerning cognitive aspects in meta-knowledge research practices. Hypotheses are suggested towards a crowd-enabled model for bibliography evaluation in order to understand the ways as humans and machines can work cooperatively and massively on scientific data to solve complex problems.

Keywords: Bibliographic data analytics, crowd-enabled model, CSCW, HCI, human computation, scientometrics, semantics, taxonomy.

1 Introduction

The functions associated with humans and machines have always been interconnected in a symbiotic process since the early 1950s. This synergy has been recently analyzed by Human-Computer Interaction (HCI) research community under the banner of human computation, a growing field focused on the machine abilities to support collaboration mechanisms aggregating efforts provided by humans to solve problems that no

A. Holzinger et al. (Eds.): SouthCHI 2013, LNCS 7946, pp. 137–156, 2013.

known computer algorithms can yet solve [1]. Computing technology has changed the nature of work supporting distinct human practices in collaborative working environments. It has been reinvented recursively and massively to meet the changing framework of social requirements and support large-scale cooperative work [2].

Since the advent of the multidisciplinary field of Computer-Supported Cooperative Work (CSCW) in the mid-1980s, social-technical factors affecting groups and crowds with different background using technology to perform complex tasks have been further explored with special emphasis on the interdependence of several actors interacting towards a common goal and changing the state of a mutual field of work [2]. Important contributions have been provided by CSCW researchers to establish an unifying theoretical framework for design [3].

Scientific data production in the field of CSCW has grown steadily for much of the past quarter century [3], disseminated by devoted and non-specific publication venues concerning their interdisciplinary scope. Established as the science of measuring and analyzing scientific and technological bibliography [9], bibliometrics is applied as a formative instrument to map the structure and impact of the field of CSCW through an integrated content and citation analysis. This bibliometric study explores a sample of 1,480 publications segmented in the form of hypothesis about the structure, growth and impact of this field towards an innovative model for analyzing and integrating meta-knowledge into bibliographic indexing systems. At a scientometric perspective of analysis, citation metadata was manually retrieved by using Google Scholar, ACM Digital Library and Web of Science [10]. The analysis is complemented with a classification of collaborative working environments in order to recognize technical trends and functional gaps. The present literature review is based on a labor-intensive method of cataloguing, reading, classifying and analyzing publications in 3 journals and 5 conferences (2003-2010). In the evaluation process, a systematic method is supported by a finer-grained taxonomy [11] to categorize functional attributes and application-level domains from 541 technology-oriented studies. Several chasms of research were identified from this comprehensive review allowing to perceive a recurring challenge on evaluating the always growing scientific literature.

In the current paradigm of CSCW-devoted research, bibliographic data available in scientific digital libraries are statically stored despite their automated indexing mechanisms. Comparisons have been presented to understand the advantages of academic digital libraries and search engines [10], which comprise bibliometric indicators (e.g., number of citations, and downloads) but discard semantic analytics behind bibliography [5]. Considering the "tedious and lengthy task" [6] of finding all journal papers, conference proceedings, posters, tutorials, book chapters, images, and videos, analyzing and classifying them manually under different analytical perspectives. A possible solution for this research gap could be established in a proposal for a crowdsourcing and human computation model that could aggregate worldwide efforts from multiple scientists and general public in the evaluation of bibliographical artifacts in order to examine information entirely accessible so that it can be possible to infer on scientometrics (e.g., co-authorship data) and semantics (e.g., knowledge maps of research topics), taking into account human needs in the computer-human interaction process. The idea relies on a lack of knowledge about similar studies intended to fill the social-technical gap of metadata handled by digital libraries, although there have been proposals with emphasis on content analysis [7].

The structure of this paper is subdivided in six distinct but related sections. Section 2 presents the known background on bibliometric approaches with an overview of the quantitative studies dedicated to HCI and contiguous fields. Section 3 discusses a set of scientometric techniques and content analysis methods, representing the analytical sample and selection criteria. Section 4 focuses on the bibliometric results in a probabilistic format. Section 5 represents a discussion about findings and limitations of this study, suggesting a crowd-enabled model as a possible solution to suppress the classification and evaluation gaps of scientific data. Section 6 presents some concluding remarks and discusses future work based on exposed limitations.

2　Background in CSCW and HCI Bibliometrics

A bibliometric study of CSCW research needs the consideration of studies with similar purposes into the wide spectrum of HCI to identify reasonable gaps and reduce the probability to duplicate scientific efforts. In this particular context, Holsapple and Luo [12] employed a citation analysis method to specify several variances on a set of journals with great influence on collaborative computing research, retrieving and analyzing a total of 19,271 citations from journal papers, conference proceedings, books and technical reports across an 8-year period (1992-1999).

In a different perspective, Serenko and Bontis [13] examined the domains of intellectual capital and knowledge management to measure the citation impact and research productivity with a methodological foundation on bibliographical analysis. The research devoted to bibliometrics in CSCW demonstrated the value of researching its configuration with an analysis of the main topics of interest, total number of citations, and Social Network Analysis (SNA) with co-authorship data. The results achieved by Horn et al. [14] demonstrated a trend of consistency in the CSCW co-authorship network between 1986 and 1999. Simultaneously, betweenness centrality, co-authoring partnership, productivity, and collaboration robustness indicators were identified for HCI and CSCW cumulative network between 1982 and 2003.

A meta-analysis of the ACM CSCW conference (1986-2002) [15] was made using Linear Discriminant Analysis (LDA). Results represented a high number of contributions by academics since 1990 in addition to a predominant research effort from USA (70-90%) face to Europe (10-30%). Central topics were focused in group issues, ethnographical and experimental studies, and development/architectural aspects of cooperative systems, whilst theoretical approaches decreased gradually. In the collaboration level, the most common function was centered in the communication and information sharing processes, followed by coordination and awareness, and a minor percentage of papers were oriented to jointly production and decision-making.

As suggested by Wania et al. [16], a bibliometric analysis can be suitable to determine how design and evaluation communities are related in the field of HCI, and how it can be used to build a comprehensive theory. In this sense, author co-citation analysis, visualization tools and multivariate techniques were used to explore relationships between communities. Results revealed seven clusters within HCI research community (i.e., CSCW, design theory and complexity, design rationale, user-centered design, cognitive engineering, cognitive theories and models, and participatory design). The CSCW cluster focuses on building systems that enable or enhance collaboration and cooperative work among groups. In the same year, Jacovi and colleagues [6] showed a citation graph analysis of ACM CSCW in its 20th birthday, attempting to analyze its structure and trends (1986-2004). Results allowed to detect a manifest division of the field associated to mutual citation of technical- and social-oriented papers and a slight emphasis on social aspects of collaboration technology, representing the ACM CSCW as a technology-oriented publication venue. This study identified a particular need to develop labor-intensive bibliometric studies supported by distinct reading and classification methods for publications to achieve accurate results. Approximately 801 citations were retrieved from a sample constituted by 465 papers using Google Scholar's citation index. Main clusters were theories and models, ethnography and user studies (83 papers), computer science (82 papers), meeting/decision support, shared media spaces and conferencing (43 papers), and cluster trends such as instant messaging and workspace awareness [6]. A bibliometric exercise for SIGCHI Conference on Human Factors in Computing Systems [17] allowed to identify the most cited first authors (1990-2006), influential sites of research, cited papers, and expected citations.

The scope of the analysis performed by Wainer and Barsottini [18] was centered in 169 papers from ACM CSCW (1998-2004). This study pointed to a steady decline of non-empirical papers, a stable portion of groupware design and evaluation, high number of descriptive studies, and a constant growth in the number of papers characterizing group dynamics/collaboration settings testing hypothesis through experiments. In the particular domain of HCI, Henry et al. [19] presented a visual examination covering CHI, which denoted a high number of accepted papers, citations and references by paper. Frequent terms counted between 1983 and 2006 included usability, graphical interfaces, ubiquitous computing, augmented reality, and information visualization.

A different analysis of CHI conference [20] emphasized the number of authors by paper, repeat authorship at CHI and ACM CSCW, frequency of the number of authors per year, and CHI authors by gender. Nevertheless, Wainer et al. [21] evaluated the vast domain of computer science showing prevalence indicators for design and modeling. A quantitative analysis [8] on the countries and organizations that contributed to the success of CHI conference was performed for 26 years of publication.

A bibliometric study of the CHI conference proceedings [22] identified influential citation factors considering author's affiliation institution and country. Meanwhile, a bibliometric exercise was made for CRIWG Conference on Collaboration and Technology [23], analyzing 246 papers (2000-2008). A total number of 336 citations were calculated, resulting in a citation average of 1,37 per paper, a h-index of 6, and no citation values for 132 studies (53%). A list with most-cited papers and authors were presented, and research topics were identified taking into account their impact. Internationalization ratio decreased in the last biennium of analysis and the countries with greatest presence in CRIWG were Brazil, Chile, Germany, Portugal and Spain.

Furthermore, an analysis of 25 years of CSCW research in healthcare [24] included 128 papers (1988- 2011) published in JCSCW, CHI, ACM CSCW, ACM

International Conference on Supporting Group Work (GROUP), and European Conference on Computer-Supported Cooperative Work (ECSCW). Table 1 shows a general analysis of HCI bibliometrics research, demonstrating a quantitative orientation face to qualitative concerns, low citation rates for this kind of study, and a large number of bibliometric studies focused in the CHI conference.

Table 1. Bibliometric studies in CSCW and HCI contiguous literature

Year	Author(s)	Temporal coverage	Sample size	Bibliometric indicators[1]	Analytical dimensions
2003	Holsapple & Luo	1992-1999	7,364 papers	12 citations	Citation count; number of papers; rankings of influential journals; research approach
2004	Serenko & Bontis	1993-2002	450 papers	150 citations	Number of papers; citation count; affiliations; countries; co-authorship; top authors; top papers
2004	Horn et al.	1982-2003	22,887 publications	51 citations	Co-authorship networks; betweenness centrality; author rankings; number of members; citations by publication source and date; visibility and stability of the CSCW community
2006	Convertino et al.	1986-2002	300 papers	1 citation	Author affiliation; geographical location; level of analysis; type of study; CSCW characteristics; analysis of references; SNA
2006	Wania et al.	1990-2004	64 authors from HCI	27 citations	Co-citation count; cluster analysis; author co-citation map
2006	Jacovi et al.	1986-2004	465 papers	22 citations	Most quoted papers; modularity; clustering; betweenness centrality; chasm analysis
2006	Oulasvirta	1990-2006	CHI proceedings	2 citations	Most cited first authors; influential sites of research; productive authors; cited papers; expected citations
2007	Wainer & Barsottini	1998-2004	169 papers	14 citations	Number of papers; research approach; references
2007	Henry et al.	1983-2006	CHI, UIST, AVI and InfoVis proceedings	30 citations	Most prolific authors; most cited researchers; betweenness centrality; citation count; number of papers; number of references; acceptance rate; sources of key papers; keywords; co-authorship networks; macro structure; HCI communities
2007	Barkhuus & Rode [30]	1983-2006	CHI proceedings	35 citations	Research approach and methods; number of papers; average number of participants
2009	Kaye	1983-2008	CHI proceedings	5 citations	Author count; gender analysis; repeat authorship; conference growth
2009	Wainer et al.	2005	147 papers	12 citations	Research approach
2009	Bartneck & Hu	1981-2008	CHI proceedings	12 citations	Number of papers; pages per year; citation count; geographical distribution; number of authors; h-index; g-index; top organizations; affiliations; best paper awards
2010	Bartneck & Hu	1983; 1985-1991; 1993-2008	5,697 papers	5 citations	Network graph of continents and countries; collaboration conditioning factors; average number of organizations; citation count
2010	Antunes & Pino	2000-2008	246 papers	1 citation	Citation count; number of papers; top cited papers; top authors; country distribution; co-authorship; special issues; analysis of references; main research areas; research objectives; topics; evaluation methods; SWOT analysis
2012	Fitzpatrick & Ellingsen	1988-2011	128 papers	2 citations	Concept analysis; distribution of core CSCW-related papers by venue, year and country

3   Methodology and Approach

The partial characterization of the state of research in CSCW is enabled through a set of bibliometrics methods and techniques [25] and taxonomy-based analytics that allow to identify and compare collaboration technologies and functional attributes from the "rapidly expanding groupware arena" [11]. Research processes are fragmented to parameterize different stages for implementing the overall work of retrieving, analyzing, cataloguing and classifying publications. The methodology followed part of the systematic review protocol suggested by Kitchenham et al. [26], adapting guidelines from other bibliometric studies [6, 14, 22, 23], theory for analyzing, and content analysis with focus on the classification model used for taxonomic assessment [11].

---

[1] Retrieved from Google Scholar's citation index in January 2013.

3.1   Research Questions

The primary goal of this paper sets up in the possibility of evaluating the current state of research in CSCW at a bibliometric level, studying a representative sample of scientific literature production in the 21st century. The bibliometric study is intended to identify trends trough a quantitative analysis on bibliographic data entirely accessible from citation indexes, leading to the following Research Questions (RQ):

RQ1: Which conferences and journals dedicated to CSCW enable to identify technical gaps, impacts and variations over time and how they can be evaluated?

RQ2: What is the taxonomy with the most-appropriate categories to support a bibliometric analysis and how can be distilled the functional attributes of collaboration systems from literature?

RQ3: How to fill the gap between quantitative and qualitative dimensions concerning the current scientometrics paradigm?

The multidisciplinary nature of CSCW makes many authors publish their scientific papers in non-dedicated CSCW conferences and journals, which make it difficult to carry out a comprehensive bibliometric study covering the vast set of CSCW publications. This argument was validated by Jacovi *et al.* [6] in that "any heuristic chosen to identify which venue or publication belongs to CSCW field is error prone and will be subject to criticism and arguments". Devoted conferences and associated journals can represent a reliable sample, since the majority of CSCW authors present their work in these venues. Furthermore, their editorial boards include the most cited researchers.

In fact, there is no knowledge about a taxonomy with the adequate granularity for a CSCW literature classification. A representative fraction of the taxonomies presented in the literature [27] relies on the evaluation of temporal, spatial and technical properties, neglecting other semantic metadata analytical dimensions. The taxonomy selected for this study [11] has several categories to characterize the functional attributes of collaboration systems but presents critical limitations concerning the limitative spectrum of analysis, inconclusive results for particular units, constantly outdated categories, lack of semantic evidences, and cognitive effort to extract taxonomic units.

3.2   Inclusion and Exclusion Criteria

This paper covers a wide range of CSCW-devoted bibliography in order to represent a broader viewpoint of its scientific variations at a socio-technical level. Concerning the electronic databases selected for the paper extraction and citation analysis, the preference criteria by Google Scholar, ACM Digital Library and WoS relapsed on multiple literature-based factors. Digital libraries such as SpringerLink and IEEE Digital Library were not included in this analysis because its metadata does not contain citation and reference metadata [19]. According to Mikki [10], WoS is a useful data source for bibliometric analysis, where the journal selection process is based on published standards, expert opinions, regular publications and quality of information about citations. Comparatively, Google Scholar index covers more papers than WoS and provides an easy access to full texts [28]. Negative aspects of Google Scholar are related with its software resources, including an inadequate clustering of identical citations that result in duplications, inflated citation counts, and incapacity to identify all authors [29]. In citation analysis level, Google Scholar, ACM Digital Library and WoS remain updated, providing seeking mechanisms comparable in terms of coverage. Scopus was not included due to the lack of access to scientific metadata and a similarity to WoS.

Selection criteria to delimit the sample were defined by the following deterministic factors: complementariness to previous bibliometric studies; up-to-date metadata; free access to proceedings (i.e., ECSCW); online access (requiring a membership) to abstracts and full papers from ACM Digital Library, SpringerLink Libraries, IEEE Digital Library, and World Scientific; reference venues for regular publication by CSCW authors [3]; and iterant presence of CSCW topics in all venues, confining a specificity face to other conferences. Updated and diversified CHI-oriented bibliometric studies [8, 17, 19, 20, 30] represent the main factors by which CHI was not included.

3.3   Bibliometric Data Seeking, Collecting and Cataloguing Methods

Metadata was extracted, catalogued and selected for analysis including a total number of 1,480 publications, distributed by 5 conferences and 3 journals (Table 2). Publications included papers, posters and tutorials, and editorials and tables of contents without a linear structure for analysis were excluded. Some limitations in cataloguing can be explained in the absence of data on research evidences at a semantic level, authorship indicators, and coverage of venues such as CHI and MobileHCI, suggesting possible lines of future work. Citation data were directly accessed from Google Scholar, ACM Digital Library and WoS in November 2011. Nevertheless, only Google Scholar provided bibliometric indicators to all publications – WoS covers 1,081 papers, and ACM Digital Library only includes citation data related with 952 papers.

Table 2. Conferences and journals selected for bibliometric analysis

Type	Name	Acronym	Time interval	Number of papers
Conference	ACM International Conference on Supporting Group Work	GROUP	2003-2010	265[2]
	ACM Conference on Computer Supported Cooperative Work	CSCW	2004-2010	286
	European Conference on Computer-Supported Cooperative Work	ECSCW	2003-2009	90
	International Conference on Computer Supported Cooperative Work in Design	CSCWD	2006-2009	391
	CRIWG Conference on Collaboration and Technology	CRIWG	2006-2009	121
Journal	Computer Supported Cooperative Work: The Journal of Collaborative Computing and Work Practices	JCSCW	2003-2010	146
	International Journal of Computer-Supported Collaborative Learning	ijCSCL	2006-2010	103
	International Journal of Cooperative Information Systems	IJCIS	2006-2010	78

3.4   Taxonomic Evaluation Method for Technology-Oriented Publications

The classification of CSCW publications with a technological nature involved a parallel cataloguing process in which a total of 541 studies available in the proceedings of GROUP (2003-2010), ACM CSCW (2004-2008), ECSCW (2005-2007) and CRIWG (2006-2008) were classified. Selection criteria were based on different time intervals, diversity in their topics of interest, and identity of publication venues.

---

[2] This number includes 26 posters and 4 tutorials presented in ACM GROUP '10.

The evaluation of papers oriented to collaboration systems was based on a previous systematic review of taxonomic proposals [27] where Mittleman *et al.*'s [11] taxonomy was selected due to its reasonable granularity, timeliness to some current technologies, and capability to validate a general semantic analysis with the characteristics of collaboration tools introduced in the literature. However, this taxonomy does not cover some collaboration support systems (e.g., surface computing, and virtual worlds) or human-centered aspects (e.g., individual, group or crowd contexts using technology).

The "comparison scheme attributes for collaboration systems" [11] allow to "compare, contrast, optimize, and select among groupware technology implementation". Its most important attribute is the core capability provided by a tool (e.g., text-sharing, promoting social interaction and engagement whilst exchanging data between different entities). Content describes the kinds of data structures that may be used to a particular collaboration scenario (e.g., a pictorial image, object, or diagram). Relationships are associations established by users among contributions. A groupware system can support a set of actions that users can take on structures or relations (e.g., categorize). Synchronicity relates to the expected delay between the time that a user executes an action and the instant at which other users answer to that action. Identifiability is the degree to which users can set who executed an action (e.g., subgroup). Access controls are related with the configuration of user's rights and privileges. Session persistence is the degree to which contributions visibility is ephemeral or permanent. Alert mechanisms can be understood as interruptions or notifications used to attract immediate attention. Last but not least, awareness indicators represent the means by which a user may know what each group member have access to a session, the nature of their roles and their current status.

In other perspective, a "classification scheme for collaboration systems" [11] comprises a finer-grained application-level examination. Jointly authored pages are technologies that provide a shared window within which multiple users may contribute, usually simultaneously (i.e., conversation tools, shared editors, group dynamics tools, and polling tools). Streaming technologies provide a continuous feed of dynamic data (i.e., desktop/application sharing, audio, and video conferencing). Information access tools are technologies that provide group members with ways to store, share, find, and classify data objects (i.e., shared file repositories, social tagging systems, search engines, and syndication tools). Finally, aggregated systems combine technologies and tailor them to support a specific kind of task (e.g., Microsoft SharePoint, and Hojoki).

Comparison and classification schemes were used to identify opportunities for collaboration systems' developers and users by categorizing trends and gaps. A literature review based on this taxonomy produce evidences about the growth of attributes such as workplace awareness to coordinate group actions and avoid duplicated efforts, alert mechanisms to capture attention with minimal levels of distraction, or access controls to ensure a secure activity. However, further research is required updating these taxonomic units taking into account the variable requirements of collaboration systems. A limitation of this taxonomy relies on the lack of social-technical evidences that can be extracted from literature to correlate categories. Its granularity restricts the evaluation focus on technical mechanisms instead of social requirements.

Concerning the literature classification process, a first stage was constituted by an intensive reading of each paper's abstract, obtaining a perception about its subject. In the taxonomy-based classification, the abstract represent a first step for categorizing a technology-oriented or conceptual/theoretical study in order to analyze the nature of a collaboration technology taking into account its functional attributes and application-level category. The manual search by taxonomic terms allowed to refocus the classification process to Mitttleman *et al.*'s [11] taxonomic units, losing a semantic analysis at a less granular perspective. For specific contexts in which search by terms was not fully efficient, a process based on the full reading of each paper to achieve taxonomic evidences was adopted following contextual aspects provided by literature. A systematic cataloguing and systematization method concluded the evaluation process.

4   Findings

In the context of this bibliometric study (2003-2010), a set of variables was examined presenting their orientation, total and average number of citations and papers without citations. Bibliometric techniques adopted in this analysis reflected simple counts of papers correlating resultant metadata to visualize the evolution of this field in the 21st century. Impact factors and technological attributes were carefully measured by biennium and publication venue using structured and unstructured evaluation techniques that provide distinct perspectives on scientific metadata, a difficult task to perform by a single evaluator or research team.

4.1   Bibliometric Indicators of CSCW Research

Distinguishing types of publication (i.e., technological, or conceptual) is difficult due to the complexity of CSCW bibliography and misinterpretations resulting from human evaluation. The distinction was adapted from Wainer and Barsottini [18], assuming that technological papers are focused on a proposal, implementation or evaluation of collaboration working environments, whilst conceptual papers relies on theoretical, social/group dynamics, empirical concerns with real-world observation (i.e., ethnography), and ways of working and coordinating together. According to the results, a technological orientation is clearly noted, experiencing an inversion for the last years.

In a narrower range of analysis to what is possible to compare simultaneously from the three levels of indexing (Fig. 1), the average number of citations in the Google Scholar is higher in comparison to another indexes in all years, which denotes a comprehensive range and allows to achieve an accurate perspective on what is happening worldwide, encompassing not only citations in scientific papers but also its reference in other scientific literature such as Ph.D. theses, M.Sc. dissertations, and book chapters. It is also noted that some conferences occur every two years, which affects citation data influencing the overall results. An analysis performed to determine the average number of citations achievable from Google Scholar allowed to identify citation indexes with accentuated values for ECSCW (2003), JCSCW (2003, 2005) and ACM CSCW (2004). In an opposite level, CSCWD and CRIWG present the lower levels.

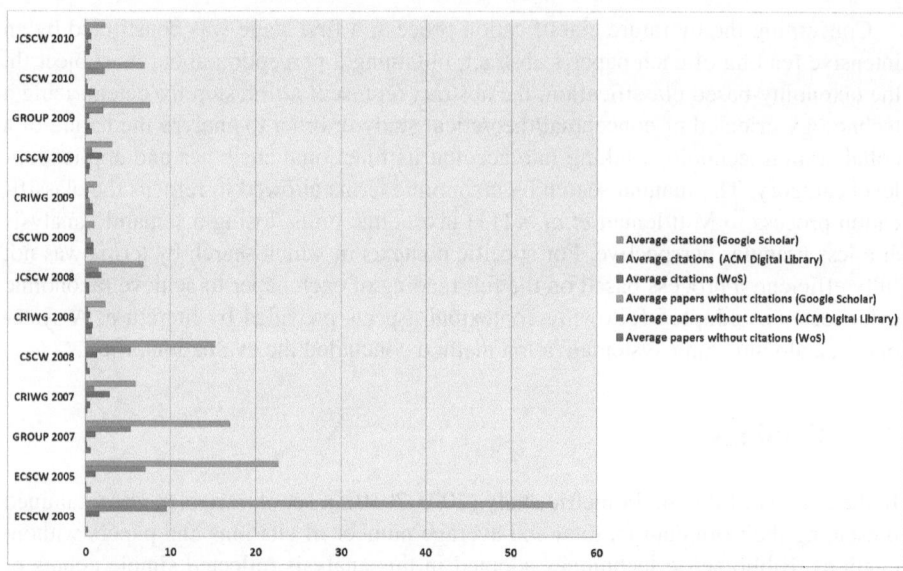

Fig. 1. Global analysis of comparable data in Google Scholar, ACM Digital Library and WoS

As shown in Fig. 2, it is possible to visualize the presence of CSCW researchers in the last biennium of the last decade (2009-2010), extracting the affiliation's country from each paper. Taking into account the results achieved with this analysis, USA was the most present country in GROUP (2009, 2010), ACM CSCW (2010), ECSCW (2009), ijCSCL (2009, 2010), and JCSCW (2009, 2010).

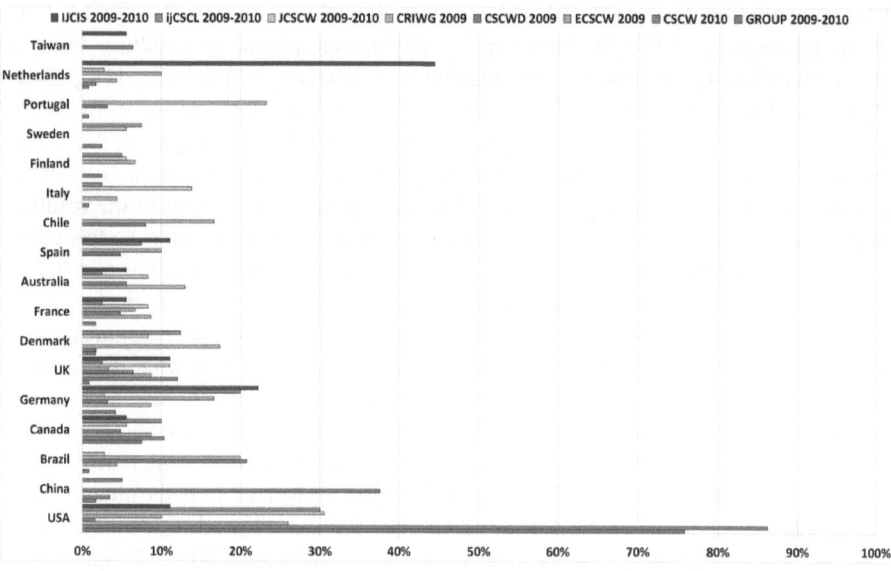

Fig. 2. Presence of CSCW researchers by affiliation's country (2009-2010)

The most present country in CSCWD (2009) was China, followed by Brazil. IJCIS represented a majority of authors from Netherlands, followed by Germany. Denmark and Australia denoted an active presence in ECSCW (2009), whilst Portugal, Brazil, Chile and Germany were the main contributing countries in CRIWG (2009). Other visible examples are Italy for JCSCW, France for ECSCW, and Canada for ijCSCL.

4.2   Taxonomy-Based Classification of Collaboration Systems

Technology-oriented classification included a total set of 541 documents in a biennial format demonstrating relationships between functional attributes and application-level domains, introduced from 4 CSCW-devoted conferences (2003-2010). The bars that represent the 2003-2004 biennium include GROUP, and ACM CSCW, whist the bars associated with the next two years (2005-2006) represent a fraction of the papers presented in GROUP, ACM CSCW, ECSCW, and CRIWG. The horizontal axis shows the percentage of occurrence of a specific taxonomic unit according to the amount of studies that discuss technological issues in CSCW bibliography.

Fig. 3 plots the results achieved with the study of the functional attributes of collaboration systems, organized by biennium and based on the comparison scheme suggested by Mittleman et al. [11]. Trends are identified with respect to text sharing/links (e.g., a blog, where users can provide shared text or links), graph (i.e., zero to many links for other objects) and list (i.e., ordered set of objects) relationships, add content, asynchronous systems, full anonymity and subgroup/pseudonym identification, inability to edit or delete contributions (which is not applicable in social interaction systems such as Facebook which contains a feature to edit comments), asynchronous systems, collaboration tools without notification/alert mechanisms, and awareness indicators.

On a different analytical perspective focused on the functional attributes of collaboration technologies by conference, general conclusions points to a prevalence of text sharing in CRIWG, its corresponding absence of awareness mechanisms, and its focus on identification issues. ECSCW denotes an interest by awareness, alert and identification mechanisms, access control, and an additional importance of text sharing associated with conferencing capabilities. ACM CSCW discards awareness in some systems but makes use of notification mechanisms and ephemeral contributions. In turn, GROUP shows a greater emphasis on text sharing with hyperlinks and asynchronous applications, representing a major venue for awareness tools in order to situate participants about the current state of work in progress.

Fig. 4 refers to the "classification scheme for collaboration tools" [11], where a preponderance of group dynamics tools (30%), and a steady increase of social tagging systems (5%), video conferencing (5%) and search engines (5%) are verified. Oppositely, audio conferencing (2%) and desktop/application sharing tools (8%) expressed a remarkable decrease. Aggregated systems (10%) showed a peak in 2005-2006 biennium, and shared file repositories (5%) denoted a decrease until the penultimate biennium, growing up in 2009. Syndication tools (6%) followed the same route, conversation systems (11%) were more addressed in the first biennia, shared editors (9%) was stable, and polling tools (13%) had great influence at a scientific level of analysis.

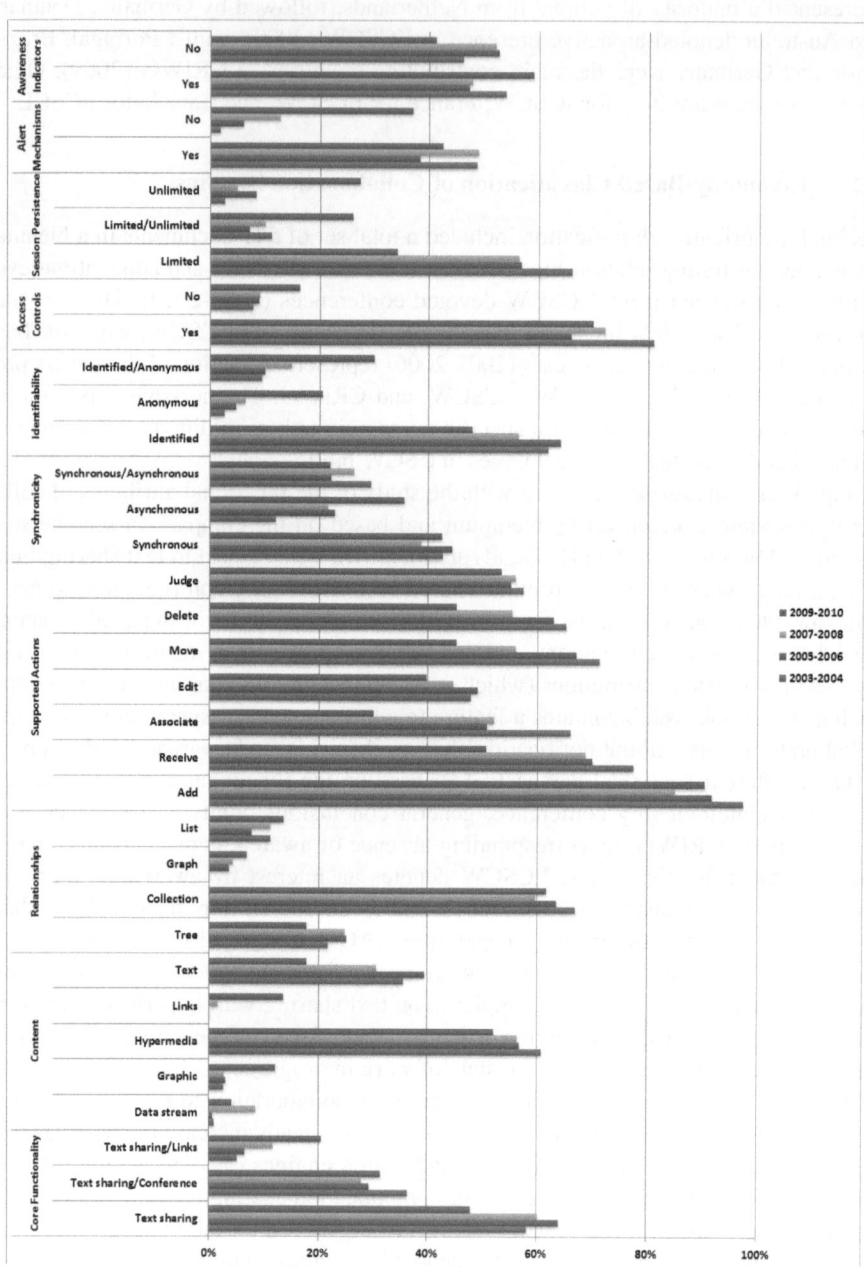

Fig. 3. Biennium analysis of the functional attributes of collaboration systems

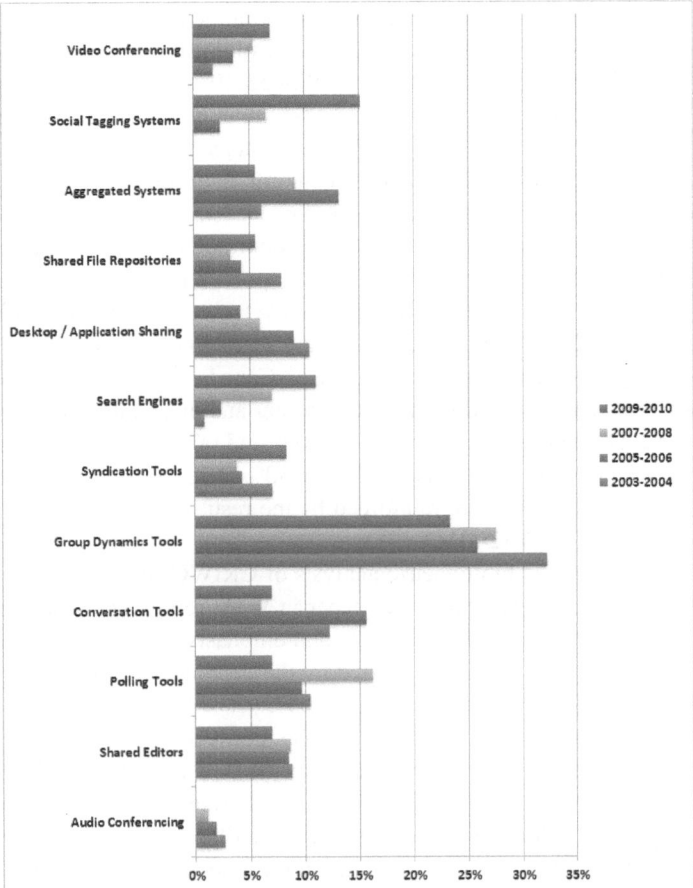

Fig. 4. Biannual analysis of application-level categories

For all publication venues, group dynamics tools represented the prevalent category. Transitioning to CRIWG, the interests are mainly focused on aggregated systems, polling tools, shared editors and desktop/application sharing tools, respectively. In the case of ECSCW, its scope relies on desktop/application sharing, followed by aggregated systems and conversation tools. ACM CSCW bet clearly in polling tools, conversation tools, shared editors and desktop/application sharing. Finally, GROUP has several studies spread over conversation systems, social tagging, aggregated systems, search engines and shared editors.

5   Discussion

Research papers devoted to collaborative computing appeared in multiple publication venues, reflecting its interdisciplinary identity. Concerning the JCSCW, it is oriented toward "design, implementation, and use of collaborative computing" and "has grown out of the computer science field with a strong sociological orientation" [12], a notion validated by the 2003-2010 dataset with a total of 53,4% sociological publications.

CSCW researchers had a high portion of co-authors outside their community upon the birth of the field in the mid-80s, maintaining connections to co-authors from non-CSCW devoted outlets (e.g., CHI) [14]. A temporal dispersion for cited studies in the ACM CSCW proceedings (2000-2002) represented a "strong bias toward citing recent papers within CSCW", which result can be corroborated by the deviation from trend in the number of citations shown in Fig. 1. It is important to note that North American (70-90%), European (10-30%) and Asian (0-10%) characterized the ACM CSCW participation (1986-2002) [15], which levels are maintained for the 2009-2010 biennium with strong representation from USA, UK, Canada and China. Its research contribution was primarily focused in the development and evaluation of architectures of computer systems, toolkits for collaborative tools, and other technology-related topics [6], and theoretical contributions declined from 30% to fewer than 10% since 1992 to 2002 [15]. These indicators were reinforced by the results presented in this bibliometric study for ACM CSCW (2004-2010).

In comparison with the bibliometric analysis of CRIWG research [23], similarities are identified in the average citation per paper in WoS, representativeness distributed by Portugal, Brazil, Chile, Spain and USA, and emphasis on prototyping and designing collaborative systems, which is verified by the percentage of technology-oriented papers (81,8%) published between 2006 and 2009.

At an application-level, advances in mobile networks and virtual worlds (i.e., Second Life) were achieved in the beginning of the new century. The 2003-2004 biennium introduced several approaches related with social interaction support tools such as Skype, Digg, Photobucket, MySpace, LinkedIn and World of Warcraft. The following year constituted a period of maturation for social network services and this explain an exponential increase of papers dedicated to technological issues, following a research trend identified by Jacovi *et al.* [6] for instant messaging. Under the banner of Web 2.0, social interaction support tools such as Facebook, Flickr and wiki-based services bring new forms cooperative work. It should be noted that services such as YouTube, Twitter, TeamViewer, Gmail, Wikispaces and Zoho emerged between 2005 and 2006. In the 2007-2008 biennium, collaboration tools like Dropbox and Google Docs introduced advances in storage capabilities and workspace awareness supported by cloud computing. Awareness indicators are still not a *sine qua non* condition in most collaboration tools, presenting a trend to increase. The year 2009 marked the creation of Google Wave, which had lost its consistency and ended its services in 2010. Although the year 2010 does not provide very specific data in our analysis, it is possible to observe a trend towards sociological purposes oriented to an understanding of the current practices and needs in collaborative working environments. Table 3 summarizes the main results obtained from the CSCW research review.

Table 3. Results and trends of the bibliometric review of CSCW research (2003-2010)

Category	Sample	Results	Trends
Bibliometrics	**Conferences** CSCWD (391[3]) GROUP (265) ACM CSCW (286) CRIWG (121) ECSCW (90) **Journals** JCSCW (146) ijCSCL (103) IJCIS (78)	**Citation analysis** <u>Average number of citations</u> ACM CSCW (30,08), JCSCW (24,22), ECSCW (21,99), ijCSCL (17,48), GROUP (15,07), IJCIS (10,33), CRIWG (3,9), CSCWD (1,45) <u>Number of papers without citations</u> CSCWD (177), GROUP (69), CRIWG (26), IJCIS (16), ijCSCL (12), JCSCW (10), ECSCW (6), ACM CSCW (5) **Type of study** <u>Conceptual/theoretical</u> JCSCW (78), ijCSCL (44), ACM CSCW (39), GROUP (34), CRIWG (22), ECSCW (15), IJCIS (14), CSCWD (1) <u>Technology-oriented</u> CSCWD (391), ACM CSCW (247), GROUP (217), CRIWG (99), ECSCW (75), JCSCW (68), IJCIS (64), ijCSCL (59) **Authorship** <u>Representativeness by country[4]</u> GROUP (USA, Canada, Germany), ACM CSCW (USA, UK, Canada, China), ECSCW (USA, Denmark, Australia, Canada, Germany, France), CSCWD (China, Brazil, Chile, UK, Taiwan), CRIWG (Portugal, Brazil, Germany, Chile), JCSCW (USA, Italy, UK, Denmark, France, Australia), ijCSCL (USA, Germany, Denmark, Canada), IJCIS (The Netherlands, Germany, Spain, USA, UK, France, Australia, Taiwan)	**Growth** <u>Citation analysis</u> JCSCW (2004-2005), IJCIS (2007-2009) <u>Type of study by venue</u> Conceptual/theoretical (GROUP, ACM CSCW, JCSCW, ijCSCL) Technology-oriented (CRIWG) <u>Type of study by year</u> Conceptual/theoretical (2005-2006, 2007-2008, 2009-2010) Technology-oriented (2004-2005, 2006-2007) **Decrease** <u>Citation analysis</u> GROUP (2003-2010), ECSCW (2003-2009), ACM CSCW (2004-2010), CRIWG (2007-2008), JCSCW (2003-2004, 2005-2009), ijCSCL (2006-2010), IJCIS (2006-2007, 2009-2010) <u>Type of study by venue</u> Conceptual/theoretical (CRIWG) Technology-oriented (GROUP, ACM CSCW, ECSCW, JCSCW) <u>Type of study by year</u> Conceptual/theoretical (2004-2005, 2006-2007) Technology-oriented (2005-2006, 2007-2008, 2009-2010) **Stagnation** <u>Citation analysis</u> CSCWD (2005-2009), CRIWG (2006-2007, 2008-2009), JCSCW (2009-2010), IJCIS (2007-2009) <u>Type of study by venue</u> Conceptual/theoretical (CSCWD, ECSCW, IJCIS) Technology-oriented (CSCWD, IJCIS, ijCSCL) <u>Type of study by year</u> Conceptual/theoretical (2003-2004, 2008-2009) Technology-oriented (2003-2004, 2008-2009)
Taxonomic classification	**Conferences** GROUP (217) ACM CSCW (215) CRIWG (72) ECSCW (37)	**Application-level categories by conference** <u>CRIWG</u> Shared editors, Group dynamics tools, Aggregated systems <u>ECSCW</u> Desktop/Application sharing, Video conferencing <u>ACM CSCW</u> Audio conferencing, Polling tools, Syndication tools <u>GROUP</u> Search engines, Social tagging systems **Functional attributes by conference** <u>CRIWG</u> Text sharing (core functionality), Tree (relationships), Receive, Associate, Edit and Delete (supported actions), Identified (identifiability), Access controls <u>ECSCW</u> Text sharing/Conference (core functionality), Data stream, Graphic, Links and Text (content), Graph and List (relationships), Move and Judge (supported actions), Asynchronous (synchronicity), Awareness indicators <u>ACM CSCW</u> Hypermedia (content), Collection (relationships), Add (supported actions), Synchronous and Synchronous/Asynchronous (synchronicity), Limited (session persistence), Alert mechanisms <u>GROUP</u> Text sharing/Links (core functionality), Anonymous and Identified/Anonymous (identifiability), Limited/Unlimited and Unlimited (session persistence)	**Growth** <u>Application-level categories</u> Social tagging systems, Search engines, Video conferencing <u>Functional attributes</u> Unlimited and Limited/Unlimited (session persistence), Asynchronous (synchronicity), Identified/Anonymous and Anonymous (identifiability), Text sharing/Links (core functionality), Links, Graphic and Data stream (content), Graph and List (relationships), Awareness indicators **Decrease** <u>Application-level categories</u> Group dynamics tools, Desktop / Application sharing, Conversation tools, Polling tools, Audio conferencing, Shared file repositories <u>Functional attributes</u> Text sharing and Text sharing/Conference (core functionality), Hypermedia and Text (content), Tree and Collection (relationships), All supported actions, Synchronous/Asynchronous (synchronicity), Identified (identifiability), Access controls, Limited (session persistence), Alert mechanisms **Stagnation** <u>Application-level categories</u> Aggregated systems, Syndication tools <u>Functional attributes</u> Synchronous (synchronicity)

---

[3] Total number of publications considered for bibliometric analysis.

[4] Data related with the last biennium of analysis (2009-2010).

5.1   Limitations

The limitations identified in this study are established in the following aspects: limitative spectrum of analysis; inconclusive results for several units; time-consuming with the laborious processes of data seeking, gathering, cataloguing, and classifying; static granularity of taxonomic schemes; lack of bibliometric perspectives (e.g., downloads, author's production and affiliation indicators); lack of more qualitative evidences that can be possible through semantic analytics; cognitive load; and lack of a case study with a massive number of humans interacting on bibliography.

In order to overcome the analytical gaps refereed above at a scientometric, human-centered perspective, a crowd-enabled model is suggested as a potential solution with emphasis on the stimulating challenge of infer about causal relations between science, technology and society through human-aware semantic analytics. To achieve this aim, a variety of Web measures will need to be compiled to establish a Scientometrics 2.0 paradigm [31]. Scientific data collection concerning research collaboration efforts is a difficult problem, and an integrated taxonomic and scientometric model represents an initial approach to track the emergence of new topics, gaps, trends and hypotheses at a massive scale taking into account the earlier findings in HCI and CSCW research.

5.2   Towards a Crowd-Enabled Model for Bibliographic Data Analytics

Human cognition as a powerful computing resource for scientometrics and semantic analytics from bibliography suggest different challenges associated with researchers and general public working on scientific data. Chi *et al.* [4] approached the research endeavor of Augmented Social Cognition as a "core value of research in HCI". This social evolution from Engelbart's prospect for a "human intellect augmentation" aims the enhancement of group abilities "to remember, think, and reason" augmenting aptitudes to acquire, produce, communicate and use knowledge, and to advance collective and individual intelligence in socially-mediated information environments [4].

Crowdsourcing is emerging as a production model in which networked people collaborate to complete complex tasks, including collaboration, ethical and legal aspects [35]. Whereas human computation replaces computers with humans, crowdsourcing replaces traditional human workers with members of the public [1]. However, CSCW and HCI research communities have advanced with few implementation proposals in that direction, showing hesitation [35]. More research is needed to characterize social dynamics in crowd-computer interaction working scenarios, identifying driving forces for mass collaboration, knowledge creation and problem-solving. Human factors need particular attention for design crowdsourcing systems with respect to their "assumed model of use" [2], confining to HCI the challenging mission of informing about principles and methodologies to improve the ways as humans interact through technology.

Citizen Science projects (e.g., Fold.it and Galaxy Zoo [1]) have engaged volunteers in collecting, analyzing and curating data. However, "few projects have reached the full collaborative potential of scientists and volunteers" [32], demonstrating a need to explore these human-centered contexts more deeply. Meta-knowledge about scientific production is founded upon shared vocabularies and practices. Aggregating efforts from cognitive operators evaluating bibliographic data can result in high quality re-sults, low cost (at the cognitive level), and production speediness [1], whilst are created social ties at an evolutionary and "mass" collaboration spectrum. This scena-rio can originate a novel working ecosystem for HCI researchers and general volun-teers within which a human crowd can contribute actively with different visions and expertise through a system that (indirectly) coordinates problem solving efforts.

If we move to the classification of HCI bibliography, crowds can be considered in-to the loop to evaluate bibliographic data under different perspectives. An open model supported by Human Intelligence Tasks (HITs) as semantically-potentiated units ex-ecuted by human computation and crowdsourcing [1] is suggested as an attempt to fill the socio-technical gaps of incompleteness, interpretation, organization and ambiguity in bibliographic metadata. A massive collaborative working ecosystem based on HITs performed by humans operating on different classification scales (e.g., folksonomies) within scientometrics and semantic analytics is required to produce meta-knowledge as a conceptual framework that can leverage the time and cognitive load improving the decision-making, learning and problem-solving efforts. A cost-effective, rapid and robust method is needed for assessing the quality of content analytics and social dy-namics [34]. Complementarily, shared mental models merit particular consideration for understanding users working massively.

Fig. 5 represents the suggested crowd-enabled model, taking into account the cur-rent status of digital libraries in which a user can only retrieve papers in a PDF format or elementary bibliometric indicators without semantic analytics behind bibliography. Bibliographic data can be processed by human crowds which members are exposed to external and internal factors (e.g., knowledge background, and motivation). Humans can use different technologies (e.g., text mining, and bibliometric tools) and methods for analysis. HITs are created by users and associated to collaboration features (e.g., metadata annotation, comment, and data classification) to produce metadata. Outputs are expected in a form of knowledge base supported by distinct visualization scales.

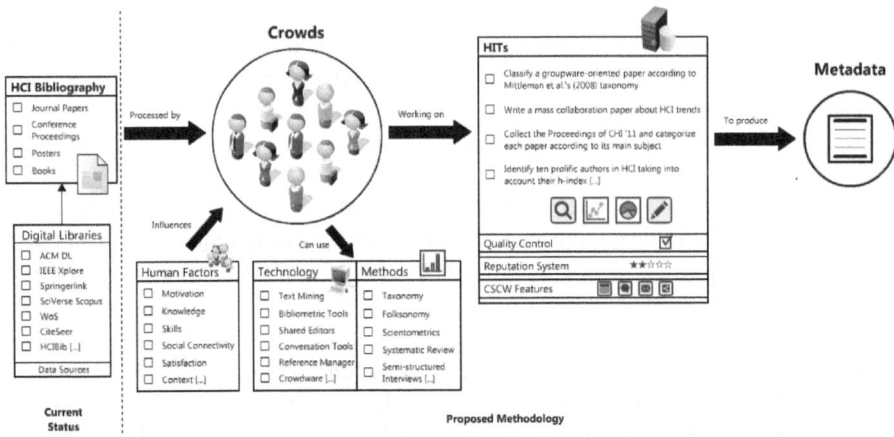

Fig. 5. Crowd-enabled model for bibliographic data analytics

6   Concluding Remarks and Future Directions

Despite efforts using statistical methods to measure the growing volumes of scientific bibliography annually published in the fields of HCI and CSCW, classification biases remain as a recurrent problem for human evaluators due to the polymorphic nature of bibliographic data. This challenging scenario requires innovative ways of analysis that can be articulated in scientometrics, bibliometrics, cybermetrics, text mining and machine learning, knowledge domain visualization and social semantic analytics through crowdsourcing and human computation mechanisms. Putting crowds into the loop of science evaluation can improve the current labor-intensive, time-consuming, difficult to repeat and sometimes subjective task of scientometricians. The cognitive power provided by human crowds can be aggregated as a powerful computing resource [1]. As result, this purpose can lead to evaluate the impact of scientific production, impact on society at an evolutionary spectrum, as well as social-technical, cultural and political repercussions in a "mass" collaboration effort. In order to overcome the circumscription of quantitative studies by scientometrics, inconsistency problems and lack of qualitative studies in CSCW, an integrated classification approach is required. Human factors in a scientometric- and semantic-based massive collaboration scenario are thus seen as a field of study to broaden knowledge frontiers through social dynamics.

Although Priem and Hemminger [31] have introduced the paradigm of Scientometrics 2.0 sustained in the evaluation of scholars, recommendation of papers and global study of science in order to monitor the growth of scientific literature using Web 2.0 tools (e.g., data repositories, social bookmarking, social networks, or microblogging), a challenging way expects HCI community to achieve comprehensive results through retrieving, cataloguing, classifying and analyzing a set of bibliographical, schematic, and video-based artifacts to paint a "big picture" of scientific meta-knowledge.

Due to the current limitations identified in this bibliometric study with a total set of 1,480 publications (2003-2010), it is important to reformulate results broadening the sample, exploring different perspectives of analysis, and providing more conclusive insights. Analyzing bibliometric data on co-authorship networks, topics or affiliations can be described as lines of future work. It is expected to examine more citation indexes (e.g., Scopus), publication venues (such as CHI, NordiCHI, and SouthCHI) and fields of research to broaden this hybrid bibliometric approach.

The crowd-enabled model for bibliographic data analytics will be validated in the future through several experiments involving humans working cooperatively on HCI-related scientific metadata. The prototype of an observatory for CSCW and HCI publications [33] is under development and will serve to identify requirements and validate a human-aware research ecosystem based on the aggregation of massive collaboration efforts around bibliographic data.

Acknowledgments. This work is funded (or part-funded) by the ERDF – European Regional Development Fund through the COMPETE Programme (operational programme for competitiveness) and by National Funds through the FCT – Fundação para a Ciência e a Tecnologia (Portuguese Foundation for Science and Technology) within project «FCOMP - 01-0124-FEDER-022701».

References

1. Quinn, A.J., Bederson, B.B.: Human Computation: a survey and taxonomy of a growing field. In: Proceedings of the ACM Conference on Human Factors in Computing Systems (CHI 2011), pp. 1403–1412 (2011)

2. Schmidt, K.: The concept of 'work' in CSCW. Computer Supported Cooperative Work 20(4-5), 341–401 (2011)

3. Grudin, J., Poltrock, S.E.: Taxonomy and theory in Computer Supported Cooperative Work. In: Kozlowski, S.W.J. (ed.) The Oxford Handbook of Industrial and Organizational Psychology. Oxford University Press, New York (2012)

4. Chi, E.H., Pirolli, P., Suh, B., Kittur, A., Pendleton, B., Mytkowicz, T.: Augmented social cognition: using Social Web technology to enhance the ability of groups to remember, think, and reason. In: Proceedings of the 35th SIGMOD International Conference on Management of Data Providence (2009)

5. Nichols, D.M., Twidale, M.B., Cunningham, S.J.: Metadatapedia: a proposal for aggregating metadata on data archiving. In: Proceedings of the ACM iConference 2012, pp. 370–376 (2012)

6. Jacovi, M., Soroka, V., Gilboa-Freedman, G., Ur, S., Shahar, E., Marmasse, N.: The chasms of CSCW: a citation graph analysis of the CSCW conference. In: Proceedings of the ACM Conference on Computer Supported Cooperative Work, CSCW 2006 (2006)

7. Sajid, N.A., Ali, T., Afzal, M.T., Ahmad, M., Qadir, M.A.: Exploiting reference section to classify paper's topics. In: Proceedings of the ACM Conference on Management of Emergent Digital Ecosystems (MEDES 2011), pp. 220–225 (2011)

8. Bartneck, C., Hu, J.: Scientometric analysis of the CHI proceedings. In: Proceedings of the ACM Conference on Human Factors in Computing Systems, pp. 699–708 (2009)

9. Nicolaisen, J.: Bibliometrics and citation analysis: from the Science Citation Index to cybermetrics. Journal of the American Society for Information Science and Technology 61(1), 205–207 (2010)

10. Mikki, S.: Google Scholar compared to Web of Science: a literature review. Nordic Journal of Information Literacy in Higher Education 1(1), 41–51 (2009)

11. Mittleman, D.D., Briggs, R.O., Murphy, J., Davis, A.: Toward a taxonomy of groupware technologies. In: Briggs, R.O., Antunes, P., de Vreede, G.-J., Read, A.S. (eds.) CRIWG 2008. LNCS, vol. 5411, pp. 305–317. Springer, Heidelberg (2008)

12. Holsapple, C.W., Luo, W.: A citation analysis of influences on collaborative computing research. Computer Supported Cooperative Work 12(3), 351–366 (2003)

13. Serenko, A., Bontis, N.: Meta-review of knowledge management and intellectual capital literature: citation impact and research productivity rankings. Knowledge and Process Management 11(3), 185–198 (2004)

14. Horn, D.B., Finholt, T.A., Birnholtz, J.P., Motwani, D., Jayaraman, S.: Six degrees of Jonathan Grudin: a social network analysis of the evolution and impact of CSCW research. In: Proceedings of the ACM Conference on Computer Supported Cooperative Work (CSCW 2004), pp. 582–591 (2004)

15. Convertino, G., George, T., Councill, I.: Mapping the intellectual landscape of CSCW. In: Proceedings of the ACM Conference on Computer Supported Cooperative Work (2006)

16. Wania, C.E., Atwood, M.E., McCain, K.W.: How do design and evaluation interrelate in HCI research? In: Proceedings of the 6th Conference on Designing Interactive Systems, pp. 90–98 (2006)

17. Oulasvirta, A.: A bibliometric exercise for SIGCHI Conference on Human Factors in Computing Systems (2006), http://www.hiit.fi/node/290 (retrieved in January 2013)

18. Wainer, J., Barsottini, C.: Empirical research in CSCW – a review of the ACM/CSCW conferences from 1998 to 2004. Journal of the Brazilian Computer Society 13, 27–36 (2007)
19. Henry, N., Goodell, H., Elmqvist, N., Fekete, J.-D.: 20 years of four HCI conferences: a visual exploration. International Journal of Human Computer Interaction 23(3), 239–285 (2007)
20. Kaye, J.: Some statistical analyses of CHI. In: Proceedings of the ACM Conference on Human Factors in Computing Systems (CHI 2009), pp. 2585–2594 (2009)
21. Wainer, J., Barsottini, C.G.N., Lacerda, D., de Marco, L.: Empirical evaluation in computer science research published by ACM. Information and Software Technology 51(6), 1081–1085 (2009)
22. Bartneck, C., Hu, J.: The fruits of collaboration in a multidisciplinary field. Scientometrics 85(1), 41–52 (2010)
23. Antunes, P., Pino, J.: A review of CRIWG research. In: Kolfschoten, G., Herrmann, T., Lukosch, S. (eds.) CRIWG 2010. LNCS, vol. 6257, pp. 1–15. Springer, Heidelberg (2010)
24. Fitzpatrick, G., Ellingsen, G.: A review of 25 years of CSCW research in healthcare: contributions, challenges and future agendas. In: Computer Supported Cooperative Work, pp. 1–57 (2012)
25. Garfield, E.: Citation indexes to science: a new dimension in documentation through association of ideas. Science 122, 108–111 (1955)
26. Kitchenham, B., Brereton, O.P., Budgen, D., Turner, M., Bailey, J., Linkman, S.: Systematic literature reviews in software engineering – a systematic literature review. Information and Software Technology 51, 7–15 (2009)
27. Cruz, A., Correia, A., Paredes, H., Fonseca, B., Morgado, L., Martins, P.: Towards an overarching classification model of CSCW and groupware: a socio-technical perspective. In: Herskovic, V., Hoppe, H.U., Jansen, M., Ziegler, J. (eds.) CRIWG 2012. LNCS, vol. 7493, pp. 41–56. Springer, Heidelberg (2012)
28. Haglund, L., Olsson, P.: The impact on university libraries of changes in information behavior among academic researchers: a multiple case study. The Journal of Academic Librarianship 34(1), 52–59 (2008)
29. Jacsó, P.: Google Scholar revisited. Online Information Review 32(1), 102–114 (2008)
30. Barkhuus, L., Rode, J.: From mice to men – 24 years of evaluation in CHI. In: Proceedings of the ACM Conference on Human Factors in Computing Systems (CHI 2007) (2007)
31. Priem, J., Hemminger, B.: Scientometrics 2.0: toward new metrics of scholarly impact on the Social Web. First Monday 15(7) (2010)
32. Rotman, D., Preece, J., Hammock, J., Procita, K., Hansen, D., Parr, C., Lewis, D., Jacobs, D.: Dynamic changes in motivation in collaborative citizen-science projects. In: Proceedings of the ACM Conference on Computer Supported Cooperative Work (2012)
33. Santos, J., Paredes, H., Fonseca, B., Correia, A.: Preliminary study of an observatory for CSCW scientific publications. In: Proceedings of the 18th International Conference of European University Information Systems organisation (EUNIS 2012): E-science and E-repositories. Virtual Libraries, Virtual Laboratories (2012)
34. Kittur, A., Chi, E., Suh, B.: Crowdsourcing for usability: using micro-task markets for rapid, remote, and low-cost user measurements. In: Proceedings of the ACM Conference on Human Factors in Computing Systems (CHI 2008) (2008)
35. Schneider, D., Moraes, K., de Souza, J.M., Esteves, M.G.P.: CSCWD: five characters in search of crowds. In: Proceedings of the 16th International Conference on Computer Supported Cooperative in Design (CSCWD 2012), pp. 634–641 (2012)

An Empirical Evaluation of a Usability Measurement Method in a Model Driven Framework

Lassad Ben Ammar and Adel Mahfoudhi

University of Sfax, ENIS, CES Laboratory
Soukra Road km 3,5, B.P: 1173-3000 Sfax Tunisia
benammar_lassad@hotmail.com,
adel.mahfoudhi@ceslab.org

Abstract. Usability is increasingly considered as a basic determinant of the Interactive Systems (IS) success. An IS that satisfies all the functional requirements can be rejected by end-users if it presents usability problems. Unusable User Interface (UI) is probably the main reason that may lead to the failure in the actual use of an IS. Therefore, several approaches dealing with the evaluation of the user interface usability have been proposed in literature. However, these approaches are focused on the final system and require a large amount of resources to perform the evaluation (end-users, video cameras, questionnaires, etc.). The ability to go back and makes major changes to the design is greatly reduced. It is widely accepted that the evaluation performed at the beginning of the development process is a critical part of ensuring that the product will be used and effective for its intended purpose. In addition, an early usability evaluation would be a significant advantage with regard to saving time and resources.

The purpose of the present paper is to investigate the integration of the usability issues at an early stage of the development process. A model based approach is presented and empirically evaluated.

Keywords: Plastic User Interface, Usability Model, Empirical Evaluation, Model Driven Engineering.

1 Introduction

Usability denotes the ease of use of a system for a particular class of users carrying out specific tasks in a specific environment. It is widely considered as a basic determinant of the acceptance of an interactive system [4]. Unusable User Interface (UI) is probably the main reason that may lead to the failure in the actual use of an interactive system [28]. For that reason, a variety of approaches have been adopted in literature in order to evaluate the usability of user interfaces ([8], [20], [26], among them). However, these methods involve activities that require a huge amount of resources (usability experts, questionnaire, several end users, usability laboratory, etc). They are focused in the final product in order to

A. Holzinger et al. (Eds.): SouthCHI 2013, LNCS 7946, pp. 157–173, 2013.

carry out the evaluation. Consequently, changes to the user interface are costly and difficult to implement.

In recent years, the emergency of a wide spectrum of interactive devices has raised new issues for user interface designers and developers. They are facing the challenge of producing not only a highly usable user interfaces but also that can be adapted in order to enable different classes of users to access information regardless of the interactive devices they are using even when the environment changes dynamically. [29] used the term *Plastic* to indicate this kind of user interfaces. Within this context, several approaches have been proposed. Those following the Model Driven Engineering[1] (MDE) [27] principles proved quite appropriate [13]. A renowned work in this context is the Cameleon projet [11] which provides a unifying reference framework for the user interface development taking into consideration the context of use wherein the interaction takes place. The main limitation of the Cameleon framework is that research efforts have focused only on the functional aspect of the user interface adaptation while neglecting usability. Usability is considered as a natural by-product of whatever approach was being used. Therefore, there is a need to expand the Cameleon framework in order to change perspective and make usability a first class entity in its development process.

The main objective of this paper is to promote the usability issue as a first class entity in the Cameleon framework. To do so, we propose to expand such framework by considering usability engineering as a part of the development process. We propose to carry out the evaluation from the conceptual models.The objective is to make usability evaluation independent from the system implementation and to reduce the development costs involved by measuring the usability late in the development process. The proposed usability evaluation method is based on a usability model which decomposes usability on measurable attributes and metrics. It is intended to isolate potential usability problems so as to determine a figure of merit of the overall interface.

The remainder of this paper is structured as follows. While Section 2 presents an outline of the usability methods quoted in the literature, section 3 provides a brief description of our proposed to integrate usability issue into an MDE method. The proposed usability model is described in Section 4, and the empirical study to evaluate the proposed usability model is illustrated in section 5. Finally, Section 6 presents the conclusion and provides perspectives for future research work.

2   Related Works

The usability evaluation is often defined in [24] as methodologies for measuring the usability aspects of a user interface and identifying specific problems. There exist several methods addressing the usability evaluation of the user interfaces. In

---

[1] Model Driven Engineering MDE: a software approach which promotes a new form of building software systems based on the construction and maintenance of models at different levels of abstraction to drive the development process

this section, the focal point is on the analysis of model-based methods since our main motivation is to integrate usability issues into a model driven development approach.

Model-based usability evaluation methods specify usability attributes and metrics required to assess the user interface in order to identify potential usability problems. Usability models are usually based on existing standards such as ISO/IEC 9126-1 [18] and ISO/IEC 9241-11 [2]. In fact, both standards are useful in providing principles and recommendations. However, they are abstract and need to be extended and / or decomposed for their use on different kinds of systems.

[3] proposed a usability model that extends the ISO/IEC 9126-1 model, which is intended to evaluate the usability of a user interface from the beginning of an MDE approach. The main limitation of this proposal is the lack of guidelines about how usability attributes are measured and how to interpret their scores. An extension of this model is proposed in [15] in order to assess web applications.

[28] reviewed the existing usability standards and models to detect their limitation and complementarities. As a result, a consolidated model (QUIM) based on the ISO/IEC 9241-11 standard is proposed. Other relevant characteristics such as Learnability and Security are extracted from ISO/IEC 9126-1 and other resources to enrich the model. The QUIM model includes metrics that are based on the system code as well as on the generated interface. This makes the application of the QUIM to a model driven development process difficult.

[5] evaluated the usability of multi-devices user interfaces in terms of effectiveness, efficiency and satisfaction. The usability evaluation is based on the experiments with end-users. This dependency is incompatible with an early usability evaluation.

[25] proposes an early usability measurement method. The usability evaluation is carried out early in the development process since the conceptual model. The main limitation of this proposal is that metrics are specific to the OO-method [16]. Therefore, they cannot be applied to other method, which is a disadvantage. They need some adaptation in order to be used (adopted) in other similar methods.

Considering the research works just mentioned, three main limitations are underlined. The first problem is the lack of measurement details. The proposals (except the proposition of Panach) specify usability attributes and metrics without defining how these metrics should be measured and how to interpret their scores. The second problem is the need for the system implementation. Most proposals carry out the evaluation at the last step of the development process which is incompatible with an automatic early evaluation. Regardless of the approach, none of them takes into account the variation of context elements during their process activities and the influence it brings to the selection of the most relevant attributes and metrics.

It becomes clear that integrating usability issues into an MDE method for plastic user interface generation is still an immature area. Therefore many more research works are needed. However, it should be noted that the aforementioned models are useful in providing guidelines about the most relevant attributes required to measure the user interface usability. They can be a useful resource from which we draw our proposal model.

3   Proposed Method to Integrate Usability into a Model Driven Development Process

3.1   Overview

As already mentioned, the main motivation of this paper is to integrate usability issues as a part of the development process of the Cameleon framework. In fact, the choice of the Cameleon framework is motivated by the fact that such framework unifies models, methods and tools for the generation of user interfaces for multiple contexts of use. The Cameleon framework structures the development process into four levels of abstraction, starting from task specification to a running interface.

- The Task and Concepts: brings together the concepts and the tasks descriptions produced by the designers for that particular interactive system and that particular context of use.
- The Abstract User Interface (AUI): this level represents the user interface in terms of interaction spaces (or presentation units), independently of which interactors are available on the targets.
- The Concrete User Interface (CUI): this level turns an Abstract UI into an interactor-dependent expression.
- The Final User Interface (FUI): this level consists of source code, in any programming or mark-up language (e.g., Java, HTML, etc.).

In the Cameleon framework, conceptual models are a primary artifact in the analysis and design of an interactive system. They are used to define the user requirements and as a basis for developing interactive systems to meet these requirements. In the software engineering field, the quality of the conceptual models is usually neglected. Research efforts have focused on the quality of the final product. However, more that half of the errors which occur during the systems development are requirement errors [14]. The correction of a post-implemented error is more than 100 times more costly to correct it during the requirement analysis [9]. Therefore, it is more effective to concentrate on the quality assurance from the conceptual models. In the present paper, we focus our interest in the usability characteristic which is largely considered as one, among other, of the most important quality characteristic. We argue that ensuring the usability of a user interface, generated according to the Cameleon framework, from the conceptual model can be an appealing way to ensure the usability of this user interface.

The conceptual models covers the abstract user interface level and the concrete one. The concrete user interface is the most affected by usability. For that reason, we opted to perform the evaluation from the concrete user interface (Fig.1).

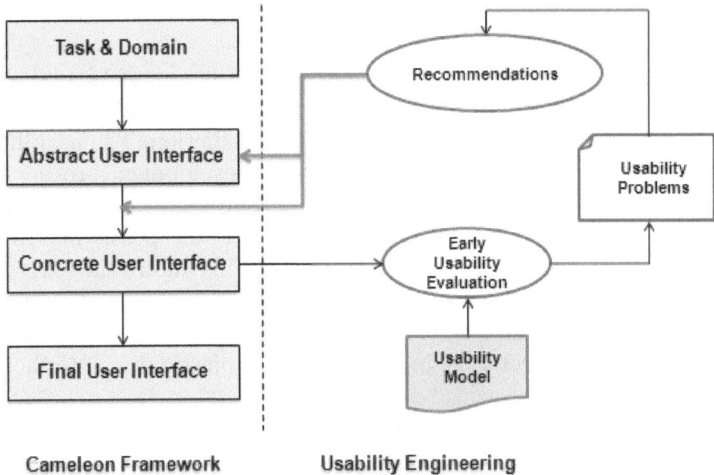

Fig. 1. Proposed Method to Early Usability Evaluation in the Cameleon Framework

As far as the early usability measurement method is concerned, it extends the one presented in [25]. In such proposition, the usability is evaluated from the conceptual model. The usability metrics presented in this proposition are adapted since they are specific for the OO-method. The applicability of our proposed method is shown in the present paper through Cameleon-Compliant method presented in [10]. Such method follows the MDE principles and use the BPMN [1] notion to define the user interface models. The BPMN notation is built on the Petri networks which allows the validation of the user interface models.

The extension covers three steps. The first is the add of some other usability attributes and metrics which are relevant in the context of plastic user interface (e.g., *Prompting* and *Informative Feedback*). These attributes are not only closely related to the user features, but also crucial to better guide a user with a low level of experience in interacting with computer. This explains the importance of their measurement in the context of plastic user interface. We also add the Attractiveness attributes. We argue that this sub-characteristic is crucial since it presents attributes that are related to the user preferences such as the color and the font style presented in the user interfaces. The second step is to adapt the concept of some usability metrics in order to be compatible with the underlying method. The last step is association of a priority index (weight) with each usability attribute in the grouping function. This step aims at promoting the most relevant usability properties with respect to the population characteristics and/or the task requirements.

Generally speaking, our proposed early usability measurement method is made up on four stages: 1) attributes specification, 2) metrics definition, 3) indicators definition, and 4) grouping function establishment.

3.2 Early Usability Measurement

The proposed early usability measurement method is a model-based approach. This category of usability evaluation method employs a usability model and a user interface model to generate a user interface prediction. The usability model is intended to be used in a plastic user interface development process from the conceptual models. For that reason, we take into account two key factors when we propose the usability attributes. The first one is the possibility to be measured quantitatively from the conceptual model. This allows the early usability evaluation and the automation of the evaluation process. The second is the relation between each usability attributes and the features of the context of use. This make the attribute relevant in the context of plastic user interface.

Attribute Specification. With regard to the Learnability sub-characteristic, we propose to associate the following attributes: *Prompting, Predictability* and *Informative Feedback*. The *Prompting* refers to the information provided to the user about the system status, possible or expected actions. The *Predictability* focuses on the available means that help the user to predict his future action. In fact, knowing the possible actions and their consequences may decrease the probability of errors. The *Informative Feedback* concerns the system's response to the user action. With respect to the user characteristics (expert, novice, etc.), learnability attributes will be considered as essential or optional in order to guarantee a high level of user satisfaction. The user without experience in similar application should be guided at all times.

The Understandability sub-characteristic can be decomposed into many attributes. The first attribute is the *Information Density* which is the user's workload from a perceptual and cognitive point of view pertaining to a set of elements. Next, *Brevity* focus on the reduction of the user's cognitive efforts (number of action steps). The short-term memory capacity is limited. Consequently, shorter entries reduce considerably the probability of making errors. Besides, *Navigability* pertains to the ease with which a user can move around in the application. Finally, *Message Concision* concerns the use of few words while keeping expressiveness in the error message. The majority of understandability attributes are related to the platform features. For example, the screen size has strong influences to the information density, the navigability and the brevity attributes.

Operability includes attributes that facilitate the user's control and operation of the system. We propose the following attributes: *User Operation Cancellability*, the possibility to cancel actions without harmful effect to the normal operation; *User Operation Undoability*, the proportion of actions that can be undone without harmful effect to the normal operation; *Explicit User Action*, the system should perform only actions requested by the user; *Error Prevention*, available means to detect and prevent data entry errors, command errors, or actions with destructive consequences. Interactive systems should allow a high level of control to users especially those with a low level of experience. Hence, the user interface is obliged to present interface components allowing such control.

The screen size of the platform being used can affect this control when it does not allow displaying button like undo, cancel, validate, etc.

The Attractiveness sub-characteristic includes the attributes of software products, which are related to the aesthetic design to make it attractive to the user. We argue that some aspects of attractiveness can be measured with regard to the *Font Style Uniformity* and *Color Uniformity*. The *Consistency* measures the maintaining of the design choice to similar contexts. The user preferences in terms of color or font style are related to the attractiveness attributes. It should be noted that some environment features (e.g. indoor/outdoor, luminosity level) affect the choice of the color in order to obtain a good contrast that gives clearer information.

Fig. 2 shows an overview of our proposal for attributes specification. The added attributes are colored red.

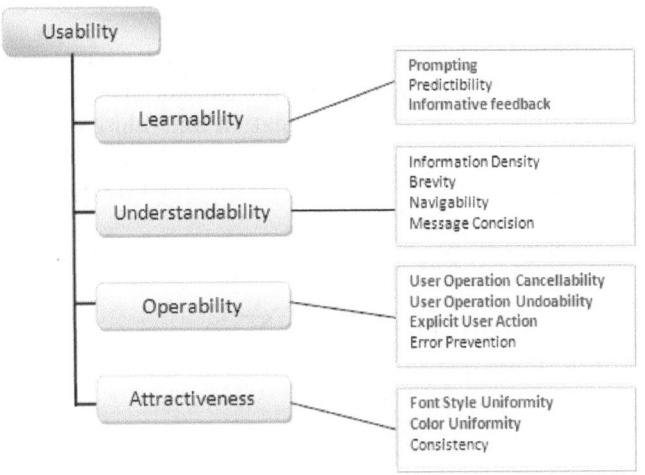

Fig. 2. Proposed Usability Model

Metric Definition. Metrics definition is crucial in order to be able to measure the usability of internal attributes. Metrics are intended to be used since the conceptual models. Therefore, they should be founded on the basis of the conceptual primitives of the underlying method. It should be noted that even though the metrics are specific to the method presented in [10], the concept of each one can be applied to any MDE method with similar conceptual primitives. As already mentioned, our proposed method is intended to evaluate the usability of plastic user interface from the conceptual models. We opted for metrics that are closely related to some context features and can be affected when these features changes. However, it should be noted that the user capacity and preferences, the screen size of the platform being used and the luminosity of the environment are the most considered features when defining the metrics. In what follows, we list the definition of some examples of these metrics. It is recommended to look at the description of the underlying method presented in [10] in order to better understand some specific terminologies.

Prompting
One way to guide the user to enter correct data is to display the required data format when it is necessary. Hence, user interface should display as maximum as possible the supplementary information to better guide the user. We propose to calculate the average of label that display supplementary information as a metric to measure the prompting attribute (PR).

$$PR = \sum_{i=1}^{n} StaticField()/n. \tag{1}$$

StaticField() returns the number of labels (UIStaticField in the proposition of [10]) that display additional information.

Information Density
It is usually recommended to have user interface which are not too dense. The information density can be measured using the number of elements per interface to keep a good equilibrium between information and white space. We propose four metrics: the number of input elements (ID1), the number of action elements (ID2), the number of navigation element (ID3) and the total number of elements per user interface (ID4).

The average of field edit per user interface (UIWindow in [10]).

$$ID1 = \sum_{i=1}^{n} xi / \sum_{i=1}^{n} yi. \tag{2}$$

x ∈ (UIFieldEdit), y ∈ (UIWindow).
The average of action elements per user interface.

$$ID2 = \sum_{i=1}^{n} xi / \sum_{i=1}^{n} yi. \tag{3}$$

x ∈ (UIFieldAction), y ∈ (UIWindow).

Brevity
Due to the capacity of the human memory which cannot retain more than three scenarios, we propose the number of step (counted in keystrokes) required to accomplish a goal or a task from the source screen (UIWindow) to the target screen.

$$MA = distance(x, y). \tag{4}$$

x,y ∈(UIWindow), distance(x,y) returns the distance between x and y.

Navigability

The navigability can be measured by counting the number of navigation elements per user interface (Navigation Breadth).

$$NB = \sum_{i=1}^{n} xi / \sum_{i=1}^{n} yi. \tag{5}$$

x $\in$ (UIFieldNavigation), y $\in$ (UIWindow).

Message Concision

Since the quality of the message is a subjective measure, we propose the number of word as an internal metric to measure the quality of the message.
The number of word in a message

$$WN = \sum_{i=1}^{n} xi. \tag{6}$$

x $\in$ (word in UIDialogBox).

Error Prevention

To prevent the user from error while entering data, we propose to use a conceptual primitive which represents a list (dropdown list, radio button, etc) when the input element have a set of limited possible values.

$$ERP = \sum_{i=1}^{n} list(x)/n. \tag{7}$$

x $\in$ (UIFieldIn with limited possible values), *list* return the number of primitive which represents a list (UIFieldList).

Indicator Definition. The previously defined metrics provides a numerical value that needs to have a meaning in order to be interpreted. The mechanism of indicator is restored in order to reach such a goal. It consists in the attribution of qualitative values to each numerical one. Such qualitative values can be summarized in: Very Good (VG), Good (G), Medium (M), Bad (B) and Very Bad (VB). For each qualitative value, we assign a numerical range. The ranges are defined on the basis of some usability guidelines and heuristics described in the literature. Next, we detail the numeric ranges associated with some metrics in order to be considered as a Very Good value.

- Prompting: Some usability guidelines recommend the use of additional information (e.g. the required data format) in order to better guide the user during entering data [7]. At least 95% of the input element labels should display information (Prompting PR).
- Predictability: usability guidelines recommend action label that should be clear, descriptive and meaningful. 95% of action labels should be non-default labels and display supplementary information in order to increase usability [25] (Action Determination AD).

- Information Density: several usability guidelines recommend minimizing the density of a user interface [22]. We define a maximum number of elements per user interface to keep a good equilibrium between information density and white space: 15 input elements (ID1), 10 action elements (ID2), 7 navigation elements (ID3), and 20 elements in total (ID4) [25].
- Brevity: some research studies have demonstrated that the human memory has the capacity to retain a maximum number of 3 scenarios [21]. Each task or goals requiring more than 3 steps (counted in keystrokes) to be reached decreases usability (Minimal Action MA).
- Navigability: some studies have demonstrated that the first level navigational target (Navigation Breadth NB) should not exceed 7 [23].
- Message Concision: since the quality of the message can be evaluated only by the end-user, the number of the word in a message is proposed as an internal metrics to assess message quality (Word Number WN). A maximum of 15 words is recommended in a message [25].
- Error Prevention: The system must provide mechanisms to keep the user from making mistakes [7]. One way to avoid mistakes is the use of ListBoxes for enumerated values. [25] recommend at least 90% of enumerated values must be shown in a ListBox to improve usability (ERP).

It should be noted that ranges are established with two different ways. For metrics which are extracted and adapted from the proposition of [25], only the concept of metrics is adapted. We opted for the same ranges of values since they are empirically validated. This is the case of Predictability, Information Density, Error Prevention, etc. For the other metrics, the value to be considered as Very Bad is estimated taken into account the value recommended as Very Good. The discussion with some usability experts is crucial in order to benefit from their experience and help us to estimate the value to be considered as a Very Bad. After that, we equitably distribute the values for the Good, Medium and Bad categories since we have the two extremes. May be some slightly adjustments are necessary. The Table 1 shows the list of indicators that we have been defined.

Table 1. Proposed indicators

Metric	VG	G	M	B	VB
AD	>0.95	$0.95 \leq AD \prec 0.85$	$0.85 \leq AD \prec 0.75$	$0.75 \leq AD \prec 0.65$	$AD \leq 0.65$
ID1	$\prec 15$	$15 \leq ID1 \prec 20$	$20 \leq ID1 \prec 25$	$25 \leq ID1 \prec 30$	$ID1 \geq 30$
ID2	$\prec 10$	$10 \leq ID2 \prec 13$	$13 \leq ID2 \prec 16$	$16 \leq ID2 \prec 19$	$ID2 \geq 19$
ID3	$\prec 7$	$7 \leq ID3 \prec 10$	$10 \leq ID3 \prec 13$	$13 \leq ID3 \prec 16$	$ID3 \geq 16$
ID4	$\prec 20$	$20 \leq ID4 \prec 30$	$30 \leq ID4 \prec 40$	$40 \leq ID4 \prec 50$	$ID4 \geq 50$
MA	$\prec 2$	$2 \leq MA \prec 4$	$4 \leq MA \prec 5$	$5 \leq MA \prec 6$	$MA \geq 6$
NB	$\prec 7$	$5 \leq NB \prec 10$	$10 \geq NB \prec 13$	$13 \leq NB \prec 16$	$NB \geq 16$
WN	$\prec 15$	$15 \leq WN \prec 20$	$20 \leq WN \prec 25$	$25 \leq WN \prec 30$	$WN \geq 30$
ERP	>0.90	$0.90 \leq ERP \prec 0.80$	$0.80 \leq ERP \prec 0.70$	$0.70 \leq ERP \prec 0.60$	$ERP \leq 0.60$

Grouping Definition. The grouping function aims at putting metrics and attributes together in order to obtain a single usability measure. We adapt the grouping function proposed by [25] by the ad of weight to each element of the usability model tree. The attribution of the priority index requires usability expert and domain expert. This step aims at promoting the most relevant usability properties with respect to the population characteristics and/or the task requirements. As an outcome, the usability model will be annotated by the priority index. The model annotation is performed at the usability requirements establishment phase which precedes each evaluation.

While executing the evaluation, metrics are applied. The obtained numerical values are converted into their corresponding qualitative one. Next, each categorical value is converted to numerical values with respect to the following hypothesis. VG $\Rightarrow$ 5, G $\Rightarrow$ 4, M $\Rightarrow$ 3, B $\Rightarrow$ 2, and VB $\Rightarrow$ 1. The final result is calculated with the formula presented by equation 8:

$$AVG = \sum_{i=1}^{n} pivi. \tag{8}$$

Where pi represents the weight of the item and vi represents the numerical values of the item.

The last step in the aggregation function is to convert the obtained numerical value into an ordinal value. We assign VB to the value between 1 and 1.5, B to the value between 1.6 and 2.5, M to the value between 2.6 and 3.5, G to the value between 3.6 and 4.5 and VG to value lower or equal to 5.

The three steps are applied for each grouping. Groupings are performed bottom-up from indicators until the overall user interface usability is reached.

4 An Experiment to Evaluate Our Proposal

We argue that measuring the internal usability is an appealing way to predict the external usability of software product. It is recommended that internal metrics have a relationship that is as strong as possible with the external metrics. The experimentation elaborated in this Section aims at investigating the relationship between the proposed metrics and those perceived by end-user.

4.1 Objectives

With respect to the GQM template [6], the goal of the experiment is to **analyze** internal measures of usability **for the purpose** of evaluating it **with regard** to their relationship with those perceived by end-users **from the viewpoint** of the researcher **in the context** of end-users evaluating the interactive system that is automatically generated from conceptual models.

The main research question conveyed through this study is:

RQ: is there a significant coherence between user's perception about the usability of the final product and value obtained with the proposed usability method?

We identify two hypotheses related to RQ:

- H0: There is not a significant difference between the usability obtained with our proposed method (EUE) and that perceived by the end-user (PU).
  H0: μ EUE= μ PU.
- H1: There is a significant difference between the usability obtained with our proposed method (EUE) and that perceived by the end-user (PU).
  H1: μ EUE $\neq$ μ PU.

4.2   Designing the Experimentation

Identification of Variables. We identify two types of variables:

- **Response variable:** variable that corresponds to the outcome of the experimentation [19]. We identify each usability sub-characteristic as a response variable.
- **Factors:** variable that affects the response variable. We identify the Evaluation Method. This factor has two alternatives: 1) early usability evaluation without end-user, 2) usability evaluation with end-user.

Objects. The object is **rent a car system**. It is specified using the conceptual models presented in [10] and the final system is (semi-) automatically generated from these models.

Subjects. The subjects were Thirteen undergraduate students from the Sfax National School of Engineering. Their age ranged between 27 and 35 years. Although the subjects did not have any experience in conceptual modeling, they had high level of knowledge in Human Computer Interaction. The number of the subjects is chosen according to the recommendation presented in [17].

4.3   Executing the Experimentation

Instruments. The instruments used to carry out the experiment were:

- *A demographic questionnaire*: A set of questions to know the level of experience of each user in interactive applications similar to the rent a car system.
- *Tasks*: A list of tasks that the user must carry out. The definition of tasks is intended to guarantee that all the users interact with the same contexts that are the most significant.
- *Survey*: A list of fourteen questions defined to capture the user's perception in a 5-point Likert scale format. Each question refers to one of the defined metrics to measure the usability of the internal attribute. PR and AD use the same question and the same thing for ID3 and NG. Using this survey, the user's impressions for each metrics is obtained. Hence, the usability values obtained by means of the proposed method can be compared with those perceived by the end-user. It should be noted that we need a specific question for each attribute that is why we could not use any existing questionnaire. Fig. 3 shows an example of questions from the survey.

MC: error message clearly explain the problem's causes.	○ ○ ○ ○ ○
ID2: the number of function button per UI is optimal?	○ ○ ○ ○ ○
MA: user is lost among screen and does not remember the source?	○ ○ ○ ○ ○

Fig. 3. Example of question from the survey

- *Spreadsheet*: It was used to accelerate the metric calculation based on the conceptual models.

4.4   Validity Evaluation

The validity evaluation is an important concept which is intended to ensure that the experimental results are valid for the target population.

Conclusion Validity. This type of validity refers to the the degree to which the conclusions made about the null hypothesis are reasonable or correct. Our evaluation was threatened by random heterogeneity of subjects. This threat appears when some users are more experienced than others. In our experiment, the experience is related to the use of interactive applications. This threat was resolved with a demographic questionnaire that allowed us to evaluate the knowledge and experience of each participant beforehand. The demographic questionnaire revealed that most users had experience with this kind of systems.

Construct Validity. One of the most basic issues in validity is the *construct validity*. It provides an answer to the following question: are we measuring what we intended to measure? We have used an inter-item correlation analysis to evaluate the construct validity of the response variable. For each item, we made use of two criteria: *Convergent validity*, which refers to the convergence among different indicators used to measure a particular construct; and the *Discriminant validity*, which refers to the divergence of indicators used to measure different constructs [12]. If the convergent validity was higher than the discriminant validity, the item is validated. The results of the validity analysis show that the *Convergent validity* value was higher than the *Discriminant validity* value (see Fig.4) for each item, except for ID3, ID4 and MA.

In order to conduct the reliability analysis on the survey, we calculate the Chronbach alpha for every question of the survey. The value obtained for the whole questionnaire was 0.966, which is a very good value for reliability. The reliability for the response variables were: 0.584 for learnability, 0.848 for understandability, 0.671 for operability, and 0.756 for the attractiveness. We argue that these values are also very good for an academic experiment.

		PR	AD	IF	ID1	ID2	ID3	ID4	MA	NB	MC	UOC	UOU	EUA	ERP	FSU	CU	CS	CV	DV	Valid
prompting	PR	1	0.5	-0.5	0.866	1	0.5	-0.945	-0.5	0.866	-0.5	0.866	0.5	0.5	-0.5	0.5	1	-0.5	0.3333	0.261	yes
Predictability	AD	0.5	1	0.5	0	0.5	1	-0.756	-1	0	-1	0.866	1	1	0.5	1	0.5	0.5	0.6667	0.294	yes
Informative Feedback	IF	-0.5	0.5	1	-0.87	-0.5	0.5	0.189	-0.5	-0.866	-0.5	0	0.5	0.5	1	0.5	-0.5	1	0.3333	0.033	yes
Information Density	ID1	0.8660254	0	-0.866	1	0.866	0	-0.655	0	1	0	0.5	0	0	-0.866	0	0.866	-0.866	0.3159	-0.04	yes
	ID2	1	0.5	-0.5	0.866	1	0.5	-0.945	-0.5	0.866	-0.5	0.866	0.5	0.5	-0.5	0.5	1	-0.5	0.1839	0.337	no
	ID3	0.5	0.5	0.5	0	0.5	1	-0.756	-1	0	-1	0.866	1	1	0.5	1	0.5	0.5	-0.179	0.687	no
	ID4	-0.9449112	-0.756	0.189	-0.65	-0.945	-0.756	1	0.76	-0.655	0.756	-0.98	-0.7559	-0.756	0.189	-0.76	-0.94	0.189	-0.071	-0.53	yes
Brevity	MA	-0.5	0	-0.5	0	-0.5	-1	0.756	1	0	1	-0.87	-1	-1	-0.5	-1	-0.5	-0.5	0.1794	-0.64	yes
Navigability	NB	0.8660254	0.866	-0.866	1	0.866	0	-0.655	0	1	0	0.5	0	0	-0.866	0	0.866	-0.866	0.3159	0.05	yes
Message Concision	MC	-0.5	0.7559	-0.5	0	-0.5	-1	0.756	1	0	1	-0.87	-1	-1	-0.5	-1	-0.5	-0.5	0.1794	-0.56	yes
User operation Cancellability	UOC	0.8660254	0.5	0	0.5	0.866	0.866	-0.982	-0.87	0.5	-0.87	1	0.86603	0.866	0	0.866	0.866	0	0.683	0.24	yes
User Operation Undoability	UOU	0.5	1	0.5	0	0.5	1	-0.756	-1	0	-1	0.866	1	1	0.5	1	0.5	0.5	0.8415	0.211	yes
Explicit User Action	EUA	0.5	-1	0.5	0	0.5	1	-0.756	-1	0	-1	0.866	1	1	0.5	1	0.5	0.5	0.8415	0.057	yes
Error Prevention	ERP	-0.5	0.5	1	-0.87	-0.5	0.5	0.189	-0.5	-0.866	-0.5	0	0.5	0.5	1	0.5	-0.5	1	0.5	-0.04	yes
Font Style Uniformity	FSU	0.5	0.866	0.5	0	0.5	1	-0.756	-1	0	-1	0.866	1	1	0.5	1	0.5	0.5	0.6667	0.284	yes
Color Uniformity	CU	1	0.5	-0.5	0.866	1	0.5	-0.945	-0.5	0.866	-0.5	0.866	0.5	0.5	-0.5	0.5	1	-0.5	0.3333	0.261	yes
Consistency	CS	-0.5	1	1	-0.87	-0.5	0.5	0.189	-0.5	-0.866	-0.5	0	0.5	0.5	1	0.5	-0.5	1	0.3333	0.068	yes

Fig. 4. Inter-Item Correlation Analysis

4.5   Data Analysis

In this Sub-Section, we compare the usability perceived by end-user with the outcomes of our proposed usability evaluation method. Fig. 5 represents the comparison for the **rent a car system**.

We can state that the trend is similar for most metrics. For example, values are similar for PR, AD, ID1, ID2, ID4, MA, UOU, UOC, ERP, CU, and CS.

On the basis of the observed values, we can state that there is a relation between the values obtained from our proposal and the user's perception.

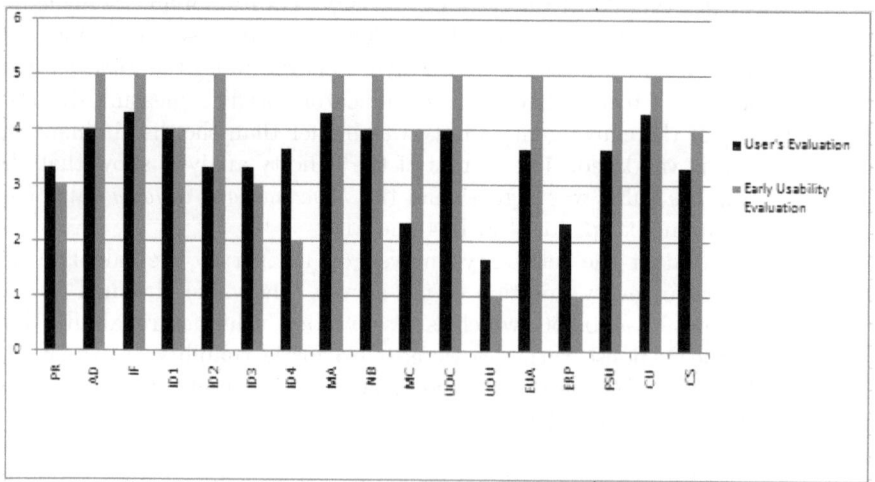

Fig. 5. Comparison of user's perception with the early usability method

The significant difference observed for some attributes can be explained by the range of values used as indicators. We may adjust some of them in order to better improve their accuracy since they are extracted from other research works that focus on other domains.

In order to study the comparison of factors in depth, we performed a statistical study called standard deviation. This test is a statistical procedure that is used to determine the mean difference between a sample and the value of a population mean. In our case, the sample was composed of the evaluation performed with thirteen subjects (the experiment) and the population mean was the level of usability obtained from metrics and indicators (early usability evaluation). The results of the standard deviation test show that there are no significant differences between the population mean and the sample for most of metrics. Only three metrics have a significant difference (IF, NB and FSU). This can be explained by the sources from which indicators are extracted. Some adjustments are recommended in order to improve the results.

The application of the grouping function to the two methods (User's Perception UP, Early Usability Evaluation EUE) provides the results shown in Table 2.

Table 2. Usability level of the underlying system

	Learnability	Understandability	Operability	Attractiveness
UP	M	M	M	G
EUE	M	G	M	VG

Considering the results, we can state that the null hypothesis is true for 52% of the proposed metrics. We argue that this results can be considered as encouraging as to build on it and conduct many more experiments to improve our study. The first experience with the empirical evaluation of our proposed method allows us to learn more about the potentialities of our method in the the prediction of the usability perceived by end-user. However, the accuracy of results and their acceptance rate is the main questions to be resolved in further experiments. The considerable contribution to the development costs of the final application is the main advantage of the early usability measurement method presented in this paper. The experimentation emphasizes the importance of the empirical evaluation to improve our proposed measurement methods. It is not enough to provide an apparently adequate set of metrics and indicators. An empirical evaluation is usually recommended to assess the accuracy of the measurements.

However, it is essential to conduct many more experiments with other types of system and try to verify if the results will be the same. It is also crucial to more adjust the indicators estimated based on the value defined on the usability guidelines and surveys.

5   Conclusions and Future Work

In the present paper, an extension of the Cameleon framework is presented. The extension aims at integrating the usability issues during the development process of user interface where features of the context of use are taken into account. To reach this objective, we propose an early usability measurement method. The objective of this paper is to show the importance of early evaluating the usability from the conceptual model. To do this we propose a model based approach that evaluate the concrete user interface. The usability model used to perform the evaluation gather usability attributes that can be quantified using usability metrics which are based on the conceptual primitives of the underlying method. However, the concept of these metrics can be adapted in order to be used in other similar approaches.

The proposed method have two objective. The first one is to detect usability problems from the design phase which allow their correction early and with a low cost than correcting them after implementation. The second objective is to predict the usability level of the generated user interface. The present paper focus on the second objective.

To better consolidate our method, we conduct an empirical evaluation. to do that, an experiment was conducted with thirteen participant in order to investigate the relationship between the value obtained by our method and the value perceived by end-users. Results show the usefulness of the contribution in the prediction of the usability perceived by end-users. It also allows us to learn more about the potentialities and limitations of our proposed method. Results show the importance of the empirical validating a proposal rather than be justified it by logical or theoretical arguments alone.

Further research works are intended to investigate the implementation of an automatic usability evaluation process. The implementation of the usability driven model transformation process is a crucial target for further research work. The accuracy of the results requires a slightly adjustment of the indicators and to conduct many more experiments in order to validate the new proposed values.

References

1. Bpmn: Business process modeling notation version 1.0. (2004),
   http://www.bpmn.org
2. ISO/IEC 9241. Ergonomic Requirements for Office Work with Visual Display Terminals (VDTs). ISO/IEC (1998)
3. Abrahao, S., Insfran, E.: Early usability evaluation in model driven architecture environments. In: Proceedings of the Sixth International Conference on Quality Software, pp. 287–294. IEEE Computer Society, Washington, DC (2006)
4. Abran, A., Khelifi, A., Suryn, W., Seffah, A.: Usability meanings and interpretations in iso standards. Software Quality Control 11(4), 325–338 (2003)
5. Aquino, N., Vanderdonckt, J., Condori-Fernández, N., Dieste, Ó., Pastor, Ó.: Usability evaluation of multi-device/platform user interfaces generated by model-driven engineering. In: Proceedings of the 2010 ACM-IEEE International Symposium on Empirical Software Engineering and Measurement, ESEM 2010, pp. 30:1–30:10. ACM, New York (2010)
6. Basili, V.R., Caldiera, G., Dieter Rombach, H.: The goal question metric approach. In: Encyclopedia of Software Engineering. Wiley (1994)
7. Christian Bastien, J.M., Scapin, D.L.: Ergonomic criteria for the evaluation of human-computer interfaces. Technical Report RT-0156, INRIA (June 1993)

8. Bevan, N., Macleod, M.: Usability measurement in context. Behaviour and Information Technology 13, 132–145 (1994)
9. Boehm, B.W.: Software Engineering Economics. Prentice Hall, Englewood Cliffs (1981)
10. Bouchelligua, W., Mahfoudhi, A., Mezhoudi, N., Daassi, O., Abed, M.: User interfaces modelling of workflow information systems. In: Barjis, J. (ed.) EOMAS 2010. LNBIP, vol. 63, pp. 143–163. Springer, Heidelberg (2010)
11. Calvary, G., Coutaz, J., Thevenin, D.: A unifying reference framework for the development of plastic user interfaces. In: Nigay, L., Little, M.R. (eds.) EHCI 2001. LNCS, vol. 2254, pp. 173–192. Springer, Heidelberg (2001)
12. Campbell, D.T., Fiske, D.W.: Convergent and discriminant validation by the multitrait-multimethod matrix. Psychological Bulletin 56, 81–105 (1959)
13. Coutaz, J.: User interface plasticity: model driven engineering to the limit! In: EICS, pp. 1–8 (2010)
14. Endres, A., Rombach, D.: A handbook of software and systems engineering: empirical observations, laws and theories. The Fraunhofer IESE series on software engineering. Pearson/Addison Wesley, Harlow, England (2003)
15. Fernandez, A., Insfran, E., Abrahão, S.: Integrating a usability model into model-driven web development processes. In: Vossen, G., Long, D.D.E., Yu, J.X. (eds.) WISE 2009. LNCS, vol. 5802, pp. 497–510. Springer, Heidelberg (2009)
16. Gómez, J., Cachero, C., Pastor, O.: Conceptual modeling of device-independent web applications. IEEE MultiMedia 8(2), 26–39 (2001)
17. Holzinger, A.: Usability engineering methods for software developers. Commun. ACM 48(1), 71–74 (2005)
18. ISO/IEC. ISO/IEC 9126. Software engineering – Product quality. ISO/IEC (2001)
19. Juristo, Moreno: Basics of Software Engineering Experimentation. Kluwer Academic Publishers, Norwell (2001)
20. Kirakowski, J., Corbett, M.: Sumi: the software usability measurement inventory. British Journal of Educational Technology 24(3), 210–212 (1993)
21. Lacob, M.E.: Readability and Usability Guidelines (2003)
22. Shneiderman, B., Leavit, M.: Research Based Web Design & Usability Guidelines (2006)
23. Murata, M., Uchimoto, K., Ma, Q., Isahara, H.: Magical number seven plus or minus two: Syntactic structure recognition in japanese and english sentences. In: Gelbukh, A. (ed.) CICLing 2001. LNCS, vol. 2004, pp. 43–52. Springer, Heidelberg (2001)
24. Nielsen, J., Molich, R.: Heuristic evaluation of user interfaces. In: Proceedings of the SIGCHI Conference on Human Factors in Computing Systems: Empowering People, CHI 1990, pp. 249–256. ACM, New York (1990)
25. Panach, J.I., Condori-Fernandez, N., Vos, T.E.J., Aquino, N., Valverde, F.: Early usability measurement in model-driven development: Definition and empirical evaluation. International Journal of Software Engineering and Knowledge Engineering 21(3), 339–365 (2011)
26. Rubin, J.: Handbook of Usability Testing: How to Plan, Design, and Conduct Effective Tests. John Wiley & Sons, Inc., New York (1994)
27. Schmidt, D.C.: Model-driven engineering. IEEE Computer 39(2) (February 2006)
28. Seffah, A., Donyaee, M., Kline, R.B., Padda, H.K.: Usability measurement and metrics: A consolidated model. Software Quality Control 14, 159–178 (2006)
29. Thevenin, D., Coutaz, J.: Plasticity of user interfaces: Framework and research agenda. In: Sasse, A., Johnson, C. (eds.) Proc. Interact 1999, Edinburgh, pp. 110–117. IFIP IOS Press Publ. (1999)

The Impact of User Diversity on the Willingness to Disclose Personal Information in Social Network Services

A Comparison of Private and Business Contexts

Anne Kathrin Schaar, André Calero Valdez, and Martina Ziefle

Human-Computer Interaction Center, RWTH Aachen University, Germany
{schaar,calero-valdez,ziefle}@comm.rwth-aachen.de

Abstract. Social media and social network sites (SNS) are a central medium for communication within the Internet. There has never been a faster possibility for information exchange across the globe with a comparable range and size of audience. So far, SNS are very popular in private communication. But can other fields of application profit from this role model? To find out more about the comparability of the two contexts (private and business) and to specify transferable design guidelines, we investigated the willingness to disclose private data in both private and business context, knowing that data disclosure is one significant success factor for SNS and communities. Therefore, an exploratory questionnaire study ($N = 151$) was designed. The focus of the study is based on the question whether there is a difference between the contexts and whether these differences are related to user diversity factors (age, gender, perceived locus of control over technology (PLoC), and personality traits according to Five Factor Model (FFM)). First results reveal that there is a significant difference between the two contexts that is hard to explain using only factors of user diversity.

Keywords: Demographic change, FFM, social network sites, self-disclosure, personality, technology acceptance.

1 Introduction

The success story of SNS on the Internet cannot be denied. A lot of effort is put into trying to replicate the approach to match up with the success of private SNS, e.g. facebook, in business cases. The problem is that although there is a lot of research in this field, there are no generally accepted design criteria or guidelines available. One research project that tries to fill this gap for the working context in Germany is the project iNec "Innovation through expert-communities in the context of the demographical change." This project consortium is an interdisciplinary team of social scientists, economists, computer scientists, and practice partners that lined up to generate a sustainable community concept accompanied by a personnel development concept.

A. Holzinger et al. (Eds.): SouthCHI 2013, LNCS 7946, pp. 174–193, 2013.
© Springer-Verlag Berlin Heidelberg 2013

This concept is designed to face the challenges of demographic change and erosion of the normal employment history: Small- and medium-sized enterprises, e.g., in Germany, are struggling with big problems. These problems are addressing particularly sustainable knowledge management and personnel development, in order to overcome of lack of qualified personnel and fast staff turnover [1].

How This Paper Is Organized. In the following subsections the scenario of this research is pointed out. Therefore, the situation of a world dealing with the effects of demographic change and erosion of the normal employment history is portrayed (see Section 1.1). Afterwards, the related work and state of the art of research within the field of SNS for the working context are presented (see Section 1.2). Following that, the approach of user-centered community development of the iNec project is introduced to underline the impact of user diversity on the acceptance of technology (see Section 1.3).

The main focus of the study and the questions addressed are presented in Section 2. Subsequently, the questionnaire instrument of this study is presented (see Section 3). The fourth section of the paper presents the central findings of the investigation on the impact of user diversity on the willingness to disclose personal information. Finishing this paper in Section 5, the results are discussed, limitations are named, and an outlook on future research is worked out.

1.1 The Effect of Demographic Change and Erosion of the Normal Employment History for the Working Context

In order to point out the necessity of suitable tools and approaches to face arising challenges, this section works out the status quo of a working world struggling with two profound social developments, namely demographic change and erosion of normal employment histories. In a first step, the effects of demographic change on the working world are presented, followed by an outline of the impact of the erosion of normal employment histories. Concluding this section, both phenomena are interlinked to define overall challenges for the working world.

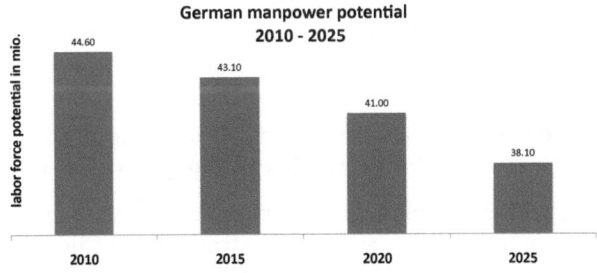

Fig. 1. Decrease of German manpower potential. Source: Graph based on data of IAB (Institut für Arbeitsmarkt und Berufsforschung).

Demographic Change. Most European countries are struggling with the demographic change which is accompanied by decreasing fertility rates and an increasing amount of elderly people [2]. This change affects all areas of European society [3]. One sector that is especially affected is the working world[4](see Fig. 1). Facing the effects of the demographic change in the working world is important, because common prosperity is interlinked with it. In Germany, the demographic change is predominantly responsible for a threatening lack of qualified personnel [5]. Many small- and medium-sized enterprises know that, because of upcoming retirements, they will lose a considerable amount of their workforce.

Another challenge that enterprises will have to face is the impact of an aging workforce on the job development. It is essential to define age appropriate workspaces, tasks, and support over time. Especially when considering technology as a solution, the impact of age on the acceptance of technology and learnability must be included in the discussion (see Section 1.3).

Erosion of the Normal Employment History. In addition to the challenges of demographic change, the working world is influenced by a phenomenon called erosion of the normal employment histories in the social sciences [6–8]. The concept of a normal or standard employment biography is a German phenomenon which stems from the times of the economic miracle in Germany during the late 1940s. The normal employment biography is based on the following aspects: a) permanent contract of employment, b) full time jobs, c) contractually standardized payment, d) social insurance payment obligation. Although the idea of this normal work biography is very present in people's minds, it has never been a social reality for the masses, but shaped the image of work until today. At least in times of globalization and an increasing need for flexibility at work, the assumption of a standardized working biography idea is no longer feasible. Today, work is characterized by part-time employment, parental leaves, stays abroad, home office, and comparably flexible working schedules [9–11]. The general transition to flexible and individually differing career paths generates special requirements in regard to inner corporate communication of enterprises in order to keep the communication both sustainable and robust.

Summing this section up, we can say that the working life is strongly affected by social changes which lead to the need for a stronger support of sustainable communication and knowledge management support in enterprises.

1.2   Communication and Knowledge Management via Social Network Services/Communities in the Working Context

The idea of using technical support in the working context to enhance job performance, knowledge management, and administration is not new. Especially technology acceptance in the context of Information and Communication Technologies (ICT) has been investigated intensively by authors like Davis or Venkatesh and others since the 1980s [12, 13].

The rise and prosperity of SNS [14–17] as one form of social media brought a new chance for networking for enterprises and high expectations regarding the benefit enterprises might get from SNS usage. The successful implementation of other social software applications like wikis and weblogs [18, 19] also supports SNS implementation activities in enterprises.

In the context of research on SNS implementation in enterprises, Richter and Koch identified six central characteristics of SNS that are useful for the working context: a) *identity management* (representation of a person via profiles), b) *management of contacts* (networking), c) *expert-search* (within an enterprise), d) *support of context- and network awareness*, and e) *support of common exchange* (in an enterprise) [20].

But there is only little knowledge about empirical values regarding SNS realization, although SNS for enterprises are considered to have a big positive impact on knowledge management. This fact is considerably interesting because knowledge is considered a key factor of production as well as a motor of innovation potential of enterprises [20].

A case study of Richter and Koch that focused on success criteria for business related SNS revealed that the integration of SNS in the daily routine is a central success criterion. Other important factors were ease of use, development of the tool according to users needs, integration of existing systems, incentives, corporate culture and the recognition of benefits. Furthermore, Richter and Koch revealed that a critical mass is essential to realize long-term usage of the system.

Summarizing this section, we can state that the idea of integrating SNS into the business context is quite popular, but the knowledge about a successful realization in the working context reveals no concrete guidelines yet. The existing knowledge is mostly focused on individual solutions that are themselves focused on particular enterprises, or overgeneralized criteria which do not lead to practical implementation.

The next section takes these considerations into account and presents an approach of user-centered community development as an approach that could provide a design process which can be generalized to a broader target group.

1.3   The Approach of User-Centered Community Design

The approach of user-centered community design addresses the challenge to find design, implementation, and schooling criteria that are suitable for the integration of SNS in the working context, and transferable to diverse enterprises. In this context the idea of the user-centered community design is focused on two central aspects: first, the *comprehension of employees' cognitive skills, their emotional-, motivational-, and knowledge-related needs* in their working environment; and second, the *understanding of aspects related to linguistics and communicative usability* in the context of social media and SNS.

The elements of the user-centered community design research approach are user characteristics (age, gender, personality, educational level, technical expertise, perceived locus of control over technology (PLoC), social media expertise etc.) as *independent factors* and motivation, matching of incentives, usability, design-criteria as *dependent factors* (see Fig. 2). The overall goal of the user-centered community design is to define general design criteria for SNS in the

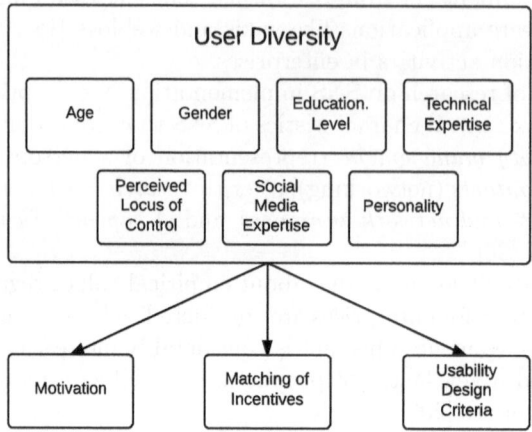

Fig. 2. User-centered community design approach. The effect of user diversity criteria on SNS/community design is evaluated to allow tailored solutions.

working context with focus on usability, motivation, and incentives concepts that can be adapted to diverse enterprises according to their personnels' profile.

2   Main Focus of the Study and Questions Addressed

In order to find out whether business SNS/communities can benefit from the knowledge about private SNS, we started this exploratory research focusing on the comparison of these two different settings (private vs. business). According to the user-centered community design approach, the focus is set on the influence of demographic data (age and gender), PLoC (sometimes referred to as *computer self-efficacy*) as well as personality (FFM) on the *willingness to disclose data* in SNS. Hence, the following research questions were relevant:

- RQ1: Is there a difference in willingness to disclose data between private and business context?
- RQ2: Does gender influence the willingness to disclose data in different contexts?
- RQ3: Does age influence the willingness to disclose data in different contexts?
- RQ4: Does the PLoC influence the willingness to disclose data in different contexts?
- RQ5: Does personality (FFM) influence the willingness to disclose data in different contexts?

In a second step, the focus is set on incentives and moderating factors that might influence the willingness to disclose data. Therefore, the following research question was addressed:

- RQ6: Is there an impact of moderating variables on the willingness to disclose data?

The research questions presented build the base for the questionnaire instrument presented in the following section (Section 3).

3   Method

In order to reach a large number of participants, the questionnaire method was chosen. The questionnaire was provided electronically. Before distribution, differently aged adults examined the questionnaire to avoid misunderstandings and possible lack of clarity. Filling in the final version of the questionnaire took between 25 and 40 minutes.

In the following sections the design of the study is presented: Section 3.1 contains the central variables of the study and Section 3.2 a description of the questionnaire's design.

3.1   Variables

As *independent variables* age, gender, personality (according to FFM [21]), and PLoC were chosen. Personality was measured according to the FFM with bipolar adjective scales (see Table 1). In order to keep the methodology similar to earlier research, PLoC was assessed using eight questions with a six-point Likert scale (range: 8–48, Cronbachs's $\alpha = .91$).

As *depended variables* we selected the evaluation of a set of personal data (name, date of birth, hobbies, etc.) that is often used in social media profiles (see Table 2). The evaluation was assessed on a dichotomous scale ($1 = I\ would\ disclose\ this\ information$, $2 = I\ would\ not\ disclose\ this\ information$). Because of the explorative character of the study, we chose this polarizing answering-scale to get a first definitive idea of users' attitude. Additionally, we asked the participants to evaluate moderating conditions for information disclosure, e.g., money as an incentive or more information about how the data is handled and possibly disseminated. All items were presented in two settings: *private* and *business*.

3.2   Questionnaire Instrument

The questionnaire used in this study is divided into six main parts: (a) demographic data, (b) PLoC, (c) personality according to FFM, (d) expertise with social media, (e) evaluation of willingness to disclose data in social media applications, (f) evaluation of moderating factors for data disclosure (e.g., money or more information). More information about the topics and the scales used are given in the sections below:

3.3   Variables Related to User-Diversity

Three areas of user-diversity are of interest to our study. We look into demographic data, the PLoC, and into the big five personality measures (FFM).

Demographic Data: Each participant was asked to state his/her age, gender, educational level as well as current profession in order to give us the opportunity to investigate the influence of these factors on the willingness to disclose information in SNS.

Perceived Locus of Control (PLoC). In order to get more information about the attitude and interaction with technology, we asked for PLoC. This factor is assessed via eight questions on a six-point Likert scale (range: 8–48, Cronbach's $\alpha = .91$).

Personality. Personality traits are evaluated according to Neo-Five-Factor-Inventory from Costa and McCrae [22]. This inventory uses the scales: *openness, conscientiousness, extraversion, agreeableness*, and *neuroticism*. In this questionnaire we used a short version of the Five Factor Inventory (FFI) [21, 23]. In our study the the items are presented as a bipolar 9-point adjective scale (see Table 1).

3.4 Evaluation of Disclosure of Different Data in Social Media Applications

The disclosure of data within SNS is an integral part for a successful usage of such applications. In order to find out what data a user is willing to disclose in social media applications, we asked for an evaluation (*"disclose"* and *"retain"*) of 15 different data items (Table 2) for both scenarios, *private* and *business*.

Some of these items are related to private contact data while others are related to business contact data. Both are assessed in both contexts.

Social Media Usage Concerns. In order to find out whether the participants have a positive or negative attitude against social media, we used an item set of 10 items (on a six-point Likert scale) asking for the level of agreement to certain statements about social media (see Table 3).

4   Results

This section presents the central findings of the current study according to the research questions (see Section 2). Section 4.1 presents the sample of the study. The following subsections present the influence of the factors age, gender, personality, and PLoC on the willingness to disclose data, for each of the contexts, *private* and *business*. After that, we present the evaluation of moderating factors for the willingness to disclose private data to get information about the suitability of incentives and the influence of moderating factors.

Employed Statistical Methods. As statistical methods, Mann-Whitney U, Kruskal-Wallis and Friedman tests are used. For normality testing, Kolomogorov-Smirnov testing was used. For testing of nominal scales, Chi-Square tests are used and Cramér's-V is reported. The level of significance was set to $\alpha = .05$. Effect sizes, if applicable, are reported using Pearson's r.

Table 1. Evaluation of the NEO Five-Factor-Inventory items on a bipolar adjective scale

Please classify yourself within the following character traits. Which trait fits you best?								
☐ **extroverted**, sociable, thirsty for interaction with other people	☐ very	☐ fair	☐ a little	☐ yes/no	☐ a little	☐ fair	☐ very	☐ **introverted**, quiet, taciturn, secluded, loner
☐ **emotional**, nervous, worried, strained, sensitive	☐ very	☐ fair	☐ a little	☐ yes/no	☐ a little	☐ fair	☐ very	☐ **easy-going**, calm, relaxed, self-content, robust
☐ **open-minded**, unbiased, inquisitive, sophisticated, imaginative	☐ very	☐ fair	☐ a little	☐ yes/no	☐ a little	☐ fair	☐ very	☐ **determined**, rigid beliefs, low interest in news, traditional
☐ **curt**, cold, critical, quick to anger, distrustful	☐ very	☐ fair	☐ a little	☐ yes/no	☐ a little	☐ fair	☐ very	☐ **sociable**, cooperative, cordial, kind, accommodating
☐ **conscientious**, reliable, careful, tidy, ambitious	☐ very	☐ fair	☐ a little	☐ yes/no	☐ a little	☐ fair	☐ very	☐ **sloppy**, casual, untidy, unpunctual, chaotic, nonchalant

Table 2. Evaluation of the data in social media profiles, dichotomous scale: "disclose" or "retain"

I would disclose the following information in a private SNS:		
☐ first name	☐ address (private)	☐ profession
☐ second name	☐ phone (job)	☐ hobbies
☐ sex	☐ phone (private)	☐ marital status
☐ date of birth	☐ mobile phone number	☐ religious affiliation
☐ address (job)	☐ email	☐ political opinion

Table 3. Exemplary items of social media usage motives on a six-point Likert scale (1=total agreement to 6=total rejection) order by level of agreement descending

I am skeptical about social media, because...	M	SD
... there is no established etiquette.	2.75	1.37
... it is an impersonal way of communication.	3.15	1.34
... it induces the impoverishment of interpersonal relationships.	3.15	1.45
... it facilitates voyeurism.	3.52	1.45
... social media is also involved in criminal and abuse contexts.	3.67	1.52
... it supports stalking.	4.04	1.43
etc...		

For all tests, case-wise deletion of missing values was applied. Because not all participants finished the survey, some results rely on smaller samples. For these cases, either the reduced sample size (i.e., N) or the absolute frequency of a measurement (i.e., n) is given.

4.1   Sample Description

The sample of this study comprises a total of $N = 151$. The sample of the study is rather young with a mean age of 27.4 ($SD = 8.0$). The educational level of the sample is quite high with 50% ($n = 75$) having "Abitur" (the highest German high school degree) and further 37% ($n = 55$) having a college degree.

Furthermore, we can report that the sample has a bias to female participation with $n = 89$ female participants and $n = 62$ male participants.

According to expertise with social media we have a rather tech-savvy sample: In the context of social media usage only 3% ($n = 4$) of the sample reported that they never use social media. The rest of the sample uses social media at least 0-10 minutes a day ($n = 13$) or most more than 4 hours a day ($n = 33$). In this context, we can also report that the participants' age correlates negatively but highly significantly with social media usage frequency ($r = -.225, p < .01$).

We can also say that the sample reveals no unanimous attitude towards the evaluation of the character of social media: 39% ($N = 132$) reported to agree (i.e., *rather agree, agree* and *agree completely*) that social media are impersonal. The statement "social media supports the impoverishment of human values," was confirmed by 44% ($N = 133$) of the participants.

For the factor *PLoC*, we can report that the sample has a perceived high PLoC ($M = 4.58, SD = .98$).

Referring to personality (all personality scales range: $1 - 9$) we can say that the level of *neuroticism* was average ($M = 4.5, SD = 1.76$). Male participants revealed lower neuroticism than females ($M_{\male} = 3.8$, $M_{\female} = 5.0$, Mann-Whitney $U = 1797, Z = -3.626, r = .3, p < .01$). *Extraversion* was slightly above average ($M = 5.9, SD = 1.55$). Males showed lower extraversion than females ($M_{\male} = 5.6$, $M_{\female} = 6.1$, Mann-Whitney $U = 2214, Z = -2.142, r = .175, p < .05$). *Openness* was above average ($M = 6.9, SD = 1.41$) for the whole sample. In comparison to the average distribution, the level of *agreeableness* was lower ($M = 3.8$, $SD = 1.57$). For the factor *conscientiousness* we can report a level above average ($M = 6.5$, $SD = 1.53$). None of theses scales was normally distributed (Kolmogorov-Smirnov test yields $D(142) > .09$ and $p < 0.01$ for all scales).

Summarizing, we can state that we have a young, predominantly female sample with a high level of extraversion which is quite tech-savvy and affine to social media, but also critical of the effects of social media towards society.

4.2 Willingness to Disclose Data in the Private and Business Context

To get a first impression whether the willingness to disclose private data in SNS depends on the setting the current SNS is used in, we made a descriptive comparison of all evaluated data. As Figure 3 and 4 illustrate, there are differences between the two settings. Especially the disclosure of *address (work)*, *phone number (work)*, *mobile phone number*, and *hobbies* revealed deviations.

The willingness to disclose work related data (address and phone number) increases enormously in the context of a business usage context (see Fig. 4): For address (work) we revealed an increase from 6% ($n = 132$) in the private context up to 71% ($n = 111$) and for the phone number (work) from 4% ($n = 131$) up to 76% ($n = 111$).

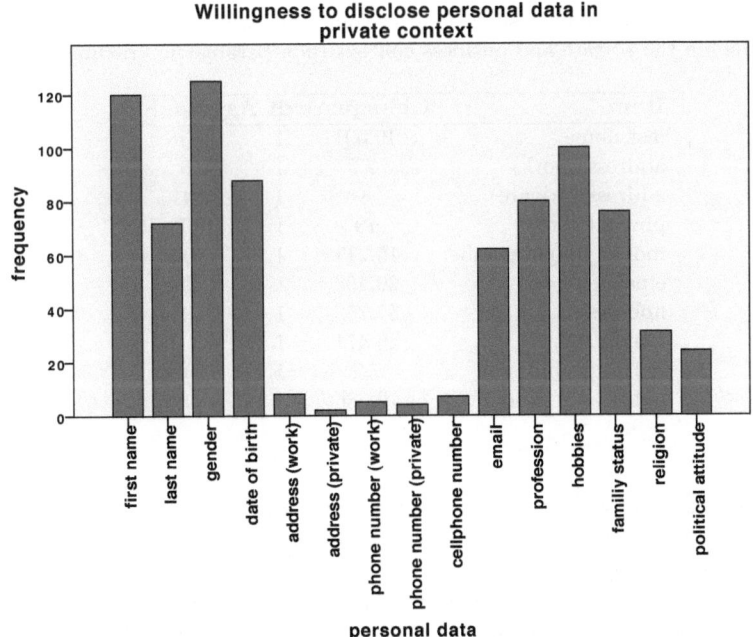

Fig. 3. Willingness to disclose personal information in the private context

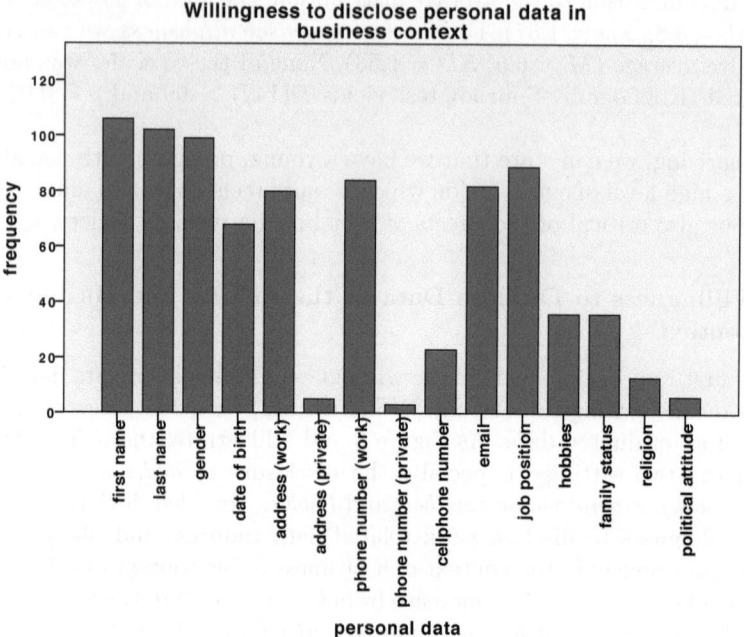

Fig. 4. Willingness to disclose personal information in the business context

Table 4. Results repeated measures analysis comparing willingness to disclose personal data in SNS in the private and business context (non-parametric Friedman Test)

Item	Chi-square	df	Asymp. Sig.
last name	40.091	1	0
address (work)	73	1	0
address (private)	4	1	0.046
phone (work)	79	1	0
mobile phone number	15.211	1	0.001
email	20.455	1	0
hobbies	37.753	1	0
family status	26.471	1	0
religious affiliation	7.2	1	0.013
political attitude	10.286	1	0.001

Interestingly, the willingness to disclose more sensitive data, like one's mobile phone number, also rises in the business context: the willingness to disclose the mobile phone number increases from 5% ($n = 130$) in the private context up to 22% ($n = 106$) in the business context. Moreover, the disclosure of one's email address increases from 47% ($n = 131$) to 74% ($n = 111$). Other aspects, like hobbies, decrease from a business oriented using context to the private one, even if not to a big extent (76% $n = 131$ *private*; 33% $n = 108$ *business*).

In addition to the descriptive analysis, non-parametric Friedman tests were implemented to find out whether the differences between the two settings are statistically significant. As Table 4 illustrates, significant differences between the two settings could be revealed for: last name, address (work), address (private), phone number (work), mobile phone number, email, hobbies, family status, religious affiliation and political attitude.

4.3   Influence of User Diversity on the Willingness to Disclose Data in SNS

In order to get more information about, the origin of these differences and taking the answering-scale into account non-parametric Chi-square tests for independence and Kruskal-Wallis tests were performed. According to the research questions 1–5 (see Section 2) the following section presents the influence of gender, age, PLoC, and personality on the disclosure of private data aspects in SNS. Results of both settings are presented together in individual subsections according to the independent variables: *age, gender, PLoC,* and *personality.*

For the analysis we formed groups:

- *Age groups* were formed as a median split (young: 14–25 years, and old: 26–55 years).
- *PLoC* was divided into two groups (low: means ranging 1–4.75; high: means from 4.76–6, median split).
- The *FFM personality traits* were each divided into three groups: low level of the current factor, medium, and high, creating 3X5 factorial levels.

Age. Due to the fact that age is often an important carrier variable for the acceptance of technology, especially ICT, we analyzed the influence of the age groups (young and old) on the willingness to disclose personal data in the context of private SNS and business oriented ones.

Non-Parametric Kruskal-Wallis tests revealed that the factor age only influences the willingness to disclose data in the context of private SNS. In this context, revealing work address ($\chi^2(1) = 4.097$, $p = .043$), work phone number ($\chi^2(1) = 5.414$, $p = .038$) and mobile phone number ($\chi^2(1) = 4.097$, $p = .043$) are influenced by age. For the disclosure of phone numbers (mobile phone as well as landline), we can report that younger participants are more willing to disclose this information. The willingness to disclose the work address was higher within the older age group (old: 76% $n = 54$; young: 69% $n = 55$).

Gender. To find out whether there are gender differences in the willingness to disclose data in SNS we have run Chi-square tests for independence. Results revealed that gender influences both the willingness to disclose one's own gender ($\chi^2(1) = 5.901$, $p = .015$, Cramér's-$V = .211$) as well as one's private phone number ($\chi^2(1) = 5.733$, $p = .017$, Cramér's-$V = .211$) significantly in the private usage context. Female participants are less willing to disclose gender or their private phone number.

For the business context, gender differences are significant for mobile phone number disclosure ($\chi^2(1) = 4.262, p = .039$, Cramér's-$V = .201$). In this context, women are less willing to disclose information.

Perceived Locus of Control (PLoC). The PLoC has no influence on the willingness to disclose personal data in private SNS. The willingness to disclose data in business related SNS only reveals a significant influence on the disclosure of a person's religious affiliation ($\chi^2(2) = 14.933, p = .011$). Members of the group "high level of PLoC" are more willing to disclose their religious affiliation, although the willingness to disclose religious affiliation was very low in general only 5% ($n = 77$) stated that they would disclose their religious affiliation.

4.4   The Influence of Personality

Addressing the research question (RQ5), we investigated the influence of FFM personality traits *openness, conscientiousness, extraversion, agreeableness*, and *neuroticism* on the willingness to disclose personal data in *private* or *business* social networks. For the analysis, non-parametric Kruskal-Wallis test was chosen.

Openness. Results show that *openness* has a significant influence on the willingness to disclose the private address in the private context ($\chi^2(2) = 19.654$, $p < .001$) as well as in the business context ($\chi^2(3) = 8.175, p = .017$). For both cases we can state that the higher the level of openness the higher the willingness to disclose one's private address in SNS.

Conscientiousness. *Conscientiousness* influences the willingness to disclose one's mobile phone number ($\chi^2(2) = 10.011, p = .007$), religious affiliation ($\chi^2(2) = 8.314, p = .016$), and political attitude ($\chi^2(2) = 12.011, p = .007$), but only in the private context. : Although the willingness to disclose the religious affiliation is generally rather low, people with a high level of conscientiousness are more willing to disclose their religious affiliation. 15% ($N = 34$) of participants with a high level of conscientious confirmed that they would disclose that information. Within the group of participants with a moderate level of conscientiousness only 10% ($N = 31$) and within the group with a low level 13% ($N = 40$) stated that they would disclose their religious affiliation. Regarding the disclosure of one's mobile phone number and political attitude, we can say that the higher ones level of conscientiousness the lower the proportion of people willing to disclose this data.

Extraversion. The level of *extraversion* has a significant influence on the disclosure of the private address in private SNS ($\chi^2(2) = 9.377, p = .009$) and business orientated ones ($\chi^2(2) = 7.385, p = .025$). Also, the willingness to disclose one's political attitude is significantly affected by extraversion in private (($\chi^2(2) = 9.324, p = .009$) as well as in business contexts ($\chi^2(2) = 9.543$, $p = .008$). For the private context we could also reveal a significant influence of extraversion on the disclosure of ones work address ($(\chi^2(2) = 12.795$, $p = .002$) and one's phone numbers (private phone number: $\chi^2(2) = 9.386$, $p = .009$; work phone number $\chi^2(2) = 13.313$, $p = .001$). On the one hand, we can summarize for influence of extraversion that an increasing level of extraversion influences the willingness to discloses data positively. But on the other hand, we have to report that there is a generally low willingness to disclose data in all cases portrayed here: The only item that reached a willingness to disclose above 30% was the disclosure of the political attitude in the private usage context (i.e., 39%).

Agreeableness. *Agreeableness* has no significant influence on the willingness to share personal data in either private or business oriented SNS.

Neuroticism. The last personality trait of the FFM scale, *neuroticism*, influences the willingness to disclose ones hobbies ($\chi^2(2) = 13.775$, $p = .001$) and the family status ($\chi^2(2) = 7.889$, $p = .019$) in the private using context. For the business context, the mobile phone usage is significantly influenced by neuroticism ($\chi^2(2) = 7.492$, $p = .024$). According to the influences of neuroticism disclosure on the willingness to disclose personal data, we can report that the higher the level of neuroticism the lower the willingness to disclose one's mobile phone number in the business related usage context. In the context of the disclosure of a persons' family status we revealed that people with a high level of neuroticism are more willing to disclose their family status. 79% ($N = 33$) stated that they would disclose their data. In comparison, only 53% ($N = 45$) of the participants with a medium level of neuroticism and 49% ($N = 51$) with a low level would disclose their hobby within a SNS. For the disclosure of one's hobbies, we revealed that people with a high level of neuroticism are more willing to disclose their hobbies than participants with a lower level: 100% ($N = 33$) of participants with a high level of neuroticism would disclose their hobbies whereas only 69% ($N = 45$) of the participants with a medium level of neuroticism and 67% ($N = 52$) of the ones with a low level are willing to disclose this information.

4.5 Moderating Factors for the Willingness to Disclose Personal Data in SNS

In order to find out whether moderating factors can influence the willingness to disclose personal data, we asked each participant to evaluate four statements (on a four-point Likert scale from 1 = totally disagree to 4 = totally agree) addressing incentives and other moderating aspects for the disclosure of personal data.

As the two figures (see Fig. 5 and 6) illustrate, *data disclosure not via Internet, money* and *positive media* were, on average not regarded to have a positive impact on the willingness to disclose data in SNS neither private nor business related ones. Only *more information* is evaluated to have a positive impact on the willingness to disclose data in SNS.

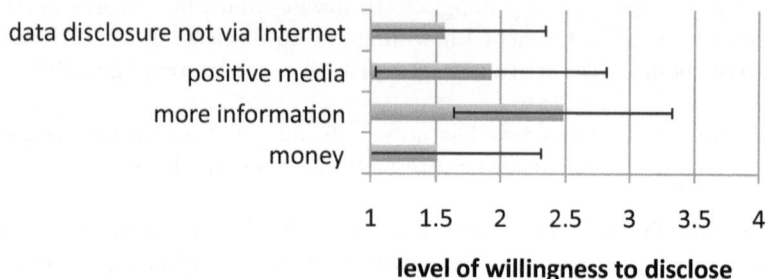

Fig. 5. Mean comparison of moderating factors for the willingness to disclose personal data in SNS in a private context (on a four-point Likert scale)

4.6 Influence of User Diversity on the Evaluation of Moderating Factors

To learn more about the influence of user-diversity on the moderating factors for data disclosure, non-parametric Kruskal-Wallis tests were executed to detect differences in the evaluation habits. Results revealed that the factors age and gender are not causing significant differences in the evaluation of the moderating factors for data disclosure.

The PLoC revealed a significant difference for money as an incentive for data disclosure in private SNS ($\chi^2(1) = 4.265$, $p = .039$). The higher a person's PLoC, the higher their willingness to disclose data for money.

The FFM personality traits revealed no significant difference for the factors extraversion, neuroticism, and conscientiousness. Agreeableness showed a significant difference in the evaluation of the incentive *money* in the context of business oriented SNS ($\chi^2(2) = 6.051$, $p = .049$), the higher the level of agreeableness the lower the evaluation that money would enhance the willingness to disclose data in the business context. The factor openness revealed a significant difference in the business context ($\chi^2(2) = 8.303$, $p = .016$) for the statement less negative press would enhance the willingness to disclose data. The higher a participant's level of openness, the lower the rejection of this statement.

Summing this section up we say that the moderating aspects *money, less negative press* and *data entry not via Internet* are not regarded to have a positive impact on the willingness to disclose personal data in SNS. The only factor regarded to have a positive impact was early information (for private SNS as well as business related ones). Also, the user diversity factors age, gender, PLoC as well as personality showed no meaningful influence on the moderating factors.

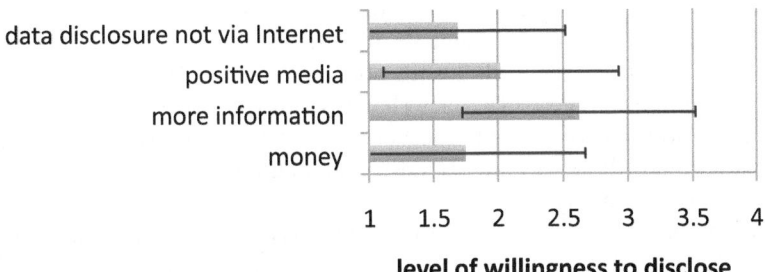

Fig. 6. Mean comparison of moderating factors for the willingness to disclose personal data in SNS in a business context (on a four-point Likert scale from $1 = disagree$ to $4 = agree$)

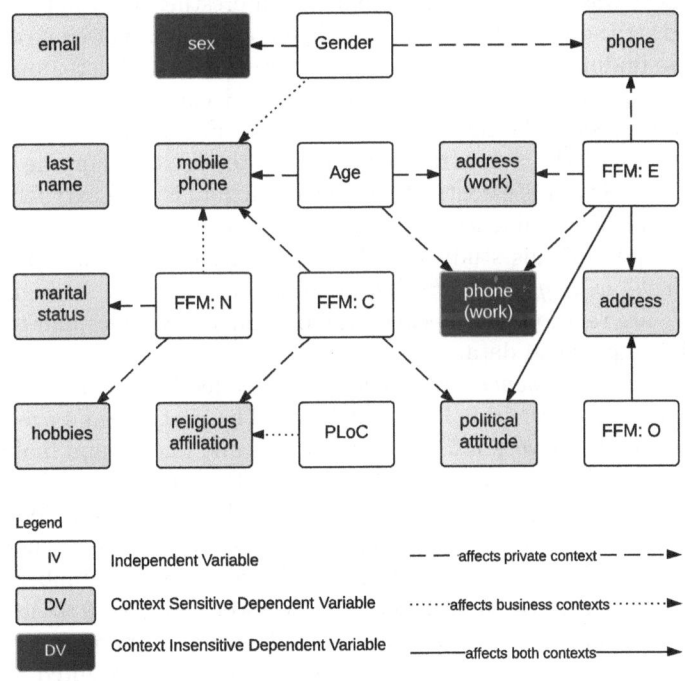

Fig. 7. Visual overview of the relationsships of IV and DV. FFM = Five Factor Model, PLoC = Perceived Locus of Control. All dependent variables denote willingness to disclose

5   Discussion

As data disclosure is a central factor for running a SNS successfully, we investigated the willingness to disclose personal data in SNS in two different settings (private and business). According to the research questions (see Section 2) this research was focussed on the influence of user diversity (age, gender, personality (FFM), PLoC) on the willingness to disclose personal data in SNS, and on moderating factors (data disclosure not via Internet, positive media, more information, money). Due to the fact that SNS in the private context are very successful, we wanted to find out whether these settings are evaluated similarly. Similarities would allow to transfer design guidelines more or less one on one into the business context.

In the context of this research, we could reveal that there is a significant *difference between data disclosure in private or business related SNS* (RQ1). Significant differences were found for the data: address (work), phone number (work), mobile number, and hobbies. For all differences we found that the working context leads to a higher level of willingness to disclose data.

A relatively high level of willingness to disclose work related data in work related context was not surprising. What was interesting was the fact that data like political attitude, marital status, or religious affiliation showed no differences. Taking these findings into account, we could argue that a direct transition from concepts of private SNS to business related SNS could be possible for some personal data except, the four mentioned above. Especially sensitive personal data seems to underlie a general unwillingness to disclose. For the context of business related SNS it is essential to define which data is necessary for successful usage and what fears influence willingness to disclose.

Another aspect of this study was the investigation of the *influence of user-diversity on the willingness to disclose personal data of SNS*: As Figure 7 illustrates, there are relationships between the dependent variables and the willingness to disclose personal data.

The factors *age* and *gender* are predominantly affecting the disclosure of data in the private usage scenario (RQ2 and RQ3). The participant's age influences data that is related to work information (address and phone) and mobile phone. Due to the fact of the relatively young sample, the experience with work and effects of working life on the private sector could lead to these differences. The willingness to disclose one's private phone number and sex is influenced by a person's gender. The same is relevant for one's mobile phone number in a business scenario. Since all these parameters show lower willingness to disclose data for women one could assume that the low willingness to share either a private phone number or one's sex could be related to avoiding unwanted approaches of male users. This finding is vaguely supported by the effect of neuroticism on willingness to disclose a mobile phone number which is also higher in women. Furthermore, extraversion, conscientiousness, and openness improve willingness to disclose data, but mostly in private contexts (RQ5). One could argue that in business settings varying personality does reflect willingness to disclose, because voluntariness of use (i.e., work) is rather low in this context.

Interestingly, *PLoC* showed only little impact on many facets of data disclosure (RQ4). This finding strengthens the idea that an SNS is more likely to be seen as a medium of communication than one of technology.

The only *incentive* (RQ6) for data disclosure that reaches a positive effect is *more information*. One could argue, since information is a central aim of SNS solutions, that this finding only replicates the importance of *perceived usefulness* from other technology acceptance research.

Designing an SNS for internal business communication requires knowledge of user diversity factors of the specific staff in order to customize required profile data within the SNS. It is necessary to communicate effectively why certain data is surveyed, and to demonstrate the effect of the availability of this data on improvement of information exchange within an organization.

Limitations and Future Research. In the context of this study, we have to name some limitations. Due to the fact that the answering options for data disclosure were limited to dichotomous answering options, we could only run non-parametric tests. In future research, the findings of this study should be investigated by using higher level scales to get a deeper insight into the willingness to disclose data. Additionally, the motives behind the willingness to disclose specific data must be investigated. The relatively young age of our sample promts us to intensify the investigation of age effects within a more age-heterogenous sample in future studies.

Assessment of incentives is particularly tricky, because incentives reported as being most effective do not actually need to be the most effective incentive, as users might not be fully aware of their motives. People might disagree with *money* being an effective motivator but behavioral studies have confirmed different findings in certain settings. In future studies, behavioral studies should be added because they are better suited to determine the impact of incentives.

Acknowledgments. We would like to thank the anonymous reviewers for their constructive comments on an earlier version of this manuscript. We would also like to thank Chantal Lidynia for her research assistance. This study has been funded by the German Ministry of Education and Research (BMBF) and the European Social Fund (ESF) within the programe "Innovationsfähigkeit im demographischen Wandel" under the reference number 01HH11045.

References

1. Davenport, T.H., Prusak, L.: Working knowledge: How organizations manage what they know. Harvard Business Press (2000)
2. Buck, H., Kistler, E., Mendius, H.G.: Demographischer wandel in der arbeitswelt: Chancen für eine innovative arbeitsgestaltung (2002)

3. Deutsche Akademie der Naturforscher (ed.): More Years, More Life: Recommendations of the Joint Academy Initiative on Aging, 1. Auflage. Nova Acta Leopoldina N.F., vol. 108. Wissenschaftliche Verlagsgesellschaft (2010)
4. Bloom, D.E., Canning, D.: Global demographic change: Dimensions and economic significance. Working Paper 10817, National Bureau of Economic Research (October 2004)
5. Institut der Deutschen Wirtschaft Köln: Die Zukunft der Arbeit in Deutschland: Megatrends, Reformbedarf und Handlungsoptionen. IW-Studien. Dt. Inst.-Verl., Köln (2008)
6. Sullivan, S.E.: The changing nature of careers: A review and research agenda. Journal of Management 25(3), 457–484 (1999)
7. Osterland, M.: Normalbiographie und Normalarbeitsverhältnis (1989)
8. Reitzle, M., Körner, A., Vondracek, F.W.: Psychological and demographic correlates of career patterns. Journal of Vocational Behavior 74(3), 308–320 (2009)
9. Hill, E.J., Ferris, M., Märtinson, V.: Does it matter where you work? a comparison of how three work venues (traditional office, virtual office, and home office) influence aspects of work and personal/family life. Journal of Vocational Behavior 63(2), 220–241 (2003)
10. Venkatesh, A., Vitalari, N.P.: An emerging distributed work arrangement: an investigation of computer-based supplemental work at home. Management Science 38(12), 1687–1706 (1992)
11. Bailey, D.E., Kurland, N.B.: A review of telework research: Findings, new directions, and lessons for the study of modern work. Journal of Organizational Behavior 23(4), 383–400 (2002)
12. Davis, F.D.: Perceived usefulness, perceived ease of use, and user acceptance of information technology. MIS Quarterly, 319–340 (1989)
13. Venkatesh, V., Morris, M.G., Davis, G.B., Davis, F.D.: User acceptance of information technology: Toward a unified view. MIS Quarterly, 425–478 (2003)
14. Kaplan, A.M., Haenlein, M.: Users of the world, unite! the challenges and opportunities of social media. Business Horizons 53(1), 59–68 (2010)
15. Correa, T., Hinsley, A.W., De Zuniga, H.G.: Who interacts on the web?: The intersection of users personality and social media use. Computers in Human Behavior 26(2), 247–253 (2010)
16. Bothorel, C., Lohr, C., Thépaut, A., Bonnaud, F., Cabasse, G.: From individual communication to social networks: evolution of a technical platform for the elderly. Toward Useful Services for Elderly and People with Disabilities, 145–152 (2011)
17. Calero Valdez, A., Schaar, A.K., Ziefle, M.: State of the (net) work address developing criteria for applying social networking to the work environment. Work: A Journal of Prevention, Assessment and Rehabilitation 41, 3459–3467 (2012)
18. Koch, M., Richter, A.: Enterprise 2.0: Planung, Einführung und erfolgreicher Einsatz von Social Software in Unternehmen. Oldenbourg Verlag (2009)
19. Holzinger, A., Kickmeier-Rust, M.D., Ebner, M.: Interactive technology for enhancing distributed learning: a study on weblogs. In: Proceedings of the 23rd British HCI Group Annual Conference on People and Computers: Celebrating People and Technology, BCS-HCI 2009, pp. 309–312. British Computer Society, Swinton (2009)

20. Richter, A., Stocker, A., Mller, S., Avram, G.: Knowledge management goals revisited – a cross-sectional analysis of social software adoption in corporate environments. In: ACIS 2011 Proceedings (January 2011)
21. Costa, P.T., McCrae, R.: Neo five-factor inventory. Psychological Assessment Resources, Odessa (1991)
22. Costa, P.T., McCrae, R.R.: Normal personality assessment in clinical practice: The neo personality inventory. Psychological Assessment 4(1), 5 (1992)
23. Rammstedt, B., John, O.P.: Measuring personality in one minute or less: A 10-item short version of the big five inventory in english and german. Journal of Research in Personality 41(1), 203–212 (2007)

Practical Neurophysiological Analysis of Readability as a Usability Dimension

Inês Isabel Pimentel Oliveira[1] and Nuno Manuel Guimarães[2]

[1] SITILabs, Lusófona University, Portugal
ines.oliveira@ulusofona.pt
[2] LaSIGE/ISCTE-IUL, University Institute of Lisbon, Portugal
nmcfg@iscte.pt

Abstract. This paper discusses opportunities and feasibility of integrating neurophysiologic analysis methods, based on electroencephalography (EEG), in the current landscape of usability evaluation methods. The rapid evolution and growing availability of low-cost, easier to use devices and the accumulated knowledge in feature extraction and processing algorithms allow us to foresee the practicality of this integration.

The work presented in this paper is focused on reading and readability, identified as a key element of usability heuristics, and observable in the neurophysiologic signals' space. The experiments are primarily designed to address the discrimination of the reading activity (silent, attentive and continuous) and the verification of decreasing readability, associated with the user's mental workload analysis. The results obtained in the series of experiments demonstrate the validity of the approach for each individual user, and raise the problem of inter-subject variability and the need for designing appropriate calibration procedures for different users.

Keywords: Usability analysis, neurophysiologic signals, EEG.

1 Introduction

The current usability evaluation methods range from interpretative to predictive, the former based on the observation and study of the actual use of an artifact during its development cycle, and the latter exploring external analyses performed by experts equipped with standards, heuristics and modeling techniques [1]. The methods capture either the behavior and perceptions of users or the interactive attributes of the artifact, and converge to evaluation conclusions based on the qualitative or quantitative analysis of empirically collected data.

Alternative, or complementary, methods based in the measurement of physical and physiological signals of the human user (e.g. eye-movements, heart rate (HR) and heart rate variation (HRV), skin conductance (SC), or electroencephalography (EEG)) have been used more frequently in contexts with critical requirements for human performance [2], and tested in dedicated labs, as opposed to the use of the former empirical methods, typically adopted by usability labs participating in the design and development of interactive artifacts for the general user or consumer.

A. Holzinger et al. (Eds.): SouthCHI 2013, LNCS 7946, pp. 194–211, 2013.

The evolution of the technological landscape leads us reassess the opportunities for expanding and improving the set of tools for usability evaluation. First, capture devices are cheaper, more reliable, less intrusive, and usable with increasing autonomy. Examples of this evolution are HR or SC measurement devices, which have become portable and wireless and even EEG systems have left the controlled conditions of clinical settings (see for example, the design of dry electrode devices [3]. Second, the capacity to process these signals evolved dramatically, both in computing power and in the understanding of the algorithms that extract meaning from the human data.

As a result of this evolution, we can envision a feasible integration of human physical and physiological information in common interactive artifacts, as a new modality. On the other hand, in the scope of usability evaluation, we can aim at incorporating those human signals in the analysis setup, namely in the common usability lab environment, thus reinforcing the mature and widely adopted empirical methods with easier to use physical measurement methods.

In this paper we assess the effectiveness of a brain signal analysis in usability evaluation, with a focus on readability - the ability of a user being able to read a text. This is not a sufficient condition for system usability, but it is, in many interactive artifacts, a necessary one. Readability is affected by interface design decisions, with a particular relevance on presentation choices. Readability has an impact in usability heuristics, discussed below.

Our focus is therefore the detection and analysis of the cognitive activity of reading. Again, readability is not a sufficient condition for a user to read but it is a necessary one. The detection of reading should be a good indicator of readability, provided that variables that create obstacles to reading such as high text complexity, foreign language, distraction, fatigue, or even cultural bias, are eliminated. In this work, we considered that a strong correlation between reading and readability should be sought in continuous attentive reading activities. This avoids the need of discrimination between recognizing word and text as grammatically appropriate character sequences, and recognizing isolated words as individual learned symbols.

The next section reviews a number of works that have used physiological signal processing in the scope of the analysis of the usability of some system or tool. In the following two sections, we scope this work along the baseline aspects: (i) reading as an activity correlated with readability, which is in turn directly affected by user interface design decisions and has an impact on heuristically defined usability criteria, and (ii) the set of computational techniques used in the processing of brain signals. The concrete experimental framework is then presented, followed by the results of a set of experiments. The implications for future work towards an effective integration of brain signal processing in usability evaluation are elaborated in the conclusion.

2   Related Work

Beer et al. refer that "the usability lab of the future" must integrate analysis tools based in physiological measures, including the EEG [4]. These signals are potentially valuable for measuring users' emotional valence and vigilance during the interaction [5]. As the data generated with these methods comes directly from the users' physical processes, without intermediation of an observer or expert, it can reveal, for example, social masks, when users avoid giving negative answers in interviews. Still, this integration is preliminary. The studies quoted below compare physiological based analysis with classical usability methods, e.g. questionnaires.

Table 1. Studies comparing physiological-based methods with classical empirical methods for analysis of specific usability dimensions

Refer-ence	Main Goals	Analysis Methods	Main Conclusions
#1 [6] 5 partic-ipants	Distinguish emotional states using 3 distinct menus: —regular &familiar —illegible —error	**Physiological**: EEG Theta, alpha and beta rhythms of the best 2 out of 10 electrodes **Classical**: —Questionnaire —Task Difficulty classification —A/V and eye tracking recordings	—Attested the correlation between EEG and inquiry data (1 user); —Attest the correlation between EEG and difficulty classification (5 users)
#2 [7] 43 parti cipants	Study the emotional response to 2 alternative prototypes for an e-government site, (with/without anthropomorphic Web Assistant)	**Physiological**: ESR[1] differen tial analysis with (max-min)/min, max and 1st peak value **Classical**: Inquiries, SMEQ[2] Scale Inquiry	—Attest the correlation between ESR and classical methods —Users preferred Web Assistant version —Differences between both sites were statistically relevant with both measures
#3 [8,9] 20 par ticipants	—Performance test to evaluate an uni versity learning system —Non moderated time limited tasks Different system experienced users.	**Physiological**: ESR and HRV[3] **Classical**: —Extended NPL[4] inquiry —TAP[5] —A/V recordings —SUS[6] questionnaire	—Attest the correlation between users performance and emotional state; —Both groups reveled emotional differences
#4 [10,11] 10 part icipants	Study mental workload differences in a set of equivalent tasks in MS Excel 2003 and 2007	**Physiological**: EEG Alpha and beta rhythms' average Normalized PSD. **Classical**: SUS questionnaire	—Attest the correlation between both types of measures software experience and alpha and beta ratio variation —Users preferred (and showed less mental workload) Excel 2007

---

[1] Electrodermal Skin Response.
[2] Subjective Mental Effort Questionnaire.
[3] Heart rate variation.
[4] National Physics Laboratory.
[5] Think Aloud Protocol.
[6] System Usability Scale.

Reference	Main Goals	Analysis Methods	Main Conclusions
#5 [12] 4 participants	Performance versus workload test in a simple game with 3 distinct difficult levels	**Physiological**: —EEG: Avg. PSD[7] (in alpha, beta, theta, delta and gamma), cross spectrum and coherence —fNIR[8]: Normalized Oxygenation Variation **Classical**: User performance (game score)	—Performance is proportional with level's difficulty —Accuracy classification depends on the used measure (better with fNIR) —fNIR may interfere with EEG sensors
#6 [13] 10 participants	Evaluate user preferences and emotional states regarding 4 car company web-sites	**Physiological**: —EEG (ERPs, PSD in beta and theta) —HR (Std, Greater and minor freq. ratio) **Classical**: —Preference questionnaire —Error and Task completion rates —Task Execution time —A/V and screen recordings	—100% of correlation between classical versus EEG results —60% of correlation between classical versus ECG results
#7 [14] 36 participants	Game UX evaluation of an immersive game using 2 input devices and consoles: —Standard gamepad in PSP2 —Wii Remote in Nintendo	**Physiological**: EEG - Normalized PSD in alpha, beta, delta, theta and gamma **Classical**: Questionnaires —GEQ (Game Experience Questionnaire) —Auto-localization, to evaluate perception aspects in VR environment	—Attest the correlation between both types of measures; —WII Remote scores better in questionnaires and also causes a greater mental activity

These studies show the potential of physiological measures in usability and user experience evaluation and demonstrate the correlation between physiological and traditional methods. The test cases are however very constrained situations, and several open issues are identified. First, capture devices are expensive, intrusive and complex to handle, making it possible to generate emotions that are not directly related with the interaction [5]. Secondly, it is difficult to generalize the results, because of the various degrees of variation, such as gender, age and culture. Finally, the interpretation of the measures is complex, even when the cause and effect are known, because it strongly depends on the social and interpersonal context [15].

3   Reading in Usability

Usability heuristics have become generalized tools to evaluate usability of interactive products, systems or services. These heuristics are empirically consolidated reflections of the structural coupling [16] requirements that a usable user interface

---

[7] Power Spectrum Density.
[8] Functional Near Infrared Spectroscopy.

implicitly meets. This coupling between a user and an artefact is maintained as long as the properties of the artifact are compatible with the user's cognitive or physical abilities. On one side we have characteristics of the artifact like legibility, language, visibility or aesthetics, and on the other we have human cognitive processes like reading, understanding, memory or different emotional reactions.

As an example, let us consider the universally acknowledged Nielsen heuristics [17] listed in Table 2. The table relates the heuristics with cognitive processes through a number of (not exhaustive and non orthogonal) determining user interface characteristics or interaction mechanisms. This tentative mapping is partially justified by the experimentations reported in the previous section (quoted in column 4).

Table 2. Relations between (de facto standard) usability heuristics and cognitive processes

Heuristic (1)	Determining UI Characteristics (2)	Cognitive processes (3)	Related work(4)
1. Visibility of system status	Legibility, visual[9] expression, feedback (e.g. icons)	Perception incl. Reading	#2
2. Match system and real world	Semiotic design (e.g. metaphors)	Understanding, Memory, **Emotion**	#2
3. User control and freedom	Multitasking, escapability, recovery (e.g. undo/redo)	Memory, Workload, Learning, **Emotion**	#3, #7
4. Consistency, standards	Visual design, Homogeneity (e.g. layout, menus)	Perception, Memory	#1
5. Error prevention	Legibility, visual feedback (e.g. data formats)	Perception incl. Reading, Memory, Workload	#1
6. Recognition rather than recall	Semiotic design, legibility (e.g. menus)	Perception incl. Reading, Memory	#1
7. Flexibility, efficiency of use	Attention requirements, Adaptability (e.g. shortcuts)	**Workload**, Memory, Learning	#3, #4, #5, #7
8. Aesthetic, minimalist design	Legibility, visual design (e.g. look)	Perception, Reading, **Emotion**	#6
9. Help users recognize, diagnose, and recover from errors	Legibility, visual feedback (e.g. error messages)	Perception, Reading, Problem solving	

The above associations express a path between usability heuristics and cognitive processes that can be observed through their external manifestations in physical and physiological signals. This path is conceptually important for an integrated perspective of the analysis and evaluation methods.

Reading, especially continuous, attentive, and silent reading, has not been analyzed in this context. In fact, reading in the common user interface is generally associated with word recognition for most of the textual elements of the user interface (e.g. labels, menus, icons or forms). Its performance can be severely affected by several design factors including: typeface and text features problems (e.g. inappropriate color and text or line spacing), poor contrast between background and text, uncomfortable

---

[9] "Visual" is mentioned here in the broad sense of an external, perceptually intelligible representation, but it can be based in any other modality like audio or haptic forms.

screen distance, design and formatting problems (e.g. too wide or too narrow text and center or right justification) [18]. Readability can therefore be considered as a usability guideline among the heuristics referred above [19].

4   Brain Signals

In this section, we briefly describe the hardware and software platform used to capture and process the brain signals. The selected and used computational techniques are also briefly enumerated, as a more detailed explanation and discussion of the processing techniques can be found elsewhere [20, 21].

The signal acquisition and selection was based in two fundamental requirements. First, the acquisition devices should be low-end devices, usable in the environment of a usability lab, as opposed to a clinical environment. The low-end devices, with a limited number of channels, do still require some level of expertise to set up an acquisition session (electrode placement and impedance adjustment) but are manageable by an experienced technician or researcher, and are in line with the expected evolution of more usable and portable acquisition devices.

Second, the signals to observe should avoid highly demanding synchronization requirements. Since the goal is to detect and discriminate reading activity, the focus of the analysis was the variation of brain waves instead of the brain responses to discrete stimuli. This focus leads to the choice of the analysis of brain rhythms (alpha (α), beta (β), delta (δ), theta (θ), and gamma (γ)), instead of ERP (Event Related Potentials), which require controlled synchronization conditions between stimuli and acquired signal (a few milliseconds). While the later signals provide the proper information for studying brain responses and are actually the main source of "input" in BCI (Brain Computer Interfaces), see [22-24], the former analysis is appropriate for cognitive process detection and better suited for future lightweight devices.

4.1   Signal Aquisition

The signal acquisition was made in an open space human-computer interaction lab with MindSet MS-1000, a sixteen (16) channel digital capture device, and its proprietary software acquisition tool named MindMeld. All sensors were attached to an ElectroCap cap and positioned accordingly with the 10-20 International System: six (6) in the frontal area, four (4) in the temporal, and the remaining six (6) in the parietal, central and occipital (two in each area).

The capture was performed at 256Hz using referential electrodes placed in ear lobes. All requirements defined by EEG capture experts and the devices fabricants were met: all users were connected to a ground wire to reduce the electrical noise peak; hair was brushed with a wooden brush to reduce electrostatic; scalp sensors place was previously cleaned with alcohol; conductive gel was applied in all electrodes and impedance was maintained below 5000kΩ in all electrodes.

4.2   Signal Processing Chain

The components of the signal processing chain we applied to the brain signals are shown in Fig. 1. In the figure, the thicker connectors mean "mandatory path"; traced connectors mean "alternative or optional", and the thinner connection shown the contribution of feature selection to the indicated steps in the chain.

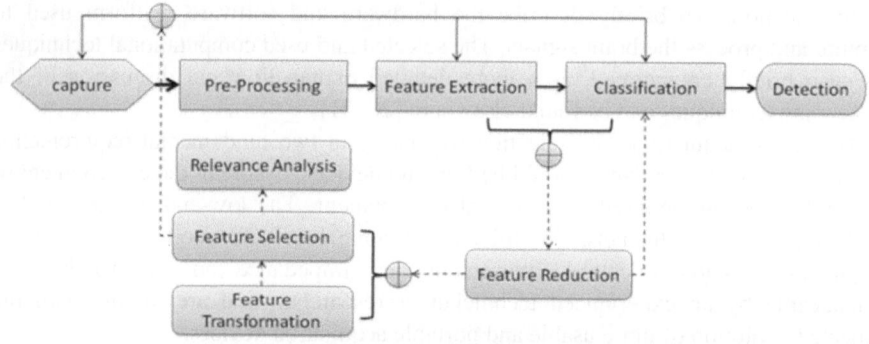

Fig. 1. The Signal Processing Chain

The sixteen (16) signals, one per channel, are pre-processed individually to reduce non EEG artifacts (e.g. electrical noise), and transformed into feature vectors, where each vector is composed by 16x5(80) real values – the estimated average power spectrum in delta, theta, alpha, beta and gamma rhythms, determined in one second periods (also called *windows*), overlapped in 0.5 seconds. A feature vector can then be classified in certain classes related to user cognitive processes, such as reading and non-reading. In the process, feature vector dimension can previously be reduced, to increase the chain and classification overall performance, through transformation and/or selection methods [25]. The feature selection can also be based on relevance analysis. This analysis ranks features according to their contribution to the discrimination of the classes under observation [21].

All the results presented and discussed in this paper were obtained using PSD (Power Spectrum Density) feature extraction and an SVM (Support Vector Machines) classifier. PSD measures the energy of the signal in a certain frequency [21]. It is a frequency feature, so to get its variation over time, the PSD is determined in one second length rectangular windows, overlapped in 0.5 seconds. SVM are supervised classifiers proven to be successful in EEG analysis [26]. SVMs divide the solution space in hyper-planes through discriminating functions. In our case we use the kernel trick that makes SVMs, originally linear, nonlinear classifiers. This kernel uses a Gaussian radial basis function (RBF), generally used in BCI research.

Preprocessing methods that were used in the results presented in this paper only include a Notch (narrow band) filter, which allows reducing electrical noise peek at 50Hz, still present after grounding users. No method has been used to reduce eye and movement artifacts. Our goal is to build a method robust enough to handle these interferences that naturally result from user interaction.

5   Experimental Procedures

An experimental session (or trial) is composed by a sequence of several distinct experiments, all related with silent reading in a screen. A session takes approximately twenty-five (25) minutes. All experiments were separated by thirty (30) second resting periods, during which users were asked about the text topic (they just read), when they stopped reading, and their overall mental and emotional state.

All the results presented in this paper were performed with six (6) users, three (3) women and three (3) man, ages between 20 and 45, without relevant neurological or sight or visual known conditions, three (3) using glasses, and one (1) left-handed. All users concluded successfully a higher educational degree and frequently read literary, technical and/or news texts in both paper and digital format. There was no previous training, but all users repeated the experiences in different days, with distinct texts and images.

All texts were written in the native language and never repeated for the same user. An event generator application was used to build and display an event script such as a slide show [20]. We built twenty-three (23) different scripts for these experiments. All content was displayed in a 15.4'' laptop LCD colored screen, with a 1280x800 resolution and 4,295E+9 colors. The laptop was set in a regular desk, with about 70-80 centimeters height. Users sat in front of the screen, at a distance between 50-60 centimeters. In general, all texts were displayed with Arial 21px font in a black foreground over a white background, unless experiments thus required. The experiments whose results are described in this paper are the following:

1. **Text versus Blank Screen:** Users read two texts (with news) for 30 seconds each, interleaved with a blank screen for 20 seconds. This was a preliminary experiment, to evaluate whether it was possible distinguishing silent reading cognitive state from another basic visual state, such as looking at a blank screen, to tune algorithms and also to study the variation between sessions and users.
2. **Text versus Drawings:** this is a similar experience, but, instead of a blank screen, it interleaves text with black and white unfilled drawings for 30 seconds. It allows assessing the possibility of distinguishing silent reading cognitive state regarding a simple visual, non verbal, stimulus.

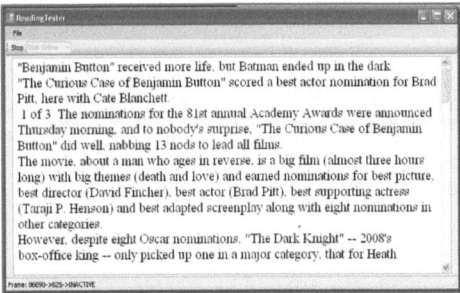 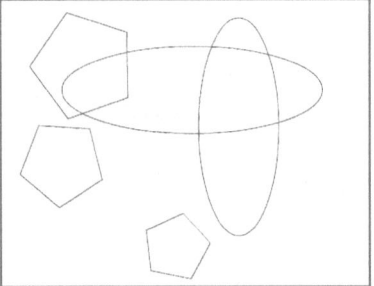

Fig. 2. Example of news and drawing display used in the first two experiments

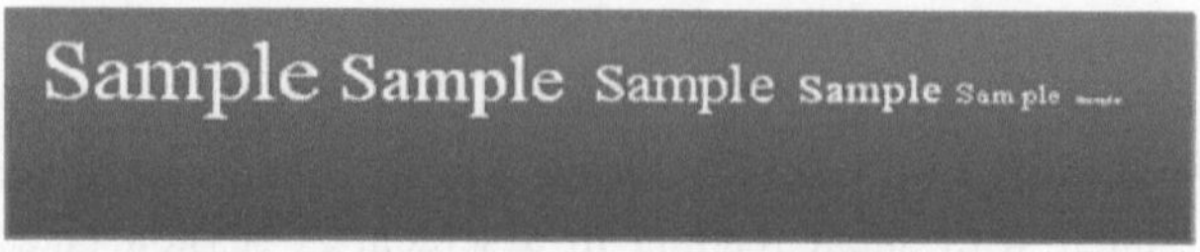

Fig. 3. Text size variation simulation used in Text Size Decrease experiment

3. **Text Size Decrease.** Users read a 70 words news text, one word at a time, each lasting one second. Every ten seconds the size of text decreases by 3px, varying between 21px and 3px.

4. **Background/Text Contrast Decrease (by varying background).** Users read news text during seventy (70) seconds while every ten (10) seconds the background is darkened about 16% in relation to white. This was preceded by the same experience without text to serve as control.

3. **Background/Text Contrast Decrease (by varying text).** Users read news text during seventy (70) seconds while every ten (10) seconds the text is lighten about 16% in relation to black.

6. **RGB Difference Background/Text Decrease.** Users read news text during seventy (70) seconds while every ten (10) seconds the RGB difference between background and text is reduced between 5 to 15%.

All these experiments concern directly and indirectly the usability heuristics (1) visibility, (4) standards, or (8) aesthetic and minimalist design, mentioned in Table 2. As previously mentioned, text visual characteristics influence readability, and consequently reading performance. This indirectly influences all other heuristics where the reading cognitive process plays a role, such as Recognition and Recall.

5.1   W3C (World Wide Web Consortium) Thresholds

To guarantee that a text can be read in a screen by users with color deficits , the W3C proposes a minimum font size for screens of 9px [28] and a contrast and RGB difference thresholds of 125 and 500 respectively [27]. The last two sizes (6px and 3px) in experiment 3 violate these W3C recommendations, and the intensity and RGB values that were used in experiments 4-6 are shown in the next tables.

Table 3. Experiment 4. Intensity values and compliance with W3C thresholds.

Experimental Step	Back. Intensity (B)	Text Intensity (T)	(B)-(T)	Compliance with W3C threshold
1	255	0	255	Yes
2	214	0	214	Yes
3	173	0	173	Yes
4	132	0	132	Yes
5	91	0	91	No
6	51	0	51	No

Table 4. Experiment 5. Intensity values and compliance with W3C thresholds.

Experimental Step	Back. Intensity(B)	Text Intensity(T)	(B) –(T)	Compliance with W3C threshold
1	255	0	255	Yes
2	255	40	215	Yes
3	255	81	174	Yes
4	255	122	133	Yes
5	255	163	92	No
6	255	204	51	No

Table 5. Experiment 6. RGB values and compliance with W3C thresholds.

Experimental Step	Background			Text			RGB Difference	Compliance w/ W3C threshold
	Red	Green	Blue	Red	Green	Blue		
1	255	255	255	0	0	0	765	Yes
2	255	247	215	20	0	40	657	Yes
3	235	239	215	20	0	120	549	Yes
4	235	223	215	20	0	200	453	No
5	195	223	215	60	0	200	373	No
6	175	223	175	80	8	200	335	No

6   Results and Discussion

The organization of this section is the following: In **section 6.1.** are presented the results regarding experiments 1-2, where is analysed silent continuous reading distinction towards other simple visual states. Here are discussed topics such as user and session generalization.

The results of the remaining experiments, which vary text or background aspects that affect readability, are discussed in **section 6.2**. Based on the work of Kimura and Masaki [10,11], we analyze the correlation between classical evaluation based measures, such as inquiries, and an EEG based measure. This measure was the beta/alpha PSD ratio, considered to be indicative of *mental workload* [10,11].

The presented results consider the following data corpus subsets:

- **Intra-user data set (A).** Includes 13 sessions of a single unique user.
- **Inter-user data set (B).** Includes 12 sessions of six users, two sessions each.

All the procedures and metrics were initially tuned using data set A. The following section discusses the results of processing these experiments using both data sets.

6.1   Silent Reading Distinction

The results of silent reading distinction (with both data set A and B) are shown in Fig. 4. F-Measure is a classification performance measure that averages precision and recall geometrically in a single value. It varies between 0%, the worst possible result and, 100%, the best, where all mental states were 100% correctly classified.

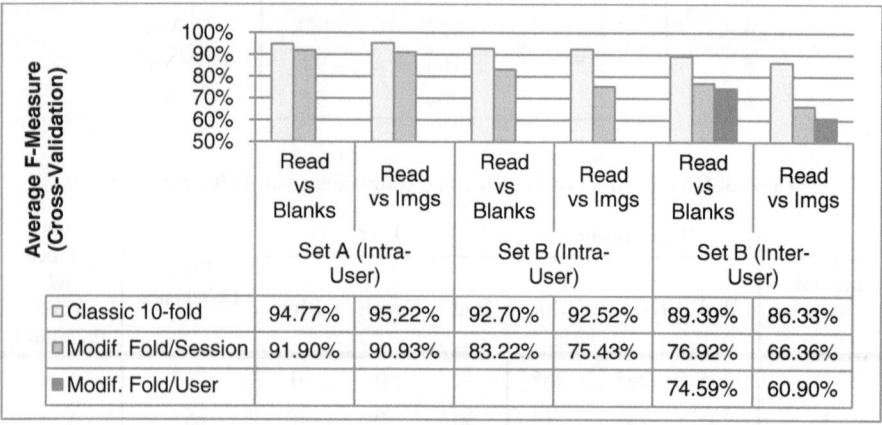

	Read vs Blanks	Read vs Imgs	Read vs Blanks	Read vs Imgs	Read vs Blanks	Read vs Imgs
	Set A (Intra-User)		Set B (Intra-User)		Set B (Inter-User)	
☐ Classic 10-fold	94.77%	95.22%	92.70%	92.52%	89.39%	86.33%
▨ Modif. Fold/Session	91.90%	90.93%	83.22%	75.43%	76.92%	66.36%
■ Modif. Fold/User					74.59%	60.90%

Fig. 4. Silent Reading Detection Results

We used both classical and modified versions of cross-validation. Cross-validation is an evaluation procedure, commonly applied while using supervised classifiers. These classifiers learn upon some correctly class labeled training data set, requiring a previous training step. This causes the results to depend on the selection of the training and test sets. Cross-validation[10] minimizes this dependency, making this selection more trustworthy. Modified schemes test the result generalization to distinct sessions and users[11].

Classic cross-validation schema results in Set A, 94,77% and 95,22%, suggest that there is a clear distinction between the silent reading mental state and alternative patterns. This also attests that the feature vectors of both classes clearly fall into different areas of the solution space, which is split in two by SVM. Session generalization results, 91,90% and 90,93%, show a slight decay of the classifier performance, but are promising towards the possibility of training the classifier with previously recorded sessions.

---

[10] Cross-validation splits randomly the available data set in similarly sized sub-sets, called folds, 10 in our case. It then performs 10 runs of train and test classification procedures, training with 9 folds and testing with the remaining one. The final result is the average of all classification iterations.

[11] The folds of these schemes coincide with sessions and users, which means that we are testing if the classifier can be trained with sessions and users, distinct from the sessions and users tested.

Inter-user Set B classic 10-fold results were above 85%, which indicates that the reading pattern is also detected in this case but session and user generalization performed poorly. User generalization can only be possible if both mental states are very similar in all users. Session generalization is also affected by this, since we have sessions belonging to distinct users.

6.2   Classical Measures Correlation

Our main goal is to successfully relate EEG based measures with classical methods measures, such as reading performance and inquiry data, while varying readability aspects such as text size and background/text contrast (Experiments 3 to 6).

We considered that a possible measure could be **mental workload** – beta/alpha ratio, which has been proved to be related with mental workload and user discomfort [10,11]. Beta rhythm (13-30Hz) has been related with mental activity and alpha (8-13Hz), to the mental rest in usability related experiments. So when user's mental workload is high the amount of alpha rhythm decreases, and the amount of beta and beta/alpha increases [10,11].

Mental Workload measure was first determined in each channel, using one seconds segments with 0.5 seconds overlapping, and then averaged twice. First it was spatially averaged in all channels to obtain the mean overall mental workload. Next it was temporally averaged in all samples belonging to a distinct experimental step, which we consider to be a reading situation where the text characteristics, such as size, contrast or color difference, remain constant. Next two sections discuss the results obtained while relating this measure with classical method measures, starting by performance based heuristics, directly determined from the text characteristics.

Performance Based Measures Correlation. We considered that the following two heuristics could approximate reading performance by changing some text or background relevant property (e.g. text size):

- **Reading performance,** inversely proportional to the considered aspect, that is:

$$\text{Reading\_performance}(\text{step}_i) = \text{aspect}(\text{step}_i)/\text{aspect}(\text{step}_1) \qquad (1)$$

- **W3C related ranking**, where the difference of the aspect regarding W3C orientations was quantified as

$$\text{W3C related ranking}(\text{step}_i) = \begin{cases} 0, \text{if diff}(\text{state}_i) < 0\% \\ 1, \text{ if } 0\% \leq \text{diff}(\text{state}_i) < 35\% \\ 2, \text{if } 35\% \leq \text{diff}(\text{state}_i) < 70\% \\ 3, \text{if } 70\% \leq \text{diff}(\text{state}_i) < 105\% \\ 4, \text{if diff}(\text{state}_i) \geq 105\% \end{cases} \qquad (2)$$

where

$$\text{diff}(\text{step}_i) = \text{aspect}(\text{step}_i)/\text{W3C threshold} - 1 \qquad (3)$$

Both heuristics consider that the initial step always assures a better readability that the following steps.

Next table shows the results of the correlation analysis between these performance heuristics and the mean workload in all sessions. The use of averaging in EEG is widely disseminated in order to reduce variability, and in this case results are not definitive but can show a trend.

Table 6. Correlation of the mean step workload with performance heuristics (inter-user Set B)

Experiment		Heuristic	Reading Performance	W3C Ranking
Text Size Decrease		CORR	☑0,794	☑0,906
		PVAL	0,033	0,005
Back./Text Contrast Decrease	Varying Back.	CORR	☒ -0,134	☒-0,097
		PVAL	0,800	0,856
	Varying Text	CORR	☒-0,196	☒-0,107
		PVAL	0,710	0,840
Back./Text RGB Difference Decrease		CORR	☑0,722	☑0,716
		PVAL	0,105	0,109

Correlation measures the probability of existing a linear relation between two measures; when it is close to 1 or -1, it is considered very strong; when is 0, it doesn't exist. In this case we are using Pearson correlation: PVAL is the p-value or the probability of the correlation being null; when it is below 0.05 or at least 0.1 it means that the conclusion is probabilistically relevant. Correlation and un-correlation evidence is signaled in the table through ☑ and ☒; the remaining values are inconclusive but point towards a possible correlation.

The results displayed show that mean mental workload is highly correlated with text size aspect variation, but the same conclusion does not hold in the remaining experiments. Both contrast experiments show significantly uncorrelated values, which means that mental workload very likely background/text contrast decrease is not linear related with the contrast difference itself. However, RGB difference shows a no significant correlation with both performance metrics.

Inquiry Based Measures Correlation. The same methodology was applied to the inquiry data that was registered both previously and during experimental sessions. This includes indicators of user fatigue and reading stop, which were approximated with the following two heuristics:

- **Fatigue State:** rates the user perceived fatigue state:

$$\text{Fatigue\_State(trial}_i) = \begin{cases} 1, \text{completely awake} \\ 2, \text{awake} \\ 3, \text{lightly tired} \\ 4, \text{tired} \\ 5, \text{very tired} \end{cases} \quad (4)$$

- **Reading (Occurrence) State**: signals whether reading has occurred or not in a certain experimental step:

$$\text{Reading\_State(step}_i) = \begin{cases} 1, \text{read} \\ 0, \text{didn't read} \\ 0.5, \text{read partially} \end{cases} \tag{5}$$

Fig. 5 presents graphically the correlation variation between the fatigue heuristic and the average mental workload in each step of experiments 3-6, also in inter-user Set B. For simplicity sake we omit the p-value (PVAL) and just display correlation values. All grayed areas signal correlations above 0.5. The significance of the correlations will be referred in context.

The obtained results show that the correlation with reported fatigue varies with the readability aspect being considered. In general texts resize experiment steps are significantly correlated, contrast steps, uncorrelated and color difference, insignificantly correlated. For example, Graphic a) shows a significant trend of a positive correlation between fatigue reported state and mental workload when text size gets smaller. This also means that minor size text reading implied a greater mental workload in users that reported being more fatigued.

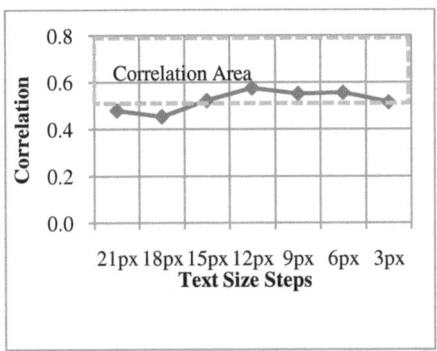

a) Text Resize Experiment

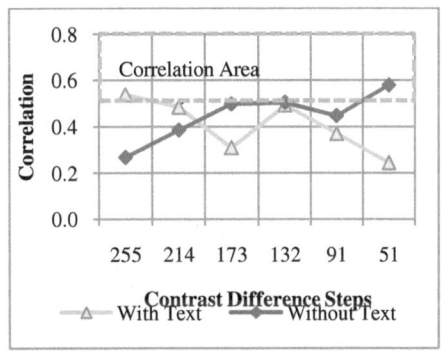

b) Back./Text Contrast (Varying Back.)

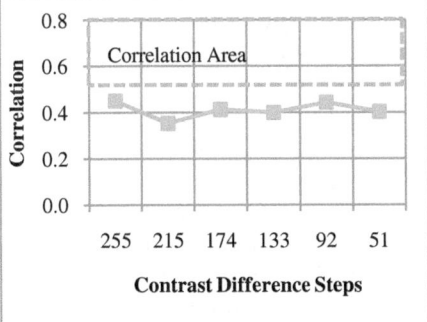

c) Back./Text Contrast (Varying Text)

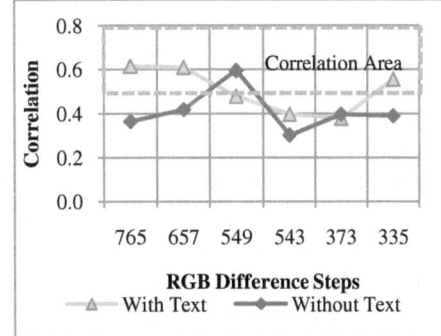

d) Back./Text RGB Difference

Fig. 5. Fatigued state-Mental workload correlation results (inter-user Set B)

Regarding RGB difference, it revealed some positive correlation in some color combinations, and contrast variation experiments were generally uncorrelated with fatigue reported state. When RGB difference lowers below the W3C defined threshold (in step 4) correlation visibly decreases, indicating this may cause a greater mental workload in more fatigue users (see Graphic d).

Additionally, graphics b) and c) show a similar correlation values in the initial steps, in line with the fact that both experiments start with the same text and background colors. And also in graphics b) and d) one can verify that there are mental workload differences when user reads or does not read, even when the backgrounds are the same.

Table 6 presents the correlation results regarding the remaining inquiry based heuristic: reading (occurrence) state. These were performed in some specific steps (usually the last) of the described experiments also in inter user Set B. In text size experiment we use the last but one step, because in the last step all users reported that they couldn't read the text[12]; in RGB difference, users declared to read in all steps.

Table 7. Read occurrence-Mental workload correlation results (inter-user Set B)

Experiment		Step	CORR	PVAL
Text Size		6) 6px	☑0,732	0,0162
Background/Text Contrast	Varying Background	6) 51	☒0,027	0,933
	Varying Text	6) 51	☒0,028	0,933
RGB Difference		NA		

These results point that there is a correlation between reading occurrence and mental workload only in text variation experiment. As it was told before this requires further study because this can be text size specific.

7   Conclusions and Future Work

The integration of low cost and feasible neurophysiologic methods in the usability analysis framework is possible and can be effective in some specific conditions. This is the main conclusion that can be drawn from the suite of experiences reported in this paper.

Based on the mapping of usability heuristics or guidelines onto specific cognitive processes, such as reading in our case, and on the appropriate feature extraction and measurement, we can observe neurophysiologic changes of the user that are directly correlated with the manipulation of typical usability conditions of an interface. In other words, the analysis of the EEG signals performed by an appropriate and computationally sensible processing chain can make convincingly discriminating decisions concerning reading states and corresponding readability analysis.

---

[12] Correlation with constant functions cannot be mathematically determined.

The effectiveness of this method for a single user is clearly demonstrated in the classification results that were presented. Its generalization for different users is still an open question, and suggests further work in, at least two directions. The first, aiming at generalization, is the increase of the corpus size that may lead to the discovery of a significant average pattern for the cognitive state under observation. The second, in the opposite direction of personalization, is the design of a calibration procedure that will lead to different baselines for different users, and therefore different classification thresholds.

This paper also discussed the relation of mental workload, an EEG based measure, and reading performance heuristics or inquiry based measures, based in readability aspects variation such as text size, contrast and color. The results obtained so far are promising, indicating that it is possible to successfully relate both types of measures in some of the experiments, and also in some legibility aspects. A greater corpus, with more users and more sessions with the same users are required to deal more effectively with EEG variability.

Acknowledgements. This work was partially supported by Fundação para a Ciência e Tecnologia (FCT), Portugal, Grants SFRH/BD/30681/2006 and PPTDC/EIA-EIA/113660/2009.

References

1. Dix, A., Finlay, J.E., Abowd, G.D., Russell, B.: Human Computer Interaction, 3rd edn. Pearson Education Limited (2004) ISBN-13: 978-0-13-046109-4
2. Schmorrow, D., Kruse, A., Reeves, L., Bolton, A.: Augmenting Cognition in HCI: 21st Century Adaptive System Science and Technology. In: Sears, A., Jacko, J.A. (eds.) The Human–Computer Interaction Handbook, 2nd edn., pp. 1172–1188. Lawrence Erlbaum Associates (2008) ISBN-13: 978-0-8058-5870-9
3. Zander, T.O., Lehne, M., Ihme, K., Jatzev, S., Correia, J., Kothe, C., Picht, B., Nijboer, F.: A dry EEG-system for scientific research and brain-computer inter-faces. Frontiers in Neuroscience 5, art. 53 (2011)
4. Beer, R., Lehman, W., Noldus, L., Patèrno, F., Schmidt, E., Hove, W., Theuws, J.: The Usability Lab of the Future, Human Computer Interaction, INTERACT 2003 (2003)
5. Ganglbauer, E., Schrammel, J., Deutsch, S.: Applying Psychophysiological Me-thods for Measuring User Experience: Possibilities, Challenges and Feasibility. In: Proc. in User Experience Evaluation Methods in Product Development (UXEM 2009) in Conjunction with Interact 2009 (2009)
6. Hu, J., Nakanishi, M., Matsumoto, K., Tagaito, H., Inoue, K., Shima, K., Torii, K.: A Method of Usability Testing by Measuring Brain Waves. In: Proc. of the International Symposium on Future Software Technology (ISFST 2000) (2000)
7. Foglia, P., Prete, C., Zanda, M.: Relating GSR Signals to traditional Usability Me-trics: Case Study with an anthropomorphic Web Assistant. In: IEEE Intnl. Instrumentation and Measurement Technology Conf., Victoria, Vancouver Island, Canada, May 12-15 (2008)
8. Stickel, C., Ebner, M., Steinbach-Nordmann, S., Searle, G., Holzinger, A.: Emotion Detection: Application of the Valence Arousal Space for Rapid Biological Usability Testing to enhance Universal Access. In: Stephanidis, C. (ed.) Universal Access in HCI, Part I, HCII 2009. LNCS, vol. 5614, pp. 615–624. Springer, Heidelberg (2009)

9. Stickel, C., Scerbakov, A., Kaufmann, T., Ebner, M.: Usability metrics of time and stress-biological enhanced performance test of a university wide learning management system. In: Holzinger, A. (ed.) USAB 2008. LNCS, vol. 5298, pp. 173–184. Springer, Heidelberg (2008)

10. Kimura, M., Uwano, H., Ohira, M., Matsumoto, K.: Toward Constructing an Electroence-phalogram Measurement Method for Usability Evaluation. In: Jacko, J.A. (ed.) HCI International 2009, Part I. LNCS, vol. 5610, pp. 95–104. Springer, Heidelberg (2009)

11. Masaki, H., Ohira, M., Uwano, H., Matsumoto, K.: A Quantitative Evaluation on the Software Use Experience with Electroencephalogram. In: Marcus, A. (ed.) Design, User Experience, and Usability, Pt II, HCII 2011. LNCS, vol. 6770, pp. 469–477. Springer, Heidelberg (2011)

12. Hirshfield, L.M., Chauncey, K., Gulotta, R., Girouard, A., Solovey, E.T., Jacob, R.J.K., Sassaroli, A., Fantini, S.: Combining Electroencephalograph and Functional Near Infrared Spectroscopy to Explore Users' Mental Workload. In: Schmorrow, D.D., Estabrooke, I.V., Grootjen, M. (eds.) FAC 2009. LNCS, vol. 5638, pp. 239–247. Springer, Heidelberg (2009)

13. Lee, H., Seo, S.: A Comparison and Analysis of Usability Methods for Web Evaluation: The Relationship Between Typical Usability Test and Bio-Signals Characteristics (EEG, ECG). In: Proc. of 2010 DRS (Design Research Society) Montreal Conference (2010) ISBN 978-2-9811985-2-5

14. Nacke, L.: Wiimote vs. Controller: Electroencephalographic Measurement of Affective Gameplay Interaction. In: Proc. of the Intnl. Conf. on the Future of Game Design and Technology Futureplay. ACM Press (2010)

15. Ward, R., Marsden, P.: Affective computing: problems, reactions and intentions. Journal of Interacting with Computers 16(4), 707–713 (2004)

16. Winograd, T., Flores, F.: Understanding Computers and Cogniton: a New Foundation for Design. Addison Wesley (1986)

17. Nielsen, J., Molich, R.: Heuristic evaluation of user interfaces. In: Proc. ACM CHI 1990 Conference, Seattle, WA (April 1990)

18. Shneiderman, B.: Designing the User Interface, Strategies for Effective Human-Computer Interaction, 3rd edn. Addison Wesley (1997) ISBN 0-201-69497-2

19. Tognazzini, B.: First Principles of Interaction Design, AskTog – Interaction Design Solutions for the Real World. NN/g – Nielsen Norman Group (January 18, 2012), AskTog: http://www.asktog.com/basics/firstPrinciples.html

20. Oliveira, I., Grigore, O., Guimarães, N.: Reading detection based on electroen cephalo-gram processing. In: WSEAS 13th Intnl. Conf. on Computers, Rhodes, Greece (2009)

21. Oliveira, I., Grigore, O., Guimarães, N., Duarte, L.: Relevance of EEG Input Signals in the Augmented Human Reader. In: ACM – Augmented Human, AH 2010, Megève, France (April 2010)

22. Wolpaw, J.R., Birbaumer, N., Heetderks, W.J., McFarland, D.J., Peckham, P.H., Schalk, G., Donchin, E., Quatrano, L.A., Robinson, C.J., Vaughan, T.M.: Brain–Computer Interface Technology: A Review of the First International Meeting. IEEE Transactions on Rehabilitation Engineering 8 (2000)

23. Millán, J.R.: Adaptative Brain Interfaces. Communications of the ACM 46(3), 74–80 (2003)

24. Zander, T.O., Gartner, M., Kothe, C., Vilimek, R.: Combining Eye Gaze Input with a Brain-Computer Interface for Touchless Human-Computer Interaction. International Journal of Human Computer Interaction 27(1), 38–51 (2011)

25. Guyon, I., Elisseeff, A.: An Introduction to Variable and Feature Selection. The Journal of Machine Learning Research 3, 1157–1182 (2003)
26. Xu, Q., Zhou, H., Wang, Y., Huang, J.: Fuzzy support vector machine for classification of EEG signals using wavelet-based features. Medical Engineering & Physics 31, 858–865 (2009)
27. W3C: CSS Techniques for Web Content Accessibility Guidelines 1.0, Obtained in December 2011, from W3 (2010), http://www.w3.org/TR/WCAG10-CSS-TECHS
28. W3C: Fonts, Obtained in December 2011, from W3 (2011), http://www.w3.org/TR/CSS2/fonts.html
29. Fisch, B.: Fisch and Spehlmann's EEG Primer: Basic Principles of Digital and Analog EEG. Elesevier (1999) ISBN 978-0-444-82148-5

Query Behavior: The Impact of Health Literacy, Topic Familiarity and Terminology

Carla Teixeira Lopes[1] and Cristina Ribeiro[1,2]

[1] DEI, Faculdade de Engenharia, Universidade do Porto
[2] INESC TEC
Rua Dr. Roberto Frias s/n, 4200-465, Portugal
{ctl,mcr}@fe.up.pt

Abstract. We conducted a user study to analyze how health literacy, topic familiarity and the terminology used in past queries affect query behavior in health searches. We found that users with inadequate health literacy have less success in web searches and show more difficulties in query formulation. These users and the ones not familiar with the topic use medico-scientific terminology less often than users with more health literacy and topic familiarity. We conclude that search engines should help these groups of users in query formulation and, since technical documents stimulate the use of medico-scientific terminology in query reformulation, mechanisms like query suggestion can have long-term benefits.

Keywords: Web search; query formulation; health literacy; topic familiarity; user study.

1 Introduction

There are mismatches between the terminology used by health consumers and the one used in standard medical vocabularies and health documents [1], and this may be an obstacle to successful health searches. The development of techniques to improve the communication between health professionals and consumers and the proposal of initiatives to help consumers understand health information are receiving a large attention nowadays. The first was recently discussed in a workshop of the 2013's Conference on Human Factors in Computing Systems (CHI) entitled "Patient-Clinician Communication – The Roadmap for Human-Computer Interaction" and the second was discussed in a panel of the Association for Information Science and Technology (ASIST) 2010 annual meeting [2].

Two user characteristics influence the amplitude of this terminology gap. One is the health literacy, that is, "the degree to which individuals have the capacity to obtain, process, and understand basic health information and services needed to make appropriate health decisions" [3]. The other is topic familiarity, i.e., user's general knowledge about the topic of a search task (e.g.: diabetes). Note that these two features are distinct. A health consumer with good health literacy is expected to be unfamiliar with several health topics.

A. Holzinger et al. (Eds.): SouthCHI 2013, LNCS 7946, pp. 212–223, 2013.

We are convinced that higher levels of health literacy (HL) and topic familiarity (TF) give users the ability to formulate medico-scientific queries in addition to lay queries and therefore a higher probability of finding the necessary information. Moreover, we think the above characteristics influence the query reformulation behavior after an initial iteration where technical documents, i.e., documents containing medico-scientific terminology, are accessed. The characterization of these behaviors may help search engines decide if and how search assistance mechanisms like query suggestion or ranking algorithms can be personalized.

2   Related Work

In the following subsection we describe the main work regarding the influence of topic familiarity on query formulation behavior. The lack of studies considering health information literacy made us describe, in the other subsection, studies that explore users' information literacy on Information Retrieval (IR) behavior.

2.1   The Influence of Topic Familiarity on Query Formulation

Several works explore the influence of topic familiarity in IR. In the health domain, Wildemuth [4] examines the search behavior of medical students that were observed on three different occasions: at the beginning of a course, at the end of the course, and six months after the course. The author concluded that individuals with less domain knowledge were less efficient in selecting concepts to include in search queries and performed worse in search modification. Moreover, although it improved performance in all occasions, system assistance during query formulation was considered more useful on users with less knowledge on the topic.

Two different studies explore the influence of topic familiarity on the use of a thesaurus for query expansion. Sihvonen and Vakkari [5] conducted a study with 15 users having knowledge on the topic and 15 users without this knowledge, concluding that the use of the thesaurus was helpful for the experts but not for the novices. This conclusion contradicts Wildemuth [4] conclusions. In the other study, Shiri [6] analyzed how topics familiarity affected users behavior on thesaurus use and concluded that "searches involving moderately and very familiar topics were associated with browsing around twice as many thesaurus terms as was the case for unfamiliar topic".

2.2   The Influence of Information Literacy on IR Behavior

Birru et al. [7] observed low literacy adults searching for health information. The search terms used to find health information were one of the analyzed items. Authors concluded that, without guidance, users had difficulty "generating original search terms that would yield specific results", which constitutes a barrier to getting specific and targeted web health information. Note that this study explores users' information literacy and not users' health literacy. As defined by the National Forum on Information Literacy, information literacy is "the ability to know when there is a need for information, to be able to identify, locate, evaluate, and effectively use that information for the issue or problem at hand" [8].

Kodagoda and Wong [9] also focused on information literacy and studies how low literacy users search for information. They compared the retrieval performance of high and low literacy users and concluded that low literacy users take more time to complete the search task, are less accurate, spend more time on each web page, are less informed by webpages, have less focused search strategies, have a greater t4endency to re-visit web pages and more likely get lost than high literacy users. In agreement with Summers and Summers [10], Kodagoda and Wong [9] concluded that low literacy users often prematurely abandon their searches, judging they reached their goal. In domains like health, where inappropriately interpreted information may have impact on the life of the user or someone they care, this can be problematic. The consequences on users' life, the importance of successful health searches for an informed health consumer and the prevalence of health web searches distinguish the health domain from others, where query behavior may have been studied in the light of users' familiarity or literacy.

To learn how to make web health contents more usable and accessible for users with low health literacy, Summers and Summers [10] compared the reading and navigational strategies of users with different health literacy skills. Among several conclusions, they found that users with low literacy often avoid search because it requires proper spelling and typing capabilities and because they have difficulties processing search results pages. Considering users' information literacy, Kodagoda et al. [11] proposed Invisque (INteractive VIsual Search and Query Environment), a system that allows users to create queries and search for information in a visual manner. The system was evaluated using three measures: search outcome (successful, unsuccessful or abandon), time spent and number of pages visited. Authors concluded that low-literacy users benefit from the system in terms of time spent and number of pages visited. However, users with higher literacy have a slightly worse performance with this system.

To the best of our knowledge, there are no works exploring the influence of health information literacy in web searches.

3   User Study

Our study involved 40 medically lay persons (25 females, 15 males) with a mean age of 22.25 years (sd = 6.42). The health literacy (HL) of these users was evaluated through an adaptation of the Short Assessment of Health Literacy for Spanish-speaking Adults [12]. This health literacy test incorporates a comprehension test with 50 multiple-choice questions and it is easy and quick to administer. It has a threshold that allows the differentiation of users with inadequate health literacy. We grouped users in three classes: Inadequate (9 users),

Elementary (13 users) and Good Health Literacy (18 users), based on the threshold proposed in the test and through hierarchical clustering for the users above the test threshold.

Initially, besides completing the health literacy test, users had to fill a questionnaire where they were asked about demographic information, how they rated their success in general web search and in health web search and their knowledge about the medico-scientific terms related with the information situations.

Users were assigned a sequence of 8 tasks using a a Latin-square like procedure that assured that all users assessed the relevance of all information situations, but only once each and of queries of both types of terminology, the same number of times. To preempt users' fatigue, each task had to be performed in different days, that is, tasks had to be separated by an interval of, at least, 24 hours. Users did not have time limits to perform each task. In each task users had to propose a treatment for a disease/condition associated with an information situation, given a set of documents provided by the researchers. The information situations were defined based on questions submitted to the health category of the Yahoo! Answers service. From the list of open questions of this category and, in a decreasing order of popularity, we selected the questions about treatments to a symptom/disease in which the underlying medico-scientific and lay terminology was different, based on a glossary of technical and popular medical terms [13]. For instance, a disease like *diabetes* would be excluded because it is expressed with the same term in both terminologies. The following information situations were defined:

1. About 3 days ago, I started having a burning feeling every time I urinated. How should I treat this?
2. For the past 5 days my head has been very itchy and I don't have lice. What can I do to stop the itching?
3. I have high uric acid (8.0 mg/dL) with reference units 3.6 - 7.7. How can I lower my uric acid level?
4. I am suffering with an inflammation on my lips and mouth area for more than a year. I have difficulties eating. What can I do to treat it?
5. My father got bit by a dog and is in the hospital with a bone infection. How is this treated?
6. I frequently get heartburn even when I stay away from spicy stuff. What can I do to prevent it?
7. I have been noticing lots of hair coming out from my head. Usually I only comb my hair once a day. What can I do to stop losing my hair?
8. I'm on the computer all day so I type a lot and use the mouse. My right pointing finger is starting to give me some joint pain. How I can treat my finger?

Using a computer, for each task, users had to: (1) provide the elements to calculate topic familiarity, (2) provide the query they would use, in a text-field similar to the ones used in search boxes, (3) assess the relevance of 30 documents provided by the researchers in an URL format, (4) answer the question included in the information situation and (5) provide two additional queries using text-fields. The documents assessed in the third step were obtained by the researchers using Google as a black-box search engine and either a medico-scientific or a lay query. A medico-scientific query is a query including one or more medico-scientific terms like *pyrosis*. A lay query is a query that only contains lay terms like *heartburn*, the lay synonym for *pyrosis*. Henceforward, tasks in which the user assesses documents retrieved with a lay query will be referred as lay sessions or lay tasks. On the other hand, tasks involving documents retrieved with medico-scientific queries will be referred as technical sessions or technical tasks.

Topic familiarity (TF) was evaluated through the combination of three elements, explicitly provided by the user in each task: familiarity with the topic, previous searches on the topic, knowledge about the medico-scientific term associated with the topic. Pairs "user, topic" are distributed by topic familiarity categories as follows: not familiar (161 pairs), somehow familiar (113 pairs) and familiar (46 pairs). Through this distribution we can also see that the majority of tasks presents a topic unfamiliar to the user. To analyze the relationship between health literacy and topic familiarity, we applied the chi-squared test of independence and found we could not reject the null hypothesis that both variables are independent ($\chi^2(4)=5.66$, p=0.23). This helps to sustain the claim that both variables are different.

The two following research questions guided this research.

1. How is health query formulation behavior affected by health literacy and familiarity with the topic?
2. How does the access to lay and medico-scientific content affect query reformulation in general and at different levels of health literacy and topic familiarity?

4   Data Analysis

To address the first research question, we characterize the queries initially formulated by users pertaining the presence of medico-scientific terminology, advanced operators, spelling errors and also the format of the query. We do it in a general way and also by health literacy and topic familiarity. We consider the query has medico-scientific terminology if it contains the disease/condition technical term as defined in the glossary of technical and popular medical terms [13]. For example, for the information situation "About 3 days ago, I started having a burning feeling every time I urinated. How should I treat this?", the query had to include the term *dysuria*. As advanced operators we consider the OR operator, phrase search (""), exclusion of terms (-) and fill the blanks (*). A query is considered to contain spelling errors if it includes at least one misspelled term. This is particularly important in health queries because medical terminology, mostly the scientific one, is hard to spell by users that are not health professionals. If the query begins by question words like 'how', 'what', 'when', 'where', 'who', 'why' or ends with a question mark, it is considered to be in a question format.

To address the second research question we analyze how the access to content with lay and medico-scientific terminology affects the subsequent queries with respect to terminology.

To compare the number of terms employed by users with different health literacy and topic familiarity levels, we have used the ANOVA test. In all the other comparisons, we have used the test of equal proportions between pairs of samples. For example, to compare the inadequate HL group with the elementary HL group regarding the use of medico-scientific terminology, we compare the proportion of queries that include this type of terminology in the first group with the proportion of queries that use it in the second group. Although we present the chi-squared value for the proportion tests, note that, when comparing two samples, the chi-squared test for equality of two proportions is the same as a z-test. In fact, the chi-squared distribution with one degree of freedom is the square of a normal deviate one. Since we are performing multiple comparisons, we applied the Bonferroni correction in these tests, dividing α by 3, the number of tests performed. We use a ** to represent significant results at 0.01 and * for significant results at 0.05. To compute the Confidence Intervals (CI) we use the t-student statistic in the mean number of terms and the chi-squared distribution in the remaining ones.

4.1   Query Formulation Behavior

The mean number of terms in the initial query was 4.1 (95% CI: [3.9, 4.3]) with a standard deviation of 1.8. From the initial queries, 7.2% (95% CI: [4.7%, 10.7%]) included medico-scientific terminology, 26.6% (95% CI: [21.9%, 31.8%]) included advanced operators, 12.5% (95% CI: [9.2%, 16.7%]) were formulated in a question format and solely 1.2% (95% CI: [0.4%, 3.4%]) contained spelling errors. As expected, the proportion of initial queries with medico-scientific terminology is significantly higher in users who already knew the term: 22.1% (95% CI: [14.5%, 32%]). Still, most of these users formulate an initial query without medico-scientific terminology. The proportion of spelling errors is higher in queries formulated with medico-scientific terminology (4.3%) than in queries without it (1%), yet this proportion difference is not statistically significant.

An analysis by health literacy shows no significant differences in the number of terms and spelling errors by health literacy level. Regarding medico-scientific terminology, we found that good HL users use it significantly more than elementary HL users ($\chi^2(1)$=10.6, p=5.7e-04**). We also found that inadequate HL users employ advanced operators less often than elementary HL users ($\chi^2(1)$=8.3, p=2e-03**) and good HL users ($\chi^2(1)$=9.4, p=1e-03**) and design their query in a question format more often than good HL users ($\chi^2(1)$=10.7, p=5e-04**).

Results regarding the use of advances operators make us suspect that health literacy and web search expertise may be related. To verify this, we decided to analyze the relation between users' health literacy and the degree of success they think they have in general web search (Fig. 1) and in health web search. In general web search, evaluated in a 5-value scale where 1 corresponds to the lowest success rate and 5 to the highest success rate, the median of the web

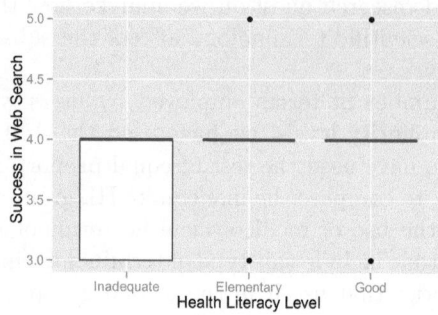

Fig. 1. Success in web search by level of health literacy

search success is 4 in all levels of health literacy. However, the proportion of answers beneath 4 is higher in the inadequate health literacy level. Through the Chi-Squared test of independence, we found that web search success and health literacy are related ($\chi^2(4)$=54.3, p=4.6e-11**) having a weak positive association with a Spearman correlation of 0.34. In terms of health web search success, assessed in the same scale as web search success, its median is lower (2) in the inadequate HL level than in the other levels (3). Plus, we found that these variables are related ($\chi^2(6)$=32.3, p=1.4e-05**) with a positive, but low, Spearman correlation (0.19).

In terms of topic familiarity, we found that the number of terms does not significantly differ between levels of familiarity with the topic. We found that users who are not familiar with the topic use medico-scientific terminology less often than somehow familiar users ($\chi^2(1)$=16, p=3.16e-05**) and familiar users ($\chi^2(1)$=7.4, p=3e-03*).

4.2   Query Reformulation Behavior

After assessing documents retrieved with medico-scientific queries, the proportion of subsequent queries using medico-scientific terminology is 19.4%, while in lay sessions this proportion downs to 7.8%, a significant difference ($\chi^2(1)$=17.2, p=1.65 e-05**). After search tasks without medico-scientific terminology the proportion of queries in question format is 13.4%, higher than in tasks with it (12.5%), but not significantly different. Since queries in the format of a question indicate user's difficulties in the search task [14], this may that indicate medico-scientific content helps in query reformulation and is probably richer in alternative terms.

Table 1 shows the proportion of queries with medico-scientific terms in query reformulation. Similarly to the initial queries, users that already know the scientific term, use medico-scientific terminology significantly more than the other users. In a global perspective, 24.7% of the post-search queries, formulated by users who knew the scientific term before the search session, use medico-scientific terminology. In contrast, in users who did not know the scientific term, only 8.9%

Table 1. Proportion of reformulated queries with medico-scientific terminology by type of session in users who previously knew/knew not the scientific term

Type of session	Know	Know not	Know > Know not?
All sessions	24.7%	8.9%	$\chi^2(1)$=27.2, p=9.02e-08**
Technical	34.0%	12.7%	$\chi^2(1)$=18.6, p=8.16e-06**
Lay	14.4%	5.2%	$\chi^2(1)$=6.4, p=0.006**

of the post-search queries include this type of terminology. This difference is statistically significant, in general, and also after lay and medico-scientific sessions, what shows the importance of knowing the scientific term to the use of this type of terminology in future queries. However, lay sessions discourage the use of medico-scientific terminology even in users who already know the scientific term. In these users the proportions lowers from 34% in medico-scientific sessions to 14.4% in lay sessions.

In reformulations including medico-scientific terminology, we also analyzed the reasons for this change. This type of terminology could have been excluded in the first query because it is part of users passive vocabulary and not of its active vocabulary. On the other hand, the documents assessed in the first iteration might have introduced new terminology to the user. Since, for each user, we are aware of his prior knowledge about the scientific term, we can use this information to distinguish both cases. As can be seen in Table 2, users who previously knew the scientific term used it in 44.3% of the post-search queries. Consequently, this is the proportion of cases where the scientific term was not included in the first query because it is part of users' passive vocabulary. From the 95% confidence interval, it is not possible to conclude that this proportion is significantly different from 50% and, therefore, significantly different from the proportion of cases due to terminology learning.

In Table 2 it is also possible to see that the first post-search queries including scientific terminology were mostly formulated by users who had the scientific term in their passive vocabulary. The opposite happens with the second post-search queries, that is, the majority of the users using medico-scientific terminology in the second query have just learned the term in the search session. Similarly to what happens with the global post-search query analysis, through the confidence intervals, we cannot conclude these proportions are significantly different from 50%.

In terms of health literacy, after medico-scientific tasks, good HL users are more likely to use medico-scientific terminology (22.2%) when compared with elementary HL (16.4%) and inadequate HL (18.1%) users. None of these differences is significant. We also found that, in all levels of health literacy, the majority of the users (proportions between 62.5% and 69.4%) formulated one of the subsequent queries with medico-scientific terminology. Moreover, although in a very low proportion, only users with elementary (1.9%) and good health literacy (1.4%) formulated both queries with medico-scientific terminology.

Table 2. Proportion of post-search queries with medico-scientific terminology formulated by users that knew the scientific term and did not use this terminology in the pre-search query

Post-search query	Scientific term known	95% CI
First	57.9%	[34%, 79%]
Second	39.2%	[26%, 54%]
Either first or second	44.3%	[33%, 57%]

An analysis by topic familiarity shows that the use of medico-scientific terminology after medico-scientific tasks increases with the topic familiarity (9.5% for not familiar, 26.8% for somehow familiar and 34% for familiar users). In terms of significant differences, we found that users who are not familiar with the topic are less prone to use medico-scientific terminology after medico-scientific sessions than somehow familiar ($\chi^2(1)$=12.9, p=1.6e-04**) and familiar ($\chi^2(1)$=15.7, p= 3.7e-05**) users.

Analyzing the number of subsequent queries with medico-scientific terminology, we found that the proportion of users with 2 medico-scientific queries increases with topic familiarity (from 0.6% to 0.9% to 4.4%) and the opposite happens with the proportion of users with 0 medico-scientific queries (from 40.4% to 23.9% to 21.7%). The majority of users in each level of topic familiarity wrote 1 medico-scientific query but, in users not familiar with the topic, this proportion is much lower than the proportions in the other groups of users.

5   Discussion

We verified that health consumers rarely use medico-scientific terminology and that, as expected, users who know the scientific term use it more often. However, even these users include it in only 1 out of 4 health queries. Moreover, we found that users with good health literacy use it more often than elementary health-literate users. In terms of topic familiarity, users who are not familiar with the topic use medico-scientific terminology less often than other users. This is in accordance with previous studies [4,7] that conclude that users with less knowledge on the topic and less literacy have less ability to include specific terms in queries.

If queries in question format indicate difficulties [14], the formulation of health queries is harder for inadequate health-literate users than for good health-literate users. Furthermore, the former class of users employs advanced operators less often than other users, which indicates they may have less search experience and less ability to fully exploit the potential of search engines. The weak positive association found between web search success and health literacy agrees with the above findings. Moreover, this is in accordance with Summers and Summers [10], who found that low health literacy users avoid searches because they have difficulties formulating queries and processing results' pages. Since users with inadequate health literacy are ill prepared for conducting health web searches, search engines should focus their attention on this group of users, providing special help mechanisms in health query formulation.

Concerning query reformulation, we found that access to documents containing medico-scientific terminology encourages the use of this type of terminology in subsequent queries. In fact, after medico-scientific sessions the proportion of subsequent queries using scientific terminology is significantly higher than after lay sessions. This happens in users who didn't know the scientific term and in users who knew it. The former learn the scientific term through the documents assessed in the search session and the latter use it from their passive vocabulary.

We found that about half of the queries reformulated to include medico-scientific terminology were a result of terminology learning. The other half had to do with forcing the use of passive vocabulary where the scientific term was included. Through the analysis that distinguishes the first and the second post-search queries, we found that users who have learned the scientific term in the search session tend to use it more in the second query than in the first. This shows that these users have reluctance to use it and only do it as a further alternative.

After the medico-scientific sessions, users who are not familiar with the topic are less prone to use medico-scientific terminology than more familiar users. For this reason and because they use medico-scientific terminology less often in the initial query, these users' health query formulation should also be given special attention by search engines.

If search engines understand the differences between low and high health literacy users and between users familiar and not familiar with a topic, they can develop strategies to better support each type of user find the information they need. Strategies include new interfaces or new features that leverage users' understanding of the information retrieved (e.g.: providing definitions of medical terms). The Invisque system [11] is an example of a visual interface developed to help low literacy users overcome search difficulties. In addition, systems can also adjust the ranking of the documents or develop query suggestion mechanisms in which the terminology of the suggested query is adjusted to users' knowledge. Queries can be a simple translation of the initial user query or can introduce new related terms. Both low and high health literacy/topic familiarity users can benefit from such a system. The former type of users probably benefit from translations from medico-scientific to lay terminology which can, for example, happen when users don't understand the terminology used by clinicians or the one included in medical reports and want to inform themselves. Moreover, they can benefit from lay queries using synonyms or related terms. On the other hand, users with more knowledge can also benefit from translations to medico-scientific terminology. Considering the query reformulation findings, the benefits of a query suggestion system might be twofold. It not only provides access to documents that wouldn't be reached without the given suggestions but also stimulates the use of different terms in subsequent queries.

Nonetheless, to guarantee that users understand the retrieved documents, it is important to adapt the query suggestions to users' health literacy and topic familiarity.

6 Conclusion

In this work we analyze how the type of terminology used in past queries affect query formulation and reformulation in users with different levels of health literacy and familiarity with the topic. If not the first, this is one of the first works dealing with health literacy in the information retrieval domain. Although some of the results are predictable, we consider important to have their empirical demonstration.

We found that, although consumers rarely use medico-scientific terminology in their queries, the ones with higher health literacy or topic familiarity do it more often. Users with low health literacy or topic familiarity were found to have more difficulties in query formulation, not only selecting and typing the appropriate medical terms but also on general aspects like the inclusion of advanced operators. The contact with documents using medico-scientific terminology encourages the use of this type of terminology in future queries. Although this is statistically significant in every user, users who did not know the medico-scientific term from the beginning seem more reluctant to use this type of terminology.

Analyzing behaviors of users with different characteristics can help search engines to define how they can provide a better experience for each type of user. This can be done in query formulation, in ranking or at the interface level. As expressed above, we believe a personalized query suggestion system that translates queries between the medico-scientific and the lay terminology can be beneficial to consumer health information retrieval.

As future work we intend to analyze which type of terminology should be used in query suggestions for users with different levels of health literacy and topic familiarity.

Acknowledgments. Thanks to Fundação para a Ciência e a Tecnologia for partially funding this work under the grant SFRH/BD/40982/2007. Thanks to Dagmara Paiva, M.D., and to Michael Luís, M.D., for their contribution on the evaluation of the medical accuracy of users' answers.

References

1. Zeng, Q., Kogan, S., Ash, N., Greenes, R.A., Boxwala, A.A.: Characteristics of consumer terminology for health information retrieval. Methods of Information in Medicine 41(4), 289–298 (2002)
2. Souden, M., Rubenstein, E.L.: Listening to patients: how understanding health information use can contribute to health literacy constructs. In: Proceedings of the 73rd ASIS & T Annual Meeting on Navigating Streams in an Information Ecosystem, ASIS&T 2010, vol. 47, Silver Springs, MD, USA, American Society for Information Science (2010)

3. USA Department of Health and Human Services: Healthy People 2010, Washington, DC (2000)
4. Wildemuth, B.M.: The effects of domain knowledge on search tactic formulation. J. Am. Soc. Inf. Sci. Technol. 55(3), 246–258 (2004)
5. Sihvonen, A., Vakkari, P.: Subject knowledge, thesaurus-assisted query expansion and search success. In: Proceedings of the RIAO 2004 Conference (2004)
6. Shiri, A.: Topic familiarity and its effects on term selection and browsing in a thesaurus-enhanced search environment. Library Review 54(9), 514–518 (2005)
7. Birru, M.S., Monaco, V.M., Charles, L., Drew, H., Njie, V., Bierria, T., Detlefsen, E., Steinman, R.A.: Internet usage by low-literacy adults seeking health information: an observational analysis. Journal of Medical Internet Research 6(3) (September 2004)
8. NFIL: What is the NFIL? (2013), http://infolit.org/about-the-nfil/what-is-the-nfil/ (cited March 4, 2013)
9. Kodagoda, N., Wong, B.L.W.: Effects of low & high literacy on user performance in information search and retrieval. In: Proceedings of the 22nd British HCI Group Annual Conference on People and Computers: Culture, Creativity, Interaction, BCS-HCI 2008, vol. 1, pp. 173–181. British Computer Society, Swinton (2008)
10. Summers, K., Summers, M.: Reading and navigational strategies of web users with lower literacy skills. Proc. Am. Soc. Info. Sci. Tech. 42(1) (January 2005)
11. Kodagoda, N., Wong, B.L.W., Rooney, C., Khan, N.: Interactive visualization for low literacy users: from lessons learnt to design. In: Proceedings of the 2012 ACM Annual Conference on Human Factors in Computing Systems, CHI 2012, pp. 1159–1168. ACM, New York (2012)
12. Lee, S.Y.Y., Bender, D.E., Ruiz, R.E., Cho, Y.I.I.: Development of an easy-to-use spanish health literacy test. Health Services Research 41(4 pt.1), 1392–1412 (2006)
13. Stichele, R.V.: Multilingual glossary of technical and popular medical terms in nine european languages. Technical report, Heymans Institute of Pharmacology, University of Gent, Gent (December 1995)
14. Aula, A., Khan, R.M., Guan, Z.: How does search behavior change as search becomes more difficult? In: Proceedings of the 28th International Conference on Human Factors in Computing Systems, CHI 2010, pp. 35–44. ACM, New York (2010)

MeD UD – A Process Reference Model
for Usability Design in Medical Devices

Derek Flood, Fergal Mc Caffery, Valentine Casey, and Gilbert Regan

Dundalk Institute of Technology, Dundalk, Co. Louth, Ireland
{derek.flood,fergal.mccaffery,val.casey,gilbert.regan}@dkit.ie

Abstract. A critical component to the success of software systems is the incorporation of the end user. Ensuring that the end user can use the system effectively and efficiently is an important consideration. Failure to do this can lead to user error which in turn can have serious or even fatal consequences. To address this issue in the medical domain, where the risk to patient and user safety is quite high, a number of standards and guidance documents promote the use of Human Factors and Usability Engineering techniques during the development of devices. In this paper we introduce MeD UD (Medical Device Usability Design) – A Process Reference Model (PRM) for evaluating usability engineering in the medical device domain. Through a process assessment utilising the MeD UD PRM, medical device organisations can improve their usability design processes to achieve more usable products, reduce the risks associated with user errors and efficiently meet the medical device regulatory requirements.

Keywords: Usability, Medical Device Software, Process Reference Model, IEC 62366:2007.

1 Introduction

The development of technology in recent years has allowed for medical devices to provide more effective and efficient patient care. These results can be attributed, in part, to the increasing role of software within medical devices. Through the use of software, complex configuration changes can be implemented easily. In 2006, it was noted that software was now incorporated into over half of the medical devices for sale on the U.S. market [1].

A side effect of the increased complexity of medical devices is the increased chance of human-error. Errors, slips and lapses can occur in every aspect of human activity. When these mistakes occur with medical devices the results can be fatal. In 2007, Ms. Myra Jean Garman took her own life to escape the pain she suffered as a result of the misapplication of a medical device. Ms. Garman, who was suffering from breast cancer, was left in severe pain after she was given twice the recommended dose of radioactive seeds on five separate occasions. The state regulators attributed the over radiation to a mistake on behalf of a physicist who had entered an incorrect magnification factor into the treatment planning computer. [2] Ms. Garman is unfortunately not an isolated incident. In New Jersey 36 cancer patients were

A. Holzinger et al. (Eds.): SouthCHI 2013, LNCS 7946, pp. 224–239, 2013.
© Springer-Verlag Berlin Heidelberg 2013

over-radiated and a further 20 received substandard treatment due to human-error during the application of a medical device [2].

Errors like these can be reduced through the use of usability engineering. Usability engineering is the *"application of knowledge about human behaviour, abilities, limitations, and other characteristics related to the design of tools, devices, systems, tasks, jobs, and environments to achieve adequate usability"* [3]. The incorporation of human aspects into the design process enables designers to develop interfaces in accordance with the users' expectations and needs which can improve the overall user experience and reduce the likelihood of human error.

Software Process Improvement (SPI) frameworks such as SPICE [4] or CMMI [5] allow organisations to improve their software development processes. These models divide the software development process into a number of discrete processes and outline the objectives to be achieved when undertaking these processes. Through an SPI assessment an organisation's weaknesses and strengths can be identified and guidance can be provided as to how they can improve their existing processes.

To assist organisations improve their usability design processes, this work outlines the MeD UD (Medical Device Usability Design) framework which has been developed specifically for the medical device domain. This framework incorporates the latest thinking from the IEC 62366:2007 [3] standard, and the US Food and Drug Administration (FDA)'s *Applying human factors and usability engineering to optimise medical device design* [6] on the topic of usability and human factors engineering.

The remainder of this paper is structured as follows: Section 2 provides the background to this work. Section 3 discusses software process improvement within the medical device domain. Section 4 describes the research methodology used during the development of MeD UD while Section 5 outlines the MeD UD framework. Section 6 discusses how the MeD UD framework is different from existing usability assessment models. Section 7 then discusses the future of this work before the paper is concluded in Section 8.

2   Background and Related Work

2.1   The Role of Software in Medical Devices

Software is omnipresent, affecting every aspect of our daily lives. It is incorporated in most household devices, including items as diverse as washing machines and DVD players, in motor vehicles, and even in wrist watches. It is no surprise therefore that medical devices are becoming more dependent on software. In 2006, Faris [1] found that software was incorporated in over 50% of medical devices for sale in the United States of America.

The choice for using software in medical devices is motivated by the ease with which it can allow complex changes to be made, without the need for expensive hardware changes. However the use of software brings with it a number of risks. In the first half of 2010 the FDA recalled 23 medical devices which were classified as Class I, meaning that there is *"reasonable probability that use of these products will cause serious adverse health consequences or death"*. It was found that of these re-calls 6 were likely to be caused by software defects [7].

Also in 2010 the FDA published a white paper [8] detailing an improvement initia-tive which they undertook to improve the quality of infusion pumps. This initiative arose out of concerns due to the quality of infusion pumps being sold in the US. Be-tween 2005 and 2009 the FDA received approximately 56,000 reports of adverse events associated with the use of infusion pumps, including numerous injuries and deaths. During this same period 87 infusion pumps were recalled, 14 of which were designated as Class I and 70 were designated as Class II, meaning that the use of the device may cause temporary or medically reversible adverse consequences or that the probability of serious adverse health consequences or death is remote.

Many of these adverse events are related to deficiencies in device design and engi-neering. Although the range of potential issues is quite large, in the report the FDA outline three of the most common types of problems reported, namely software de-fects, user interface errors and mechanical or electrical failures.

In 2007 the European Council amended the Medical Device Directive (MDD) [9], which governs the approval and marketing of medical devices in the European Union (EU). This amendment came into effect in March of 2010. As part of this amendment the EU recognized the importance of software and revised the directive to include the provision that software can now, in its own right, be classified as a medical device. As a result software can now be subjected to the same regulations and standards as other medical devices [10].

2.2   Medical Device Regulations, Standards and Guidance Documents

In order to sell a medical device within the European Union (EU), the medical device organisation must demonstrate that they are compliant with the regulations set forth by the EU. Similarly, to sell medical devices within the US the organisation must demonstrate compliance with the FDA regulations [11]. In order to help organisations achieve compliance with these regulations the EU and FDA have published guidance documents that address specific aspects of the regulations and also recommend com-pliance with harmonised and consensus international standards. Medical device or-ganisations may chose not to follow these guidelines and standards and still receive approval to market their device; however they must provide strong justification for not doing so.

One of the most fundamental requirements of a medical device organisation to achieve regulatory compliance is the implementation of a Quality Management Sys-tem (QMS). A QMS ensures that the processes used during the development and pro-duction of a medical device are defined and monitored to ensure high quality products are developed. The requirements of a quality management system have been outlined by the International Organisation for Standardization (ISO) in ISO 13485:2003 [12]. This standard is referred to by the European regulations and has recently been ac-cepted by the FDA as adequate fulfilment of the requirements of a QMS.

As part of the QMS, organisations must perform risk management activities. To improve the quality of the medical devices, the organisation should identify all risks possible and take appropriate action to help mitigate these risks. ISO 14971:2007 [13] describes the requirements of a risk management process for medical device development. This standard identifies 6 key stages; risk analysis, risk evaluation, risk control, evaluation of overall residual risk acceptability, risk management report, and production and post-production information.

IEC 62304:2006 – *Medical device software – Software life cycle processes* [14] provides specific guidance on how to perform software development activities for software that is to be incorporated in a medical device. This is an EU harmonised standard and is recognised by the FDA as a consensus standard. It is therefore used to develop medical device software for both the European and US markets.

2.3 Usability

The ISO [15] define usability as *"The extent to which a product can be used by specified users to achieve specified goals with effectiveness, efficiency and satisfaction in a specified context of use."* In this definition, the ISO identify three factors that should be considered when designing usable products; **user, goals** and **context of use**. A deep understanding of each of these factors is essential for the development of a usable application as they can all affect the way in which it is used.

- **User:** - refers to the person that will interact with the application. By understanding the user of the system application designers can avoid a number of issues that can make a system difficult to use. For example, consider the development of a mobile application for the management of diabetes. Diabetic patients can suffer from retinopathy which limits the patients' vision thus making it difficult to see. During the design of a mobile application for diabetic patients knowledge of this may encourage developers to increase the size of fonts and objects displayed.

- **Goals:** - refers to the intended outcome of the user. An understanding of the task to be completed can be critical to the success or failure of a product. During the development of a new application the designer must understand what the user is trying to accomplish as well as why they are doing it in such a way. In some cases it can be found that application designers are restricted in the improvements they can make by regulations.

- **Context of use:** - refers to the location in which the application is to be used. This can include the physical and social elements of the environment in which the application is to be used. The environment can limit the methods of input and output putting extra constraints on the developer. For example medical devices that are to be used in a noisy environment should contain alarms that can alert the user through the background noise, either through the use of a flashing light or a loud alarm.

The ISO definition also outlines three measurable attributes that reflect the overall usability of the application:

- **Effectiveness:** Accuracy and completeness with which users achieve specified goals;
- **Efficiency:** Resources expended in relation to the accuracy and completeness with which users achieve goals;
- **Satisfaction:** Freedom from discomfort, and positive attitudes towards the use of the product.

A number of other models of usability have been proposed over the years. One of the most widely acknowledged was originally proposed by Nielsen [16]. In his model, Nielsen outlines five attributes of usability that should be considered:

- **Efficiency:** Resources expended in relation to the accuracy and completeness with which users achieve goals;
- **Satisfaction:** Freedom from discomfort, and positive attitudes towards the use of the product.
- **Learnability:** The system should be easy to learn so that the user can rapidly start getting work done with the system;
- **Memorability:** The system should be easy to remember so that the casual user is able to return to the system after some period of not having used it without having to learn everything all over again;
- **Errors:** The system should have a low error rate, so that users make few errors during the use of the system and that if they do make errors they can easily recover from them. Further, catastrophic errors must not occur.

Unlike the ISO, Nielsen does not consider effectiveness to be an attribute of usability, but instead an attribute of utility. In this model, Nielsen considers utility to be the ability of the system to allow the user to accomplish their task and is independent of usability.

There are a number of techniques that can help application developers to develop usable products, such as user centred design. User centred design focuses on the needs, demands and requirements of the end user. Holzinger et al. [17] outlines one such process that has been proven on many projects.

The protocol outlined in Fig. 1, adopted from [18], shows how user centred design can be performed, highlighting the role of the user throughout the development of the medical device. The process begins with the identification of end-users who are represented throughout the rest of the process. To aid in the development of a usable system, after analysis the processes recommends the development of low-fidelity prototypes that are tested with real users to determine which approaches work best. After this a high-fidelity prototype is developed which provides a rich user experience for the user to evaluate. The process then recommends development, once a suitable design has been found. This is then tested further to ensure it is usable before it is released.

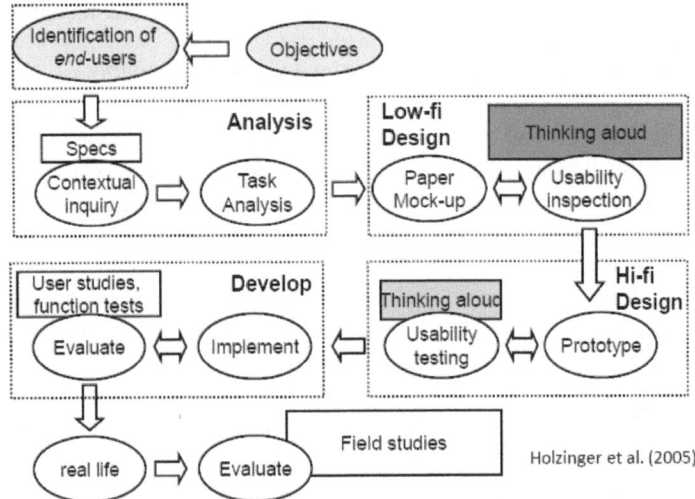

Fig. 1. A Method for User Centred Design

This approach makes extensive use of the Think Aloud protocol, which allows analysts to understand how users approach a task by requiring them to describe what they are thinking while completing the task. This approach helps to reduce the costs as think aloud is a low cost method that can be applied throughout the development process from analysis to test.

2.4   The Usability of Medical Devices

Compliance with the standards outlined above can help to prevent software from failing through the elimination of software defects. Conformance with these regulations and standards do not provide protection against human error. More than 300 patients were over radiated by powerful CT scanners, which had obtained FDA approval, used to detect strokes in four hospitals in the US. In one hospital, which detected the errors after 18 months when patients started losing their hair, found that the overdose was displayed on-screen however the technicians administering the scans did not notice [2].

Similarly during an analysis of infusion pumps recalled by the FDA between 2005 and 2009, user errors were identified as one of the most common cause of the recalls [8]. It was found that on some devices the screen failed to make clear the units of measurement (pounds vs. kilograms) when entering patient data for calculating the dosage, leading to incorrect dosages being applied.

Although human error is an inevitable part of product usage, product designers have a responsibility to minimise the probability of human error occurring. To help developers achieve this goal usability practitioners have developed a series of heuristics and guidelines that have evolved from common issues that have been found with other devices. For example, Jacob Neilsen has developed a set of 10 general purpose heuristics that should help prevent usability errors. These heuristics were based on an analysis of 249 usability problems observed in 11 projects [19]. A number of heuristics such as these have emerged for a range of domains including the World Wide Web and mobile applications.

Within the medical device domain ANSI/AAMI HE75:2009 [20] has been developed to provide a range of human factors design principles for medical devices across 25 sections ranging "from general considerations for human interface design to specific medical considerations such as surgical tools, mobile devices and connectors" [21].

In addition to the guidelines and design principles outlined above, the FDA and ISO recognise the importance of usability in a guidance document and international standard respectively. For medical devices sold within the US, the FDA have produced the Guidance document *Applying human factors and usability engineering to optimise medical device design* [6] which details a process for applying usability engineering during medical device development.

IEC have produced IEC 62366:2007 - *Medical Devices – Application of usability engineering to medical devices* [3] which is a FDA recognised consensus standard and is harmonized with the EU Medical Device Directive. IEC 62366 details the requirements for applying usability engineering to the design and development of medical devices. The standard focuses predominantly on risk management and risk control but also outlines some of the key requirements for performing usability engineering activities, such as user and context identification and analysis.

3   Software Process Improvement

There are many reasons why organisations undertake software process improvement evaluations. General purpose software process improvement frameworks, such as CMMI [5] and ISO/IEC 15504-5:2012 [4], can be used to help organisations to identify areas in which their software development processes can be improved.

In addition to this SPI models can be used to determine the state of a software development organisations practices for the purpose of supplier selection. In the late 1980s the US air force commissioned the development of a model to provide an objective evaluation of software subcontractors. This model, developed by the SEI at Carnegie Mellon University, became known as CMM and later CMMI.

3.1   Software Process Improvement within the Medical Device Domain

The models described above have been developed for general purpose software process assessment and as such do not provide sufficient coverage to achieve medical device regulatory compliance [22]. To address this issue a medical device specific SPI framework, titled Medi SPICE, has been developed.

The objective of undertaking a Medi SPICE assessment is to determine the state of a medical device organisation's software processes and practices. This is in relation to the regulatory requirements of the industry and best practice with the goal of identifying areas for undertaking process improvement [22]. It can also be used as part of the supplier selection process when an organisation wishes to outsource or offshore part or all of their medical device software development to a third party or remote division [23].

Medi SPICE is based upon the latest version of ISO/IEC 15504-5:2012 [4] and ISO/IEC 12207:2008 [24]. It is being developed in line with the requirements of ISO/IEC 15504-2:2003 [25] and contains a Process Reference Model (PRM) and Process Assessment Model (PAM). It also incorporates the requirements of the relevant medical device regulations, standards, technical reports and guidance documents.

The Medi SPICE PRM consists of 44 processes and 15 subprocesses which are fundamental to the development of regulatory compliant medical device software. Each process has a clearly defined purpose and outcomes that must be accomplished to achieve that purpose.

Medi SPICE also contains a PAM which is related to the PRM and forms the basis for collecting evidence that may be used to provide a rating of process capability. This is achieved by the provision of a two-dimensional view of process capability. In one dimension, it describes a set of process specific practices that allow the achievement of the process outcomes and purpose defined in the PRM; this is termed the process dimension. In the second dimension, the PAM describes capabilities that relate to the process capability levels and process attributes, this is termed the capability dimension [26].

3.2   Capability Maturity Models in Healthcare

Electronic health records pose serious risks to patient safety due to the volume of information they contain and the limited time available by medical practitioners to process these records. For this reason usability plays a major role in the presentation and organisation of medical health records and with healthcare organisations.

In 2011 the Healthcare Information and Management Systems Society (HIMSS), through the HIMSS usability task force [27] introduced a healthcare usability maturity model to allow *"health leaders and individuals to assess their levels of usability and then build to more advanced levels."* The proposed model contains five different aspects of usability within the healthcare organisation; focus on users, management, process & infrastructure, resources and education.

The maturity model defines five levels at which an organisation can operate, summarised in the following table, taken from [27]:

Table 1. Healthcare usability Maturity Model Phases

Phase	Title	Description
1	Unrecognised	Lack of awareness of usability. No practices, policies or resources
2	Preliminary	Sporadic inclusion of usability. Very limited resources
3	Implemented	Recognized value of usability. Small team doing usability
4	Integrated	All benchmarks of usability implemented including, a dedicated user experience team
5	Strategic	Business benefits well understood, usability mandated, budget and people part of each year's budget, results used strategically throughout the organisation

4   Research Methodology

The aim of this work is to develop a software process improvement framework for medical device organisations' usability engineering processes. To meet this aim, the authors have developed a PRM incorporating existing usability engineering standards and guidance documents and will subsequently develop an ISO/IEC 15504-2 compliant PAM. The research methodology used is depicted in Fig. 2.

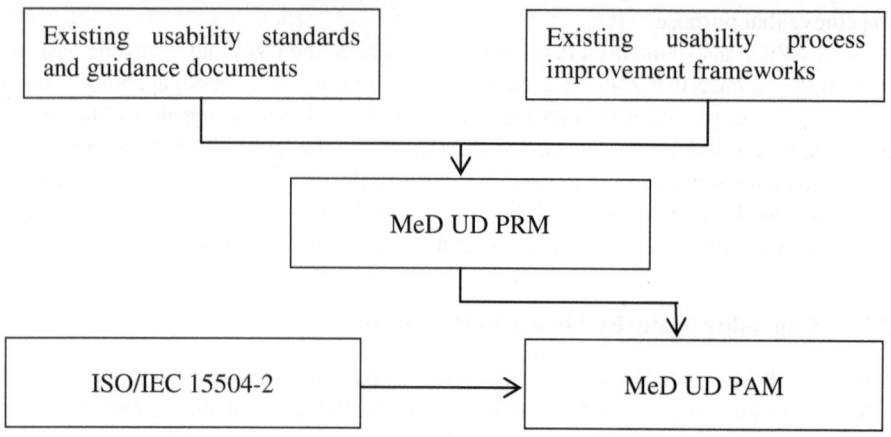

Fig. 2. Research Methodology

It can be seen that the MeD UD PRM incorporates both existing usability standards and guidance documents and existing usability process improvement frameworks. Both the ISO and the FDA have produced significant guidance documents relating to the incorporation of human factors and usability engineering into the development of medical devices. An overview of these documents is provided in the following section.

4.1   Usability Standards and Guidance Documents

The IEC have produced the international standard IEC 62366:2007 – *Medical Devices – Application of usability engineering to Medical Devices* to help during the implementation of a usability engineering process. This standard specifies "a process for a manufacturer to analyse, specify, design, verify and validate usability, as it relates to safety of a medical device" [3].

The standard places a strong focus on the identification and elimination of risks associated with the use of the medical device. As part of the usability engineering process, the standard highlights the importance of the identification of Hazards and Hazardous situations, a critical component of the risk management process.

In addition to this the standard in Section 5.7 Note 2, also recommends an iterative development cycle, specifying the need to perform usability validation throughout the design and development of the medical device.

As part of the usability engineering process, IEC 62366 specifies the need to perform usability verification, ensuring the user interface meets the requirements of the usability specification, and usability validation, ensuring that the primary operating functions can be accomplished through the user interface.

The standard not only requires usability to be incorporated into the medical device, it specifies that usability engineering should also be applied to the development of the User Manual and other supporting documentation as well as to training users in the use of the medical device and all material necessary to support this training.

While the standard does outline the requirements of the usability engineering process, it does not specify specific methods for achieving these requirements. This approach allows the organisation to select the most appropriate methods for the development of a particular medical device which meet the requirements of the standard.

For medical device manufacturers wishing to distribute their products within the United States of America, the FDA have produced the guidance document *"Applying human factors and usability engineering to optimise medical device design"* [6].

This document also emphasises the need for the incorporation of usability and human factors engineering throughout the entire development lifecycle. While IEC 62366 specifies that validation should be performed, the FDA guidance document provides guidance on how to perform validation, including the use of laboratory and clinical validation.

In addition the FDA guidance document outlines some of the methods that can be used to identify hazards and hazardous situations including, contextual analysis, interviews and focus groups, functional task analysis, Heuristic evaluation and Expert review.

4.2   Usability Process Improvement Frameworks

In addition to considering existing standards and guidance documents, during the course of this work a number of existing usability frameworks were considered. Trump [28] is an ISO/IEC 15504 compliant software process improvement method for human centred activities in the system lifecycle. The model is based on ISO 13407 *Human centred design processes for interactive systems* [29].

Trump has been developed to evaluate how well organisations are performing human centred design as part of system development and support projects. It can also be used to help organisations plan what human centred design activities to perform [28]. In addition to this the trump model can be used to help organisations evaluate their existing human-centred design activities.

Within this model there are 7 processes relating to the incorporation of human-centred activities into the software development process. The incorporated processes (descriptions taken directly from [28]) are:

- **Ensure Human Centred Design (HCD) content in system strategy:** - Establish and maintain focus on stakeholder and user issues in each part of the organisation which deal with system markets, concepts, development and support;
- **Plan and manage the HCD Process:** - Specify how the human centred activities fit into the whole system lifecycle process and the enterprise;

- **Specify stakeholders and Organisational requirements:** - Establish the requirements of the organisation and other interested parties for the system. This process takes full accountability of the needs, competencies and working environment of each relevant stakeholder in the system;
- **Understand and Specify the context of use:** - Identify, clarify and record the characteristics of the stakeholders, their tasks and the organisational and physical environment in which the system will operate;
- **Produce design solutions:-** Create potential design solutions by drawing on established state of the art practice, the experience and knowledge of the participants and the results of the context of use analysis
- **Evaluate designs against requirements:** - Collect feedback on the developing design. This feedback will be collected from end users and other representative sources
- **Introduce and operate the system:** - Establish the human-centred aspects of the support and implementation of the system.

An alternative to the Trump Assessment model is KESSU UD by Jokela [30]. Like Trump, KESSU UD is based on ISO 13407 but it also incorporates ISO/TR 18529 [31]. The model has been developed as an objective model for facilitating discussions with development staff during and after usability maturity assessments. The model has also been used as a basis for project planning and communicating the essence of usability to development managers and practitioners.

The KESSU UD model consists of seven processes described below;

- **Identification of user groups:** - During this processes the expected user groups are defined and categorised in a meaningful way. For example potential user groups on an infusion pump could be medical professionals, patients and home carers
- **Context of use analysis:** - The goal of this process is to define the potential user groups tasks, and the environment in which these tasks will be performed. For example a context of use for the aforementioned infusion pumps could be a noisy hospital ward in which a nurse could administer morphine to a patient.
- **User requirements determination:** - This process defines the usability and User Interface (UI) design requirements. The requirements shall be used to drive decision making during the design of the final system.
- **User task redesign:** - This process is used to design how users will carry out their task with the product under design.
- **Usability feedback:** - This process facilitates the qualitative evaluation of the product.
- **Usability verification:** - The usability verification process is used to measure the product under development against the usability and design requirements.
- **Interaction design:** - During this process the elements of the system that the user will interact with (Buttons, Radio Boxes, Text Displays, etc.) are designed. This also includes user documentation and training.

5   Med UD

The MeD UD framework, illustrated in Fig. 3 below, consists of 5 processes spanning the entire development process. The processes defined within the MeD UD framework are performed during the requirements gathering, implementation and testing phases of the software development life cycle. The following provides a high level overview of the processes of the MeD UD Process Reference Model:

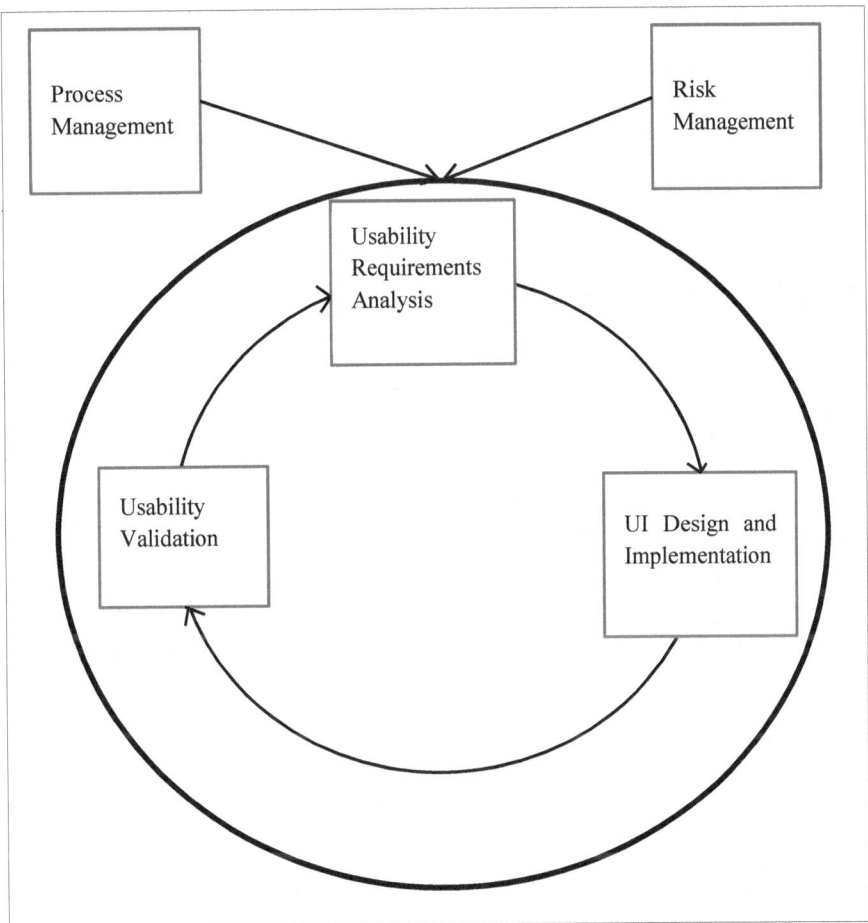

Fig. 3. The MeD UD Framework

- **UD1 – Usability requirements analysis**: - The aim of this process is to define the usability requirements relating to the medical device. In defining these requirements the user, task, context and interaction are all considered. As part of the usability requirements all user groups are identified and analysed. During this analysis user profiles are created for each target user group and key characteristics, including users' level of training are considered.

In addition to this all context(s) of use are identified and analysed. This analysis should include any environmental hazards that may be contained within the context and their impact on the medical device and the interoperability of the medical device with other devices in the environment.

The usability requirements analysis should also identify and analyse the expected user interaction with the medical device. A significant aspect to this process is the identification of the primary operating and frequently used functions.

- **UD2 - Risk management:** - The second process is concerned with risk management. As user error during the use of the medical device carries significant risk, risk management activities relating to the use of the medical device should be carried out. This should be conducted in line with ISO 14971 (ISO, 2007), the risk management standard for the medical device domain, and focus on the risks associated with usability.

- **UD3 - User interface design and implementation**: - This process aims to mitigate against user risks through the development of the interface and supporting documentation. The interface should be developed in accordance with the usability specification. The supporting documentation should be developed in line with the user profiles so that it can be easily understood by the end user. The documentation should also include information relating to training in the use of the medical device.

- **UD4 - Usability validation**: - The Usability validation process aims to ensure that all usability requirements have been met. Validation is performed on a medical device representing the finished product that has been successfully verified against the usability specification.

    Prior to the validation, a validation plan is prepared. The validation should be performed in a realistic environment and should be sensitive enough to capture all use related problems whether or not the user is aware of such problems. The process covers both simulated use validation testing and clinical validation.
    - **Simulated use validation testing:** - During simulated use testing the participants should be representative of actual end users and the environment should be sufficient to enable generalisation to the anticipated actual use. The validation should include both subjective and objective measures.
    - **Clinical validation**: - The aim of clinical validation is to ensure adequate validation of the medical device within a clinical environment while ensuring the safety of participants and patients during the evaluation.

- **UD5 - Process management**: - This process ensures the appropriate management of the usability engineering process through process management. The process should be managed and documented in line with the requirements of the quality management system. To ensure adequate documentation all results of the usability process should be maintained in the usability engineering file.

6   Discussion

The proposed MeD UD assessment model is different from existing process assessment models for usability in a number of ways. Firstly, as the MeD UD assessment model has been developed based on guidelines from both the FDA and ISO it contains a strong emphasis on risk management in line with ISO 14971.

As part of the risk management process of MeD UD there is a requirement for organisations to identify the hazards relating to usability and the sequence or combination of events that can lead to a hazardous situation. This is not an explicit requirement in either the Trump or KESSU UD assessment models.

In addition to this the MeD UD also requires the specific documentation of the usability engineering process. This kind of documentation is mandated by the medical device regulations and as such is required in a usability assessment model for the medical device domain. In other domains such strict documentation is not required to market their products and is therefore not included within general usability assessment models to the same extent as in MeD UD.

The MeD UD assessment model has been developed to compliment Medi SPICE by focusing on the requirements for a usability engineering process. Should organisations wish to focus only on their usability processes they could undertake a MeD UD assessment rather than undertaking a full Medi SPICE assessment.

7   Future Work

The next step of this work will be to validate the PRM. The PRM will be validated by experts from both academia and industry. As well as this it is intended to validate the model with experts within the software process improvement community.

Once the PRM has been validated, the PAM will be developed. In order to do this, the transformation method developed by Barafort et al. [32] will be utilised. This transformation method identifies key requirements for the PAM, in this case the PRM presented above and through a goal oriented approach produces a ISO/IEC 15504 compliant PAM.

In order to further develop and test the MeD UD framework, a MeD UD assessment will be performed within at least two medical device organisations. The goal of these assessments will be to identify the maturity of the organisation with regard to their software processes for usability and to assist them improve these processes. These assessments will also be researched and based on the results finding reports produced and submitted for expert review. The MeD UD PRM and PAM will be updated and amended based on feedback from these expert reviews.

8   Conclusions

The misapplication of a medical device can have serious or even fatal consequences on both the user and the patient. For this reason, human factors and usability engineering practices are used to minimise the risks associated with the use of a medical device by ensuring that users can operate the device in a safe, effective and efficient manner.

A range of standards and guidance documents have emerged which can help developers implement these practices. These documents provide guidance on all aspects of development from the process to use to detailed guidelines on the most suitable components, and style of these components, to be used on a medical device.

In this paper the MeD UD framework is introduced. The MeD UD framework is a process improvement framework for improving human factors and usability engineering processes within the medical device domain. The framework consists of five processes across all aspects of the product development cycle.

Acknowledgements. This research is supported by the Science Foundation Ireland (SFI) Stokes Lectureship Programme, grant number 07/SK/I1299, the SFI Principal Investigator Programme, grant number 08/IN.1/I2030 (the funding of this project was awarded by Science Foundation Ireland under a co-funding initiative by the Irish Government and European Regional Development Fund), and supported in part by Lero - the Irish Software Engineering Research Centre (http://www.lero.ie) grant 10/CE/I1855.

References

1. Faris, T.H.: Safe and Sound Software: Creating an Efficient and Effective Quality System for Software Medical Device Organizations. ASQ Quality Press (2006)
2. Bogdanich, W.: As Technology Surges, Radiation safeguards lag. New York Times (January 26, 2010)
3. IEC 62366:2007, Medical Devices – Application of usability engineering to medical devices
4. ISO/IEC 15504-5:2012, Information technology - Process Assessment - Part 5: An Exemplar Process Assessment Model. Geneva, Switzerland, ISO (2012)
5. CMMI Product Team, Capability Maturity Model® Integration for Development Version 1.2. Software Engineering Institute, Pittsburch PA (2006)
6. Food and Drug Administration (FDA), Draft Guidance for Industry and Food and Drug Administration Staff - Applying Human Factors and Usability Engineering to Optimize Medical Device Design (2011)
7. Sandler, K., Ohrstrom, L., Moy, L., McVay, R.: Killed by Code: Software Transparency in Implantable Medical Devices. Software Freedom Law Center (2010)
8. Food and Drugs Administration (FDA), Infusion Pumps Improvement Initiative (2010), http://www.fda.gov/medicaldevices/productsandmedicalprocedur es/GeneralHospitalDevicesandSupplies/InfusionPumps/ ucm205424.htm (accessed December 7, 2012)
9. European Council, Council Directive 2007/47/EC (Amendment). Official Journal of The European Union, Luxembourg (2007)
10. McHugh, M., McCaffery, F., Casey, V.: Standalone Software as an Active Medical Device. In: O'Connor, R.V., Rout, T., McCaffery, F., Dorling, A. (eds.) SPICE 2011. CCIS, vol. 155, pp. 97–107. Springer, Heidelberg (2011)

11. Burton, J., McCaffery, F., Richardson, I.: A risk management capability model for use in medical device companies. In: International Workshop on Software Quality (WoSQ 2006). ACM, Shanghai (2006)
12. ISO 13485:2003, Medical devices — Quality management systems — Requirements for regulatory purposes. 2nd edn. Geneva, Switzerland, ISO (2003)
13. ISO 14971 – Medical Devices – Application of risk management to medical devices, Switzerland, ISO (2007)
14. IEC 62304:2006, Medical device software—Software life cycle processes. Geneva, Switzerland, IEC (2006)
15. ISO/IEC, ISO 9241: Ergonomic requirements for office work with visual display terminals (VDT) s - Part 11 Guidance on usability (1998)
16. Nielsen, J.: Enhancing the explanatory power of usability heuristics. In: Proc. ACM CHI 1994 Conf., Boston, MA, April 24-28, pp. 152–158 (1994a)
17. Holzinger, A.: Biomedical Informatics: Computational Sciences meets Life Sciences. BoD, Norderstedt (2012)
18. Holzinger, A., Geierhofer, R., Ackerl, S., Searle, G.: Cardiac@View: The User Centred Development of a new Medical Image Viewer. In: Zara, J., Sloup, J. (eds.) Central European Multimedia and Virtual Reality Conference, pp. 63–68. Czech Technical University (CTU), Prague (2005)
19. Nielsen, J.: Usability Engineering. Morgan Kaufmann Publishers Inc. 358 (1993)
20. Association for the Advancement of Medical Instrumentation. ANSI/AAMI HE75:2009, Human factors engineering – Design of medical devices (2009)
21. North, R.A., Patterson, P.A.: A Guide to Navigating the Expanded Human Factors Standard. Biomedical Instrumentation & Technology 44(3), 245–247 (2010)
22. McCaffery, F., Dorling, A.: Medi SPICE Development. Software Process Maintenance and Evolution: Improvement and Practice Journal 22, 255–268 (2010)
23. Casey, V.: Virtual Software Team Project Management. Journal of the Brazilian Computer Society 16, 83–96 (2010)
24. ISO/IEC 12207:2008, Systems and software engineering - Software life cycle processes. Geneva, Switzerland, ISO (2008)
25. ISO/IEC 15504-2 - Software engineering — Process assessment — Part 2: Performing an assessment. 2003: Geneva, Switzerland (2003)
26. Casey, V., Mc Caffery, F.: Medi SPICE and the development of a Process Reference Model for inclusion in IEC 62304. In: The 7th International Conference on Software Paradigm Trends, ICSOFT 2012, Rome Italy, July 24-27 (2012)
27. HIMSS Usability Task Force, Promoting usability in Health Organisations: Initial Steps and Progress towards a Healthcare Usability Maturity Model Health. Information and Management Systems Society (2011)
28. Earthy, J.: Usability Maturity Model: Processes. Lloyds Register of Shipping (1999)
29. ISO/IEC. 13407 Human-Centred Design Processes for Interactive Systems, ISO/IEC 13407: 1999 (E) (1999)
30. Jokela, T.: The KESSU Usability Design Process Model Version 2.1. Oulu University (2004)
31. ISO/TR 18529, Ergonomics of Human–system Interaction—Human-centred Lifecycle Process Description. International Organization for Standardization, Geneva (2000)
32. Barafort, B., Renault, A., Picard, M., Cortina, S.: A transformation process for building PRMs and PAMs based on a collection of requirements – Example with ISO/IEC 20000. In: SPICE 2008, Nuremberg, Germany (2008)

Dictionary of the Slovenian Sign Language on the WWW

Luka Cempre, Aleksander Bešir, and Franc Solina

Computer Vision Laboratory,
Faculty of Computer and Information Science,
University of Ljubljana
Tržaška cesta 25, 1000 Ljubljana, Slovenia
{lukaslo,alex.besir}@gmail.com, franc.solina@fri.uni-lj.si
http://sszj.fri.uni-lj.si

Abstract. The article describes technical and user-interface issues of transferring the contents and functionality of the CD-ROM version of the Slovenian sing language dictionary to the web. The dictionary of Slovenian sign language consist of video clips showing the demonstration of signs that deaf people use for communication, text description of the words corresponding to the signs and pictures illustrating the same word/sign. A new technical solution—a video sprite—for concatenating subsections of video clips necessary for their smooth display on most available platforms was developed. The contents of the dictionary which were re-edited are combined also with other resources available on the web. Added were also new exercises for learning the sign language.

Keywords: sign language, multimedia dictionary, web application, video player, video sprite.

1 Introduction

The fastest way in which deaf people can communicate is by using sign language using their hands. Facial expressions and body posture which accompany signing can modify the basic meaning of a hand gesture. Sign languages have emerged naturally in deaf communities alongside or among spoken languages already in the ancient past [1]. Like spoken languages different sign languages and dialects evolved around the world.

Only after the year 1500 first attempts were made to formally educate deaf children. First books about signing and attempts to formalize sign languages appeared. An important breakthrough was the realization that hearing is not a prerequisite for understanding ideas. One of the most important early educators of the deaf and the first promoter of sign language was Charles Michel De L'Epée (1712–1789) in France. He founded the fist public school for deaf people. His teachings about sign language quickly spread all over the world.

A gesture in a sign language equals a word in a written language. A sign language is therefore a set of signs or hand gestures. Similarly, a sentence in

A. Holzinger et al. (Eds.): SouthCHI 2013, LNCS 7946, pp. 240–259, 2013.

a written language equals a sequence of gestures in a sign language. However, sign language in a given geographical region is not related to the grammar of the spoken language in the same region. For example, in Spain and Mexico they use a totally different sign language although they share the same spoken and written language. On the other hand, in South Africa they use one sign language although they speak eleven different languages [1]. Different sign languages are related mainly due to the influence of formal education and learning of sign languages. Slovenian sign language was derived from the French Sign Language through the Austro-Hungarian sign language in 1840 when the first school for deaf children opened in Slovenia [1]. Sign languages continuously evolve and new signs, such as for example scientific terms are being added to the sign vocabulary [2].

Spoken language is in essence linear—only one sound can be made or received at a time. Sign language, on the other hand, is visual and visual perception allows processing of simultaneous information. Therefore, simultaneous expressions can be used, for example, classifiers which allow a signer to spatially show a referent's type, size, shape, movement, or extent take advantage of the spatial nature of sign language. Gestures in a sign language often emulate the movement or the shape of objects described by the corresponding sign. This principle is called iconicity [1]. Sign languages vary also in word-order typology, for example, Austro-Hungarian Sign Language is of Subject-Object-Verb type while ASL is Subject-Verb-Object. Influence from the surrounding spoken languages is not improbable [1].

To communicate proper nouns and un-common words, sign languages use finger spelling or a manual alphabet [1]. Since the majority of signing employs full words, a signed conversation can proceed with the same pace as a spoken conversation. The Slovenian sign language (SSL), which is used in Slovenia and serves also as the object of this work, consists of approximately 4000 different gestures for common words.

Usually, printed sign language dictionaries, textbooks and manuals relay on illustrations using drawings or photographs which are augmented by text descriptions, for example, such as in the introductory textbook for learning Slovenian sign language [3]. Multimedia technology therefore seems an ideal medium for presentation, reference and learning of such gestural knowledge since it can incorporate also video material. The first multimedia sign language manuals and dictionaries which started to appear in the 90-ties were on CD-ROMs. The American Sign Language Dictionary on CD-ROM was published in 1994 [4]. Our efforts to develop a dictionary of the Slovenian Sign Language started at about the same time [5, 6] and culminated with the publication of the Dictionary of the Slovenian Sign Language on CD-ROM in 2001 [7]. Several other CD-ROM based sign language courses or dictionaries appeared at that time, such as the Czech sign language course [8], British Sign Language [9], etc.

Multimedia CD-ROMs are usually dependent on the type and version of the computer operating system. Due to the fast evolution of operating systems practically all CD-ROMs developed in the not too distant past are therefore practically not usable anymore. The potential users of our dictionary, which worked perfectly under Windows 7, can not use it on current hardware and software platforms. Our motivation for the work reported in this article was therefore to reuse the contents of the Slovenian Sign Language Dictionary and transfer it to a new technological platform which would make the knowledge even more readily available to potential users. At the same time we wanted to reedit the contents and to expand the functionality of the dictionary. World Wide Web experienced in the past decade a tremendous growth in speed as well as in technical prowess and hence presents the obvious choice as the most appropriate medium for such contents. The decision to transfer the material of the CD-ROM version of the dictionary to the web was therefore clear. Another reason for transferring the dictionary to the web is also the appearance of tablet devices which generally do not support CD-ROMs but offer connectivity to the Internet.

Another venue for teaching sign language which was made available by advances in computing is using a virtual human avatar, generated by computer graphics methods, instead of video recordings of an actual human performing signs [10]. This approach, although appealing, has so far not resulted in any large sign language corpus. Namely, besides proper hand movements, the accompanied face expressions are also important for understanding of a sign language. Therefore, any signing avatars should be produced using the highest quality computer graphics which is still too computationally expensive for such applications.

The largest research interest in computing in relation to sign language is oriented towards sign language recognition [11]. Sign language recognition has the well defined goal to translate signs performed by a signing person into text and offers an exciting environment for testing various recognition methods in computer vision.

Sign language support should be incorporated in various communications channels. Using a small window for the signing interpreter is quite common on TV and video material. Now, it is important to include such possibilities also on web pages. Since it is difficult to include this option in the design of web pages from the very beginning and since it can be also distracting to the general public, development of transparent sign language videos which appear only on request were proposed [12]. In this way, the original web page design is preserved but an additional web layer for sign language video is available.

The rest of the article continues as follows: Section 2 is a recapitulation and analysis of the original Slovenian Sign Language Dictionary on CD-ROM that guided us in the design of the enhanced version of the dictionary for the web. The contents and functionality of the new web-based version of the dictionary is described in Section 3. Section 4 presents the technical details of the web-based implementation. In Conclusions we discuss the first user experiences and directions for possible future work.

2   Dictionary of the Slovenian Sign Language on CD-ROM

We developed our first concept of a CD-ROM based multimedia sign language dictionary for the deaf in 1995 [5, 6]. We demonstrated this concept also at the New Talent Pavilion, MILIA'95, in Cannes, France. The only other similar dictionaries at that time were for the American Sign Language [4, 13]. A pilot application of our sign language dictionary consisting of less than 100 words was made in 1996 [14], while the final application, which included also a method for synthesis of signs from several video clips, was finished in 1999 [15]. This was a well received technical achievement since our CD-ROM-based Dictionary of the Slovenian Sign Language of the deaf was selected among the top 15 products in the Student Europrix'99 MultiMediaArt Competition [16]. The final version of the Slovenian Sign Language Dictionary was eventually officially published on CD-ROM in 2001 [7].

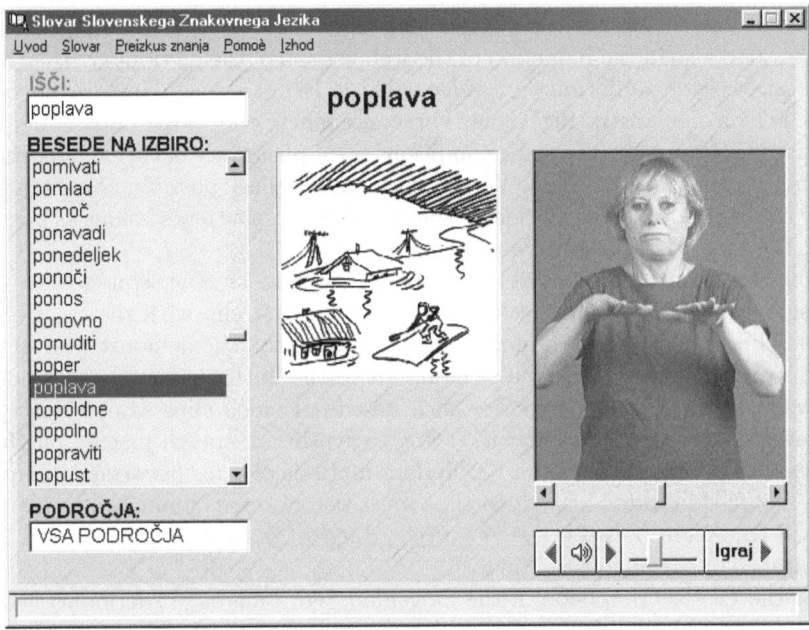

Fig. 1. Word "poplava" ("flood" in English) is on the CD-ROM version of the Slovenian sign language dictionary illustrated with a drawing and a video clip showing the corresponding gesture

The CD-ROM version of the Slovenian Sign Language dictionary includes about 2500 most frequent words or signs. Each word or sign (see Fig. 1) is illustrated with a drawing and the corresponding sign is demonstrated on a video clip. Words are arranged in alphabetical order and also in thematic subgroups so that related words can be found easier. Several signed words are assembled out of two basic signs. For example, the sign for a "farmer" (Slov. "kmet") is assembled out of signs for "rural" (Slov. "kmečki") + "person" (Slov. "oseba"). Similarly, the sign for a "farm" is assembled out of signs for "rural" (Slov. "kmečki") + "landscape" (Slov. "pokrajina"). To save storage space on the CD-ROM and to include more words in the dictionary, we decided to exploit this feature of assembling signs also by concatenating their corresponding video clips. Therefore, the number of video clips in the dictionary can be smaller than the number of words and space for data storage on the CD-ROM could be saved to include more words in the dictionary. This feature of assembling signs turned out quite useful also now, during the transfer of the dictionary to the web, since we were able to expand the sign language vocabulary just by assembling preexisting signs.

Concatenation of video clips presumes a uniform appearance of all video clips so that when we observe an assembled sign, we get the impression that the sign was captured continuously. A uniform appearance of video clips requires that the same person is signing on all video clips. The demonstrator of sign language in the described dictionary was Ms. Ljubica Podgoršek who is the most well known interpreter of sign language in Slovenia and who graciously collaborated also in the redaction of the web version of the dictionary. To achieve the best possible uniformity of video clips it is not enough just to have the same person demonstrating signs. For consistency, the video clips should be captured under exactly the same conditions (i.e. appearance of the demonstrator, lightning, camera setup etc.). We achieved the highest possible consistency of video clips by videotaping the entire sign vocabulary in as few sessions as possible using the same sign demonstrator.

Concatenation of video clips into "natural" looking signing sequences can not be achieved just by concatenating the end of the first clip with the start of the second clip. Namely, in each individual sign video clip, the demonstrator always starts and ends the gesture with the hands in the initial or neutral position at the waist level. "Gluing" together such un-edited video clips would look quite un-natural and in effect similar to trying to synthesize speech just by playing a sequence of prerecorded words. Redundant motions of arms between subsequent signs recorded in individual video clips must therefore be eliminated to assure a smooth transition between the video recordings of individual signs and give an appearance of continuous signing.

For the CD-ROM version of the Slovenian Sign Language Dictionary we developed a new method for concatenating sign video clips which we describe elsewhere [15, 17]. We used computer vision methods to track the position of both hands in all video clips and during entire video sequences. Based on the position of hands we defined four different criteria for concatenation of video clips. Which criteria is used depends on the type of signs (i.e. one-handed or two-handed, general position of the hands etc.) that need to be concatenated. This approach of synthesizing sign language by concatenation of video clips was later used or further developed by several other creators of sign language dictionaries [18–20].

Words which are not in the dictionary or proper names can be shown by spelling and using video clips which contain the signs for individual letters. The complete finger alphabet forms a distinct part of our sign language dictionary showing only still images of gestures for individual letter signs.

2.1 Other Sign Language Initiatives in Slovenia in the Past Ten Years

In 2003 the Association of deaf and hearing impaired people in Slovenia and the Association of interpreters of the Slovenian Sign Language also issued a CD-ROM version containing videos of the most used signs in the Slovenian sign language [21]. However, due to similar issues described above, this CD-ROM is now also technically obsolete.

The Association of interpreters of the Slovenian Sign Language has also developed a light web version of Slovenian sign language dictionary with around a hundred words related to politics [22]. Words are organized alphabetically where for each word a short description is given and a video clip of the performed sign can be played. To play these videos the website uses flowplayer, the HTML5 video player for the web. Unlike the sign video clips that we use, where the demonstrator does not pronounce the corresponding word, the sign language demonstrator on these video clips pronounces the signed word.

On the web page of the Association of deaf and hearing impaired people in Slovenia [23] is available a richer video dictionary of Slovenian sign language, containing signs from the Slovenian and the International sign language. Signs are organized alphabetically and according to selected topics but no other explanation or additional information about the chosen words is available. The website uses jw-player, HTML5 and Flash video player.

2.2 Web-Based Sign Language Dictionaries for Other Languages

The largest web presence has the American sign language (ASL) which is used in more than 50 countries [4]. **Handspeak** [24] is a website with a powerful ASL dictionary which has over 6000 words (glosses) and is still growing. Words are ordered as in a traditional dictionary and the website offers a word search option. One of the more powerful tools on this website is that you can describe a sign with handshape and movement and then search for a word (the dictionary works both ways). When looking for a word, the user of the handspeak dictionary sees only a video and a short word definition, sometimes but only rarely, synonyms and notes would show up. Missing videos can be spotted which makes this dictionary a bit unreliable. The website also includes general information about american sign language such as courses, using sign language with kids, fingerspelling etc.

Signing Savvy [25] is one of the most well known web-based ASL dictionaries. It contains more than 7000 searchable words but is unfortunately payable. It contains also a section for the youngest with 80 basic words.

ASLPro [26] is from a web developer's point of view a poorly designed website filled with ads, but has a powerful collection of videos which were poorly converted into flash (the videos still include play, stop, forward buttons inside the video). The dictionary is divided into four major parts: (1) "The main dictionary" with all the words; (2) "Religious Signs" with a lot of words and names used in different religions, churches and holy books; (3) "Conversational Phrases" which include videos of common phrases used in shops, occupations, nature and similar; and, finally, (3) "ASL for babies" with the most common signs that could be taught to a baby. Every word or phrase is only represented by a video. The website also includes a quiz that is similar to the first of our three quizzes on our website where you have to pick the corresponding word after seeing a sign.

British Sign Language [27] is a web-site that is, such as our web dictionary, also derived from a CD-ROM dictionary. The online dictionary includes 500 words. Every word is presented with an image in gif format (instead of a video) which are not easy for the eyes since only around 2 frames per second are available and hence just a few frames to present a single word. Each word, however, includes a really good description of how it is signed and, if available, related words. The website has also a section for phrases but, unfortunately, only one phrase is shown online, all others are offered only on a CD. The full content of the dictionary is therefore still available only on a payable CD-ROM. Similar to our website, the British Sign Language website offers words grouped by their meaning. A list of several online sign language resources is available [28].

3   Web-Based Dictionary of the Slovenian Sign Language

Our first attempt to move the Slovenian sign language dictionary to the web using the Java programing language goes back to 2000 [29]. This effort was only partially successful. The most severe problems which remained unresolved were with the playback of concatenated video clips. After another decade of intensive development of web technology we believe that the technology is now ripe to transfer the dictionary and its entire functionality to the web, in particular, since due to technical obsolescence, the original CD-ROM version is practically not usable anymore.

At the same time we decided to redesign also the graphical user interface, to combine the original information contained in the dictionary with other resources available on the web and, finally, we had to solve the problem of smooth playback of concatenated video clips.

We used this opportunity also to correct some mistakes and to add new words to the dictionary whose sign could be assembled out of two or more existing video clips. Since many words in the sign dictionary are assembled out of two or more basic signs, it was possible to add new words into the dictionary without the need to record new video clips. Ms. Ljubica Podgoršek selected more than 100 new words for the web-based dictionary that we could assemble out of existing sign video clips.

Currently, the web version of the sign dictionary includes 2514 words and 1801 video clips. The difference is due to sign synonyms when the same sign can have different meanings (486 words) and because some words are assembled out of two or more video clips (245 words).

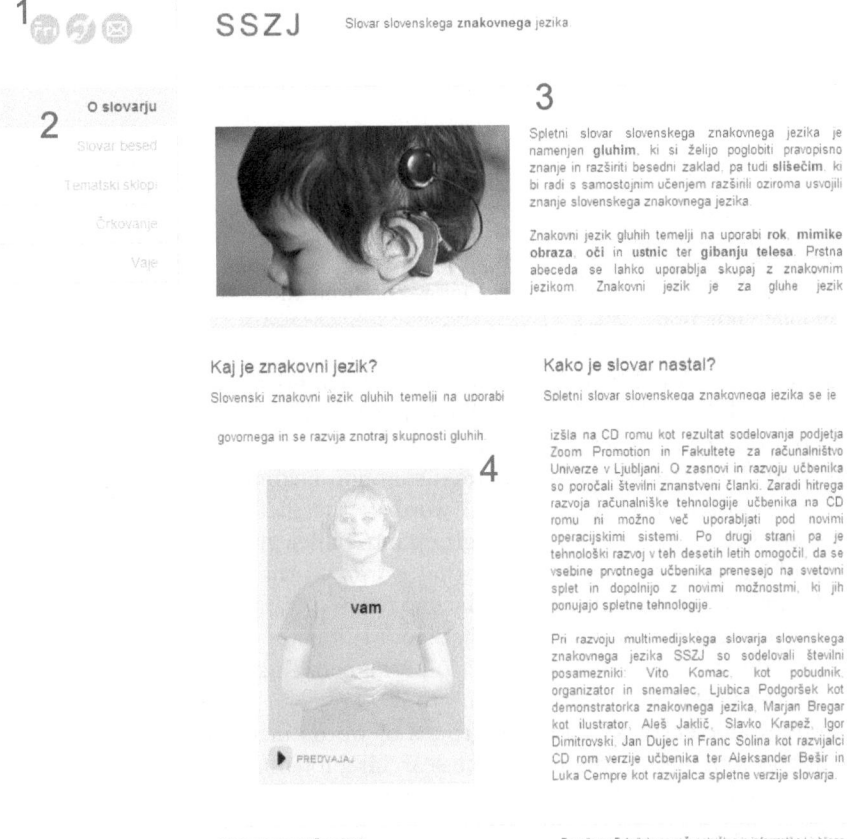

Fig. 2. On the left side of all web pages of the dictionary are links for navigation: (1) link to the Computer vision laboratory where the dictionary was implemented, link to other resources for the deaf, and email contact of the administrator of the dictionary; (2) five links to the main parts of the dictionary: home page, alphabetical list of words, thematic groups of words, signs for individual letters, exercises. On the right side are the contents of the web pages. On the right side of the home page shown here are: (3) some general information about sign language, about the sign dictionary and acknowledgements to all contributors, (4) a player for video clips used for showing the demonstration of all signs included in the dictionary which was developed specially for this purpose.

3.1 Graphical User Interface

We aimed for a rather minimalistic design of the whole web dictionary so that the video player would clearly stand out of the pages. The new home page of the dictionary is shown in Fig. 2. On the left side of all pages are links for navigating the dictionary, while on the right side are the contents of web pages.

Fig. 3. An AJAX powered search field for words from the alphabetical list offers an autocomplete function

The core functionality for searching the alphabetical word list is the ajax powered search field (Fig. 3) which offers an autocomplete function. This makes the search of words easier since it instantly shows the user all the remaining words from the dictionary which share a common begining.

The description of each individual word in the dictionary is structured as follows (see Fig. 4): (1) the thematic group into which the word belongs and the number of basic signs needed to show that word, (2) the description of the word from the web dictionary of slovenian language [30], (3) the video player showing the corresponding demonstration of the sign, (4) images acquired through search for the word with google images, and (5) permanent link to the web page giving the users the possibility to directly link to it.

There are currently 38 thematic groups of words in the dictionary (Fig. 5). Thematic grouping of words makes the searching for related words much faster. The most common words in each thematic group are presented with their corresponding sign videos visually organized into a grid (Fig. 6).

The page dedicated to the alphabet and spelling (Fig. 7) contains a link to the thematic group "alphabet", where video clips for each letter sign can be seen, and a link to the still images of hands signs for the letters in the alphabet. On the bottom of the page words can be spelled out with the help of these hand signs.

Exercises for learning the slovene sign language were substantionally expanded. There are three types of exercises (see Fig. 8):

- after seeing a video clip with a sign, select the correct word among five choices,
- after seeing a video clip with a sign, write down the interpreted word,
- for the given word, demonstrate the sign yourself and then compare you sign with the correct sign in the video clip.

For each exercise you can limit the selection of words to selected thematic groups and select the number of repetitions.

pikapolonica

Beseda je del tematskega sklopa živali.   **1**

Besedo izrazimo z eno kretnjo.

Razlaga besede iz SSKJ: **2**   **3**

pikapolónica -e ž (ó) *hrošč s sedmimi črnimi pikami na rdečih sprednjih krilih:* otrok si je na dlani ogledoval pikapolonico

Več iz SSKJ...

Označi razlago kot neprimerno

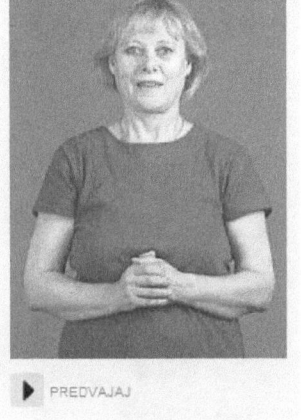

▶ PREDVAJAJ

Slike besede iz iskalnika Google Images: **4**

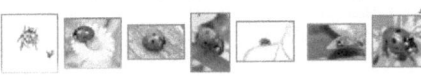

Zgornje slike so pridobljene kot rezultat pri iskanju besede na Google Images. Slike so zato lahko nepovezane z besedo ali neprimerne (prijavi neprimerne slike).

Permalink povezava do besede: **5**

🔗 sszj.fri.uni-lj.si/?stran=slovar.index&beseda=1286

Permalink je stalni internetni naslov, ki vodi do te strani slovarja. Kopirajte ga, če želite komu poslati povezavo do te besede ali če si besedo shraniti med zaznamke.

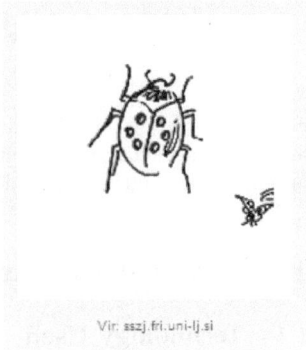

Vir: sszj.fri.uni-lj.si

Fig. 4. Description of the word "pikapolonica" ("ladybird" in English). (1) In which thematic group belongs the word—animals and how many signs are needed for demonstration—one. (2) description of the word, (3) window for the video demonstration, (4) pictures found with Google Images, (5) permalink to the word, on bottom right is the selected picture, the illustration of the word by artist Marjan Bregar in this case.

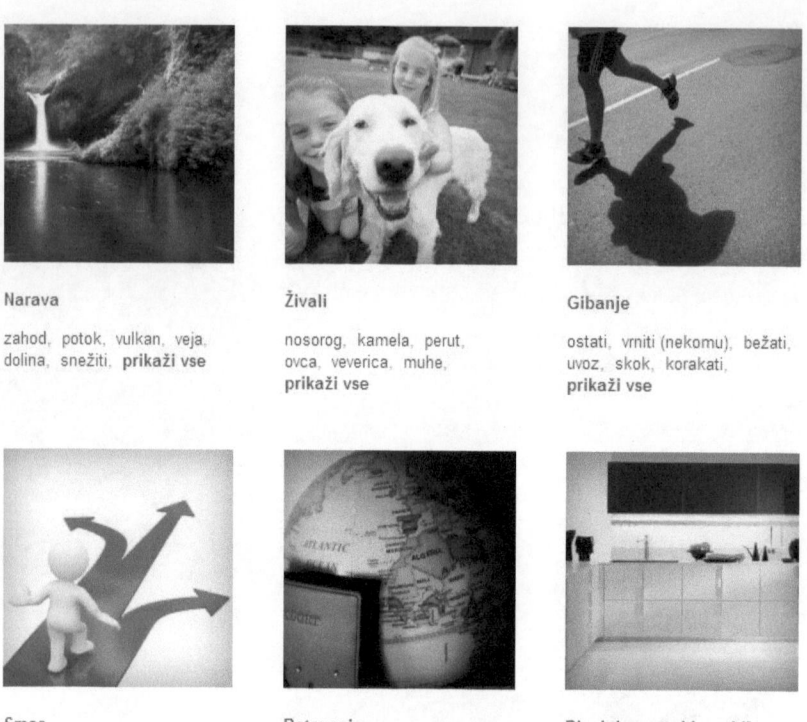

Narava

zahod, potok, vulkan, veja,
dolina, snežiti, **prikaži vse**

Živali

nosorog, kamela, perut,
ovca, veverica, muhe,
prikaži vse

Gibanje

ostati, vrniti (nekomu), bežati,
uvoz, skok, korakati,
prikaži vse

Smer

asfalt, ob, poleg, prehod,
kol, smer, **prikaži vse**

Potovanje

razgled, traktor, kamp,
potovati, tračnice, nahrbtnik,
prikaži vse

Bivalni prostori in pohištvo

hladilnik, jedilnica, nikjer,
omara, tapeta, pomivati,
prikaži vse

Fig. 5. Words in the dictionary are organized into 38 thematic groups to make the searching and learning of related words easier. Themes from left to right and from top to bottom are: nature, animals, movement, direction, travel, living areas and furniture.

4   Technical Details of the Web-Based Implementation

4.1   Technology Used

Prior knowledge, experience, ease of use and programming speed lead us to the decision to implement the web-based dictionary on the PHP platform. A development server running Apache HTTP service was set up. For the main data storage we used the MySQL database management system and we took great care to design a well organized database scheme. When the application's back-end was ready, we focused on how the dictionary's proper front-end should be structured and what its platform dependancies would be.

Since one of our main goals was to make the web-based implementation of the dictionary accessible to as many users as possible, this consideration lead to the conclusion that platform dependancies should be minimized. The first step towards achieving this goal was to avoid the use of rich multimedia browser

Tematski sklopi > Osebe

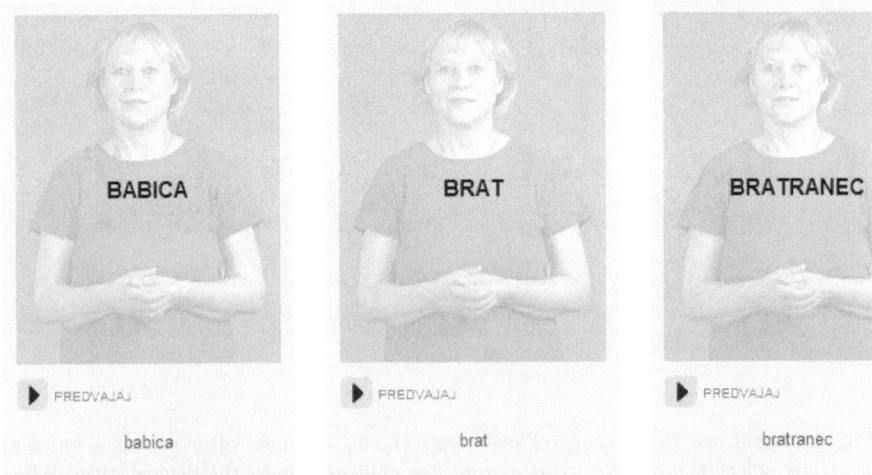

Fig. 6. Words on pages dedicated to individual thematic groups are organized alphabetically into a rectangular grid of sign videos

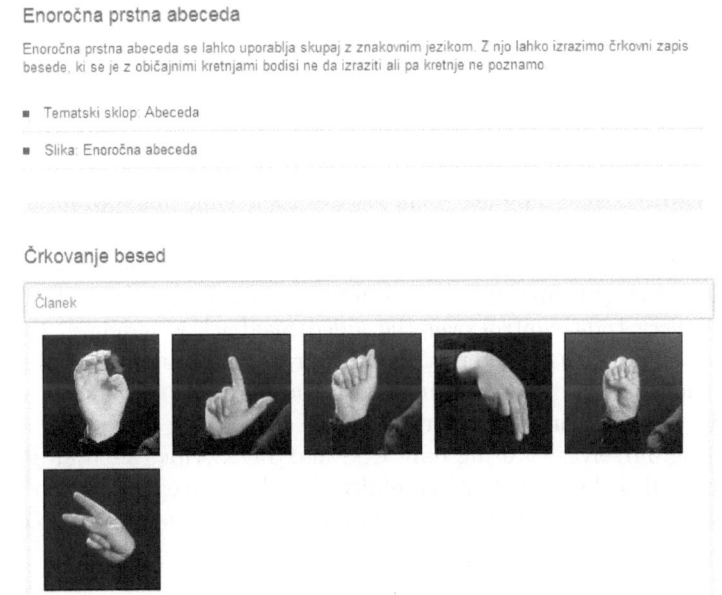

Fig. 7. Page dedicated to the hand alphabet and spelling. The word "članek" (Engl. "article") is spelled with the help of one hand signs for letters.

Vaje

S pomočjo preprostih vaj, ki so del tega spletnega slovarja, lahko utrdite ali preverite svoje poznavanje
slovenskega znakovnega jezika. Na voljo so trije tipi vaj - pri vsakem lahko v naslednjem koraku sami izbirate
tematske sklope, ki jih že poznate.

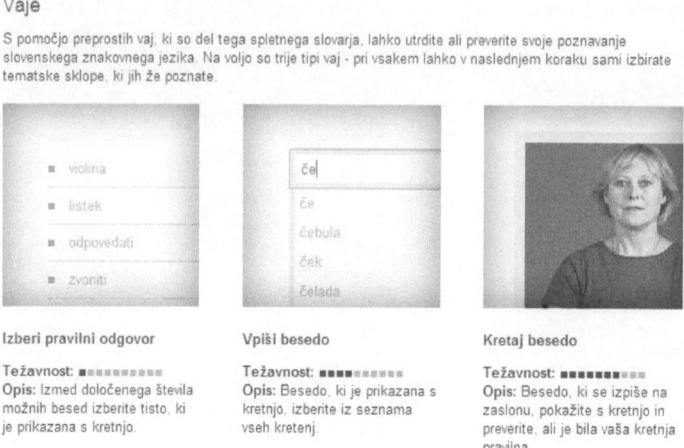

Izberi pravilni odgovor	Vpiši besedo	Kretaj besedo
Težavnost: ■■■■■■■■■■	**Težavnost:** ■■■■■■■■■■	**Težavnost:** ■■■■■■■■■■
Opis: Izmed določenega števila možnih besed izberite tisto, ki je prikazana s kretnjo.	**Opis:** Besedo, ki je prikazana s kretnjo, izberite iz seznama vseh kretenj.	**Opis:** Besedo, ki se izpiše na zaslonu, pokažite s kretnjo in preverite, ali je bila vaša kretnja pravilna.

Fig. 8. There are three types of exercises: (1) on the left: after seeing a video clip of a sign, select the correct word among five choices, (2) in the center: after seeing a video clip of a sign, write down the correct word, (3) on the left: for the given word, demonstrate the sign and compare it with the correct demonstration of that sign.

plugins such as Flash or Java which are not included or even available on some popular platforms. We ended up limiting ourselves to using only the universally supported CSS syntax for page design and JavaScript code for the interactive parts of the dictionary.

4.2   Implementation of a Custom JavaScript Video Player

Video clips with a sign language demonstrator showing the appropriate sign is an integral part of a sign language dictionary. Since we decided to illustrate signs assembled out of two or more basic signs also by concatenating their corresponding video sign clips and at the same time eliminating redundant motions of hands, a very tight control over the video playback is required. Namely, to play a video clip from a predetermined arbitrary start point till a predetermined arbitrary end point and then continue with the playback of the next video clip in the same way without any interruption.

Restricting ourselves to using only CSS and JavaScript raised an important issue which had to be considered carefully. A video player for playback of sign videos had to be chosen. We considered and studied several available options and came to the following conclusions:

– players implemented as web browser plugins (Flash, Java, JavaFX, etc.) cannot be used, as they would make the dictionary platform dependent since some mobile platforms, tablet PCs and other handheld devices are not provided with these plugins.

– HTML5 is nowadays almost universally supported, making it a potentially good option. However, HTML5 video players are not fully controllable by JavaScript, making it impossible to implement the playback of compound words, which are concatenated out of two or more basic sign video clips which need to start and end playing at arbitrary points.
– Converting the videos to Animated GIF format was also considered. However, compared to the HTML5 option, the playback is even less controllable.
– A custom video player should be implemented, which would be fully controllable using JavaScript functions and would further provide JavaScript with the information about which video frame is currently being played. This would allow the playback of assembled words which are concatenated out of two or more basic video clips.

The last conclusion lead us to the idea of converting video files to a custom format which could be controlled by JavaScript. After some brainstorming, discussion with other developers and testing a series of prototypes we were able to develop a working JavaScript controllable video player.

4.3   A New Format for Video Clips

First, we extracted all picture frames from the original video files script and saved them internally as a series of JPEG images using a Python script. Because the original videos are not of the best quality we did not want to degrade them even further and have therefore used the highest JPEG quality (Q=100) that uses a compression rate 2.6:1. The quality of the new video format from the viewer's perspective remained almost the same and any differences are barely noticeable. Since the original video files were recorded with a frame frequency of 15 frames per second we obtained 15 JPEG files for each second of the original video. Next, we merged the individual JPEG images of each video clip into a single larger (actually only wider) JPEG image. In this way, all the original video clips were converted into corresponding JPEG images which were assembled out of video frames of the original video clip. An example of such an image can be seen on Fig. 9. To differentiate this format from the original video clip we decided to name this type of images a *video sprite*.

In addition to the original aim of the new format for video clips, to gain a more precise control of video playback, another beneficial effect turned up—the resulting images or video sprites were considerably smaller than the original videos. On average, the new file size was reduced to 60% of the original file. This reduction in size is especially important since our application runs on the web and video clips can be downloaded from our server much faster.

Our JavaScript video sprite player creates an HTML element with a fixed size (which is the same as the size of a single video frame) and attaches it as a CSS directive, which determines the element's background image. The selected background image is the video sprite version of the target video. Due to the fixed HTML element size, only the first frame from the video sprite is seen.

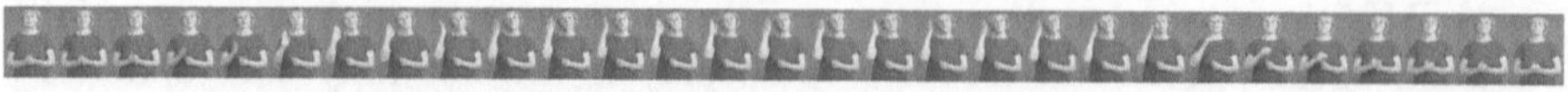

Fig. 9. Each original video clip was converted into a single JPEG image file which contains all video frames of the original clip. We named this format a *video sprite*.

Using JavaScript we can wait until the video sprite is fully downloaded (because the video sprite is actually a single JPEG image) and react afterwards. Next, the JavaScript code starts shifting the HTML element's background image to the left 15 times per second, creating the illusion of video playback.

The described implementation makes it possible to fully control video playback from JavaScript. By loading two more video sprites and using them as background images for the same HTML element at appropriate times, it becomes possible to stack basic sign videos together at preselected points to sign a compound word. The solution that we implemented has been tested on different software and hardware platforms. The results of the playback of a single and merged videos have been satisfying and to an observer look almost the same as the ones from the CD-ROM version of dictionary on almost all platforms. Video playback was tested on PC laptops and PC desktop computers on most widely used browsers including Google Chrome, Mozilla Firefox, Internet Explorer and Opera running on the operating systems Microsoft Windows XP, 7 and 8 and Linux Ubuntu (with the exception of Internet Explorer). Video playback was tested also on an Apple MacBook Pro using the Safari browser running under OSX. The final testing was performed also on tablets and mobile devices where video performed as expected on Apple iPad and iPhone running the Safari browser under iOS operating system, on Android Samsung Galaxy Tab under Android browser, on a "low budget" Android tablet MpMAN MP824 under Opera and on mobile device HTC Desire Z, running Android 4.0, using a 3G network connection to the Internet. A slower performance of the video playback was noticeable only on a LG KC910i most likely due to a much slower hardware, but signs in the video clips were still recognizable.

4.4   How Images That Illustrate the Dictionary Words Are Found

The original CD-ROM version of the dictionary includes a large set of images for illustrating the meaning of words included in the dictionary (as seen on Fig. 1). These images make the learning process faster and easier, especially for younger learners, considering also that deaf people in general are not as proficient readers as the hearing population. Taking into consideration the fact that the spoken and written language is not their primary language. These original illustrations which were drawn expressly for the dictionary by Marjan Bregar[1] were included also in the current web version of the dictionary. However, not every word in

---

[1] Marjan Bregar is a renowned slovenian cartoonist and illustrator, best known for his series of cartoons in the 1950s and 1960s featuring Peter Mozolc in the weekly satirical newspaper *Pavliha*.

the CD-ROM version was illustrated and also new words were added to the web version of the dictionary. How could we fill the missing illustrations? Employing a professional illustrator for a self contained dictionary made sense but on the web exist so many public repositories with rich collections of multimedia that creating new material for that purpose would be unnecessary and superfluous. How could we combine the words from our dictionary with this vast collection of images on the web?

We decided to test a simple and straightforward approach by using Google Image Search API. When a user selects a word in the dictionary, the API is used to perform an image search query using the selected word and the first five resulting images are shown. The results are generally relevant, but there are cases in which the resulting images do not appropriately illustrate the word's meaning. To eliminate such cases we created a simple tool that allows the dictionary's editors to manualy remove inappropriate results. We also created a way in which the users can report image inconsistencies that the editors may have missed.

This simple approach enlarged the initial set of illustrations significantly and demonstrated its usefulness, but almost a third of all search queries produced inappropriate results. Based on these initial and encouraging results we are in the process of improving our search for illustrations:

- replacing Google Image Search API (which is deprecated since of 26 May 2011) with the new and improved Google Custom Search API,
- using beside Slovenian words also their English translation as search queries,
- enabling the users of the dictionary in a crowd sourcing manner to vote on the appropriateness of illustrations so that gradually the best illustrations for the selected words would emerge, and
- giving the users the option to manually enter new image sources.

5   Discussion

A multimedia sign language dictionary can serve multiple functions. Primarily, it supports the learning process of sign language in special educational institutions for the deaf as well as enables normal hearing people who are in daily contact with deaf people to learn to communicate with them in sign language. Another goal of a sign language dictionary is to standardize a given sign language. Since communities of deaf people are often isolated from each other there is a great tendency to develop local dialects which are then not easily understood by other communities of deaf people. A dictionary can unify the meaning of signs and at the same time define a standard way of performing a sign. A dictionary can also partially fill the lack of qualified sign language instructors. The web version of the multimedia dictionary of the Slovenian Sign Language addresses these needs in Slovenia. The dictionary of the Slovenian sign language can now be freely accessed over the Internet from different computing platforms, including tablet computers.

Statistics for the web based Slovenian Sign Language dictionary usage which have been tracked since its opening on 25 June 2012 are encouraging. After the initial buzz the web dictionary was receiving direct traffic and referral traffic from the Facebook page of the dictionary [31] and emails that had been sent to different associations for impaired hearing. In the first month the website was receiving around 5 to 20 unique daily visitors, 70% of which were new and 30% returning. All together 240 unique visits were tracked in July most of which were either referred to the website or came to it by entering the url address directly. 16% of the traffic came to dictionary through a search engine such as Google, Yahoo, Najdi.si etc. Since then, the statistics have gone up because of the increased ranking on major search engines. Our website has been ranking first for the main phrase "slovar slovenskega znakovnega jezika" (Engl. "Dictionary of the Slovenian sign language") on Google. In November 2012 almost 900 unique visitors have seen our website with the Slovenian sign language, half of which have been referred to it via search engines. About 50% of the visitors were returning and an average visit duration was 7 minutes. It should be mentioned that the population of Slovenia is about two million which gives a rough estimate of the total number of speakers of Slovenian language and at the same time the corresponding number of users of the Slovenian sign language.

In the future, we would like to improve the learning experience of the dictionary users. We are cooperating with instructors of deaf children to find better ways of designing the exercises offered with the dictionary. We would like to enable registration of individual users so that the system could track their progress and suggest the next best exercises that they should take for faster learning.

Although a full usability study of the Slovenian sign language dictionary is still missing we received valuable feedback from instructors in schools for deaf children. As a result of this feedback, a distinctive dictionary interface for children who can not read yet is in preparation. In general, we would like to make the user interface more visual and less dependent on text. Pre-lingually deaf children, whose familiarity with their local spoken language is that of a second language learner, written text is in general much less useful than is commonly thought. As is the use of computers in learning of the alphabet by hearing children now common due to their easy accessibility, we would like find a way how to systematically and interactively teach deaf children new signs by expanding the functionality and improving the user interface of the dictionary. Combining several signs into sign sentences brings up also the problem of generation of sign language from written text [10]. Since the grammar of sign languages in general differs from the corresponding natural language, for example Slovenian sign language versus written Slovenian language, the synthesis of sign language from text must be tackled in the context of language translation.

Another desirable feature that we would like to implement is to make the dictionary two-way, so that the user could describe a sign and get the corresponding word. A simple way of describing a sign is just to repeat or demonstrate it. This brings us again to the problem of sign language recognition and interpretation [11].

Since the community of users who regularly use the dictionary is rather stable we would like to engage them also in some type of crowd sourcing to improve the dictionary. As the first step in that direction, the users will be able to vote which of the images selected with the help of Google image search offers the best illustration of the currently selected word.

6   Conclusions

The Slovenian sign language on the WWW project started with the rather humble goal: to make the contents of the original, more than 10 years old CD-ROM version of the sign dictionary accessible again, primarily to children in the school for deaf. Due to technical obsolescence the original CD-ROM version was not usable anymore. However, during the project we realized that we could use the Internet not only as the medium for distribution of the dictionary contents but to also to combine the original contents of the sign dictionary with other sources of information available on the Internet. For the textual description of meaning of individual signs/words we use the Dictionary of the Slovenian language on the web. For pictures that illustrate the words we use Google image search.

At the same time we decided to make a redaction of the dictionary contents. The nature of the sign language where new words can be included by combining existing signs (videos) allowed us to expand the dictionary contents with new words without making new video clips. The user interface is very important, in particular for deaf children. We would like to make a specific interface for children with less stress on text and the possibility to manipulate and combine video clips into whole sentences.

Since the sign dictionary constructs some words/signs by merging two or even three signs/words, concatenating of video clips from arbitrary start and end points on all possible platforms is necessary. To achieve this goal we devised our own method for playing video clips on the web which is based on a new format for video clips that we named video sprite.

We hope that the solutions and experiences that we gained during this project will help other developers of web-based sign dictionaries for other sign languages.

Acknowledgments. This work was supported by the Slovenian Research Agency, research program Computer Vision (P2-0214). We thank Ms. Ljubica Podgoršek for selecting and demonstrating all signs and for her continuous help in improving the contents and functionality of the dictionary.

References

1. Wikipedia: Sign language, http://en.wikipedia.org/wiki/Sign_language (accessed March 4, 2013)
2. Quenqua, D.: Pushing sciences limits in sign language lexicon. The New York Times (December 3, 2012),
   http://www.nytimes.com/2012/12/04/science/
   sign-language-researchers-broaden-science-lexicon.html?ref=science&_r=0

3. Podboršek, L., Kranjc, K.: Naučimo se slovenskega znakovnega jezika 1: učbenik za slovenski znakovni jezik. Zavod za gluhe in naglušne, Ljubljana (2012)

4. Sternberg, M.L.A.: The American Sign Language Dictionary on CD-ROM. Harper Collins, New York (1994)

5. Jaklič, A., Vodopivec, D., Komac, V.: Learning sign language through multimedia. In: Proceedings of International Conference on Multimedia Computing and Systems, Washington, pp. 282–285 (1995)

6. Jaklič, A., Vodopivec, D., Komac, V., Gašperič, M.: Multimedia learning tools for the hearing impaired. In: Proceedings of the World Conference on Educational Multimedia and Hypermedia, ED-MEDIA 1995, Graz, pp. 354–359 (1995)

7. Komac, V., Gašperšič, M., Jaklič, A., Krapež, S., Igor, D., Solina, F., Podboršek, L.: Učbenik slovenskega znakovnega jezika (CD-ROM). Zoom Promotion: Fakulteta za računalništvo in informatiko, Ljubljana (2001)

8. The Union of the Deaf, Brno: Czech sign language course, http://www.kurzznakovereci.cz (accessed March 5, 2013)

9. british-sign.co.uk, http://www.british-sign.co.uk (accessed March 5, 2012)

10. Elliott, R., Glauert, J.R.W., Kennaway, R., Marshall, I., Sáfár, E.: Linguistic modelling and language-processing technologies for Avatar-based sign language presentation. Universal Access in The Information Society 6, 375–391 (2008)

11. Ong, S.C.W., Ranganath, S.: Automatic Sign Language Analysis: A Survey and the Future beyond Lexical Meaning. IEEE Transactions on Pattern Analysis and Machine Intelligence 27, 873–891 (2005)

12. Debevc, M., Kosec, P., Holzinger, A.: Improving multimodal web accessibility for deaf people: sign language interpreter module. Multimedia Tools and Applications 54, 181–199 (2011)

13. The Communication Technology Laboratory at Michigan State University: Personal Communicator CD-ROM (1995)

14. Krapež, S.: Slovar znakovnega jezika za gluhe/Sign language dictionary for the hearing impaired. Dipl. ing. thesis, University of Ljubljana, Faculty for Computer and Information Science (1996)

15. Krapež, S., Solina, F.: Synthesis of the sign language of the deaf from the sign video clips. Electrotechnical Review 66(4-5), 260–265 (1999)

16. EuroPrix99 Multimedia Art, Europe's Best in Multimedia (1999), http://www.europrix.org

17. Solina, F., Krapež, S., Jaklič, A., Komac, V.: Multimedia dictionary and synthesis of sign language. In: Rahman, S.M. (ed.) Design and Management of Multimedia Information Systems, pp. 268–281. Idea Group Publishing (2001)

18. Chuang, Z.J., Wu, C.H., Chen, W.S.: Movement Epenthesis Generation Using NURBS-Based Spatial Interpolation. IEEE Transactions on Circuits and Systems for Video Technology 16, 1313–1323 (2006)

19. Chiu, Y.H., Wu, C.H., Su, H.Y., Cheng, C.J.: Joint Optimization of Word Alignment and Epenthesis Generation for Chinese to Taiwanese Sign Synthesis. IEEE Transactions on Pattern Analysis and Machine Intelligence 29, 28–39 (2007)

20. Wang, R., Wang, L., Kong, D., Yin, B.: Making smooth transitions based on a multi-dimensional transition database for joining chinese sign-language videos. Multimedia Tools and Applications 60, 483–493 (2012)

21. Žele, A.: Multimedijski praktični slovar slovenskega znakovnega jezika (CD-ROM). Zveza društev gluhih in naglušnih Slovenije, Združenje tolmačev za slovenski znakovni jezik, Ljubljana (2003)

22. Zavod Združenje tomačev za slovenski znakovni jezik: Terminološki slovar SZJ – politični žargon, `http://tolmaci.si/islovar/index.php/islovar/index/Z` (accessed 8 December 2012)
23. Zveza društev gluhih in naglušnih Slovenije: Slovarji, `http://www.zveza-gns.si/slovarji` (accessed December 8, 2012)
24. Lapiak, J.: Handspeak: sign language resource, `http://www.handspeak.com` (accessed December 8, 2012)
25. Signing Savvy, `http://www.signingsavvy.com` (accessed March 4, 2013)
26. ASLpro.com, `http://www.aslpro.com` (accessed March 5, 2013)
27. BritishSignLanguage.com: A Guide to British Sign Language, `http://www.britishsignlanguage.com` (accessed December 8, 2012)
28. Sign Languages, `http://www.yourdictionary.com/languages/sign.html` (accessed March 5, 2012)
29. Dujec, J.: Slovar slovenskega znakovnega jezika gluhih v programskem jeziku Java. Diplomska naloga, Univerza v Ljubljani, Fakulteta za računalništvo in informatiko (2000)
30. Znanstvenoraziskovalni center Slovenske akademije znanosti in umetnosti, Inštitut za slovenski jezik Frana Ramovša, ZRC SAZU Ljubljana: Slovar slovenskega knjižnega jezika (2000), `http://bos.zrc-sazu.si/sskj.html` (accessed 8 December 2012)
31. Facebook: Slovar slovenskega znakovnega jezika, `http://www.facebook.com/SlovarSlovenskegaZnakovnegaJezika?fref=ts` (accessed December 8, 2012)

A Usability Requirements Analysis
for Wireless Interaction and Connectivity
for Elderly Hearing Aid Users

Matjaž Debevc[1], Ines Kožuh[1], and Hilmar Meier[2]

[1] University of Maribor, Slovenia
{matjaz.debevc,ines.kozuh}@um.si
[2] Sonova, Switzerland
hilmar.meier@phonak.com

Abstract. Recent studies have shown an increase in the number of elderly smartphone users with hearing aids. The question arises as to how to optimize smartphone use for elderly people who have hearing aids, and in particular how to allow remote control and streaming audio from different audio devices. In our usability requirements analysis, which included 27 participants, we examined two different types of implementation for connecting smartphones to a hearing aid. First, a direct connection between one specific brand of smartphone and a hearing aid is examined. Second, an indirect connection between the usual smartphone and a hearing aid via wireless adapter is investigated. The research findings showed that participants liked the concept of using the smartphone as a streaming device, although opinions were divided as to whether to use a direct or an indirect connection. In conjunction with the indirect connection, we also examined the style of wearing of the adapter. Most of the participants preferred the shirt and belt clip implementation.

Keywords: hearing aids, hearing instruments, mobile applications, user studies, evaluation.

1 Introduction

Promoting and encouraging elderly people to use hearing aids (HAs) has become a global concern that requires further action. The World Health Organization estimates that in 2004 over 275 million people around the world had a hearing impairment, which is roughly 4% of the world's population [1, 2]. Of this 4%, the majority are elderly people and are affected due to the typical age-weakening hearing loss in high frequencies known as presbycusis [3].

Unfortunately, elderly people often reject the idea of using a HA, despite clearly suffering from hearing loss. One reason for the decline is the fact that HA users often have difficulty listening to audio devices, especially telephones [4]. The intelligibility of speech via audio devices is considerably lower than the intelligibility in face-to-face speech. This is mainly caused by a lack of visual contact, and compounded by the absence of lip-reading, limited telephone bandwidth, compression algorithms and background noise.

A. Holzinger et al. (Eds.): SouthCHI 2013, LNCS 7946, pp. 260–271, 2013.
© Springer-Verlag Berlin Heidelberg 2013

On the other hand, it is evident that demographical, structural and social trends tend towards elderly people, which may have a dramatic effect on the design and development of usable hearing aids and human-computer interfaces. It is expected that the EU-25 countries will experience a demographic shift. In 2000, an estimated 15.7% of the population was older than 64. This is expected to increase to 17.6% in 2010, and 20.7% in 2020 [5].

Considering these trends, hearing loss may play a crucial role. In the study by Davis [6] it was reported that about four million Europeans have a severe or profound degree of hearing loss, about 20 million have moderate, and 76 million have mild hearing loss.

The fact that concerns us is that the production of HAs meet less than 10% of global demand. In developing countries, fewer than 1 out of 40 people who need a hearing aid have one. The majority of hearing aid users are elderly people, due to typical age-weakening hearing loss [3]. About 55% of people over 60 years are deaf or hard of hearing, 30% of people between 60 to 80 years have mild deafness and 60% of people over 80 years have moderate deafness. An estimated 70–80% of adults between 65 and 75 years of age suffer from presbycusis. Presbycusis leads to a lower quality of life and depression among elderly people, and can lead to a decrease in social contact and, subsequently, a more isolated lifestyle. It is estimated that at least 900 million people will suffer from presbycusis by 2050 [7].

One of the possibilities for solving the aforementioned problems is to increase the use of HAs and the quality of speech both to and from audio devices. We propose connecting audio devices to a HA via smartphone. This plays an increasingly important role in the social environment for the elderly people, as well as in younger culture [8]. By connecting HAs with a smartphone, it is also possible to enable a more user-friendly method of remote controlling a HA, improve the fine-fitting process and allow for the connection for different audio devices at once.

This concept is based on the actual use of existing small and handy communication and information devices. However, the problem is that an additional device is needed for every audio device. It means that users need several different devices to be able to use them in various environments.

Thus, we developed a concept that would enable the connection of various audio devices by one device: a smartphone. The reason is that it is one of the most commonly used devices.

In this paper, we will review existing solutions and introduce the concept of using a smartphone in connection with HAs, which would allow the remote control of HAs, streaming audio from a home phone, TV, radio, hi-fi, car radios, computers, watch / door alarms and wireless microphones (Fig. 1). In addition, with the help of a usability requirements analysis, we verified how users perceived different ways of connecting smartphones and HAs. First, we investigated connections without any interface adapters between HAs and the smartphones currently on the market. Second, we examined two possible solutions for connecting HAs and smartphones. In the first one, we explored the concept of a direct link between one specific brand of smartphone and a HA. In the second one, we examined the concept of an indirect connection with a connection adapter between a smartphone and a HA.

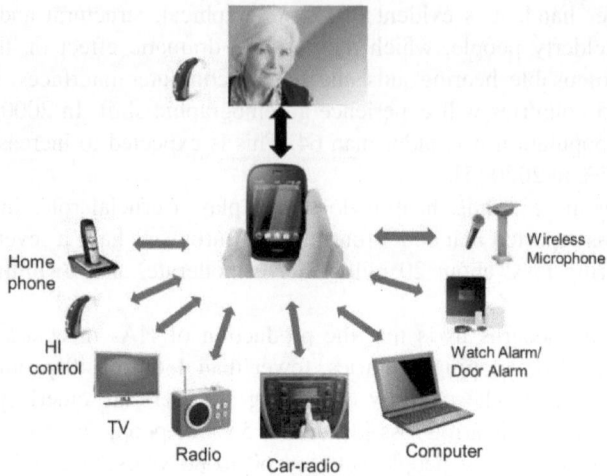

Fig. 1. Hearing aid connected to audio devices via smartphone

We also investigated which style of wearing would be more appropriate in the case of using a connection adapter. To the best of our knowledge, connecting audio devices via smartphones directly to a hearing aid has not been widely studied and analysed yet, although the analogy has been used in some exercise campaigns, e.g. the Starkey T2 Remote application [9].

2   Background and Related Work

The most common connection between smartphones and other devices is to use Bluetooth. In 2008, more than half of the phones placed on the market had Bluetooth capabilities [10]. In recent years, most of the HA manufacturers (e.g. Phonak, Starkey, Siemens and Oticon) and mobile phone producers (e.g. Samsung, Nokia) have aspired to enhance the functionalities of mobile phones for a connection to HAs.

Unfortunately, since Bluetooth uses a significant amount of energy and requires a larger device than we wanted, there has yet to be a successful implementation of Bluetooth connection directly to HAs [11]. Therefore, manufacturers have recently produced mostly indirect solutions for connecting HAs with mobile phones. It works in a way that additional adapters are in use, which follow the Bluetooth signal from smartphone to adapter and then transfer the signal with the help of another wireless system to the HA. Such a wireless systems can be integrated within the HA because of its small size, such as the Hearing Instruments Body Area Network (HiBAN) by Phonak.

Such indirect devices help the smartphone and a HA interact. In general we divide them into:

- connectivity devices and
- interaction devices.

A connectivity device (e.g. iCom from Phonak) connects hearing aids wirelessly to telephones, MP3 players, frequency modulation (FM) systems, and computers. The device functions as a wireless headset, allowing for the benefit of hands-free functionality. Usually these devices connect to other 3rd party systems, like mobile phones via Bluetooth.

The interaction device (e.g. remote control SoundPilot2 from Phonak) provides the possibility of controlling the volume and programming of hearing aids. It also allows for other control interactive functionality.

With regard to the growing number of functionalities and possibilities for the better control of digital HAs, there is a growing demand for visual feedback with the help of a visual display. Within both connectivity and interaction devices, we further classify devices into devices with the systems that provide the following features:

- audio feedback,
- visual feedback,
- audio and visual feedback.

Recently, combined connection and interaction in a single device (e.g. ComPilot from Phonak) is provided, which includes the wireless listening of audio devices, HA remote control, and audio feedback.

Other devices that use Bluetooth technology and are currently on the market include iCom and ComPilot by Phonak, as well as Tek and Oticon Streamer by Siemens [12]. These devices basically use Bluetooth for communication with mobile phones. Afterwards, a signal is divided into several parts in a way that a discrete signal is sent to each HA separately. The HA needs an FM receiver to connect the devices in order to work, such as the Phonak ComPilot. Unfortunately, users can face several limitations. For instance, the Phonak ComPilot can only be used for HAs produced by Phonak and not for HAs produced by other companies. A solution for this problem was developed by Artone, where telecoil [10] is used to establish a connection between HAs and devices. Whether a telecoil is integrated within the HA, an adapter receives a signal from other devices via Bluetooth and the adapter sends it further to a HA via induction to the telecoil.

In the middle of 2012, Apple acquired a patent, in which Apple's operating system iOS will bring compatibility for "Made for iPhone" hearing aids [13]. Apple's patents for a "Hearing assistance system for providing consistent human speech" and the related "Providing notification sounds in a customizable manner" both equip portable devices, such as the iPhone, with digital hearing aids and will create a direct link of communication between the HA and the smartphone using 2.4 GHz band low-power protocol of the Bluetooth Low Energy communications standard [14].

Due to current issues regarding direct connections between HAs and smartphones, our aim was to verify the usability requirements analysis of how users would accept the following possible solutions of connections between smartphones and HAs:

- a direct connection with a specific brand smartphone and
- an indirect connection with an interface device to every smartphone existing on the market within a 50 cm distance.

In addition, our aim was to verify which style of wearing for adapters users would accept in case of an indirect connection between smartphones and HAs.

3   Research Setting

3.1   Design of the Research

Research Questions. Within the scope of the aim, we propose examining the following research questions:

RQ1: Are there statistically significant differences in users' perception of two concepts: 1) a direct connection between a HA and streaming audio and 2) an indirect connection between a HA and streaming audio from specific devices?

The first research question seeks to ascertain whether there are statistically significant differences between users' perception of a direct connection, where a specific brand smartphone is used, and an indirect connection between a HA and streaming audio, where an interface device is used to connect a HA and every smartphone existing on the market. We expect to find statistically significant differences between both concepts.

RQ2: Are there statistically significant differences in assessment of the concept of using a smartphone for a connection between a HA and streaming audio from specific devices between two groups:

    a)   participants younger than 66 years and

    b)   participants 66 or more years old?

We assume to find statistically significant differences in perceiving the concept of using a smartphone for connecting a HA and streaming audio between two aforementioned groups.

RQ3: What are the preferred styles of wearing of adapters needed for an indirect connection?

Measures. We developed and applied a non-standardized questionnaire that comprised two main sections: a questionnaire on the general information about the participant and a questionnaire on the participant's views on low fidelity prototyping of remote controllers. We combined closed and open-ended questions. The responses for close-ended questions were given via a 5-point Likert scale (from totally dislike to totally like).

Within the first section, we provided eight questions to gather demographic data and illustrate the users' profiles (age, gender, occupation, hearing status, duration of HA use, subjective opinion on the frequency of computer use, the use of a smartphone, the sort of applications used with a smartphone).

The second section comprises 14 questions. First, participants were asked to provide their subjective opinion on how useful the concept of connecting audio devices, such as TVs, radios, computers, FM systems, was via smartphone with a HA. They were also asked to express their subjective opinion about direct and indirect connection, as well as provide reasons for their opinion via open-ended questions. Second, they were asked to assess how they liked six possible styles of wearing of adapters for indirect connections: headset, shirt clip, belt clip, wristband, neck loop, pen and belt clip (Fig. 2). In addition, they were also asked to rank three of them based on which they preferred the most.

Preparation for Implementation of the Research. We planned our visits in HA stores. We prepared invitations for cooperation in the study, where the aims of our research were clearly stated. Invitations were sent to HA stores and associations for the deaf and hard of hearing in Slovenia and Switzerland. We asked audiologists and secretaries of the associations to disseminate information about the study. They set the dates for the implementation of the research.

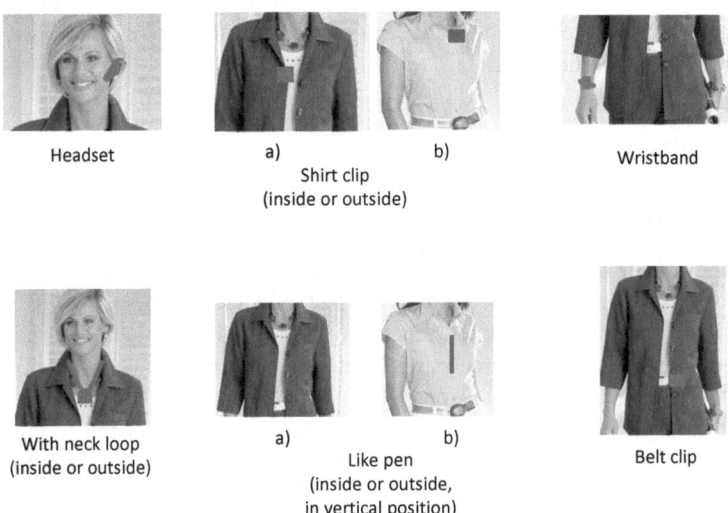

Headset

a) Shirt clip (inside or outside) b)

Wristband

With neck loop (inside or outside)

a) Like pen (inside or outside, in vertical position) b)

Belt clip

Fig. 2. Styles of wearing for hearing aid interface device

3.2   Procedure

The study was conducted in Slovenia and Switzerland in the middle of 2011. The participants were recruited from a group of existing clients of audiology centres. Members of the hearing society in Slovenia and Switzerland attended. Evaluators visited the audiology and society centres at an agreed-upon period to meet with the participants.

The evaluator first presented, in detail, the objectives of the study and provided an information sheet. After signing the consent form, a paper questionnaire was distributed. The research lasted 30 minutes.

3.3   Statistical Analysis

Descriptive statistics were used to analyse data. The relationships between variables were inspected by calculating the Spearman's Rho coefficient. Statistically significant differences between two independent age groups were verified by the Mann-Whitney U test. Median scores of the same sample for two variables were inspected with a Wilcoxon Signed-ranks test. All analyses were performed with SPSS version 20.0.

3.4   Participant Profile

Twenty-seven participants (9 female, 18 male) aged from 48 to 85 years (M = 61.52, SD = 18.25) attended the study. Most of them did not boast any technical experiences; only seven participants (25%) already had a smartphone. All participants used HAs. The preferred use of audio device among the participants was watching TV, telephone conversations, listening to radio, and the use of computer and wireless microphones. Most participants (30%) reported the TV as the most frequently used audio device. Telephones were in second place, with 22% of participants. And the radio was in third place, with 15% of participants.

4   Results

4.1   Preferred Type of Implementation

The findings of the analysis have shown that the mean score for the solution of using a smartphone was 3.96 (Mdn = 5.0, SD = 1.51). Nineteen participants (70.3%) liked the solution of using every smartphone existing on the market, five participants (18.5%) did not like it and three participants (11.1%) were undecided. To find an answer on the first research question, we analysed the results further. Among those who liked the concept of using a smartphone, the mean score for the solution with a direct connection between a smartphone and a HA was 3.63 (Mdn = 3.64, SD = 1.07) and the average score for the solution with indirect connections was 3.84 (Mdn = 3.92, SD = .90) which is also shown in Fig. 3.

The Wilcoxon Signed-rank test indicated no statistically significant difference in liking the concept of connection between a direct (Mdn = 3.64) and an indirect one (Mdn = 3.92), Z = - .77, p > .05.

We conducted a further analysis of the data gathered with open-ended questions to interpret and find reasons for data gathered with quantitative close-ended questions.

Reasons for Assessment of the Concept: Connection Smartphone-HA. We considered the question of how useful the users believed the connection between smartphone and a HA to be. We classified the responses into two categories. Within the first category were set users who liked the concept of using a smartphone and in the second category were those who did not like it.

Most participants who liked the concept of using a smartphone pointed out the advantage of using just one device for different hearing situations. The main issues raised included simplicity and ease of use. To a lesser extent, concerns about the user interface and the automatic connection between a HA and other devices via smartphone was mentioned.

The following comments illustrate these points:

"Perfect – there is no need to have so many devices with so many charging and connection cables when travelling abroad."

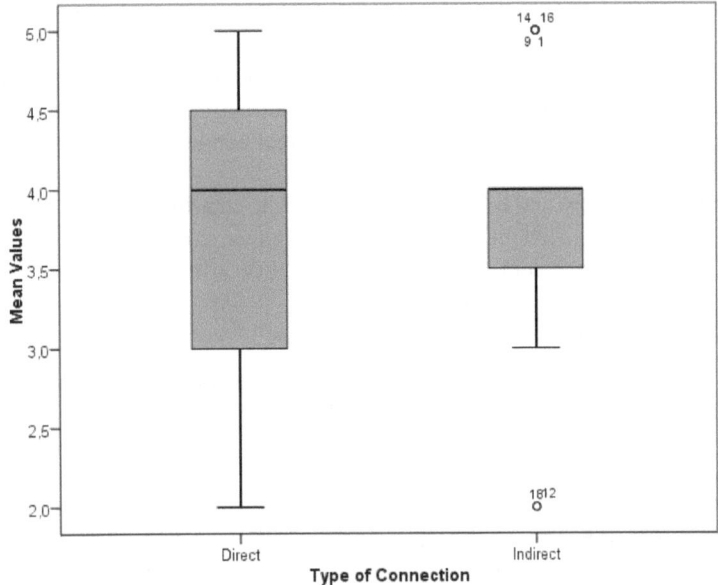

Fig. 3. Preferred type of implementation

Most participants who liked the concept of using a smartphone pointed out the advantage of using just one device for different hearing situations. The main issues raised included simplicity and ease of use. To a lesser extent, concerns about the user interface and the automatic connection between a HA and other devices via smartphone was mentioned. The following comments illustrate these points:

"Perfect – there is no need to have so many devices with so many charging and connection cables when travelling abroad."

"The concept is perfect, but the user interface should be as easy as possible."

Participants who did not like the concept of using smartphone for connecting mainly spoke about their concern about being able to use smartphones in general and also for the purposes of connectivity. The following comment from a participant illustrates these points:

"I do not want to have more devices and cables."

Reasons for Assessment of the Concept: Direct Connection Smartphone-HA. We also examined the reasons behind participants' opinion of using a direct connection with a smartphone for connecting and controlling a HA with other devices. The responses were classified into two categories regarding their liking the concept of direct connection. Participants who liked the concept mainly spoke about its practicality and usability for this type of connection. This point is illustrated in the following comment:

"To have only one way in terms of direct connection is not so bad as long as it is also easy to handle."

Participants who did not like the concept of a direct connection provided several reasons why. They were mainly concerned as to whether they would be obliged to use the specific brand of smartphone. To a lesser extent, participants spoke about their concern whether old smartphones would support direct connection. They would not be willing to change their smartphone to use a direct connection. The following comments reflect the aforementioned points:

"I do not want to rely and be dependent on just one smartphone producer."

"Here is the layout problem. The question is whether smartphones offer such functionalities. Next, the problem may be habits and ordinariness. Why and how should we replace good old smartphones with new ones?"

Reasons for Assessment of the Concept: Indirect Connection Smartphone-HA. We classified responses into two categories. Within the first category were set users who liked the concept of an indirect connection and within the second those who did not like the concept. The analysis of participants' opinions on an indirect connection showed that those who liked it stressed the flexibility, the practicality of the adapter and a chance of not being obliged to use the specific brand of smartphone. The following comment from a respondent is an example of these points:

"I would like to have the freedom of choice for my smartphone!"

Most participants who did not like the concept of an indirect connection declared their concerns about requiring additional devices when using an adapter. To a lesser extent, they spoke about their discomfort with using adapters and the need for an additional save bag. The following comment represents these points:

"An additional device is very problematic. There are problems with too many adapters."

4.2   Preferred Type of Implementation Regarding Age

The participants' age was reported to be associated with the concept of using a smartphone, $r = -.386$, $p < .05$, and a direct connection, $r = -.389$, $p < .05$. It means that as the participants' age increased, the concept of using a smartphone and a direct connection was rejected more often.

To answer the second research question, participants were classified into two groups split by the median age (66 years). In the first group there were 13 participants younger than 66 years and in the second group there were 14 participants who were 66 or older. Statistically significant differences were reported between the groups both with the concept of using a smartphone (the mean ranks were 17.65 (group 1) and 10.61 (group 2), $U = 43.5$, $p < .05$) and a direct connection (the mean ranks were 17.77 (group 1) and 10.50 (group 2), $U = 42.0$, $p < .05$). The results indicate that people under the age of 66 caused statistically significant higher satisfaction with the concept of using a smartphone for connecting and controlling a HA with other devices ($p = .02$), which can be seen in Fig. 4. Concomitantly, being under 66 years had an impact on higher satisfaction with the concept of a direct connection between a smartphone and a HA ($p = .017$). The differences between both age groups in an indirect connection were statistically non-significant.

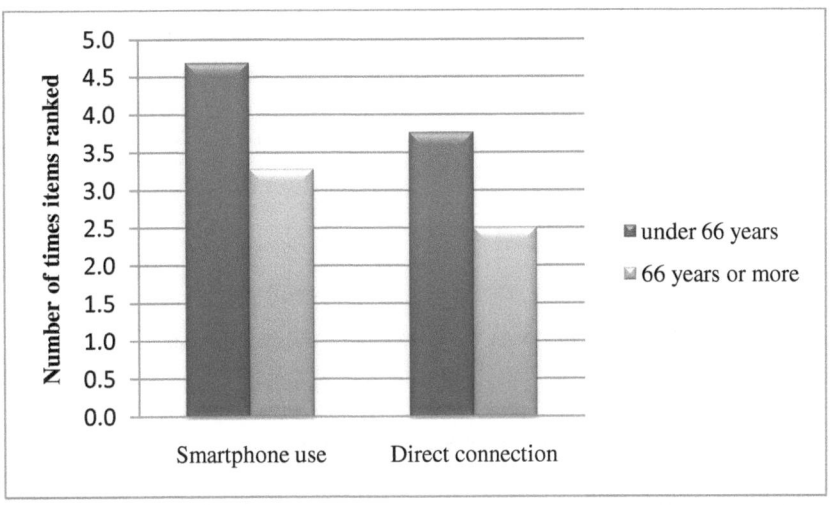

Fig. 4. Preferred type of implementation in two age groups

4.3   Preferred Styles of Wearing

To answer the third research question, we examined the preferred styles of wearing. Participants were shown figures of possible styles of wearing of adapters needed for an indirect connection. The participants were asked to find the three most appropriate ways of wearing and to allocate them in order, from the most desirable to the third, less desirable, but still useful, style of wearing. Fig. 5 shows that the most frequent choice was "shirt clip" (25.9%), "belt clip" followed with 18.5% and, surprisingly, "pencil" also garnered 18.5%.

5   Discussion and Conclusion

In this paper, we introduced the concept of using a smartphone in connection with a HA, which would allow for the remotely controlling the HA in various hearing situations, in particular in connection with different audio devices. We examined elderly participants' opinions, where we verified how they perceived different ways of connections between smartphone and a HA.

The research findings have shown that participants liked the concept of using a smartphone in connection with HAs, which would allow for the remote controlling of HAs in connection with streaming audio devices. Although an indirect connection between the HA and the usual smartphone with the use of adapter was assessed as slightly better than a direct connection between a specific-brand smartphone and a HA, the differences were not statistically significant.

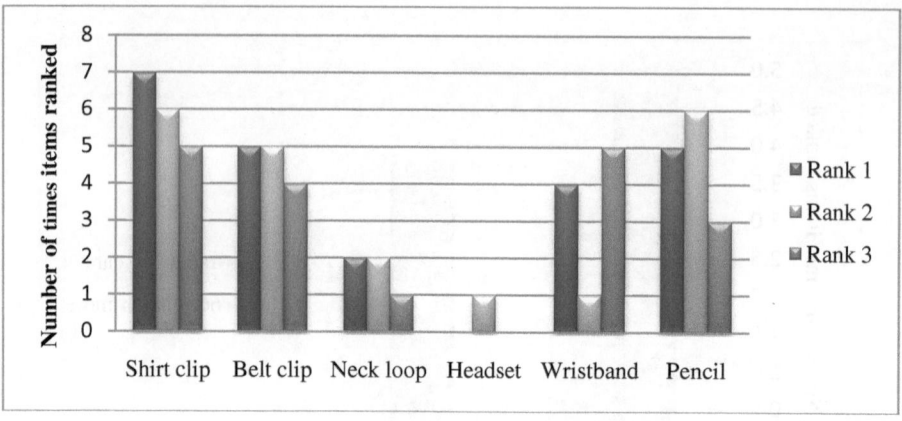

Fig. 5. Preferred styles of wearing

When being favourable for indirect connection, participants liked the concept of having shirt and a belt clip as well as a pencil when asked about their most preferred styles of wearing of adapters for indirect connections between a smartphone and a HA.

Age was reported to be an important factor in users' perception of a direct connection between a smartphone and a HA. Participants younger than 66 years slightly preferred the concept of using a direct connection than participants aged 66 or more.

Our study has several limitations. Firstly, the sample size of the study is relatively small. Twenty-seven participants were involved in the study, aged from 48 to 85 years. We mainly focused on elderly people who constitute the most numerous group of HA users in Slovenia. Secondly, the participants assessed concepts, and not concrete products, with their subjective opinion. The research findings may differ if an assessment of concrete products was performed.

Despite those limitations, the findings of the study can be transferred also to younger users with hearing loss, among whom the use of smartphones seems to be more prevalent. In future work we aim to develop a prototype for a functional smartphone and an adapter that will enable connections between a smartphone and a HA. Investigating design and usability of such devices will be imperative.

Acknowledgments. We would like to acknowledge Sonova, Stäfa, Switzerland for its funding and support and specially thank to pro audito schweiz for their interest in and support of this research.

References

1. Manchaiah, V.K.C., Zhao, F.: Storytelling in different cultural context: applications to hearing loss public awareness. Journal of Behavioral Health 1(4), 322–329 (2012)
2. Cavender, A.C., Ladner, R.E.: Hearing Impairments. In: Harper, S., Yesilada, Y. (eds.) Web Accessibility: A Foundation for Research, pp. 25–36. Springer, New York (2008)

3. Sprinzl, G.M., Riechelmann, H.: Current Trends in Treating Hearing Loss in Elderly People: A Review of the Technology and Treatment Options – A Mini-Review. Gerontology 56(3) (2010)
4. Qian, H.: A Phone-Assistive Device Based on Bluetooth Technology for Cochlear Implant Users. IEEE Transactions on Neural Systems and Rehabilitation Engineering 3, 282–287 (2003)
5. Arch, A., Abou-Zhara, S.: How Web Accessibility Guidelines Apply to Design for the Ageing Population. In: Proceedings of Accessible Design in a Digital World Conference, York, UK (2008)
6. Davis, C.D.: Visual Enhancements: Improving Deaf Students' Transition Skills Using Multimedia Technology. Career Development for Exceptional Individuals 22(2), 267–281 (1999)
7. RNID Market Report: Presbycusis (Age-Related Hearing Loss) Market Opportunities for Pharmaceutical and Biotechnology Companies. RNID market report (2004), http://www.mid.org.uk/VirtualContent/84925/presbycusis.pdf
8. Kobayashi, M., Hiyama, A., Miura, T., Asakawa, C., Hirose, M., Ifukube, T.: Elderly user evaluation of mobile touchscreen interactions. In: Campos, P., Graham, N., Jorge, J., Nunes, N., Palanque, P., Winckler, M. (eds.) INTERACT 2011, Part I. LNCS, vol. 6946, pp. 83–99. Springer, Heidelberg (2011)
9. Coleman, M.: There's a hearing app for that. Hearing Journal 64(11), 12–16 (2011)
10. Coad, G., Irving, S., Searchfield, G.D.: Performance and Listener Preference of Four Mobile Phone-to-Hearing Aid Interface Units. Health Care and Informatics Review Online 14(2), 27–35 (2010)
11. Sandrock, C., Schum, D.J.: Wireless Transmission of Speech and Data to, from, and between Hearing Aids. Hear J. 60(11), 12–16 (2007)
12. Bloom, S.: Connectivity: Early steps point the way toward wireless wonders to come. Hearing Journal 62(10), 17–20 (2009)
13. Apple Inc., Providing Notification Sound. In: A Customizable Manner, USPTO Patent Application 20120213393 A1 (2012)
14. Gomez, C., Oller, J., Paradells, J.: Overview and Evaluation of Bluetooth Low Energy: An Emerging Low-Power Wireless Technology. Sensors 12, 11734–11753 (2012)

Investigating an Accessible and Usable ePub Book via VoiceOver: A Case Study

Valentina Bartalesi Lenzi and Barbara Leporini

ISTI - CNR
Via G. Moruzzi, 1 - 56124, Pisa
{valentina.bartalesi,barbara.leporini}@isti.cnr.it

Abstract. In this paper we investigate the opportunities and limitations for blind and visually impaired people when reading an ePub document via Voice-Over for mobile devices. The ePub format is based on an (x)html structure; organizing and handling its source code is therefore very important in order to guarantee satisfactory interaction with the eBook. In this work we analyze the main accessibility and usability issues when interacting with an ePub document via VoiceOver, in order to evaluate possible solutions to source code difficulties. We have considered several accessibility requirements for the use of eBooks in order to focus on the potential technical solutions which were evaluated. From this perspective, we considered two eBooks in order to apply our methodology. Comments and suggestions were provided by eight blind users who evaluated the eBooks via iPhone and iPad devices.

Keywords: eBook accessibility, eBook usability, ePub format, blind users.

1   Introduction

Electronic books, and in particular ePub publications, are increasingly used to be read especially on mobile devices. As a result, people who have difficulties in reading paper-printed books may have new opportunities, provided that the digital versions are accessible. This is particularly important for the blind [1].

EBooks obtained by web-based conversion tools do not currently enable users with vision impairments to fully appreciate and interact with all the content. The content, in fact, is usually not well structured, because: (i) the images do not have meaningful textual descriptions, (ii) data tables do not have text explanation and are not organized in a logical way, (iii) and the index of contents as well as navigational features are not available (e.g. heading levels used in the web page content). On the other hand, the ePub format is based on an (x)html structure. So in our study we decided to investigate which tags included in the source (x)html code influence the reading experience for the resulting ePub version. In particular, the aim was to solve some issues encountered by people using the Apple VoiceOver[1] screen reader when interacting with an ePub document. We focused on VoiceOver because we were interested in developing

---

[1] http://www.apple.com/accessibility/voiceover/

A. Holzinger et al. (Eds.): SouthCHI 2013, LNCS 7946, pp. 272–283, 2013.

an accessible eBook for mobile devices, like the iPad and iPhone. Indeed, these devices offer a combination of screen reader and gestures to make the operating system and applications accessible to blind people through a touch-screen. We choose two PDF eBooks for our case study: (1) *"Storia illustrata di Firenze"* (Illustrated History of Florence) [2] and (2) *"Breve storia illustrata della Toscana"* (Brief Illustrated History of Tuscany) [3]. To convert the PDF versions into the ePub format we used the tool Book4All [4] which was designed to support operators in adapting e-documents to a more suitable version for blind users, e.g. (x)html or Daisy format. For this purpose, we implemented a specific module in order to export the PDF files also into the ePub format. This module was used to apply and test specific technical solutions in order to obtain a suitable eBook. In short, thanks to the ePub module developed we could evaluate the quality of our proposed accessibility solutions.

The paper is organized as follows: Section 2 reports related works about eBook accessibility for blind and visual impaired people describes the ePub format and introduces the web-based conversion tools. Section 3 reports some usability and accessibility issues encountered when reading an eBook. Section 4 presents our case study and describes our methodology, our proposed technical solutions, some considerations, and a short discussion on the proposed solution. Some comments and suggestions provided by eight blind users are also briefly described. Finally, conclusions and future work close the paper.

2   Background

2.1   Related Work

In order to overcome limitations of the printed material for blind people who cannot satisfy their information needs, electronic documents represent an important solution. In this direction several attempts have been made to develop formats that can be accessible for people with visual impairments. Daisy consortium[2], for example, develops, maintains and promotes open international DAISY (Digital Accessible Information System) Standards for accessible multimedia. This standard is designed to make e-books accessible for everyone in both audio and text format. Digital talking books can be used through readers which can play the audio and simultaneously display the corresponding text. Some studies investigate how the reading can be improved [5]. Adjouadi et al. [6] introduced a new automatic book reader for blind people: a fully integrated system with a high reading accuracy. Scientific contents present additional difficulties in reading through a screen reader. Kanahori et al. [7] proposed an integrated system for scientific documents including mathematical formulae, using a speech output interface. Using this system, visually impaired people can read printed scientific documents by means of speech output.

Several information systems are more and more proposed to access and generate material in electronic format. This has increased the need to customize web tools on the base of users' characteristics and preferences. Bottoni et al. [8] proposed a system

---

[2] http://www.daisy.org/

to support the users interactivity for editing, annotating, and indexing e-documents. In [9] the authors propose an approach to automatically generate an e-text for a specific topic hierarchy, starting with a subject indicated by the user. In [10] The authors propose and describe a method and a first developed tool prototype for making e-documents accessible and usable for visually-impaired users. The method is based on some automatic transformations that require the support of operators to obtain more meaningful results. Bianchetti et al. [11] proposed a rule-transformation model aimed at eliminating the post-processing and enabling even for authors without PDF accessibility knowledge to create high quality accessible PDF documents. That concept have been implemented as an add-in for Microsoft Word 2007 and Word 2010. [12] reports a study on text-customization needed by visually-impaired users for reading PDF documents. The results encourage to better exploring this field and including text customization functionalities in the reading tools. Velazquez et al. [13] proposed a first prototype of the TactoBook system, a computer-based software translator designed to enable blind users to read eBooks in braille format. The so converted eBooks can be read on a compact, lightweight, and highly-portable tactile terminal. The work described in [14] presents a study conducted on the importance and usefulness of eBook content adaptation with respect to a simple digital version. The adaptive eBook resulted more accessible and usable in terms of content navigation. [15] discusses a range of commonly available eBook formats and e-readers taking into account their accessibility features. Finally, for what concerns, in particular, the state of the art of the reader devices actually available, in [16] an evaluation in a usability and accessibility perspective is presented. Our approach is aimed at exploring new opportunities to use the common ePub format.

2.2   The ePub Format

EPub (electronic Publication) is the distribution and interchange format standard for digital publications and documents based on Web Standards [17]. EPub defines a means of representing, packaging and encoding structured and semantically enhanced Web content — including XHTML, CSS, SVG, images, and other resources — for distribution in a single-file format. Thus publishers can produce a single digital publication file to be distributed. EPub 2 was initially standardized in 2007. In October, 2011, ePub 3 was approved as a final Recommended Specification. The ePub 3 format supports HTML elements like headings (H1-H6), ordered and unordered lists (such as ol, ul, li, dl, dd, dt), tables (table, th, td), images (img), blockquote and links.

We chose the ePub as the format because this can be read by many kinds of hardware and software readers independently from the operative system. An ePub document can also be easily read by blind users via assistive technologies both through desktop and mobile platforms (i.e. VoiceOver-based devices). Furthermore, the ePub format is an open and free standard, without royalties, so anyone (editors, private users, cultural associations etc…) can use it without any particular grant. Finally, it is easy to produce ePub documents both through specific software and by hand.

The eBook in ePub format appears as a single file with ".epub" extension. Technically speaking, it is a compressed zip format archive containing a numbers of given files and folders. Some files describe the book content (file list, eBook structure, title, author, etc...), the other ones contain the book text. The description files are XML files, while the text is marked-up in XHTML. CSS are used to format the text. All these languages are open source and standard.

2.3   Conversion Tools

Many easy-to-use tools exist for converting eBook formats. Mobipocket Desktop[3], for example, is a tool for Amazon Kindle users. Another conversion tool is Calibre [18], a more general software that can convert among a large number of formats, that supports Kindle, Sony PRS line, Nook and a large number of other devices.

Converting between eBook formats presents some limitations. Using a tool like Calibre, for example, it is not possible to edit the book before the conversion. Calibre is simply able to transform the content from one format to another but it is not an editing tool. If there are typos in the text, a dedicated editing tool such as Sigil[4] or Book Designer[5] must be used. Another issue in using Calibre is formatting lost. Not all eBook formats support the same formatting. Bold and italics are preserved in most cases but complex page layout may not. In summary, tools like Calibre are only able to shift from a format to another carrying the input format properties, they don't add to the output anything that was not already in the input. So if the input is poorly formatted, the output will be too.

3   Accessibility and Usability Issues

The main problems encountered by blind and visual impaired people when access to the eBook contents via assistive technologies [10] may be especially due to:

- Lack of context. When navigating with a screen reader (or a magnifier) the user is only able to access small portions of a text at any one time and may lose the overall context of the current content shown on the screen. Thus having an overview of the available sections and sub-sections, for instance, might a problem for a blind and visually-impaired reader.
- Information overload. Often several unchanging portions of the content (such as the page header, the number of the page, etc.) may overload the system, as the user has to read through all the items nearly every time the text is read, thus slowing down content exploration. Therefore, a well organization of the contents becomes a fundamental step to simplify the reading (e.g., avoiding repetitive and superfluous contents or providing mechanisms to quickly skip them).
- Excessive sequencing in reading the information. The commands for navigation and reading may force the user to access the content sequentially. For instance, long tables can make reading frustrating. A mechanism to quickly kip them or extracting their contents into a linked external source could be a possible solution.

---

[3] http://www.mobipocket.com/en/downloadsoft/
productdetailsreader.asp
[4] http://code.google.com/p/sigil/
[5] http://www.thebookdesigner.com/

Due to these problems, reading an e-document can be somewhat laborious, especially according to the functionalities offered by the various kinds of screen readers or text-to-speech technology. The Amazon Kindle, for example, provides a text-to-speech system for eBook content (actually only for English texts) and some voice menus. On the contrary, the iBooks app allows blind users to read the eBook content via Voice-Over-based device which offers various opportunities to navigate through the content. In Adobe Digital Editions text-to-speech and Braille output are available for all titles through the third party screen readers, e.g. Jaws[6] (version 12 and 13), NVDA[7] and Window-Eyes[8], on a Windows computer, or VoiceOver, on a Mac.

Based on the issues discussed above, the most important eBook requirements we considered when reading through a screen reader or text to speech technology for blind people can be summarised in:

1. reading the eBook content in the correct logical order;
2. a correct interpretation of the content of tables and lists;
3. a correct detection of the images by reading their alternative descriptions, if any, and their captions;
4. informing the user about the type of the elements (e.g. titles, lists, etc.);
5. providing a mechanism to easily and quickly navigate within the content structure (i.e. a content of index and the opportunity to skip from a section to another one).

Unfortunately not all these aspects are well considered and implemented when converting documents by means of automatic tools, for example from PDF to ePub. The contents are not usually correctly read by the screen readers unless some specific features and mechanisms are applied. When preparing an ePub eBook, for example, the corresponding HTML code, in fact, is often not standard or not well-formed. In the same way, the indexes created by conversion tools are often incomplete and with broken links. In this sense, VoiceOver when reading an ePub is not able to inform the users about the presence of images or titles: it just reads the caption and text, but does not inform the user about what they are referred (i.e. it is a caption of an image or it is a section title). In addition, even though a heading level (i.e. <h1>, <h2>, etc.) is applied to a title, no gesture is available to skip from a title to another one (as indeed it appends in a Web page for example). These are all aspects we considered those accessibility and usability aspects in our study.

4   The Case Study

4.1   Methodology

In order to investigate blind user interaction with an eBook through a mobile device, we selected two Italian PDF eBooks "Illustrated History of Florence" and "Brief Illustrated History of Tuscany" provided for our case study by an Italian publisher.

---

[6] http://www.freedomscientific.com/products/fs/
jaws-product-page.asp
[7] http://www.nvda-project.org/
[8] http://www.gwmicro.com/Window-Eyes/

The eBooks were chosen according to the aspects we intended to evaluate. In particular we took into account the presence of:

1. several chapters, so as to have a table of contents;
2. several images and captions, in order to understand how to handle them via VoiceOver and small screens;
3. different types of lists, to evaluate how easily the VoiceOver is able to interact with them.

In our case study we identified the aspects which need specific (x)html tags and attributes in order to ensure a certain level of accessibility and usability in the ePub format. Moreover our study also took into account the CSS analysis. In addition, during the case study and the tests, we observed how different usage of the tags affects the user interaction via VoiceOver. In order to test our proposed solutions, we developed a new function of the tool Book4All in order to convert the document from PDF to ePub. We designed and developed this specific module by passing through the IBF intermediate format (i.e. as described in [4]). In this way we could make any necessary modifications to the code generated as output at any time. As a result we were able to test different technical solutions to apply to the output in ePub format by adding and removing specific tags and attributes. We tested the output by using the iBooks App running on iPad and iPhone devices. Figure 1 shows two pages from the "Illustrated History of Florence" eBook.

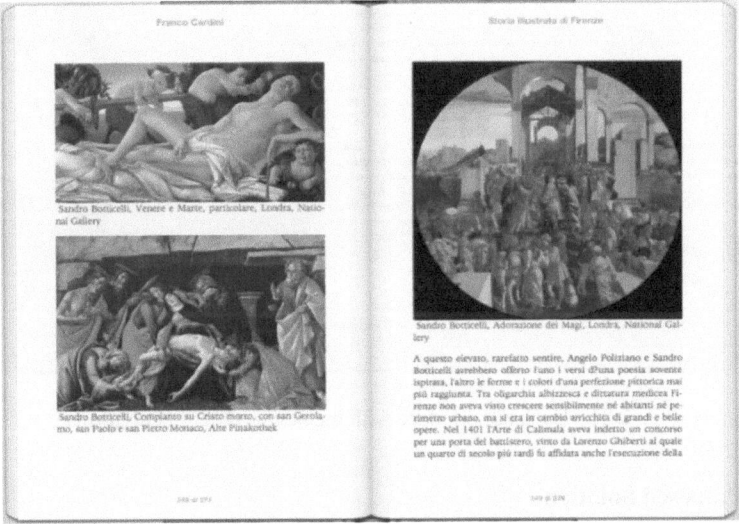

Fig. 1. Two pages with images, captions and text from the "Storia illustrata di Firenze"

Book4All is a software originally designed to convert PDF files into two accessible formats for blind users: XHTML 1.0 and DAISY 3.0. Book4All is both a conversion and an editing tool. Using this tool an operator can adapt an electronic document to a more flexible and usable version. For example, the operator can: (i) insert an ALT attribute to the images, (ii) give a description of the image, (iii) add a title before tables and lists which describes these elements, (iv) redesign tables with correct tags, and so on.

In order to simplify the operator's work, the tool automatically extracts useful data from the PDF source. All the content is organised and tagged in an xml-based intermediate format. This data is then used by the operator to prepare the content which will be used to generate different final formats. In particular, it is possible to edit contents, add images and table descriptions and finally to export the result in one of the supported formats. Examples of editing are inserting additional descriptions for the image, checking and modifying the logical structure of the document i.e. the titles and headings previously chosen by the tool, and so on. Once the operator has finished to edit the intermediate content, the information can be exported in different versions: an accessible (x)html format, Daisy and, more recently, also in ePub format. Figure 2 shows the Book4All interface with the ePub export button.

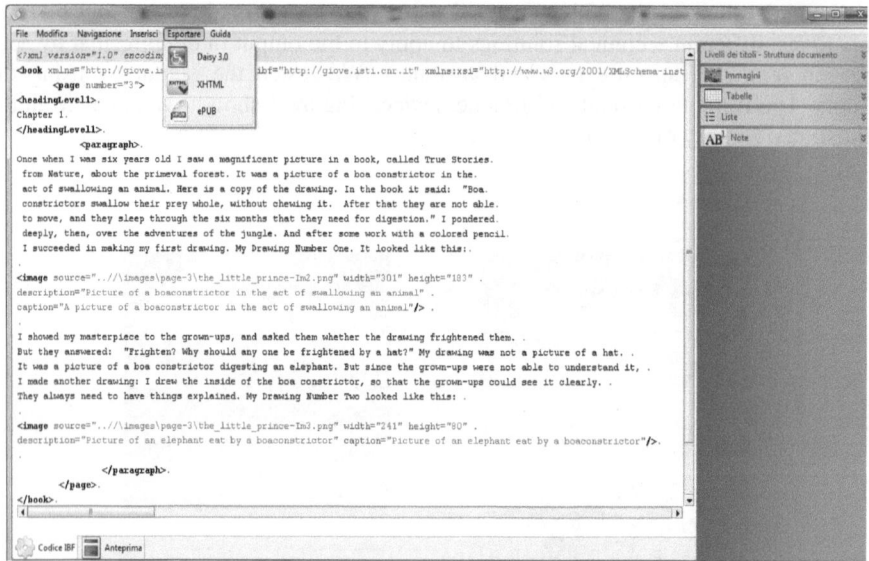

Fig. 2. The Book4all interface with the new export in ePub format

4.2 Proposed Solution

As mentioned before, the main purpose of our study is to investigate how the (x)html source needs to be implemented so that the resulting ePub format is suitable for a reading via VoiceOver. In particular, we took into account those tags and attributes which are related to the elements we analysed: tables, images, headings and links. For each case, we propose a possible (x)html code solution that was tested as ePub output format via the Book4All tool.

Tables and Lists. The tables and lists produced by automatic tools for converting PDF to ePub are not generally correctly read by the screen readers because the corresponding HTML code is often not standard or not well-formed. Our semi-automatic tool allows the operator to rebuilt tables and lists with correct and standard HTML tags. In this way, the screen reader correctly reads the content of tables and lists. Unfortunately, it is not able to inform the user about the semantics of the elements. E.g. it does not say "table" when a table is encountered. To solve this problem we suggested to the operators to add a title before tables and lists for describing these elements. This information can be added via a hidden label that can be detected by VoiceOver but it is not visible to everyone. This means that the layout of the eBook is not modified, while the screen reader is able to announce additional information to a blind user. Technically this solution can be obtained through a specific class in the CSS file which makes not visible the text included in that class (as it is for a Web page [19]).

Images. Concerning images, we have noticed that VoiceOver presents two kinds of behaviour when reading in a sequential way:

1. in presence of a succession of more than one image with captions (i.e. no text except the captions), VoiceOver firstly detects the <img> tags and so it reads ALT attributes and then all the captions (e.g. Image-ALT-text1, Image-ALT-text2, Caption 1, Caption 2). This can make confusion to the users;

2. in presence of text between more than one image in the same page, VoiceOver correctly reads all the contents, including ALT attributes, in a right sequential order.

To improve the eBook accessibility, Book4All adopts two different behaviours in order to take advantage of the above issues.

When in the same page there are two images in succession, we inserted each image (<img> tag) and caption (<span> tag) in an single anchor tag (<a> tag). Even if this approach is not semantically correct, because there are no real links on the images, it allows the reader to have a consistent content lecture and a consequent understanding. Indeed, using the anchor tag, VoiceOver reads text, images and captions in the order in which they appear in the page. Unfortunately, it isn't able to read the image tags and their ALT attributes. In order to solve this problem, we suggested to the operators to insert, for each image, an informative content caption that could be helpful also for blind people. Then we used the hidden tag procedure in order to inform the user about the presence of an image: our tool automatically inserts, before the captions, a span tag with the text "Image:" that is not displayed thanks to the use of a dedicated CSS class. In this way VoiceOver reads the hidden text and the user understands if he/she is in presence of an image.

For what concerns the case in which more images are in the same page with text between them, our tool doesn't insert the tag <a>. VoiceOver in fact is natively able to correctly read the page elements. In this case, the operator should take care of writing a detailed text for the ALT attribute and another simpler one for the caption.

Figure 3 shows how VoiceOver can read a content concerning images when two images are sequential and when they are separated by a text block.

What VoiceOver reads	Related HTML code
Image: Sandro Botticelli, Venus and Mars, particular with Mars sleeping, London, National Gallery	```<p>` ` <a>` ` <img` ` src="../images/page194/Venere.png"></img> ` ` <span id="hidden">Image:</span>` ` <span>Sandro Botticelli, Venus and Mars,` ` particular with Mars sleeping, London, National` ` Gallery</span>` ` </a>` `</p>```
Image: Sandro Botticelli, Lamentation over the Dead Christ, with san Gerolamo, san Paolo e san Pietro, Monaco, Alte Pinakothek	```<p>` ` <a>` ` <img` ` src="../images/page194/Compianto.png"></img> ` ` <span id="hidden">Image:</span>` ` <span> Lamentation over the Dead Christ, with san` ` Gerolamo, san Paolo e san Pietro, Monaco, Alte` ` Pinakothek </span>` ` </a>` `</p>```
...text content...	
Image: The painting is part of a cycle on the life of Saint Peter, and describes when Jesus directs Peter to find a coin in the mouth of a fish in order to pay the temple tax. The Tribute Money, fresco in the Brancacci Chapel, Santa Maria del Carmine, Florence ...text content...	```<p>` ` <img src="../images/page16/Ghirlandaio.png"` ` alt="The painting is part of a cycle on the life` ` of Saint Peter, and describes a scene from` ` the Gospel of Matthew, in which Jesus directs` ` Peter to find a coin in the mouth of a fish in` ` order to pay the temple tax"></img> ` ` <span id="hidden">Image:</span>` ` <span>The Tribute Money, fresco in the Brancacci` ` Chapel, Santa Maria del Carmine, Florence</span>` `</p>```

Fig. 3. How VoiceOver can read a content concerning images

Titles and Headings. Finally, regarding the content structure as well as titles we used Heading Levels. In Book4All we used the H1 tags as criterion to split the eBook content and to create the sections and the index of the eBook. When reading a web page or a structured PDF document, a blind user exploits the headings to move through the sections and sub-sections. Unfortunately we noticed that in the ePub format it is not possible to manually navigate the content using the Heading Levels, differently from HTML documents. Furthermore, VoiceOver is not able to recognize the Heading Levels tags as titles and does not inform the users about that. This situation causes a limitation to content access by visual impaired people. This especially occurs because the VoiceOver screen reader does not offer a gesture or a way to do that. A possible suggestion could be to add the hidden word "Title 1" before the section title (i.e. H1 tags) to inform the reader about it. We implemented and tested this kind of solution in the Book4All tool. However, the screen reader technology should overtake this limitation. For instance, a possible way could be to use a different voice or a short sound to inform the user that the paragraph is indeed a title.

4.3   Evaluation

The two eBooks obtained through Book4All were tested on both Apple and Android-based devices. These eBooks were made available on an online server for the participants to evaluate. Participants were asked to explore the contents as well as to perform some specific actions aimed at testing the added features: i.e. (1) using the table of contents to move to a given chapter; (2) reading a given section which contained two consecutive figures; and (3) Paying particular attention to the section titles in order to identify any differences compared to traditional books.

In order to identify possible participants, we contacted the Italian Association for the blind. Eight blind users answered to our invitation: 5 males and 3 females aged from 27 to 66. They worked on the evaluation from home and tested the eBooks on their VoiceOver mobile devices (2 iPhone4, 4 iPhone4s, 2 iPhone 5 and 2 iPad). The users e-mailed us some comments and suggestions. Users appreciated especially that information provided in a hidden way for the images and headings. Five of out eight users noticed the screen reader announcing for the "heading" word before each section title. Other suggestions are related to use this "type of technique" to (i) add other additional information, such as the number of items that are in a list (before the reading of the list); (ii) give useful information about a table (before the reading of the table); (iii) add invisible links, detectable by the assistive technology, in order to skip large text portion while reading (e.g. a big table, a quoted text, and so on). Concerning descriptions for the figures and images, six of the eight users declared that they prefer a small description available along the text (i.e. assigned to the alt attribute), whereas a longer description with more details should be available on demand (e.g. by clicking on a link or via a specific command). Three participants claimed the lack of a specific command to obtain a list of available headings within the text, as it happens using Jaws in Windows OS.

4.4   Discussion

Our study has revealed that some interaction issues still exist for VoiceOver users although the (x)html source used for generating the pub version is correct. Some aspects should be better managed by the assistive technologies. In particular, VoiceOver for mobile devices does not support very well an ePub format in terms of specific aspects.

Based on the issues experienced when interacting with an ePub document via VoiceOver, we focused on three reading aspects: (1) interaction with the book logical structure, (2) appropriateness of the images (alternative descriptions and captions), and (3) information provided for the type of elements. We have proposed a possible solution to overcome the observed problems, which we applied to a case study of two eBooks. Summarizing, we proposed to use:

1. hidden content to label images, lists, tables and titles to announce useful information;

2. an anchored link <a>to embed each image when more than one are in a sequence. This type of solution is not particularly "elegant", but at the moment it seems to overcome the issue encountered for a sequence of images.

Concluding, based on the experienced interaction problems and potential technical solutions we identified for reading an ePub, we can suggest:

(1)   the assistive technologies - such as VoiceOver - should appropriately support a good interaction with the structure of the contents (i.e. gestures to detect and navigate among headings, tables, lists, and so on);

(2)   the (x)html source code and the resulting ePub version have the appropriate elements (e.g., tags and attributes) to provide useful semantic information to the assistive technologies so that blind people are able to get more suitable information when reading a book;

(3)   the applications used for reading an eBook - such as iBooks - are able to pass all needed information available in the book code and offer suitable accessible functions to interact with an eBook.

5   Conclusions

In this paper we presented a study on the ePub document generation in order to identify possible issues and solutions encountered by blind users when reading an eBook. On the basis of a case study conducted with two eBooks, we have experienced some accessibility and usability issues when reading the content via iBooks App and VoiceOver assistive technology for mobile devices. We observed that VoiceOver is not completely able (1) to detect the sequence of images and their captions (when more than one image is available in succession), and (2) to announce the information about the type of the element (such as image, table and heading). To improve blind user interaction, we proposed a potential solution to be applied to the (x)html source code. In particular, we identified the tags and attributes affecting the interaction with the eBook via VoiceOver.

To test our methodology, we developed a new ePub generation module for the Book4All tool, which we used during our case study. Through a preliminary evaluation with eight users we received a positive response with regards the two eBooks considered in our case study.

Our study suggests that both developers of assistive technologies, eBook code architecture and reading applications as well keep in mind to support a suitable interaction for people with special needs. Concerning future work, we will plan to organize a more structured user testing and to consider other mobile platforms.

Acknowledgements. This study is part of the collaboration with Pacini Editore and I.Ri.Fo.R. Regionale della Toscana on the accessibility for publishing.

References

1. Edmonds, C.: Providing access to students with disabilities in online distance education: Legal and technical concerns for higher education. American Journal of Distance Education 18(1) (2004)

2. Cardini, F.: Storia illustrate di Firenze. Pacini Editore, Pisa (2009)

3. Poloni, A., Verga, M., Volpi, A., Rogari, S.: Breve storia illustrata della Toscana. Pacini Editore, Pisa (2012)

4. Calabrò, A., Contini, E., Leporini, B.: Book4All: A tool to make an e-book more accessible to students with vision/visual-impairments. In: Holzinger, A., Miesenberger, K. (eds.) USAB 2009. LNCS, vol. 5889, pp. 236–248. Springer, Heidelberg (2009)

5. Brzoza, P., Spinczyk, D.: Multimedia Browser for Internet Online Daisy Books. In: Miesenberger, K., Klaus, J., Zagler, W.L., Karshmer, A.I. (eds.) ICCHP 2006. LNCS, vol. 4061, pp. 1087–1093. Springer, Heidelberg (2006)
6. Adjouadi, M., Ruiz, E., Wang, L.: Automated Book Reader for Persons with Blindness. In: Miesenberger, K., Klaus, J., Zagler, W.L., Karshmer, A.I. (eds.) ICCHP 2006. LNCS, vol. 4061, pp. 1094–1101. Springer, Heidelberg (2006)
7. Kanahori, T., Suzuki, M.: Scientific PDF Document Reader with Simple Interface for Visually Impaired People. In: Miesenberger, K., Klaus, J., Zagler, W.L., Karshmer, A.I. (eds.) ICCHP 2006. LNCS, vol. 4061, pp. 48–52. Springer, Heidelberg (2006)
8. Bottoni, P., Ferri, F., Grifoni, P., Marcante, A., Mussio, P., Padula, M., Reggiori, A.: E-Document management in situated interactivity: the WIL approach. Universal Access in the Information Society 8(3), 137–153 (2009)
9. Chen, G., Li, Q., Jia, W.: Automatically Generating an E-textbook on the Web. World Wide Web 8(4), 377–394 (2005)
10. Contini, E., Leporini, B., Paternò, F.: A Semi-automatic Support to Adapt e-Documents in an Accessible and Usable Format for Vision Impaired Users. In: Miesenberger, K., Klaus, J., Zagler, W.L., Karshmer, A.I. (eds.) ICCHP 2008. LNCS, vol. 5105, pp. 242–249. Springer, Heidelberg (2008)
11. Bianchetti, R., Erle, M., Hofer, S.: Mainstreaming the Creation of Accessible PDF Documents by a Rule-Based Transformation from Word to PDF. In: Miesenberger, K., Karshmer, A., Penaz, P., Zagler, W. (eds.) ICCHP 2012, Part I. LNCS, vol. 7382, pp. 595–601. Springer, Heidelberg (2012)
12. Henry, S.L.: Developing Text Customisation Functionality Requirements of PDF Reader and Other User Agents. In: Miesenberger, K., Karshmer, A., Penaz, P., Zagler, W. (eds.) ICCHP 2012, Part I. LNCS, vol. 7382, pp. 602–609. Springer, Heidelberg (2012)
13. Velazquez, R., Hernandez, H., Preza, E.: A portable eBook reader for the blind. In: Proceedings of Annual International Conference of the IEEE, pp. 2107–2110 (2010)
14. AbdelRazek, M., Modayan, A.: Adaptive eBook framework. In: Proceedings of IEEE 2012, pp. 324–329 (2012)
15. Ranti Junus, S.G.: E-books and E-readers for Users with Print Disabilities. Library Technology Reports 48(7) (2012)
16. Huthwaite, A., Cleary, C.E., Sinnamon, B., Sondergeld, P., McClintock, A.: Ebook readers: separating the hype from the reality. In: Proceedings of 2011 ALIA Information Online Conference & Exhibition, Sydney Convention & Exhibition Centre (2011)
17. International Digital Publishing Forum (IDPF), http://idpf.org/epub
18. Calibre Manual, http://manual.calibre-ebook.com/conversion.html
19. Leporini, B., Paternò, F.: Applying Web Usability Criteria for Vision-Impaired Users: Does It Really Improve Task Performance? International Journal of Human-Computer Interaction 24, 17–47 (2008)

Route Descriptions in Advance and Turn-by-Turn Instructions - Usability Evaluation of a Navigational System for Visually Impaired and Blind People in Public Transport

Elke Mattheiss and Elmar Krajnc

FH Joanneum, University of Applied Sciences, Kapfenberg, Austria
{elke.mattheiss.itm10,elmar.krajnc}@fh-joanneum.at

Abstract. Wayfinding in public transport is still a great challenge for visually impaired and blind people. The presented evaluation study was conducted in the context of the research project Ways4All, which aims to develop an accessible system to facilitate the use of public transport for visually impaired and blind people. The study aims to assess the indoor and outdoor navigation modules of the mobile application developed in Ways4All. In a field study with 16 participants usability and accessibility issues of the system were identified. Furthermore it was investigated whether visually impaired and blind people wish to have a route description in advance, besides the turn-by-turn instructions provided by the system. The data analysis shows that the majority of visually impaired and blind people like to have the possibility to process a route description before they actually navigate. On the basis of the user feedback and the occurring issues, recommendations for the system design were created.

Keywords: Usability evaluation, accessibility, visually impaired, public transport, outdoor navigation, indoor navigation.

1 Introduction

One of the greatest challenges for visually impaired and blind (VIB) people is to find their way in an unknown or complex environment. That is why different kinds of navigational aids have been proposed in a number of research as well as commercial projects.

According to Golledge [1] wayfinding is "the process of determining and following a path or route between an origin and a destination". A recent review of research about wayfinding and spatial cognition can be found in [2]. The author claims that wayfinding and navigation are usually used interchangeably in previous research. Furthermore spatial cognition is described as serving the function of wayfinding, by putting spatial knowledge, like cognitive maps, into action. Therefore supporting VIB people to form cognitive maps can ease navigation.

A. Holzinger et al. (Eds.): SouthCHI 2013, LNCS 7946, pp. 284–295, 2013.

The research project Ways4All Complete[1] aims to facilitate the wayfinding of VIB people in public transport. The project is concerned with the conception of an accessible system, which includes above other functionalities an indoor and outdoor navigation. The system provides the users with turn-by-turn instructions from the starting point to the destination.

The focus of the present paper is on the usability evaluation of the indoor and outdoor navigational system, i.e. to which extent visually impaired users are able to achieve specified goals with the application[2]. Furthermore we investigate the question if VIB users of the Ways4All system would like to be provided in advance with route information in addition to the turn-by-turn instructions.

2   Related Work

Relevant research work from the areas nonvisual wayfinding as well as accessibility of indoor and outdoor navigational systems, and public transport are presented in the following sections.

2.1   Wayfinding of VIB People

The wayfinding of VIB people has been a topic in research for a long time. Overall research suggests that also VIB people form cognitive maps and have a spatial representation of their environment [2]. To assist VIB people in wayfinding, the use of tactile maps was often discussed in literature. For example Espinosa and colleagues [3] suggest using tactile maps besides direct experience in wayfinding to let VIB people learn spatial representations.

Passini and Proulx [4] state, based on previous research, that VIB people are able to learn simple routes and travel unaided, especially with previous visual experience, mobility courses, and repeated exposure to the route. Also Quinones and colleagues [5] found in an interview study with two visually impaired participants, that participants create detailed mental maps of locations they frequently visit. However, in unknown environments, like public buildings, wayfinding remains a challenge for most VIB people. In an experiment Passini and Proulx [4] compared the journey of 15 congenitally totally blind with a control group of sighted participants through a complex architectural setting. After two guided tours participants were supposed to describe their planned journey and then take the tour on their own, while thinking aloud about what they are doing. The results suggest that the blind participants plan their journey in more detail. Furthermore blind people use reference points like architectural elements (e.g. door frames) detectable with their cane, which are not even noticed by sighted participants, who use visual reference points.

Efforts to assist wayfinding for VIB people can basically have either a technological or an environmental emphasis [4]. That means VIB people can either be

---

[1] www.ways4all.at

[2] cf. ISO 9241-11:1998 Ergonomic requirements for office work with visual display terminals (VDTs) -- Part 11: Guidance on usability

provided with perceptual and guiding tools, or the environment can include an information system, which is accessible to them.

Technological wayfinding tools for visually impaired people, which are the focus of the present paper, have a long history. Already in 1985 Preiser [5] proposed an electronic guidance system built into the floor, which allows VIB people to follow a route by using a cane equipped with a receptor. This system also allowed including verbal messages at specific places along the route.

Investigations about requirements for systems supporting different wayfinding tasks [6] revealed that only few visually impaired people carry special navigation technology when they navigate to frequently visited places. They rather use landmarks like distinct physical objects (e.g. trees), smells, or sounds for route information. However, wayfinding issues occur also for regular routes, when they get lost because of having made a detour or when the environment changed (e.g. landmarks change or obstacles appear). For unfamiliar routes visually impaired people tend to prepare thoroughly, find directions made by sighted people often inadequate, and rather ask others in their vicinity than relying on the Global Positioning System (GPS) when getting lost. Quinones and colleagues [6] state that a navigational system should therefore not only provide turn-by-turn instructions but also supply information about the environment like landmarks and functional elements to support visually impaired people to build mental maps of their surrounding. Furthermore the system should be incorporated in an existing technology, like a mobile phone, that users carry with them.

2.2   Indoor and Outdoor Navigational Systems for VIB People

In recent years a wide range of papers were published targeting the topic of indoor and outdoor navigation for VIB people. Previous research on personal guidance systems with GPS [7] showed that VIB users prefer synthesized speech indicating the current distance to the next waypoint to other displays involving tones or pointing in a direction. Another finding relates to the use of headphones, which was deprecated by many participants.

An example for an *outdoor navigational system* is the lightweight navigation system for low vision users called iWalk [8], which runs on smart phones and uses GPS. With iWalk users can query input based on speech recognition and get provided with turn-by-turn walking directions. A high color palette and large font should assure the accessibility for the target group. Stent and colleagues [8] also state that they plan to add public transit information to the system in the future.

Other systems related to outdoor navigation are a mobile-cloud pedestrian crossing guide to detect the status of an intersection light with real-time image processing [9], and a GPS-based application named CrossingGuard providing information about intersection geometry [10]. The comparison between more detailed and baseline information given by CrossingGuard reveals, that users feel more comfort at unfamiliar intersections with detailed information.

Many of the proposed *indoor navigational systems* are based on Radio Frequency Identification (RFID) technology. For example Willis and Helal [11] describe a navigation and location determination system for blind people based on a RFID tag grid. In the proposed system spatial coordinates and all information about the surrounding space is stored in the RFID tags, which provides independence from a remote spatial database. The authors describe the navigation infrastructure in indoor (e.g. government buildings) as well as outdoor (e.g. college campuses) space.

A location-aware tour-guide based on RFID in the context of exhibitions is described in [12]. The user interface is based on a device with hardware buttons and was evaluated with over 100 blind visitors of an international exhibition. The system includes information about the service areas, key places, and crossroads, to support users in building a mental map of the surrounding ambient. Bellotti and colleagues [12] conclude that the system was widely appreciated, because it enabled the users to have new, engaging experiences, but that the results would be better if the localization technology were more precise.

In contrast to other researchers Ivanov [13] did not use a RFID tag grid to avoid the high costs related to the installation of a high number of tags. The authors propose an indoor navigational system for navigating from room to room, by reading out two tags above and under the door handle. One tag provides navigational information and the other contains voice messages (e.g. "go straight 5.5 meters, turn left, right side of corridor, count 5 doors"). An evaluation of this low cost system with eight blind users showed that all participants were able to reach the target reference point, and only one participant needed assistance.

2.3   Public Transport Accessibility for VIB People

Usage of public transport can be challenging for people with and without disabilities. This is why mobile applications to support the navigation of public transport are becoming increasingly important and the usability of such systems should be considered in design as well as evaluation [see e.g. 14].

There is some research work with special focus on accessibility in the area of public transport. Related to that it is crucial to consider the requirements of VIB people in the design of public transport stations. Padzi [15] list standard guidelines like incorporation of guiding blocks in the walking surfaces, floors with a slip-resistant surface, large enough symbols and letters in signs, tactile Braille letters, adequate level of illumination, and signals in visible as well as audible form.

Besides sticking to general guidelines researchers also worked on the design and development of navigational systems to facilitate the usage of public transport for VIB users. For example Guentert [16] described a tool to assist blind people in changing trains inside of train stations. Moreover the author compared two prototypes. One prototype provided the user with piece-by-piece directions, like standard GPS, while changing trains. The other one provided a description of the whole station, before the users actually had to change, to give them the possibility to build a comprehensive cognitive model of how the station is organized. The author claimed that by these means blind people might gain a better understanding about their environment and therefore travel more independently. In a small user study Guentert [16] found that participants preferred the prototype with a description of the whole station. Also, when asked about their mental picture of the station they were able to recall the basic structure.

3   The Ways4All System

The technical system developed in the Ways4All project, aims to support VIB people in wayfinding while using public transport. For the implementation of the assistive system it was necessary to make infrastructural modifications to vehicles and buildings. The current version of the application consists of several modules; for the present paper only indoor and outdoor navigation are relevant.

The *outdoor navigation* provides the users with turn-by-turn instructions for outdoor navigation based on GPS tracking. In addition to the indication of distances and turn instructions, also information especially relevant for VIB people is provided (e.g. height of the pavement, lights with acoustic signals).

The *indoor module* provides the users with turn-by-turn instructions for the navigation inside the station. The localization of the users works with RFID tags installed along the guiding blocks for the blind. Users have to attach a RFID receiver to their ankle (see Fig. 1), which reads the location from the RFID tags when the user passes them.

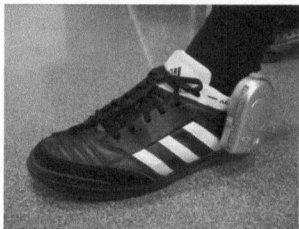

Fig. 1. RFID reader for the indoor navigation

A central part of the overall system is the *mobile application* running on Android-based touch mobile phones, allowing the users to make use of the technical infrastructure. The application was developed using a user-centered design process [17]. That means that the target group was involved repeatedly beginning from an early stage of development (e.g. by means of user analysis and paper prototypes). The original user application was also already adapted based on the user feedback gathered by various preliminary usability studies [e.g. 18]. The latest adaptions to the user interface before the field evaluation were done based on lab usability tests conducted with four VIB people. The main technical adaptation was the integration of the Ways4All application and Android 4 functionalities.

Fig. 2 shows screenshots of the current user interface of the Ways4All application. On the main menu all functionalities of the application is listed. When the speech output is activated the elements are read out load, when the user moves his/her finger over the screen (talking finger technique). Selecting an element works by tapping twice on it. The menu of the outdoor navigation contains four elements, which enable to select a route, get (audible) information about the GPS status, start the navigation, and display/repeat the last instruction. In the menu of the indoor navigation, users can select a route with the first and second element depending on which station is loaded.

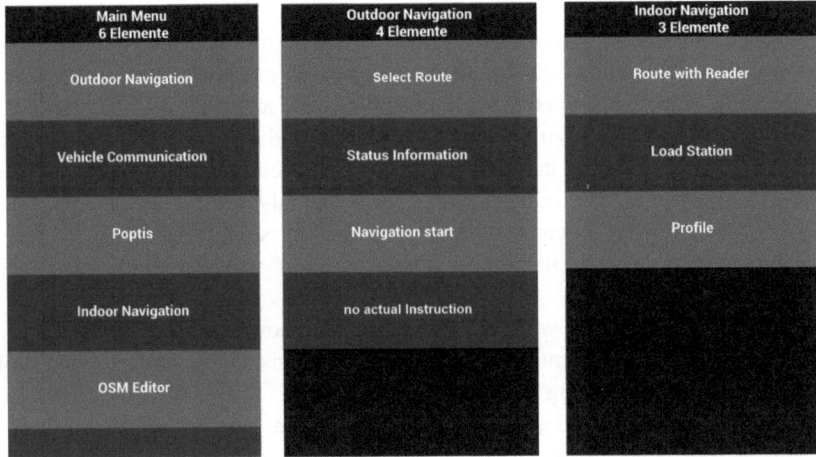

Fig. 2. Ways4All screens: a) main menu, b) outdoor navigation, c) indoor navigation

4   Research Method

The indoor and outdoor module of the Ways4All system was evaluated in a field test. Participants had to use the system while navigating along test routes and to think aloud about any occurring issue. The participants were tested individually with one test facilitator. Two different test facilitators were involved in the study.

As previous research suggests that VIB people plan their journey in more detail [4], want information about their environment [6], and prefer to get the big picture of the route [16], half of the participants where provided with a description of the route before they had to navigate. The other half received only the turn-by-turn instructions, to investigate their opinion towards the system. The evaluation plan is described in detail in the following sections.

4.1   Participants

For the evaluation 16 participants were recruited with the aid of a center for the blind involved in the project. Because the Ways4All system should be suitable for people with different severity levels of visual impairments, people with residual vision as well as completely blind were invited to participate. By these means we were able to evaluate the graphical user interface as well as the operation with speech output implemented in the application. The 13 male and 3 female participants were between 18 and 69 years old. Most of the participants used the public transport every day, and one participant used it once a week. Asked to rate their prior knowledge about the outdoor and indoor routes on a scale from one (very good) to five (very bad) revealed that most of the participants had a low knowledge about the routes (indoor route: mean = 4.07, standard deviation = 1.52; outdoor route: mean = 3.88, standard deviation = 1.27). The testing took about 75 minutes and participants received a financial compensation in form of a voucher.

4.2   Study Design

To investigate the systems usability and the influence of route information given in advance a between-subject factorial study design was used. The varied factor is the given *pre-information* (yes versus no) about the route and environment. Half of the participants were provided with a short description of the route and the environment before they actually had to take the route, to give them the possibility to create a mental model about it. The other participants were only provided with the system's turn-by-turn instructions. Because directions of sighted people are often considered as inadequate by VIB people [6] the descriptions were validated with the first test participant [cf. 16].

The experimental groups were balanced as far as possible according to sex, age, and especially visual impairment (visual versus non-visual operation of the mobile phone) to avoid an influencing effect of these factors.

To assess the usability and accessibility of the system, various measures were used, including an assessment of occurring usability issues, perceived usability and task load, and user feedback.

4.3   Material

The evaluation was executed with the Ways4All application running on a Samsung Galaxy S3 GT-19300 with Android 4.0.4. The assistive application TalkBack was activated to make the mobile phone accessible for blind users.

Written instructions and test protocols were prepared to ensure the same study conditions for all participants. Indoor and outdoor module of the system were assessed separately by gathering user feedback. For both modules questions for a structured interview were prepared targeting the opinion of the participants' towards the modules. Additionally quantitative measures of usability and task load were applied. Established questionnaires to measure usability (System Usability Scale (SUS), adapted from [19]) and task load (NASA-Task Load Index (NASA-TLX), adapted from [20]) were translated in German and used. The SUS consists of ten statements and participants have to indicate on a 5-point scale how much they agree to each statement. The NASA-TLX includes six different kinds of task load (mental load, physical load, temporal load, effort, frustration, and performance) and participants have to state on a scale from 1 to 21 how much load they experienced during the task.

4.4   Procedure

Prior to the field tests, participants were introduced to the study and the Ways4All system. Also some initial feedback was gathered after this short introduction.

Prior to taking the route participants were told the target of the route. One experimental group was additionally provided with pre-information of the route and environment. This description includes the turns participants have to take (similar to the turn-by-turn instructions), but also some additional information about the surrounding area (e.g. garage exits, hall with pillars).

The used procedure for the field test was a mixture of *behavior observation and thinking aloud test*. On the one hand participants were instructed to verbalize any issues or insecurities they face. On the other hand the test facilitator observed the participant closely and records all occurring issues in the test protocol. The test facilitator corrected detours and operational errors, if the participants did not correct it immediately by themselves. As some participants already knew parts of the test route, they were explicitly instructed to use the Ways4All system even if they knew where to go. The indoor module was tested on a test route inside a metro station; the outdoor navigation took place in the surrounding area of this station. Both routes took the participants about 5 to 10 minutes and included several turns.

After each module test participants were asked questions to assess their opinion towards the modules. At the end of the module tests participants answered some final interview questions and the compensation was paid.

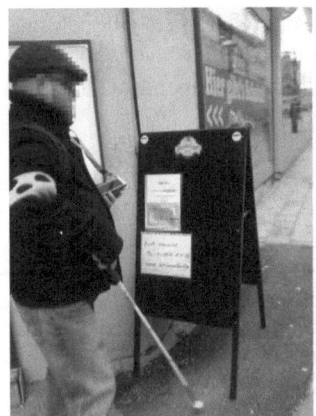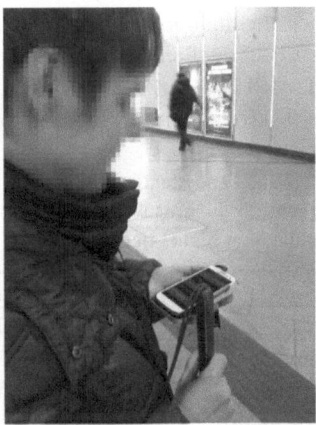

Fig. 3. Participants navigating during the a) outdoor route, b) indoor route

5   Results and Discussion

In this section the results of the 16 conducted field tests are presented. First some general issues with the system are described. Then the results regarding the provision of route information in advance is discussed in detail.

5.1   Usability and Accessibility of the Ways4All System

The main issues, which occurred during the testing, relate to technical problems with the GPS reception and the range of the RFID tags. Because of insufficient GPS reception and not read RFID tags, participants were sometimes provided with incorrect or no information. Therefore it is essential to foster fallback mechanisms and redundant information in the system, in case of information is missed.

Only few usability issues with the user interface were identified. In general participants had no problems with operating the application and evaluated it as rather simple because of the small number of options.

However, the sensitivity of the touch device seemed to be an issue for some blind participants. When they accidentally pushed the back button of the mobile phone, they left the application and were annoyed to be forced to start over again. It should be harder to leave the application, especially because it cannot be assumed that user frequently access other functionalities of the mobile phone while they navigate.

The visually impaired participants who operated the application in a visual way, raised the issue that some information (e.g. the GPS status) is presented only audible, but not visually. Also the graphical design seems to be not ideal and the contrast between font and background color should be maximized.

As can be seen from Table 1 participants rated the usability of the outdoor module in average higher than the usability of the indoor module. Also in most of the task load categories the indoor module was rated higher than outdoor module. This is probably due to the technical problems with the RFID tags, which occurred during many of the tests. However, the results should be considered with caution because of the small sample size and the large standard deviations.

Table 1. Mean values and standard deviations (SD) for the usability (SUS ratings between 1 "low usability" and 5 "high usability") and task load (NASA-TLX ratings between 1 and 21, higher values indicating higher demand) scale

	Outdoor navigation	Indoor navigation
SUS	mean=4.08, SD=0.57	mean=3.21, SD=1.11
Mental demand	mean=7.50, SD=5.61	mean=9.69, SD=7.61
Physical demand	mean=5.44, SD=5.43	mean=4.63, SD=6.11
Temporal demand	mean=4.38, SD=5.12	mean=6.06, SD=6.96
Effort	mean=5.13, SD=6.29	mean=8.75, SD=6.77
Frustration	mean=5.81, SD=5.68	mean=10.63, SD=8.03
Performance	mean=6.31, SD=5.42	mean=8.88, SD=6.91

5.2   Pre-information about Route

Participants were asked if they would like to get information about the route in advance in addition to the turn-by-turn instructions. This kind of information which users can process before they actually take the route (e.g. at home) seems to be very important for VIB people, in outdoor as well as indoor navigation, because the majority of participants expressed the wish to be provided with such an information. In Table 2 the detailed answers of the participants are listed.

The eight participants who were provided with a pre-information were asked, if the pre-information helped them to find their way to the destination. Most of them answered with yes both in outdoor (5 participants) and indoor (4) navigation. One participant said that s/he would have found the destination also only on the basis of the pre-information and without the turn-by-turn instructions. Another participant

Table 2. Participants answers to the question if they would like to have a pre-information about the route in outdoor and indoor navigation (the number of participants are indicated in square brackets)

Outdoor navigation	Indoor navigation
yes [6]	yes [10]
yes, I would process it at home [2]	yes, like in Poptis [1]
yes, I always wanted that [1]	yes, I always wanted that [1]
yes, but should be optional [1]	yes, but I can do it without [1]
yes, but only for short routes [1]	yes, because the tags do not work [1]
yes, but in a visual way (map) [1]	yes, but in a visual way (map) [1]
yes, it doesn't hurt [1]	no, because I don't need it [1]
yes, for complicated routes, but no, for easy routes [1]	
no, in general, but yes in unknown area [1]	
no, because I don't need it [1]	

stated that it helped but was not necessary, because the turn-by-turn instructions worked fine. However, one participant claimed after the outdoor navigation that this kind of double information could also be misleading, and two participants said regarding the pre-information of the indoor navigation that it helped only a bit. Latter is probably due to the length of the indoor route description, because - in contrast to the outdoor route description - it was too long to memorize.

A closer look at the mean values in the usability and task load scales does not show a clear trend about whether participants with and without pre-information rate the usability and task load differently.

6   Conclusions

Although participants had to face some technical problems with the Ways4All system the average rating of the usability is rather high and the ratings of the task load rather low. Also most participants appreciated the system and would like to use it when the technical issues are solved. Similar to the conclusion in [12] it is probable that the results would be better, if the localization technology were more accurate.

Regarding the pre-information, the study yielded a clear preference of the users. As most participants would appreciate a pre-information about the route, Ways4All should provide the users with a route description in advance, in addition to the turn-by-turn instructions. This result goes in line with [16], where also a preference for an overall picture was noted. However, close attention has to be paid to how the information is presented. The description should be optional and serve as a possibility to prepare for a trip at home. The description should not be too long and provide an overview of the route.

7   Limitations and Outlook

Because of the small number of participants, the main focus of the present work was to identify usability issues with the Ways4All system and conclude from them implications for the system design. This involves mainly qualitative data, and a quantitative approach including testing for statistical significance was out of scope.

Besides that, technical problems with the GPS reception in the outdoor tests, and the RFID tags in the indoor tests, has attracted much of the participants' attention. A large proportion of the users' feedback was related to the technical issues. That is why the participants may have neglected other aspects of the application. Also performance measures like the task completion time and the number of detours could not be considered, because of technical problems.

Therefore, a further study with a stronger quantitative approach should be conducted, when the system is adapted according to the user feedback and the detected issues. Furthermore, in following research projects we want to develop solutions, which can be better customized by the user (e.g. overview versus turn-by-turn navigation) and also other mobile platform beside Android should be covered then.

Acknowledgments. The project Ways4All Complete ran from January 2010 to March 2013. The overall project manager was the University of Applied Sciences FH-JOANNEUM in Kapfenberg, Austria. Project participants were Salzburg Research mbH, Graz University of Technology, Österreichische Arbeitsgemeinschaft für Rehabilitation (ÖAR), Hilfsgemeinschaft der Blinden und Sehschwachen Österreichs, Digital Concepts, SPI Intelligence Services GmbH, Österreichische Blindenwohlfahrt, Wiener Linien GmbH & Co KG, and ÖBB. The project was subsidized by the Austrian Federal Ministry for Transport, Innovation and Technology (BMVIT) and the Austrian Research Promotion Agency (FFG).

References

1. Golledge, R.G.: Human wayfinding and cognitive maps. In: Golledge, R.G. (ed.) Wayfinding Behavior: Cognitive Mapping and other Spatial Processes, pp. 1–45. Johns Hopkins University Press, Baltimore (1999)
2. Devlin, A.S.: Environmental perception: Wayfinding and spatial cognition. In: Clayton, S.D. (ed.) The Oxford Handbook of Environmental and Conservation Psychology, 41–64. Oxford University Press, New York (2012)
3. Espinosa, M.A., Ungar, S., Ochaita, E., Blades, M., Spencer, C.: Comparing methods for introducing blind and visually impaired people to unfamiliar urban environments. Journal of Environmental Psychology 18, 277–287 (1998)
4. Passini, R., Proulx, G.: Wayfinding without vision: An experiment with congenitally totally blind people. Environment and Behavior 20(2), 227–252 (1988)
5. Preiser, W.: A combined tactile-electronic guidance system for visually impaired person in indoor and outdoor spaces. In: Proceedings of the International Conference on Building Use and Safety Technology, pp. 49–53 (1985)

6. Quinones, P.-A., Greene, T., Yang, R., Newman, M.: Supporting visually impaired navigation: a needs-finding study. In: Proceedings of the 2011 Annual Conference Extended Abstracts on Human Factors in Computing Systems', CHI EA 2011, pp. 1645–1650. ACM, New York (2011)

7. Loomis, J.M., Marston, J.R., Golledge, R.G., Klatzky, R.L.: Personal guidance system for people with visual impairment: A comparison of spatial displays for route guidance. Journal of Visual Impairment & Blindness 99(4), 219–232 (2005)

8. Stent, A.J., Azenkot, S., Stern, B.: Iwalk: A lightweight navigation system for low-vision users. In: Proceedings of the 12th International ACM SIGACCESS Conference on Computers and Accessibility, ASSETS 2010, pp. 269–270. ACM, New York (2010)

9. Angin, P., Bhargava, B.K.: Real-time mobile-cloud computing for context-aware blind navigation. International Journal of Next-Generation Computing 2(2) (2011)

10. Guy, R., Truong, K.: CrossingGuard: Exploring information content in navigation aids for visually impaired pedestrians. In: Proceedings of the 2012 ACM Annual Conference on Human Factors in Computing Systems, CHI 2012, pp. 405–414. ACM, New York (2012)

11. Willis, S., Helal, S.: RFID information grid for blind navigation and wayfinding. In: Proceedings of the 9th IEEE International Symposium on Wearable Computers (ISWC), pp. 34–37. IEEE (2005)

12. Bellotti, F., Berta, R., Gloria, A.D., Margarone, M.: Guiding visually impaired people in the exhibition. In: Mobile Guide, Turin, Italy (2006),
http://mobileguide06.di.unito.it/pdf/Bellotti&al.pdf

13. Ivanov, R.: Indoor navigation system for visually impaired. In: Proceedings of the 11th International Conference on Computer Systems and Technologies and Workshop for PhD Students in Computing on International Conference on Computer Systems and Technologies, CompSysTech 2010, pp. 143–149. ACM, New York (2010)

14. Peischl, B., Ziefle, M., Holzinger, A.: A mobile information system for improved navigation in public transport: User centered design, development, evaluation and e-Business scenarios of a mobile roadmap application. In: International Conference on Data Communication Networking, e-Business and Optical Communication Systems, pp. 217–221. SciTec Press, Rome (2012)

15. Padzi, F., Ibrahim, F.: Accessibility of visually impaired passengers at urban railway stations in the klang valley. International Transaction Journal of Engineering, Management, & Applied Sciences & Technologies 3(3), 277–292 (2012)

16. Guentert, M.: Improving public transit accessibility for blind riders: a train station navigation assistant. In: The Proceedings of the 13th International ACM SIGACCESS Conference on Computers and Accessibility, ASSETS 2011, pp. 317–318. ACM, New York (2011)

17. Krajnc, E., Feiner, J., Schmidt, S.: User centered interaction design for mobile applications focused on visually impaired and blind people. In: Leitner, G., Hitz, M., Holzinger, A. (eds.) USAB 2010. LNCS, vol. 6389, pp. 195–202. Springer, Heidelberg (2010)

18. Krajnc, E., Knoll, M., Feiner, J., Traar, M.: A touch sensitive user interface approach on smartphones for visually impaired and blind persons. In: Holzinger, A., Simonic, K.-M. (eds.) USAB 2011. LNCS, vol. 7058, pp. 585–594. Springer, Heidelberg (2011)

19. Brooke, J.: SUS: A "quick and dirty" usability scale. In: Jordan, P.W., Thomas, B., Weerdmeester, B.A., McClelland, I.L. (eds.) Usability Evaluation in Industry, pp. 189–194. Taylor & Francis, London (1996)

20. Hart, S.G.: Nasa-task load index (NASA-TLX); 20 years later. In: Proceedings of the Human Factors and Ergonomics Society Annual Meeting, vol. 50(9), pp. 904–908 (2006)

Elements of Play for Cognitive, Physical and Social Health in Older Adults

Fares Kayali[1], Naemi Luckner[1], Oliver Hödl[1], Geraldine Fitzpatrick[1],
Peter Purgathofer[1], Tanja Stamm[2], Daniela Schlager-Jaschky[3], and Erika Mosor[3]

[1] Vienna University of Technology, Institute of Design and Assessment of Technology, Austria
{fares,naemi,oliver}@igw.tuwien.ac.at,
{geraldine.fitzpatrick,peter.purgathofer}@tuwien.ac.at
[2] FH Campus Wien, Department of Health / Medical University of Vienna,
Department of Rheumatology, Vienna, Austria
tanja.stamm@meduniwien.ac.at
[3] FH Campus Wien, Department of Health, Vienna, Austria
erika.mosor@aon.at, danhar@drei.at

Abstract. An increasingly older demographic emphasizes the need to deal with a likewise increasing number of people with cognitive disabilities like dementia or Alzheimer's disease. While no cure exists the preventive potential of activities in the areas of reminiscence, cognitive, social and physical activity has been recognized. This paper looks at the possibilities of technological interventions in this field from a game design perspective. The paper follows the core research question "Which elements of play can be used in a playful holistic application combining reminiscence, cognitive, social and physical activities to prevent or postpone the development of cognitive disabilities such as dementia for older adults?" Examples are qualitatively analysed and lead to the identification of the elements auto-biographical play, musical play, kinaesthetic play, object-based play, adaptive play, collaborative play and role playing. The list of these elements is expendable and lays the foundation for a holistic design space.

Keywords: aging well, play, game elements, dementia prevention, serious games, reminiscence.

1 Introduction

Due to steady advances in both disease prevention and treatment our society benefits from a longer life expectancy but also faces new challenges [1]. There is a growing demographic of older adults who despite of the advances made in other fields, still face the risk of cognitive disabilities such as dementia or Alzheimer's disease. The ever growing number of people who have one of these disabilities puts a great strain on care institutions who have trouble accommodating more and more patients. The exploding costs of care expenses demand new approaches for therapy and especially prevention. This demographic shift is accompanied by a change of the understanding of health and health care. Movements like the quantified self use technology to

A. Holzinger et al. (Eds.): SouthCHI 2013, LNCS 7946, pp. 296–313, 2013.
© Springer-Verlag Berlin Heidelberg 2013

integrate personal health, data feedback and consequently self reflection of one's health into everyday life. Governments try to encourage self responsibility of patients, hospitals discharge people into outpatient care earlier. It can be observed that there is a shift from a care society to a participation society, which empowers patients and encourages people to take on more responsibility for their well being.

This paper looks at how to support people with their goal to age well, in particular taking account of the three major challenges accompanying aging: cognitive loss; physical decline; and social isolation. These challenges are not discrete but closely interrelated. Cognitive disabilities cannot be prevented entirely but their onset can be postponed and their progression can be slowed by engaging in beneficial behaviour, thus enabling a longer prosperous life. For example, as also summarised in Grosinger et al [2]: low levels of social connections and infrequent participation in social activities affects the risk of cognitive decline [3]; and physical activity helps to improve cognitive performance [4], is particularly key to promoting health and well being among older people [5] and "regular physical activity is a key component of successful aging" and "may also slow down the course of Alzheimer's disease" ([6], pp.401) but physical activities typically decrease with age [7]. Beneficial behaviour therefore includes a mixture of cognitive, physical and social exercises. Also the values of reminiscence to promote well aging in older adults need to be taken into account, including identity-forming and self-continuity, enhancing meaning in life and coherence, preserving a sense of mastery, and promoting acceptance and reconciliation [8].

The starting premise of this paper is that games can provide a platform to combine all dimensions of these exercises to make them more engaging and to sustain these activities long term and so contribute to a prolonged independent life and also a lessened strain on care facilities. It seems promising to take a holistic approach and combine the four areas into one intervention. However, while there are a number of games that focus on one or more of these areas, there are no principled approaches to doing so nor an understanding of key elements of play that can support these. The aim of this paper is to identify elements of play to combine these diverse areas, to increase motivation and to sustain long term engagement. This leads to the following research question:

"Which elements of play can be used in a playful holistic application combining reminiscence, cognitive, social and physical activities to prevent or postpone the development of cognitive disabilities such as dementia for older adults?"

The goal of this paper is to open up the design space for possible technological interventions in this context. We will identify holistic and playful concepts across the areas of reminiscence, social activity, cognitive activity and physical activity, which are beneficial to delay or avoid the development of cognitive disabilities. This will be achieved through relating literature review of the current state of the art with a theoretical analysis of qualitative examples.

2   Research Approach

This paper builds on existing literature on games and dementia as well as a review of selected serious game examples to answer the above question. Based on the concepts of reminiscence, cognitive, social and physical activity discussed in the literature review we make a selection of games and serious toys, which are then qualitatively analysed. Relevant elements of play to prevent cognitive disabilities are extracted, discussed and are then interpreted in the context of a holistic application.

This paper is written in the context of the project Lebensnetz, a playful approach to prevent the development of cognitive disabilities. The paper's findings are informed by preliminary insights from four focus groups held as part of the project. The focus groups were comprised of 8-10 persons each and were held between October and November 2012 in Vienna, Austria. The first focus group involved experts from academia, health and care institutions, the second was held with members of the older adults target audience, the third with the families of older adults and the fourth was attended by care personnel. The focus groups were audio-recorded, transcribed and thematically analysed and will be the focus of another publication (under preparation). While not the core focus here, we will still draw on insights from the focus groups, and relate them to the findings of this paper. The key contribution of the paper is the identification of elements of play supporting holistic activities and directed at an older adults target audience.

The elements of play are identified through a qualitative analysis of the four selected game examples. The resulting differentiation of play elements in a holistic context and relating them with the current state of the art forms the core research result of this paper.

3   Literature Review

In this section we first elaborate on adult play and discuss the use of games and game elements in technological interventions targeted at older adults. We then move on to individually identify how reminiscence, social, cognitive and physical activity can support aging well.

3.1   Older Adults and Play

When designing games for older adults, age related changes have to be taken into account [9]. Some abilities tend to decline as people get older, including short-time memory, speed, executive functions and visual perception [10]. Barriers can for example be created by using too little contrasts or colours that are hard to discriminate. In this context, thinking about accessibility is of great importance [11]. McLaughlin et al. [12] also raise the issue of stereotype threat. Stereotype threat is the fear of failing at something because of stereotypes about the group a person belongs to, for example, "computer games are made for kids".

These changes can be addressed by carefully choosing physical interaction methods, feedback systems, an accessible interface and adaptive difficulty of the gameplay. Older adults tend to have less experience using computers than younger people. To facilitate learning a game Whitlock et al. [13] propose training support before getting started and during the learning process.

Quandt et al. [14] explored the experiences of older gamers and found that most of them got into playing as part of their jobs, were introduced by the children's generation or because of life-changing events like illnesses. They found that gaming impacts social acceptance of older gamers, creating frustration or resignation on their partner's side, but building a common ground for the interaction between different generations.

Concentrating on the interests of older gamers Pearce [15] conducted a study consisting of an online survey, interviews and discussion groups. She concluded that the PC is the platform of choice for older gamers (though Grosinger et al. [2] found a reluctance to spend too much time at the PC and instead found good acceptance among older people for using tablet computers; Murata et al. [16] also argue that a tablet computer tends to have fewer age-related usability issues for pointing tasks). They favour single-player games but are interested in mature companionships with other gamers. The older generation of gamers leans towards intellectually challenging games over speed and reflex-oriented games and are less interested in levelling and skill acquisition but just want to have fun.

The insights on adult play from the focus groups only partially overlap with Pearce's study. While many say they play in various contexts (e.g. with their grandchildren), most deny playing games (although they do play card and board games) and explicitly say they do not play digital games and many even avoid using a PC all together. It was also a common statement in the older adults focus group that they don't like to play alone but rather like to play together with their peers. Most said that the aspect of gaming they enjoy most is to play in a social context which fosters togetherness and spawns discussions. While Pearce [15] found that old adults play for fun rather than to hone skills and to overcome challenges focus group members were very conscious about the need to train their cognitive skills and regarded games as a possible means to do so.

Overall, the insights on adult play lead to the assumption that play can provide a motivating context for a technological intervention but that using a classic videogame might turn away many. For a project that is meant to encourage various beneficial activities the concept of gamifying these activities instead of making a full game out of them thus is tempting. Standard gamification techniques such as giving out awards, badges and points come into play here and can form an important part of a system's feedback [17]. For a meaningful system that sustains engagement in the long term it is necessary to move beyond these techniques though. In this context game elements are understood not only as a score and feedback layer but as mechanics, which further meaningful interaction or engagement with a cause [18]. Consequently we understand elements of play as ways users can interact with these game elements.

Especially in the context of health it is necessary that approaches do more than just reward the right kind of behaviour. If positive results receive positive feedback this conversely also means that if players make no progress they are penalized. This is not desirable because it might not be the patient's or user's fault that he or she has taken some steps backward and even then these kind of players need to be encouraged even more. Referring to Bartle's [19] distinction of player types this means that game elements should not only appeal to the success oriented "achievers" and "killers" who focus on rewards, scores and competitive play but also to the "explorers" and "socialites" who play less goal oriented. This opens up the spectrum between intrinsic and extrinsic motivation. External rewards might lead to more immediate engagement with a system but the more powerful intrinsic motivation can only be triggered through a deeper embedding of game mechanics where the game enables players to interact with the desired cause in a meaningful way. The term "gameful design" is used to describe such approaches (see [20] and [21]). For a project that should encourage beneficial activities across a wide range of areas, this means that these activities should not only be rewarded in a game-like sense but that the activities themselves shall be designed from a game design perspective to make them engaging and playful.

3.2 Physical Activity

Digital games, especially designed for older adults and for the benefit of their health, are becoming increasingly popular [22]. These games are often designed as exergames which require bodily interaction to play the game [23]. In their paper they define and compare Sony PlayStation Move, Nintendo Wii, and Microsoft Xbox 360 Kinect as the three major solutions for these kind of games.

Especially Microsoft's Kinect is used in games for preventative health care or rehabilitation as no handheld devices are needed and the tracking is not limited to certain body parts or specific gestures [24]. However, the full-body effort needed with Kinect can also be a disadvantage for people in wheelchairs and older adults who might not be able to move a lot. In any case it is important to clarify whether the primary purpose of an exergame is the training or rehabilitation of particular body parts or if the physical interface is mainly used as a game controller with the intention to increase physical activity.

3.3 Cognitive Acitivity

In his book about play Stuart Brown ([25], p.34) sees important parts of cognition related to playing as "discriminating relevant from irrelevant information, monitoring and organizing our own thoughts and feelings, and planning for the future". Playing games without doubt requires concentration and, depending on the genre, uses cognitive abilities to various degrees. A higher amount of cognitive activity is needed in genres like puzzle or adventure games. There is mixed evidence though about whether playing these kinds of games can help delay or stop cognitive decline in older adults. Nouchi et al. [26] has shown positive short term effects in cognition and executive function for an audience with an average age of 69 using a commercial brain training game. Likewise Brem et al. [27] also used a commercial brain training game to evaluate if cognitive decline after hip surgery is slowed in people with an average

age of 45. They found that the use of a video game can stop cognitive decline during prolonged hospital stays but could not substantiate positive effects on memory. Stern et al. [28] used a custom made game to train cognitive function and basic motor ability. While a training effect in cognitive functions could be observed it could not be fully isolated from the preconditions and training effects of motor abilities. Basak et al. [29] could show that using a commercial real time strategy game which involves complex tasks and decisions positively influences executive functions like task switching, working memory, visual short-term memory, and reasoning in the short term.

Overall the studies cited show some potential of games to be used to train cognitive abilities in older adults. All the discussed studies were conducted using short terms ranging from 4 to 12 weeks and thus only short term effects can be confirmed while long term effects and potential are unknown. However, there are enough positive reports from off-the-shelf games to suggest that game activities are a good means of cognitive training.

Reminiscence. Reminiscence is a cognitive activity that is used to remember and re-live one's past. A playful approach to reminiscence can hold great value to older adults because it stimulates their cognitive functions while being entertaining. Various definitions of reminiscence exist emphasizing different aspects of the process of re-calling past experiences. Parker ([30], p.517) distils the essence as "a selective process in which memories are evoked and reconstructed, probably with varying degrees of intensity and emotional involvement". Reminiscence can take place in a silent interpersonal or an oral intrapersonal setting, both of which are caused by conscious or intentional as well as non-conscious or spontaneous triggers [31].

There are different ways to look at reminiscence and its purpose. Bluck et al. [32] describe the directive, self, and social functions that reminiscence serves. The directive function can help dealing with the present and future by remembering the past. It can facilitate processes like problem-solving and predicting an outcome. The self function helps create and preserve a sense of self. Social functions work towards interacting and engaging with others, sharing memories, empathizing and building relationships. Wong and Watt [33] define six types of reminiscence: integrative, instrumental, transmissive, narrative, escapist, and obsessive reminiscence. Of these six categories, only integrative and instrumental reminiscence support successful aging by achieving a sense of self-worth, self-continuity and mastery.

Reminiscence therapy is used in people with dementia ([34], [35], [36], [37], [38]). People who suffer from dementia show short-time memory loss that makes participation in social activities and interaction increasingly difficult. Concentrating on a person's long-term memory can potentially facilitate communication and social interaction and lead to an improved integration into the community and well-being. [35]

Some studies [39] point out that the effectiveness of reminiscence for the prevention and treatment of dementia has not been proven. Several other studies ([30], [31], [32], [33], [34]) indicate that reminiscence can have a positive effect on cognitive functions and hence has positive implications for people with dementia. Parker ([30], p.523) suggests that "decline in short- and long-term memory leads to an increased reliance upon remote memory systems" and that "increased use of remote memory in older adults improves general cognitive functioning". Lai et al. [34] conducted a study in nursing home residents with dementia trying to detect impacts of reminiscence on their well-being. They concluded that reminiscence helps to improve the psychosocial well-being of the participants. Wang [36] found that cognitive functions of participants increase while depressive symptoms are reduced as a result of using group reminiscence therapy.

3.4   Social Activity

Older adults need to feel that activities they engage in offer benefits to be interesting [12]. Video games provide social opportunities that are seen as important in the lives of seniors or as Hirsch et al. ([40], p.74) put it "An elder's quality of life is dependent on a rich set of social relationships among a variety of individuals." Games improve interaction with friends, family and younger generations, but also with people from other social circles and decrease social distance [41]. Games can not only be played together, but also discussed in hindsight and used as conversation starters.

Koster [42] presented a collection of social mechanics that can be found in games. He named helping, status, handicapping, roles, trust, community and teamwork among his list of 40+ social mechanics. Helping takes on an important role in playful interaction. Users can work together in a team, or can show one another what they already know. Status can be derived from helping others or succeeding in a difficult task. Handicapping is a tool to balance knowledge and capabilities of players in order to provide a pleasurable gaming experience for everyone. If a player is extremely experienced and the other doesn't know the game, the experienced player gets a handicap, making the game harder for him/her while favouring the inexperienced player. Playing can build up trust between the players out of a need for them to work together and overcome challenges.

Games create a safe environment to take on different roles in a social surrounding. Players can try out the roles of comrades as well as enemies and change between roles during a game [43]. The change of roles in social activities can be seen as empowering people. They can take control and steer the game in a direction they want to go in or take on roles they see themselves in.

Research ([44], [2]) indicates that the social factor of games constitutes a motivating and engaging environment. Competition and team building as well as personal and social involvement are rewarding and create a sense of accomplishment.

4   Qualitative Examples

Based on the four areas of reminiscence, cognitive, social and physical activity, interesting examples are chosen which predominantly build on one of these areas each. Most examples overlap into other areas as well. The analysis of the examples shall help us in learning about how features can come together in a holistic application. In this chapter we first introduce each example and describe the elements directed at hindering cognitive disabilities. In the following discussion chapter we then pull together and interpret the possible use and meaning of these elements in a holistic context.

4.1   Example 1 (Reminiscence): Music Memory Box

The Music Memory Box (created by [45]) is a collection of personal objects in a box whose placement triggers the box to play different songs. The project was chosen for analysis because it constitutes an unusual and art-based approach, which also is highly personalized. The objects carry RFID chips and were either selected or designed and crafted in a user-centered design process by Meineck together with her user Barbara (see the below picture). Each object represents a certain family member. The songs triggered by the objects were selected by Barbara as well. This makes the Music Memory Box a very personal object and allows Barbara to directly relate to it. As she triggers the playback of individual songs the combination of objects and music also helps her to trigger associated memories.

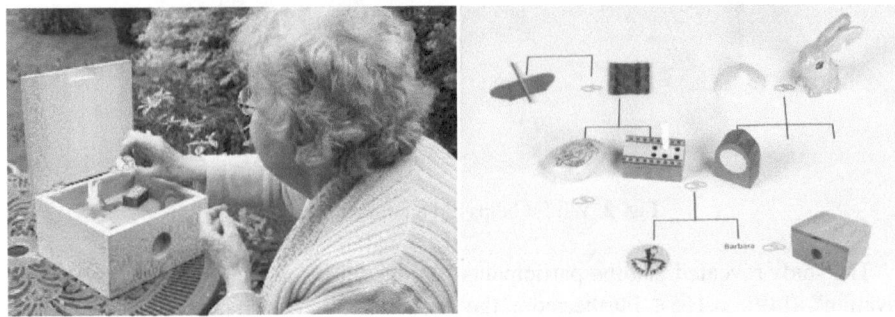

Fig. 1. The Music Memory Box filled with objects, which represent a family tree

While the Music Memory Box is not a game but a serious toy, it nonetheless invites playful exploration of its contents both in a tangible (by using objects) and digital (through triggering music playback) way. The elements of play in this case are the objects which allow access to the music and in a metaphorical sense to the player's memories. Each of the objects in the box was made to represent and to trigger memories of a member of Barbara's family tree. Studies show that music is useful in coping with dementia ([46], [47]), that music is preserved longer than other memories in people with dementia [48] and thus can be a good anchor point to access memories.

4.2   Example 2 (Physical Acitivity): Wii Fit

Nintendo's Wii Fit is a collection of exergames that are played with the whole body using (1) the Wii balance board, a floorboard that measures the movement of the whole body, (2) the Wiimote, a wireless movement controller operated by hand, and (3) the Nunchuck, an extension of the Wiimote to play with both hands. We have chosen this as an example because first, since its introduction in 2006 Nintendo's Wii became a popular, easy-to-play and low-cost game environment that older people can use. Use of the Wii in care homes has been documented in [44]. The purposes of the games from a health perspective are muscle building, yoga positions, aerobics and balance. Especially the latter have been used for balance training with old adults and furthermore evaluated [49]. In the study they have used basic step, soccer heading, ski slalom, and table tilt, letting the participants 3 times per week, 30 minutes each session over a period of 3 months. All games are intended to exercise static and dynamic balance, motor response and give visual and auditory feedback.

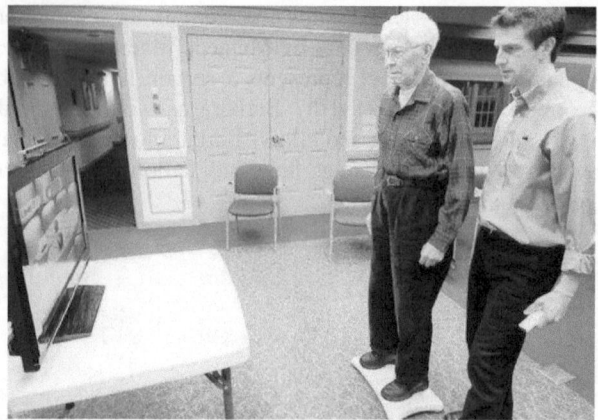

Fig. 2. Wii Fit helps old adults with balance

The study revealed that the participants "enjoyed playing and found the games motivating" ([49], p.165). Furthermore the authors observed a general improvement regarding the balance of the participants. However, the authors suggest a close supervision and guidance for a better progress and a reduction of the risk of an injury. Apart from that the majority of all participants reported they were playing the games also together with their grandchildren which indicates additional social benefits and increase of motivation.

The underlying study shows the suitability of a gaming approach to support health and improve well-being of old adults. The importance of specific aspects are identified which are important when the players are old adults and are usually negligible with young people. These are body and health-related issues on the one hand, and the need of supervision on the other hand.

4.3   Example 3 (Cognitive Acitivity): Eldergames

An example of a game to support cognitive activity is Eldergames. The Eldergames project ([50], [51]) was chosen because it focuses on furthering cognitive activity but embeds it in a social context. It is a table installation with a screen surface. Up to four players can sit around the table and play together but it can also be played alone or with remote players. The interface is controlled with a pen which is tracked through four cameras, each mounted to a metal bar in the four corners of the table. Game-play centres around a memory game. Mistakes in the memory game can be compensated by short minigames which focus on training isolated cognitive aspects like reasoning or divided as well as selective attention. Another module of the project allows monitoring performance of the target audience.

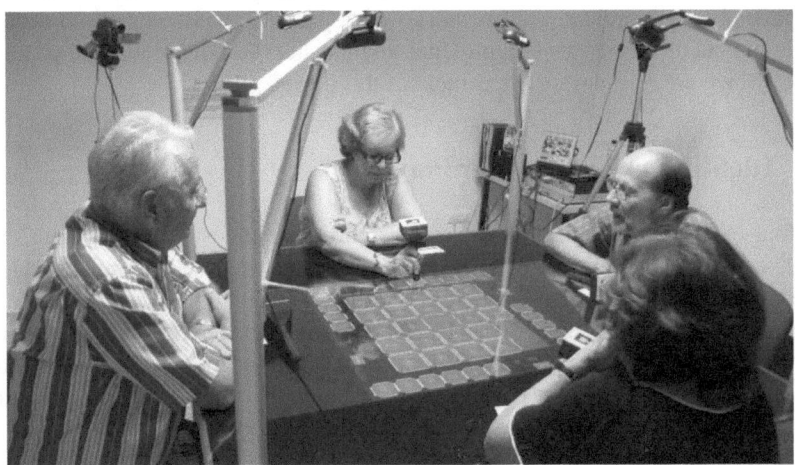

Fig. 3. A test group playing the memory game module of the Eldergames project

Acceptance and usability evaluations [52] showed a good overall response but pointed out individual areas for improvement like better feedback and instructions as well as a more balanced and adjustable difficulty level.

In Eldergames augmented reality [53] is used to bridge digital games with physical objects. The physical nature of the project not only helps in lowering the technological barrier of entry but the table setup also naturally facilitates social contact and social play. The project also showed that rather simple games can still help further cognitive engagement. It also showed that a bridge to known analogue games (like memory) is helpful in making the game accessible.

4.4   Example 4 (Social Activity): DanceAlong

The DanceAlong project [54] is an augmented dancing environment aimed at older adults. It is introduced as an example for encouraging social activity among large groups of players. DanceAlong was developed to provide entertaining means of exercise and social engagement to the target group. Participants can choose from a list of song clips of old movies and dance along with the actors. The setup consists of a dedicated dancing area and two big screens with the projection of the movie scene in the front and the back of the dance floor. Participants dance along mirroring the dance moves they see on screen.

The game is designed to promote positive social interaction. Interviews conducted by the authors showed that older people tend to interact within a set group of acquaintances and seldom leave their social circle. They also found that dancing is mentioned as a desired activity by many older people but hindered by various factors like the lack of a partner, no space to dance or a lack of dance events. DanceAlong is a group activity with no need for one particular dancing partner and encourages interaction beyond social circles using memories of a shared past. It doesn't only focus on socializing but also involves reminiscence and physical components in the game-play, both of which are relevant for the context of this paper.

5   Identifying Elements of Play

The four examples, though chosen for their particular focus on either reminiscence, social, cognitive or physical activity, are interesting because they all overlap into some of the other areas. These overlaps and the elements of play, which manage to bring different areas together, are what we are most interested in. We think that a holistic approach, which combines all four of the mentioned areas, holds potential to increase the preventive effect of such an application. The following interpretation of the analysis describes elements of play directed at a older adults target audience and puts them in a holistic context. We identify a series of elements of play as we go through the four qualitative examples again.

Autobiographical play happens when games trigger memories and let players relive moments of their past. The Music Memory Box' focus is on reminiscence and what can be learnt from this project is to make use of the even stronger relation people have with personal objects. It also shows that it is beneficial to have assistance with collecting materials and making selections. Similar systems can be designed to facilitate collaborative use, to enable families and friends to interact with the system together and to contribute content. Thus autobiographical play allows reminiscence to be combined with social activity. In the focus groups we also learned that at care homes personnel fills out a biography sheet together with older patients to be able to better relate to them. A system focused on autobiographical play for example could use these sheets to enter data. Another possibility brought up during the focus groups is to combine autobiographical and make-believe play by using a game to create part real part imaginary biographies. Langer ([55], p.158) describes the potential of recalling the past: "Perhaps older memories are more meaningful to the elderly; this type of information was worthy of encoding in the past and is worthy of retrieval in the present."

Musical play, as opposed to music making, describes playful interaction with musical contents [56]. Both the Music Memory Box and DanceAlong revolve around musical play. The before cited studies show music helps remembering things and can be used as a preventive measure. Research in reminiscence [31] shows that reminiscence can be triggered by various cues, such as music. In the Music Memory Box musical play triggers reminiscence and supports social activity because the box can be played and listened to together and can be used as a starting point to share memories. DanceAlong encourages reminiscence and physical activity through music contents.

Collaborative play happens when two or more players play together and try to reach a common goal. DanceAlong tries to provide the means for collaborative play for a broad audience of participants. Everyone willing to dance along can be included. This approach is beneficial for the use of the game at big events where it acts as conversation starter and entertainment and motivates interaction and mingling. In the focus groups we also found that weekly singing is a very popular social activity at care homes. The game could be filled with any kind of content, but choosing songs from the players pasts is a powerful tool. Collaborative play was also found to be a beneficial factor in the above cited study on Wii Fit.

One of the functions of reminiscence is the social function as described by Bluck et al. [32] which facilitates the sharing of memories and, moreover, engaging in and building of relationships. This function is particularly used to achieve the goal of DanceAlong to act as a nexus to connect different social circles. The process of reminiscence is also amplified by the social context of the game. Stories and conversations among the participants can lead to additional memories of the individual.

Role play has players take on a different roles or perspectives than their own. This can also mean going back to past experiences. Another effect of reminiscence according to Bluck et al. [32] is the self function. Playing the game and remembering the past is a role play activity. Players are put in the roles of celebrities of their youth and might get a sense of self that they might not have had in a long time. This might lead to a feeling of renewed youth and empowerment. Connecting to memories and experiences on a deeply individual level is a personal benefit that serves as an additional complement for the otherwise social game. A similar correlation between reminiscing and role playing can also be attributed to the Music Memory Box.

Kinaesthetic play [57] means that physical bodily interaction is used to control a game rather than a controller interface. This can make the game more immersive for players and at the same time makes gameplay easier to grasp for observers. Kinaesthetic play also adds another sensory layer to a holistic concept. Dancing is a physical activity and not always easy to do alone as was mentioned in interviews conducted for the DanceAlong project. Establishing a social, open environment for players to participate in, is the goal of DanceAlong. The game designers decided on letting the players just mirror the dance moves on the screen in contrast to letting them use controllers, track their movements or give feedback on the correctness of the movements. This design decision is beneficial for the target group and the interaction with each other and the game. The dance floor is open for as little or as many dancers as want to join in. Participants are not restrained by possible mistakes and players with physical restrictions are not excluded from the activity. Thus DanceAlong serves as a strong example for connecting the areas of reminiscence and social activity with physical activity.

Wii Fit's focus is physical activity and aninteresting aspect of the above described study is that participants occasionally played together with their grandchildren when they had no official guidance of the study-team, instead of playing alone as intended by the study design. This tendency to willingly play within a social context should be considered when designing games mainly addressed at old adults. Involving relatives or other possible players might be an important part of the game-play. Additionally such co-players can even assist and take care of old adults playing games if there are any health-related issues to be aware of. Similarly to the DanceAlong project, the use of kinaesthetic play seems to encourage others to take part and thus bridges physical with social activity. Additionally kinaesthetic play can be tightly intertwined with cognitive activity. Games in particular often prompt players to correctly recall and reproduce certain moves, like dance moves in DanceAlong or exercises in WiiFit.

Object-based play is interacting with a game through the use of dedicated physical objects. In the Eldergames project a tangible interface facilitates social activity by prompting four players to sit around a table to play together. Play itself centers on small cognitive activities. The interface acts as a bridge between these activities and the social context. The use of a table and its acceptance by test users points to the use of objects rather than using screens and classic interfaces like keyboard and mouse. The focus groups showed insecurity towards PC technology as well and thus building a dedicated play object like in Eldergames might help overcome this barrier of entry. The Music Memory Box also strongly relies on the use of objects which shall trigger music and associated memories and also facilitate to play with the box together. Object-based play and tangible interaction can help to better identify with a technological solution and also ease entry. It is helpful in a social context because it makes other players' actions easier to trace and comprehend. Focus groups interviews also showed a conscience among older adults that they need to train their cognitive abilities and they do so by e.g. solving crosswords or playing Sudoku. Thus a system that comes close to these analogue activities should be well accepted.

Table 1. Elements of play and their function to bridge activities in a holistic context

Element of play	Found in	Reminiscence	Social act.	Cognitive act.	Physical act.
auto-biographical play	Music Memory Box	X	X		
musical play	Music Memory Box, DanceAlong	X	X		X
collaborative play	DanceAlong, Wii Fit	X	X		
role play	DanceAlong, Music Memory Box	X		X	
kinaesthetic play	DanceAlong, Wii Fit		X	X	X
object-based play	Eldergames, Music Memory Box	X	X	X	
adaptive play	Eldergames		X	X	

Adaptive play helps to establish a level playing field. The older adults demographic is very heterogeneous and diverse. Thus for cognitive tasks the difficulty level will always be an issue. What is easy for one person might be too difficult for another. Especially in a social play context difficulty must be adjusted to keep the game motivating for all who participate. Both the level of difficulty and/or the complexity of tasks should challenge a player to make the game satisfying while at the same time they should be low enough not to trigger feelings of anxiety or being overwhelmed. A digital solution can us adaptive difficulty to help level the playing field in a social context and thus act as a second way to bridge cognitive and social activity. For example the game can be made easier for some players so that they don't fall behind. In the focus groups it was mentioned that when playing board games together in the care home people often change the rules slightly to help each other during the course of the game.

6   Conclusion

In this paper we identify several elements of play and describe them with respect to their use to establish a holistic context across the areas of reminiscence, social activity, cognitive activity and physical activity.

This paper first gives an overview of using game elements as motivating components in applications for older adults which support one or more of the above activities. By studying examples we identify a series of elements of play which act as bridges between different activities (see Table 1). Aside from these particular elements of play, the main contribution of this paper is to open up the design space and subsequently study further examples of holistic elements of play.

In the focus groups we found that digital games might not always be accepted by an older demographic but we could find evidence that play still is attractive to them. Hence we suggest that a playful application which uses elements of play to engage people increases the acceptance of an application aimed at our target audience.

The elements of play we extract from the four analysed examples are autobiographical play, musical play, kinaesthetic play, object-based play, adaptive play, collaborative play and role playing. All of them serve an important purpose in bridging two or more of the areas of reminiscence, cognitive, social and physical activity. These elements of play are not mutually exclusive and can be used together to establish a holistic context for applications with the purpose of preventing cognitive disabilities. In this paper we derive the described elements of play from a qualitative analysis and from literature. The next step would be an evaluation of the elements with users.

Future work will also include finding more of these elements and designing a system which manages to engage people across all four areas. We think that a playful and holistic approach can result in higher acceptance than a game or focused intervention in this context. Furthermore such an approach can have preventive effects against cognitive disabilities. These assumptions need to be evaluated through studies after such a system has been designed. This paper provides a foundation for a holistic design space as well as a set of elements of play that can be used in different play contexts.

List of Images

References

1. WHO World Health Organisation, Active Ageing: A Policy Framework (2002), http://whqlibdoc.who.int/hq/2002/WHO_NMH_NPH_02.8.pdf (accessed December 12, 2012)
2. Grosinger, J., Vetere, F., Fitzpatrick, G.: Agile Life: addressing knowledge and social motivations for active aging. In: Proceedings of OzCHI 2012 (2012)
3. Zunzunegui, M.-V., Alvarado, B.E., Del Ser, T., Otero, A.: Social Networks, Social Integration, and Social Engagement Determine Cognitive Decline in Community-Dwelling Spanish Older Adults. The Journals of Gerontology Series B: Psychological Sciences and Social Sciences 58(2), 93–100 (2003)
4. Voelcker-Rehage, C., Godde, B., Staudinger, U.M.: Cardiovascular and coordination training differentially improve cognitive performance and neural processing in older adults. Frontiers in Human Neuroscience 5(26), 17–26 (2011)
5. Brassington, G.S., Atienza, A.A., Perczek, R.E., DiLorenzo, T.M.: Intervention-related cognitive versus social mediators of exercise adherence in the elderly. AJPM 23(2), 80–86 (2002)
6. Rolland, Y., Abellan van Kan, G.: Physical activity and Alzheimer's disease: from prevention to therapeutic perspectives. Journal of the American Medical Directors Association 9(6), 390–405 (2008)
7. Schutzer, K.A., Graves, B.S.: Barriers and motivations to exercise in older adults. Preventive Medicine 39, 1056–1061 (2004)
8. Bohlmeijer, E., Roemer, M., Cuijpers, P., Smit, F.: The effects of reminiscence on psychological well-being in older adults: a meta-analysis. Aging & Mental Health 11(3), 71–89 (2007)
9. Holzinger, A., Searle, G., Nischelwitzer, A.K.: On Some Aspects of Improving Mobile Applications for the Elderly. In: Stephanidis, C. (ed.) HCI 2007. LNCS, vol. 4554, pp. 923–932. Springer, Heidelberg (2007)
10. Whitlock, L.A., McLaughlin, A.C., Allaire, J.C.: Video Game Design for Older Adults: Usability Observations from an Intervention Study. In: Proceedings of the Human Factors and Ergonomics Society Annual Meeting, vol. 55(1), pp. 187–191 (2011)
11. Miesenberger, K., Ossmann, R., Archambault, D., Searle, G., Holzinger, A.: More Than Just a Game: Accessibility in Computer Games. In: Holzinger, A. (ed.) USAB 2008. LNCS, vol. 5298, pp. 247–260. Springer, Heidelberg (2008)
12. McLaughlin, A., Gandy, M., Allaire, J., Whitlock, L.: Putting Fun into Video Games for Older Adults. Ergonomics in Design: The Quarterly of Human Factors Applications 20(2), 13–22 (2012)
13. Whitlock, L.A, McLaughlin, A.C., Allaire, J.C.: Training Requirements of a Video Game-Based Cognitive Intervention for Older Adults: Lessons Learned. In: Proceedings of the Human Factors and Ergonomics Society Annual Meeting, vol. 54(27), pp. 2343–2346 (2010)

14. Quandt, T., Grueninger, H., Wimmer, J.: The Gray Haired Gaming Generation: Findings From an Explorative Interview Study on Older Computer Gamers. Games and Culture 4(1), 27–46 (2008)
15. Pearce, C.: The Truth About Baby Boomer Gamers: A Study of Over-Forty Computer Game Players. Games and Culture 3(2), 142–174 (2008)
16. Murata, A., Iwase, H.: Usability of touch-panel interfaces for older adults. Human Factors 47(4), 767–776 (2005)
17. Schell, J.: Design outside the box. Presentation at Design Innovate Communicate Entertain Summit, p. 4 (2010)
18. Deterding, S., Sicart, M., Nacke, L., O'Hara, K., Dixon, D.: Gamification. using game-design elements in non-gaming contexts. In: Proceedings of the 2011 Annual Conference Extended Abstracts on Human Factors in Computing Systems, pp. 2425–2428. ACM (2011)
19. Bartle, R.: Hearts, clubs, diamonds, spades: Players who suit MUDs. Journal of MUD research 1(1), 19 (1996)
20. McGonigal, J.: Reality is broken: Why games make us better and how they can change the world. Penguin Press HC (2011)
21. Deterding, S., Dixon, D., Khaled, R., Nacke, L.: From game design elements to gamefulness: defining gamification. In: Proceedings of the 15th International Academic MindTrek Conference: Envisioning Future Media Environments, pp. 9–15. ACM (2011)
22. Gerling, K.M., Schulte, F.P., Masuch, M.: Designing and evaluating digital games for frail elderly persons. In: Proceedings of the 8th International Conference on Advances in Computer Entertainment Technology, ACE 2011, November 1-8, p. 62. ACM Press, New York (2011)
23. Tanaka, K., Parker, J., Baradoy, G., Sheehan, D., Holash, J., Katz, L.: A Comparison of Exergaming Interfaces for Use in Rehabilitation Programs and Research. Canadian Game Studies Association 6(9), 69–81 (2012)
24. Boulos, M.N.K.: Xbox 360 KinectExergames for Health. Games for Health Journal 1(5), 326–330 (2012)
25. Brown, S.L., Vaughan, C.C.: Play: How it shapes the brain, opens the imagination, and invigorates the soul. Avery Publishing Group (2009)
26. Nouchi, R., Taki, Y., Takeuchi, H., Hashizume, H., Akitsuki, Y., Shigemune, Y., Sekiguchi, A., Kotozaki, Y., Tsukiura, T., Yomogida, Y.: Brain training game improves executive functions and processing speed in the elderly: A randomized controlled trial. PloS one 7(1), e29676 (2012)
27. Brem, M., Lehrl, S., Rein, A., Massute, S., Schulz-Drost, S., Gelse, K., Schlechtweg, P., Hennig, F., Olk, A., Jacob, H.: Stop of loss of cognitive performance during rehabilitation after total hip arthroplasty—Prospective controlled study. Significance 60, 19 (2009)
28. Stern, Y., Blumen, H., Rich, L., Richards, A., Herzberg, G., Gopher, D.: Space Fortress game training and executive control in older adults: a pilot intervention. Aging, Neuropsychology, and Cognition 18(6), 653–677 (2011)
29. Basak, C., Boot, W., Voss, M., Kramer, A.: Can training in a real-time strategy video game attenuate cognitive decline in older adults? Psychology and Aging 23(4), 765–777 (2008)
30. Parker, R.G.: Reminiscence: A Continuity Theory Framework. The Gerontologist 35(4), 515–525 (1995)
31. Webster, J.D., Bohlmeijer, E.T., Westerhof, G.J.: Mapping the Future of Reminiscence: A Conceptual Guide for Research and Practice. Research on Aging 32(4), 527–564 (2010)

32. Bluck, S., Alea, N., Habermas, T., Rubin, D.C.: A Tale of Three Functions: The Self-Reported Uses of Autobiographic Memory. Social Cognition 23(1), 91–117 (2005)
33. Wong, P.T., Watt, L.M.: What types of reminiscence are associated with successful aging? Psychology and Aging 6(2), 272–279 (1991)
34. Lai, C.K.Y., Chi, I., Kayser-Jones, J.: A randomized controlled trial of a specific reminiscence approach to promote the well-being of nursing home residents with dementia. International Psychogeriatrics 16(1), 33–49 (2004)
35. Alm, N., Dye, R., Gowans, G., Campbell, J., Astrell, A., Ellis, M.: A Communication Support System for Older People with Dementia. Computer 40(5), 35–41 (2007)
36. Wang, J.: Group reminiscence therapy for cognitive and affective function of demented elderly in Taiwan. International Journal of Geriatric Psychiatry 22(12), 1235–1240 (2007)
37. Bornat, J.: Reminiscence and oral history: parallel universes or shared endeavour? Ageing and Society 22(2), 219–241 (2001)
38. Flood, M., Phillips, K.D.: Creativity in older adults: a plethora of possibilities. Issues in Mental Health Nursing 28(4), 389–411 (2007)
39. Thorgrimsen, L., Schweitzer, P., Orrell, M.: Evaluating reminiscence for people with dementia: a pilot study. The Arts in Psychotherapy 29, 93–97 (2002)
40. Hirsch, T., Forlizzi, J., Hyder, E., Goetz, J., Kurtz, C., Stroback, J.: The ELDer project: social, emotional, and environmental factors in the design of eldercare technologies. In: Proceedings on the 2000 Conference on Universal Usability, pp. 72–79 (2000)
41. Ijsselsteijn, W., Nap, H., De Kort, Y., Poels, K.: Digital game design for elderly users. In: Proceedings of the 2007 Conference on Future Play 2007, p. 17 (2007)
42. Koster, R.: Social Mechanics, The Engines Behind Everything Multiplayer. Slides Presented at the Game Developers Conference, San Francisco, California (2011)
43. Salen, K., Zimmerman, E.: Rules of Play: Game Design Fundamentals. The MIT Press (2003)
44. Harley, D., Fitzpatrick, G., Axelrod, L., White, G., McAllister, G.: Making the Wii at home: game play by older people in sheltered housing. In: Leitner, G., Hitz, M., Holzinger, A. (eds.) USAB 2010. LNCS, vol. 6389, pp. 156–176. Springer, Heidelberg (2010)
45. Meineck, C.: Music Memory Box (2012), http://www.chloemeineck.co.uk (accessed December 12, 2012)
46. Clark, M.E., Lipe, A.W., Bilbrey, M.: Use of music to decrease aggressive behaviors in people with dementia. Journal of Gerontological Nursing 24(7), 10–17 (1998)
47. Sung, H., Chang, A.M.: Use of preferred music to decrease agitated behaviours in older people with dementia: a review of the literature. Journal of Clinical Nursing 14(9), 1133–1140 (2005)
48. Cuddy, L.L., Duffin, J.: Music, memory, and Alzheimer's disease: is music recognition spared in dementia, and how can it be assessed? Medical Hypotheses 64(2), 229–235 (2005)
49. Agmon, M., Perry, C.K., Phelan, E., Demiris, G., Nguyen, H.Q.: A pilot study of Wii Fit exergames to improve balance in older adults. Journal of Geriatric Physical Therapy 34(4), 161–167 (2011)
50. Gamberini, L., Alcaniz, M., Barresi, G., Fabregat, M., Ibanez, F., Prontu, L.: Cognition, technology and games for the elderly: An introduction to ELDERGAMES Project. Psychnology Journal 4(3), 285–308 (2006)
51. Gamberini, L., Fabregat, M., Spagnolli, A., Prontu, L., Seraglia, B., Alcaniz, M., Zimmerman, A., Rontti, T., Grant, J., Jensen, R.: Eldergames: videogames for empowering, training and monitoring elderly cognitive capabilities. Gerontechnology 7(2), 111 (2008)

52. Gamberini, L., Martino, F., Seraglia, B., Spagnolli, A., Fabregat, M., Ibanez, F., Alcaniz, M., Andrés, J.: Eldergames project: An innovative mixed reality table-top solution to preserve cognitive functions in elderly people. In: 2nd Conference on Human System Interactions, HSI 2009, pp. 164–169. IEEE (2009)

53. Alcañiz Raya, M.L., Gòmez, J.A., Gamberini, L., Martinelli, M., Prontu, L., Seraglia, B., Varotto, D.: Design and development of a mixed reality solution for gerontechnology applications. Gerontechnology 7(2), 66 (2008)

54. Keyani, P., Hsieh, G., Mutlu, B., Easterday, M., Forlizzi, J.: DanceAlong: Supporting Positive Social Exchange and Exercise for the Elderly Through Dance. In: CHI 2005 Extended Abstracts on Human Factors in Computing Systems, pp. 1541–1544 (2005)

55. Langer, E.: Counterclockwise: Mindful Health and the Power of Possibility. Ballantine Books (2009)

56. Kayali, F., Pichlmair, M.: Playing Music, Playing Games - Simulation vs. Gameplay in Music-based Games. Paper presented at the Vienna Games Conference 2008 'Future and Reality of Gaming', FROG (2008)

57. Westecott, E.: Bringing the Body back into Play. In: The [player] Conference Proceedings, Copenhagen, Denmark (2008)

Understanding the Digital Game Classification System: A Review of the Current Classification System and Its Implications for Use within Games for Health

Hannah Ramsden Marston[1] and Stuart T. Smith[2,3]

[1] Institute of Movement & Sport Gerontology, German Sport University Cologne, Germany
h.marston@dshs-koeln.de, marstonhannah@hotmail.com
[2] Neuroscience Research, Randwick, New South Wales, Australia
[3] Centre for Research and Education in Active Living, University of Tasmania
Stuart.Smith@utas.edu.au

Abstract. This paper discusses and identifies the current video game classification systems employed throughout North and South America, Europe, Eurasia, Far East and Australasia. Ten main systems are employed, and although there are similarities, there are differences across the systems concerning: content descriptors, rating process and age categories. This paper proposes a series of recommendations for the classification of off-the-shelf games used by clinicians within the healthcare sector, for ease of use and clarity while implementing games for rehabilitation use. It is suggested; a worldwide classification system would facilitate a greater understanding and eradicate issues which occur by clinicians, support networks and patients utilizing this innovative approach to aid rehabilitation. For such a system to be established, a number of regional organizations, industry professionals, academics and end-users would be required to outline a format, and establish an appropriate system to be utilized.

Keywords: Classification System, Health, Rehabilitation, Digital Gaming.

1 Introduction

The use of off-the-shelf videogames is fast arising in popularity as a rehabilitation and training aid within many clinical environments. This entertainment medium, which during its short life span has quickly expanded in both hardware and software technology formats, initially perceived as a leisure pass time, [1] suggest this medium has the potential to assist people with rehabilitation. In recent years, several studies have been conducted to identify the suitable use and implementation of both commercial and high-end video game technologies for health issues such as rehabilitation of motor function following a stroke and fall prevention in older adults [2].

Conversely, a recent review focuses upon the utilization of current videogame console systems in the provision of training and rehabilitation programs to older

A. Holzinger et al. (Eds.): SouthCHI 2013, LNCS 7946, pp. 314–331, 2013.

adults within their own homes. The review proposes several scenarios whereby the consoles have been used within a clinical environment. In particular, it concentrates upon the functional independence of older adults; injury and disability resulting from a stroke and fall and the additional opportunities provided by internet-enabled game consoles. Which in turn suggests this technology can serve a wider purpose for example; rehabilitation and training but also facilitate and improve the healthcare services distributed to older adults [2].

In addition to console-based videogames, online gaming environments such as Second Life [3] are providing positive approaches to psychological rehabilitation, for example with soldiers returning from war zones and are suffering from post-traumatic stress disorder (PTSD). The environment can aid soldiers and their families to understand the causes and symptoms [3-4]. Likewise, exergames have shown to be a positive facet in combating subsyndromal depression (SSD), based upon a 12-week intervention utilizing the Nintendo Wii™ Sports, 35 minutes per session, three times a week. The respective authors reported the results displayed a substantial improvement towards 'depressive symptoms, mental health-related quality of life, and cognitive performance'. However, the results did not show an improvement towards the 'physical health-related quality of life' [5]. To ascertain and build upon the initial findings, the researchers stipulate further investigation is required via randomized control trials [5]. The studies which have been reported in the respective review [1] do not outline the specific segments of the games which have been the most beneficial for health rehabilitation in the respective studies.

The method of interaction is varied in current game technologies and has enabled both proficient and novice users the opportunity to experience new forms of gaming into their lives. Due to the nature of the consumer markets, this has motivated development companies to identify innovative approaches to enhance videogame interaction which has led to the integration of leading-edge elements such as; video capture and inertial sensing devices which have the capability to measure physical movement of individuals. Until recently, such technology could only be found in expensive and dedicated laboratory facilities. It is becoming evident that the use of off-the-shelf game technology within the health sector [see 1] is going to increase, in particular with users unfamiliar with such modes of interaction. There is a possibility that health consumers, their personal and clinical support networks may lack a full understanding of video game technology and how it may best be applied to healthcare.

The aim of this review is to provide an outline of videogame technology that has hitherto been neglected in the games for health literature, that being the classification of commercially available videogames. This review outlines the history, development and procedures undertaken by the 10 rating systems currently in use across three regions (North and South America, Europe, Eurasia, Far East and Australasia). Following this, recommendations are proposed offering guidance for the development of a rating system that will be appropriate for the classification of video games for use in health-related contexts across all regions.

1.1   The Devise and Development of Off-the-Shelf Game Classification Organization

At present, off-the-shelf games are classified by one of 10 organizations depending upon their regional distribution; for North America, The Entertainment Software Rating Board (ERSB) [6], Europe, The Pan European Game Information (PEGI) [7], Australia, The Australian Classification Board (ACB) [8-9], New Zealand, The Office of Film and Literature Classification (OFLC) [10], Japan, The Computer Entertainment Rating Organization (CERO) [11] (CERO), and Singapore, The Media Development Authority (MDA) [12], the Unterhaltungssoftware Selstkontrolle (USK) in Germany [13], the Game Rating Board (GRB) in South Korea [14], Russia [15], and finally the Department of Justice, Rating Titles and Qualifications in Brazil (DJCTO/DEJUS) [16]. It is possible, many games are required to be rated by all 10 organizations. Consequently, all off-the-shelf games which are available on the market have to be rated.

The demise of a classification for videogames was in response to a hearing in the US congress directed by US Senators Lieberman and Kohl, initially resulting in two competing systems in 1994. It was suggested to the industry that a more appropriate rating system would be more suitable. Subsequently, the industry was given one year to devise a self-regulated system or the U.S. federal government would establish a system for implementation [17] and with this in mind, the industry sponsored the developments, resulting in the Software Publishers Association (SPA) and the Interactive Digital Software Association (IDSA, which is now known as the Entertainment Software Association).

The SPA organization created the Recreational Software Advisory Council (RSAC) which was given the role of creating a category system primarily focusing on content. A survey was designed to assess the level (1-4) of content (nudity/sex, violence, and offensive language) quantity and included 'expert media researchers' [17] such as Dorothy Singer and Don Roberts. Consequently, the IDSA formed the Entertainment Software Rating Board (ERSB) which created a system focusing on an age-based classification mirroring that used for film ratings. Initially, four categories were created K-A (Kid through Adult), T (Teen; ages 13 and older), M (Mature; ages 17 and older), and AO (Adults Only; ages 18 and older). Initially the K-A category was utilized but then was split into two categories; EC (Early Childhood; ages 3 and older) and E (Everyone; ages 6 and older). An additional category was added in 2005, E10+ (Everyone 10 and older) and this information was placed on to the front of all packaging. Content descriptors which informed the consumer of the content within the game(s) were placed on to the back of products; however, the level of detail was not consistent to that by the RASC classification system. Overtime, the ERSB classification became the leading system due to the RASC system categories being difficult to understand on the products and for the lack of age inclusion [18].

1.2   Why Is There a Need for a Classification System Aimed at the Health Sector?

The evolvement of hardware and software technologies in the mid-1990s has brought this medium to the attention of researchers focusing upon the devise of classification systems (primarily ERSB, PEGI and MAPP) utilized for the purpose of entertainment media (videogames, internet, music and television). However, the literature outlines that the systems in place are not necessarily reliable although, the systems do provide substantial information. It is suggested further work could be conducted to rectify this issue.

Studies have shown parents perspective of the current entertainment mediums are not satisfactory in providing adequate information, adding to the primary focus of age-based ratings, and content descriptors do not represent the context of the medium in full [20-21].

In addition the notion of "forbidden fruit" has being documented showing games which have been categorized under a label such as mature (M) or adult only (AO) is more alluring to younger audiences, especially boys, [19-18,22] who may want to play violent videogames as a means of proving their "manhood" [18] . Bijvank et al. [22] suggested; "Playing videogames with restrictive labels might be a way for boys to vicariously obtain satisfaction through thrills and antisocial behavior" (pg. 874). The principle work of Bijvank et al. has concentrated on the impact of violence and content exposure [20-22] through video games in addition to, television program content portrayed [23] to young audiences.

1.3   Rating Organizations for Off-the-Shelf Games

Ten classification systems are presented in Table 1 which provides a brief description of how each classification is executed for that particular region/country. The data presented includes, age categories, content descriptors, rating process, who is employed to rate the games and the icons.

Table 1. Presents the rating organizations for videogames

Classification System	Region	Age Categories	Content Descriptors
ERSB http://www.esrb.org/ratings/index.jsp	North America	Early childhood (EC, 3+), Everyone (E, 6+ and 10+), Teen (T, 13+), Mature (M, 17+), Adults only (A), 18+)	Submit online questionnaire detailing pertinent content (all content, context, rewards system & player control). A DVD showing all pertinent content, game play, missions, cut scenes, extreme instances of content and all content that is not playable but exists in the game code must be disclosed. Minimum of 3

Rating process/Raters	Icons
Submit online questionnaire detailing pertinent content (all content, context, rewards system & player control). A DVD showing all pertinent content, game play, missions, cut scenes, extreme instances of content and all content that is not playable but exists in the game code must be disclosed. Minimum of 3 raters, have experience with children	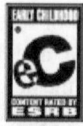 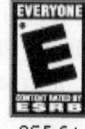 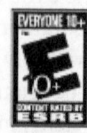 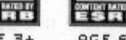 AGE 3+ AGE 6+ AGE 10+ 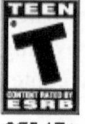 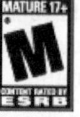 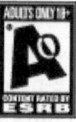 AGE 13+ AGE 17+ AGE 18+

raters, have experience with children,

Classification System	Region	Age Categories	Content Descriptors
PEGI http://www. pegi.info/en/ index/id/26# question_1	Europe, South Africa, UAE	3, 7, 12, 16 and 18 years. * will work within a country law (Portugal). Parental control system; block/ restrict content (2, 3, 5, 7 & 9)	OK label (online content, rated at a 3)

Rating process/Raters	Icons
4 stages. A form is submitted and reviewed. Both content and the game review are assessed prior to giving a suitable PEGI rating. A content declaration is required by the developer/ publisher, giving a complete overview of the game. With this information, it allows the reviewer to concentrate on the particular game elements which may affect the decision of the rating. Netherlands Institute for the Classification of Audio (NICAM) – categorizes games between 3 &7, Video Standards Council (VSC) categorizes games between 12-18.	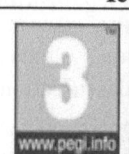 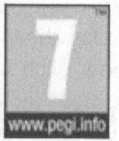 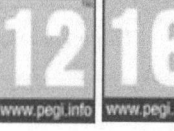 

Classification System	Region	Age Categories	Content Descriptors
Australian Classification Board (ACB) http://www.classific ation.gov.au/Inform ationcentre/Pages/N ewGuidelinesforthe ClassificationofCo mputerGames.aspx	Australia	G, PG, M, MA 15+, R 18+ and RC	No information specified

Rating process/Raters	Icons
Using the National Classification Code (NCC) and guidelines prior to release and advertisement. The classification board assigns a rating and reviews can be sought via the Classification Review Board. Three main areas cover the rating system; (1) the context of the game, (2) impact of the assessment and (3) the decision to employ 1 of the 6 classification systems employed for off-the-shelf games. Raters are present on the classification board.	**MA** 15+ RESTRICTED — Not suitable for people under 15. Under 15s must be accompanied by a parent or adult guardian **G** — General **M** — Recommended for mature audiences **PG** — Parental Guidance Recommended for Younger Viewers.

Classification System	Region	Age Categories	Content Descriptors
Computer Entertainment Rating Organization (CERO) http://www.cero.gr.jp/	Japan	The scheme uses a lettering/color scheme. A & black (all ages), B & green (12+ years), C & blue (15+ years), D & orange (17+ years), and Z & red (18+). Additional icons can be added for educational/database, CERO regulations compatible – used for trial version and rating scheduled – used for promotion items which publishers use for advertisements	26 content descriptors: sex, violence, antisocial (human trafficking, suicide/self-injury, drugs, prostitution, gambling, language). 9 content icons.

Rating process/Raters	Icons
Includes games for household and mobile phones. It covers expressions hidden in commands/tricks. CERO receives an ethics reviewing request. The items subjected to reviewing include 24 items, each expression has an upper limit and if exceeded then they are banned expression, (expressions found within the 26 content descriptors). An age classification is decided based upon evaluating results; CERO notifies the publishers of the result; and The publisher indicates an age classification mark on the product. Raters a recruited from female/male, in various occupations ranged between 20-60 years. Recruited from the public and trained by CERO.	Content icons 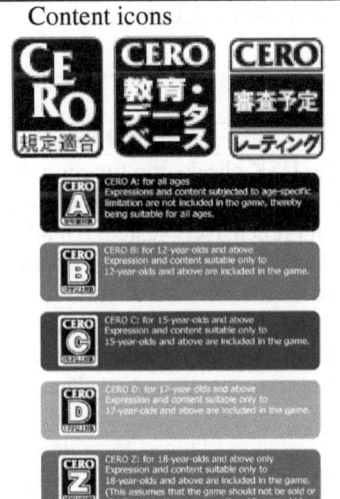

Classification System	Region	Age Categories	Content Descriptors
Departamento de Justiça, Classificação, Títulos e Qualificação (DJCTQ or DEJUS). Department of Justice, Rating, Titles and Qualification	Brazil	6 ratings. L; for all audiences, 10; for people aged 10 plus, 12 and 14 are similar to the ERSB's Teen category, 16; is similar to the ERSB's Mature and suitable for people 16+ and 18 is the equivalent to ERSB's Adult Only.	No information specified

Rating process/Raters	Icons
A completed form outlining the type of platform(s), content, genre, and contact details, including copyright. An overview of the game, and additional material to be classified. A justification for the desired classification based on the content. Evidence of payment to the Development of National Film Industry. Finally the submission of the game will be submitted and within 20 days a response will be given as to the rating decision. No information was sourced relating to the raters.	

Classification System	Region	Age Categories	Content Descriptors
Unterhaltungssoft ware Selbstkontrolle (USK) http://www.usk.de/en/	Germany	These are: 0, 6, 12, 16 and 18. Within each category.	The content descriptors and the age categories are closely linked. For example; the 16 category will include 'acts of violence' and the games will feature armed combat, a framework story.

Rating process/Raters	Icons
The USK checks the functionality of the game and all documentation submitted initially. The game is comprehensively tested. All additional information is collated as supplied by the publisher allowing a full evaluation relevant to child protection issues. A report is written. The USK hands the responsibility for the classification to the Classification Committee whereby the tester presents the game. The USK nor the tester issues an age suggestion. Each member of the committees has the opportunity to play the game in full which 'is a unique approach worldwide'. Classifications are determined by an advisory council comprising g if 16 people from an array of	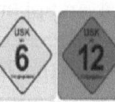 

backgrounds (churches, youth associations, research institutes, federal government and federal state ministers, ministers of education and cultural affairs of the federal states.

Classification System	Region	Age Categories	Content Descriptors
Media Development Authority (MDA). http://www.mda.gov.sg/Industry/Video/Guidelines/Pages/VGClassificationGuidelines.aspx	Singapore	A game can be assigned an M18 (mature 18) and enforceable by law. In certain circumstances, if titles carry 'contentious elements' an age advisory label is required. If games contain content which exceeds 'acceptable social standards & could be potentially harmful to society'.	Includes violence, nudity, sex, language and drug use.

Rating process/Raters	Icons
The board will take into account: generally accepted social mores, need to protect the young, racial/religious harmony, national interest, treatment of theme and content, evaluation of impact, creative educational merit. Third-party modifications are not rated by the board. No information is specified regarding the raters	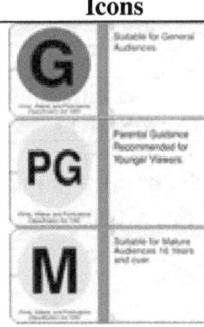

Classification System	Region	Age Categories	Content Descriptors
New Zealand http://www.censorship.govt.nz/industry/industry-games.html	New Zealand	G, PG, M, MA 15+, R 18+ and RC. There are 5 classifiable themes within each rating category	No information specified.

Rating process/Raters	Icons
Conducted under the act this contains the NCC. The act covers 4 points: (a) the standards of morality, decency and propriety generally accepted by reasonable adults;(b) the literary, artistic or educational merit (if any) of the publication, film or computer game; (c) the general character of the publication, film or computer game, including whether it is of a medical, legal or scientific character; (d) the persons or class of persons to or amongst whom it is published or is intended or likely to be published. Decisions made under the code should address the following: (a) adults should be able to read, hear, see and play what they want; (b) minors should be protected from material likely to harm or disturb them; (c) everyone should be protected from exposure to unsolicited material that they find offensive; (d) the need to take	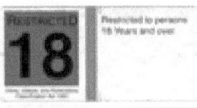

account of community concerns about: (i) depictions that condone or incite violence, particularly sexual violence; and (ii) the portrayal of persons in a demeaning manner. Office of Film & Literature Classification (OFLC). An expert gamer will play the game while an officer from the office examines the game against the criteria located in the Classification Act.

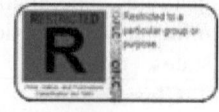

Classification System	Region	Age Categories	Content Descriptors
Game Rating Board. http://www.grb.or.kr/english/default.html	South Korea	A – for all, 12+, 15+, 18+ and T for testing	There are 7 content descriptors: sexuality, violence, fear/horror/threatening, language, alcohol/tobacco/drug, crime/anti-societal/anti-governmental messages, gambling

Rating process/Raters	Icons
3 processors to the rating process. Within the first process there are 6 stages. Stage 1: application submitted online, stage 2: all documents checked, stage 3: in-depth review/technical test and game is examined by tester/reviewer. Stage 4: decision of rating/content descriptors. Stage 5: there are 3 options at this level; rating pending, rating decision or provisional rating declined. Stage 6: the rating is issued with a certificate. The additional 2 processors provide an informative overview of how to appeal against a rating. The rating board comprises of 15 individuals from the areas of education, law NGO member who meet every Wednesday and Friday to discuss the forthcoming ratings.	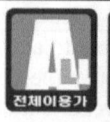 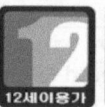 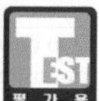 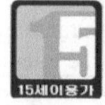 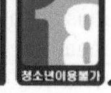      

Classification System	Region	Age Categories	Content Descriptors
Federal Law of 28.07.2012 N 139-FZ. Article 12.	Russia	0+, 6+, 12+, 16+, 18+	Content which is banned includes: the encouragement of children to commit a threat to their life, drug, alcohol consumption, gambling, prostitution, and vagrancy, the incitement of violence towards animals or humans. Foul language, denying family values and

Rating process/Raters	Icons
	being disrespectful towards parents and pornographic material.
Category '0+' is aimed at children 6 and under. Reviewing a translated document via a web link, it seems the document outlines that products are assigned a classification by an expert. However the definition of 'expert' is not specified. The assessment of suitability will include: the subject, genre, contents and artistic design, perception of information for each age category, the probability of certain content being harmful to the health/development of children.	No icons available. On products there may also be a text warning in adidtion to the figures. The text warning is "for childre older than six years". There is a minimum of 5% sizing for the icons which will be employed on the product.

2   Discussion

Overall there have been five continents comprising of ten regional/countries which have been reviewed in respect to the approval of off-the-shelf games. The main features identified from the classification systems are: (1) the process of application, (2) content descriptors, (3) age categories, (4) execution of rating a game, and (5) code of conduct. It is important to note, not all of the information was available via the documentation for example reviewing the information for Brazil and Russia did not report an in-depth analysis in comparison to the ERSB or PEGI. Although these features are utilized across the regions, there are also, discrepancies across the classification systems forming a variance of how videogames are rated and categorized for the market? This leads to the question, where does 'games for health' stand within the market place for the future use within clinical/home settings and users?

2.1   Games for Health

Since the release of the PlayStation® Eye toy (1999) and more recently the Nintendo™ Wii (2005) and Microsoft™ Kinect (2010) consoles; researchers have focused their efforts, to applying these technologies for the benefit of health rehabilitation in conjunction with commercial software (Wii Sports/Resort). The commercial software will have to have undergone an inspection by the regional classification board prior to being released in the respective region(s). However, with this notion becoming popular and results albeit utilizing small populations suggest this approach could be fruitful; additional work is needed in this area. Several recommendations were proposed by [1] relating to future work conducted in the realm of commercial technologies and health rehabilitation.

Alternatively, researchers, clinicians and entertainment manufactures may need to consider obtaining approval for the use of specific hardware and content for the purpose of health rehabilitation. For example; the development of drugs by pharmaceutical companies are required to complete a process comprising of several stages which are necessary for the release of a new drug on to the market. The process can be lengthy and may take several years before the approval is granted via government bodies such as the Food and Drug administration (FDA) [24] in America which also approves medical devices into three categories (1-3). Category three is the most regulated, and is defined as a device which can support or sustain life or has the ability to prevent impairment or has the potential to cause harm relating to illness or injury [25]. Additionally, Class II devices require both special and general control requirements which refer to labeling or mandatory performance standards. Class I devices require little regulation but do require general control requirements. This includes manufacturing of site registration, listing the device, premarket notification and quality system regulations [26, 27].

For the approval of medical devices, a Premarket Approval Application (PMA) is completed similar to that submitted for a New Drug Application (NDA). A private license is granted for marketing a medical device. However, a class 3 device which fails the PMA requirements is deemed 'adulterated' and cannot be marketed [25].

Approval of medical devices in Europe is granted by the European Council Medical Device Directive [26-28]. Altogether there are four classifications and the higher the category, the more invasive and risky it is to prospective individuals. To classify a device, several factors are considered; (1) length of use, (2) invasive or surgically invasive, (3) is the device implantable or active, and (4) contains a therapeutic substance.

It is proposed with future studies and the identification of results via the integration of commercial hardware for health rehabilitation, video game consoles may have to be processed through this application, to be certified and be legally covered which in turn will enable appropriate information to be sought by the public and the health sector to identify such devices which have been suitably passed to be categorized as a medical device.

2.2   Content Descriptors

As previous studies have shown the parent's perspective of content descriptors is not sufficient and the studies conducted by [20-21] identified 45 observations of content which could have had a justified content descriptor in 29 games, which were absent. The respective authors concluded games rated at category M (ERSB) include a variety of unlabeled content which may be exposed to audiences who are impressionable and influence behavior, perceptions and attitudes.

Thompson & Haninger [21] contend the level of violence in E-rated games is extensive, although the content descriptors do reiterate this level of intensity, further caution is required. The results showed genres which required the gamer to kill/injure a character were rewarded and overall, there was intentional violence implemented into genres such as sports, racing, and action which may not have been published on the packaging. This leads onto the suggestion that content descriptors provided by the ERSB, are misleading and may not cover the full spectrum of the game content.

It is suggested, the assignation of content descriptors can be inconclusive and the ERSB do not provide sufficient detail relating to content descriptors. Furthermore,

[20] note, the ERSB assigns descriptors to some games but not all which contain the same content thus, leading to confusion for parents who are seeking a comprehensible indicator. With this in mind, [20] propose the ERSB should provide greater transparency about the descriptors and their rating standards.

Conversely, the MDA specifically outlines game content which is not allowed within games and if it is implemented then it is possible the game will not be classified and will be banned. For a game to be rated M18 (Mature 18), six areas will be reviewed: (1) theme, (2) violence, (3) sex, (4) nudity, (5) language, and (6) drug use. Indicators are placed on to the products which may contain this type of content within the game. Similar content areas are focused upon under Federal Law in Russia. However, there are no specific labels assigned to the products and the level of content varies depending upon the specific age category. Moreover, the Russian Federal Law focuses upon content which does not encourage children to inflict violence and self-harm to themselves, animals and other humans. Vagrancy/begging and the denial of family values including being disrespectful towards elders is assessed. The DJCTO/DEJUS in Brazil also has no content descriptors for the classification of games and reviewing the translated documentation (Russia and Brazil) there were no specific content descriptors examined.

Based upon existing studies not all content is presented and appropriately categorized, especially in games such as Grand theft Auto (GTA) whereby; the gamer has the potential to unlock hidden content via codes or completing tasks. Consequently, this facet changed the initial rating by the ERSB from M to AO [20]. With this in mind, the concept of establishing a suitable health rating system to be comprehensible by the public is crucial, especially the design/implementation of content descriptors to ensure the content which has been implemented into the game is projected correctly on to the packaging. It is suggested, this notion would provide all interested parties will feel safe in utilizing commercial games for use in the health sector.

2.3   Age-Based Labeling

The implementation of a rating system by age is clearer to understand by parents than content descriptors. On the contrary, [19] reported age-based ratings are simpler to understand than detailed descriptors to base a decision. However; the authors state "the system fails if there is no true consensus on what is age appropriate" [19] (pg 42), resulting in the limited use of the rating system by parents. An age appropriate system will vary depending on the region although the alignment with the current rating systems, the content has to be deemed appropriate by parents not by the organization(s). In Table 1 nine of the ten classifications have icons which are placed onto the products with the exception of Russia. Although they have an age classification system, the respective document provided no visual icons. Taking into account the information presented in the translated document, there was no detailed outline as to how parents or guardians are advised to the classification of games across Russia. The classification system implemented in Brazil is closely associated to that of the ERSB.

It has been noted the application of age-based ratings allures younger users to play or watch content, known as forbidden fruit [18-19, 22]. Although the purpose of the rating systems is to provide guidance to parents, earlier studies have shown some parents do not follow the age-based categories, nor, pay close attention to the information. Therefore, it is questionable, whether there should be an overhaul of the rating systems? Gentile et al., [19] concluded the perceptions by parents in the respective study, requires change, and consideration should taken into account to establish a universal rating system across all entertainment mediums, which was recommended by The American Academy of Pediatrics. This notion could be suitable for these mediums. However; it is questionable whether a universal system would be appropriate for games with the primarily purpose of health rehabilitation. Equally, it is questionable whether this would eradicate the confusion and contradictions of content descriptors and age-based ratings which is currently being witnessed?

2.4   Rating Process

Rating the actual game content is utilized by similar processors across all regions. There are however, regional differences during this process. Likewise, the region of Australasia uses a color coding system which identifies games that are restricted in one country but not in another (New Zealand). The PEGI system uses a similar classification unless the law of a particular country varies for example; Portugal which has a different age rating to that of other European Union (EU) countries. The age classification implemented by the ERSB is similar to that of PEGI, but again varies. The age rating is more detailed, than PEGI and Australasia, including additional systems, starting approximately at the Teen level and Adult Only (18+). In Japan, a color scheme, with a letter from the alphabet, follows a similar ethos to PEGI and Australasia. However, the rating system employed in Singapore has two categories; Mature 18 (M18) and if caution is required a separate label is assigned stating 'suitable for 16 & above'. If games do not fall into either of these categories but are approved for distribution, the games are not required to carry any rating label. Although there are no age-based labels used, the MDA do suggest that parents are required to seek out more information about the game content prior to purchasing.

Likewise, seven of the ten organizations do not report actual game playing when reviewing a game for a classification rating. However, the three classification boards that do execute game play are South Korea, New Zealand and the USK in Germany. Additionally the USK report that the whole game is played and allows all of the advisory committee to play the game prior to making a final decision. The USK website states this facility is unique worldwide. All ten organizations use different approaches; the ERSB employs adults who have experience with children. Two administrations are used by PEGI one for rating games aimed at children and one aimed at teenagers/adults. PEGI do not stipulate the experience of the raters employed, but in comparison to Australasia who use the expertise of a gamer(s) to play the game, in conjunction with an officer from the OFLC, who examines the content against a set criterion.

Furthermore, the CERO recruits various people between the ages of 20-60 years who are employed in a variety of occupations. The MDA board assigns ratings to games, and consists of individuals from both the education and business sectors. The raters recruited by the USK are individuals who are associated in professions concerned with the welfare of children. For example; the church, youth organizations, research institutes, Federal government and Federal State Ministers of education and cultural affairs. Furthermore 50 individuals, State wide have been appointed from areas such as teachers and journalists. Similar raters are utilized by the GRB in South Korea but also comprises of individuals from the legal profession and non-governmental organizations (NGO). The rating process in South Korea comprises of six stages, the first stage comprises of the application being submitted, at stage 2 all of the documents are checked and then at stage 3 the game undergoes an in-depth examination by a tester/reviewer. Stage 4 comprises of a rating decision based on the content descriptors, followed by stage 5 which has three parts (rating pending, rating decision/provisional or rating declined). Stage 6 is the issuing of a certificate. The rating system in Russia is executed by an expert. However, in the translated document, there was no specific detail relating to the assignation of the expert. Similarly, in Brazil the translated document outlined no detail of how the product is rated or by whom.

Taking into account the approaches of content and age based ratings from 10 organizations there are several differences; (1) labeling of content descriptors and age-based categories, (2) similar age-based coding with the exception of Singapore, (3) rating process of games varies across all organizations; and (4) Japan provides informative labels displaying additional game/rating standard.

Consequently, off-the-shelf games for entertainment are regulated; but a regulation of games for rehabilitation does not exist. Therefore the authors suggest, with collaboration amongst academics, industry professionals, health practitioners, patients and their support network(s) a universal classification system should be devised to display critical information which would inform prospective users the suitability of a game for rehabilitation. Similarly, the Australian government have designed and implemented a tick symbol which is placed onto food packaging to display the nutritional value to consumers. It is suggested, what has been employed here, could be taken and built upon within a suggested health rating system. Additionally, researchers and clinicians should contemplate particular areas of a game which could be more beneficial to the patient whereby a positive effect is being noted during the rehabilitation.

Taking into account the information presented in this paper, the authors are proposing several recommendations building upon previous literature to initiate a discussion of a classification system for games aimed at the health sector. Several recommendations are proposed which have been highlighted from earlier studies, but also taking into account the information from the different regions in a bid to start a discussion and process for stream lining a game classification which is presented in Table 1.

- Adopt/devise a national classification system for all entertainment mediums [18-19], with the additional section relating to games for health.
- In future studies, clinicians and researchers should attempt to identify which areas of the game(s) are most beneficial to the patient during the rehabilitation.
- Suitable content descriptors to represent different health conditions.
- Adopt the notion of the PEGI, Australasia or Japan color schemes used for the age-based rating categories which would provide consumers an easier way to understand the category. However, based upon parents differing viewpoints, it is suggested adopting the labeling system employed in Singapore maybe more cohesive.
- Consideration should be taken into account if age-based rating were to be maintained. The organization/regulation should abide by each country's law. This has been demonstrated with the roll out of PEGI in Portugal.
- Conduct interviews with parents to gain further insight to understand and establish how parents perceive age and content categories [18-19]. It is anticipated this would facilitate building upon knowledge for re-categorization and can be broadened to include patients, clinicians to aid in the design of health categories.
- Conduct initial consultation and guidance by the prospective board in relation to health and the potential for law suits by the public based upon the game(s) being suitable for health rehabilitation. In conjunction; the need for future longitudinal studies of health and games should be considered, following a similar process to that by the FDA approval of medication.
- A consistent approach to the rating of games for use within a clinical/health environment. This could take on experience and guidance from clinicians, support networks, patients, academics and industry professionals who have substantial experience in a variety of environments in particular randomized control trials (RCTs). It is suggested undertaking a similar approach to that of the USK (Germany) whereby, the whole game is played by the raters/reviewers would be suitable to understand and assign a suitable health classification.
- Implementing a tick symbol similar to that utilized in Australia for healthy food, is a possibility to indicate the suitability of software for utilization in the health sector. This could be implemented as an initial stage of the process while the design and devise of a fully entertainment medium classification is being produced.
- Current and future commercial game hardware systems will apply for approval from respective government agencies to be classified as an appropriate medical device. This would mean games companies applying to the FDA and the European Council Medical Device Directive.

The proposed recommendations have taken into account the information which has previously being published by the respective authors, in conjunction with the work by [1].

It is suggested, if there was an overhaul of the classification system as proposed by [18-19] enabling the new system to follow the existing system implemented by the MDA organization in Singapore, whereby games which contain themes, require a M18 or an advisory notice. Additionally, removing the age-based rating could be justified based upon the studies which have outlined, parents do not actually take on board the age-based ratings. Furthermore, it has been established that parents find the content descriptors confusing, and in some instances, some games do not carry the necessary descriptors as they should, [18-19] it is questionable whether this should really be continued.

On the contrary, adopting a similar system to that used in Singapore would enable parents to decide for themselves which games are suitable for their children based upon their own information seeking and parental values. However, the primary objective of a new system is to target games which have been identified suitable for use in the health sector. Therefore, suitable content descriptors are needed which may aid prospective users to initially identify the suitability of the product for a particular health complaint/condition. This detail would need to be thoroughly discussed and an appropriate design label(s) created if it was decided to be included.

Similarly, raising the awareness to the research and industry communities regarding the subject of approval is at present not a necessity but the authors feel this is an area which may encounter future concerns from a legal stand point. In particular, if there are specific claims about a piece of hardware/software. For example, software/hardware which is said to facilitate the prediction and prevention of falls, the authors question whether approval from the appropriate authorities is required for 'medical devices' and whether there should be some level of certification to actually display to users the proposed equipment is appropriate for this particular rehabilitation.

It is suggested, further investigation would include the legal profession, government bodies, researchers, clinicians and manufactures to identify and understand the potential if any, of future actions brought forward from individuals who have used the hardware/software for a specific health complaint. With this in mind, one approach for all groups concerned is to initially conduct a series of discussions based upon the investigations being conducted to gain clarity for the published studies, and to identify if at any point there could be legal action or approval required.

3   Conclusions

Employing a universal rating system in addition to a health sub-category has the potential to be cohesive throughout all health settings. Integrating similarities between the classification organizations could provide ease of use and adoption. However, it is suggested a similar format to that of Singapore which presents itself in a simple and cohesive format maybe the most suitable or a combination of the ratings systems to ensure all necessary information is presented.

Nevertheless, agreeing upon a universal rating structure would entail representatives from each of the rating organizations, in conjunction with academics, clinicians, patients and their support networks, having to agree upon a new set of criteria with the assistance of industry professionals and the rating organization boards. This would take time and lengthy discussions amongst many interested parties. During the process of a new classification system additional consultation with the FDA and the European Council Medical Device Directive bodies should be considered to determine the legal/approval standpoint of commercial game products for health. Consequently, the impact of an aging society and the issues and recommendations which have been identified in this paper are important facets for the future use, sustainability and the integration of technology into the lives of older adults.

References

1. Marston, H.R., Smith, S.T.: Interactive Videogame Technologies to Support Independence in the Elderly: A Narrative Review. Games for Health Journal 1(2), 139–152 (2012)
2. Smith, S.T., Schoene, D.: The use of exercise-based videogames for training and rehabilitation of physical function in older adults: current practice and guideline for future research. Aging Health 8(3), 243–252 (2012)
3. Linden Labs, Second Life, PTSD education, http://secondlife.com/destination/t2-ptsd-education (accessed January 2012)
4. Games: Improving Health, ESA, http://www.theesa.com/games-improving-what-matters/ESA_FS_Health_2011.pdf (accessed January 2012)
5. Rosenberg, D., Depp, C.A., Vahia, I.V., Reichstadt, J., Palmer, B.W., Kerr, J., Norman, G., Jeste, D.V.: Exergames for Subsyndromal Depression in Older Adults: A Pilot Study of a Novel Intervention. Am. J. Geriatr. Psychiatry. 18(3), 221–226 (2011)
6. Entertainment Software Rating Board (ERSB), http://www.esrb.org/index-js.jsp (accessed January 2012)
7. Pan European Game Information (PEGI), http://www.pegi.info/en/index/id/28/ (accessed January 2012)
8. Australian Classification Board (ACB), http://www.classification.gov.au/ (accessed January 2012)
9. Australian Classification (Publications, Films and Computer Games) Act 1995 (2008). Guidelines for the Classification of Computer Games. Attorney-General's Department, Canberra (2011), http://resources.news.com.au/files/2011/05/25/1226062/865826-guidelines-for-computer-games-classification.pdf
10. Office of Film & Literature Classification, New Zealand (OFLC), http://www.censorship.govt.nz/industry/industry-games.html (accessed January 2012)
11. Computer Entertainment Rating Organization (CERO), http://www.cero.gr.jp/
12. Media Development Authority (MDA), http://www.mda.gov.sg/Industry/Video/Guidelines/Pages/VGClassificationGuidelines.aspx
13. Unterhaltungssoftware Selskontrolle (USK), Germany, http://www.usk.de/en/classification/
14. Game Rating Board (GRB), South Korea, http://www.grb.or.kr/english/default.html
15. Russia Federal Law, Article 12 (July 28, 2012), http://base.consultant.ru/cons/cgi/online.cgi?req=doc;base=LAW;n=133372;from=108808-0;div=LAW;rnd=0.05636497470550239

16. Departamento de Justiça, Classificação, Títulos e Qualificação(Department of Justice, Rating, Titles and Qualification) (DEJUS), Brazil,
    `http://portal.mj.gov.br/classificacao/data/Pages/MJ6BC270E8PTBRNN.htm`
17. Chalk, A.: Inappropriate Content: A Brief History of Videogame Ratings and the ERSB, The Escapist Magazine (July 20, 2007),
    `http://www.escapistmagazine.com/articles/view/columns/the-needles/1300-Inappropriate-Content-A-Brief-History-of-Videogame-Ratings-and-the-ESRB`
18. Gentile, D.A.: The rating systems for media products. In: Calvert, S., Wilson, B. (eds.) Handbook of Children, Media, and Development, pp. 527–551. Blackwell Publishing, Oxford (2008)
19. Gentile, D.A., Maier, J.A., Hasson, M.R., Lopez de Bonetti, B.: Parents' Evaulation of Media Ratings a Decade After the Television Rating Were Introduced. Pediatrics (2011), doi:10.1542/peds.2010-3026
20. Thompson, K.M., Tepichin, K., Haninger, K.: Content and Ratings of Mature-Rated Video Games. Arch. Pediatr. Adolesc. Med. 160(4), 402–410 (2006)
21. Thompson, K.M., Haninger, K.: Violence in E-Rated Video Games. JAMA 286(5), 591–598 (2001), doi:10.1001/jama.286.5.591
22. Bijvank, M.N., Konijn, E.A., Bushman, B.J., Roelofsma, P.H.M.P.: Age and Violent-Content Labels Make Video Games Forbidden Fruits for Youth. Pediatrics 123, 870 (2009), doi:10.1542/peds.2008-0601.
23. Cantor, J.: Ratings for Program Content: The Role of Research Findings. The ANNALS of the American Academy of Political and Social Science 557(1), 54–69 (1998)
24. Food and drug administration (FDA),
    `http://www.fda.gov/Drugs/default.htm` (accessed April 2012)
25. Food and Drug Administration (FDA). Medical devices,
    `http://www.fda.gov/MedicalDevices/ProductsandMedicalProcedures/DeviceApprovalsandClearances/PMAApprovals/default.htm`
26. Mackenzie, J.H.: Regulation in the Medical Devices Industry in the US and Europe. Business Briefing: Medical device Manufacturing and Technology (2004),
    `http://www.touchbriefings.com/pdf/954/qualimedd_techEDITED.pdf` (accessed April 2013)
27. Hills, B.J.: The EU Medical Devices Approval Process: Device Classification and the Technical File (2011),
    `http://www.gatewayfda.com/medical-devices/the-eu-medical-devices-approval-process-device-classification-and-the-technical-file/` (accessed April 2013)
28. European Medicines Agency (EMA),
    `http://www.ema.europa.eu/ema/index.jsp?curl=pages/home/Home_Page.jsp&mid` (accessed April 2012)

A Preliminary Evaluation
of a Participation-Centered Gameplay
Experience Design Model

Luís Lucas Pereira and Licinio Roque

Department of Informatics Engineering
University of Coimbra, Portugal
{lpereira,lir}@dei.uc.pt

Abstract. In this paper we report on evaluation experiments from a Participation-Centered Gameplay Experience Design and operationalising instrument following a Design Science Research approach. The proposed model aims to contribute to an informed game design process by giving center stage to the notion of participation - the way players take part in the gameplay activity - from which a gameplay experience emerges and is interpreted by players. In order to achieve such an outcome, the model proposes six lenses for participation: Playfulness, Challenge, Embodiment, Sociability, Sensemaking and Sensoriality, to be able to rationalize and reflect on different forms of playing. To operationalise the model we present a design instrument consisting of a set of guiding questions, designed to elicit the main gameplay experience features, which strengthen each form of participation. We report on the evaluation of the model and instrument based on their introduction and use by 15 teams of game design students during their conceptualization phases, on 8 different project themes. We further present an analysis of students classification of the instruments, on understandability, productiveness and relevance, crossed with an analysis of the notebooks produced during the concept creation, to discuss and decide different ways to improve the model.

Keywords: Game Design, Gameplay Experience, Design Methods, Evaluation, Design Science Research, Participation-Centered Design.

1 Introduction

The Gameplay Experience is the ultimate goal of playing a videogame. Designing a videogame consists of enabling and inhibiting forms of player participation according to an idealized experience [1]. When designing a game, a player experience is always invoked, regardless of whether it is considered explicitly or implicitly, in the designer's decision-making process. It is our basic conjecture that the explicit consideration of the participatory qualities of the gameplay experience could help orient the game design activity towards configuring the design elements most capable of enabling the intended forms of participation.

A. Holzinger et al. (Eds.): SouthCHI 2013, LNCS 7946, pp. 332–348, 2013.

If on one hand the aim of a videogame object is to support an experience, on the other, the design of this experience is not directly within the designer's reach in view of the non-deterministic nature of our relation with technology and of the subjectivity associated with the experience [1]; This challenge is compounded with the difficulty in addressing (characterizing, thinking, streamlining) the videogame, mainly because of its multiple character. From the previous perspective arises the research motivation to focus on the issue of player participation in the game play experience.

In this paper we report the results from a first evaluation of a Participation-Centered Gameplay Experience Design Model aimed at supporting the design and analysis of videogames, in order to achieve a rationalization between what the designer intended the playing experience to be and the experience potentially achieved, as interpreted by players. This model will be further developed through the characterization of forms of player participation in the game play activity.

One key feature of this model is the goal of assist the process of game design at different stages design intention, artefact configuration and gameplay experience evaluation providing a unified vision for the activity of game design through the notion of participation. For model operationalisation we developed a set of guiding questions designed for reflection on the player's participation elicited by the gameplay experience. In a Design Science Research context, the game design guiding questions correspond to a design artifact and, as a result, we discuss which ones should be improved based on the evaluation report.

Section two presents the research context for the creation of the proposed game design model. Section three we present the initial proposal of the game design model and in section four we report on the process of creating and evaluating the Participation-Centered Gameplay experience Design Guidelines (PGxDG) instrument to operationalise the model, with a discussion of issues found during design experiments. In section five we discuss further research on the model and instrument and on section six we present our conclusions.

2   Background

2.1   Game Design Models

The variety of forms that a video game may take, along with the diverse nature of its elements, may result in a complex and obscure design process. If one adds to this the qualities of the different experiences that a video game may support, then analyzing and streamlining the decision-making processes leading to an intended experience becomes a challenging task. In the text "I Have No Words & I Must Design" Greg Costikyan[2] states that "as game designers, we need a way to analyze games, to try to understand them, and understand what works and what makes them interesting", suggesting that a critical language is needed in order to achieve that.

Game Design Models as abstract representations provide vocabulary and set of concepts that help to think, analyse and design games in a more formal way [3]. Based on his experience as game designer, Church [4] states that models give a way to talk about the underlying components of a game. Instead of just saying, That was fun, or I dont know, that wasnt much fun, we could dissect a game into its components, and attempt to understand how these parts balance and fit together. In the essay Formal Abstract Tools Church [4] proposes a potential framework taking the form of a set of design tools. These design tools are modular concepts that aim to contribute to a terminology for moving the game design discussion forward, going beyond the discussion of fun. Others contributions to analyse and design games in a formal way are the MDA framework [5], Patterns in Game Design [6], the PLEX framework [7].

The game design models referenced contribute to a formal understanding of game design, through diverse approaches, still, a common feature of these models is the fact that they do not include an explicit relationship between the analysis of game design and evaluation of the gaming experience. The model of game design that we propose, and for which we developed a guiding instrument that is evaluated in this paper, aims to contribute to the practitioner's reflection-in-action on the gameplay experience from the definition of design intentions to the characterization of the game object, but also as a framework for developing participation indicators for evaluating the player's experience, as illustrated in [8].

2.2 Gameplay Experience and Participation

User Experience is hard to define and characterize in a formal manner because of its holistic and multi-dimensional nature [9] [10]. In the game studies field, gameplay experience has often been characterized through concepts like fun [25] [11], flow [12][13] or immersion [14][15]. In addition to the often ambiguous definition of these concepts, their usefulness for design purposes is questionable, at least in the sense that they do not allow us to think of the experience enabled by the videogame medium in a way which is both clear, comprehensive, and generative of new experiences.

Play is experienced through participation. When a player interacts with a game, the formal system is manifest through experiential effects. [16] Participation is seen as a key feature of the videogame medium [17][18]. The player takes part in determining the activity. The experience emerges through actual player participation, through the interpretation of the context of the game and how the player acts in it. Design is the process by which a designer creates a context to be encountered by a participant, from which meaning emerges. [16]

We consider the design of a videogame as the creation of a special kind of context [1]. This context consists of elements that promote and inhibit certain forms of participation, from which experience and meaning emerges. In order to design a videogame it is then necessary to consider how the elements composing the game medium will be translated by the player, so as to support the intended forms of participation and, consequently, a game playing experience. Thus, we find the concept of participation to be very influential in the ideation of gameplay experience and, consequently, in the design of games as participatory media. It is therefore relevant to think of the design activity in terms of player participation and to develop measurable indicators of participation as essential instruments towards a more informed design.

3 Methodology

Design artifacts in the form of conceptual frameworks are a usual type of knowledge production in Human-Computer Interaction research community. Our overall research aim deals with the creation of conceptual instruments to support the design and evaluation activities on the videogame medium. On the theoretical nature of this contribution, the proposed model was developed through the synthesis of concepts that aim to inform and interpret the design and evaluation of videogames.

To address this research challenge called for a methodology that would enable us to experiment with different approaches to design, as part of a process to explore the relation between the design solutions proposed and the results achieved. [19][20]. Design Research is a research method that accurately fits these needs. [21]. Design Research "involves the analysis of the use and performance of designed artifacts to understand, explain and very frequently to improve on the behavior of aspects ... .Such artifacts include - but certainly are not limited to - algorithms (e.g. for information retrieval), human/computer interfaces and system design methodologies or languages" [22]. One type of design research consists of an iterative process, which includes several phases - Awareness of Problem, Suggestion, Development, Evaluation, and Conclusion [22]. Design Research starts with an Awareness of Problem from which it is generated a proposal for a new research effort. The problem is the lack of methodological guidance for Game Design and Gameplay Experience Evaluation. Research outputs of DSR include constructs, models, methods, instantiations, and better theories [22].

In the context of our study, we are interested in using Design Science Research to achieve a model to support Game Design activities. From the suggestion phase of Design Research results a tentative design of the research outputs, mainly the proposed Participation-Centered Gameplay Experience Design and Evaluation Model. In the next section we will present the initial design of the model to characterize Gameplay Experience. Once completed the model, in the development phase we achieved the first version of a derived artifact a set of design guidelines based on proposed model to support game design activity, in the form of questions for reflection.

In this paper we report on the first evaluation of the proposed game design guidelines, corresponding to the artifact evaluation step the DSR process. The evaluation process is described in section 5 and aims to understand if this instrument can help novice designers orienting game design activities and to draw implications for the revision of the gameplay experience model underlying the production of the guidelines instrument. This evaluation centered on assessing how understandable and influential the modeled concepts were in learning and design practice.

4   A Participation-Centered Gameplay Experience Design Model

In this section we present an initial proposal for a model to guide the activity of game design. The model is instrumental in our attempt to address the question of: how to reframe the design of a videogame from the perspective of players participation? This model is intended to have a guiding role, assisting the designer in considering how the player takes part in the game. To achieve that we consider six perspectives on participation: Playfulness, Challenge, Embodiment, Sensemaking, Sociability and Sensoriality (fig. 1). These dimensions seek to assist the designer in thinking, in a comprehensive manner, about the range of possibilities at her disposal to define or give a certain character to a game. The perspectives considered result from the synthesis of the literature on the nature of play activity, the conceptualization of the gameplay experience and the motivation of the players.

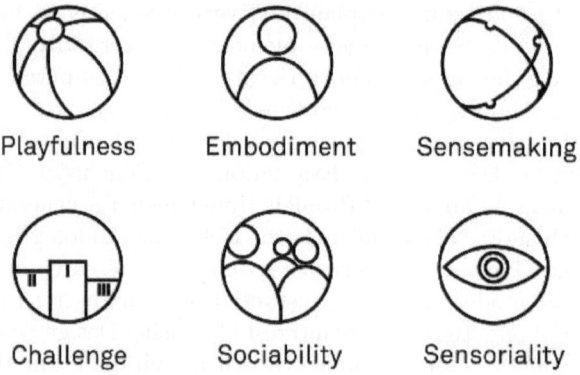

Fig. 1. Six perspectives to rationalize the participation of players

We will present the references that support each perspective. The number of perspectives considered comes from the criteria used in the conceptualization of the model. This number was reduced to a minimum to ease the model appropriation and rationalization that still allowed us to approach the design of the medium and the gameplay experience in a wide and inclusive way. In turn, we expect these six forms of participation can also be used to characterize gameplay activities, so as to confront actual player participation with the intention originally set. These lenses are mostly complementary and when successfully integrated they should provide an holistic perspective. Moreover, it can be quite complex to establish a rigid boundary between these views of interaction as, often, different forms of participation share common aspects when realized in a game artifact.

With the purpose of operability of the model thus presented in the context of design activities, we identified three operative focus: defining design intentions, characterizing game artifacts and mapping and analyzing player participation. Those three focuses derive directly from the conceptual base that supports the proposition of the model centered in the concept of participation: bearing in mind that the videogame, as an artifact, mediates the players participation from which the potentially intended playing experience emerges. In the following subsections we will describe the three focuses along the six participation perspectives.

4.1 Focus of Analysis

Intention. The first operational level concerns Intention: What is the participation ideal that the videogame is suggesting? It is often from a design intent that the conception of a gameplay experience emerges. As already noted, we assume that a design exercise departs from a proposed experience ideal, by configuring certain forms of participation. At the intent level of operation we generate and organize the proposed forms of participation and, implicitly, the kind of experiences to be enabled. This focus analyses and rationalizes the character or style of the proposed or idealized game, meaning, the essence or value of the game activity.

Artifact. The second operational level concerns the Artifact: How does the artifact supports the idealized forms of participation? At this level we envision an object as medium that enables an interaction context calling for the intended forms of participation. In other words, we aim to align the features of the artifact with a model of player interaction supportive of the intended player participation. This focus analyses and rationalizes the artifact videogame as network of mediators that support the participation, helping us to think about the nature of the mediators them selves used in the artifact.

Participation. Finally, the third operational level concerns Participation: What characteristics of the actual player activity are consistent with or revealing of the participation idealized? This level of operation is meant to focus observation, analysis and evaluation of actual player participation, in particular, to examine if the game activity meets the design intent, and to point towards the indicators and metrics we can define that would be revealing of progress towards that intent. This focus allows characterizing player participation, measuring the level of alignment between the real appropriation of the game by the player and the idealized.

4.2 Six Perspectives on Participation

Playfulness. The videogame as a context of free, informal, and unstructured participation. Think of the videogame as a toy with interpretative flexibility, allowing for player exploration and improvisation. Player participation is based on interaction with the game led by an intrinsic motivation. This lens is based on the concept of paidia (free-form, spontaneous, child-like type of play) [23]. Evidence for the plausibility of this lens is found in the literature in the context of player motivations Discovery, Customization, Escapism [24], Easy Fun [25] ; player profiles Explorers [26]; and the characterization of the gameplay experience Creation, Exploration, Discovery [27].

Challenge. The videogame as a context of structured participation, of a formal challenge, or according to a proposed target. Think of the videogame as a goal driven context, defined by rules. Player participation is assessed in terms of how relevant his performance is in overcoming the challenge, given the purpose of the game. Player performance is usually linked with the mastery of physical or mental abilities. This lens is based on formal perspectives of games, what Callois [23] describes as ludus (rule-based, structured play) and agón (competitive activities). Evidence for the plausibility of this lens are found in the literature in the context of player motivations Advancement, Competition [24], Hard Fun [25]; player profiles Achievers, Killers [26]; and the characterization of the gameplay experience Difficulty, Competition [27], and challenge-based immersion [14].

Embodiment. The videogame as a context of physical participation, both virtual and actual. Think of the videogame as a context for physical performance. Player participation is based on the physical relationship established between the player and the videogame, whether that happens through the virtualization and representation of the players body in the game itself, thereby projecting the players body in the virtual physical space of the game, or just by interpreting player movement as an interface with the game. This lens is related to immersion in relation to the players embodied interaction with screen-and-speaker world, partly by providing salient somatosensory and proprioceptive support for the feeling of embodiment presence in the game world. [28]; Evidence of the plausibility of this lens can be found in the literature on player motivations Altered States [25]; and the characterization of the gameplay experience Sensation [27], sensory immersion [14].

Sociability. The videogame as a context of social participation, of establishing relationships between players. Think of videogame as a context for legitimizing forms of interaction between players, of role configuration. Player participation is based on the establishment of relationships, whether of competition or cooperation, or through any another type of communication. This lens is based on the perspective of games as social systems [30]. Evidence for the plausibility of this lens can be found in literature on the context of player motivations Socializing, Relationship, Teamwork [24], The People Factor [25]; player profiles Socializers [26]; and the characterization of the gameplay experience Camaraderie[27].

Sensemaking. The videogame as a context of significant participation, of creation of meaning. Think of the videogame as a means of expression. Player participation is based on interpreting and acting on the semantic space represented in the videogame. This lens is related to the "significant function" of play phenomena [29]. Evidence for the plausibility of this lens can be found in the literature in the context of player motivations Role-Playing [24], Easy Fun [25]; and the characterization of the gameplay experience Simulation, Fantasy [27], imaginative immersion [14].

Sensoriality. The videogame as a context of multisensory involvement. Think of the game as a source of stimulation for the senses. Player participation is then based on engaging in perception, filtering, acceptance or reproduction of a stimulus. This lens is grounded on the sensorial dimension of an experience [9] and is strongly related to Embodiment lens. We decided to include two different lenses because they put in perspective different characteristics of the artefact: space and movement (Embodiment), and style and atmosphere (Sensoriality). Evidence of the plausibility of this lens can be found in the literature on player motivations Altered States [25]; and the characterization of the gameplay experience Sensation [27], sensory immersion [14].

5 From Model to Instrument: Participation-Centered Gameplay Experience Design Guidelines (PGxDG)

5.1 The Making of the PGxDG Instrument

To assist in idea generation, reasoning and analysis of decisions in the game design process, and to operationalise the proposed model, we developed PGxDG instrument based on 5 guiding questions for each participation lens in the model. The choice of making guidelines in the open-ended form of questions is to promote creativity and reasoning.

The questions on table 1 are the first set of draft question designed to elicit designer's reflection along the model perspectives and correspond to the first iteration of a design process for an instrument to support game design. These questions were defined in order to explore the topics behind each participation lens, based on the literature, and with the aim of stimulating reflection with varying depth by participants on the design process. We limited the construction of the instrument to the selected five questions per perspective with the intention to keep it effective, yet simple enough to avoid overloading the design exercise. Questions were grouped in sections to preserve and explore the context of each lens.

To evaluate the model globally, i.e. whether or not it is helpful in practice, we are, at first, interested in understanding if the proposed questions are effectively understood by users of the proposed model, and whether or not they are perceived as productive, i.e., if they help to generate meaningful contributions in the definition of a game design concept. With this first iteration of the models evaluation in the context of game design learning activities, we wanted to gather data that could help improve the design instrument, for its effectiveness with the target user group.

Table 1. Proposal of Participation-Centered Game Experience Design Guidelines

	Label	Operational Questions
Playfulness	PL1	What type of game characteristics incentive free participation?
	PL2	What kind of restriction constrains free participation of the players?
	PL3	Which interactive elements enhance free participation?
	PL4	To what extent players can express themselves through free participation?
	PL5	To what extent the game promotes improvisation by the players?
Challenge	CH1	What are the goals and how do they organize the participation of the players?
	CH2	What are the possible outcomes of the game?
	CH3	How does the game value the participation of the players?
	CH4	What type and level of skills are required by the game?
	CH5	What is the flexibility in the ways to achieve the proposed goals?
Embodiment	EM1	How to characterize the game space?
	EM2	What is the perspective of players regarding the game space?
	EM3	What is the representation of players in the game space?
	EM4	How do the players physically interact with the game?
	EM5	How to characterize possible movements in the game space?
Sensemaking	SM1	What is the theme of the game and its underlying messages?
	SM2	What is the role of players in the represented semantic context?
	SM3	How is the semantic context represented?
	SM4	What are the significant procedures in the game?
	SM5	How do each of the other perspectives help build that semantic context?
Sensoriality	SS1	What is the style and atmosphere that the game offers?
	SS2	What are the main feelings that the game is intended to invoque?
	SS3	What are the elements responsible for sensory stimuli?
	SS4	How do different stimuli relate to each other? (work together)
	SS5	To what extent the sensory environment results from participation of players?
Sociability	SO1	What is the social configuration proposed by the game?
	SO2	What kind of interactions between players are proposed by the game?
	SO3	What kind of roles are proposed by the game?
	SO4	How does the participation of a player influences the participation of others?
	SO5	What kind of perception players have of each other? (visibility)

5.2   Evaluation Context and Method

The evaluation of the participation-Centered design instrument presented serves
two purposes: To understand if the instrument itself can be helpful for orienting
game design activities, in particular in the context of learning to perform game
design; To draw implications for the revision of the gameplay experience model
behind the production of instrument itself, by assessing how understandable and
influential the concepts in the model were in learning and design practice. This
evaluation was carried out in the context of an elective course on Game Design
and Development, part of a Masters on Informatics Engineering study program.
In it, game design students must conceive and develop a videogame demo in
one semester, going through concept definition, detailed design, implementation,

and gameplay experience evaluation. The model and instrument were presented during the concept definition phase, in which the guidelines questionnaire was used as support for their initial design process. The class in which we rehearsed the use of the instrument is constituted by 60 game design students, organized in 15 teams of 3 to 6 members, ages ranging from 22 to 30, predominantly male (95%) and come from an Informatics Engineering background (95%). All students have an understanding of English as second language.

The starting point for each of the projects was a set of themes (Petri Dish, Internet Memes, Dance it, Move it, Play 360, Sound Emotion, Roses Miracle, and Multiplayer Surreal) which were assigned to groups based on stated preferences and breadth of coverage of the themes. Projects briefs drafted and presented had little detail on how the design should be developed. With the several theme proposals, we intended to promote diversity in the projects conceptual domain, so that, on one hand, we could provide opportunity to analyze and discuss different aspects of game design during course debates, and, on the other, to create opportunities for students to explore how the participation-Centered model of gameplay would be employed in a diversity of project domains, that could promote exploration of its multiple dimensions.

Throughout the use of the model, we also gave game design students a questionnaire for them to rate the guiding questions, to be ranked on a Likert scale ("Strongly Agree", "Agree", "Undecided", "Disagree" and "Strongly Disagree") regarding understandability of each question ("read and understood the question"), and productivity of the question towards the design (can we find answers in the design intention). A further option was given in the productivity scale - "Not Applicable" - which was intended to signal for analysis any questions that designers found were not applicable to their specific design case. Finally, students were asked to rate the relevance of questions ("helped us think even if it did not produce a direct response") by feely distributing 10 relevance points through all questions (at most 1/3 of questions got points).

In order to make the design process more structured and auditable, we made available to each group an A2 board with the guiding questions. This printout had 6 areas - the participation model perspectives - to be used as notebook to write notes and ideas during their design sessions. Through this instrument we hoped to help the students collect ideas, possibly enabling analysis of ideas generated by which questions, which of these lead to greater and lesser number of meaningful answers, and to verify if the result was coherent with students own perception as derived from the validation questionnaires. After the themes were attributed and the game design model was presented and the design supporting instruments were given and their use staged during a kickoff design session, teams were asked to proceed autonomously to outline their concepts, in the form of a 7 minute presentation, for the next week, at which time questionnaires and notes were collected for analysis.

5.3   Results

The results described in this section come from two data sources:

(a) the survey intended to evaluate the students perception of the questions proposed, their understandability and usefulness;
(b) the analysis of the notes resulting from the 15 exercises of game concept definition;

The surveys were answered individually producing 60 surveys that were subsequently analyzed. Of the 15 work groups, 14 delivered useful notebook sheets.

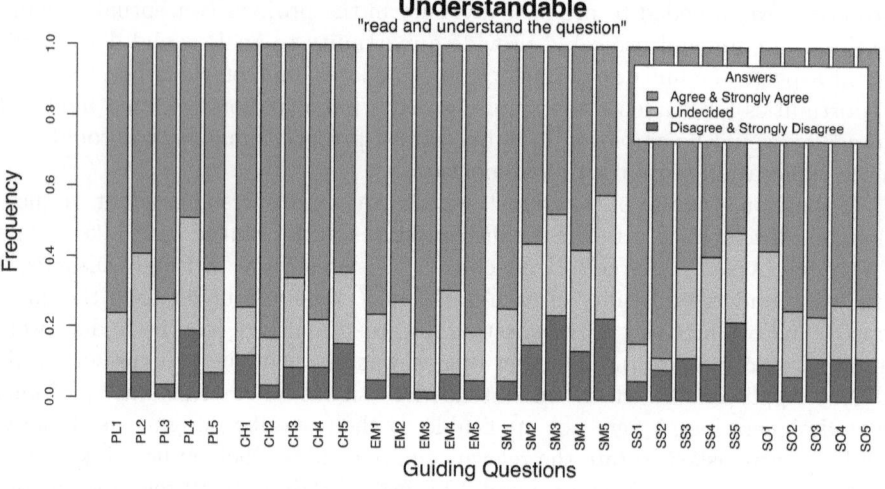

Fig. 2. Instrument classification: "understandable"

The graphs on Fig. 2 and Fig. 3 represent the results of the guiding questions classification regarding, respectively, their understanding and productivity. Taking into account the type of answer to these questions and the evaluation we intended to do, we opted to group the results over three categories: positive (Strongly Agree and Agree); neutral (Undecided) and negative (Disagree and Strongly Disagree). Therefore, on the Fig. 2 and Fig. 3 graphs, each bar represents the classification result for each guiding question (tagged according to Table 1), where the frequency of answers for the three groups is represented.

On the Fig. 4 graph, a count of the guiding questions classified as not applicable is presented. On the Fig. 5 graph, we represent a count of the guiding questions classified in terms of relevancy points attributed. On this relevancy classification, 13 surveys werent considered because the lack of validity of the answers.

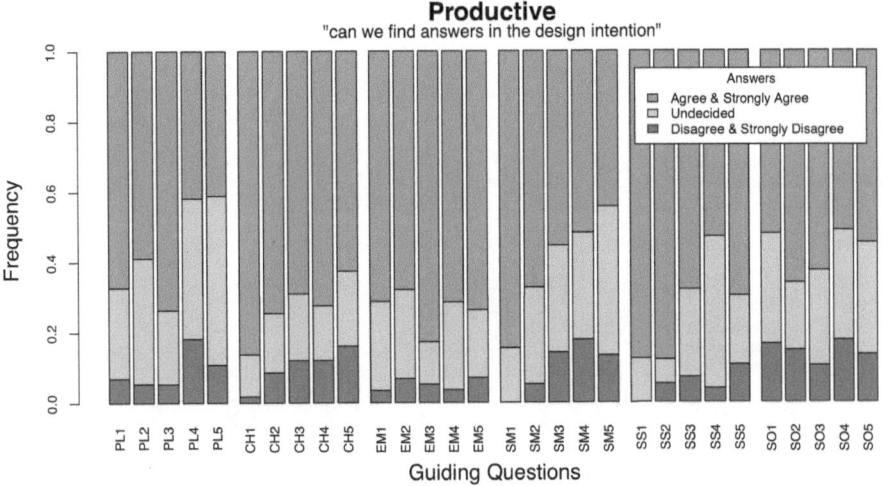

Fig. 3. Instrument classification: "productive"

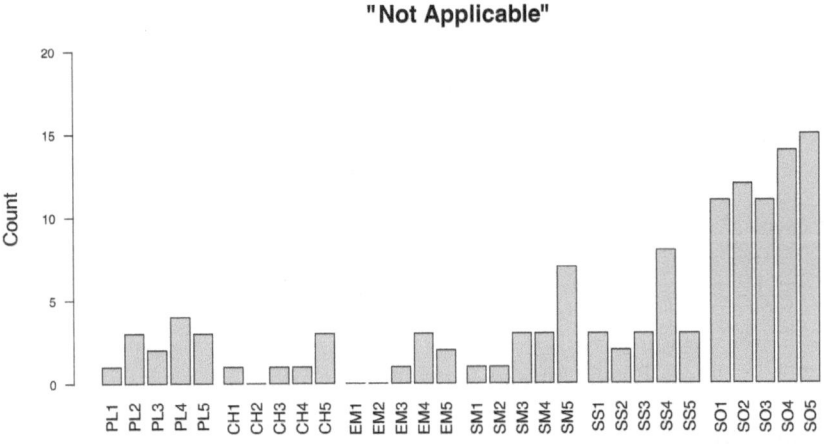

Fig. 4. "Not Applicable" questions

The analysis of the notes resulting from the exercise of game concept definition was made through the counting of coherent answers to guiding questions found in each participation area of the notebook, as classified by the researchers. The number of coherent answers given to each guiding question is represented in Fig. 6.

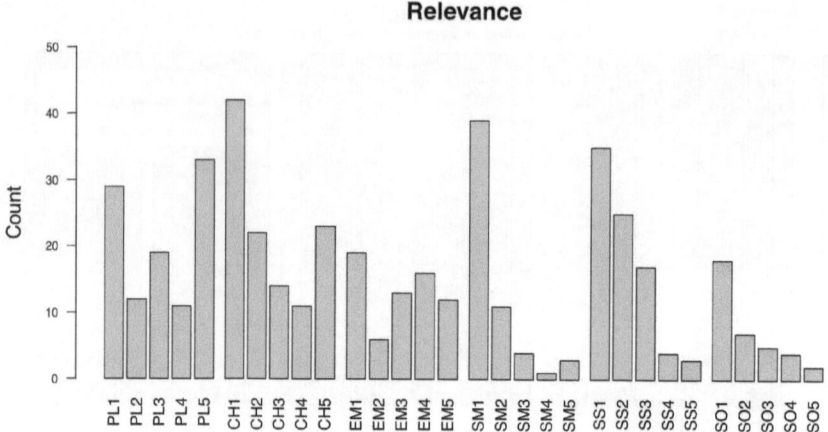

Fig. 5. Instrument classification: "relevance"

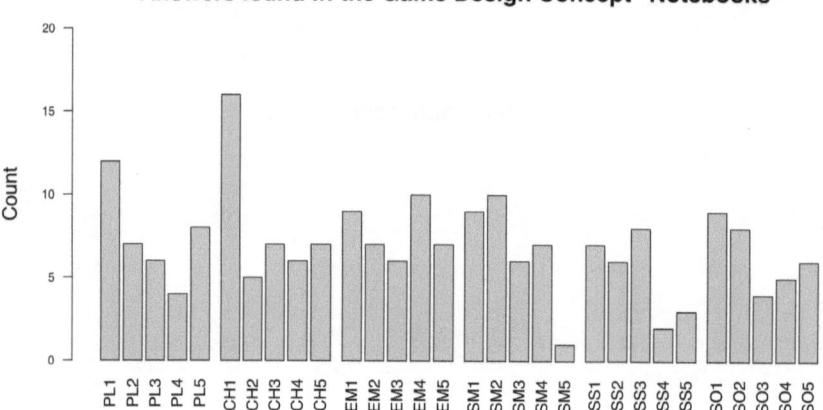

Fig. 6. Answers found in "Notebooks"

5.4   Discussion

The objective of the model usage evaluation was to gather information that would allow us to: a) improve the model; b) identify potential problems regarding the proposed guiding instrument; and c) its usefulness regarding the concept definition for a gameplay experience and proposed artefact characteristics.

Understandability. As for the results analysis about the understanding of the questions by model users, we identified as candidates for reformulation those guiding questions that had a number of negative answers (Disagree and Strongly Disagree) above 10%. With this criteria we identified questions PL4, CH1, CH5, SM2, SM3, SM4 and SM5, SS3, SS4, SS5, SO1, SO3, SO4, SO5. The questions

SM3, SM5, SS5 deserved special attention because they presented a challenge to approximately 25% of the population, along with the questions PL4, CH5, SM2, SM4 that registered approximately 20% of negative answers.

Question CH1 denotes some controversy, although it counts more than 1% of negative answers, it also counts a significant number of positive answers (Strongly Agree and Agree), 75%. We consider that a possible reason for this is the fact that this question has a double intention (What are the goals and how they organize the participation of the players?). The same kind of controversy happens on the questions SO3, SO4 and SO5, deserving a more detailed analysis against other classifications.

On the guiding questions from each participation perspective as a whole, the questions belonging to the Sensemaking perspective seemed to be the more problematic in terms of understanding them. This might relate to a difficulty in decoding the more abstract terminology adopted, such as, semantic context instead of narrative, story or plot. We opted to use a distinct terminology, from the one usually employed in the game design literature, to contribute to a more divergent thinking, while trying to avoid potential pre-conditioning on the game conception exercise if typical solutions were hinted on. Still regarding the participation perspectives, groups of guiding questions belonging to the Embodiment perspective were those that demonstrated the best results on the understanding classification given by the model users.

Productiveness. As for the analysis of the results on the questions' productivity we opted for two criteria. We have identified as candidates for reformulation the questions that possessed a rate of negative answers (Disagree and Strongly Disagree) above 10%, and a number of positive answers (Strongly Agree and Agree) below 66%. With these two criteria we identified the following candidates: PL2, PL4, PL5, CH3, CH4, CH5, SM3, SM4, SM5, SS4, SS5, SO1, SO2, SO3, SO4, SO5. Questions PL4, CH5, SM4, SO1 and SO4 deserve special attention by having approximately 20% of negative answers. As well as the questions PL4, PL5 and SM5 that display only about 43% of positive answers.

As a whole, the questions belonging to the Sensemaking and Sociability perspectives record the worst results in productivity, a results coherent with the understanding classification, which might denote a consequence relationship. On the Sociability group it is noticeable a high number of not applicable classifications as Fig. 4 graph shows. We attribute this distinct classification to the game concepts defined as single player, which leads us to a future reflection on whether this sociability perspective of participation runs out or not in a single player game. As a whole, questions belonging to the Embodiment perspective, again, show the best results, similar, again, to the understanding classification.

Relevance. Through the analysis of Fig. 5 it is possible to notice that the questions generally considered less relevant by model users were SM3, SM4, SM5, SS4, SS5 and SO3, SO4, SO5, which is consistent with the understanding and productivity classifications.

Game Design Concept Notes. From the analysis of Fig. 6 we can conclude that the guiding questions for which less answers could be indentified on game concept notebooks were PL4, SM5, SS4, SS5 e SO5, fact that is coherent with the classifications displayed on the surveys/questionnaires. Again, it's on the Sensemaking and Sensoriality participation perspectives that we find the worst answer counts, therefore, the main candidates for reformulation of this design instrument.

Analysis of the notebooks show that coherent answers were actually produced for the guiding questions associated with the Challenge perspective, which seems to contradicts some of the criticism related to productivity on this section. This analysis of notebooks also shows that the questions associated with the Sociability perspective appear partially answered on the notebooks, somewhat questioning the negative perception shown on questionnaire classifications for this perspective - on the productivity scale, relevance and, most of all, on the "not applicable" classification.

6   Future Work

In this paper we presented an evaluation of a questionnaire for stimulating a participation-Centered gameplay experience design. Further work will focus on tuning this instrument by answering to specific problems identified on this analysis. Moreover, it is still unclear to the researchers to what extent the analysis of the impact of using this instrument can be transferred to reform the model itself. Possibly this will require further content analysis of the text in notebooks produced during the conceptualization phase, and an ethnography of the design process that can reveal further impacts downstream, as teams re-iterate design models while moving from concept to prototype.

In terms of research methodology, the exercise of evaluation presented in this paper represents a first cycle of design research, where we evaluate the interpretation and perception of usefulness of the first version of the game design instrument. For the next cycle of design research a new version of this instrument will be drafted based on the results of this evaluation and further evaluation activities will be undertaken, encompassing the evaluation of the gaming experience.

For further evaluation and development of the model we will also need to consider issues related to its scope, analyzing in which way these perspectives are adequate or comprehensive in characterizing players participation. To that end our current major concern is to determine how to observe and measure player's participation in game play contexts through the proposed lenses. For each proposed dimension we want to identify a set of indicators and metrics for evaluating players participation.

7 Conclusion

In this paper we presented a participation-Centered gameplay experience model to guide game design activities. We developed a design instrument in the form of guiding questions as a methodological instrument to help apply the proposed model in game design activities. The proposed instrument was introduced in a set of design exercises, conducted with 15 teams of game design students during a one week process of concept definition. Having outlined the basic structure, the model and instrument is being tested, evaluated and improved in consecutive iterations, following a Design Science Research approach. Current evaluation being reported generally shows the model dimensions are being explored in design exercises with consistent outputs being achieved under the several lenses, although some particular aspects of the design instrument need further work, specifically, a set of guiding questions were identified as troublesome in understandability, productivity and general perception of relevance. Overall this preliminary evaluation of the game design instrument and model allowed us to collect detailed and valuable information to improve this instrument for next iterations of design research.

Acknowledgements. This work was supported by the Fundação para a Ciência e Tecnologia (Foundation of Sciences and Technology) (SFRH/BD/45114/2008) and the CISUC ICIS project CENTRO-07-0224-FEDER-002003.

References

1. Roque, L.: A sociotechnical conjecture about the context and development of multiplayer online game experiences. In: DiGRA 2005 Conference: Changing Views Worlds in Play (2005)
2. Costikyan, G.: I have no words I must design: Toward a critical vocabulary for games. In: Computer Games and Digital Cultures Conference Proceedings, Tampere, Finland (2002)
3. Salen, K., Zimmerman, E.: The game design reader. MIT Press (2006)
4. Church, D.: Formal abstract design tools. Game Developer 6(8), 44–50 (2009)
5. Hunicke, R., LeBlanc, M., Zubek, R.: MDA: A formal approach to game design and game research. In: Proceedings of the AAAI Workshop on Challenges in Game AI, pages 0404 (2004)
6. Bjork, S., Holopainen, J.: Patterns in game design. Cengage Learning (2005)
7. Korhonen, H., Montola, M., Arrasvuori, J.: Understanding playful user experience through digital games. In: International Conference on Designing Pleasurable Products and Interfaces, pp. 274–285 (2009)
8. Pereira, L.L., Roque, L.: Gameplay Experience Evaluation Centered on Participation: the Fátima Game Design Case. In: Proceedings of the 2013 ACM Annual Conference Extended Abstracts on Human Factors in Computing Systems Extended Abstracts (2013)
9. McCarthy, J., Wright, P.: Technology as experience. MIT Press (2004)
10. Hassenzahl, M.: Experience design: Technology for all the right reasons. Synthesis Lectures on Human-Centered Informatics 3(1), 1–95 (2010)

11. Fullerton, T., Swain, C., Hoffman, S.: Game design workshop: a playcentric approach to creating innovative games. Morgan Kaufmann (2008)
12. Csikszentmihalyi, M.: The flow experience and its significance for human psychology. Cambridge University Press (1988)
13. Chen, J.: Flow in games (and everything else). Communications of the ACM 50(4), 31–34 (2007)
14. Ermi, L., Mayra, F.: Fundamental components of the gameplay experience: Analysing immersion. In: Worlds in Play: International Perspectives on Digital Games Research, p. 37 (2005)
15. Thon, J.: Immersion revisited: on the value of a contested concept. In: Extending Experiences-Structure, Analysis and Design of Computer Game Player Experience, pp. 29–43 (2008)
16. Salen, K., Zimmerman, E.: Rules of play: Game design fundamentals. The MIT Press (2004)
17. Aarseth, E.: Cybertext: perspectives on ergodic literature. Johns Hopkins Univ. Pr. (1997)
18. Raessens, J., Goldstein, J.: Computer games as participatory media culture. In: Handbook of Computer Game Studies. MIT Press (2005)
19. Cross, N.: Engineering Design Methods: Strategies for Product Design, 4th revised edn. John Wiley and Sons Ltd., Chichester (2008)
20. Schon, D.A.: The Reflective Practitioner: How Professionals Think in Action. Ashgate Publishing Limited, Aldershot (1991)
21. Hevner, A.R., Chatterjee, S.: Design research in information systems: theory and practice. Springer, New York (2010)
22. Vaishnavi, V., Kuechler, W.: Design Science Research in Information Systems (2004), http://desrist.org/desrist (last updated September 30, 2011) (retrieved August 1, 2012)
23. Caillois, R.: Man, play, and games. Univ. of Illinois Pr. (2001)
24. Yee, N.: Motivations for play in online games. CyberPsychology & Behavior 9(6), 772–775 (2006)
25. Lazzaro, N.: Why we play games: Four keys to more emotion without story. Design 18, 1–8 (2005)
26. Bartle, R.: Hearts, clubs, diamonds, spades: Players who suit muds. Journal of MUD Research 1(1), 19 (1996)
27. Costello, B., Edmonds, E.: A tool for characterizing the experience of play. In: Proceedings of the Sixth Australasian Conference on Interactive Entertainment. ACM (2009)
28. Gregersen, A., Grodal, T.: Embodiment and Interface. In: Perron, B., Wolf, M.J.P. (eds.) The Video Game Theory Reader 2, Routledge, London (2009)
29. Huizinga, J.: Homo ludens: A study of the play-element in culture, vol. 3. Taylor & Francis (2004)
30. Klabbers, J.: The magic circle: Principles of gaming & simulation. Sense Publishers (2006)

Increase Physical Fitness and Create Health Awareness through Exergames and Gamification

The Role of Individual Factors, Motivation and Acceptance

Philipp Brauner[1], André Calero Valdez[1], Ulrik Schroeder[2], and Martina Ziefle[1]

[1] Human-Computer Interaction Center
[2] Computer-Supported Learning Research Group
RWTH Aachen University, Germany
{brauner,calero-valdez,schroeder,ziefle}@comm.rwth-aachen.de

Abstract. Demographic change and the aging population push health and welfare system to its limits. Increased physical fitness and increased awareness for health issues will help elderly to live independently for longer and will thereby reduce the costs in the health care system. Exergames seem to be a promising solution for promoting physical fitness. Still, there is little evidence under what conditions Exergames will be accepted and used by elderly. To investigate promoting and hindering factors we conducted a user study with a prototype of an Exergame. We contrasted young vs. elderly players and investigated the role of gamer types, personality factors and technical expertise on the performance within the game and changes in the attitude towards individual health after the game. Surprisingly, performance within the game is not affected by performance motivation but by gamer type. More importantly, a universal positive effect on perceived pain is detected after the Exergame intervention.

Keywords: Exergame, Health Awareness, Design For All, Gamer types, Physical Fitness, User Acceptance, Gamification.

1 Introduction

Todays society is facing a tremendous demographic change that will push the health and welfare system to its limits. One central issue is the rising number of elderly and frail people that depend on the support of others. Currently, 3.2 jobholders support one elderly person. According to current projections this dependency ratio will fall by over 50% to 1.85 jobholders supporting one elderly person within the next 40 years. Furthermore, the share of elderly people being 80 years and older will rise from 5% in 2008 to 14% in 2060[1]. As these very old people demand special medical attention and increased support by others, this leads to additional stress in the health and welfare system in many societies. In

A. Holzinger et al. (Eds.): SouthCHI 2013, LNCS 7946, pp. 349–362, 2013.
© Springer-Verlag Berlin Heidelberg 2013

order to keep the health-care system affordable, new and innovative approaches must be developed. One central goal should be to focus on prevention instead of treatment. Some preliminary results suggest that "Exergaming" – a combination of the words "Exercise" and "Gaming" – is a suitable tool to offer prevention instead of treatment by increasing physical and cognitive fitness of elderly [2,3].

Various Exergames exist in various different domains. However, only few of them are targeted at the growing population of elderly people. To build commercially successful and clinically useful Exergames the factors promoting or hindering the acceptance and usage of these games must be identified. To understand these factors we conducted a formal user study. Although focused on acceptance and performance aspects of Exergaming, we also investigated whether these games raise the awareness of the importance of individual health. In the following section we will very briefly review related work, in section 3 we will describe the Exergame we used in the study. The results of the study are presented in section 4, which is followed by a discussion of the findings in section 5. The paper concludes an outlook for subsequent research.

2   Related Work

Exergames seem to be a useful approach to meet the challenges raised by the threatening cost explosion in the care sector. By including people – especially the older ones – to keep physically fit, the demands for increased care costs and the shortcomings in the care personnel could be met.

The popularity of Exergames however is not only supporting the health status of persons, even though this is a key factor in this context. They also help to establish a health related behavior, an awareness of healthy living habits and a sensitivity of the individual responsibility to care for themselves, especially at older age[4]. This novel shift from former public care – which traditionally was mostly limited to health insurances and medical personnel – to individual care responsibility is an important step into a cognitive reframing of peoples mindset. Understanding health issues and the importance of prevention in combination with a playful approach increases the health motivation to promote bodily interaction to play the game.

The potential power of Exergames are based on old psychological principles, as e.g. performance feedback and rewards[5], self-control and self-efficacy[6], fun [7] and motivation principles, such as the Premack principle[8]. According to Premack the intrinsic motivation of humans can be harnessed by coupling a less desirable activity with more desirable activities. In the context of physical exercises and raising health awareness would be coupled with joyful activities such as playing a (computer-) game within an enjoyable setting.

Beyond these positive effects of games, the design process of Exergames also needs to consider some specifics of seniors. Beyond the well-known decrease in short-time memory, speed, executive functions and visual perception[9], it should be taken into account that older adults have an outdated understanding of technology and a reduced experience in using current technology[10]. Still it has been found that the interest in novel technology in older adults is high[11]. Contrary to young users, technology is not merely interesting because it is just novel, but technology interest in older seniors heavily depends on how useful technology is for them and how much the technology meets seniors high standards for aesthetic design and fun. The fear of being stigmatized by technology also influences seniors interest in technology[12].

There are limited valid psychometric instruments to describe people regarding their gaming preferences. One approach is the Bartle Player Type that origins from the analysis of massive multiplayer online games (MMOGs). The Bartle test was revised by Yee[13] and developed into a scale with the three main dimensions *Social*, *Achievement* and *Immersion* and 10 sub-dimensions that describe different gaming motives. People who score high on the social scale like to play games for building and maintaining relationships either within the game or outside to game. Achievers are driven understanding the game mechanics and optimizing their strategy accordingly, by competing against others or by advancing in a game and collecting money or resources. Players, who dive into a new role, customize their appearance and enjoy discovering new areas within a game score high on the Immersion scale.

Unknown in this regard is what motivational concepts can be leveraged to harness the desire to play an Exergame especially in regard to the very old.

3   Method

In this section we detail the methodology underlying this paper. First we describe the game "FruitSalad" which had been developed for this work. Then the experimental setup, the independent and dependent variables are outlined and the formation of the participant group and their characteristics are outlined.

3.1   Game Development

To investigate human factors affecting the acceptance of Exergames we first developed a prototypic game by using a participatory, user-centered and iterative design process. The game is similar to an already existing prototype "GrabApple" [14] that uses a Kinect sensor for detecting the users movements and also places the user inside a virtual garden to pick up apples from a tree. The difference between "GrabApple" and our custom-tailored "FruitSalad" lies in the target group. "GrabApple" is de-signed as a casual game to promote physical fitness, while "FruitSalad" explicitly targets elderly people and therefore focused on high contrast images, sounds that are perceivable even with hearing impairments and game play that leverages the cognitive abilities of the elderly. Also the "FruitSalad" game is – besides its gaming nature – designed as a tool in which different factors can be modified, varied and examined.

Regarding the development process, we started with a paper prototype and gathered feedback from potential users about the game concept and the visual appearance. As previous studies revealed that elderly users like games with a gardening theme[15], we designed a game in which fruits and vegetables had to be collected from trees and soil. The game starts with a brief introduction screen that explains how the in-game avatar is controlled and how the game can be paused at any given time by performing a specific gesture. For detecting the users body movements and performed gestures we used a Microsoft Kinect sensor. To allow the users to see themselves in the garden and to get direct feedback on their body movements and picking activities, the player is presented as a virtual avatar within a garden.

Currently the game consists of three consecutive levels: The first two are training levels for practicing the movements to grab a fruit from the tree (level 1) and to pick up a carrot from the soil (level 2). In the third level, the users have to pick up fruits and vegetables from both trees and soil (Fig. 1 shows an in-game screenshot (left) and a user playing the game during the study (right)).

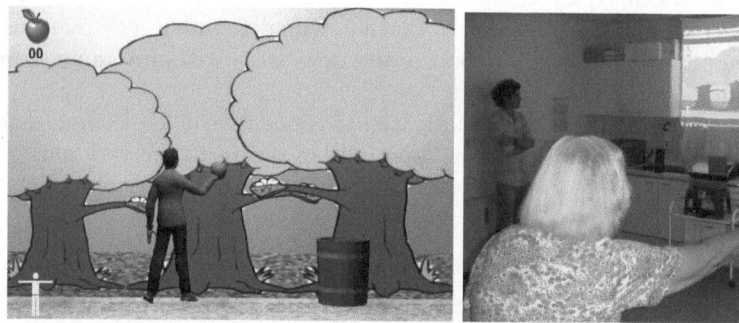

Fig. 1. In-game screenshot of the game (left) and a user playing the game (right)

3.2   Experimental Setup

To understand what factors influence the liking of Serious Games for promoting body movements and task performance within Exergames we carried out a controlled experiment. Although the game supports serving multiple fruits and vegetables at the same time, we limited this to exactly one element at a given time and thereby reduced confounding effects in this study. Participants were instructed with a predefined script and were interviewed prior and after the experiment. For deriving hypotheses a research model with crucial factors had been formed (see Fig. 2). The independent and dependent variables are listed in the following.

Independent Variables. On the side of independent variables, we examined gender and age (contrasting a younger and an older group) as typical "carrier variables" which need to be detailed regarding other individual moderator variables. As moderation variables we surveyed the individual extent of performance motivation, gaming motivation and inclination towards games, technical expertise (usage frequency and perceived ease of use of technology) and technical

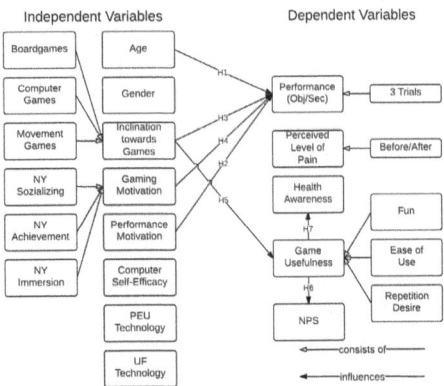

Fig. 2. Research model and Hypotheses. NY = Nick Yee Player Types, PEU = Perceived Ease of Use, UF = Usage Frequency, NPS = Net Promoter Score.

self-efficacy. Based on findings from previous studies we suspected that technical expertise influences task performance as well as liking of the developed game prototype. To validate this assumption we measured the technical expertise of the participants with three scales: First, the usage frequency of a set of technical devices (computers, TVs, ...). Second, the perceived ease of use of these devices was assessed.. Third, the participants subjective technical expertise (STC)[16]. The latter scale consists of questions such as "I can solve many technical difficulties I encounter on my own". This scale is closely related to self-efficacy can explain difference in learnability, performance differences and differences in product liking [17,18]. Also, as individual attitudes towards gaming could impact the liking and performance, we assessed gamer types by a revised Bartle Player Types scale by Yee[13] and the inclination towards different game types in general. We measured performance motivation by a scale from Schuler[19].

Dependent Variables. As dependent variables we measured the task performance (seconds per object) for each of the three levels, the participants perceived pain level before and after the experiment and the evaluation of the games usefulness in terms of "easy to use", "fun" and "wish to play the game again". As an overall rating of the developed prototype we additionally inquired the Net Promoter Score (NPS)[20]. The single 10-level Likert scale asks how likely the user will recommend the game to its peers. While consisting of a single item, this scale can effectively predict the success of a product.

Hypotheses. We assumed that age had a negative effect on performance, as younger players are expected to have a higher fitness level (H1). We also expected that people with high performance motivation are more inclined to use Serious Games for increasing physical fitness than people with a lower performance motivation (H2). Furthermore both inclinations towards gaming in general (H3) as well as gaming motivation (H4) in particular should influence performance.

General inclination towards gaming should also affect the evaluation of the games usefulness (H5), which in turn should influence NPS (H6) and changes in health awareness (H7). Gender, technical expertise and changes in perceived level of pain are used as controlling variables (see Fig. 2).

3.3   Description of the Sample

In total 71 persons volunteered to take part. The age range was 20 to 86 years ($M = 48.3$; $SD = 21.6$). 50.3% of participants were female (36 females, $M_{female} = 48.2 years$; $SD_{female} = 20$; 35 males: $M_{male} = 48.5$; $SD_{male} = 23.7$). Overall, 30% reported to suffer from a chronic illness (mainly asthma and allergies, but also diabetes and cardiovascular diseases, which was found to increase with age ($r = 0.23$; $p = .057$). To investigate the age-related effects we partitioned the subjects by age in three distinct groups: Young ($< 30 years$, $n = 21$), middle ($30 - 65 years$, $n = 29$) and old ($> 65 years$, $n = 21$). Gender was equally distributed across the age groups ($\chi^2(2, N = 71) = 2.914$, $p = .233 > .05$).

3.4   Performance Motivation, Gamer Types, Inclination to Gaming

Performance motivation was equal across both genders ($F(1, 63) = .271, p = .605, n.s.$) and the three age groups ($F(2, 63) = .008, p = .992, n.s.$). We analyzed the interdependencies of the game preferences and the player types. While these scales correlate to a great extent ($r = .407$, $p < .01$), only limited dependencies between gender and age on these scales were found.

We found no significant gender effects on Bartles Achievement scale ($r = -.227$, $p = .063 < .1$, $n.s.$), Social scale ($r = -.071$, $p = .563, n.s.$) and the Immersion scale ($r = -.187$, $p = .112$, $n.s.$). Gender did also not affect the inclination towards classical board and card games ($r = .053$, $p = .660$, $n.s.$), computer games ($r = -.173$, $p = .149$, $n.s.$) and movement games, such as geocaching or sports ($r = -.194$, $p = .105$, $n.s.$).

Age did not affect the achievement ($r = -.127$, $p = .302$, $n.s.$) and social scale ($r = -.029$, $p = .812$, $n.s.$). However, with increasing age people were significantly less inclined to immerse into a game ($r = . - 239$, $p = .046 < .05$). With age the inclination towards board games seem to decrease ($r = -.214$, $p = .073 < .1$, $n.s.$). Liking of computer games decreases with age ($r = -.633$, $p < .001$). Also, movement games seem to be preferred more by the young than by the older ($r = -.386$, $p < .001$). The general, inclination towards games seem to decrease with age ($r = . - 386$, $p = .001 < .05$). It is an interesting finding that Bartles Achievement score and the performance motivation score did not correlate ($r = .000$ sic!), $p = .997$, $n = 67$) showing that both individual facets do measure independent constructs.

In summary, the young are more inclined than the old to play games in which they can immerse and which are either computer based or physical movement. Furthermore, the inclination towards gaming is independent of gender.

4   Results

This section is structured as follows. First, the effects of age and gender on task performance and evaluation of the usefulness of the game are reported. Then we describe the effects of the game playing on perceived physical fitness (comparing ratings before and after the study). Finally, we relate individual factors (technical expertise, performance motivation, health status) in order to understand the power of using of serious games in a health context.

4.1   Employed Statistical Tests

The data was analyzed using bivariate correlations, χ^2-tests, uni- and multivariate analyses of variance (ANOVA/MANOVA), multiple linear regressions, and repeated measure analysis. Type 1 error rate/significance level was set to $\alpha = .05$. (within the less restrictive level of $\alpha = .1$, findings are referred to as marginal significant). Type II error rates/power were set to $(1 - \beta) = .8$ (Power results are only reported if below this threshold). Pillais values were used for omnibus F-tests in the MANOVAs. Ordinal-scaled data were analyzed with the Wilcoxon Rank test and the Friedman test. Furthermore multiple linear regression analysis (enter method) was used. Predictors with low standardized beta values were removed between runs. F-Values and degrees of freedom are omitted, because all reported models explained more variance than respective scale means. Only significant predictors are used in the reported models. Models that show high inflation factors $(VIF >> 1)$ are also not reported. Effect sizes are reported as Cohens d and as Pearsons r for non-parametric tests. Because parametric tests are robust against small violations in assumptions, non-parametric test are only used to verify the effects. In our case only slight changes in effects sizes could be reported when switching from parametric to non-parametric tests, and only if variances differed to a large extent. Missing values were deleted listwise on a per test basis. If a smaller sample is used for a test, sample size is reported.

4.2   Evaluation of the Game, Raising of Health Awareness

The participants of the user study evaluated the prototype very well. All participants (100%, $n = 70$) had no difficulties to control the in-game avatar and over 94% of the users ($n = 66$) stated that they had fun playing the game. Likewise, 78% of the participants stated that they would like to play the game again. The majority of the users stated that this Exergame would increase their motivation to exercise on a regular basis (27% of the users disagreed, while 72% agreed).

No significant gender ($n.s.$) or age ($n.s.$) differences were found regarding the aforementioned questions. Although no significant overall effect of age was found, we exploratory peeked into the relationship of age and game rating and carried out four one-way ANOVAs. These showed that age influences the perceived fun of the game ($F(2, 67) = 3.14$, $p = .049 < .05$) with elderly having more fun ($M = 4.8$) than the middle aged ($M = 4.3$) and young ($M = 4.0$) users. Also, the desire to play the game again depends on age ($F(2, 67) = 3.74$, $p = .029 < .05$), with elderly being more inclined to replay the game again ($M = 4.4$) than middle aged ($M = 3.6$) and young users ($M = 3.6$). No age differences showed up regarding the difficulty of the game ($n.s.$) and the motivation to exercise more often ($n.s.$). See Fig. 3 for details.

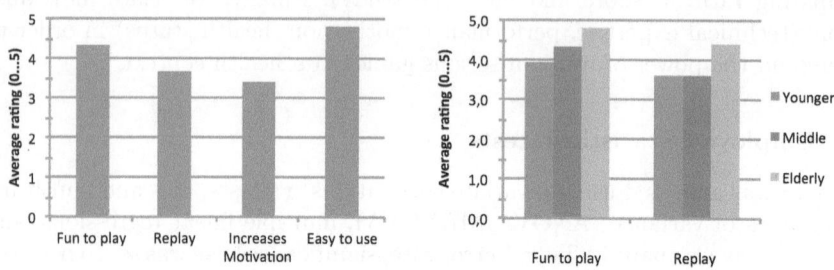

Fig. 3. Overall rating of the game and age differences in the rating of the game

4.3   Effects on Task Performance

Task performance in our study refers to the amount of apples and carrots participants could pick per second. Participants picked on average, 0.12 ($SD = .16$) apples per second in level 1 (stretching task), 0.16 ($SD = .26$) carrots per second in level 2 (bending task) and 0.22 ($SD = .37$) carrots and apples in level 3 (stretching and bending). The tasks were slightly different across the levels. Still, as level 1 and 2 are subsets of level 3, the performance is comparable and we found that the average task performance in level 3 is higher than in the previous levels ($F(2, 63) = 85.5, p < .05$).

In the first level task performance differs significantly between men and women ($F(169) = 4.17, p = .45 < .05$), with men being faster ($M = .18 objects/sec.$, $SD = .07$) than women ($M = .14 objects/sec.$, $SD = .06$).

As expected, age has a strong impact on task performance with younger participants being faster than older participants. On average young participants picked $M = 0.3$ ($SD = 1.16$) objects/sec. in level 3 of the game, whereas old participants were half as fast with $M = 0.15$ ($SD = .26$) objects/ sec. Participants from the middle-aged group scored $M = 0.26$ ($SD = .86$) objects/sec. The difference between the age groups is significant ($F(2, 68) = 12.87, p = .000 < .0$). A post-hoc test shows that the performance of the elderly differed significantly from both younger groups (see Fig. 4).

Gender did not affect learnability, but there was a marginal significant influence of age ($F(3, 63) = 2, p = .1$), showing that age groups did not learn equally fast. Though, as pictured in Figure 4, all age groups considerably increase their performance from the first trial (bending) to the last trial (mix).

There is a significant main effect of performance motivation on task performance in the first level ($F(1, 67) = 4.701, p = .034 < .05$). In the beginning (level 1) participants with low performance motivation were faster ($M_{low} = 0.16 objects/sec.$, $SD = .35$) than participants with high performance

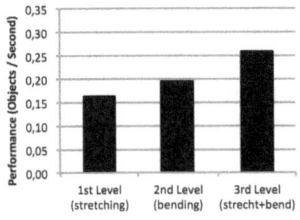
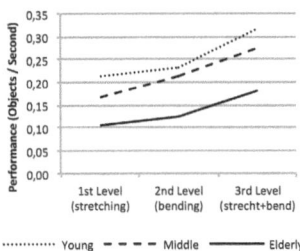

Young ············· Middle - - - - Elderly ———

Fig. 4. Performance for the three levels (left). Performance increases with levels indicating learnability of the game. Performance increases differ for the age groups (right).

motivation (M_{high} = $0.11 objects/sec.$, SD = .16), which is counter intuitive on a first sight. Though, this effect fades out after the first level. While participants with lower performance motivation are, on average, still faster than participants with high performance motivation, this effect is no longer significant for the second ($F(1, 66)$ = 2.334, p = .131 > .05, M_{low} = $0.18 obj/sec.$, M_{high} = $0.15 obj/sec.$) and the third level ($F(1, 66)$ = 1.399, p = .241 > .05) of the game (M_{low} = $0.25 obj/sec.$, M_{high} = $0.21 objects/sec.$).

When looking at correlational data for performance many variables influence performance. In particular age (r = −.65), computer self-efficacy (r = .49), Technology PEU (r = .51), Technology UF (r = .26), general inclination towards gaming (r = .56) and gaming motivation (r = .31) correlated significantly with performance (i.e. in level 3). Since almost all of these measures correlated with each other we first tried to disentangle their individual influences by running a linear regression on age.

Age is most strongly predicted with a double predictor model using both Technology PEU and UF explaining over 50% more variance (adjusted r^2 = .50) than the scale mean ($F(2, 54)$ = 29.53, p < .01) with PEU being a four times stronger predictor (standardized slope = -.85) than UF (standardized slope = .26). Adding computer self-efficacy (CSE) to the model could only increase explained variance to 55%. Age seems to be a satisfactory explanation of the three concepts CSE, PEU and UF.

In order to understand what independent variables have the strongest impact on performance multiple linear regression analysis was performed using the enter method with the variables that showed an impact either in correlational or ANOVA analysis on performance. Each level was individually analyzed.

Interestingly, analysis of both initial levels (bend and stretch) showed that age alone was the strongest predictor for performance. In level 1 age showed a standardized slope (β) of -.6 (B = −0.002, SEB = 0, t = −6.18, p < .01, constant B = 0.26, SEB = 0.016, t = 15.73, p < .01). The model was able to predict 35% more variance (adjusted r^2 = .35) than the scale mean ($F(1, 69)$ = 38.14, p < .01). No other predictor showed a similarly high rate of prediction. All models using more than one predictor were unable to increase the explained variance against the scale mean. For level 2 results were very similar (standardized slope

$\beta = -.59$, constant $B = 0.29$, $F(1, 68) = 35.89$, $p < .01$) with age being the only predictor explaining 34% more variance than the scale mean. For level 3 a two-predictor model was found to increase explained variance. Age and gaming motivation were able to explain 43% more variance (adjusted $r^2 = .43$) than the scale mean ($F(2, 64) = 25.67$, $p < .01$) with age being a twice as strong predictor as gaming motivation (see Tab. 1). Excitingly, performance motivation showed no influence in any linear regression.

Table 1. Linear Regression table for performance in Level 3

Model	B	SE B	β	t
(constant)	0.326	0.026		12.556**
Age	-0.002	0	-.593	-6.344**
Gaming Motivation	0.023	0.008	.254	2.714*

$* = p < .05$, $** = p < .01$.

4.4 Effects on Perceived Health Status (Pre-Post Comparison)

Using repeated measures analysis we found that perceived health status improved during the intervention. On a scale from 0 (no pain) to 4 (severe pain) the level of pain decreased significantly from $M = 0.69$ ($SD = .86$) to $M = 0.37$ ($SD = .75$) ($F(1, 64) = 19.186$, $p < .01$). Adding the age group into the repeated measures as a between subjects effect improves the model ($F(2, 63) = 3.859$, $p < .05$) showing that the decrease in level of pain is strongest in the oldest user group (see Fig. 5).

Since level of pain was highest in the old participants group multiple linear regression analysis was conducted to disentangle the effect of initial level of pain and age on the change between before and after the intervention. The change in level of pain could be predicted using a two-predictor model with both initial level of pain (before intervention) and age, explaining 32% more than the scale mean (adjusted $r^2 = .323$). The initial level of pain was twice as strong in predicting the change than age (see Table 2). This shows that the intervention is helpful to decrease the level of pain and in particular for the elderly.

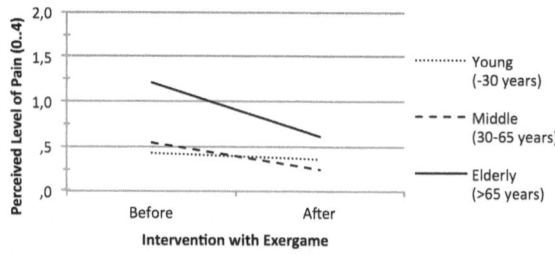

Fig. 5. Perceived Level of Pain for the three age groups before and after the intervention

Table 2. Linear regression table for change in level of pain

Model	B	SE B	β	t
(constant)	0.278	0.152		1.826*
Level of Pain (before)	-0.002	0	-.593	-3.87**
Age	-0.008	0.003	-.28	-2.563**

$* = p < .05, ** = p < .01.$

4.5   Influence on Liking of the Game

Liking of the game differs significantly across the age groups ($F(2, 69) = 3.153$, $p = .049 < .05$). On average older adults like the game more (M = 4.75, SD = .71) than middle aged adults (M = 4.23, SD = 1.07) and young adults (M = 3.95, SD = 1.16). Furthermore, we found no significant difference between the group with low (M = 4.2, SD =1.1) and the group with high performance motivation (M = 4.4, SD = 1.0) ($F(1, 66) = .709$, $p = .403 > .05$) on liking of the game. Participants with high performance motivation are slightly more inclined to play the serious game again (M = 3.9, SD = 1.3) than participants with low performance motivation (M = 3.3, SD = 1.7). However, this difference is not significant ($F(1, 66) = 2.807$, $p = .099 > .05$). Regarding the recommendation score (NPS) both groups differ significantly ($F(1, 67) = 4.69$, $p = .034 < 0.05$). The participants with low performance motivation are less likely to recommend the serious game (M = 6.3, SD = 2.2) than the participants with high performance motivation (M = 7.4, SD = 1.8).

4.6   Qualitative Results

Most participants reported that they enjoyed playing the game. However, they criticized the premature ending of the game and they would have liked to play more levels. In contrast to many other studies several participants demanded to play the game again after the experiment had finished. We learned that the pause gesture used in the game (raising both arms horizontally) to pause and resume the game was found confusing for some users. The gesture was added to the game to allow users to rest for a few seconds without reducing their game score. We observed however, that the pause function was never triggered by intention, but that a few users triggered the function accidentally and repeatedly.

5   Discussion

We examined the usefulness of Exergames regarding their potential to increase physical activity and to decrease the level of physical strain by comparing the reported scores before and after the experiment. Assuming that fun and personal involvement increases participants overall motivation to play again, we assessed also the NPS score, thus the willingness of participants to recommend the proto-type to its peers. This measure reflects the "intention to use" evaluation which had been originally used in Davis' technology acceptance model[21].

In order to understand, which individual characteristics might modulate not only the willingness and the effort to play, but also the performance level and the individual feeling after the experiment, we studied users of both gender in a wide age range (20-86 years of age) As psychometrically the performance motivation, the Bartles game typology, and the technical self-efficacy had been measured, we were able to relate these individual traits to performance and the evaluation of the general useful-ness of Exergames.

Recapitulating the main outcomes, results were very promising. Though per-formance level did reveal a significant effect of age (with a higher performance in the younger group), all age groups showed a significant increase in performance over the three game levels, thus showing a sustainable physical activity and an increasing motivation to optimize performance. The game was specifically de-signed for elderly, still it was unclear whether and to what extend elderly like the game. We assumed that only a share of the participants actually enjoy the game. Hence, an astounding finding it that most participants from the oldest age group reported fun during playing and willingness to play again. More so, the level of reported health strain/pain was reduced to the largest extent in the older groups, corroborating the appropriateness of the gaming approach also in the senior group.

The fact that we did not find a significant correlation between the levels of per-formance motivation (measuring the general willingness of individuals to engage for performance increase) and the Bartles gaming score (measuring the individ-ual inclination to engage in games) was not expected. On the present data basis we cannot fully resolve this finding. On the one hand we could have examined an extraordinarily highly motivated group in both components, thus reflecting a kind of ceiling effect. On the other hand this also could reflect a specificity of the power of Exergames for older adults. Pearce found that old adults play for fun rather than to hone skills and to overcome challenges, but need a gaming environment in which they might feel their own effort as a mediator to fun and achievement[22]. In the health context it therefore seems of high impact to foster the whole spectrum between intrinsic and extrinsic motivation. The number of successfully grabbed fruits might be the external rewards that increase the im-mediate engagement with the gaming surrounding, but the intrinsic component to feel well during the game and to feel to be a successful player is also an exigent component what may have caused the high evaluations of fun and the wish to play again in the senior group. Both components are therefore to be considered for Exergames in the health context.

Beside the gestures in the game (picking fruits and vegetables, placing them into a basket) the application may also requires a set of meta-gestures to control the state of the game (pause/resume), to skip a level, to get to configuration menus etc. In the current prototype we implemented a gesture for the action pause/resume. This gesture however was frequently triggered unintentionally by some users. Especially elderly users had difficulties to understand the connection between their current posture from within the game and the trigged pause screen. Therefore, games must consider that gestures should be intuitive and unequivocally distinguishable from each other[23].

The Exergame was evaluated very well regardless of age and gender. All participants stated that they had fun playing the game and they found the game easy to use. Regardless of age and gender users got faster with each level of the game. Although slower in the first level of the game, women quickly increased their performance in the 2nd and 3rd level to a greater extend then men.

6 Summary and Outlook

The current game prototype offers various starting points for further improvements. First, many users complained that the game ended too soon. Therefore additional levels have to be developed. To sustain long-term motivation we also need an understanding which kind of motivation forms might be especially suitable for the senior group. Also, as we only know the effects of the single play mode so far, we should also examine the usefulness of collaborative play, which could also enhance older adults needs of social activities and the interaction with friends, family and younger generations, but also peers[12].

Acknowledgements. The authors thank all participants for their willingness and enthusiasm taking part in the study. We also thank Tatjana Hamann, Ralf Philipsen, Nedim Szen, Martin Moos and Christopher Rausch for their research support. We would like to thank the anonymous reviewers for their valuable feedback on an earlier version of this manuscript.

References

1. Giannakouris, K.: Ageing characterises the demographic perspectives of the European societies. Eurostat, Statistics in Focus (2008)
2. McGonigal, J.: Reality Is Broken: Why Games Make Us Better and How They Can Change the World. The Penguin Group (2011)
3. Tanaka, K., Parker, J., Baradoy, G., Sheehan, D., Holash, J.R., Katz, L.: A Comparison of Exergaming Interfaces for Use in Rehabilitation Programs and Research. Loading 6(9), 69–81 (2012)
4. Gerling, K.M., Schulte, F.P., Masuch, M.: Designing and evaluating digital games for frail elderly persons. In: ACM International Conference Proceeding Series. Cent. Inf. Tecnol., Ydreams (2011)
5. Catania, A.C., Skinner, B.F.: The Selection of Behavior. The Operant Behaviorism of BF Skinner: Comments and Consequences, vol. 563. Cambridge University Press (1988)
6. Bandura, A.: Self-efficacy: Toward a unifying theory of behavioral change. Psychological Review 84, 191–215 (1977)
7. Bisson, C., Luckner, J.: Fun in Learning: The Pedagogical Role of Fun in Adventure Education. Perspectives. Journal of Experiential Education 19(2), 108–112

8. Premack, D.: Toward empirical behavior laws: I. Positive reinforcement. Psychological Review 66(4), 219 (1959)
9. Whitlock, L.A., McLaughlin, A.C., Allaire, J.C.: Video Game Design for Older Adults: Usability Observations from an Intervention Study. In: Proceedings of the Human Factors and Ergonomics Society Annual Meeting, vol. 55(1), pp. 187–191 (September 2011)
10. Ziefle, M., Bay, S.: How older adults meet complexity: Aging effects on the usability of different mobile phones. Behaviour Information Technology 24(5), 375–389 (2005)
11. Arning, K., Ziefle, M.: Effects of age, cognitive, and personal factors on PDA menu navigation performance. Behaviour Information Technology 28(3), 251–268 (2009)
12. McLaughlin, A., Gandy, M., Allaire, J., Whitlock, L.: Putting Fun into Video Games for Older Adults. Ergonomics in Design: The Quarterly of Human Factors Applications 20(2), 13–22 (2012)
13. Yee, N.: Motivations for play in online games. Cyberpsychology & Behavior: the Impact of the Internet, Multimedia and Virtual Reality on Behavior and Society 9(6), 772–775 (2006)
14. Gao, Y., Mandryk, R.L.: GrabApple: The Design of a Casual Exergame. In: Anacleto, J.C., Fels, S., Graham, N., Kapralos, B., Saif El-Nasr, M., Stanley, K. (eds.) ICEC 2011. LNCS, vol. 6972, pp. 35–46. Springer, Heidelberg (2011)
15. De Schutter, B., Vandenabeele, V.: Meaningful Play in Elderly Life. In: 58th Annual Conference of the International Communication Association Communicating for Social Impact (2008)
16. Beier, G.: Kontrollüberzeugungen im Umgang mit Technik [Locus of control when interacting with technology]. Report Psychologie 24(9), 684–693 (1999)
17. Brauner, P., Runge, S., Groten, M., Schuh, G., Ziefle, M.: Human Factors in Supply Chain Management Decision making in complex logistic scenarios. In: Proceedings of the 15th HCI International, Las Vegas. Springer, Heidelberg (to be published, 2013)
18. Arning, K., Ziefle, M.: Understanding age differences in PDA acceptance and performance. Computers in Human Behavior 23(6), 2904–2927 (2007)
19. Schuler, H., Prochaska, M.: LMI: Leistungsmotivationsinventar;[Dimensionen berufsbezogener Leistungsorientierung]. Hogrefe (2001)
20. Reichheld, F.F.: The number one you need to grow. Harvard Business Review 12, 47–54 (2003)
21. Davis, F.D.: Perceived Usefulness, Perceived Ease of Use, and User Acceptance of Information Technology. MIS Quarterly 13(3), 319 (1989)
22. Pearce, C.: The Truth About Baby Boomer Gamers: A Study of Over-Forty Computer Game Players. Games and Culture 3(2), 142–174 (2008)
23. Brauner, P., Bay, S., Gossler, T., Ziefle, M.: Intuitive gestures on multi-touch displays for reading radiological images. In: Proceedings of the 15th HCI International, Las Vegas. Springer, Heidelberg (to be published, 2013)

Design of a Game-Based Pre-hospital Resuscitation Training for First Responders

Marco Kalz[1], Birgit Schmitz[1], Henning Biermann[2], Roland Klemke[1],
Stefaan Ternier[1], and Marcus Specht[1]

[1] Centre for Learning Sciences and Technologies (CELSTEC), Open University of the
Netherlands, P.O. Box 2960, 6401 DL Heerlen, The Netherlands
[2] University Hospital Aachen, Department of Anaesthesiology, Pauwelsstr. 30, 52074 Aachen,
Germany
{marco.kalz,birgit.schmitz,roland.klemke,marcus.specht}@ou.nl,
hbiermann@ukaachen.de

Abstract. This paper reports about the design of a game-based training intervention for pre-hospital resuscitation training. Our underlying assumption is, that survival chances in cardiac arrest situations could be significantly improved, if bystanders would be better educated and prepared to help. Based on a discussion of problems of current training concepts and related educational theories a game-based learning intervention is proposed. The focus of the intervention is the improvement of procedural knowledge and self-efficacy of participants. The game is designed on the basis of the ARLearn platform. The game context and game-design is discussed. Last but not least we discuss short-term and long-term evaluation scenarios.

1 Introduction

Cardiac arrest is one of the leading causes of death worldwide. In Europe alone it is estimated that approximately 350 000 people die from cardiac arrest each year [1]. Traditional interventions have not sufficiently decreased mortality rates and increased the rate of cardiopulmonary resuscitation (CPR) especially by first responders. This rate of first-responder CPR is critical to increase survival rates since the professional medical emergency services need approximately 8 – 10 minutes to arrive at an incident. In the Euregio Meuse-Rhine (EMR) the rate of bystander resuscitation is approx. at 27% [2]. In other countries and regions there is a rate between 65% and 75% of bystander resuscitation before the professional services arrive. The project "EMuRgency - New approaches for Resuscitation Support and Training" is a socio-technical innovation project with the target to increase the rate of bystander resuscitation and on the long run increase survival chances and the quality of life in our region [3]. In this project we are developing a number of services and innovative educational interventions to increase awareness, knowledge and willingness to help for inhabitants of the region. For this purpose the consortium is currently testing a notification-system for first responders and has developed technology-enhanced learning solutions to provide flexible access to resuscitation training for different stakeholder groups.

A. Holzinger et al. (Eds.): SouthCHI 2013, LNCS 7946, pp. 363–372, 2013.

Besides classical E-Learning interventions for institutions, a mobile application for CPR training is currently in development. In addition, we are designing a game-based learning solution for schools and universities as a more authentic way of training CPR skills. In this paper we introduce the design and implementation of this game-based learning solution. Based on a discussion of current approaches to train first responders we analyse the training from the perspective of the situated learning theory and discuss related work. Then we introduce ARLearn as the technological basis of the game-based learning intervention. The game-setting and game-design is explained next and the study design for the evaluation is introduced. Last but not least we discuss limitations and provide a research outlook.

2   Background and Related Work

Traditional training approaches for pre-hospital resuscitation training are mostly based on lecture-centric phases in combination with training of motor-skills on a manikin in a group-training context. In many European countries this training is part of a mandatory first-aid-training before being allowed to get the driver license. While this is on the one hand a window of opportunity to train large parts of a population in basic resuscitation skills and knowledge from an educational perspective this training format delivers only short-term knowledge and competence building whose retention times is normally not longer than 3 to 6 months [4]. From the perspective of the situated learning theory [5] this result is not surprising. The situated learning theory is a general theory of knowledge acquisition or an epistemology that has a central assumption that learning should take place in the same context in which it is applied. Herrington and Oliver [6] deduct the following guidelines for the design of educational interventions from the situated learning theory:

- Provide authentic context
- Provide authentic activities
- Provide access to expert performances & narratives
- Provide multiple roles and perspectives
- Support collaborative construction of knowledge
- Provide coaching & scaffolding at critical times
- Promote reflections to enable abstractions to be formed
- Promote articulation to enable tacit knowledge to be made explicit
- Provide integrated assessment of learning within a task

These design guidelines point into the direction of using simulations and game-based approaches for resuscitation training to increase authenticity on the one and on the other hand allow the application of knowledge to the problem context in which it could occur.

Earlier research explored the use of simulations and game-based approaches to train resuscitation skills to diverse audiences. Perkins [7] has discussed the potential of simulation for resuscitation training. The possibility to test and re-test processes and activities without involvement of any risks for a patient is seen as one of the most important benefits to use simulations in resuscitation training. The author then presents results of a literature review about the use of simulations in resuscitation training. In this review, different types of simulation approaches are identified, namely integrated clinical (hardware) simulators and online (software) simulators. These simulations have delivered positive effects in terms of learning outcomes and learning experience, mostly for medical professionals (and not laymen) and focus on advanced life support (and not basic life-support). In general, simulations are costly and need efficient integration into a related curriculum. While such investments might pay off in a clinical context, for the training of laymen such an investment is unrealistic, also because the skills to be trained are not comparable to the ones needed in advanced life support (ALS) for nurses or emergency doctors working in a hospital.

As an alternative to the full simulation environments authors have proposed game-based approaches for resuscitation training. Charlier [8] argues that game-based approaches to train basic life support (BLS) are a promising option for CPR motor skills training in schools. According to the author traditional approaches are mostly focusing on summative assessment due to scarce resources and material, while formative assessment might be much more beneficial for learners. She proposes a combination of peer-assessment and game-based assessment and presents a board-game designed as a proxy to assess first aid competences of learners. Creutzfeldt, Hedman, & Felländer-Tsai [9] propose alternatively the use of gaming in multiplayer virtual worlds as a pre-phase to traditional CPR training. In their study they could show that preparatory activities conducted in virtual worlds contributes positively to CPR performance and skills. Based on the design principles of the situated learning theory and the results of earlier research we have designed and implemented a game-based approach for pre-hospital resuscitation training. In the next part we introduce the AR-Learn platform as technological basis to implement the intervention.

3   Technology

We are designing the intervention with the ARLearn-platform. ARLearn is a platform for location-based mobile learning. The platform consists of an authoring interface that enables game-designers to bind a number of content items and task structures to locations and to use game-logic and dependencies to initiate further tasks and activities [10]. The platform has been recently used for several similar pilot studies in the cultural heritage domain [11] and the training of volunteers for hostage-taking incidents in international organizations [12].

The cloud-based ARLearn service is hosted on Google App Engine as an open source project that permits others to reuse and contribute. ARLearn has been developed in an iterative design process, starting with a mock-up version, for which we gathered feedback on general approach, user interface and authoring/teaching aspects from two cultural science teachers and two technology-enhanced learning researchers.

Various kinds of clients connect to this game engine. The Android client allows for game play in the real world, while the StreetView-based client (called StreetLearn) offers a virtual environment [13]. Media items (including multiple-choice questions, video objects, and narrative items) are a central concept in ARLearn. They can be positioned on a map or made available depending on the game logic. A video can thus be bound to a coordinate, it can appear at a certain moment as a message in the player's inbox, or appear or disappear based on actions taken in the game.

An ARLearn game is a reusable game logic description that can be instantiated in numerous game-runs. Within a game, an author defines items, dependencies between items, game score rules and progress rules. A run defines users grouped in teams. While playing, users generate actions (e.g., "read message", "answered question") and responses. This output is also managed within the realm of a run. Basic elements of the object model are media items that hold information or add a function to the game. Media items can be positioned on a map or used for messages that users can receive at a specified point in time or in relation to a defined event. Specialisations of Media items allow to ask questions (MultipleChoice) or to include multi media (Audio- and VideoObjects). Dynamic items such as a transport task let users perform pickup and drop actions: A pickup item can be taken by users and can be dropped at a dropzone. Actions can lead (through dependencies) to new available items, increased scores or increased game progress. Items have a simple life-cycle with three states: Initially, an item can be visible or invisible (initial state). Invisible items can become visible (active state). When the item is no longer needed, it can become invisible again (used state). Items can define dependsOn and disappearsOn conditions for the state transitions. A simple dependency mechanism is put in place to support these conditions:

- Action-based dependencies are triggered by specified actions.
- Time based dependencies bind time offsets to other dependencies.
- Boolean dependencies allow to combine other dependencies to logically.

The following motivation guided the decision to use the ARLearn platform to realise the game-based learning intervention:

- The ARLearn platform is multi-user enabled
- The ARLearn platform is location-aware, which allows for realistic game-play settings
- Commonly used smartphones can be used to play ARLearn games, which simplifies game distribution.
- The event-based game model of ARLearn allows to design realistic game processes, which simulate mission critical real-life situations and conditions
- The game-design should be re-usable so that the game can be easily adapted to other locations and contexts

The ARLearn toolkit is used for the design and implementation of the game-based resuscitation training. With the authoring environment all elements and roles are designed and dependencies are fixed. For the run of the game the players use mobile devices with the ARLearn client installed. In the next chapter we discuss the game-design that we have implemented with ARlearn.

4   Game-Design and Setting

4.1   Setting and Game Context

The game is envisioned as an extension of classical group-based resuscitation courses. These courses are mostly focused on transfer of factual knowledge and the training of skills on a CPR-puppet. The skills-training is focused on motoric skills and the right compression depth, frequency and rhythm. An underrepresented part in these trainings are learning activities related to procedural knowledge, the willingness to help and self-efficacy. Thus the game is designed to increase procedural knowledge, to train processes in an emergency situation and to influence the willingness to help and self-efficacy. The game-context is a first-aid course or a dedicated basic-life-support training. To play the game 3 – 4 mobile devices with the Android platform are needed and a computer for the debriefing session. It is expected that the players play three rounds of the game to allow improvement and reflection. A CPR manikin is placed in the vicinity of the training location and this location is used as the place for notifying the participants about the CPR case and leading them to the victim. The game is organized in messages that occur on the main screen of the ARLearn application. Each message triggers an activity of the players or provides input in form of video/audio messages.

The mobile devices with the ARLearn platform are used for several purposes.

- They enable the different users to play in a realistic environment, being guided to an actual AED device.
- They provide the possibility to send controlled notifications to users emulating communicative behaviour.
- They allow to monitor and record user behaviour and reuse this data a for later reflection and feedback session.
- ARLearn further allows augmenting the situation with location dependent information, process information and notifications, as well as instructive, situation-dependent educational materials.

4.2   Game-Design

The game-design is oriented on the design recommendations for situated learning scenarios. The tasks involved in the game are aiming to produce a more authentic context for learners than the typical classroom lecture criticized earlier in the paper. The game-design is shown in figure 1. The game can be played with 2 or 3 players and there are 3 different roles foreseen: A CPR player, a player who documents the performance with video recording and an optional player who is responsible to find and get an Automated External Defibrillator (AED) to the victim.

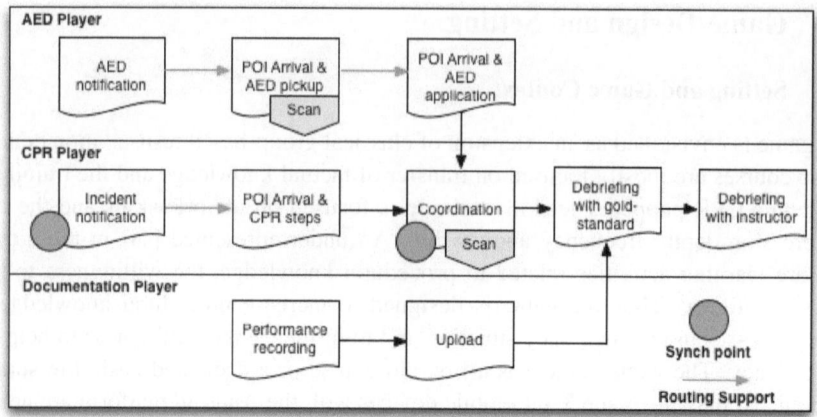

Fig. 1. Game-design resuscitation game

The game is organized in three phases: An introduction phase, a game-phase and a debriefing phase.

- Introduction Phase

The gamemaster gives a brief introduction about content and place of the game. The game is being explained, the rules and the aim. Groups are formed. Each group is provided with cellular phones.

- Game Phase

The game is initiated with a notification-message that informs the CPR player that a victim is in the direct surrounding of the team. The CPR player starts to identify the location of the victim accompanied by the documentation player. During the routing-phase the stress level of the player can optionally be increased with sounds or visuals that represent the decrease of oxygen in the body of the victim. After identifying the victim, the CPR player has to perform the steps required in case of a witnessed cardiac arrest, namely securing of the area, calling for help, controlling the breath and finally starting cardiopulmonary resuscitation (CPR) with a CPR doll. The documentation player records this process. As an option, the AED player receives the location of a nearby AED and he has to find the device and bring it to the location of the victim. Here the players have to scan a barcode to communicate to the system that the AED has arrived at the victim. Now the CPR player and the AED player have to coordinate their action in terms of continuing CPR and at the same time preparing the application of the AED. The documentation player is responsible for recording the performance in the best quality possible. The game is over after approximately 8 – 10 minutes after which the emergency medical services arrive.

- Debriefing Phase

When the game is over, the debriefing phase is started. The player meet at a location nearby and they enter the debriefing phase. The first part of the debriefing is based on a self-assessment. The team watches the performance and compares this to a gold-standard video that shows the ideal performance and situation. The results of the self-assessment are presented to a tutor who discusses the performance and provides tailored feedback to the self-assessment.

While we have presented here only one round of the game the players can change roles and play the game again. In this case the self-assessment will be done based on the three performances compared to the gold-standard. Since AED handling might not be part of all CPR trainings this part is optional.

4.3   Game Components

The game-components are based on the concept of role-playing. Research has shown that 'repeated practices in realistic role-playing scenarios with situations and environments students are most likely to encounter' can increase confidence and the willingness to respond to an emergency [14]. The game enables students to experience the diverse roles involved in case of emergency.

The game content is related to the Chain of Survival, i.e. (a) to prevent cardiac arrest, (b) to buy time, (c) to restart the heart and (d) to restore quality of life. It comprises three phases, an introduction phase, a mobile gaming phase and a debriefing phase. In the Introduction Phase, players are presented a short introduction to the game, e.g. how to read QR codes with a telephone. They will then be provided with telephones and the game phase will start immediately. In the Game Phase, students play in teams of two. When opening the actual game, they already have the first message available, which relates to their role. The two initial roles are: role of bystander and role of AED support. The learners are randomly assigned to one of these roles.

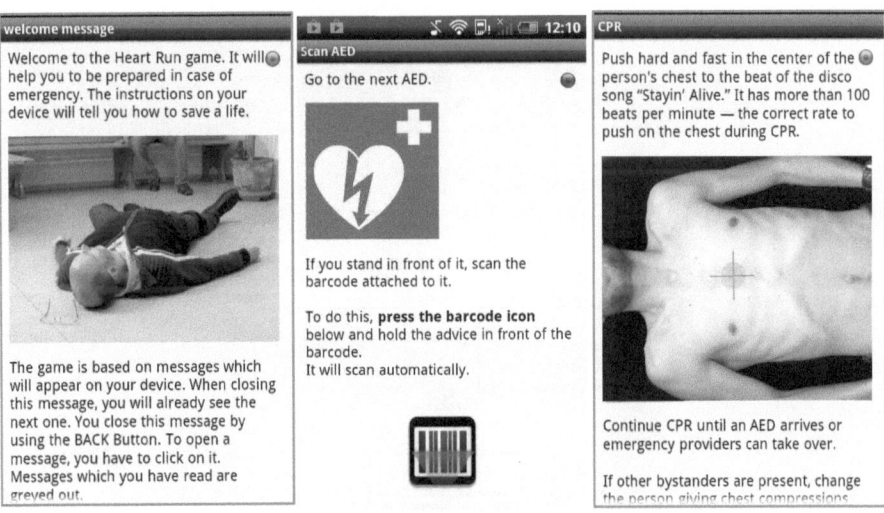

Fig. 2. Screenshots game-based resuscitation training

Also, in the course of the game phase, the player gets an unexpected alert message that requires immediate action. This time, no information is given on how to proceed. This part of the game has a third role integrated, the documenter. Immediately after the alert message has arrived, every player immediately needs to start action: find the next AED and get it (role of AED support), go somewhere and provide BLS (role of bystander), record the scene of action with the integrated camera of the smart phone and upload it to the system (role of documenter).

With the first message the game starts to count down 10 minutes. After this time, the game automatically ends with the message that the ambulance has now arrived and will take over the victim. Within the Debriefing Phase students revise and share the knowledge they acquired within the course of the gaming phase. To do so, their recording as well as an ideal type of action (gold-standard video) is presented. Learners are then required to compare both versions and reflect on things to improve. The game can be played several times, with participants switching roles. This way, the game allows students to perceive the emergency situation from different perspectives.

5   Evaluation Planning

Our hypothesis is, that participants who follow the game-based learning intervention show equal knowledge and performance results compared to the control group but better retention of knowledge and self-efficacy compared to the control group. We are currently preparing a study to evaluate effects of the game-based learning intervention. The study design is shown in figure 3.

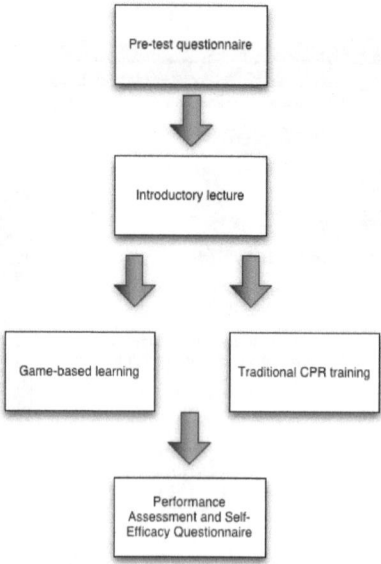

Fig. 3. Study-design game-based resuscitation training

All participants will first be provided with a baseline questionnaire to test their knowledge about CPR and their self-efficacy to act in case of an incident. According to Maibach, Schieber & Carroll [15] self-efficacy is a factor that is not directly linked to knowledge but can be the most important one in case of an incident. It can be best influenced through performance mastery and observational learning. After the pre-questionnaire all participants will be provided with an introductory lecture that will treat the basic knowledge about resuscitation. Participants will then be randomly assigned to the treatment group or the control group. The treatment group will follow the game-based learning intervention while the control group will receive a traditional CPR training with a doll and a control device that provides feedback about the depth and speed of compressions. In addition, a tutor will be present to give feedback to the learners.

The treatment group will follow the game-based learning intervention as discussed earlier. As a next step, all participants will be involved in a performance test on a CPR doll. Afterwards, all participants will fill out a post-questionnaire again related to their CPR knowledge and perception of their self-efficacy. The questionnaire will be again send out to the participants after 6 months after the intervention.

6   Discussion

This paper has introduced a game-design for a pre-hospital resuscitation training intervention for laymen. While the game-design is already worked out in detail, we have not yet decided with which means we can increase the stress of participants (e.g. emotional video footage, counters etc.). If the results of the first study confirm our hypotheses we will in the future implement a second study that will realize a factorial design in which a treatment group will receive 4 different implementations of the game-design that differ in terms of the stress-components involved. Another alternative for future research is the altering of the debriefing method used.

The game-design implemented will be published for others to be reused. We believe that the game-based training concept is a promising direction for pre-hospital resuscitation training for first responders. On the one hand, the method is easy to implement, on the other hand we expect more authenticity of the training without the costs of high-fidelity simulations often used in training scenarios for medical professionals. Furthermore, we aim to extend the game towards a longer-term involvement of players aligned with the EMuRgency project's goal to set up a community of trained volunteers for resuscitation.

Acknowledgements. This publication was partly financed by the European Regional Development Fund (ERDF), regions of the Euregio Meuse-Rhine and the participating institutions under the INTERREG IVa program (EMR.INT4-1.2.-2011-04/070, http://www.emurgency.eu).

References

1. Lippert, F., Raffay, V., Geogiou, M., Steen, P., Bossaert, L.: European Resuscitation Council Guidelines for Resuscitation 2010 Section 10. The ethics of resuscitation and end-of-life decisions. Resuscitation 81, 1445–1451 (2010)
2. Fries, M., Beckers, S., Bickenbach, J.: Incidence of cross-border emergency care and outcomes of cardiopulmonary resuscitation in a unique European region. Resuscitation 72, 66–73 (2007)
3. Kalz, M., Klerkx, J., Parra, G., Haberstroh, M., Elsner, J., Ternier, S., Musaddaq, A., Schilberg, D., Jeschke, S., Duval, E., Specht, M.: EMuRgency. A smart region invests in technology and community education for cardiac arrest. In: Workshop Horizon 2020: Smart cities Learning in Conjunction with the Alpine Rendez-Vous 2013, Villard-de-Lans, France, January 28-February 1 (2013)
4. Soar, J., Mancini, M.E., Bhanji, F., Billi, J.E., Dennett, J., Finn, J., Morley, P.T.: Part 12: Education, implementation, and teams: 2010 International Consensus on Cardiopulmonary Resuscitation and Emergency Cardiovascular Care Science with Treatment Recommendations. Resuscitation 81, e288 (2010)
5. Lave, J., Wenger, E.: Situated learning: Legitimate peripheral participation. Cambridge University Press (1991)
6. Herrington, J., Oliver, R.: An instructional design framework for authentic learning environments. Educational Technology Research and Development 48(3), 23–48 (2000)
7. Perkins, G.D.: Simulation in resuscitation training. Resuscitation 73(2), 202–211 (2007)
8. Charlier, N.: Game-based assessment of first aid and resuscitation skills. Resuscitation 82(4), 442–446 (2011)
9. Creutzfeldt, J., Hedman, L., Felländer-Tsai, L.: Effects of pre-training using serious game technology on CPR performance–an exploratory quasi-experimental transfer study. Scandinavian Journal of Trauma, Resuscitation and Emergency Medicine 20, 79 (2012)
10. Ternier, S., Klemke, R., Kalz, M., Van Ulzen, P., Specht, M.: ARLearn: augmented reality meets augmented virtuality. Journal of Universal Computer Science. Special Issue on Technology for Learning Across Physical and Virtual Spaces 18(15), 2143–2164 (2012)
11. Ternier, S., De Vries, F., Börner, D., Specht, M.: Mobile augmented reality with audio. Supporting fieldwork of Cultural Sciences students in Florence. In: Presentation at the In SuEdu 2012 workshop at the SEFM 2012, the 10th International Conference on Software Engineering and Formal Methods, Thessaloniki, Greece (2012)
12. Gonsalves, A., Ternier, S., De Vries, F., Specht, M.: Serious games at the UNHCR with ARLearn, a toolkit for mobile and virtual reality applications. In: Specht, M., Sharples, M., Multisilta, J. (eds.) Proceedings of 11th World Conference on Mobile and Contextual Learning (mLearn 2012), Helsinki, Finland, October 16-18, pp. 244–247 (2012)
13. Van Rosmalen, P., Klemke, R., Westera, W.: Alleviating the Entrance to Serious Games by Exploring the Use of Commonly Available Tools. In: Proceedings of the 5th European Conference on Games Based Learning, Athens, October 20-21, pp. 613–619 (2011)
14. Chamberlain, D.A., Hazinski, M.F.: Education in Resuscitation. In: An ILCOR Symposium Utstein Abbey Stavanger, Norway, June 22-24 (2001)
15. Maibach, E.W., Schieber, R.A., Carroll, M.F.: Self-efficacy in pediatric resuscitation: implications for education and performance. Pediatrics 97(1), 94–99 (1996)

The Resigned, the Confident, and the Humble: A Typology of Computer-Related Attribution Styles

Monique Janneck[1] and Sascha R. Guczka[2]

[1] Luebeck University of Applied Sciences, Luebeck, Germany
monique.janneck@fh-luebeck.de
[2] University of Hamburg, Hamburg, Germany
sascha.guczka@uni-hamburg.de

Abstract. Attribution, i.e. the systematic ascription of causes and effects in situations of failure or success, has so far received little attention in HCI research. In this paper we investigate specific computer-related attribution styles by means of a diary study and an online survey. By using cluster analysis we developed a typology of nine distinct attribution styles that come into effect in success or failure situations when using computers. Also, we were able to distinguish attribution styles that can be assumed to be favorable or unfavorable regarding computer mastery. Methodical issues in computer-related attribution research and implications for research and practice are discussed.

Keywords: Attribution, computer-related attitudes, computer mastery, computer failure, user types.

1 Introduction: Attribution Research

How do people explain things that happen to them? When and how do they feel in control? These are some of the questions that *attribution research* is dealing with.

The central concepts of attribution research refer to the explanations people find for why things happened the way they did (so-called *causal attributions*) and the extent of *control* that people feel they have over external events. Four attributional dimensions have been identified: *locus, stability, controllability,* and *globality* [e.g. 1, 2].

Let's take a failed exam as an example to explain these concepts:

- *Locus* describes whether the candidate believes that it was his/her own fault (internal attribution – "I did not study enough") or tends to blame other people or circumstances (external attribution – "the exam was too difficult / the examiner was unfair").

- *Stability* refers to the temporal aspect ("This time I failed" vs. "I always fail").

- *Controllability* describes the influence the candidate believes to have on the situation ("I could have studied more" vs. "Studying more would not have helped").

- Finally, *globality* refers to the generalizability of the situation ("I just don't like this subject" vs. "I never do well in written exams").

A. Holzinger et al. (Eds.): SouthCHI 2013, LNCS 7946, pp. 373–390, 2013.
© Springer-Verlag Berlin Heidelberg 2013

Attribution processes are highly relevant for people's behavior, emotions, and motivation [e.g. 3]. E.g., if the unsuccessful student manifests an external attribution ("the examiner was unfair") he or she might feel less distressed, but might also not work as hard as would be necessary to pass the exam in the second attempt. Contrary, internal attribution might cause self-doubts and self-reproach, but finally lead to an increased effort – provided the candidate feels the situation is somewhat controllable.

Recurring attributional patterns in different situations and contexts are called *attributional styles*. Certain attributional styles might have detrimental effects on motivation, coping, and accomplishments or even go along with psychiatric illness. E.g., patients with depression often attribute negative situations as internal, stable, and uncontrollable ("I am to blame but there is nothing I can do to change the situation") while positive situations are attributed as external, specific, and instable ("I was simply lucky this time") [e.g. 1, 4].

Attribution styles are considered as part of one's *self-concept*, which represents all of a person's self-referred attitudes [e.g. 5]. Therefore, attribution styles can be seen as rather stable over time.

In this paper we investigate the impact of attribution processes on Human-Computer Interaction: How do people explain how computers work? When and how do they feel in control when interacting with computers? We assume that just like in other areas of life attribution processes will influence behavior, emotions, and motivations related to the use of computer technology. Furthermore, specific computer-related attribution styles might affect computer use and the acquisition of computer skills in a more or less favorable way: E.g., users that tend to blame themselves for computer errors (internal locus) but have no idea how to avoid them (low feeling of controllability) might feel helpless when using computers or even avoid computer use altogether.

Thus, knowledge of computer-related attribution styles and processes in our view will help to understand users and difficulties they have when using computers or even to design adaptive systems that respond to different types of users in a specific, appropriate way.

Even though attribution theory is a long-known and well-researched concept, so far there has been little research on computer-specific attributions. Existing studies often deal with gender differences in computer use and do not address genuine computer-related attribution styles and processes. Nevertheless there are some interesting results:

Several authors found that girls tend to explain successful computer use with external factors (simple tasks, being lucky) while attributing failures internally to a lack of competencies. Contrary, boys tend to attribute success internally to their own skills and failures to external circumstances (e.g. bad usability) [e.g. 6, 7, 8]. Male attribution styles correlate positively with media competencies and computer skills [9].

Taking into account that women are still gravely underrepresented in computing these findings hint at how relevant attribution styles might be for successful Human-Computer Interaction: Having favorable or unfavorable attribution style, respectively, might account for differences regarding computer mastery, computer anxiety, or simply different styles of using computers.

2   Research Questions and Methods

Prior to investigating specific computer-related attribution styles a methodical question needs to be answered: How should we measure attribution processes?

Most studies in attribution research have been using *questionnaires*. A number of standardized questionnaires exist, e.g. the Attribution Style Questionnaire (ASQ, [10]). However, they mostly focus on clinical psychological research and diagnostics (attribution styles of mentally ill patients) and psychometric properties are partly poor.

To our knowledge, there is only one computer-specific questionnaire, the FEcA [11]), which is only available in German. It tries to capture attributions by asking participants to imagine specific situations ("Imagine that you learned how to use a new software on your own") and then measuring the responding thoughts. In our view, however, it's unclear whether the situations imagined by the participants seem 'real' and are actually relevant to them or whether there would be other attribution processes in real-life situations. In any case, one can assume that imagination does not have the same effect as actual experiences, as attributions are especially strong if something happens unexpectedly.

Diary studies are a research method widely and successfully used in work and organizational psychological research [cf. 12], but are also used in HCI [e.g. 13, 14]. In diary studies participants record their experiences, feelings, behaviors etc. over a certain time by means of a more or less pre-structured survey form (ranging from free reports to standardized questionnaires). The main advantage of diary studies is that real situations are recorded in a prompt and detailed manner [15, 12]: This is especially important in attribution research since recalling attributions after some time has already passed may result in distorted perception [16]. Furthermore, in diary studies longitudinal data can be collected.

However, diary studies are complex and time-consuming and require a lot of discipline and effort from the participants. Therefore, drop-out rates are usually high [12].

In this paper we explore diary studies versus questionnaires as a 'classical' research paradigm in attribution research: In our first study, we asked participants to record computer-related experiences and related emotions, cognitions, and behaviors over a period of several weeks by means of a standardized diary. In our second study, we used an adapted version of FEcA to collect data on computer-related attributions by means of an online questionnaire.

Therefore, in this paper we investigate theory-related as well as methodical questions:

- Can we identify stable, specific computer-related attribution styles which influence people's cognitions and behaviors?
- Are diary studies an appropriate research instrument to measure computer-related attributions, compared to questionnaires?

In the next sections procedures and results of study 1 and study 2 will be presented, followed by a general discussion.

3   Study 1

3.1   Procedure and Sample

In the diary study, participants were asked to record situations of success and failure when using computers (both private and workplace use) by means of a standardized diary form (see figure 1). It was up to the participants to decide whether success or failure had taken place.

The diary pages contained a short description of the situation and several questions regarding the attributional dimensions of *locus*, *stability*, *controllability* and *globality*. Items were phrased on the basis of the Sport Attributional Style Scale (SASS, [17]). Furthermore the context of the situation (location, reasons for computer use, other persons involved, duration of computer use etc.) and some socio-demographic data was recorded.

Please describe the breakdown that just happened:		
What caused the breakdown?		
1. I would locate the cause of the breakdown...		
internally (I am to blame)	1 3 4 5 6 7	externally (the system is to blame)
2. The cause of this breakdown is...		
a singular event	1 3 4 5 6 7	recurring
3. The cause of the breakdown is..		
controllable	1 3 4 5 6 7	uncontrollable
4. The cause of this breakdown is likely to promote other breakdowns...		
just in this situation	1 3 4 5 6 7	in other situations as well
5. This breakdown was...		
not important	1 3 4 5 6 7	very important

Fig. 1. Part of a diary page

The diary was handed out in paper and not electronically to avoid conjuring up further attribution processes [12]. Each diary contained ten forms each for success and failures.

Participants were high school and college students as well as employees to cover a wide range of age groups and use situations. Participants were able to contact the experimenter at all times. However, we refrained from systematic reminders and also rewards, since those are known to influence participants' responses in diary studies [12].

A total of N=19 diaries were returned, corresponding to a return rate of 38%, which is satisfactory for a diary study [16]. 11 participants were female (58%). Mean age was 25.4 years (range: 17-58 years). On average they had 11 years (range: 5-20 years) of experience in private computer use and 10 years (range: 2-25 years) experience of using computers at school or at the workplace, respectively. Participants self-rated their computer skills at a medium 3.6 on a Likert scale ranging from 1 (low) to 5 (expert).

3.2   Results

Participants reported a total of 152 situations (on average 8 per person). 58 were successes (on average 3.05 per person) and 94 (on average 4.95 per person) failures (table 1). About 60% of failures were reported in workplace situations, but only 43% of success situations.

The situations were categorized regarding the application context by two independent raters (application software, hardware, Internet/Networking, operating system, other). Interrater reliability was substantial at 81.5% (Cohen's Kappa was calculated as commonly accepted measure for interrater reliability and was high at 0.72, [18]). Participants mainly reported situations related to application software (51%) and Internet/Networking issues (20%; see table 1).

Table 1. Descriptive data regarding success and failure situations

			Success situations	Failure situations	All situations
Situations		N (avg.)	58 (3.05)	94 (4.95)	152 (8)
Context	Work	n (%)	25 (43.1%)	57 (60.6%)	82 (53.9%)
	Private	n (%)	33 (56.9%)	37 (39.4%)	70 (46.1%)
Category	Application software	n (%)	38 (65.5%)	40 (42.6%)	78 (51.3%)
	Internet/ Networking	n (%)	7 (12.1%)	24 (25.5%)	31 (20.4%)
	Operating system	n (%)	3 (5.2%)	16 (17%)	19 (12.5%)
	Hardware	n (%)	3 (5.2%)	12 (12.8%)	15 (9.9%)
	Other	n (%)	7 (12.1%)	2 (2.1%)	9 (59%)
			58 (100%)	94 (100%)	152 (100%)

The attributional dimensions are only moderately intercorrelated, thus supporting the construct validity of the research instrument. Merely *locus* and *controllability* show correlations above r > 0.5. However, this is theoretically plausible: If people see internal causes for a situation they normally also experience higher controllability.

Attribution of Success. As an explorational instrument for discovering structures in raw data we used hierarchical *Cluster Analyses* [19]. The first part in the Cluster Analysis was to measure each subject's individual level of attribution per dimension (location, globality, stability, controllability) collected over each situation. After that a matrix was built, containing the distance between the subjects regarding each dimension (the distance was calculated via euclidian measures). The next step consisted of clustering each subject or group of subjects together while keeping the inner cluster variance low, using Ward's method for computing the cluster linkage criterion. To rule out which cluster solution stands out we considered the variance changes and the plotted structure (dendrogram) for each data set [20]. We only included diaries that contained at least three success situations (n=9).

In the following, low values for *locus* mean that those persons attribute reasons for success mainly internally, while high values indicate that they believe external factors to be responsible. Low *stability* values mean that causes are believed to change over time, high stability value indicate recurring events. High levels of *globality* indicate that similar attributions take place in different contexts, while low levels of globality indicate that attributions are not generalized to other situations.

Finally, high levels of *controllability* indicate low perception of control (and vice versa), which is counterintuitive, but is due to the wording of the corresponding item.

For attribution of success, four clusters could be identified (fig. 2).

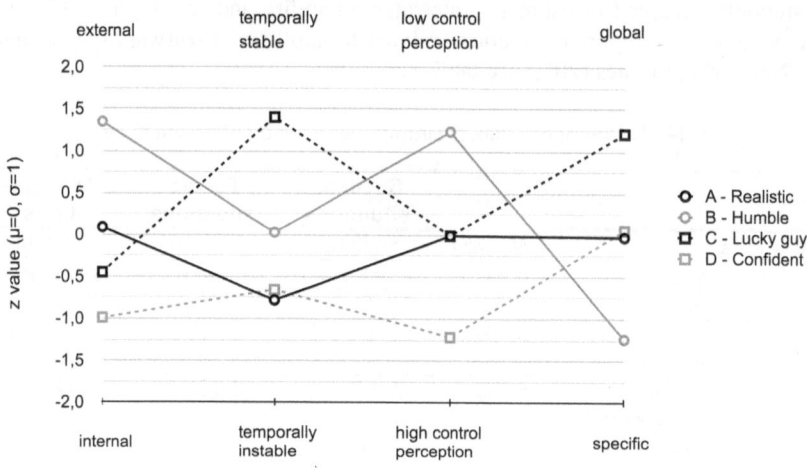

Fig. 2. Clusters for success situations

The four clusters can be characterized as follows. We used stereotypical names and exemplary statements to illustrate the kind of attitude and behavior that might be associated with the respective style:

- Cluster A: *"Realistic"* – *"Sometimes I am successful, sometimes not"*. Persons from cluster A have medium values in all dimensions except for stability, where they have the lowest values, which can be interpreted as a realistic, but not overly optimistic view of their own achievements.
- Cluster B: *"Humble"* – *"This time I was lucky"*. Persons from cluster B attribute success to external factors and experience only low levels of control when using computers.
- Cluster C: *"Lucky guy"* – *"Everything I do turns out right"*. Even though persons from cluster C don't have the highest values concerning internality, they feel more in control that persons from cluster B and also attribute more stable over time and also more globally, thus displaying a sense of faith that things will go right.
- Cluster D: *"Confident"* – *"I am competent and responsible for my own success"*. Persons with this attribution pattern see internal reasons for their success and experience high controllability. This can be seen as a favorable attribution style.

Table 2 shows the mean values for the clusters. ANOVAs were calculated showing significant differences between clusters. Effect sizes (Cohen's f, [21]) are high.

Table 2. Descriptive statistics for success clusters

Cluster Success	A n=3	B n=2	C n=1	D n=3	F value	p	f
Locus	2.067	3.219	1.571	1.076	8.769	0.02*	0.419
Stability	3.314	4.086	5.4	3.432	6.08	0.040*	0.512
Controllability	1.772	2.867	1.771	0.706	12.79	0.009**	0.419
Globality	3.390	2.229	4.571	3.467	3.933	0.087	0.499

Attribution of Failure. n=11 participants had reported a minimum of three failure situations in their diaries and were included in the analysis. For attribution of failures, three clusters were identified (fig. 3).

Again, clusters are characterized by means of stereotypical statements:

- Cluster X: *"Shrugging"* – *"Every failure is unique"*. Persons in cluster A have medium values regarding locus, stability, and controllability, and low levels of globality, thus believing that different situations have unique causes.

- Cluster Y: *"Confident* – *"I know it was my fault, but next time I will do better"*. Persons from cluster B mainly see internal reasons for their failures, but experience high levels of controllability and also believe that failures will not persist over time or in different situations, thus displaying confidence that they will be successful in the future.

- Cluster Z: *"Resigned"* – *"I never understand what computers do"*. Persons from cluster C have high values in all dimensions, thus showing a fatalistic attribution pattern: They perceive computer-related failures as uncontrollable and expect this to happen over and over again – a rather unfavorable attribution style that can be compared to the so-called pattern of "learned helplessness" that is observed in patients suffering from depression [cf. 1].

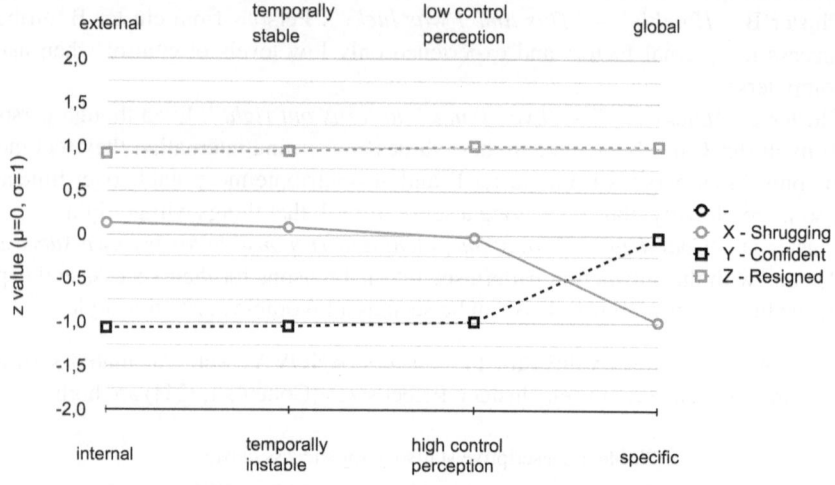

Fig. 3. Clusters for failure situations

As for success situations, differences between clusters were significant, with moderate effect sizes (table 3).

Table 3. Descriptive statistics for failure clusters

Cluster Failure	X n=7	Y n=1	Z n=3	F value	p	f
Locus	3.324	1.429	4.58	13.18	**0.029***	0.213
Stability	3.057	1.457	4.285	32.61	**0.000****	0.233
Controllability	2.926	1.2	4.798	29.14	**0.000****	0.173
Globality	2.026	2.886	3.812	20.96	**0.001****	0.231

4   Study 2

4.1   Procedure and Sample

In the second study, we conducted an online survey using an adapted version of the FEcA questionnaire [11] to measure computer-related attributions in a larger sample and compare the results to the clusters identified in the diary study. The questionnaire contained descriptions of twelve situations of computer-related successes or failures that participants were asked to imagine. The items are given in table 4.

Table 4. Questionnaire items

Success situations	1	You are trying to use an unknown software function you never used before while layouting a presentation on your computer. It works instantly.
	2	You figured out by yourself how to use a new computer application.
	3	You quickly manage to use a formerly unknown user interface on another person's computer.
	4	You would like to print some labels. By following the step-by-step instructions you are able to print the labels without any problems.
	5	You are conducting a literature search in your library. Even though the software is totally new to you, you learn to use it quickly.
	6	After having had problems with your mail application for some time, it's now working normally again.
Failure situations	1	You accidentally delete a page when writing a paper on your computer. Despite many efforts you are not able to restore this page.
	2	A file that you saved on an external storage device can't be opened any more.
	3	Your computer screen freezes while you are working on an important task. You try to solve the problem but a first attempt fails.
	4	A friend showed you an unusual but helpful software function. Later, when you're trying to use that function by yourself, it doesn't work.
	5	You are trying to print a handout for a presentation. The printer doesn't respond. You are not able to solve the problem.
	6	You are waiting to receive an important e-mail. However, even though trying several times, you can't access your mailbox.

Participants were asked to name the cause they assumed for each success or failure situation. Also, they were asked to rate the situation according to the four dimensions of *locus*, *stability*, *controllability*, and *globality*, using seven-point Likert scales. Furthermore, some sociodemographic data as well as data regarding general computer use and experiences was collected.

96 persons participated in the survey. However, 33 questionnaires were incomplete and thus excluded from the study, resulting in a final N=63. 37 participants were female (58.7%). Mean age was 29.6 years (range: 20-61 years). On average they had 15 years (range: 5-28 years) of experience in private computer use and 12 years (range: 2-30 years) experience of using computers at school or at the workplace, respectively. Participants self-rated their computer skills at a medium 3.7 on a Likert scale ranging from 1 (low) to 5 (expert). It can be noted that female participants had significantly less experiences in private computer use and also scored significantly lower in their self-ratings of computer skills.

Again, a cluster analysis was conducted to identify specific attribution patterns. A similar clustering method as in study 1 was used, with one exception: Since the number of participants was larger in this study we were able to look for outliers before grouping together subjects in the cluster analysis. This was done by using the single linkage method [19]. So for success analysis we were able to include n=52 participants, for failure analysis n=57 participants.

4.2   Results

Attribution of Success. Table 5 shows mean values, standard deviations, and Cronbach's α (as a standard measure of reliability) for the four scales. Reliability scores were acceptable except for *globality*.

Table 5. Descriptive statistics for success situations

Success	M	SD	α
Locus	4.06	2.05	0.54
Stability	5.50	1.58	0.61
Controllability	3.49	2.07	0.70
Globality	5.18	1.78	0.48

As was observed in study 1, *locus* and *controllability* correlate at r=0.55. Furthermore, *stability* and *globality* correlate at r=0.48.

Just as in study 1, four clusters could be identified for attribution of success (fig. 4). Clusters A, B, and D were identical with the clusters in study 1. Cluster C was not present in this study, but a new cluster (E) emerged from the data.

The clusters can be characterized as follows:

- Cluster A: *"Realistic"* – *"Sometimes I am successful, sometimes not"*. Persons from cluster A have medium values in all dimensions except for stability and globality, where they have the lowest values. Thus, they show a "realistic" attribution style expecting causes and influences to change over time and in different situations.

- Cluster B: *"Humble"* – *"This time I was lucky"*. Persons from cluster B attribute success to external factors and experience only low levels of control when using computers.

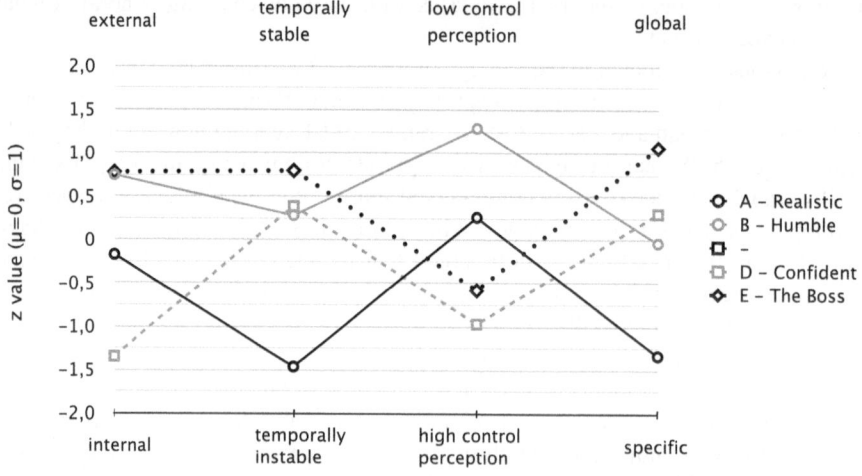

Fig. 4. Clusters for success situations

- Cluster D: *"Confident"* – *"I am competent and responsible for my own success"*. Persons with this attribution pattern see internal reasons for their success and experience high controllability. This can be seen as a favorable attribution style.

- Cluster E: *"The Boss"* – *"Success depends on the system, but I control it"*. Even though persons from cluster C also tend to attribute success to external factors, they still feel in control of the situation and also have the highest values of stability and globality. This can be interpreted as a 'boss-like' attitude knowing that there may be external factors for success but there still is a possibility to exert control over these factors.

Again, ANOVAs were calculated showing highly significant differences between clusters. Effect sizes are high (table 6).

Table 6. ANOVA results for success clusters

Cluster Success N=52	A n=20	B n=11	D n=15	E n=6	F value	p	f
Locus	4.04	4.94	2.89	4.97	46.7	< 0.001***	1.17
Stability	5.20	5.82	5.86	6.00	4.356	0.009*	0.704
Controllability	3.82	5.02	2.38	2.83	38.47	< 0.001***	1.56
Globality	4.78	5.44	5.61	6.00	8.49	< 0.001***	0.95

Attribution of Failure. Table 7 shows mean values, standard deviations, and Cronbach's α for the four scales. Reliability scores were acceptable except for *locus*.

Table 7. Descriptive statistics for failure situations

Failure	M	SD	α
Locus	4.13	2.30	0.45
Stability	4.75	1.88	0.66
Controllability	4.03	2.15	0.60
Globality	4.48	1.93	0.68

Regarding intercorrelations, again locus and controllability correlate at r=0.67 and stability and globality correlate at r=0.57.

For failure situations, cluster analysis identified four distinct clusters (fig. 5), while the diary study had revealed only three (cf. fig. 3). Clusters X, Y, and Z were replicated from study 1, while cluster W emerged as a new pattern.

The clusters can be characterized as follows:

- Cluster W: *"Realistic"* – *"This time I failed, but don't worry about it"*. Persons in this cluster see internal as well as external reasons for failures and believe that these change over time and depend on the specific situation, but still feel rather in control. This is a new pattern that was not present in study 1.
- Cluster X: *"Shrugging"* – *"Every failure is unique"*. Persons in cluster A have medium values regarding locus, stability, and controllability, and low levels of globality, thus believing that different situations have unique causes.

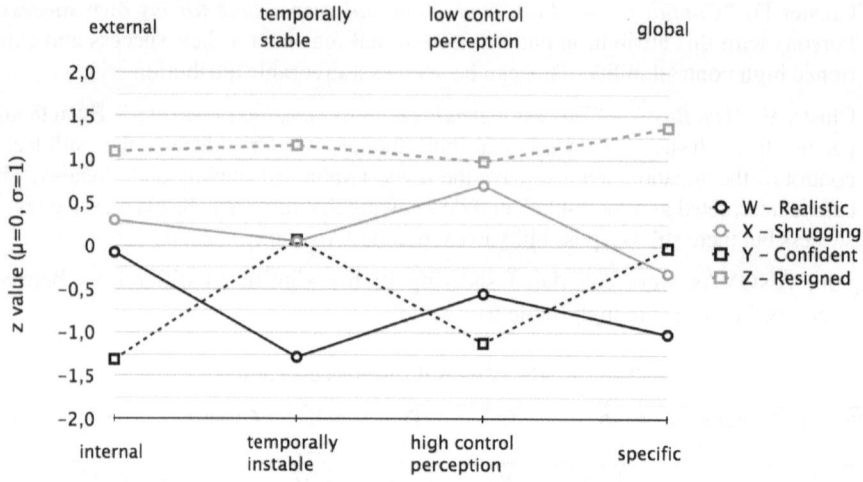

Fig. 5. Clusters for failure situations

- Cluster Y: *"Confident"* – *"I know it was my fault, but next time I will do better"*. Persons from cluster B mainly see internal reasons for their failures, but experience high levels of controllability and also believe that failures will not persist over time or in different situations, thus displaying confidence that they will be successful in the future.
- Cluster Z: *"Resigned"* – *"I never understand what computers do"*. Persons from cluster C have high values in all dimensions, thus showing a fatalistic attribution pattern: They perceive computer-related failures as uncontrollable and expect this to happen over and over again. This unfavorable style was also identified in study 1.

Again, differences between clusters were significant, with high effect sizes (table 8).

Table 8. ANOVA results for success clusters

Cluster Failure N=57	W n=12	X n=19	Y n=11	Z n=15	F value	p	f
Locus	3.89	4.15	3.03	4.70	15.7	< 0.001***	0.786
Stability	3.60	4.88	4.89	5.94	31.05	< 0.001***	1.111
Controllability	3.46	4.61	2.94	4.86	22.09	< 0.001***	1.233
Globality	3.64	4.30	4.58	5.89	19.5	< 0.001***	1.213

Relations With Other Variables. Finally, we investigated whether attribution styles are related to sociodemographic variables. Non-parametrical Kruskal-Wallis tests were calculated since the data was not normally distributed. Results are shown in table 9.

Table 9. Relations between attribution styles and other variables

	Attributional style in success situations			Attributional style in failure situations		
	χ2	df	p	χ2	df	p
Sex	51.0	3	< 0.001***	1.39	3	0.7078
Age	8.59	3	0.0353*	0.23	3	0.9725
Computer skills	0.98	3	0.8058	0.45	3	0.9295
Education	3.74	3	0.2907	4.30	3	0.2305
Private computer use	5.22	3	0.1567	1.02	3	0.7959
Workplace computer use	6.95	3	0.0736	0.58	3	0.9008

Regarding attribution of success, highly significant differences between men and women were found. Women tend to attribute more often in the realistic style, men in the humble or lucky guy style (table 10). There were no differences regarding attribution of failures.

Table 10. Gender differences in attribution styles variables

%	Realistic	Humble	Confident	The Boss
w	43.2	8.1	21.6	8.1
m	15.4	30.8	26.9	11.5

5   Discussion

5.1   Interpretation of Results and Comparison of the Two Studies

In this paper we investigated computer-related attribution styles by means of a diary study and an online survey. In the diary study, participants reported real use situations over a period of several weeks. In the online questionnaire, participants were asked to imagine several computer-related situations and rate the attributions they invoked.

Results of both studies indicate that indeed people diesplay stable, specific computer-related attribution styles, thus supporting our first research question.

Furthermore, both studies showed very similar results even though using different methods for data collection. A total of nine attribution styles were identified. Six of them were identical in both studies. In the survey study, two additional patterns emerged ('E' and 'W'), while one style ('C') could not be replicated. The slight differences are probably due to differences in sample characteristics. Furthermore, especially in the diary study the sample was small, and thus results might not be as reliable. The typology resulting from our studies is shown in table 11.

Distinct attribution styles were identified for success and failure situations. Therefore it seems feasible to separate these two aspects as it is generally done in attribution research. Nevertheless, two similar attribution styles were identified for both failure and success: "Realistic" and "confident".

Table 11. Typology of computer-related attribution styles

Cluster			Diary	Survey
S u c c e s s	A	*"Realistic"* – "Sometimes I am successful, sometimes not"	x	x
	B	*"Humble"* – "This time I was lucky"	x	x
	C	*"Lucky guy"* – "Everything I do turns out right"	x	
	D	*"Confident"* – "I am competent and responsible for my own success"	x	x
	E	*"The Boss"* – "Success depends on the system, but I control it"		x
F a i l u r e	W	*"Realistic"* – This time I failed, but don't worry about it".		x
	X	*Shrugging"* – "Every failure is unique"	x	x
	Y	*"Confident"* – "I know it was my fault, but next time I will do better".	x	x
	Z	*"Resigned"* – "I never understand what computers do"	x	x

In the clinical field attribution research often focuses on the question whether attribution styles are beneficial or detrimental regarding people's motivation, behavior, cognition and so on. Likewise, computer-related attribution styles can be categorized as favorable or unfavorable. Among the more favorable are "confident", "realistic" and "the boss". Persons with these attribution styles experience ample control over the situation when using computers. On the other side, "resigned" and "humble" are clearly unfavorable styles associated with very low levels of controllability. "Lucky guy" and "shrugging" cannot be distinctly categorized. More research is needed to find out how these people actually interact with computers.

Regarding the results it is feasible to assume that individual attributions styles will have a beneficial or inhibiting effect on computer use, e.g. regarding feelings of self-efficacy, learning to use new hardware or software or dealing with errors. How exactly these mechanisms take effect was beyond the scope of this investigation.

Regarding the context of computer use our studies revealed some interesting hints. In the diary study the use situations were categorized in terms of private vs. workplace use and also system category (e.g. application software, Internet/ Networking etc.). Due to the low number of participants it was not possible to measure whether these categories were related to specific attribution styles. However, it is interesting to note that failure situations were reported mainly from the workplace, while successes occurred predominantly in private use. An explanation would be that private computer use is generally more positively connotated, as it is usually voluntary and tasks are probably more enjoyable. It would be interesting to take a closer look at how general mood and dispositions influence computer-related attributions.

Likewise, there were differences regarding system categories: Failure reports regarding Internet/Networking, operating system und hardware were disproportionally frequent. Again, it would be interesting to investigate whether this is related to attribution processes.

In the diary study, sociodemographic variables (sex, age, computer skills) could not be analyzed in detail, since the sample was too small. In study 2, the relation of sociodemographic variables to attribution styles could be explored more systematically. Quite interestingly, neither computer skills nor experiences in using computers are related to attribution styles, which supports the notion that attribution styles are deeply rooted in one's self-concept and unlikely to change quickly.

Gender was the only relevant factor that we observed in the survey study. However, unlike other studies regarding gender differences in computer use [e.g. 6, 7, 8] we did not find that women's attribution styles were generally less favorable than men's: Quite contrary, the "humble" style which can be seen as one of the more unfavorable styles was shown more often by men. Perhaps the more complex approach of measuring attributions that we used brings forth more differentiated results regarding personal characteristics. In that respect it would also be interesting to include personality measures in further research.

An important question to ask is whether – especially negative – attribution styles can be changed. Even though attribution styles constitute part of the *self-concept* and thus can be considered as rather stable over time, e.g. [22], they are nevertheless subject to ongoing evaluation and reappraisal (e.g. as a consequence of positive experiences of computer mastery). Especially cognitive restructuring approaches might be used to change negative attribution styles. Popular examples include the 'Luck School' [23] or the Mindset approach [24].

5.2 Methodical Issues

Our second research question concerned the methodical issue of whether diary studies might be a suitable research instrument to investigate computer-related attribution styles. Again, the answer is yes: The method seems rather promising. Participants were able to record a high number of subjectively relevant situations in their everyday use context. Despite the relatively low number of participants, distinct clusters could be identified: Cluster differences are significant and effect sizes are high. In a larger sample, we would expect even bigger differences between clusters. Furthermore, cross-validation would be possible.

The biggest problem of diary studies – a high drop-out rate – was also obvious in our study. This is due to the strain the method puts on participants: They need to motivate themselves to participate over a long period of time without continuous interaction with the experimenter, remind themselves to fill out the diary, take the diary with them to different locations etc. In future studies we will try to recruit a larger sample from the very beginning to be able to include more diaries in the analysis.

We chose paper-based diaries to avoid interferences between the subject of evaluation and the method of data collection [12]. Nevertheless, it would be interesting to explore whether mobile appliances, e.g. Smartphone applications, might be suitable for data collection and make it easier for participants to record their use experiences, thus reducing drop-out rates.

In our view, a main advantage of diary studies is that people report actual experiences instead of merely imagining fictitious situations. This was also noted by the participants in the questionnaire study: Several persons said that the situations described in the questionnaire had all appeared very similar to them, that the descriptions were ambiguous or not vivid enough. This might also have affected the psychometric properties of the questionnaire, as internal consistencies were relatively low.

Nevertheless, we reached very similar results with both methods. Therefore, both instruments seem feasible for attribution research, depending on the focus of the study, the sample, resources etc.

5.3   Implications and Future Work

At the beginning of this paper we asked: How do people explain how computers work? When and how do they feel in control when interacting with computers? Answering these questions might help us to understand users better and ultimately design better technical artifacts.

To this end, including attribution styles as personal traits in *usability studies* could help to understand and interpret results: E.g., a "confident" person might not report bugs that were experienced during a test because s/he is convinced to have caused these problems her-/himself but would also be able to correct them. Likewise, the number of errors reported could be related to attribution styles. Last but not least, participants with more unfavorable attribution styles will probably experience more stress during usability studies. Short scales measuring the four attribution dimensions like the ones we used in our studies could easily be included in usability tests to systematically measure attributions. We are currently preparing a respective pilot study.

Furthermore we assume that knowing attribution styles and processes are relevant for *interface design*. For example, "enabling user control" is often seen as design principle and product quality of interactive systems. However, according to attribution research, "controllability" is also a personal variable depending on a person's attribution style. It would be interesting to investigate whether e.g. different visualization techniques or information architectures either bring forward specific attributions or are experienced differently by people with different attribution styles. E.g., persons with unfavorable attribution styles such as "resigned" might benefit from a more playful presentation of information on the screen. Even the wording of error and system messages might play a role: It is known from clinical research that patients show better compliance with their doctors' directives if they match their attribution styles (e.g. appeals on patients' self-responsibility are successful only when they have an internal locus) [cf. 4].

Last but not least we suspect that attribution styles influence how people *learn to use* (new) systems. Again, it might be possible to design *adaptive systems* to support different attribution styles (similar to the gradual increase in complexity throughout the learning process suggested by Carroll [25]).

At large we believe that attribution research is a complex field that will inform research and practice in Human-Computer Interaction in the future in manifold ways.

References

1. Abramson, L.Y., Seligman, M.E.P., Teasdale, J.: Learned helplessness in humans: Critique and reformulation. Journal of Abnormal Psychology 87, 49–74 (1978)
2. Weiner, B.: Achievement motivation and attribution theory. General Learning Press, Morristown (1974)
3. Försterling, F.: Attribution. An introduction to theories, research and applications. Psychology Press, Hove (2001)
4. Kneckt, M.C., Syrjala, A.M., Knuuttila, M.L.: Locus of control beliefs predicting oral and diabetes health behavior and health status. Acta Odontol Scand 57, 127–131 (1999)
5. Marsh, H.W., Byrne, B.M., Shavelson, R.: A multifaceted academic self-concept: Its hierarchical structure and its relation to academic achievement. Journal of Educational Psychology 80, 366–380 (1988)
6. Campbell, N.J.: High School Student's Computer Attitudes and Attributions: Gender and Ethnic Group Differences. Journal of Adolescence Research 5, 485–499 (1990)
7. Nelson, L.J., Cooper, J.: Gender Differences in Children's Reactions to Success and Failure with Computers. Computers in Human Behavior 13, 247–267 (1997)
8. Sølvberg, A.M.: Gender differences in computer-related control beliefs and home computer use. Scandinavian Journal of Educational Research 46(4), 409–426 (2002)
9. Kay, R.H.: The relation between computer literacy and locus of control. Journal of Research on Computing in Education 22(4), 464–474 (1990)
10. Peterson, C., Semmel, A., von Baeyer, C., Abramson, L., Metalsky, S.M.: The Attributional Style Questionnaire. Cognitive Therapy and Research 6, 287–300 (1982)
11. Dickhäuser, O., Stiensmeier-Pelster, J.: Entwicklungeines Fragebogens zur Erfassung computerspezifischer Attributionen. Diagnostica 46, 103–111 (2000)
12. Ohly, S., Sonnentag, S., Niessen, C., Zapf, D.: Diary studies in organizational research: An introduction and some practical recommendations. Journal of Personnel Psychology 9(2), 79–93 (2010)
13. Czerwinski, M., Horvitz, E., Wilhite, S.: A diary study of task switching and interruptions. In: Proc. CHI 2004, pp. 175–182. ACM, New York (2004)
14. Sohn, T., Li, K.A., Griswold, G.W., Hollan, J.D.: A diary study of mobile information needs. In: Proc. CHI 2008, pp. 433–442. ACM, New York (2008)
15. Alaszewski, A.: Using diaries for social research. Sage Publications Ltd., London (2006)
16. Reis, H.T., Gable, S.L.: Event-sampling and other methods for studying everyday experience. In: Reis, H.T., Judd, C.M. (eds.) Handbook of Research Methods in Social and Personality Psychology, pp. 190–222. Cambridge University Press, New York (2000)
17. Hanrahan, S.J., Grove, J.R., Hattie, J.A.: Development of a questionnaire measure of sport-related attributional style. International Journal of Sport Psychology 20, 114–134 (1989)
18. Cohen, J.: A coefficientofagreementfor nominal scales. Educational and Psychological Measurement 20, 37–46 (1960)
19. Abonyi, J., Feil, B.: Cluster Analysis for Data Mining and System Identification. Birkhäuser, Boston (2007)
20. Gillet, N., Vallerand, R.J., Rosnet, E.: Motivational clustersandperformance in a real-lifesetting. In: Motivation and Emotion, vol. 33, pp. 49–62. Springer (2009)
21. Cohen, J.: Statistical power analysis for the behavioral sciences, 2nd edn. Erlbaum, Hillsdale (1988)

22. McCrae, R.R., Costa, P.T.: Self-concept and the stability of personality: Cross-sectional comparisons of self-reports and ratings. Journal of Personality and Social Psychology 43(6), 1282–1292 (1982)
23. Wiseman, R.: The Luck Factor. Hyperion Books, New York (2003)
24. Dweck, C.: Mindset: The New PsychologyofSuccess. Random House, New York (2006)
25. Carroll, J.M.: The Nurnberg funnel: designing minimalist instruction for practical computer skill. MIT Press, Cambridge (1990)

Next Generation Tele-Teaching: Latest Recording Technology, User Engagement and Automatic Metadata Retrieval

Franka Grünewald, Haojin Yang, Elnaz Mazandarani,
Matthias Bauer, and Christoph Meinel

Hasso-Plattner-Institute,
University of Potsdam, Germany
{firstname.lastname}@hpi.uni-potsdam.de

Abstract. With the latest technological development in the last decade, new opportunities for learning environments and educational systems, such as tele-teaching, arose. Nowadays recording technology includes easy and fast workflows, high definition video recording, multiple sources and diverse output formats. With the amount of tele-teaching content growing, issues with sufficient metadata start existing. One solution is the user engagement. User engagement is based on the theory of the culture of participation and includes the usage of web 2.0 technology to activate students. This also has positive didactical side-effects. Another solution is the automatic creation of metadata. Therefore we have developed an automated framework by using video OCR (*Optical Character Recognition*) and ASR (*Automated Speech Recognition*) technologies. Indexable keywords are further extracted from those OCR and ASR transcripts.

Keywords: Tele-Teaching, Lecture Recording, Collaborative Learning, Video Analysis.

1 Introduction

The development of new technologies, especially of the World Wide Web in the early 90s changed the educational paradigm massively. The Internet has opened a new era of knowledge and opportunities for learners [1]. Technologies, like e-learning, tele-teaching, distant learning or online learning make it possible for everyone to learn and acquire new knowledge independent from lecture-halls and course schedules. Recorded lectures have proven to be important for distant media-supported learning and teaching, because whether at home or at the office, everyone can access recorded online courses via Internet. Students may access lectures whenever and wherever they like to, for example off campus, on their way to work or at home. Furthermore the recorded courses help students to follow the courses as often as they like and especially to prepare for the exam [2]. Not only students from the corresponding university, but everyone who likes to learn, such as employees or students from other universities, can continue their professional occupation by accessing to recorded lectures via Internet.

A. Holzinger et al. (Eds.): SouthCHI 2013, LNCS 7946, pp. 391–408, 2013.

1.1 Videolecturing with tele-TASK

Since 2004 the Hasso Plattner Institute (HPI) in Potsdam, Germany has been offering online-lectures. According to [3] 40% of the students are following the course in the lecture halls while the other 60% are watching the e-lectures live online or later on-demand. The high usage shows that our videolecture offerings are accepted among the students. That is the reason why this is part of the qualitative enhancement of the education at HPI. The lecture recordings at HPI are supported by the tele-Teaching Anywhere Solution Kit, short tele-TASK.

The tele-TASK system was initially designed in 2002 at the University of Trier [2]. Since 2001 it has been enhanced and optimized. Today it is used for all video recordings at HPI including lectures, seminars, reports and presentations of events.

Existing teleteaching systems restrict the operators and users. On the operator side (i.e. professor, presenter) the systems are often tied to an operating system or a required bandwidth. Another typical restriction is the usage of a specified presentation tool i.e. PowerPoint [4]. On the users side (i.e. students, learners) some systems require very complicated installations and operation steps which often also frustrate computer science students. Beside a simple usage, another important requirement is the possibility of transmission of the videos with low internet connectivity. This is the base to enable everyone to access the system and have the possibility to learn. Another issue of existing solutions is that they are not portable. They have to be built in a lecture hall and configured and can not be moved to another venue easily. Also some of these solutions have to be accessed through a network connection. More information about these solutions can be found on the web[1]. The use of standards, the option of using any operating system and presentation tool and the wish for mobility were requirements for the development of a new simple distance education system.

tele-TASK is the result of all these considerations and requirements; it supports all usual platforms, different net bandwidths and arbitrary presentation tools [2]. Special installations, configurations, or even knowledge on the part of end users are not required.

Fig. 1 shows that the tele-TASK-system comes as a compact mobile box containing a computer with a ready-to-use software, a video camera, a microphone and cables. So the recording can easily take place everywhere and be handled by the presenter himself or with the support of someone handling the camera.

With this system for lecture recording two video streams and one audio stream can be recorded at once. On the one hand, the system records a video of the lecturer but also of the (for example Powerpoint) presentation of his laptop, which is also visible for the students via an overhead projector. On the other hand, an audio stream of the presenter's speech is recorded. All three media streams are synchronously recorded and can be distributed via different modern technologies, which are described below.

---

[1] Some of the available solutions can be found at http://www.epiphan.com/, http://opencast.org/ and http://autoview.autotrain.org/

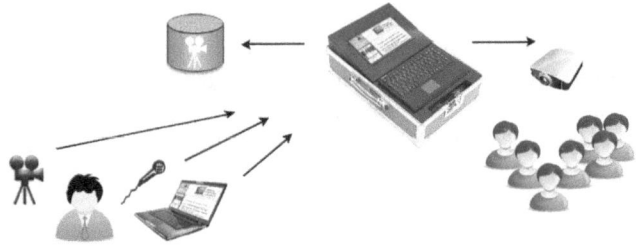

Fig. 1. The tele-TASK - tele-Teaching Anywhere Solution Kit - Workflow

1.2 Distribution of the tele-TASK Recordings

The recorded content generated by the tele-TASK system can be broadcasted live or made available offline in the form of digital media (USB flash drive, DVDs). But, the Internet is the primary channel of distribution. The portal www.tele-task.de, but also YouTube and iTunes U are utilized channels. A short description of the main channel, the portal, and its underlying web-application will follow next.

The tele-TASK portal includes a lot of different features. The following listing reflects only a part of the supported features of the portal. The video-lecturing portal tele-TASK offers different search options, a frequently updated list with featured videos, recently inserted videos, personally added tags to lectures, user-generated video annotations, assembling of personal playlists, voting for viewed lectures as well as automatically generated slide-rolls and lecture structures for navigation.

The technical basis for the hosting of the video data generated with the tele-TASK system is a Python based web-engine. The open source web-framework Django[2] is used here.

Everyone around the whole world can access a high percentage of the lectures held at the HPI displaying the presenter in an audio and video stream as well as his presentation (screen of his laptop) at the same time.

Weekly 2000 people (unique visits) from all over the world are visiting the tele-TASK archive with more than 4200 lectures and 14000 podcasts free of charge via a web-browser. The enormous number of hits counting about 29 millions from the start of the portal until now makes the success of the tele-TASK portal visible.

The large video archive and the web portal of tele-TASK are the basis for further research and development at the HPI. Several topics are currently in the research focus and some of them will be further elaborated in this paper. Those are web 2.0 technologies for activating users based on a culture of participation and automated lecture video indexing using content-based textual metadata, which are generated by applying multimedia analysis, as e.g., video OCR and ASR technologies.

---

[2] http://www.djangoproject.com

The remainder of the paper is organized as follows. We start in Section 2 with a description of the technologies and workflow of the lecture recording of the tele-TASK system. We present in Section 3 web 2.0 technologies used in our web portal for activating users. The automated lecture video analysis and retrieval will be described in Section 4. The paper ends with a short conclusion and future work in Section 5.

2   Lecture Recordings - Technologies and Workflow

We are trying to give distance learners a richer experience of the learning contents by recording the lectures as videos. Not only the slides, but also the lecturer himself is being recorded as a video. For doing so we developed a portable recording system that is capable of recording two videos at the same time. In the following section we are going to give a brief overview of the applied technologies and the workflow at our institute for the entire process of recording lectures, the post-production steps and media analysis and the publishing. For all of these steps we have developed individual software or hardware solutions.

2.1   Recording System

The tele-TASK recording system is a specialized computer in a portable attache-like box. It contains a built-in mini PC with an SSD hard drive and several other components, such as grabbers for the presentation and for the video capturing the lecturer. The spoken words of the lecturer's are transmitted to the recording system with a wireless microphone that is to be attached to the shirt or tie. The microphone's receiver is built in the recording system. But it is also possible to connect another audio source, such as an existing lecture hall sound equipment. When plugging in an external audio source, the built-in wireless microphone will be deactivated automatically. The recording system can be operated by the built-in keyboard with integrated touchpad or with the operator's fingers on the touchscreen display. It is also possible to connect other USB input devices such as a wireless keyboard. The current operating system running on the machine is Windows 7. Soon we will start our work on a Windows 8 based version adapting the recording software to the new paradigms. The recording software has been written in C# 4.5 and uses DirectShow. The codecs being used are H.264 for video and AAC for audio.

2.2   Server Infrastructure

In order to make the whole process of recording, postproduction and publishing as fast and as easy as possible, there are a few specialized servers required. A brief overview of the server infrastructure follows.

For running the web portal, a web server including a database server are used. In our institute we are using a Debian server with Apache and MySQL as database management system and a self-developed web portal based on Django and Python. For streaming the videos, an Adobe Flash Media Server[3] and - to maintain the operative readiness of the last generation recording system - a Helix Streaming Server[4] are used.

A self-built transcoding server is used for the automatic conversion to other formats, cutting and publishing of e-lectures over night. After pushing the recordings to the storage server, a nightly process converts the recordings to other formats so that the largest possible number of users can find the e-lectures in their preferred format.

Another important step in the chain of giving the users a rich learning experience is the analysis server. This server was developed and is continually improved in order to provide slide detection and extraction out of the lecture videos, automatic speech recognition (ASR) and optical character recognition (OCR). The analysis results are stored in the tele-TASK database and are used in the web portal for enriching the delivery of the e-lectures. So it is possible to generate an entire list of content including hyperlinks to the distinct position in the e-lecture without any human intervention.

2.3   Workflow

At the Hasso Plattner Institute in Potsdam, Germany most of the lecture series are being recorded with tele-TASK. Being a relatively small institute with about 460 students and only three lecture halls makes it easy for us to equip every lecture hall with a recording system. Besides we have several systems on hand to record presentations in seminar rooms or external events.

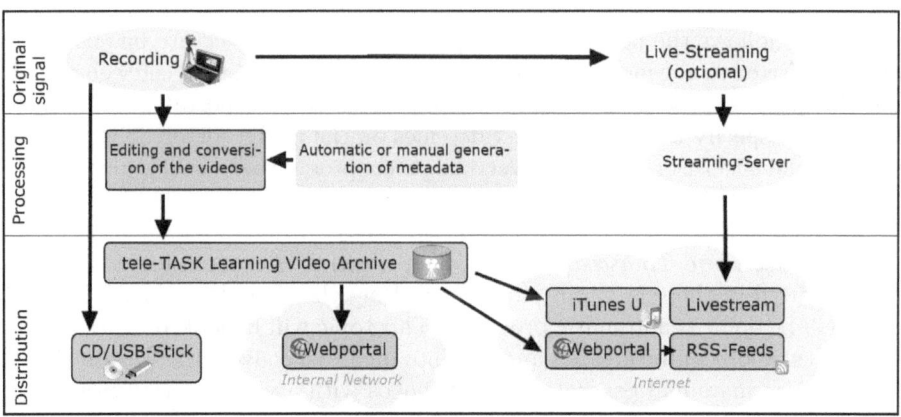

Fig. 2. Overview of the Recording and Distribution Workflow in tele-TASK

---

[3] http://www.adobe.com/products/adobe-media-server-family.html
[4] http://www.realnetworks.com/helix/streaming-media-server/

Recording takes place in the lecture halls or seminar rooms. As the systems in the lecture halls always stays there, the necessary time for preparing a lecture recording is very short. Around five minutes before the official start one member of our institute's media technology team or a student assistant should be in the lecture hall. Then he or she will boot the recording system, check if all signals such as camera, presentation and wireless microphone are connected properly and either select a predefined profile or input the lecturer's name and lecture title. But this is still possible during and after the recording. If everything is fine the recording can be started. During the recording process it is possible to create and name chapter marks on the fly. These can be edited at any time, even after the recording is finished.

Live Streaming of the lecture can also be offered by our recording system. In order to do so, the lecture recording, the path to the streaming server and the credentials have to be specified on the recording system or loaded from a profile saved earlier. Then, as soon as the recording starts, also the live streaming of the two videos (lecturer and presentation) is started. Students can watch the live stream on the tele-TASK web portal with the tele-TASK online video player. The possible options for the distribution are displayed in fig. 2.

Postproduction starts, when the recording is finished. It is possible to transfer the recordings to the media server via SFTP or to copy it to a USB device. For optional further steps of post-production we developed a post-production tool, which is installed on the computers of our media technology team. Here they can use their big screens and do exact cuts and set chapter marks. After everything is done, they can publish the e-lecture on the web portal.

Publishing follows the postproduction process. After the e-lecture has been cut and transferred to the media server, a lecture has to be created in the web portal. For this purpose a staff member has to log on to the web portal, create a new lecture and specify the path of the video files on the media server. It is possible to make the e-lecture, as well as every single chapter, either visible, unvisible or only visible to the registered students.

Video Analysis and Transcoding start when the video data and metadata have been inserted in the tele-TASK web portal. Here the slide detection, OCR and ASR will be done as automatic processes. This topic will be looked at in Section 4. Besides, a job can be created and put into queue to convert the lecture videos into other formats and generate podcast videos with a video overlay technique. These jobs will be processed by the self-built transcode server. The results of the transcoding processes are published automatically on the web portal to extend the offered possibilities of learning with the e-lecture. We invented the video overlay podcasts because - in order to maintain flexibility and offer smooth resizing - all e-lectures are being recorded as two video files. These are played back with the tele-TASK video player from within the web portal. But when it comes watching the e-lecture on a small mobile device, like a smartphone or iPod, it is much more handy to deliver a single video with an overlay (lecturer is in a corner overlying the slides). So this video can be downloaded easily and played with the native player app of the student's device. But there is much more to it than just simply playback the e-lectures. We intend to offer the students a more community-based learning approach.

3   Hands on for Students - Using Web 2.0 Technology and a Culture of Participation to Activate Users

Students using tele-teaching should be encouraged to actively collaborate with their fellow students and actively engage with the content for two reasons. First, especially when using lecture videos there has always been the problem that quite a bit of self-discipline is required from the students to follow the teacher. There is the issue, that students just lean back and consume the video without being involved. Looking at research about didactics though, it is obvious, that especially the active engagement with the material and the exchange with other learners are important for learning. Activating and engaging the students in the learning process and the collaboration among students should thus be the goal for every online learning platform. The community can benefit too, when the single user becomes more active. Knowledge will then be shared and connected.

The second reason why students should be engaged is the big mass of tele-teaching content that was produced in the last decade. The problem of how to filter and search through it arose. Metadata is the main problem in this case. Manual administration beyond the basic metadata is not possible anymore. Automatic metadata retrieval, that will be explained in Section 4, is one solution. User generated metadata is another approach to add more descriptive metadata. Search, recommendation and filtering functionalities within large learning video sets can be enhanced with those two methods. This section will deal with user generated metadata.

3.1   Community Functionalities in tele-TASK

In an e-lecture environment the community functionalities can be separated in time-independent and time-bound activities. Time-independent activities include the tagging of whole videos, the creation of playlists, a function most well-known from the music platform iTunes, chat functions and forums. Time-bound activities are the annotation functionalities that utilize a timeline approach. Those include setting time markers to memorize certain positions within the video as well as textual or multimedia annotations within the video. Another categorization would be synchronous and asynchronous functions. Chats and live-annotation in groups would be the only synchronous activities here.

In the tele-TASK project we already implemented several of the previously mentioned functionalities. These include rating of lecture videos, tagging of whole lectures, lecture-series or lecture-scenes, creation of playlists, adding of links to lecture-videos as well as a digital manuscript functionality incorporating video annotation. An overview of all functionalities that is available in the users' backend of the portal can be seen in fig. 3.

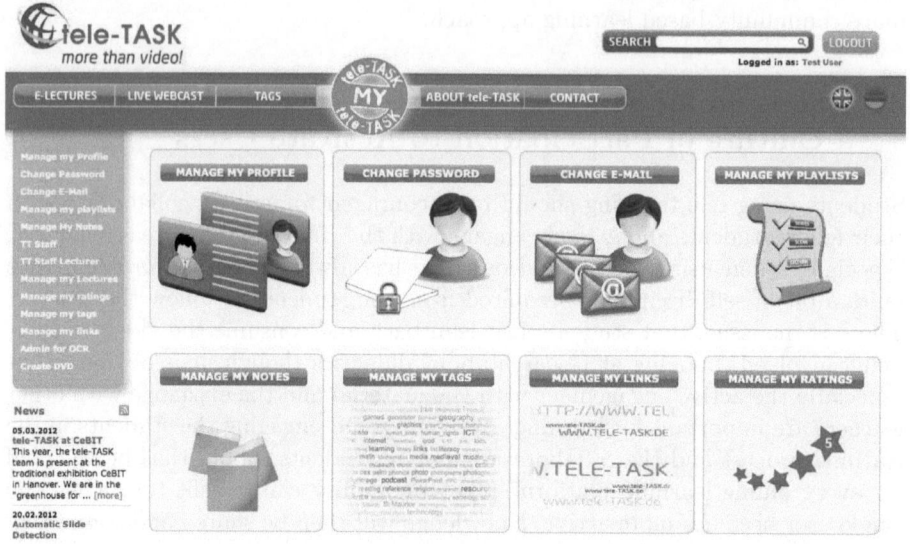

Fig. 3. Overview Web Interface of Community Functionalities in tele-TASK

Our focus in current research is on the digital annotation functionality [5], because it has been proven to be very beneficial for students [6–8]. Digital textual annotations enable the user to browse the video content according to his own notes and quickly find a certain point within the lecture again at a later point in time. Also it is possible not only to use descriptive free-text metadata as annotation, but also links and other media formats, like images [6].

Apart from the additional metadata they can utilize, also the process of annotation itself is beneficial for the students. Digital annotation leads to a deepened understanding of the topic [7], because it includes interpretation, reflection and weighting of the content [6]. Time-based annotation furthermore serves as anchored discussion as opposed to forums and thus encourages more participation as well as discussions among students [7].

Although all those community functionalities are theoretically very beneficial for the users, our experience and also other research have shown that several problems exist in this context that will be further elaborated in the next section.

3.2   Problems with Community Functionalities

Especially smaller e-learning communities often suffer from several issues concerning their community. Their member base is mostly not as large as in the huge private and free-time-oriented Web 2.0 platforms. That means that a smaller number of people actually participate and therefore the knowledge connection and sharing may not be as effective, because the key success factor for the community features is the interaction among users . Additionally, individuals in e-learning environments are less active than people in leisure and private communities. Hence, the participation is generally low. Experience with our own portal as well as a study about the Web 2.0 video service YouTube [9] showed this.

Recent research revealed, that a culture of participation needs to be integrated in order to engage users in content creation. Collaboration is no purpose in itself. Instead incentives need to be created for the users in order to encourage them to join in working cooperatively.

3.3   A Culture of Participation in tele-Teaching

Several studies and research papers focus on the phenomenon of participation in online platforms and particularly e-learning communities. Hostetter and Bush showed 2008 that group learning supports the individual motivation and eagerness to engage. They also found a strong correlation between social presence and user satisfaction. However, it was not possible, to link the learning outcomes to the feeling of social presence [10]. Kimmerle and Cress showed that a group-awareness tools can be utilized to provide a self-presentation opportunity and this triggers the willingness of individuals to participate in group activities. [11]

The term culture of participation was substantiated by Gerhard Fischer [12]. He suggested design guidelines for socio-technical systems to stimulate participation. The motivation to participate is based on intrinsic motivation. Therefore he suggests three major components. Those are meta-design, where the infrastructure enables collaborative design, social creativity, where a group of students is enabled to solve problems by collaboration and different levels of participation, which means that diverse degrees of engagement are supported. Fischer only briefly discusses learning as field of application. [12]. Dick and Zietz extended the framework for a culture of participation suggested by Fischer. They analyzed different motivation techniques. Out of this they concluded that system designers should make their users more aware of their contributions and actions within the system in order to motivate them instead of making them more active. [13] In the next paragraph the current state of the culture of participation in our tele-teaching environment is analyzed.

3.4   Status Quo of the Culture of Participation

Based on observations in our own tele-teaching web portal we would like to collect existing functionalities and methodologies and analyze their relevance for the culture of participation. The design guidelines of Fischer [12] and Dick [13] are used for the analysis. The results are collected in Table 1.

Summarizing one can say, that the culture of participation in tele-teaching environment needs a lot of improvement, especially in the fields of group-awareness, judgement and negotiation possibilities.

Table 1. Realization of the Design Guidelines for a Culture of Participation

Design Guideline	Realization in a Sample Tele-Teaching Platform
support different engagement levels	level 0: watching videos only, level 1: passive utilization of some functionality, level 2: using tagging and rating, creating links,..., level 3: creating playlists or user groups level 4: might be triggered within a didactical scenario
support human-problem interaction	A connection of the annotation functionality together with a suitable learning scenario might encourage this interaction.
underdesign for emergent behaviour	A chat function and the previously mentioned scenario are examples for the possibility to discuss and negotiate. Apart from that e-lecture environments are rather closed spaces.
reward and recognize contributions, group-awareness	Learning Scenarios may be used to honor and acknowledge the participation of people within a group of learners. Awareness mechanism are currently not supported.
feeling that behavior is being judged	Judgement cannot come up, since the previously mentioned awareness is not implemented and participation is still rather low.
co-evolution of artefacts and the community	A cross-pollination between the evolving community and the resources for system development is not possible due to security reasons from the universities side.

Digital annotation is the most profitable functionality in connection with e-lectures, because it supports the deep discussion of single aspects of the video among students. Therefore the next section will explain how a culture of participation can be fostered there and the participation improved.

3.5 An Approach to Improve Active Engagement by Establishing a Culture of Participation

This section will deal with possible solutions to reach the criteria for a culture of participation as described in the previous section.

Digital lecture video annotation is also possible in groups. It supports creating a user group, where each member may annotate the video at any point of time. It also allows group members to view each other's annotations. Five issues need to be tackled in order to incorporate a culture of participation in this area: 1) engage more students as coordinators and collaborators, 2) involve students as meta-designers, 3) foster group awareness, 4) incorporate rewards from the group and 5) create scenarios to support problem-solving and online discussion.

For the first point engagement, a first option would be the usage of a learning scenario incorporating student presentations. Fellow learners could comment on the recorded talks. The second point is to give learners the freedom to act as meta-designer. The annotation environment needs to be designed in a more open and free manner. It should be possible to include more than simple textual annotations or pre-defined files. A more open wiki-like annotation interface should be offered with freedom to include files as well as structure and design besides textual annotation. The utilization of the annotation environment as tool for the

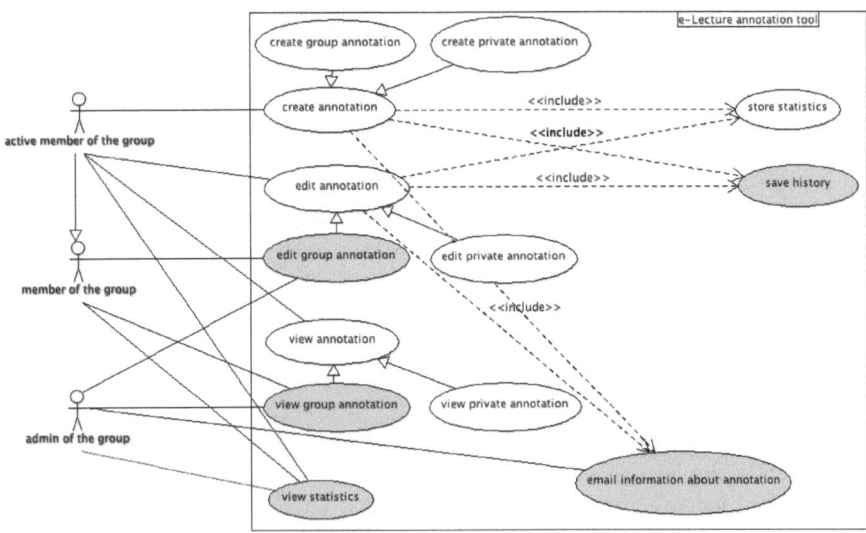

Fig. 4. Use case diagram of collaborative annotation with highlights of the culture of participation

collaborative creation of a manuscript that can serve as basis for exam preparation or as summary of the topic is one imaginable scenario. Several steps need to be taken to enable group awareness and reward. When a group of people works at the same annotation, it must be ensured that it is obvious which student accounted for which contribution. If changes are made, these are stored in a history. Because each and every step of each group member can be tracked and the users are notified of changes, people are aware that their contribution is being judged. Also, all contributions are counted in statistics that are visible for all group members. Textual group feedback and a voting system for the best group members are other options how group reward can be implemented. Some of the features of the group annotation are visualized in fig. 4. An open and flexible annotation system can also be the basis for scenarios incorporating problem-solving and online discussion. In order to start it, the teacher may spread some seeds. One scenario is the teacher asking questions within the lecture where it is the students' task to discuss them and document their discussion with the digital annotation. When annotating a live lecture students might even post questions at the same time as the lecture is actually taking place. At the end of the lesson the teacher then takes a few minutes to answer the questions.

As not the whole search and recommendation functionalities can rely on administrative and user-generated metadata, automatic metadata harvesting needs to be implemented too. The next section will deal with this topic.

4   Automated Lecture Video Analysis and Retrieval

Information storage and retrieval involve the processes to prepare, store and to find knowledge from data resources. For video retrieval, a number of methods have been proposed in the previous research works.

In order to perform an efficient video retrieval process, visual and semantical content-based approaches have been intensive studied in the last two decades. The commonly used techniques include shot boundary detection, key-frame selection, high-level and low-level feature-based video indexing, face detection, video OCR, and visual concept detection etc. The amount of lecture videos on the web has become huge, therefore an automated indexing and retrieval approach is highly desirable so that efficient lecture video search and browsing can take place.

Text and speech in video are the most important high-level semantic features, which directly depict the video content. We have thus developed a framework for automated lecture video indexing using video OCR and ASR technologies.

The studies described in [14] and [15] are based on "out-of-the-box" commercial speech recognition software. Concerning such commercial software, to achieve the satisfied results for a special working domain an adaption process is often necessary and the custom extension is rarely possible.

A conventional solution for video OCR is to first convert a video to a set of video shots, then apply an OCR engine to obtain texts. Therefore, our video OCR system consists of two parts: slide shots detection and video texts extraction. [16–18] applied a lecture video segmenter to extract the lecture slide images. The standard OCR engine and lexical filtering processes are utilized to generate the indexable texts. Since they do not apply text detection and text segmentation processes, the OCR recognition accuracy of their approach is therefore lower than our system's.

In our system a slide video segmenter has been firstly adopted in order to extract the unique slide frames from the lecture video. Then the video text detection and recognition methods are applied on each slide shot. The occurrence duration of the detected text line is determined by reading the time information of the corresponding segment. More details about the baseline algorithm of the slide video segmentation and text extraction can be found in [19]. We will thus give a general overview of the system in the next three subsections.

4.1   Video Segmentation

By segmenting videos into a set of representative key frames, we are able to index the video. The global pixel-differencing metric has been widely used for the general video segmentation task. However, regarding slide videos, we can see that the major contents of the slide such as text lines, tables, figures etc., can all be considered as the *Connected Components* (CCs). Therefore, we have developed a novel slide segmenter by using CCs instead of image pixels as the basis element. The algorithm consists of two steps: in the first step, we try to capture all changes from adjacent frames by using CC-based differencing metric.

In this way, we are able to control the valid size of CCs, in order to remove the high frequency image noise from the analysis. Since the segmentation results from the first step may contain the progressive build-up of a complete final slide over sequence of partial versions, the process continues with the second step which is intended to find the real slide transitions based on the segmented frames from the first step.

Due to the fact that the proposed segmentation method is defined for slide frames, it might be not robust, when videos with varying genres having been embedded in the slides and are played during the presentation. To fix this issue, we have extended the method by using a *Support Vector Machine* (SVM) classifier and image intensity histogram features, which are intended to distinguish the slide frames and the other video frames. Our experimental results show that the achieved classification accuracy of this approach is over 91%.

4.2   Video OCR

Texts embedded in lecture video are directly related to the lecture content, therefore they provide a valuable source for indexing. Our video text extraction framework consists of the following processing steps:

Text detection: this process determines whether a single frame of a video file contains text lines, for which a tight bounding box is returned. We have developed a two-stages approach that consists of a fast edge based detector for coarse detection and a *Stroke Width Transform* (SWT) [20] based verification procedure to remove the false alarms [21].

Text segmentation: in this step, the text pixels are separated from their background. This work is normally done by using a binarization algorithm. We have developed a image skeleton-based binarization approach [21]. The adapted text line images are converted to an acceptable format for a standard print-ocr engine.

Text recognition: we applied a multi-hypotheses framework to recognize texts from extracted text line images. The subsequent spell-checking process will further filter out incorrect words from the recognition results.

After the text recognition process, the detected text line objects and their texts are further utilized in the lecture outline extraction method [22].

4.3   Speech Recognition

In addition to OCR, ASR is an effective method for gathering semantic information from the spoken language. Combining both OCR and ASR offers the chance to improve the quality of automatically generated metadata dramatically. Thus, we decided to build a acoustic model by applying the CMU Sphinx Toolkit[5] and the German Speech Corpus by Voxforge[6] as a baseline. We collected hours of speech data from our lecturers and the corresponding transcripts in order to improve speech recognition rates for our special use case. A in-depth discussion

---

[5] http://cmusphinx.sourceforge.net/
[6] http://www.voxforge.org/

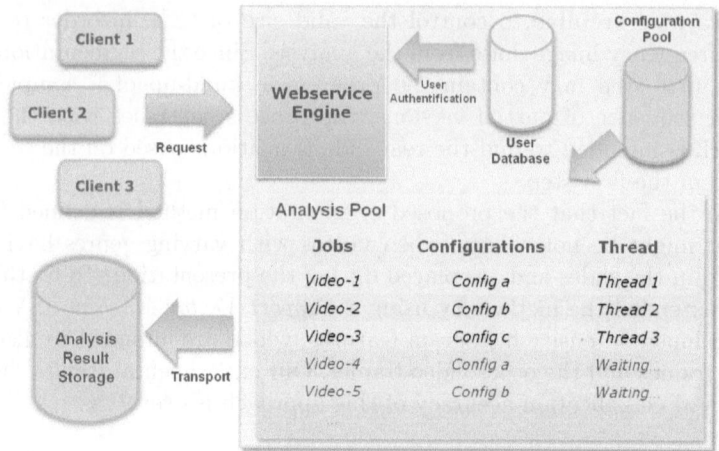

Fig. 5. Architecture of web service-based multimedia analysis framework

and the actual stand of our ASR approach for lecture videos can be found in [23].

4.4 Web Service-Based Analysis Workflow

In order to integrate the multimedia analysis engine to our lecture video portal, we have developed a SOAP (*Simple Object Access Protocol*) web service-based analysis workflow. Fig. 5 shows the framework architecture.

We have implemented a service client in our video portal that enables us to start the analysis for each lecture video. The analysis management engine validates the user data for each request from the client. The xml-based request data delivered by the service function contains the following information: media id, date time, media URL, analysis type, configuration type and language.

The analysis engine manages four major processes: media download, video transcoding, video analysis for each request, and analysis result transmission to the video portal server. The analysis engine is designed fully configurable and multi-thread safe.

After the analysis, the results will be automatically sent to the destination place on the portal server. Subsequently, we send HTTP-POST requests for saving the corresponding results to the portal database. The GUI (*Graphic User Interface*) elements of the slide segments and lecture outlines have been developed based on the plugin architecture in the video portal platform. Therefore, once the analysis result data is saved, the corresponding GUI elements will be created automatically by refreshing the web page.

For our purpose, we apply this framework to analyze the lecture videos from our institute. However, using it for the videos from other sources (e.g., YouTube[7],

---

[7] http://www.youtube.com

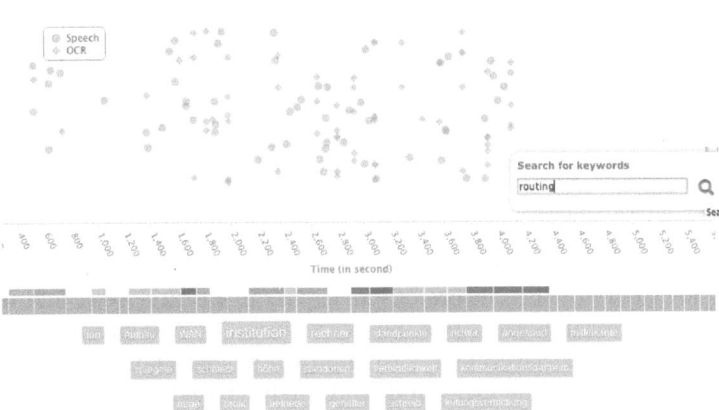

Fig. 6. Web GUI of keyword browsing and search function

Berkeley-Webcast[8] etc.), we would only need to adapt the configuration file of the analysis engine.

4.5   Keyword Extraction from OCR and ASR Data

In our framework, the keywords are extracted from OCR and ASR transcripts. In the first step, all OCR and ASR words will be arranged to an appropriate video segment. This enables us to efficiently calculate the weight factor for each keyword in the later stage. Since our system only considers nouns as the keyword, we thus capture nouns from the transcripts by applying Stanford POS Tagger (*Stanford Log-linear Part-Of-Speech Tagger*) [24] secondly.

Subsequently, we use the *stemming algorithm* to capture words with variant forms but a common meaning. This process leads to improve recall rate of the retrieval.

Since the OCR transcript might contain spelling mistakes, we have to perform a dictionary-based filtering for sorting out the error words. In order to avoid the out-of-vocabulary issue, the standard dictionary will be extended by adding technical terms of our lectures.

Then, the weight factor of each remaining word is calculated by TFIDF (*Term Frequency Inverse Document Frequency*) scores [25]. TFIDF ranks candidate keywords according to their statistical frequencies, which dose not reflect the location information of the keyword, while the location might be important for ranking keywords extracted from the web pages or lecture slides. In our framework, the OCR text line objects have been classified into several classes (cf. [22]). Therefore, we are able to apply the classified text line types to improve the

---

[8] http://webcast.berkeley.edu

keyword weighting result. Fig. 6 demonstrates the web GUI of keyword browsing and search function in our lecture video portal.

5   Conclusion and Future Work

In this paper we have shown the current status of today's video lecturing systems and environments. We briefly introduced our own tele-teaching solution tele-TASK. Furthermore our recording system and underlying web portal were introduced. The video recording workflow, latest technological developments and implementation were presented. Afterwards we discussed the issue of user participation. The theory of the culture of participation was described and discussed focusing on our research area. Possibilities to improve the current state of user activation were shown. Several ways to improve the metadata base were demonstrated next. Those include OCR and ASR analysis used to extract lecture outline, keywords and slides from the lecture recordings. In all three parts of this paper there is potential for numerous future work.

In the near future we are going to adapt our software to Windows 8 and fulfil a change in the paradigms of UI design, software architecture and deployment as well as the usage of codecs and filters. Also we are dealing with the question which and how many formats we can offer during live streaming of a lecture. Another part of our work is to minimize the time between recording a lecture and publishing it on the web portal. Future research will be done in the field of camera tracking with focus on unusual event detection.

Web 2.0 technology engaging users will be further enhanced to include more open features enabling the users to learn in their own style. This is a need identified within the theory of the culture of participation. Another need for users is more automatized support for their learning activities and progress. Semantic technologies as well as recommendation systems will be leveraged here.

As an upcoming improvement, implementing context- and dictionary-based post-processing will improve the recognition accuracy of OCR and ASR engines. The content-based video search can be further developed using automatically extracted keywords.

Since it is desired that the community functionalities as well as the content-based video browsing applications become frequently used functionalities within our tele-teaching portal, the usability and utility need to be evaluated within a user study. Questionnaires as well as usability tests and log-file analysis are currently planned. We are furthermore just conducting a study aiming to prove the usefulness of the indexing tools and annotation tools. In the study users are asked to find the start and end point of the segment in the video where a certain keyword is the topic. We measure the time needed and the precision and thus compare which of the tools - video only, slide preview and video, content structure and video, keywords and video or all - is most beneficial for users. A second task aims at finding out if those indexing or annotation tools can support learners in better concentrating on the lecture videos and keeping more of the content in mind. The tasks are accompanied by questionnaires that aim at finding out general opinions about the tools.

References

[1] Moritz, F., Siebert, M., Meinel, C.: Improving Search in Tele-Lecturing: Using Folksonomies as Trigger to Query Semantic Datasets to extract additional metadata. In: Proceedings of the International Conference on Web Intelligence, Mining and Semantics, WIMS 2011. ACM Press, New York (Mai 2011) ISBN 9781450301480

[2] Schillings, V., Meinel, C.: tele-TASK - Teleteaching Anywhere Solution Kit. In: Proceedings of ACM SIGUCCS, Providence, USA (2002)

[3] Wolf, K., Linckels, S., Meinel, C.: Teleteaching Anywhere Solution Kit (tele-TASK) Goes Mobile. In: Education, pp. 366–371 (2007)

[4] Ottmann, T., Müller, R.: The "Authoring on the Fly" system for automated recording and replay of (tele) presentations 8 (2000)

[5] Grünewald, F., Meinel, C.: Implementing a Culture of Participation as Means for Collaboration in Tele-Teaching Using the Example of Cooperative Video Annotation. In: DeLFI 2012 - Die 10. e-Learning Fachtagung Informatik. Gesellschaft für Informatik, Hagen (2012)

[6] Hofmann, C., Hollender, N., Fellner, D.W.: Workflow-Based Architecture for Collaborative Video Annotation. In: Ozok, A.A., Zaphiris, P. (eds.) OCSC 2009. LNCS, vol. 5621, pp. 33–42. Springer, Heidelberg (2009)

[7] Zupancic, B.: Vorlesungsaufzeichnungen und digitale Annotationen Einsatz und Nutzen in der Lehre, Albert-Ludwigs-Universität Freiburg, Dissertation (2006)

[8] Hermann, C., Ottmann, T.: Electures-Wiki – Toward Engaging Students to Actively Work with Lecture Recordings. IEEE Transactions on Learning Technologies 4(4), 315–326 (2011)

[9] Cha, M., Kwak, H., Rodriguez, P., Ahn, Y., Moon, S.: I Tube, You Tube, Everybody Tubes: Analyzing the World's Largest User Generated Content Video System. In: Proceedings of the 7th ACM SIGCOMM Conference on Internet Measurement, IMC 2007, San Diego, California, USA, pp. 1–13 (2007)

[10] Hostetter, C., Bush, M.: Measuring Up Online: The Relationship between Social Presence and Student Learning Statisfaction. Journal of Scholarship of Teaching and Learning, 6(2), 1–12 (2006)

[11] Kimmerle, J., Cress, U.: Group awareness and self-presentation in computer-supported information exchange. International Journal of Computer-Supported Collaborative Learning 3(1), 85–97 (2007),
http://dx.doi.org/10.1007/s11412-007-9027-z,
doi:10.1007/s11412–007–9027–z. ISSN 1556–1607

[12] Fischer, G.: Understanding, Fostering, and Supporting Cultures of Participation. Interactions 80(3), 42–53 (2011),
http://l3d.cs.colorado.edu/~gerhard/
papers/2011/interactions-coverstory.pdf

[13] Dick, H., Zietz, J.: Cultures of Participation as a Persuasive Technology. i-com (2), 9–15 (2011)

[14] Hürst, W., Kreuzer, T., Wiesenhütter, M.: A qualitative study towards using large vocabulary automatic speech recognition to index recorded presentations for search and access over the web. In: Proc. of IADIS WWW / Internet (ICWI), pp. 135–143 (2002)

[15] Repp, S., Waitelonis, J., Sack, H., Meinel, C.: Segmentation and annotation of audiovisual recordings based on automated speech recognition. In: Yin, H., Tino, P., Corchado, E., Byrne, W., Yao, X. (eds.) IDEAL 2007. LNCS, vol. 4881, pp. 620–629. Springer, Heidelberg (2007)

[16] Adcock, J., Cooper, M., Denoue, L., Pirsiavash, H.: TalkMiner: A Lecture Webcast Search Engine. In: Proc. of the ACM International Conference on Multimedia, MM 2010, pp. 241–250. ACM, Firenze (2010)

[17] Wang, F., Ngo, C.-W., Pong, T.-C.: Structuring low-quality videotaped lectures for cross-reference browsing by video text analysis. Journal of Pattern Recognition 41(10), 3257–3269 (2008)

[18] Hunter, J., Little, S.: Building and Indexing a Distributed Multimedia Presentation Archive Using SMIL. In: Constantopoulos, P., Sølvberg, I.T. (eds.) ECDL 2001. LNCS, vol. 2163, pp. 415–428. Springer, Heidelberg (2001)

[19] Yang, H.-J., Siebert, M., Lühne, P., Sack, H., Meinel, C.H.: Lecture Video Indexing and Analysis Using Video OCR Technology. In: Proc. of the 7th International Conference on Signal Image Technology and Internet Based Systems (SITIS), pp. 54–61 (2011)

[20] Epshtein, B., Ofek, E., Wexler, Y.: Detecting Text in Natural Scenes with Stroke Width Transform. In: Proc. of International Conference on Computer Vision and Pattern Recognition, pp. 2963–2970 (2010)

[21] Yang, H., Quehl, B., Sack, H.: A framework for improved video text detection and recognition. Multimedia Tools and Applications 1-29 (2012), http://dx.doi.org/10.1007/s11042-012-1250-6 ISSN 1380–7501. – 10.1007/s11042-012-1250-6

[22] Yang, H., Grünewald, F., Meinel, C.: Automated Extraction of Lecture Outlines From Lecture Videos - A Hybrid Solution for Lecture Video Indexing. In: 4th International Conference on Computer Supported Education, Porto, Portugal, pp. 13–22 (2012)

[23] Yang, H., Oehlke, C., Meinel, C.: An Automated Analysis and Indexing Framework for Lecture Video Portal. In: Popescu, E., Li, Q., Klamma, R., Leung, H., Specht, M. (eds.) ICWL 2012. LNCS, vol. 7558, pp. 285–294. Springer, Heidelberg (2012)

[24] Toutanova, K., Klein, D., Manning, C., Singer, Y.: Feature-Rich Part-of-Speech Tagging with a Cyclic Dependency Network. In: Proc. of Conference of the North American Chapter of the Association for Computational Linguistics: Human Language Technologies, HLT-NAACL 2003, pp. 252–259 (2003)

[25] Salton, G., Buckley, C.: Term-weighting approaches in automatic text retrieval. Information Processing and Management, 513–523 (1988)

Towards the Personalization of CAPTCHA Mechanisms Based on Individual Differences in Cognitive Processing

Marios Belk[1], Panagiotis Germanakos[1,2], Christos Fidas[1],
Andreas Holzinger[3], and George Samaras[1]

[1] Department of Computer Science,
University of Cyprus, CY-1678 Nicosia, Cyprus
[2] SAP AG, Dietmar-Hopp-Allee 16, 69190 Walldorf, Germany
{belk,pgerman,christos.fidas,cssamara}@cs.ucy.ac.cy
[3] Institute for Medical Informatics,
Statistics & Documentation, Research Unit HCI4MED
Medical University Graz, A-8036 Graz, Austria
andreas.holzinger@medunigraz.at

Abstract. This paper studies the effect of individual differences on user performance related to text-recognition CAPTCHA challenges. In particular, a text-recognition CAPTCHA mechanism was deployed in a three-month user study to investigate the effect of individuals' different cognitive processing abilities, targeting on speed of processing, controlled attention and working memory capacity toward efficiency and effectiveness with regard to different levels of complexity in text-recognition CAPTCHA tasks. A total of 107 users interacted with CAPTCHA challenges between September and November 2012 indicating that the usability of CAPTCHA mechanisms may be supported by personalization techniques based on individual differences in cognitive processing.

Keywords: Individual Differences, Cognitive Processing Abilities, CAPTCHA, Efficiency, Effectiveness, User Study.

1   Introduction

One of the most important security concerns on the World Wide Web today is to protect Web-based systems and services against automated software agents whose purpose is to degrade the quality of a provided service. Examples include among others the automated creation of fake email accounts that are used later on for spam, generation of massive scale advertising, manipulation of online voting systems, access of private information, generation of hyperlinks in forums to improve their Web-sites' search engine ranking, dictionary attacks of passwords, etc.

A "Completely Automated Public Turing test to tell Computers and Humans Apart" (CAPTCHA) [1, 2] is a widely used security mechanism to protect Web applications, interfaces, and services from such malicious software by verifying that the entity interacting with a system is actually a human being, and not a machine. A typical example of a CAPTCHA mechanism requires from a legitimate user to type letters

A. Holzinger et al. (Eds.): SouthCHI 2013, LNCS 7946, pp. 409–426, 2013.

or digits based on a distorted image that appears on the screen (Figure 1). Such a challenge is based on the assumption that a distorted text-based image can be easily recognized by the human brain but present significant difficulty for an optical character or image recognition system.

CAPTCHA challenges over the World Wide Web are performed primarily with the use of text-recognition CAPTCHA [3, 4, 5]. The reCAPTCHA project [4], which is currently the most popular and widely used CAPTCHA online, estimates that over 200 million reCAPTCHAs are completed daily, and it takes an average of 10 seconds to complete one. In addition, major Web service providers such as Google, Facebook, Microsoft and many others utilize text-recognition CAPTCHA to protect their premises against automated attacks [3].

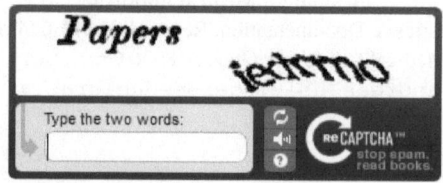

Fig. 1. Example of a text-recognition reCAPTCHA

Current text-based CAPTCHA implementations suffer from an important drawback; making the characters of the CAPTCHA hard to be recognized by computer systems, also increases the difficulty for humans, and thus decreases usability of interaction. The problem is further strengthened by the improvement of current character recognition systems that are more capable of breaking CAPTCHA mechanisms [6, 7], and as a consequence, the characters' distortion and complexity is increased making it even more difficult to be recognized by humans. Various studies have been reported that underpin the necessity for increasing usability of current CAPTCHA implementations. A study in [8] raised the usability issues of CAPTCHA and proposed a framework for evaluating various designs. A recent study which investigated users' perceptions toward CAPTCHA challenges underpins the necessity for user friendly CAPTCHA challenges as current implementations do not provide an acceptable trade off solution with regard to usability [9].

Within this realm, given that individuals share different characteristics, needs and preferences, supporting usability of CAPTCHA systems with adaptation and personalization technologies [10] may improve the system's usability and user experience by providing users with adaptive and personalized CAPTCHA challenges according to their unique characteristics. Given that current text-based CAPTCHA implementations require from individuals to recognize specific characters among irrelevant, noisy information, and process this information on a cognitive level, we suggest that individual differences in cognitive processing should be taken into consideration in the design of current text-recognition CAPTCHA mechanisms. In this respect, the purpose of this paper is to investigate the effect of specific individual characteristics of users targeting on cognitive processes (i.e., speed of processing, controlled attention and working memory capacity), toward efficiency and effectiveness of different varia-tions of text-recognition CAPTCHA challenges in terms of complexity (i.e., low, medium and high level of complexity illustrating respectively, 5, 7 or 9 characters with increased character distortion and noise).

2   Individual Differences in Adaptive Interactive Systems

Overarching aim is to drive this research towards the design and the deployment of adaptive and personalized CAPTCHA mechanisms that will assist users to accom-plish efficiently and effectively usable CAPTCHA tasks. In this respect we provide an overview of adaptive interactive systems to elicit how these could be of value for designing adaptive CAPTCHA mechanisms.

An adaptive interactive system [10] is any interactive system which is capable to automatically or semi-automatically adapt its information architecture and functio-nality as a response on implicit or explicit gathered data which are related with the users themselves, their interaction with the system or the context of use in which interaction takes place. The utter goal is to increase the functionality of the system and improve the users' experience by providing personalized and bootstrapped functionalities.

One distinctive feature of an adaptive interactive system is its user model. The user model is a representation of static and dynamic information about an individual, and it represents an essential entity for an adaptive interactive system aiming to provide adaptation effects (i.e., the same system can look different to users with different user models). For example, an information retrieval system can adaptively select and pri-oritize the most relevant items to the user's goals and/or interests. A security task in a commercial Web system can present the content adaptively to the user's level of knowledge towards security terms (e.g., provide novice users with personalized secu-rity information awareness by using additional explanations).

Adaptive interactive systems build and maintain a data model throughout computer human interaction which entails information considered essential in order to adapt content and functionalities to the unique characteristics of a user. According to the nature of information that is being modeled, we distinguish models that represent information about the user (user's knowledge, interests, goals, background and perso-nality traits) and about the user's context of use (user's location, platform, physical environment) [10].

A considerable amount of research efforts have been undertaken focusing on mod-eling and utilizing personality traits (e.g., cognitive factors) for personalization in adaptive interactive systems. Several works [11, 12, 13] have distinguished users based on their cognitive characteristics, and provided different adaptation effects ac-cordingly. A study in [11] distinguished imager and verbal users, and wholist and analyst users based on Riding's Cognitive Style Analysis [14], as well as based on the users' cognitive processing abilities. Each user was provided with adaptive presentation of content (graphical or verbal), different navigation organization (stressing analytic or holistic navigation approaches) and different amount of user control and content based on the users' cognitive processing abilities. In a similar approach in [12] users were distinguished in field-dependent and field-independent based on Witkin et al. [15] and provided different navigation organization, amount of user control, and navigation support tools for these groups. Results of these studies indicate that cognitive characteristics have significant impact in the adaptation and personalization process of Web environments by increasing usability and user satisfaction during navigation as well as learning performance.

Such findings suggest that individual differences in human cognition are important to take into account in the personalization process of an adaptive interactive system. Accordingly, modeling and adapting CAPTCHA mechanism based on users' cognitive factors could improve CAPTCHA solving efficiency and effectiveness, and minimize users' cognitive loads and erroneous interactions by providing different levels of complexity according to the cognitive characteristics of each individual.

In this context, a number of theories in human cognition exist that aim to describe and explain [16, 17, 18] the functioning of the human mind in terms of more basic processes, such as *speed of processing* which indicates the time needed by the human mind to record and give meaning to information [19, 20], *controlled attention* which refers to cognitive processes that can identify and concentrate on goal-relevant information and inhibit attention to irrelevant stimuli [19, 21], and *working memory capacity* which refers to a cognitive system for temporary storage of information and information manipulation [22, 23]. Various research works argue that these cognitive processes have an effect on comprehension, learning and problem solving [24-29]. They are mainly used in mental tasks, such as arithmetic tasks; remembering a number in a multiplication problem and adding that number later on, or creating a new password and using that password later for authentication, or recognizing the distorted text of a CAPTCHA mechanism.

To this end, given that the aforementioned cognitive factors have a main effect in problem solving and other tasks (e.g., individuals with increased working memory capacity accomplish tasks more efficiently), we suggest that such characteristics should be utilized as part of an adaptive interactive system specialized in personalizing CAPTCHA-related tasks to the cognitive abilities of each user. Main aim of this paper is to investigate how individuals with differing cognitive processing abilities perform in various CAPTCHA challenges. Such an endeavor could support the development of an adaptation engine that would embrace cognitive characteristics as its core user model and accordingly adapt the level of complexity in each CAPTCHA solving task to improve usability of interactions.

3   Method of Study

3.1   Procedure

A Web-based environment was developed within the frame of various university courses which was used by the students throughout the semester as an online blog for posting comments related to the course, as well as for accessing the courses' material (i.e., course slides, homework) and for viewing their grades. The participants were required to solve text-recognition CAPTCHA challenges with different levels of complexity throughout the semester, primarily before posting comments on the online blog. In particular, a text-recognition CAPTCHA challenge with low, medium or high level of complexity was provided to each user. For example, in case a user solved a CAPTCHA with medium level of complexity at time 0, the system would provide the same user to solve a CAPTCHA with different level of complexity (low or high complexity) at time 1 in the future with the aim to engage the whole sample with all available levels of CAPTCHA complexity.

With the aim to increase the internal validity of the study, the different levels of complexity were designed specifically to ensure that the relationship among the three different CAPTCHA types regarding their complexity level was linear. In particular, the criteria for developing the different levels of complexity were based on the number of characters presented, and the percentage of text distortion and noise illustrated in each CAPTCHA challenge. The low complex CAPTCHA entailed 5 characters and 40% text distortion and noise, while the medium and high complex CAPTCHAs entailed respectively 7 and 9 characters, and 50% and 60% text distortion and noise, as illustrated in Figure 3.

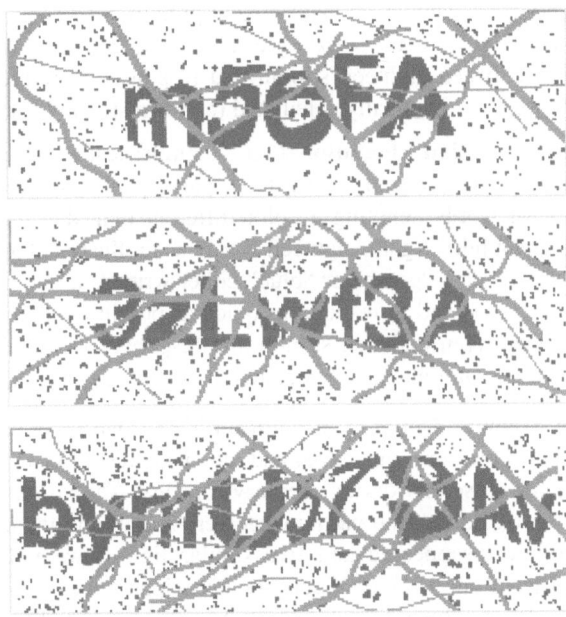

Fig. 2. Text-recognition CAPTCHA with Increasing Complexity

The text-recognition mechanism was developed using available open-source software that produced distorted images of random characters[1]. The text-recognition CAPTCHA mechanism also contained a refresh button that initialized the CAPTCHA with a new sequence of characters. Both client-side and server-side scripts were developed to monitor the users' behavior during interaction with the CAPTCHA mechanism. In particular, the total time (efficiency) and total number of attempts and refresh events (effectiveness) required for successfully solving the CAPTCHA challenge were monitored on the client-side utilizing a browser-based logging facility that started recording time as soon the CAPTCHA challenge was presented to the users until they successfully completed the CAPTCHA process. For user identification, the Web-site utilized the participants' username since the course's Web-site required user authentication for accessing the course's material.

Controlled laboratory sessions were also conducted throughout the period of the study to elicit the users' cognitive factors (speed of processing, controlled attention and working memory capacity) through a series of psychometric tests [23, 26]. The psychometric tests utilized in the study are described next.

Users' Speed of Processing Elicitation Test. The test required participants to read a number of words designating a color written in the same or different ink color (e.g., the word "blue" written in blue ink color). Eighteen words were illustrated to the participants illustrating the words "red", "green" or "blue" either written in red, green or blue ink color. The participants were instructed to press the R key of the keyboard for the word "red", the G key for the word "green" and the B key for the word "blue". The reaction times between eighteen stimuli and responses were recorded and their mean and median were automatically calculated (as suggested in [26]).

Users' Controlled Attention Elicitation Test. A similar test to the previous one was utilized, but instead of denoting the word itself, participants were required to recognize the ink color of words denoting a color different than the ink (e.g., the word "blue" written in green ink). Again, eighteen words were illustrated to the participants illustrating the words "red", "green" or "blue" either written in red, green or blue ink color, and the participants had to respond as quick as possible utilizing the keyboard. The reaction times between eighteen stimuli and responses were recorded and their mean and median were automatically calculated (as suggested in [26]).

Users' Working Memory Capacity Elicitation Test. Two tasks addressed storage capacity in short-term memory, the verbal and the visual test [23], whose results were combined to indicate a user's working memory capacity. The *visual test* illustrated a geometric figure on the screen and participants were required to memorize the figure. Thereafter, the figure disappeared and five similar figures were illustrated on the screen, numbered from one to five (Figure 4). Participants were required to provide the number of the figure illustrating the same shape as the initial figure through the keyboard. The test consisted of twenty one figures (seven levels of three trials each). As participants correctly identified the figures, the test provided more complex figures indicating an enhanced working memory capacity.

---

[1] Securimage v. 3.0, http://www.phpcaptcha.org

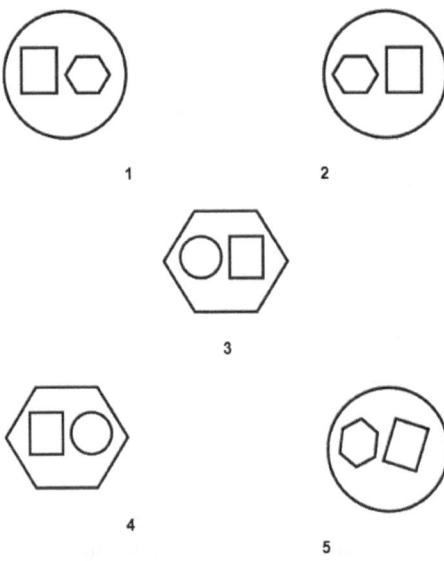

Fig. 3. Visual Working Memory Test

The *verbal test* showed a series of statements and required the participants to respond whether they are true or false. In addition, participants were required to remember the last word of each sentence and then write the last word of the sentence. The test included six levels of difficulty, e.g., in level three, participants were required to respond true/false to three successive sentences and had to remember and provide the last word of each sentence. For example, for the sentences "Knives are sharp", "The sun is shining", and "Fish have fur" the participant should respectively respond true, true and false, and then provide the word "sharp", "shining" and "fur" to the system (Figure 5). The level each participant reached indicated his/her working memory capacity.

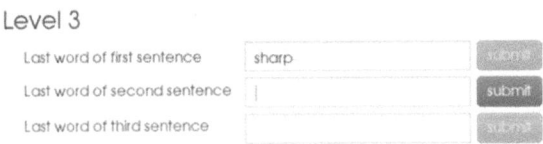

Fig. 4. Verbal Working Memory Test

3.2   Participants

A total of 107 undergraduate students (52 male, 55 female, age 17-26, mean 22) participated in the study. A total of 1172 CAPTCHA sessions have been recorded during a three-month period.

3.3   Hypothesis

The following hypothesis was formulated for the purpose of our research:

H_1. There is significant difference with regard to time (efficiency), total number of attempts and total number of refresh events (effectiveness) needed to solve a CAPTCHA mechanism among users with different cognitive processing abilities.

3.4   Analysis of Results

For the analysis, we separated participants into different categories based on their cognitive processing characteristics (limited, intermediate, enhanced) of each cognitive factor (speed of processing, controlled attention, working memory capacity), which are summarized in Table 1.

Table 1. User Groups based on Cognitive Processing Abilities

	Speed of Processing		Controlled Attention		Working Memory Capacity	
	F	%	F	%	F	%
Enhanced	59	55.1	33	30.8	46	43
Intermediate	19	17.8	18	16.8	27	25.2
Limited	29	27.1	56	52.3	34	31.8
Total	107	100	107	100	107	100

CAPTCHA Solving Efficiency. A series of three by three way factorial analyses of variance (ANOVA) were conducted aiming to examine main effects of users' cognitive processing differences (i.e., limited, intermediate, enhanced) and CAPTCHA complexity (i.e., low, medium, high) on the time needed to accomplish

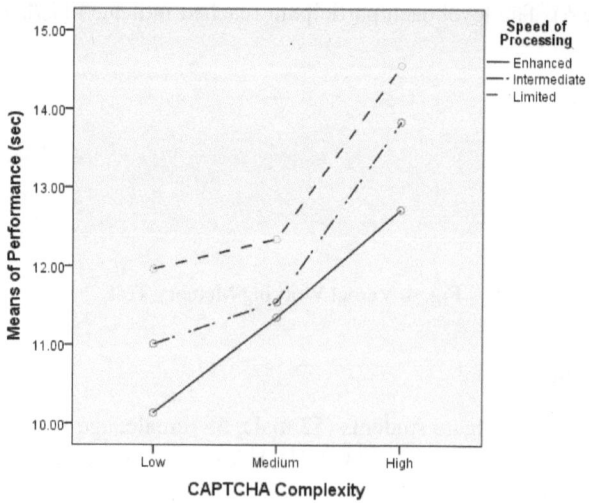

Fig. 5. Means of Performance for Speed of Processing User Groups

the CAPTCHA task. Figure 6 and Figure 7 respectively illustrate the means of performance per cognitive factor group in regard with the speed of processing (SP) and controlled attention (CA) dimension, and CAPTCHA complexity level. Table 2 and Table 3 respectively summarize post-hoc tests with CAPTCHA performance comparisons between each cognitive factor's user group (SP and CA).

The results revealed that there is a significant main effect on the time needed to solve a CAPTCHA challenge with regard to both speed of processing (SP) and controlled attention (CA) factors, and CAPTCHA complexity level. Users with enhanced SP solved significantly faster all three complexity types of CAPTCHA compared to the limited user group (p<.001).

Table 2. Multiple Comparisons between the Speed of Processing User Group

		Mean Difference	**Std. Error**	**Sig.**
Enhanced	Intermediate	-0.60	0.38	0.117
	Limited	-1.07	0.27	0.000
Intermediate	Enhanced	0.60	0.38	0.117
	Limited	-0.46	0.36	0.202
Limited	Enhanced	1.07	0.27	0.000
	Intermediate	0.46	0.36	0.202

On the other hand, users with intermediate SP did not perform significantly different compared to the limited user group (p=.202) and the enhanced user group (p=.117). Based on Figure 6, given that the means of performances of enhanced SP users in the high complex CAPTCHA, and limited SP users in the medium complex CAPTCHA were not significantly different, an adaptive CAPTCHA mechanism embracing these user characteristics could provide a highly complex CAPTCHA mechanism to users with enhanced SP, and a medium complex CAPTCHA mechanism to users with limited SP, thus having increased security for enhanced SP users, but at similar levels of usability in terms of efficiency compared to limited SP users. Similarly, given that users with limited and intermediate SP did not perform significantly different in low and medium levels of CAPTCHA complexity, in order to increase security, a medium level of complexity could be used at a minimum cost to usability.

Regarding the controlled attention (CA) dimension, results similarly indicate that users with enhanced CA perform significantly faster compared to users with limited CA (p=.001), however with no significant differences compared to users with intermediate CA (p=.111). On the other hand, no significant differences were observed between the limited and intermediate user groups across all three types of CAPTCHA complexity level (p=0.444).

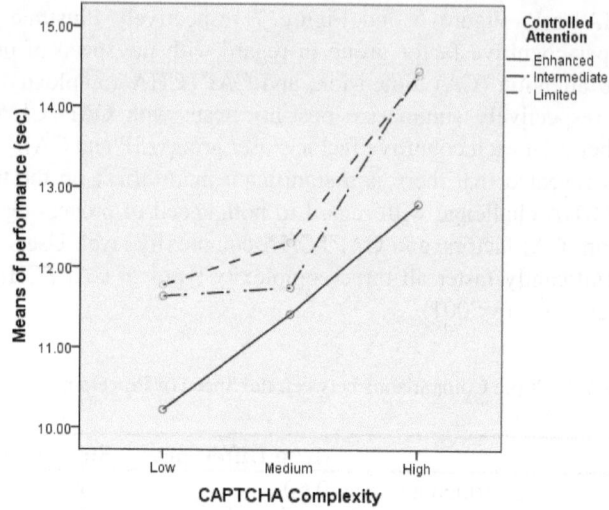

Fig. 6. Means of Performance for Controlled Attention User Groups

From a user-adaptation point of view, an adaptive CAPTCHA mechanism could recommend a CAPTCHA with medium complexity to users with limited and intermediate CA, given that these groups did not perform significantly different in the low and medium complex CAPTCHA. Regarding users with enhanced CA, a highly complex CAPTCHA for increased security could be provided since they did not perform significantly different in highly complex CAPTCHA compared to medium complex CAPTCHA interactions of the other two user groups, thus increasing security at minimum cost to usability for users with enhanced CA.

Table 3. Multiple Comparisons between the Controlled Attention User Group

		Mean Difference	**Std. Error**	**Sig.**
Enhanced	Intermediate	-0.63	0.39	0.111
	Limited	-0.93	0.27	0.001
Intermediate	Enhanced	0.63	0.39	0.111
	Limited	-0.29	0.39	0.444
Limited	Enhanced	0.93	0.27	0.001
	Intermediate	0.29	0.39	0.444

Regarding the working memory capacity (WMC) dimension, results also revealed a main effect of working memory capacity of users on the time to solve CAPTCHAs with different levels of complexity. Figure 8 illustrates the means of performance per WMC user group and CAPTCHA level of complexity. Table 4 summarizes the post-hoc tests with CAPTCHA performance comparisons between users with different working memory capacity.

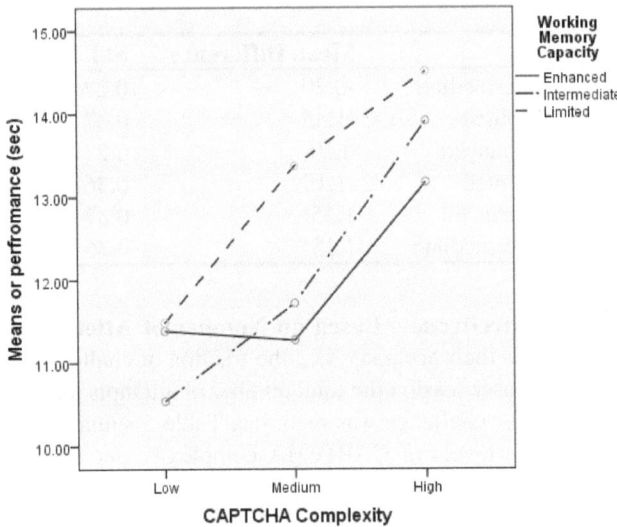

Fig. 7. Means of Performance for Working Memory Capacity User Groups

Accordingly, users with limited WMC performed significantly slower than users with intermediate WMS (p=.002) and enhanced WMC (p<.001). However, in the case of low level of CAPTCHA complexity we observe that users with enhanced WMC performed similarly as in the case of limited WMC users. A within analysis of the enhanced WMC group in this case revealed that the majority of users had limited and intermediate speed of processing which might have affected their performance. Such an observation is in line with previous theory suggesting that enhanced speed of information processing facilitates access to information that is sustained in the working memory system, and thus decreased speed of processing of users might have negatively affected their efficiency of information manipulation in the working memory system [23]. On the other hand, no significant differences between users with enhanced and intermediate WMC were observed.

To this end, as in the case of SP and CA factors, results suggest that individual differences in working memory capacity should be considered in CAPTCHA designs since a main effect of working memory capacity of users on time to solve CAPTCHA challenges has been observed. Results suggest that a CAPTCHA challenge with medium complexity could be provided to users with intermediate and enhanced WMC since no significant differences in performance were observed compared to the low complex (and less secure CAPTCHA), increasing thus security at a minimum cost to usability. In the case of limited WMC users, results suggest providing a less secure CAPTCHA to increase usability. However, regarding the intermediate and enhanced WMC groups, significant differences in their performance has been observed between the medium and high levels of CAPTCHA complexity, suggesting that a less complex (medium level), but more usable CAPTCHA challenge would significantly benefit the users.

Table 4. Multiple Comparisons between the Working Memory Capacity User Group

		Mean Difference	Std. Error	Sig.
Enhanced	Intermediate	-0.20	0.27	0.455
	Limited	-1.35	0.37	0.000
Intermediate	Enhanced	0.20	0.27	0.455
	Limited	-1.15	0.36	0.002
Limited	Enhanced	1.35	0.37	0.000
	Intermediate	1.15	0.36	0.002

CAPTCHA Solving Effectiveness Based on Number of Attempts. The effectiveness of a solver measures their accuracy, i.e., the fraction of challenges they answered correctly [30]. For each user session the total number of attempts made for successfully solving the CAPTCHA challenge was recorded. Table 5 summarizes the means of attempts across all three levels of CAPTCHA complexity per cognitive processing group (i.e., SP, CA, WMC groups). Shapiro-Wilk tests revealed that these distributions do not follow the normal distribution. On average, users with limited CA and limited WMC needed more attempts to solve the CAPTCHA challenges than the other two groups (intermediate and enhanced groups). The Kruskal-Wallis test revealed that the differences between controlled attention users was statistically significant ($H(2)=9.167$, $p=0.001$), as well as in the case of working memory capacity users ($H(2)=6.464$, $p=0.039$). In the case of the speed of processing user group, no significant differences have been observed between number of attempts of each user group, as the Kruskal-Wallis test revealed ($H(2)=3.744$, $p=0.154$), suggesting that this cognitive dimension might not significantly affect the effectiveness of CAPTCHA.

Table 5. Means of Attempts per User Group [35]

	Speed of Processing		Controlled Attention		Working Memory Capacity	
	Mean	Std. Dev.	Mean	Std. Dev.	Mean	Std. Dev.
Enhanced	2	1.37	1.71	1.07	1.82	1.06
Intermediate	1.71	1.1	1.38	0.81	1.51	0.98
Limited	1.6	1.05	2.1	1.42	2.21	1.66

Furthermore, the majority of CAPTCHA sessions (59.6%) of the sample were solved at the first try across all three cognitive groups. As expected, in the case of the low complexity CAPTCHA, 71.4% of the cases were solved at the first try, whereas in the case of medium and high complexity, the percentage decreased to 57.1% and 54.3%, respectively.

To this end, initial findings indicate that differences in controlled attention and working memory capacity might affect the effectiveness of CAPTCHA challenges since users of the intermediate and enhanced user groups needed less attempts than the ones of the limited user groups [35]. Such a result might be based on the fact that enhanced controlled attention and working memory capacity is needed to effectively focus a person's attention on the distorted characters among the added noise of current text-recognition CAPTCHAs.

CAPTCHA Solving Effectiveness Based on Number of Refreshes. Given that the CAPTCHA mechanism also contained a refresh button that initialized the CAPTCHA with a new sequence of characters in case the characters could not be recognized by the user, the solving effectiveness of CAPTCHA could also be inferred through the number of refreshes each user made in each session. Table 6 summarizes the means of refreshes across all three levels of CAPTCHA complexity per cognitive processing group (i.e., SP, CA, WMC groups). Given that the majority of sessions (72.8%) did not include a refresh event, our analysis includes sessions that needed at least one refresh event. Shapiro-Wilk tests revealed that these distributions do not follow the normal distribution.

Table 6. Means of Refreshes per User Group

	Speed of Processing		Controlled Attention		Working Memory Capacity	
	Mean	**Std. Dev.**	**Mean**	**Std. Dev.**	**Mean**	**Std. Dev.**
Enhanced	1.22	0.42	1.38	0.65	1.14	0.37
Intermediate	1.13	0.35	1.17	0.40	1.40	0.69
Limited	1.64	0.84	1.38	0.66	1.39	0.65

On average, users with limited processing abilities initiated more refresh events than the other two user groups, however, these differences were not significant as the Kruskal-Wallis test revealed (*SOP:* H(2)=3.571, p=0.168; *CA:* H(2)=0.503, p=0.778; *WMC:* H(2)=0.830, p=0.660). In this respect, no safe conclusions can be drawn at this point in time whether cognitive processing abilities have a main effect on CAPTCHA effectiveness in terms of refresh rates. This may be due to the fact that the number of initiated refresh events was limited. Nevertheless, as the sample increased, users with limited cognitive processing abilities tended to initiate more refresh events than users with intermediate and enhanced cognitive processing abilities. In this respect, further studies need to be conducted with a greater sample over a longer period of user interactions in order to reach to more concrete conclusions about the effect of cognitive processing abilities on the effectiveness of CAPTCHA in terms of refresh events.

3.5   Validity and Limitations of the Study

The validity of a study is primarily affected by its internal, external, and ecological validity. Internal validity reflects the accuracy of data and the conclusions drawn based on this data, external validity indicates whether the data and the conclusions drawn can be generalized to a wider extend [31], and ecological validity requires that the experimental design, procedure and setting of the study must approximate the real-life context that is under investigation [32].

With the aim to increase internal validity we recruited a sample of participants already familiarized with CAPTCHAs prior to the study. Thus, the participants involved rather experienced and average than novice users with respect to CAPTCHA and therefore, the research design was setup in order to avoid inference errors. There has also been an effort to increase ecological of the research since the CAPTCHA tasks were integrated in a real Web-based system and the participants were involved at their own physical environments without the intervention of any experimental equipment or person. In addition, participants were required to solve the CAPTCHA challenges as a secondary task throughout the semester during real-life tasks (the primary task was to post comments on the online blogging tool). Finally, given that future studies will contribute to the external validity of the reported research, we argue that providing personalized CAPTCHA mechanisms, adapted to users' cognitive processing abilities, as well as other individual characteristics [3, 9, 33, 34, 35] could improve the overall user experience with regard to CAPTCHA tasks.

The limitations of the reported study are related to the fact that participants were only undergraduate students with an age between 17 to 26 years. Furthermore, a single assessment of users' cognitive factors through the psychometric tests might not fully justify the users' cognitive classification since other factors (e.g., emotions, urgency, etc.) might influence the users' interactions with the test. In this respect, further studies need to be conducted with a greater sample of varying profiles and ages in order to reach to more concrete conclusions about the effect of individuals' cognitive processing abilities on their performance in CAPTCHA challenges.

4   Conclusions

The research reported aimed to increase our understanding on supporting usable CAPTCHA designs through user modeling, and adaptivity for assisting users to accomplish efficiently and effectively usable CAPTCHA tasks. Accordingly, a three-month ecological valid user study was designed which entailed credible psychometric-based tests for eliciting the users' cognitive characteristics and a text-recognition CAPTCHA, with the aim to investigate whether individuals with different cognitive processing abilities perform differently in terms of efficiency and effectiveness in text-recognition CAPTCHA challenges with different levels of complexity.

Preliminary results reveal that cognitive processing abilities of individuals primarily affect solving efficiency of text-recognition CAPTCHA mechanisms. In particular, results demonstrated that users with enhanced controlled attention and speed of processing performed significantly faster than users with limited processing abilities across all three levels of CAPTCHA complexity. Furthermore, users with limited and intermediate cognitive processing abilities performed similarly in the low and medium complexity CAPTCHA, however a decreased performance of these users was observed in the high complex CAPTCHA type. Such a result suggests that medium complexity CAPTCHA should be provided to users with limited and intermediate cognitive processing abilities since no significant differences were observed with the lower complex CAPTCHA. Such a recommendation would increase security (medium complexity instead of low) and preserve usability in terms of efficiency at equal levels. In addition, since users with enhanced cognitive processing abilities performed slightly slower in the high complex CAPTCHA compared to the less complex CAPTCHAs of the limited and intermediate user groups, a highly complex CAPTCHA could be used in the case of users with enhanced cognitive processing abilities, thus increasing even more the security of CAPTCHA at a minimum cost of usability.

Regarding the working memory dimension, significant differences in performance have been observed between users with enhanced and limited working memory capacity (primarily in the cases of medium and high complexity CAPTCHA) suggesting that users with limited working memory capacity should be provided with less complex CAPTCHA for increasing usability. Furthermore, results revealed that speed of processing abilities might affect performance in regard with working memory capacity since a within-group analysis of enhanced WMC users revealed that the majority of them had limited and intermediate levels of processing speed, thus providing a possible explanation to the fact that enhanced WMC users performed with no significant differences in the low complex CAPTCHA, compared to limited WMC users.

Regarding effectiveness (total number of attempts), initial findings indicate that controlled attention and working memory capacity affect the effectiveness of CAPTCHA challenges since users with limited cognitive processing abilities needed more attempts than the other two user groups. On the other hand, no main effect of speed of processing on the effectiveness of solving CAPTCHAs has been revealed since the differences among user groups were not significant. This result further strengthens the validity of our theoretical background since speed of processing primarily affects efficiency of interaction, whereas in the case of effectiveness, enhanced controlled attention and working memory capacity are primarily needed to effectively focus a person's attention on the distorted characters among the added noise of CAPTCHAs. Furthermore, regarding effectiveness in terms of total number of refresh events, at this point in time, no safe conclusions can be drawn whether there is a thorough significant relationship between users' cognitive processing abilities and effectiveness in regard with CAPTCHA mechanisms since the majority of sessions did not include refresh events. Nevertheless, the analysis indicates that users with limited cognitive processing abilities initiated more refresh events to solve the CAPTCHA challenges compared to users with intermediate and enhanced cognitive processing abilities.

To this end, recent research [3, 9, 33, 34, 35] suggests that an effective CAPTCHA solution should embrace both security and usability aspects as its purpose is to provide safety of operation to Web application providers but as well usability and transparency to its end users, aiming to minimize the added cognitive effort of a casual user interacting with it. Both security and usability are important, and every CAPTCHA solution should be a balancing act between the two, aiming to achieve maximum security, but at a minimum cost to usability. Based on the presented results we suggest that following a user-centered design approach, it is necessary that designers of CAPTCHA mechanisms should clearly bear in mind individual differences of users while interacting with the system, and accordingly provide a balanced usable and secure solution. In sum, the findings of the study suggest that all three cognitive factors (speed of processing, controlled attention, working memory capacity) should be taken into consideration when designing CAPTCHAs for improving the efficiency of interactions since significant differences in all three cognitive-based user groups where observed in CAPTCHAs with different complexity. With the aim to improve effectiveness of CAPTCHA interactions, the results suggest considering controlled attention and working memory capacity of users since significant differences have been observed in CAPTCHA interactions within these cognitive-based user groups.

A practical implication of this work would be to allow users explicitly declare their preferred CAPTCHA mechanism in their Web browser preference settings, and this information would be further utilized by the Web browser to present a personalized CAPTCHA challenge. Such a scenario assumes that the Web browser and the CAPTCHA mechanism of the service provider communicate under a common standard and protocol in order to personalize the CAPTCHA challenge according to the user profile stored on the Web browser. A more sophisticated approach could be based on a recommendation engine that would implicitly present the "best-fit" CAPTCHA mechanism based on historical usage data of the user in regard with efficiency and effectiveness of CAPTCHA tasks. In this respect, the high-level research goal of such an attempt would focus around two main issues; appropriate user modeling dealing with what information is important to be incorporated in the user model and how it can be represented and extracted, and appropriate adaptation procedures dealing with what adaptation types and mechanisms are most effective to be performed and how they can be translated into adaptive user interface designs in order to improve the system's usability and to provide a positive user experience with regard to CAPTCHA mechanisms.

Studies like the reported one can be useful for improving usable security on the World Wide Web through adaptivity in user interface designs with regard to CAPTCHA mechanisms, aiming to organize and present information and functionalities related with CAPTCHA tasks in an adaptive format to diverse user groups, by using different levels of abstractions through appropriate interaction styles, terminology, information presentation and user modeling techniques.

Acknowledgements. The work is co-funded by the PersonaWeb project under the Cyprus Research Promotion Foundation (ΤΠΕ/ΠΛΗΡΟ/0311(ΒΙΕ)/10), and the EU projects Co-LIVING (60-61700-98-009) and SocialRobot (285870).

References

1. von Ahn, L., Blum, M., Langford, J.: Telling Humans and Computers Apart Automatically. Communications of the ACM 47, 56–60 (2004)
2. von Ahn, L., Blum, M., Hopper, N.J., Langford, J.: CAPTCHA: Using hard AI problems for security. In: Biham, E. (ed.) EUROCRYPT 2003. LNCS, vol. 2656, pp. 294–311. Springer, Heidelberg (2003)

3. Bursztein, E., Bethard, S., Fabry, C., Mitchell, J.C., Jurafsky, D.: How Good are Humans at Solving CAPTCHAs? A Large Scale Evaluation. In: IEEE Symposium on Security and Privacy, pp. 399–413. IEEE Computer Society, Washington, DC (2010)
4. von Ahn, L., Maurer, B., McMillen, C., Abraham, D., Blum, M.: reCAPTCHA: Human-Based Character Recognition via Web Security Measures. Science 321(5895), 1465–1468 (2008)
5. Pogue, D.: Time to Kill OffCaptchas - How the Bot-proofing of the Internet is Bringing Humans Down. Scientific American (2012)
6. Yan, J., El Ahmad, A.S.: A Low-cost Attack on a Microsoft CAPTCHA. In: 15th ACM International Conference on Computer and Communications Security, pp. 543–554. ACM Press, New York (2008)
7. Baecher, P., Büscher, N., Fischlin, M., Milde, B.: Breaking reCAPTCHA: A Holistic Approach via Shape Recognition. In: Camenisch, J., Fischer-Hübner, S., Murayama, Y., Portmann, A., Rieder, C. (eds.) SEC 2011. IFIP AICT, vol. 354, pp. 56–67. Springer, Heidelberg (2011)
8. Yan, J., El Ahmad, A.S.: Usability of CAPTCHAs or Usability Issues in CAPTCHA Design. In: ACM International Symposium on Usable Security and Privacy, pp. 44–52. ACM Press, New York (2008)
9. Fidas, C., Voyiatzis, A., Avouris, N.: On the Necessity of User-friendly CAPTCHA. In: ACM International Conference on Human Factors in Computing Systems, pp. 2623–2626. ACM Press, New York (2011)
10. Brusilovsky, P., Kobsa, A., Nejdl, W.: The Adaptive Web: Methods and Strategies of Web Personalization. Springer, Heidelberg (2007)
11. Germanakos, P., Tsianos, N., Lekkas, Z., Mourlas, C., Belk, M., Samaras, G.: Towards an Adaptive and Personalized Web Interaction using Human Factors. In: Angelides, M., Mylonas, P., Wallace, M. (eds.) Advances in Semantic Media Adaptation and Personalization, pp. 247–282. Taylor & Francis (2009)
12. Triantafillou, E., Pomportsis, A., Demetriadis, S., Georgiadou, E.: The Value of Adaptivity based on Cognitive Style: an Empirical Study. Educational Technology 35, 95–106 (2004)
13. Graf, S.: Kinshuk: Advanced Adaptivity in Learning Management Systems by Considering Learning Styles. In: International Workshop on Social and Personal Computing for Web-Supported Learning Communities, pp. 235–238 (2009)
14. Riding, R.: Cognitive Style Analysis - Research Administration. Learning and Training Technology (2001)
15. Witkin, H.A., Moore, C.A., Goodenough, D.R., Cox, P.W.: Field-dependent and field-independent Cognitive Styles and their Educational Implications. Review of Educational Research 47, 1–64 (1977)
16. Demetriou, A., Spanoudis, G., Shayer, S., Mouyi, A., Kazi, S., Platsidou, M.: Cycles in Speed-Working Memory-G Relations: Towards a Developmental-Differential Theory of the Mind. Intelligence 41, 34–50 (2013)
17. Hunt, E.B.: Human Intelligence. Cambridge University Press, New York (2011)
18. Demetriou, A., Spanoudis, G., Mouyi, A.: Educating the Developing Mind: Towards an Overarching Paradigm. Educational Psychology Review 23(4), 601–663 (2011)
19. MacLeod, C.M.: Half a Century of Research on the Stroop Effect: An Integrative review. Psychological Bulletin 109, 163–203 (1991)
20. Posner, M.I., Raicle, M.E.: Images of Mind. Scientific American Library, New York (1997)
21. Stroop, J.R.: Studies of Interference in Serial Verbal Reactions. Experimental Psychology 18, 643–662 (1935)

22. Baddeley, A.: Working Memory: Theories, Models, and Controversies. Annual Review of Psychology 63, 1–29 (2012)
23. Baddeley, A.: Working Memory. Science 255(5044), 556–559 (1992)
24. Conway, A.R.A., Cowan, N., Bunting, M.F., Therriault, D.J., Minkoff, S.R.: A Latent Variable Analysis of Working Memory Capacity, Short-term Memory Capacity, Processing Speed, and General Fluid Intelligence. Intelligence 30, 163–183 (2002)
25. Shipstead, Z., Broadway, J.: Individual Differences in Working Memory Capacity and the Stroop Effect: Do High Spans Block the Words? Learning and Individual Differences (in press)
26. Demetriou, A., Christou, C., Spanoudis, G., Platsidou, M.: The Development of Mental Processing: Efficiency, Working Memory and Thinking. Monographs of the Society for Research in Child Development 67(1) (2002)
27. Unsworth, N., Spillers, G.: Working Memory Capacity: Attention Control, Secondary Memory, or Both? A Direct Test of the Dual-component Model. Memory and Language 62, 392–406 (2010)
28. Cowan, N.: The Magical Mystery Four: How is Working Memory Capacity Limited, and Why? Current Directions in Psychological Science 19(1), 51–57 (2010)
29. Klingberg, T.: The Overflowing Brain: Information Overload and the Limits of Working Memory. Oxford University Press, New York (2009)
30. Bursztein, E., Martin, M., Mitchell, J.: Text-based CAPTCHA Strengths and Weaknesses. In: 18th ACM International Conference on Computer and Communications Security, pp. 125–138. ACM Press, New York (2011)
31. Cook, T., Campbell, D.: Quasi-experimentation: Design and Analysis Issues for Field Settings. Houghton Mifflin Company, Boston (1979)
32. Brewer, M.: Research Design and Issues of Validity. In: Reis, H., Judd, C. (eds.) Handbook of Research Methods in Social and Personality Psychology, pp. 3–16. Cambridge University Press, Cambridge (2000)
33. Belk, M., Fidas, C., Germanakos, P., Samaras, G.: Do Cognitive Styles of Users Affect Preference and Performance Related to CAPTCHA Challenges? In: ACM International Conference on Human Factors in Computing Systems, pp. 1487–1492. ACM Press, New York (2012)
34. Holzinger, A., Lugmayr, A., Bogner, M.S.: Security and Usability Workshop. In: IEEE International Conference on Availability, Reliability and Security. IEEE Computing Society, Washington, DC (2009)
35. Belk, M., Germanakos, P., Fidas, C., Spanoudis, G., Samaras, G.: Studying the Effect of Human Cognition on Text- and Image-recognition CAPTCHA Mechanisms. In: International Conference on Human-Computer Interaction - HCI International. LNCS, Springer, Heidelberg (in press, 2013)

Personality Influences on Etiquette Requirements for Social Media in the Work Context
When Jaunty Juveniles Communicate with Serious Suits

André Calero Valdez, Anne Kathrin Schaar, and Martina Ziefle

Human-Computer Interaction Center,
RWTH Aachen University, Germany
{calero-valdez,schaar,ziefle}@comm.rwth-aachen.de

Abstract. Today social media is used extensively in both private and professional contexts, with using habits and conventions shaped by the private using context. It is unknown how in the users perception professional social media usage might differ from the private context and which implicit or explicit etiquette criteria apply. With an empirical questionnaire approach (N=99, ages 20-59) we examined the impact of perceived formal correctness, formal politeness and workflow compatibility of social media applications (email, blog and chat) on the acceptance of social media in the working context. We additionally analyzed the impact of personality on users perceptions toward social media etiquette. Therefore we examined correlations between two Five Factor Model (FFM or Big Five) personality traits (conscientiousness and agreeableness) and requirements for formal correctness, formal politeness and compatibility. Linear regression shows that requirements for social media etiquette are strongly influenced by conscientiousness, age and social media expertise. Differences in etiquette are evaluated in regard to formal addressing, correct spelling, acronym and emoticon usage, work disruption and perceived urgency. Furthermore differences in etiquette between different media are explained.

Keywords: Social media, technology acceptance, etiquette, personality, user centred-design.

1 Introduction and Motivation for Research

Using social media in a professional context has been an integral part of company strategies for some years now. Although social media has arrived in nearly every business sector, the implementation alone is no guarantee for its success. Company efforts in social media are visible on the Internet through activities on Facebook, twitter, blogs and others[1].

Invisible to the public eye are all activities in the field of internal communication. The typical fields of application for internal usage of social media are

A. Holzinger et al. (Eds.): SouthCHI 2013, LNCS 7946, pp. 427–446, 2013.

social networks sites with included wikis[2], blogs and other networks functions that are used for internal knowledge management. Knowledge management was devised along fundamental changes in the work environment. The shift from physical labour to knowledge work turned knowledge into a central resource of these days [3]. As Peter Drucker wrote, "knowledge is the only meaningful economic resource"[4]. Considering that the majority of baby boomers are going into retirement within the next decade, the importance of retaining expert knowledge within organizations and companies is crucial for their survival. The progressively aging workforce in combination with the increasing shift towards a knowledge society implies considerable requirements for the challenge of how expert knowledge of older workers can be efficiently used and distributed within a company[5]. Since effects like propinquity and social exchange are important for effective cooperation[6], companies put a lot of effort into technical solutions like social media that can support knowledge storage and exchange by leveraging social exchange.

The fundamental problem in this context is the circumstance that the bare technical solution is by far not enough: Professional communication has its own rules. Communication partners share knowledge of both explicit communication rituals as well as implicit and tacit communication habits and rules [7]. Those are not necessarily cognizant to communication partners, though implicitly well-established within and across companies and working groups. Similar to private communication professional communication is governed by an own etiquette and unspoken rules.

In the context of social media in the work environment we face the problem that a technology with private communication habits looms into an official sector. Especially in German language areas a gap between the usage of formal and informal language exists, due to the fine-grained variance in honorific addresses [8].

In order to find out more about acceptance parameters in the context of professional social media usage we executed this explorative study to examine the influence of a perceived need for formal correctness (like spelling), formal politeness (like honorific addresses) and the compatibility of social media into the workflow. These factors have been found to convey a sense of politeness in the chat medium in prior research [9]. Additionally we analyzed the impact of two personality (conscientiousness and agreeableness) traits on communication style preference. These factors were selected, because prior research has shown that these moderate the influence of communication between superiors and subordinates [10].

The following section presents related work and how it motivates this study. Section 3 presents the main focus of the study and the central questions addressed. Section 4 contains the methodology of the study with a description of the variables used and the questionnaire instrument. The sample is described in section 5. The central findings of the study are presented in section 6 and discussed in section 7 with a conclusion and the naming of some limitations.

2 Related Work

In the following subsections we present the different elements relevant to our study. Section 2.1 presents the status quo of social media usage in company internal communication. Section 2.2 gives more insights into the relevance of etiquette for computer-mediated communication. Section 2.3 introduces blog and chat as possible social media applications for internal business communication. Section 2.4 presents what we mean by user personality and the FFM items used for this study [11].

2.1 Social Media in Internal Communication and Its Acceptance

Social media in internal communication is mostly used for knowledge management. A recent study about the implementation of social media in German, Austrian, and Swiss companies revealed that the goals of social media implementation in the working context are predominantly congruent with the goals of knowledge management [12].

According to Richter et al. the main benefit of social media usage in a company's context can be seen in goal orientated communication, efficient knowledge transfer, the foundation of networks of experts, foundation of an open corporate culture, and an enhancement of transparency and innovation of the company [12]. But pure implementation of social media does not imply any success. Acceptance, mediated by perceived ease of use and usefulness for the potential users, is the key to a successful installation and realization of any technology. Acceptance also depends on how much a technology considers individual abilities, communication needs and requirements [13–17]. This is particularly true for social media [18].

The integration of the users specific needs was identified as one central criterion for acceptance of any Web 2.0 usage [19]. In this context it is crucial that individual preferences have to be satisfied before any collective usage should commence, although a collective usage of social media is the key feature for its professional usage. In this context the need for an understanding of the individual communication preferences becomes relevant. Ignoring individual needs and comforts would risk acceptance of the potential users.

Summing this section up we can say that proper social media integration supports the goals of knowledge management by improving internal communication of companies.

2.2 Ettiquette and Its Relevance for Communication

Human communication underlies several rule systems. Starting from rules of phonology, semantics, syntax rules, pragmatics, prosodic rules stretching over to idiosyncratic rules as well [20]. Some of these rules are in place to enable content transmission, others to enrich transmission with messages of relationship, emotion but also belonging.

In 1978 Brown and Levinson first described politeness theory in order to understand how possibly aggressive parties are able to communicate by applying a diplomatic protocol [21]. Furthermore people apply this protocol in everyday life situations to enable them to live and work together effectively. "Etiquette is not always about being pleasant, it is about being appropriate" [22]. This appropriateness needs further assessment when regarding it to language use in social media.

Cultural specific aspects are also important to acknowledge when looking at acceptance of any technology [23]. Since language is heavily culture dependent, cultural depend analyses must be performed.

In this work we consider etiquette for written online communication. This means we consider formal correctness, formal addressing and work disruption. Work disruption means how one feels to be disrupted by communication and how urgency of a particular medium influences work disruption.

In the following subsection the two social media applications chat and blog are presented in short to illustrate the range of services of social media that may be present in internal communication and how they relate to human communication.

2.3   Media

The three central media that we look at in this work are *chat*, *blog* and *email*. All three of them are compared. These media were selected, because they appear in many social platforms designed for internal communication. In order to have a similar understanding of what exactly chat and blog refer to and why they are different from email, we briefly describe their characteristics.

Chat. Chat as one application of the social media portfolio offers the opportunity to start up a conversation with someone instantly. Although chat represents an electronic mean of communication it even shows some oral communications habits [24]. Examinations of chat communication revealed that chat is medially classified as a written and connectional as an oral form of communication [24]. When looking at many chat transcripts one can find that upper and lower case usage as well as proper punctuation marks are usually missing [25]. Kilian states that people economize finger-to-key-motions, which causes the absence of this formal correctness. Another reason for mistakes and fuzziness in the field of spelling is the fact that the chat is a synchronous channel of communication: The synchronicity of communication induces a feeling of time pressure, which explains frequent mistakes as well as using abbreviations and acronyms (e.g. "afk" ∼ away from keyboard) and emoticons (smiley). Emoticons are additionally used to compensate for the missing opportunity to communicate with gestures and facial expressions. Emoticons are substitutions of important para- and nonverbal communication facets which are naturally present in face-to-face communication [26]. It is important to note, that chat communication changes depending on the circumstances it is used in, because emoticons and abbreviations might not be adequate for the working context.

Blogs. Weblogs (or Blogs) are a new medium for publication on the Internet. Via content management systems the opportunity for publication on the Internet arises for every one. Articles that are published in a Blog, appear in a chronological order on a web page. A blog offers a comment function that allows a reader to voice his opinion in regard to the published article. This opportunity enables discussions and exchange, and has even been used in learning environments [27]. Additionally a blogger has the chance to refer to other web pages via Hyperlinks. Especially through the comment function and the opportunity to refer to other web content the blog is a suitable medium for group communication [28]. The blog language is predominantly colloquial. In contrast to chat communication, communication in blogs takes orthographical rules into consideration more intensively. The reason for the higher consideration of spelling can be seen in the asynchronicity character of blog communication. Blog communication and the blogosphere, according to Schmidt, claim to adhere to formal correctness of language, correctness in terms of content as well as actuality of content [29].

It remains to be seen whether applying blogs to a work context is a suitable approach to improve knowledge exchange. In particular rules for blog etiquette and their importance need to be established.

2.4   Personality

Differential psychology has established measures of differences in personality that have been validated in many studies [30]. The most used model that emerged from prior research is the five-factor model (FFM) that measures the factors (1) neuroticism, (2) extraversion, (3) openness to new experiences, (4) conscientiousness and (5) agreeableness. Prior research suggests that personality traits influence usage behavior of social media in regard to private usage [31, 32]. How personality factors relate to social media in the professional context and the work environment has not been established yet.

3   Main Focus of the Study and Questions Addressed

For this research it was of interest whether the personality traits "conscientiousness" and "agreeableness" influenced the perceived importance of etiquette in social media usage in the work context. When looking at existing models of technology acceptance for social media, the influence of personality traits has been investigated recently only for private social networks [33–35]. Since users pick the interactions themselves within private social networks, it can be assumed that questions of etiquette are managed in a similar fashion as in private real life.

In the work environment habits of interaction are not voluntary but necessary and obligatory. This circumstance is framed by work and/or organizational requirements. Normal forms of politeness should remain similar in social network communication, but social media mediated communication brings new questions to the table. In particular it is of interest whether certain ways of using social media are accepted differently from social media in general.

Is social media used as a written medium or regarded as an oral medium? Do written or oral forms of politeness apply? How is it perceived in the work environment and is the perception of usefulness of social media influenced by the diversity of users with different amounts of experience with social media usage? Is social media different from established forms of computer-mediated communication (e.g. email)?

- RQ1: Does conscientiousness influence etiquette for social media?
- RQ2: Does agreeableness influence etiquette for social media?
- RQ3: Does the medium play a role for etiquette?
- RQ4: Does age play a role in etiquette?
- RQ5: Does social media experience play a role?

From these research questions the following hypotheses where formulated.

- H1: Conscientiousness has a positive effect on desire for etiquette.
- H2: Agreeableness has a negative effect on desire for etiquette.
- H3: Social Media Usage has a negative effect on desire for etiquette.
- H4: Age has a positive effect on the need for etiquette.
- H5: Chat is the medium with the least requirements in etiquette.
- H6: Private social media and work social media experience have different effects on etiquette.

4   Methodology

The main goal of this study was to find out whether the personal wish for an adequate etiquette has an influence on the attitude towards social media usage in the working context. To reach a larger number of participants the questionnaire method was chosen. The questionnaire was delivered electronically. The questionnaire instrument was revised by a sample of adults of different ages before the study was executed in order to check phrasing and comprehensibility of questions. Filling out the questionnaire took the testing sample between 15 and 25 minutes. Participants were approached through the researchers individual networks. Participation was voluntary and thus the sample is self-selected.

4.1   Variables

As independent variables we have chosen age, gender, social media expertise as well as the factors conscientiousness and agreeableness of the Five Factor Model (FFM). Dependent variables were the evaluation of formal correctness, formal politeness and compatibility with the workflow for email, chat and blog as social media components. The research model is visualized in Figure 1.

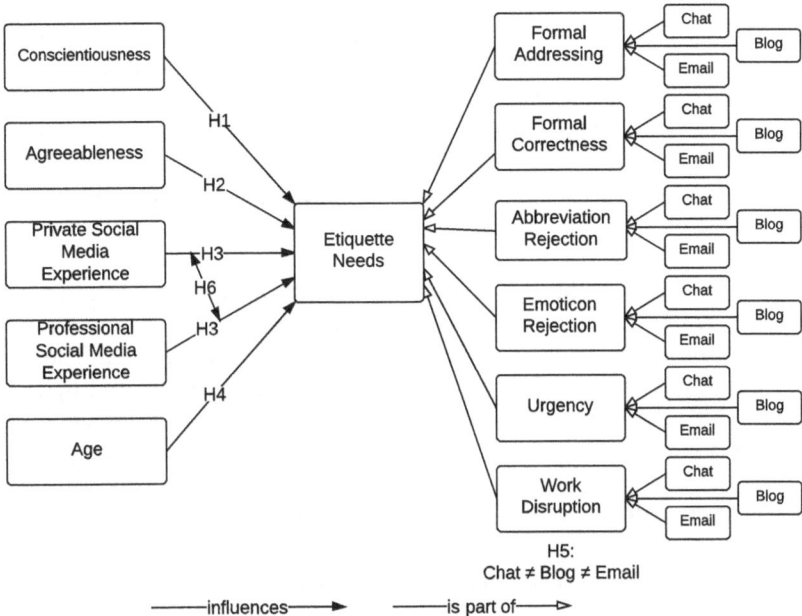

Fig. 1. The research model of this work. Ettiquette needs consists of four subscales, which each consist of items for the three media.

4.2   The Questionnaire

The questionnaire was divided into four main parts: (a) demographic data, (b) social media expertise, (c) FFM personality traits (conscientiousness and agreeableness) as well as (d) evaluation of etiquette preferences related to formal correctness, formal politeness and compatibility (with the workflow) in the context of e-mail, chat and blog. The last part measures the willingness to use both chat and blog.

Demographic Data. In order to get more information about the participants of this survey we asked them to answer questions about their age, gender and field of work (technical or non technical).

Social Media Experience: Private and in the Working Context. The private social media experience was measured by a question asking whether a person uses social media with dichotomous answering options. Additionally we asked for the frequency of social media usage and how much one likes to use it. According to usage frequency answers had to be selected out of a 7-point scale (daily, 2-3x/week, once a week, 2-3x/month, once a month, 2-3x/year, never). Asking for the degree of liking social media ("I use social Media...") , the participants could choose answering option from 1 = very unwillingly to 6 = very willingly.

In the context of the professional usage of social media participants had to indicate whether they use social media for professional reasons (answering options "yes" and "no"). Additionally we asked the participants whether their company had their own internal social media application (answering options "yes" and "no"). In addition to this general information also the frequency of usage was assessed (7= daily to 1 = never) as well as the extent to which users like using the application (1=very unwillingly to 6 very willingly), addressing the hedonic component of using social media.

FFM Personality Traits Conscientiousness and Agreeableness. The personality traits "conscientiousness" and "agreeableness" were measured by a German item set for the Big Five [11]. These constructs refer to the original FFM variables of the used factors. Each factor had to be evaluated by 10 items on a six-point Likert scale from (1=totally disagree to 6= totally agree). Items that did not reach sufficient Kaiser-Meyer-Olkin measures in principal component analysis were dropped from the full scale (remaining items see Table 1). The scales were calculated as the means of the remaining items.

Table 1. Items for agreeableness and conscientiousness (translated) and Cronbach's α for each scale

Scale and Reliability	Item-Text
Agreeableness, $\alpha = .716$	I put an effort into always being kind. I am a polite person. I am socially engaged. I am a generous person. It is easy for myself to defer my needs for others. I would never take my bad mood out on someone.
Conscientiousness, $\alpha = .887$	I have principles and I adhere to them. Even having to pay a small fine is uncomfortable for me. I put an effort into assuring that rules are complied to. I am very duteous. I complete my tasks with high precision. I was neat and tidy even as a child. If I have decided, I will not stray. I always do things with a plan in mind.

Etiquette in Email, Blog and Chat. The attitude towards etiquette in the context of e-mail, blog and chat had to be evaluated by a six-point Likert scale (1 = totally disagree – 6 = totally agree) with 11 items over the three different forms of communication (33 items total – see Table 2). All scales showed high reliability (alpha values ranging from .74 to .92). Scales were calculated as sums and then normalized by item count.

Table 2. Etiquette items for e-mail, blog, and chat (translated) and Cronbach's α for each scale

Scale and Reliability	Item-Text (one for email, chat and blog each)
Formal addressing, $\alpha = .918$ for 3x3 items	Formal salutations are important for me. An honorific address is important for me. I want to be addressed with my full name.
Formal correctness, $\alpha = .820$ for 2x3 items	Messages that disregard a correct spelling bother me. I pay attention to correct spelling and punctuation marks.
Abbreviation Rejection, $\alpha = .831$ for 1x3 items	I wish abbreviations like fyi (for your interest), brb (be right back), afk (away from keyboard) would be disposed.
Emoticon Rejection, $\alpha = .775$ for 1x3 items	Using emoticons (like smilies etc.) is okay for me. (negative item).
Urgency, $\alpha = .789$ for 2x3 items	I want a quick response to my message. I feel forced to response to messages quickly.
Disruption, $\alpha = .789$ for 1x3 items	Arriving messages interrupt my workflow.

5 Sample Description

In order to allow retesting we report demographic data, social media expertise and personality traits of the sample in the following sections.

5.1 Demographic Data

A total of 99 participants answered the questionnaire in an age range between 20 to 59 years (M=28.8 years, SD=10). The gender distribution was quite balanced with 46 male and 53 female participants. Regarding the field of work the majority of the participants work non-technical jobs (n=70). Only 29 reported to have a job that belongs to a technical field.

5.2 Social Media Experience: Private and in the Working Context

In the private sector the majority (89%, n=80) of our participants use social media. Only 11 out of 99 reported not using social media for private purposes. We can also report that those who use social media are doing this regularly: Figure 2 illustrates that over 80% of the sample use it daily.

The question how much someone likes using social media, on a six-point Likert scale (from 1=*"very unwillingly"* to 6=*"very willingly)"* was answered form 36% with very much, further 46% reported to like using social media. Only 18% rather liked or disliked using social media (see Fig.2).

In the context of a professional usage of social media, we found that 31% (N=25) are currently using social media in the working context. For the working

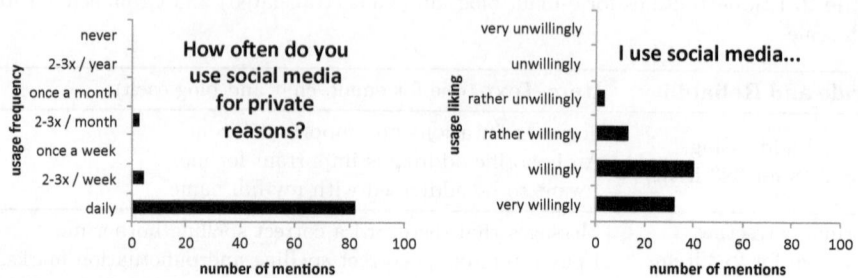

Fig. 2. Usage frequency and liking of usage of social media

context we additionally asked if the company of our participants uses own social media like internal blogs, or social networks. In our sample a total of 27 participants reported that their companies offer such technologies. When looking at individual liking of social media usage we could see that replies are not as homogenous. In our sample 20 out of 28 stated liking using social media usage ("*very willingly*" – "*rather willingly*").

Summarising we can say that participants of the study were found to be quite familiar with social media in a private context. In contrast, for the job context, we can report that only the minority is yet using social media at work. Those who have the opportunity to use company-owned social media revealed a heterogeneous using frequency and degree of liking to use it.

5.3   FFM Personality Traits Conscientiousness and Agreeableness

In addition to the assessment of demographic data and individual expertise with social media in the private and the working context we asked each participant to answer the FFM personality scales for the two selected factors, *agreeableness* and *conscientiousness*, in order to relate personality effects to the acceptance of social media and its etiquette.

Testing both scales with Kolmogorov-Smirnoff revealed that only *agreeableness* is distributed normally in this sample ($p > .05$) (see also Fig. 3). People of this sample score rather high on conscientiousness.

6   Results

Results were analyzed using bivariate correlation analysis and then in a second step with linear regression analysis. A level of significance was chosen with 95%. Test for differences of means was performed with t-tests, supported with ANOVA and ANCOVA analysis. Effect sizes for non-parametric tests are reported as Pearson's r-values with explained variances if applicable (r^2). For all used scales Cronbach's alpha for the tested sample is reported. For linear regression analysis B-values with standard errors as well as standardized slopes (β) are reported.

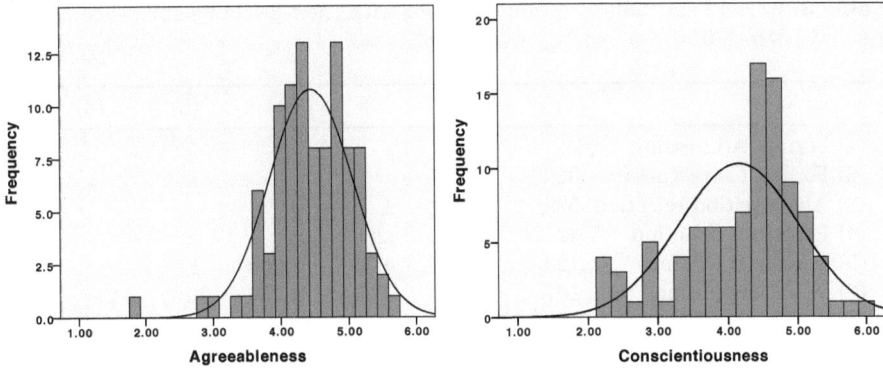

Fig. 3. Histogram and normality plot of agreeableness (left) and conscientiousness (right). The sample leans slightly to the higher end of the scale of agreeableness. Although tested as distributed normally, the conscientiousness distribution peaks at the higher middle ranges of the scale.

Missing values were deleted list-wise. Note that the semiotic meanings of the scales are different, which should be kept in mind when reading the results. The scales "formal addressing" and "formal correctness" represent a desire for these items, while "abbreviation" and "emoticon rejection" represent a reluctance to use these items. The "urgency" scale represents the perceived need for urgency in response to social media and "disruption" describes the perceived disruptiveness of social media.

6.1   Interaction of Personality and Etiquette

Factors that regarded to etiquette were first analyzed using correlation analysis (Spearman's ρ for ordinal data). Agreeableness showed no correlational interaction with all established measures like age, conscientiousness, formal addressing, formal correctness, abbreviation rejection, emoticon rejection, urgency, disruption, social media usage or social media liking ($p > .05$). Apparently, this personality trait is not at all influential for the usage and evaluation of social media.

In contrast, conscientiousness showed highly significant correlations with formal addressing ($r = .329, p < .01$) meaning that the more conscientious a person is, the more s/he required formal addressing. Similar interactions hold for abbreviation rejection ($r = .322, p < .01$) emoticon rejection ($r = .351, p < .01$) and disruption ($r = .301, p < .01$). This translates to conscientious people disliking usage of abbreviations and emoticon usage. They also feel disrupted in their workflow when using social media in the workplace.

Interestingly no interaction of conscientiousness with formal correctness could be revealed ($p = .057$), showing that the degree of conscientiousness does not necessarily influence whether users put high regard on correct spelling when using social media. This measure remains only slightly under the level of sig-

Table 3. Correlation table for etiquette items with their level of significance (2-tailed $*p < .05$, $**p < .01$)

Variable	(1)	(2)	(3)	(4)	(5)	(6)
(1) Formal Addressing	1					
(2) Formal Correctness	.329**	1				
(3) Abbreviation rejection	.539**	.332**	1			
(4) Emoticon rejection	.421**	-.058	.266*	1		
(5) Perceived Urgency	.129	.080	.058	-.206	1	
(6) Work Disruption	.107	-.035	.036	-.036	.185	1

nificance. All etiquette scales show interaction effects, with the exception of emoticon rejection and formal correctness (see Table 3).

Urgency only showed an interaction with emoticon rejection ($r = -.231$, $p < .05$), while work disruption showed no correlation with any other measure.

6.2   Interaction of Demographics and Social Media Usage

Private social media usage frequency interacts with age ($r = -.627$, $p < .01$), social media liking ($r = .339$, $p < .01$), formal addressing ($r = -.362$, $p < .01$) and abbreviation rejection ($r = -.264$, $p < .05$). Older people less often use social media. The more you use social media, the more you like it and the less you require formal addressing. Individual rejection of abbreviations also is lower when using social media often. Also it was found that liking interacts with disruption ($r = -.252$, $p < .05$), meaning that persons who like to use social media do not feel disturbed by using them.

In regard to professional social media usage only effects between frequency and liking were measurable ($r = .546$, $p < .01$). Meaning that the more you use social media for work purposes, the more you like it. Age interacts with formal addressing ($r = .402$, $p < .01$), abbreviation rejection ($r = .353$, $p < .01$) and emoticon rejection ($r = .226$, $p < .05$). Meaning that the older the users are, the more they appreciate correct formal addressing and the less they accept the usage of emoticons and abbreviations in social media interaction. Gender, in contrast, showed no significant effect on any of these scales ($p > .05$).

6.3   Interaction Effects and Linear Regression Analysis

This section presents the results of all linear regression analyses performed (see Fig. 4). Considering all the interactions described in the previous sections leaves the impression that formal correctness is a measure on its own that should rather be interpreted as an independent variable than any dependent variable. There are no interactions with any independent variables (age, gender, social media expertise, personality factors) but strong interactions with all dependent variables (formal correctness, politeness and compatibility with the work flow).

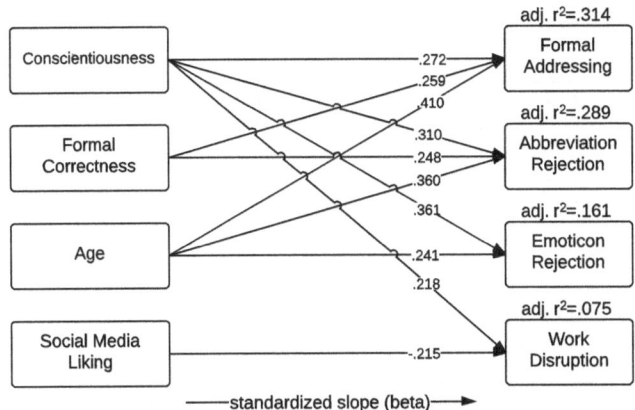

Fig. 4. Linear regression results for etiquette needs, showing both increase in explained variance (adjusted r^2) and standardized slopes (β) for all predictors and outcome variables

Linear regression analysis (multiple linear regression, enter-method) reveals that the linear model for formal addressing can explain 31% more variance than the scale mean by using age, conscientiousness and formal correctness as predictors (adjusted $r^2 = .314$, $p < .01$, see Table 4). Adding social media usage frequency or liking decreased the explained variance. This means that age is the strongest predictor for the need of formal addressing. Older, more conscientious, and more "correct" people show a stronger impact of formal address (they want to be addressed properly).

Variance in rejection of abbreviation rejection can be explained to 29% more using a linear model than using the scale mean, by using age, conscientiousness and formal correctness as predictors (adjusted $r^2 = .289$, $p < .01$, see Table 6). This means that rejection of abbreviations is most strongly predicted by age. Older, more conscientious, and more "correct" people reject usage of abbreviations more strongly.

Variance in rejection of emoticon rejection can be explained by 16% more using a linear model than using the scale mean by using age and conscientiousness as predictors (adjusted $r^2 = .161$, $p < .01$, see Table 6). Emoticons and in particular their rejection are thereby mostly determined by conscientiousness. The more conscientious you are the less you accept usage of emoticons. Age plays a smaller role. Interestingly, the need for correct spelling (i.e. formal correctness) does not imply rejection of emoticons.

Perceived urgency does not correlate with any independent variables and is thus omitted from linear regression analysis. Work disruption can be predicted using conscientiousness and social media liking, allowing to predict 8% more variance than the scale mean (adjusted $r^2 = .075$, see Table 7).

Table 4. Linear regression table for *formal addressing* with factors conscientiousness, age, and formal correctness

Model	B	SE B	β
(Constant)	-1.241	0.769	
Conscientiousness	0.382	0.146	.272**
Age	0.044	0.011	.410**
Formal correctness	0.283	0.113	.259**

$** (p < .01)$

Table 5. Linear regression table for *abbreviation rejection* with factors conscientiousness, age, and formal correctness

Model	B	SE B	β
(Constant)	-1.755	0.819	
Conscientiousness	0.480	0.158	.310**
Age	0.042	0.012	.360**
Formal correctness	0.295	0.123	.248**

$** (p < .01)$

Table 6. Linear regression table for *emoticon rejection* with factors conscientiousness and age

Model	B	SE B	β
(Constant)	-0.095	0.590	
Conscientiousness	0.428	0.119	.361**
Age	0.023	0.010	.241**

$** (p < .01)$

Table 7. Linear regression table for *work disruption* with factors conscientiousness and social media liking

Model	B	SE B	β
(Constant)	4.075	0.978	
Conscientiousness	.290	0.137	.218*
Social media Liking	-0.311	0.149	-.215*

$* (p < .05)$

6.4 Differences between Media

All scales when applied to individual media retained high Cronbach's alpha values ($> .75$) if they consisted of multiple items. When comparing means for the measures between the different media, some differences become apparent (see Table 8).

One effect is the difference of formal addressing between email and chat. Repeated measures ANOVA shows that a very strong effect due to the difference in medium for formal addressing $(F(1, 85) = 125.216, p < .01, r = .771)$. No between subject effects could be found to increase the effect size, while maintaining significance. When comparing email and blog a medium effect still holds $(F(1, 76) = 35, 467, p < .01, r = .564)$.

Another difference is the desire for formal correctness, which scores higher for blog and email than for chat (see Figure 5). Repeated measures ANOVA analysis between email and chat shows a strong effect on formal correctness due to the difference in media between email and chat $(F(1, 95) = 139.624, p < .01, r = .771)$. Adding either age or conscientiousness as between subject effects breaks this ANOVA analysis and leaves no statistically significant effect $(p > .05)$.

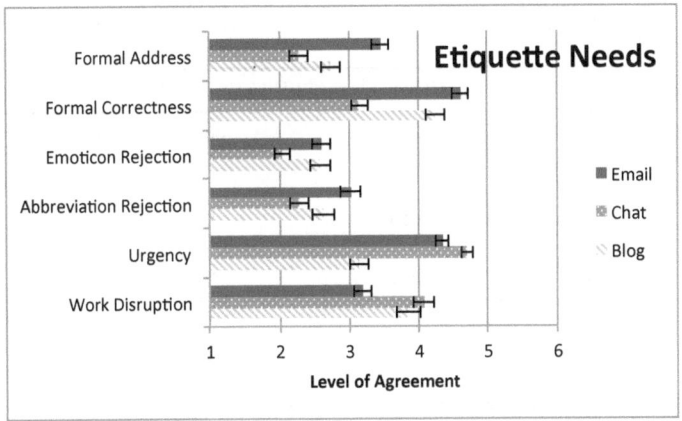

Fig. 5. Comparison of means with standard errors between media for formal address, formal correctness, emoticon rejection, abbreviation rejection, perceived urgency, and work disruption

When looking at emoticon rejection email and blog both show higher rejection than chat. Repeated measure ANOVA shows a medium effect between blog and chat $(F(1, 96) = 22.196, p < .01, r = .432)$. This effect becomes a small effect when using gender as a between subject effect (gender * medium, $F(1, 82) = 5.164, p < 0.5, r = .243$). This means that participants rejected emoticons less in chat applications than in blog, with males seeing this difference slightly stronger than females.

A similar effect is found for rejection of abbreviation usage in emails and chat. The difference in chosen medium has a medium sized effect $(F(1, 77) = 28.66, p < .01, r = .521)$ and when combined with conscientiousness a smaller effect $(r = .337, F(1, 25) = 3.206, p < .05)$. This means that participants desire a formal addressing more in email than in chat, but require more correctness in blogs than in email or chat. Furthermore rejection of abbreviations is more present in email than in chat. In general one must say, that rejection of emoticons and abbreviations was rather low ($M < 3$, scale range: $1 - 6$).

Perceived urgency is most prominent in chat and email, and least in blog. The difference between chat and blog is a strong effect when using repeated measure ANOVA ($F(1, 81) = 135.321, p < .01, r = .79$). The effect remains high in size when comparing email and blog ($F(1, 82) = 107.519, p < .01, r = .753$). No between subject effect could be found for any of the measured scales. But perceived urgency in general is different for the two sexes (the only scale, that showed a gender bias). Men perceived all three media combined as more urgently ($M\sigma = 3.07$, $M\male = 2.70$) than women ($t(93.157) = 2.396, p < .05$).

Experienced disruption of work is lowest for email. Blog and chat are perceived as rather disruptive to work. The difference between email and chat is a medium effect ($F(1, 92) = 30.90, p < .01, r = .496$). No between subjects effects were found.

Table 8. Effect sizes (r) for differences between media

Variable	Email vs. Chat	Email vs. Blog	Chat vs. Blog
Formal Addressing	.710	.564	*
Formal Correctness	.771	*	*
Emoticon Rejection	*	*	.432
Abbreviation Rejection	.521	*	*
Urgency	*	.753	.790
Work Disruption	.496	*	*

* (no significant difference)

6.5   Effects on Acceptance

Interestingly no measured scales had any influence on the willingness to use of either chat or blog. Only perceived urgency correlated with the willingness to use a chat application ($r = .296, p < .01$).

7   Discussion and Limitations

The results from this study reveal that conscientiousness and age have an effect on several measures of etiquette in social media applications (supporting H1 and H4). In particular people that are older and more conscientious tend to require a formal addressing (i.e. formal salutation, full name address, honorific address) in social media applications. Conscientious people are also more likely to feel disrupted by social media applications.

The desire for formal correctness (i.e. correct spelling and capitalization), seems to be an influence that is not itself influenced by any demographic or personality data (from this study). It also has a strong influence on the desire for formal addressing.

Similar effects were found for the rejection of using acronymic abbreviations and emoticons. Age and conscientiousness were the biggest influence factors.

The hypothesized effect of agreeableness on any measures has not been found (not supporting H2).

The usage of social media does go hand in hand with decreasing desire for formal addressing and the willingness to accept abbreviations in communication (confirming H3). But since social media usage is directly correlated with age, linear regression shows that age and conscientiousness are the predominant factors in this analysis. People with more social media experience also perceived social media usage as less disruptive.

Differences in media were also found (confirming H5). In particular it was found that chat has less requirements than email in regard to etiquette and blog and email require more formal correctness than chat. This strengthens the hypothesis that chat is perceived more as an oral medium applied synchronously rather than asynchronously. The blog on the contrary is perceived more as a publication medium than a communication medium considering that the desire for formal correctness is by far higher than in chat. Nonetheless requirements are the highest when using email. Interestingly email was perceived as the least disruptive but equally urgent as chat messages.

Differences between private social media and work social media were of the nature that experience with work social media did not influence any measures at all, where private social media experience did change desires for etiquette (confirming H6).

Summarizing we can say that personality, age and experience do play a role in etiquette needs in regard to social media usage at the workplace. User diversity must be considered when applying social networking solutions in the work environment. Social media is (at least in this sample) significantly but not extensively different from other forms of communication. In particular perceptions of synchronicity, publicity and immediacy carry over to social media etiquette. Nonetheless individual preferences apply as well.

Application. The findings in this study can be applied, when trying to bring older and younger users to use one internal social network. In particular younger users must be instructed to regard formal addressing and usage of abbreviations and emoticons when communicating with older users. This is particularly true when posting or commenting on blog entries.

It is also important to regard the need for more formal correctness of users that score higher on conscientiousness. If employees of a company diverge strongly on this measure, stricter rules might help keeping everyone on board.

When trying to define rules for emoticon and abbreviation usage one must consider, both age and conscientiousness of future users. Different rules for different media might also be of use, as for example rejection of emoticons in chat messages is rather low generally.

Urgency is perceived more strongly in men, which means that using a chat application might appeal more to men then to women, because the synchronicity (and thus urgency of a message) might be the reason they use chat in the first place (although this was not statistically validated as a difference in acceptance between genders).

Limitations. The results of this study must be considered as culture-specific and only represent a German perspective. German clearly deciphers between a formal honorific address (Sie ~ honorific you) and an informal address (Du ~ informal you). Furthermore correct German requires capitalization of all nouns in sentences. This could mean that in different languages effects could be less strong than in this German sample. However, it could be interesting to identify further language-specific or culture specific formal addressing components and to specify whether the meaning of formal addressing, especially in the older user group, is also equally high in other language cultures.

Another limitation refers to the fact that the sample examined here does not represent the whole workforce. Rather, the sample was relatively young and non-technical in their educational background. Addressing a bigger sample could improve results and shed more light on some of these findings.

A full big-five assessment could improve the understanding what other factors influence etiquette requirements. In particular openness could influence rejection of emoticons or abbreviations negatively. The inclusion of more personality factors could also lead to the identification of personal user profiles and their preferences for different types of social media as well as media-specific etiquettes.

The measure of urgency, which only correlated negatively with emoticon rejection, could imply a hidden desire to comply socially over a social network since both measure the willingness to communicate more directly (either more quickly or more emotionally).

Further research is required to thoroughly understand these factors.

Acknowledgments. We would like to thank the anonymous reviewers for their constructive comments on an earlier version of this manuscript.

This study has been funded by the German Ministry of Education and Research (BMBF) and the European Social Fund (ESF) within the program "Innovationsfähigkeit im demographischen Wandel" under the reference number 01HH11045.

References

1. Kaplan, A.M., Haenlein, M.: Users of the world, unite! the challenges and opportunities of social media. Business Horizons 53(1), 59–68 (2010)
2. Holzinger, K., Holzinger, A., Safran, C., Koiner-Erath, G., Weippl, E.: Use of wiki systems in archaeology: Privacy, security and data protection as key problems. In: Proceedings of the 2010 Intern. Conf. on e-Business (ICE-B), pp. 1–4 (July 2010)
3. Maier, R.: Knowledge Management Systems: Information and Communication Technologies for Knowledge Management. Springer (2004)
4. Drucker, P.F.: The information executives truly need. Harvard Business Review 73(1), 54–63 (1995)
5. Erlich, A., Bichard, J.A.: The welcoming workplace: designing for ageing knowledge workers. Journal of Corporate Real Estate 10(4), 273–285 (2008)

6. Calero Valdez, A., Schaar, A.K., Ziefle, M., Holzinger, A., Jeschke, S., Brecher, C.: Using mixed node publication network graphs for analyzing success in interdisciplinary teams. In: Huang, R., Ghorbani, A.A., Pasi, G., Yamaguchi, T., Yen, N.Y., Jin, B. (eds.) AMT 2012. LNCS, vol. 7669, pp. 606–617. Springer, Heidelberg (2012)

7. Preece, J., Nonnecke, B., Andrews, D.: The top five reasons for lurking: improving community experiences for everyone. Comp. Hum. Beh. 20(2), 201–223 (2004)

8. Hickey, R.: The german address system. Diachronic perspectives on address term systems: Pragmatics and beyond New Series 107, 401–425 (2003)

9. Westbrook, L.: Chat reference communication patterns and implications: applying politeness theory. Journal of Documentation 63(5), 638–658 (2007)

10. Tepper, B.J., Duffy, M.K., Shaw, J.D.: Personality moderators of the relationship between abusive supervision and subordinates' resistance. Journal of Applied Psychology 86(5), 974–983 (2001)

11. Satow, L.: Big-five-persönlichkeitstest (B5T): Test- und Skalendokumentation. (July 2012), http://www.drsatow.de

12. Richter, A., Stocker, A., Mller, S., Avram, G.: Knowledge management goals revisited – a cross-sectional analysis of social software adoption in corporate environments. In: ACIS 2011 Proceedings (January 2011)

13. Davis, F.D., Bagozzi, R.P., Warshaw, P.R.: User acceptance of computer technology: A comparison of two theoretical models. Management Science 35(8), 982–1003 (1989)

14. Venkatesh, V., Morris, M.G., Davis, G.B., Davis, F.D.: User acceptance of information technology: Toward a unified view. MIS Quarterly 27(3), 425–478 (2003)

15. Arning, K., Ziefle, M.: Understanding age differences in PDA acceptance and performance. Computers in Human Behavior 23(6), 2904–2927 (2007)

16. Ziefle, M., Schaar, A.K.: Gender differences in acceptance and attitudes towards an invasive medical stent. Electronic Journal of Health Informatics 6(2) (2011)

17. Calero Valdez, A., Schaar, A.K., Ziefle, M.: State of the (net) work address developing criteria for applying social networking to the work environment. Work: A Journal of Prevention, Assessment and Rehabilitation 41, 3459–3467 (2012)

18. Schaar, A.K., Calero Valdez, A., Ziefle, M.: Social media for the eHealth context. a requirement assessment. Adv. in Human Aspects of Healthcare 10, 79 (2012)

19. Richter, A., Koch, M.: Functions of social networking services. In: Proc. Intl. Conf. on the Design of Cooperative Systems, Carry-le-Rouet, France. Springer (2008)

20. Rothwell, J.D.: In the company of others: An introduction to communication. McGraw-Hill Humanities/Social Sciences/Languages (1999)

21. Brown, P., Levinson, S.C.: Politeness: Some universals in language usage, vol. 4. Cambridge University Press (1987)

22. Hayes, C.C., Miller, C.A.: Human-Computer Etiquette, vol. 5. Auerbach Publications (2010)

23. Alagöz, F., Ziefle, M., Wilkowska, W., Valdez, A.C.: Openness to accept medical technology - a cultural view. In: Holzinger, A., Simonic, K.-M. (eds.) USAB 2011. LNCS, vol. 7058, pp. 151–170. Springer, Heidelberg (2011)

24. Wirth, U.: Chatten. Plaudern mit anderen Mitteln. In: Siever, T., Schlobinski, P., Runkehl, J. (eds.) Websprache.net. Sprache und Kommunikation im Internet: Sprache Und Kommunikation Im Internet, 1st edn. Gruyter (June 2005)

25. Kilian, J.: T@stentöne. Geschriebene Umgangssprache in computervermittelter Kommunikation. Historisch-kritische Ergänzungen zu einem neuen feld der linguistischen Forschung. In: Beisswenger, M. (ed.) Chat-Kommunikation: Sprache, Interaktion, Sozialität & Identität in synchroner computervermittelter Kommunikation: Perspektiven auf ein interdisziplinäres Forschungsfeld. Ibidem-Verlag, Stuttgart (2001)

26. Dresner, E., Herring, S.C.: Functions of the nonverbal in CMC: emoticons and illocutionary force. Communication Theory 20(3), 249–268 (2010)

27. Holzinger, A., Kickmeier-Rust, M.D., Ebner, M.: Interactive technology for enhancing distributed learning: a study on weblogs. In: Proceedings of the 23rd British HCI Group Annual Conference on People and Computers: Celebrating People and Technology, BCS-HCI 2009, pp. 309–312. British Computer Society, Swinton (2009)

28. Koo, C., Wati, Y., Jung, J.J.: Examination of how social aspects moderate the relationship between task characteristics and usage of social communication technologies (SCTs) in organizations. International Journal of Information Management 31(5), 445–459 (2011)

29. Schmidt, J.: Weblogs: Eine kommunikationssoziologische Studie. Uvk Verlags GmbH (2006)

30. Digman, J.M.: Personality structure: Emergence of the five-factor model. Annual Review of Psychology 41(1), 417–440 (1990)

31. Rosen, P., Kluemper, D.: The impact of the big five personality traits on the acceptance of social networking website. In: AMCIS 2008 Proceedings (January 2008)

32. Devaraj, S., Easley, R.F., Crant, J.M.: Research Note–How does personality matter? relating the five-factor model to technology acceptance and use. Information Systems Research 19(1), 93–105 (2008)

33. Hughes, D.J., Rowe, M., Batey, M., Lee, A.: A tale of two sites: Twitter vs. facebook and the personality predictors of social media usage. Comput. Hum. Behav. 28(2), 561–569 (2012)

34. Correa, T., Hinsley, A.W., de Ziga, H.G.: Who interacts on the web?: The intersection of users' personality and social media use. Comput. Hum. Behav. 26(2), 247–253 (2010)

35. Amichai-Hamburger, Y., Vinitzky, G.: Social network use and personality. Comput. Hum. Behav. 26(6), 1289–1295 (2010)

Role of Information Scent and Link Position in a Successful Navigation on Web

Vamshi Velagapuri and Suvarna Rekha

Cognitive Science Lab,
International Institute of Information Technology,
Hyderabad, India
vvelagapuri@students.iiit.ac.in,
suvarna.rekha@research.iiit.ac.in

Abstract. How people navigate on the web is a question since the beginning of the hypertext days. Computational cognitive models such as CoLiDeS, CoLiDeS+, SNIF-ACT, MESA etc. tried to address user navigation on the web. When it comes to the visual search of navigation cues the models have certain assumptions like serial evaluation, top down order, working memory considerations. Two experiments were designed to address the issue of how people attend the links and the role information scent in a successful navigation. The results strengthen the fact that people select the link with the maximum scent in a successful navigation. When presented a set of navigational links, the amount of time spent on a link and the number of times it is being attended has not significantly correlated with the information scent it carries. Furthermore serial evaluation of the links is not observed for the menu size used.

Keywords: Information scent, Link position, Web usability, Web navigation, Cognitive modeling, Visual search.

1 Introduction

1.1 Hypertext

The WWW is a world view of documents referring to each other by links [1]. The non hierarchical, non linear and unbounded nature of the associations among the documents makes it look like a spider web thus called Web. The documents consist of text and images with sensitive parts called hyperlinks referring to other documents. This view is known as the hypertext paradigm.

1.2 Navigation

Navigation is the act of moving from one hypertext page to the other. Typically users navigate from the homepage following the links that lead to the information they want. Newell and Simon [2] call it the *Problem Space* where learners know only the goal and the available actions in a situation. Users in this problem space lack the

A. Holzinger et al. (Eds.): SouthCHI 2013, LNCS 7946, pp. 447–456, 2013.

additional useful knowledge as ways to decompose a goal into sub goals, or effectively rank order available actions interns of their contribution to accomplishing a goal. A new user in this problem space has no methods to progress and has to engage in search process.

Two variants of search process namely hill climbing [2], backward chaining [2] search were proposed. In Hill Climbing search strategy users tend to choose the methods which appear to lead them to the nearest state to the goal. But there can be a state which is on the successful path and may not appear to be leading to the goal at a particular stage. In order to account for this another model called Back Chaining was proposed where goals are divided into sub goals and further recursively. A final solution is constructed using the states that lead to a successful path in the bottom up manner.

Engelbeck [2] identified a special case of Hill Climbing Strategy called the label following where the users who are new to the system are comparing the action description and goal description and selecting the state based on the semantic similarity of the both. Information Foraging Theory [3], [4], [5], proposes that people traverse the path in which scent increases with respect to the cost of choosing the path. People leave the path when there is a drop in the rate of gain in information scent beyond a threshold level. The theory puts weight on the relation of navigation cues (information scent) to the user's information goal which determines the browsing actions.

2   Related Work

In the recent years several of computational cognitive models for web navigation were proposed predicting the user behavior given a goal. The models were grouped broadly either to *Hill Climbing (forward search)* or *backward chaining*.

Comprehension-based Linked model for Deliberate Search (CoLiDeS) [6], [7] claims that comprehension of the images and text is the core process underlying the web navigation. The model proposes that people compare the mental representation of the screen objects with the goal object and subsequently select a particular hyperlink or image. CoLiDeS has four cognitive processes at the core namely parsing, focusing on, comprehension, and selection. During the parsing and focusing phase the user focuses on higher level screen objects and selects the one which is more relevant to the goal and further process the screen elements in the selected area. The primary assumption of the model is that users act on the hyperlink, image, or the screen object they perceive as being most similar to the representation of their current goal. CoLiDeS+ [8] incorporates the structural information by bringing in a new concept called *path adequacy*. Path Adequacy is computed as the semantic similarity between the user-goal and the navigation path. Only if the incoming information increases the path adequacy, the link is chosen, else it backtracks to the other links on the page. Both CoLiDeS and CoLiDeS+ use the Latent Semantic Analysis [9] to compute the degree of similarity. In comprehension and selection phases model assumes that user attends all the links and selects the one which is more relevant. However the model has no explanations for the order in which people attend the links once the area which contains the navigation links was selected for further processing.

Another model based on the backward chaining search process called SNIF-ACT 1.0 [10] that explains the user behavior on web along with the visual search of screen objects. The model evaluates all the links on the page in the left-right and top-down order. The next version of the model SNIF-ACT 2.0 evaluates the links as in the previous model but will terminate the search when a threshold condition is satisfied.

Method for Evaluating Site Architecture (MESA) [11] is another model that was proposed considering the human cognition limitations in serial evaluation of the links considering the limited working memory. The model is neutral to the order in which links are evaluated and the model may results in selecting the less relevant links as it goes deep into the navigation.

The assumption of SNIF-ACT 1.0 that users evaluate all the links before selecting the intended one was proven to be a wrong strategy in another study [12]. Link position & link interest emerged as determining factors when users with low domain knowledge were asked to form new goals of learning and were asked to navigate [13]. Selection of the goal item is directly linked to the other items in the list, as users attended smaller subset of items periodically before choosing the goal item as opposed to multiple evaluations of all the items [12]. It is further observed that users at time deliberately select the low information scent links as opposed to the assumptions of CoLiDeS, CoLiDeS+, at times they tend to select any link when way finding becomes difficult [14]. The threshold reach termination of the link selection process proposed by SNIF-ACT 2.0, MESA was challenged by the idea of frustration reach considering the natural web behavior [10].

3   Research Framework

The proposed cognitive models do not take into consideration of the eye tracking data to match user behavior on screen to model behavior. Models like CoLiDeS+ whose goals are in providing support mechanisms to the user need to be aware of the user behavior during the phases of parsing and focusing on. Two experiments were designed to investigate the user behavior with the following research questions in the mind.

1. Do users conform to the assumption CoLiDeS made on selecting the link which has more information scent?
2. Whether the amount of time spent in attending the link correlate to the information scent it carries.
3. Whether the position of the link has any influence on the way in which people attend the links.
4. What role does information scent distribution in a successful navigation path play in understanding the ways of avoiding user disorientation?

4   Navigating a Large Hierarchical Website

An experiment was designed to investigate the information scent distribution of the chosen links as one navigating towards the goal.

4.1   Stimuli

The study required a large hierarchical website where a meaningful hierarchy exists. For that a website with the content focusing on human biology consisting of 70 pages with approximately 15000 words was developed. Each page has a "Back" link to its parent and links to its children. No additional navigational tools like breadcrumbs, navigation bars were provided. Maximum depth of the website is 7 and the average depth is 3.

4.2   Participant Description

28 participants of which 25 males and 3 females from undergraduate and graduate school with a mean age 22 years participated in the experiment voluntarily. Preliminary information such as age, sex, education, and familiarity with the medium were recorded from the participants.

4.3   Task Description

Three tasks were given to the participants. Each task requires browsing through the website and answering Yes/No at the end for whether the information is found or not without comprehending much from the information the task demanded. Tasks were designed not to make the participants to comprehend the content but the answers were readily available on the goal page. They were allowed to quit at any point of time during the task completion, when the information is not traceable according to them. Following is list of tasks participants were provided with.

1. Blood oxygenation occurs in the heart (True/False)
2. Coronary arteries supply blood to the heart (True / False)
3. The Skull consists of cranium and facial bones (True/False)

4.4   Measures

While the participants were performing the tasks, the sequence of links selected and time spent on each page were logged for further analysis. Latent Semantic Analysis [9] is used in calculating the semantic similarity between the task and the links visited. LSA is a statistical procedure of analyzing the relationship between a set of documents and terms they contain using. An LSA value of +1 denotes identical texts and -1 denotes oppositely meaning texts; in other words values around +1 denote high semantic similarity and values near 0 indicate two unrelated texts whereas values around -1 indicate high semantic dissimilarity.

4.5   Results

A graph was plotted using the total number of pages visited on x-axis and the number of times the LSA values were decreased. The graph reveals that lesser the pages visited steeper the LSA values accounting for the successful navigation. Pearson correlation coefficient yielded a positive correlation with $r(26) = .915$, $p = 0.01$. Participants who have visited more number of pages have recorded more times decrease in LSA values indicating disorientation. Further to investigate the visual search of navigational links on a page we have designed the subsequent experiment.

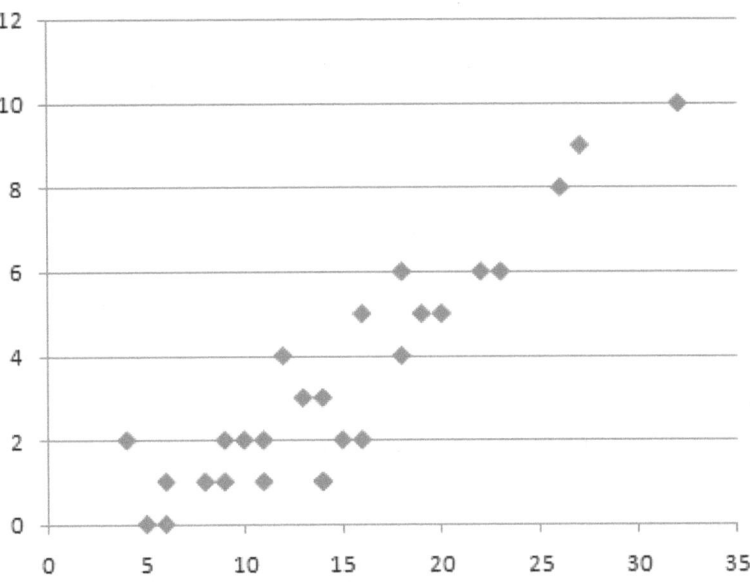

Fig. 1. Scatter graph showing the relation between the numbers of times LSA values decreased (y-axis) given the total no of pages visited (x-axis)

5   Visual Search on the Homepage Navigation Links

The experiment was designed to understand the role of position of the link and the information scent it carries in attending and selecting it, further to investigate user behavior pattern in choosing a link from navigational section. Our tasks and stimuli were adapted from a recent study and used with the permission of authors [17].

5.1   Stimuli

The stimuli consist of a home page with a navigation section related to the topic of human biology. Since the purpose of the experiment is to explore how users attend the navigational links, the non hyperlink text is removed in line with the parsing phase of

CoLiDeS [6], [7]. The home page consists of only five links to avoid further working memory constraints in line with MESA [11]. Following links were presented in the navigational section: *respiratory system, nervous system, digestive system, circulatory system* in the same vertical order. The navigational section was placed at the left hand side of the screen by considering the ease of use [15].

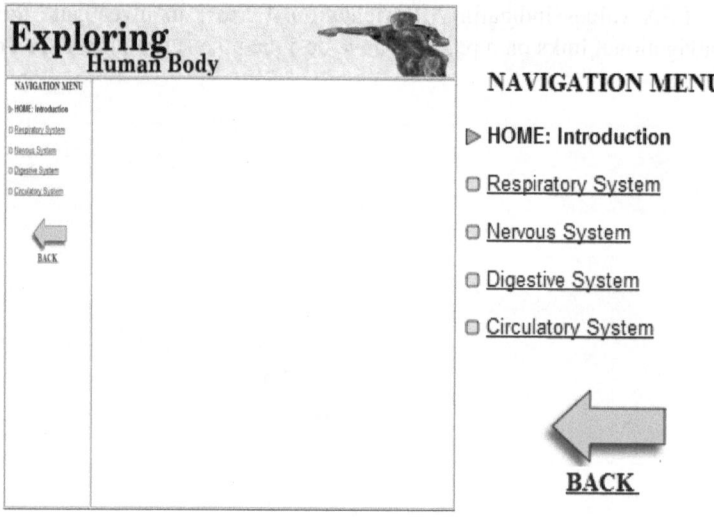

Fig. 2. Home page and navigational links

5.2   Participants

16 undergraduate students of which 11 male and 5 female with a mean age of 23 were participated voluntarily.

5.3   Tasks

Following four tasks were given to the participants. Each task ends in selecting an appropriate navigational link on the homepage.

1. The muscles of the esophagus contract in waves to move the food down into stomach. What name is given to these contractions?
2. In a respiratory system, what name is given to the valve that drops down when we swallow in order to protect our lungs and trachea?
3. Lymphatic system contains immune cells called lymphocytes, which protect our body from antigens. They are produced by lymph nodes. Name at least three locations in the body where lymph nodes are present?
4. What specific name is given to those motor neurons that act on the muscles of the face and the neck?

5.4   Equipment/Software

Eye moment recording was done using Tobii X60 Eye Tracking machine. Tobii Studio and SPSS were used for the analysis of fixation data.

5.5   Measures

Following measures were taken while the users were performing the search task for the correct navigation link given a task.

LSA Values for each of the link with respect to the task description were calculated from the tool provided by http://lsa.colorado.edu.

In order to facilitate for a better comparison across all the tasks, LSA values of the four links were normalized using the highest LSA value link for that task as key. A normalized LSA value of 1 for a given link and a particular task implies the link is closest for this goal semantically.

Mean fixation duration for each link was calculated for each task, from the fixation durations from all the participants. This will yield a set of 16 mean fixation duration values for 4 tasks and 4 active links. In a similar way *Mean fixation count* was also calculated by taking the number of times a link is being visited.

Number of times the link is selected, position from the top with the topmost link being indexed as 1 and the bottom most one as 4 were computed for further analysis.

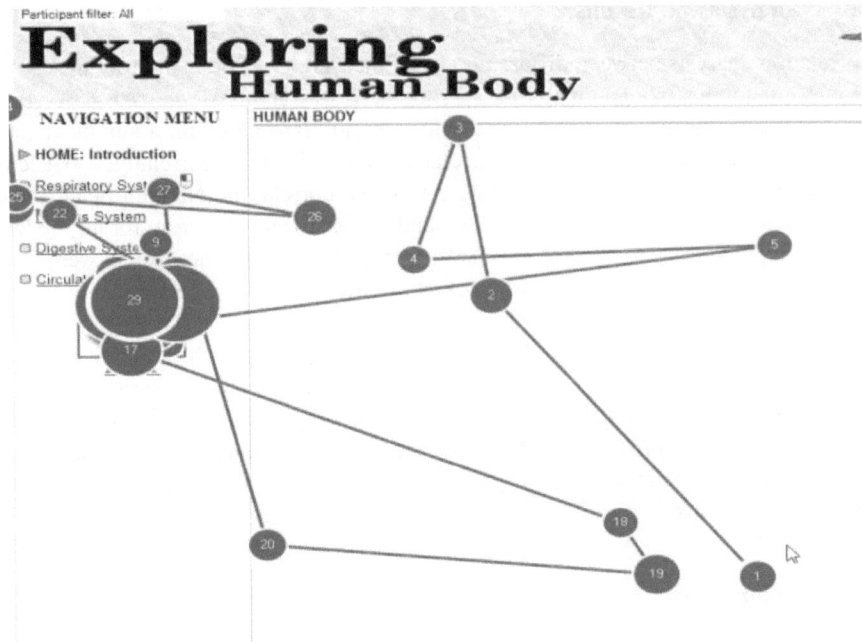

Fig. 3. Saccade and fixation moments on the stimuli for a task from one of the participant

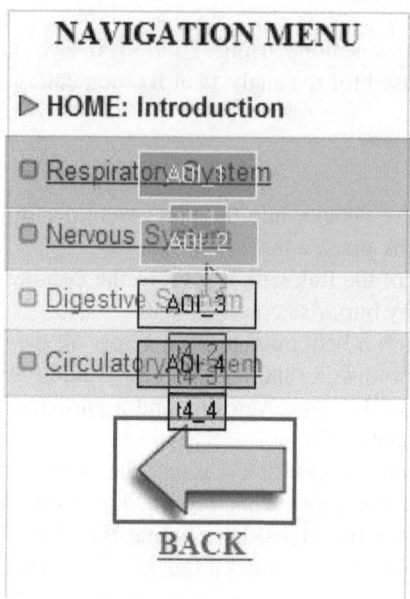

Fig. 4. Navigational links marked with the areas of interests

5.6   Analysis and Results

Correlation analysis between different pairs of measures was done in order to see how people attend the navigational links. From here onwards *Normalized LSA values* represent the information scent a link carries. *Normalized LSA values* and the *number of times the link is being clicked* correlated with a Pearson correlation coefficient value of $r(16) = .576$, $p = .02$ showing a positive correlation. No significant results were found when *Normalized LSA values* and *mean fixation duration* for all the tasks are correlated with $r(16) = -.037$, $p = 0.89$. Similarly no significant results were found between the *mean fixation count* with respect to the *Normalized LSA value* of the link with $r(16) = -.136$, $p = .611$.

Another set of correlation studies were done to evaluate whether the position of a link has any effect on the link selection. For the smaller menu like the one used in the experiment, *position of the link* and *total number of fixations* were correlated at Pearson coefficient $r(16) = -.083$, $p = .759$ and *position of the link* with *mean fixation duration* was correlated at $r(16) = -0.71$, $p = .793$ showing the statistically insignificant results.

6   Discussion

The results from the first experiment (3.4) suggest that the participants who reached the goal in lesser number of pages recorded a continuous increase in the LSA values if not successively. Participants who visited more number of pages to complete the task have either kept on deviating from the successful path accounting for the continuous decrease in LSA values or constantly selecting the higher and lower LSA value link, though not successively. In either case providing a support tool which suggests the correct link quickly, may increase both the efficiency and effectiveness. For this the key components of how users do visual search in a navigational section needs to be known for a better representation of the suggested link.

In the link selection criteria, results from the second experiment (4.6) confirm the assumption made by CoLiDeS [6], [7] that web users select the link with the highest semantic similarity to the goal. Information scent the link carries has no significant influence on the number of times it is visited and the time spent on it. The analysis with the positioning of the links reveals no effect on the way users attend the links for smaller menu size which was used in the experiment. This will contradict the assumptions of the serial evaluation of the links. Further detailed study has to be done in order to see how users attend the links if there are many, considering the limitations of the working memory.

Coming back to the idea of providing a guidance mechanism, the study eliminates some of the ways in which we can position the suggested link(s) such as increasing or decreasing order of LSA values. Given the results that users have not spent time based on the semantic similarity, and having known that the highest similarity link is chosen often, providing a suggestion mechanism for the maximum information scent link may yield in better performance and less disorientation. Further studies have to be carried in the light of how people attend given more number of links considering the working memory limitations as well the role of support mechanisms in a pleasant and successful navigation.

Acknowledgments. The authors wish to thank Dr. Saraschandra Karanam for helping us with the stimuli and tasks along with Prof. Bipin Indukhya and Prof. Herre van Oostendorp for helping us with the experiment design. The authors were grateful to the reviewers for their critical comments and recommendations.

References

1. Berners-Lee, T.J.: The world-wide web. Computer Networks and ISDN Systems 25(4), 454–459 (1992)
2. Engelbeck, G.E.: Exceptions to generalizations: Implications for formal models of human-computer interaction. Unpublished masters's thesis, University of Colarado, Department of Psychology, Boulder, Co. (1986)
3. Pirolli, P., Card, S.K.: Information Foraging. Psychological Review 106(4), 643–675 (1999)
4. Polson, P.G., Lewis, C.H.: Theory-based design for easily learned interfaces, ICS Technical Report #88-16
5. Pirolli, P.L.T.: Information foraging theory: Adaptive interaction with information, vol. 2. Oxford University Press, USA (2007)

6. Kitajima, M., Blackmon, M.H., Polson, P.G.: A Comprehension-based Model of Web Navigation and Its Application to Web Usability Analysis. In: McDonald, S., Waern, Y., Cockton, G. (eds.) People and Computers XIV - Usability or Else (Proceedings of HCI 2000), pp. 357–373. Springer (2000)
7. Juvina, I., Oostendorp, H., van, K.P., Pauw, B.: Toward Modeling Contextual Information in Web Navigation. In: XXVII Annual Conference of the Cognitive Science Society, Stresa, Italy (2005)
8. Juvina, I., van Oostendorp, H.: Modeling Semantic and Structural Knowledge in Web Navigation. Discourse Processess 45(4-5), 346–364 (2008)
9. Landauer, T.K., Dumais, S.T.: A Solution to Plato's Problem: The Latent Semantic Analysis Theory of Acquisition, Induction, and Representation of Knowledge. Psychological Review 104(2), 211–240 (1997)
10. Landauer, T.K., Dumais, S.T.: A Solution to Plato's Problem: The Latent Semantic Analysis Theory of Acquisition, Induction, and Representation of Knowledge. Psychological Review 104(2), 211–240 (1997)
11. Pirolli, P., Fu, W.T.: SNIF-ACT: a model of information foraging on the World Wide Web. In: Brusilovsky, P., Corbett, A.T., de Rosis, F. (eds.) UM 2003. LNCS, vol. 2702, pp. 45–54. Springer, Heidelberg (2003)
12. Miller, C.S., Remington, R.W.: Modeling Information Navigation: Implications for Information Architecture. Human-Computer Interaction 19(3), 225–271 (2004)
13. Brumby, D.P., Howes, A.: Good enough but I'll just check: Web-page search as attentional refocusing. In: 6th Internal Conference on Cognitive Modeling (2004)
14. Salmerón, L., Kintsch, W., Kintsch, E.: Self-regulation and link selection strategies in hypertext. Discourse Processes 47(3), 175–211 (2010)
15. Vigo, M., Harper, S.: Challenging Information Foraging Theory: Screen Reader Users are not Always Driven by Information Scent (2013)
16. Holzinger, A., Scherer, R., Ziefle, M.: Navigational user interface elements on the left side: intuition of designers or experimental evidence? In: Campos, P., Graham, N., Jorge, J., Nunes, N., Palanque, P., Winckler, M. (eds.) INTERACT 2011, Part II. LNCS, vol. 6947, pp. 162–177. Springer, Heidelberg (2011)
17. Karanam, S., van Oostendorp, H., Indurkhya, B.: A study on the role of non-hyperlink text on web navigation. Computer Science 13(3), 5–22 (2012)

The Minimal Group Paradigm in Virtual Teams

Monique Janneck[1], Petra Saskia Bayerl[2], and Jana-Eva Dietel[3]

[1] Luebeck University of Applied Sciences, Luebeck, Germany
monique.janneck@fh-luebeck.de
[2] Erasmus University, Rotterdam, The Netherlands
pbayerl@rsm.nl
[3] University of Hamburg, Hamburg, Germany
janadietel@yahoo.de

Abstract. As established by Social Identity Theory (SIT), belonging to specific groups is part of our identity and constitutes the feeling of "who I am" and "who I am not". Social groups are thus an essential part of life – not only for social interactions but also for defining part of our self-conception. Early experiments found that even minimal, entirely random in-group/out-group categorizations are sufficient to cause a status gain of the in-group, while simultaneously discriminating the out-group. In this paper we transfer this so-called Minimal Group Paradigm (MGP) to online collaboration. Two empirical studies with a total of N=190 participants were conducted to replicate the Minimal Group Paradigm in different virtual settings (informal vs. work) and with different degrees of information available about the supposed group members. Overall, results show that indeed in-group favoritism could be elicited in totally anonymous virtual settings without any real interaction. Yet, the Minimal Group effect varied according to the complexity of the clues: in-group favoritism was stronger in settings with less information available. Implications for research and practice are discussed.

Keywords: Social Identity Theory, Minimal Group Paradigm, Virtual Teams.

1 Introduction

For decades, research has studied social groups: their formation and development, how people behave, perform, and influence each other in groups, how intergroup relations are established etc. Likewise, for quite some time, research has been conducted on virtual groups, i.e., people communicating and interacting online and/or via electronic media, e.g. [1, 2, 3]. However, these two branches of research are not always tied together [cf. 4], as many 'classical' social psychological theories and findings on groups, intragroup behavior, and intergroup relations have not been systematically investigated in virtual settings.

One of these theories – which is also one of the most influential approaches in social psychology – is the *Social Identity Theory*. It deals with how people integrate memberships in social groups into their self-concept and develop a feeling of identity

A. Holzinger et al. (Eds.): SouthCHI 2013, LNCS 7946, pp. 457–476, 2013.

related to groups. Research showed that social identity influences a person's behavior in a decisive way and can also explain intergroup relations and especially conflicts and aggression between groups.

While one might generally assume that mechanisms identified in 'real-life' face-to-face groups also apply to online settings, to our knowledge there has been no systematic research regarding if and how social identity is established and displayed in virtual groups. This makes it hard to predict intergroup dynamics in virtual settings. In this paper we fill this gap reporting on an experimental investigation of Social Identity Theory in online settings. In a first step, we aimed to replicate a famous experiment, the so-called Minimal Group Paradigm – which showed that the principles of Social Identity Theory even apply to arbitrarily composed groups – with respect to virtual teams.

This paper is structured as follows: in the next section, we review Social Identity Theory and the Minimal Group Paradigm in more detail. Afterwards, research questions and methods are presented. Subsequently, the results of two experimental investigations are depicted, followed by a general discussion, pointers for further research and implications for HCI practice.

2   Social Identity Theory

Social Identity Theory (SIT) was developed in the 1970s by Tajfel and Turner [5, 6, 7, 8] and became one of the most influential social psychological theories dealing with behavior of and within groups. Social Identity Theory explains two important phenomena related to groups: in-group favoritism and out-group discrimination. In in-group favoritism group members tend to evaluate their own group and people belonging to it more favorably. This usually goes hand in hand with the devaluation of members of other groups (i.e., out-group discrimination), which may result even in outright hostile behavior against out-group members.

This process is based on the fact that social identity is an integral part of one's self-concept and closely related to the membership in social groups. For social identity to be established an individual needs to belong to a certain group and also needs to recognize that he/she belongs to this group. In this approach a wide definition of groups is used, holding that a group is made up of people who feel that they belong to this group and are recognized as such by other group members.

SIT relies on three basic concepts:

1. *Social Categorization*: Social categorization refers to "the process which transforms individuals into groups" [9, p. 21]. Categorization is a fundamental cognitive process enabling humans to process complex information rapidly by sorting it into pre-existing categories, often resulting in some form of oversimplification [10]. Often social categorization processes are based on stereotypes.
2. *Social Comparison*: Humans tend to continuously evaluate themselves by comparing their own characteristics and achievements to other individuals. As people naturally strive to uphold a positive self-concept, devaluating others is a possibility to shed a better light on oneself.

3. *Social Differentiation*: Processes of social categorization and comparison are used to establish distinct borders between members of different social groups, enabling individuals to develop their own identity as a member of one group and non-member of other groups, often accompanied by a feeling of pride and superiority related to one's own group(s).

The core concepts of Social Identity Theory can be summarized as follows:

- People strive to establish and uphold a positive self-concept and self-esteem.
- Part of one's self-concept is constituted by one's memberships in distinct social groups.
- Groups are evaluated by comparing one's own groups (so-called in-groups) with other social groups (out-groups).
- Evaluating in-groups more positively than out-groups in social comparison processes helps to uphold a positive self-concept ('if my group is successful, so am I'). Thus, out-group discrimination can be seen as a self-protective mechanism.

2.1   The Minimal Group Paradigm

The Minimal Group Paradigm (MGP) refers to a famous experiment conducted by Tajfel et al. [11] which has been replicated in numerous follow-up studies. The MGP demonstrates that social categorization processes and intergroup bias can be elicited even in randomly assigned groups without any actual social importance. The experimental set-up categorized participants in two random, abstractly defined groups (e.g. "red and blue group" or "Klee and Kandinsky group"). Participants did not know each other nor did they have any contact with other (in-group or out-group) members, but they knew which group they had been assigned to. Participants were instructed that they were taking part in an experiment on decision behavior and were asked to distribute a certain amount of money among members of the two groups. To that end they received tables showing different possibilities for distribution to choose from (e.g. "25$ to a member of the red group and 19$ to a member of the blue group", as shown in table 1). It was not possible to award the money to oneself or choose any other distribution than those in table 1.

Most participants chose distributions that maximized the difference between the two groups in favor of their in-group. This means that they preferred combinations awarding their in-group members higher amounts of money than the out-group

Table 1. Distribution Matrix for Minimal Group Paradigm experiment

Matrix for Blue Group	A	B	C	D	E	F	G	H	I	J	K	L	M
Amount given to member no. 4 of red group	25	23	21	19	17	15	13	11	9	7	5	3	1
Amount given to member no. 17 of blue group	19	18	17	16	15	14	13	12	11	10	9	8	7

members even, if that meant giving lower sums to their own group: For example, members of the blue group tended to choose options G–M (highlighted in grey in table 1) because these were especially disadvantageous for the red group even though options A–F could have "earned" their own group distinctly higher amounts of money.

These experiments show that random social categorization is sufficient to shape human behavior, namely to elicit in-group favoritism and out-group discrimination. These results are rather remarkable given that "group members" did not know nor interact with each other and also had no tangible advantage resulting from their actions. In other words: Social identity and social categorization seem to be powerful processes that can be triggered even with a very small stimulus.

2.2   Virtual Groups

The minimal group experiments have been replicated in numerous studies with different settings and contexts with different levels of group identification, anonymity, and interaction (e.g. unionists deciding about wage differences between different groups of workers, members of groups, or supporters of different political parties). Thus the Social Identity Theory and the Minimal Group Paradigm are now 'classical', well-established social psychological theories regarding social groups.

However, these theories were established long before virtual teams and online communities [cf. 12] interacting via electronic communication devices came into existence. Nowadays, membership in virtual groups is commonplace in people's everyday private and professional lives, for instance as members of social networks and online communities, registered customers of online shops, or members of organizational teams distributed across sites. This raises the question, whether the assumptions of the Social Identity Theory hold true for virtual settings as well. As interaction is often more anonymous or fleeting, group memberships may be more mutable and cursory (e.g. abandoning membership in one newsgroup or forum to adopt a new one). Also people have more possibilities to 'construct' multiple identities online, which means there might be other mechanisms underlying the processes of establishing and upholding group coherence and social identity. Nevertheless, it is feasible to assume that Social Identity plays an important role for group coherence, group dynamics, distribution of resources etc. in virtual teams as well, as was demonstrated in the original MGP experiments.

To our knowledge there has been no systematic research regarding the Minimal Group Paradigm in virtual teams so far, although previous studies have considered the formation of in-group/out-group formation in virtual settings. In their lab experiment involving computer simulations, Nan et al. [13] found that collocated vs. remote players each formed in-groups of their own. However, their main focus was on group performance. Zhu et al. [14] investigated the effects of group identity on the performance of actual working groups, but did not investigate how social identity is established and formed. Dabbish et al. [15] and Farzan et al. [16] investigated the sense of belonging in online communities, but were mainly concerned with commitment to groups, a unique concept different from social identity.

A few studies suggest that social identity is also present and effective in online settings, but these are mostly of qualitative nature, dealing with case studies from different fields [17, 18]. Rohde et al. [18], for instance, show that technical access barriers might elicit feelings of identification and even out-group discrimination on an online learning platform, whereas Janneck and Finck demonstrated that feelings of identity influence technology appropriation and coherence in web-based communities [17].

3   Research Questions and Methods

In this study we aim to replicate the original Minimal Group Paradigm in a setting involving virtual teams. Based on the scarce research evidence in the area and the fact that the MGP experiments were mostly based on anonymous settings with no face-to-face contact between participants, we assume that similar effects will be present in online teams.

To this end, we conducted two online experiments with a total of N=190 participants. In both experiments participants were presented with a number of fictional online user profiles of people they were supposed to work with in a virtual team and others supposedly belonging to a different team. In a control condition no such categorization was applied. The experiments varied regarding the setting (private vs. professional profiles) and the amount of information given in the profiles, as will be explained in more detail further on.

Instead of allocating resources, as in the original MGP, participants in both experiments were asked to rate all profiles on a variety of aspects using a 7-step semantic differential. The items either had a social focus (such as agreeable–disagreeable, friendly–unfriendly, likable–dislikable, attractive–unattractive, sociable–unsociable, polite–impolite) or a work focus (such as successful–unsuccessful, competent–incompetent, efficient–inefficient, reliable–unreliable). Factor analysis showed that all 12 aspects loaded on one factor, so all items were combined into an overall profile rating.

A separate item measured the overall likability of the profile ("The profile appeals to me") on a scale from '1:not at all' to '7:very much'.

For socio-demographic data, we collected experience with virtual teamwork (rated on a scale from '1:no experience' to '7:a lot of experience') as well as information on rater gender and age.

4   Study 1

4.1   Procedure and Sample

For study 1 a total of 16 fictional user profiles were used. The profiles had a private, leisure-time character (see figure 1). They contained a photograph and basic information such as age, hometown, hobbies, etc. Photographs were taken from a research

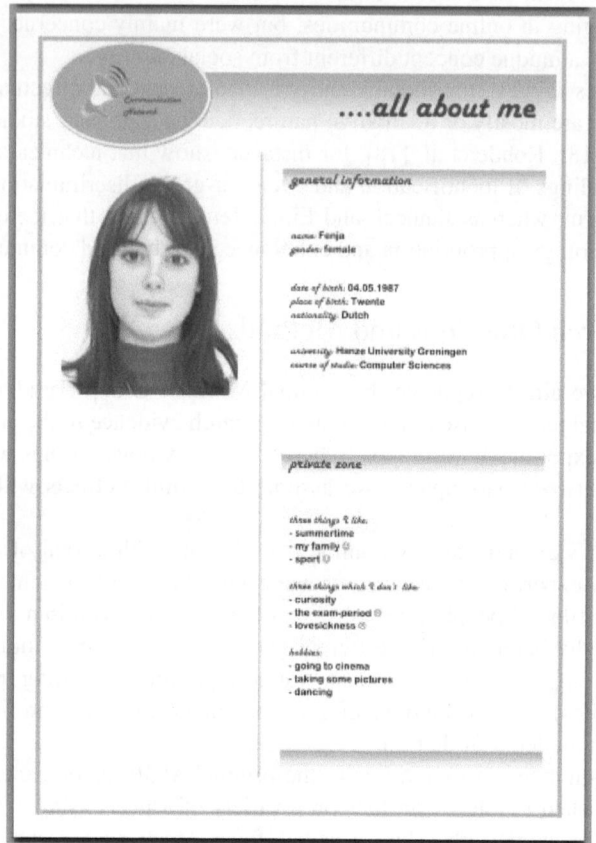

Fig. 1. Sample Profile (study 1, orange group)

database (PICS, The Psychological Image Collection at Sterling) and are normed for scientific purposes. The profiles were divided into different groups by color (orange / blue).

The online survey was distributed via national and international mailing lists. Participants were mostly university students from a variety of different countries. As an incentive an iPod Shuffle was raffled among participants.

The participants received the following instruction:

"Please imagine the following scenario: You will be working on a project assignment as a member of a virtual team. You don't know the other team members personally and will communicate with them only via electronic media. Your team's task will be to plan and prepare a workshop to present the project results. Please look at each user profile carefully. You will be asked to rate them regarding different aspects, e.g. how much you would like to work together with this person."

Participants were assigned at random to one of the following conditions:

1. *Experimental condition* (N=56; 24% male, 76% female; age: M=24.2, SD=3.5): In addition to the instructions shown above, participants were told they belonged to one of the groups (orange or blue).
2. *Control* (N=38; 45% male, 55% female; age: M=25.3, SD=3.8): No association with groups was provided.

4.2   Hypotheses

As predicted by the Social Identity Theory and the Minimal Group Paradigm, we assumed that color-coding is sufficient to yield in-group/out-group differentiation processes.

1. *H 1.1*: Participants in the experimental condition will evaluate user profiles of members belonging to their own team more favorably than profiles of members belonging to the other team.
2. *H 1.2*: User profiles belonging to the in-group in the experimental condition are evaluated better than the same user profiles in the control condition.

4.3   Results

Experimental Condition
Mean values were calculated for all profiles belonging to one 'group' (blue/orange). Unpaired t-tests were calculated to measure differences between the ratings.

Results show that indeed the profiles of the supposed "out-group members" were rated consistently and in most cases significantly more negatively than the profiles of members belonging to the assigned "in-group" (table 2). Thus, hypothesis 1.1 was confirmed.

Control Condition
Ratings of "in-group" profiles were compared to the ratings of the same profiles in the control condition, where no group membership had been assigned. Again, mean values were calculated for all profiles and unpaired t-tests were used.

Results show that the same profiles were rated consistently and in most cases significantly more positive when the raters had been told that they were on the same team with this person as compared to the neutral condition (table 3). Thus, hypothesis 1.2 was confirmed as well.

Summary of Study 1
According to the results of study 1, the Minimal Group Paradigm seems to apply to virtual teams as well: In-group/out-group differentiation processes were yielded in randomly assigned virtual groups without any personal contact.

Table 2. In-group vs. out-group ratings

Study 1: In-group vs. out-group						
Item	Group	M	SD	T	df	p
correct	in-group	4.61	1.60	1.416	55	.082[+]
	out-group	4.50	1.59			
successful	in-group	4.15	1.37	2.287	55	**.013***
	out-group	3.98	1.37			
team player	in-group	4.44	1.52	3.149	55	**.002****
	out-group	4.16	1.37			
efficient	in-group	4.16	1.33	1.446	55	.077[+]
	out-group	4.06	1.37			
competent	in-group	4.30	1.40	1.603	55	.058[+]
	out-group	4.19	1.43			
hard-working	in-group	4.01	1.29	.603	55	.275
	out-group	3.97	1.39			
dynamic	in-group	4.13	1.36	.773	55	.222
	out-group	4.05	1.29			
friendly	in-group	4.71	1.60	3.161	55	**.002****
	out-group	4.48	1.50			
respectful	in-group	4.62	1.54	3.607	55	**.001****
	out-group	4.39	1.47			
likable	in-group	4.53	1.55	3.129	55	**.002****
	out-group	4.27	1.43			
familiar	in-group	4.15	1.52	3.002	55	**.002****
	out-group	3.88	1.40			
reliable	in-group	4.40	1.44	2.957	55	**.003****
	out-group	4.20	1.43			
polite	in-group	4.48	1.53	1.525	55	.067[+]
	out-group	4.36	1.52			
good	in-group	4.54	1.53	2.733	55	**.004****
	out-group	4.34	1.49			
Overall likability	in-group	3.00	1.13	1.76	55	**.042***
	out-group	2.90	1.07			
Work together	in-group	4.01	1.50	2.30	55	**.013***
	out-group	3.75	1.28			

Quite interestingly, significant differences were found especially regarding the social dimensions of the semantic differential (like friendliness, respect, reliability…) rather than task-related dimensions (like efficiency, competency…). We assume that this might be due to the presentation of the profiles, since they evoked a personal, leisure-time impression rather than a professional appearance. This issue was addressed in study 2.

Table 3. In-group vs. control ratings

Item	Group	M	SD	T	df	p
Study 1: In-group vs. control						
correct	in-group	3.93	1.60	2.50	93	**.014***
	control	3.70	1.91			
successful	in-group	4.15	1.37	2.02	93	**.047***
	control	3.52	1.71			
team player	in-group	4.44	1.52	2.00	93	**.048***
	control	3.74	1.86			
efficient	in-group	4.16	1.33	1.79	93	.076[+]
	control	3.59	1.79			
competent	in-group	4.30	1.40	1.93	93	.057[+]
	control	3.67	1.81			
hard-working	in-group	4.01	1.29	1.66	93	.100
	control	3.51	1.68			
dynamic	in-group	4.13	1.36	1.63	93	.107
	control	3.61	1.75			
friendly	in-group	4.71	1.60	2.14	93	**.035***
	control	3.92	1.99			
respectful	in-group	4.62	1.54	2.16	93	**.034***
	control	3.84	1.99			
likable	in-group	4.53	1.55	2.30	93	**.024***
	control	3.71	1.90			
familiar	in-group	4.15	1.52	1.76	93	.082[+]
	control	3.54	1.84			
reliable	in-group	4.40	1.44	2.07	93	**.041***
	control	3.70	1.87			
polite	in-group	4.48	1.53	1.83	93	.070[+]
	control	3.82	1.96			
good	in-group	4.54	1.53	2.08	93	**.040***
	control	3.80	1.94			
Overall appear-ance	in-group	3.00	1.13	2.32	93	**.023***
	control	2.37	1.51			
Work together	in-group	4.01	1.50	1.64	93	.105
	control	3.47	1.67			

5   Study 2

5.1   Procedure and Sample

In order to replicate the results of study 1 in a different context and to further explore the Minimal Group Paradigm in virtual teams, a second online experiment was conducted, this time using a work-related context and more professionally appearing user profiles. A total of 12 profiles were used, containing name, age, location, professional experiences, areas of expertise, and a few words regarding private interests.

Furthermore, profiles either contained a photograph (again taken from PICS database) or no photograph, to investigate whether the richness of the profiles would affect ratings.

Each profile belonged to one distinct department ("Human Resources" vs. "Research & Development") of a fictional internationally operating company. Profile were color-coded (orange for "Human Resource" profiles vs. blue for "Research & Development" profiles) to enable better recognition. Examples of profiles are given in figure 2 and 3.

The participants were randomly assigned to one of these groups or the control group. They were instructed as follows:

"You work in a large international company with branches in several cities. For a new project a team needs to be created with members from several departments. The project work will primarily be done 'virtually', i.e., using electronic media such as e-mail, video-conferencing, etc. As part of the project team you can participate in the selection of the team members. Your task: On the next pages you will see personal profiles of twelve potential team members. Please consider them carefully and rate them according to a short survey."

Harry Klint	
Research & Development	
Location: Berlin	
Task: Market research	
Age: 36	
Areas of expertise:	Statistics
	Brand development
Private Interests:	Chess
	Contemporary Arts

Fig. 2. Sample profile without photograph (study 2, R&D group)

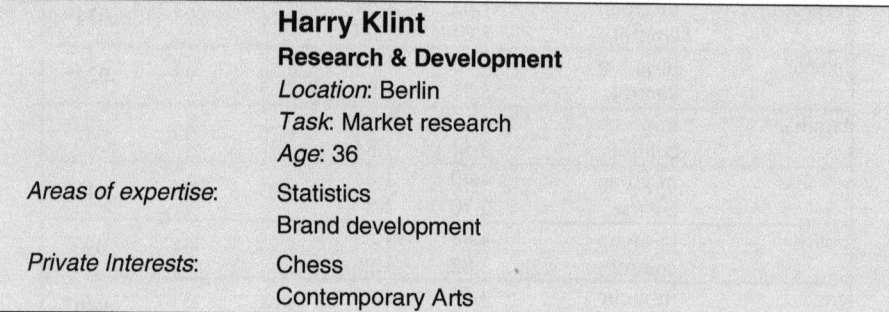

	Sarah Weil	
	Human Resources	
	Location: London	
	Task: Human resource development	
	Age: 34	
Areas of expertise:	Assessment Center	
	Advanced Training	
Private Interests:	Gospel Choir	
	Cooking	

Fig. 3. Sample profile with photograph (study 2, HR group)

Participants in the experimental conditions were also told which department they belonged to. To check whether the experimental manipulation had been successful participants were asked after completing all questionnaires, if they remembered what department they had supposedly belonged to. Participants who did not answer correctly were excluded from the calculations.

In total 274 people participated. Of these 106 had to be excluded, because they failed the manipulation check. Another 72 did not complete the experiment. This resulted in a total of N=96 participants (24% male, 76% female, age: M=30.2, SD=8.2) (HR: n1=31; R&D: n2=36; control: N3=29). Again, mostly undergraduate and graduate students participated who were recruited through online study panels. As an incentive, all participants could take part in a drawing of Amazon vouchers. The semantic differential was slightly altered and shortened to reduce the duration of the experiment. Furthermore, participants were asked, which group they generally preferred.

5.2   Hypotheses

Again, we assumed that the experimental assignment to one of the groups would be sufficient to yield in-group/out-group differentiation processes. Furthermore, we wanted to investigate whether the richness of the profile (i.e. photo vs. no photo) would affect ratings. As we did not make prior assumptions, the null hypothesis is stated in that respect.

1. *H 2.1*: Participants in the experimental condition will evaluate user profiles of members belonging to their own team more favorably than profiles of members belonging to the other team.
2. *H 2.2*:User profiles belonging to the in-group in the experimental condition will be evaluated more positively than the same user profiles in the control condition.
3. *H 2.3*: Group preferences will not be affected by the richness of the profile (i.e. containing photo vs. no photo).

5.3   Results

Figure 4 shows the results of the group preferences stated by the members of each group (one-item measure asking about the preferred group).

The R&D group shows a clear effect of in-group favoritism. However, members of the control group also favored the R&D group. This effect vanishes in the HR group, whose members stated almost balanced group preferences. Figure 4 shows how many members of the respective groups (in absolute numbers) chose the HR / the R&D group, respectively, when asked for their group preferences. Thus, apparently the profiles were not neutral, but the R&D profiles generally appealed to the participants more than the HR profiles, independent of their assignment to groups.

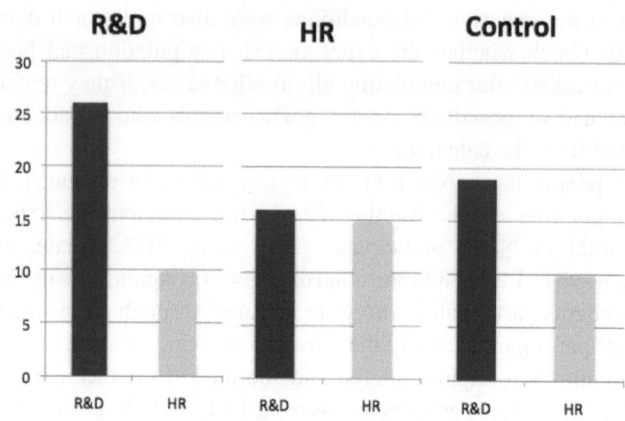

Fig. 4. Group preferences

Table 4. Rating of HR profiles by HR members vs. control

Study 2: HR group vs. control – profiles with photographs						
Item	Group	M	SD	T	df	p
correct	HR group	**5.55**	.86	.800	68	.426
	control	5.36	1.05			
successful	HR group	4.98	.93	-.128	69	.898
	control	5.01	.90			
efficient	HR group	**5.32**	.86	.235	67	.815
	control	5.27	.88			
competent	HR group	**5.31**	.87	.056	67	.955
	control	5.29	.96			
dynamic	HR group	**5.10**	.86	.479	69	.640
	control	5.01	.88			
friendly	HR group	**5.09**	.82	1.234	68	.221
	control	4.85	.80			
sociable	HR group	**4.57**	.79	.917	68	.362
	control	4.40	.69			
likable	HR group	**4.89**	.86	.993	69	.324
	control	4.69	.88			
agreeable	HR group	**5.02**	.81	1.088	69	.280
	control	4.79	.92			
reliable	HR group	**5.27**	.85	.169	69	.866
	control	5.27	.88			
polite	HR group	**4.98**	.85	.222	67	.825
	control	4.85	.77			
attractive	HR group	4.01	.92	-.191	67	.849
	control	4.05	.95			
Overall appearance	HR group	**4.88**	.66	.167	67	.868
	control	4.85	.88			

Table 5. Rating of R&D profiles by R&D members vs. control

Study 2: R&D group vs. control – profiles with photographs						
Item	Group	M	SD	T	df	p
correct	R&D group	**5.45**	.87	.373	70	.710
	control	5.36	1.05			
successful	R&D group	**5.07**	.90	.285	70	.776
	control	5.01	.90			
efficient	R&D group	5.27	.86	-.020	69	.984
	control	5.27	.88			
competent	R&D group	**5.53**	.87	1.063	69	.292
	control	5.29	.99			
dynamic	R&D group	**5.19**	.93	.864	69	.390
	control	5.01	.81			
friendly	R&D group	**4.89**	.79	.205	69	.838
	control	4.85	.80			
sociable	R&D group	**4.54**	.81	.790	70	.432
	control	4.40	.69			
likable	R&D group	**4.72**	.80	.173	69	.863
	control	4.67	.88			
agreeable	R&D group	4.71	.71	1.088	69	.280
	control	4.79	.92			
reliable	R&D group	**5.27**	.97	-.424	69	.673
	control	5.23	.89			
polite	R&D group	**5.07**	.88	.669	67	.506
	control	4.76	.78			
attractive	R&D group	3.86	.96	-.853	67	.397
	control	4.05	.95			
Overall appearance	R&D group	4.46	1.02	-1.697	68	.094
	control	4.85	.88			

To separate this general effect from the calculations on ratings and group preferences, we did not compare the R&D with the HR group, but analyzed how HR [or R&D, respectively] profiles were rated by the HR [R&D] members compared with the control group. Again, un-paired t-tests were used in all calculations.

As is shown in table 4 and table 5, in-group members of both the HR and the R&D group rated profiles of their alleged "team members" consistently more positive than members of the control group. However, the differences are very small and not significant. Thus, there is only scarce support for hypotheses 2.1 and 2.2.

To investigate our second research question regarding the influence of profile richness, we conducted the same comparisons (HR / R&D profiles rated by HR / R&D members vs. control group) with the profiles containing no photographs.

Again, in-group members of both groups rated profiles of "their team members" consistently more positively than members of the control group (tables 6 and 7). Quite surprisingly, the differences between ratings increased considerably in the no-photo condition. This is especially true for the HR group, which shows several statistically significant differences between in-group and control group (table 6). Regarding the

Table 6. Rating of HR profiles without photographs by HR members vs. control

Item	Group	M	SD	T	df	p
Study 2: HR group vs. control – profiles w/o photographs						
correct	HR group	**5.24**	.83	1.097	69	.276
	control	5.01	.96			
successful	HR group	**4.67**	.82	-.098	69	.922
	control	4.64	.87			
efficient	HR group	**4.83**	.65	.186	67	.853
	control	4.80	.92			
competent	HR group	**4.96**	.82	.343	68	.733
	control	4.89	.91			
dynamic	HR group	**5.28**	.78	1.725	69	*.089*[+]
	control	4.91	1.01			
friendly	HR group	**5.04**	.82	1.999	68	*.050**
	control	4.62	.89			
sociable	HR group	**4.96**	.90	1.805	68	*.076*[+]
	control	4.56	.80			
likable	HR group	**4.93**	1.01	2.272	69	*.026**
	control	4.40	.94			
agreeable	HR group	**4.92**	.91	1.653	69	*.103*[+]
	control	4.57	.87			
reliable	HR group	**4.98**	.71	.826	69	.412
	control	4.81	1.00			
polite	HR group	**5.00**	.80	1.092	69	.279
	control	4.76	1.01			
attractive	HR group	**3.85**	.83	.173	69	.863
	control	3.81	.78			
Overall appearance	HR group	**4.67**	.86	1.375	67	.174
	control	4.37	.92			

R&D profiles the differences were smaller, which emphasizes again that apparently the R&D profiles were generally more appealing than the HR profiles.

Thus, the null hypothesis stated in H 2.3 must be rejected: Apparently, the richness of the profiles did affect ratings: Profiles containing less information (i.e. no photo) yielded stronger effects of in-group favoritism than those with photographs.

Summary of Study 2

Findings of study 2 again show effects of in-group favoritism. However, the results are not as clear as in study 1: Apparently, as a general effect, the R&D profiles were more appealing to all participants than the HR profiles. Therefore, when asked for their group preferences, members of all groups (R&D, HR, and control) favored the R&D group. However, as hypothesized, R&D members showed the strongest preference, while HR members showed the least preference with the control group in-between. Therefore, we assume that mechanisms of social identity and in-group favoritism took effect, but were somewhat overshadowed by the general effect that some profiles were more appealing than others.

Table 7. Rating of R&D profiles without photographs by R&D members vs. control

Study 2: R&D group vs. control – profiles w/o photographs						
Item	Group	M	SD	T	df	p
correct	R&D group	**5.06**	.74	.257	70	.798
	control	5.01	.96			
successful	R&D group	**4.79**	.79	.786	70	.434
	control	4.65	.80			
efficient	R&D group	**4.93**	.63	.716	69	.477
	control	4.80	.93			
competent	R&D group	**4.94**	.69	.235	69	.815
	control	4.89	.91			
dynamic	R&D group	**5.40**	.62	2.519	70	**.017***
	control	4.91	1.01			
friendly	R&D group	**4.78**	.86	.741	70	.461
	control	4.63	.89			
sociable	R&D group	**4.84**	.85	1.298	69	.199
	control	4.56	.80			
likable	R&D group	**4.63**	.82	1.054	69	.296
	control	4.40	.94			
agreeable	R&D group	**4.71**	.77	.737	70	.464
	control	4.57	.87			
reliable	R&D group	**5.03**	.78	1.012	69	.315
	control	4.81	1.00			
polite	R&D group	**5.00**	.94	1.008	68	.317
	control	4.75	1.01			
attractive	R&D group	3.74	.89	-.388	70	.699
	control	3.81	.78			
Overall appearance	R&D group	4.35	.95	-.101	71	.920
	control	4.37	.92			

Comparing the ratings of in-group members vs. control group members slightly confirmed this result: Members of the HR group (or the R&D group, respectively) rated the profiles of their alleged group members consistently better than members of the control group. However, differences were only marginal and not significant.

Quite interestingly, profiles with or without photographs were rated differently: Again, in-group members rated profiles (without photographs) of their "team members" better than members of the control group. However, differences were considerably larger than regarding the profiles with photographs: Apparently removing the photographs from the profiles increased the effect of in-group favoritism. Again, like in study 1, especially social dimensions of the semantic differential (such as dynamic, friendly, sociable, likable...) showed statistically significant differences in ratings, even though the study had a clear workplace focus.

6   Discussion

6.1   Interpretation of Results and Methodical Issues

The aim of this paper was to investigate the Minimal Group Paradigm with regard to virtual teams. In a series of two experiments participants were asked to rate fictional online user profiles of people they were supposed to work with in a virtual team and others belonging to a different team. In a control condition no such categorization was applied.

Results show that, as predicted by Social Identity Theory, subjects preferred members of their supposed in-group to those belonging to the alleged out-group or compared to neutral ratings done by a control group, respectively. These findings were especially clear in study 1. In study 2 there seems to be an overlay effect of general attractiveness of one set of profiles, thus reducing the impact of the in-group effect. This is a clear limitation of our study.

It is hard to explain why the R&D profiles were seen as more appealing, as all profiles were completely fictitious and had been crafted according to the same pattern. Characteristics like gender, age, etc. were balanced across the profiles. One explanation might be that participants identified themselves more with the R&D sector, since they were mostly college students or from a university context.

A second methodical issue concerns the high number of participants that had to be excluded from study 2 because the manipulation check revealed that they did not remember correctly, which group they had been assigned to or were unsure about their supposed group membership. More than half of the actual participants had to be excluded from the study, resulting in a rather small sample concerning the complex design.

In the first study, we did not include a manipulation check. However, the clear effects in the data suggest that the experimental manipulation was successful and people were aware of their alleged group membership. Apparently, the simple color-coding done in study 1 was easy for the participants to remember and recognize, while the classification based on different departments ("Human Resources" vs. "Research & Development") may have been too complex. Furthermore, including profiles with and without photographs might have distracted participants from the actual classification, as those two types of profiles looked very differently. This suggests that the implicit categorization processes proposed in SIT may be suppressed in online contexts, when too much or too complex information about (potential) in-group/out-group members is presented.

Our second study was aimed at exploring, whether the context of interaction influences social categorization and in-group favoritism: While study 1 used clearly private profiles, study 2 used a workplace context and work-related profiles. Since the two contexts were investigated in separate studies, we are unable to test whether context may be an important influencing factor. From classical research on the Minimal Group Paradigm, which was conducted in work-related as well as leisure contexts, no such differences are known. However, it is interesting to note that just like in study 1 the largest differences in ratings were observed regarding the more 'social' dimensions of the semantic differential that we used (like friendliness, respect, sociability...) rather than task-related dimensions (like efficiency, competency...), even though the context was clearly work-related.

This finding may not be immediately evident. In a work-context, identities are defined over professional or work roles, which to a large extent are based on role and task-specific attitudes, beliefs and values [e.g. 19, 20]. It might thus be feasible to expect that work-related features play a stronger role in study 2, i.e., would show a bigger difference across conditions. Maybe, when actually judging people, in-group favoritism is more easily triggered concerning 'soft' characteristics and traits than more 'objective' competencies and skills. Clearly differences in contexts such as leisure versus work should be investigated in more detail. We think that this effect, if replicated, is of considerable practical relevance especially in work contexts: E.g. it might be advisable to include more informal, 'social' information, for instance, in intranets or groupware platforms to increase social identity and group coherence in working groups. As a result, team members might identify more with their virtual team, which might have a beneficial effect on group dynamics and efficiency.

A very interesting result of our study concerns the difference between profiles with and without photographs. Contrary to what one might expect, for instance based on approaches such as Media Richness Theory [21, 22] or Social Presence Theory [23], profiles without photographs yielded stronger effects of in-group favoritism than the 'richer' profiles with photographs.

Again, simple, unambiguous clues might be more likely to trigger social categorization processes [cf. 9, 10]. This seems especially relevant for online contexts such as large public online communities and forums, where interaction is more anonymous and less personal information is available.

According to the *Social Identity Model of Deindividuation Effects* [24, 25], anonymous situations in computer-mediated communication may cause deindividuation, since information about interaction partners is scarce. Such deindividuation situations might increase feelings of group cohesion and group norms [24, 25]. A surplus of information, and here especially visual information, may provide enough pointers for reducing the anonymity necessary for social categorization and comparison, thus reducing the formation of strong in-group/out-group perceptions.

A similar line of reasoning is provided by Hogg [26], who states that group formation implies a process of depersonalization, weakening the individual perception of being a unique person, but strengthening similarities among group members. Therefore, the display of photographs might have a reverse effect of emphasizing individual differences and thus weaken effects of group identity.

To sum up results, carefully speaking there is some evidence that the Minimal Group Paradigm also applies to virtual teams. There is also evidence that simple, basic clues – such as color – invoke stronger effects than more complex categorizations. However, further research is needed to explain how exactly in-group favoritism is triggered in Minimal Virtual Teams.

6.2   Implications and Future Work

In this paper we describe initial investigations regarding the question whether there is such a thing as a Minimal Virtual Group. Compared to face-to-face interactions, online settings do possess additional complexities, due to the possibility of varying type and richness of information on a person or group (e.g., text to picture or video, asynchronous or synchronous). We see the main contribution of our study in a closer investigation of the effects of disparate types of information for social group judgments (e.g. photo, no photo) as well as comparing different aspects of judgments (social vs. task-related).

Our study thus goes beyond demonstrating the possibility of introducing MGP effects online, but investigated possible *moderators* of this effect in online settings. Our study demonstrates that even simple design choices about which information users have at their disposal might have considerable effects on how users behave online. Therefore, in our view our results indicate some interesting implications for applications in HCI and design.

Our research suggests that minimal and arbitrary clues are sufficient to trigger effects of in-group favoritism and out-group discrimination – maybe even better than complex information. Since it appears to be quite easy to trigger processes of social identity online this might be an underlying mechanism that has so far been ignored in most studies concerned with online communities or computer-supported group work. Including this variable in future studies might help to analyze virtual group dynamics and also conflicts within or between teams.

In our study we used color to trigger categorization, which is already known as a powerful medium to influence people's perception and behavior [cf. 27]. Other clues might have similar effects, e.g. icons or generally visualization techniques. Therefore, designers of interactive systems might make use of such clues to help people form social identities online.

However, while we deliberately caused in-group/out-group effects, this might not always be desirable. For instance, it is plausible to assume that similar effects might occur in online forums, e-learning or CSCW systems that are supposed to encourage a common identity rather than segregating users into smaller subgroups. Conversely, most groupware systems have a rather complex structure with diverse user roles: Being assigned a different user role or using a different sub-forum might be enough to trigger possibly unwanted effects of intra-group differentiation [cf. e.g. 28].

The findings of our study can thus guide designers of HCI technologies and social media by alerting them to the issue and possibly investigating whether such effects take place. This is especially relevant when designing for online communities, where the design of user profiles is an important task.

In our future research, we are especially interested in exploring how different designs of IT artifacts affect social identity processes; e.g., does a complex, hierarchical thread structure in a user forum lead to the formation of several subgroups compared to a 'flat' structure? Do different levels of access rights influence group formation and cohesion? Answering questions like these will inspire the design of innovative and sociable cooperative and interactive systems.

References

1. Hogg, M.A.: Blackwell Handbook of Social Psychology. Blackwell Publishing (2002)
2. Koschmann, T., Hall, R., Miyake, N. (eds.): CSCL 2: Carrying forward the conversation. Lawrence Erlbaum Associates, Hillsdale (2002)
3. Lutters, W., Sonnenwald, D.H., Gross, T., Reddy, M. (eds.): Proc. ACM International Conference on Supporting Group Work. ACM Press (2010)
4. Kraut, R.: Applying Social Psychological Theory to the Problems of Group Work. In: Carroll, J.M. (ed.) HCI Models, Theories, and Frameworks, pp. 325–356. Morgan Kaufmann, San Francisco (2003)
5. Tajfel, H.: Differentiation between social groups: Studies in the social psychology of intergroup relations. Academic Press, London (1978)
6. Tajfel, H., Billig, M.G., Bundy, R.P., Flament, C.: Social categorization and intergroup behavior. European Journal of Social Psychology 1, 146–178 (1971)
7. Tajfel, H., Turner, J.C.: An integrative theory of intergroup conflict. In: Austin, W.G., Worchel, S. (eds.) The Social Psychology of Intergroup Relations, pp. 33–47. Brooks/Cole, Monterey (1979)
8. Tajfel, H., Turner, J.C.: The social identity theory of intergroup behavior. In: Worchel, S., Austin, W.G. (eds.) Psychology of Intergroup Relations, pp. 7–24. Nelson-Hall, Chicago (1986)
9. Hogg, M.A.: Intragroup processes, group structure and social identity. In: Robinson, W.P. (ed.) Social groups and social identities: Developing the legacy of Henri Tajfel, pp. 65–93. Butterworth-Heinemann, Oxford (1996)
10. Tajfel, H., Wilkes, A.L.: Classification and quantitative judgment. British Journal of Psychology 54, 101–114 (1963)
11. Tajfel, H.: Social identity and intergroup relations. Cambridge University Press, Cambridge (1982)
12. Preece, J.: Online Communities: Designing Usability and Supporting Sociability. John Wiley, Ney York (2000)
13. Nan, N., Johnston, E.W., Olson, J.S., Bos, N.: Beyond Being in the Lab: Using Multi-Agent Modeling to Isolate Competing Hypotheses. In: CHI Extended Abstracts, pp. 1693–1696. ACM Press (2005)
14. Zhu, H., Kraut, R.E., Kittur, A.: Organizing without formal organization: Group Identification, Goal Setting and Social Modeling in Directing Online Production. In: CSCW 2012: Proceedings of the ACM Conference on Computer Supported Cooperative Work. ACM, New York (2012)
15. Dabbish, L., Kraut, R.E., Patton, J.: Communication and commitment in an online game team. In: CHI 2012: Proceedings of the ACM Conference on Human Factors in Computing Systems. ACM, NY (2012)
16. Farzan, R., Dabbish, L., Kraut, R.E., Postmes, T.: Increasing Commitment in Online Communities via Building Social Attachment. In: CSCW 2011: Proceedings of the ACM Conference on Computer-Supported Cooperative Work. ACM Press, New York (2011)
17. Janneck, M., Finck, M.: Making the community a hospitable place – identity, strong bounds and self-organisation in web-based communities. International Journal of Web Based Communities 2(4), 458–473 (2006)
18. Rohde, M., Reinecke, L., Pape, B., Janneck, M.: Community-Building with Web-Based Systems - Investigating a Hybrid Community of Students. Computer Supported Cooperative Work 13, 471–499 (2004)

19. Ibarra, H.: Provisional selves: experimenting with image and identity in professional adaptation. Administrative Science Quarterly 44(4), 764–791 (1999)
20. Slay, H., Smith, D.: Professional identity construction: Using narrative to understand the negotiation of professional and stigmatized cultural identities. Human Relations 64, 85–107 (2011)
21. Daft, R.L., Lengel, R.H.: Organizational information requirements, media richness and structural design. Management Science 32, 554–571 (1986)
22. Daft, R.L., Lengel, R.H.: Information richness: A new approach to managerial behavior and organization design. Research in Organizational Behavior 6, 191–233 (1984)
23. Short, J., Williams, E., Christie, B.: The social psychology of telecommunications. Wiley, London (1976)
24. Postmes, T., Spears, R., Lea, M.: Breaching or building social boundaries? SIDE-effects of computer-mediated communication. Communication Research 25, 689–715 (1998)
25. Postmes, T., Spears, R., Lea, M.: Intergroup differentiation in computer-mediated communication: Effects of depersonalization. Group Dynamics: Theory, Research, and Practice 6, 3–16 (2002)
26. Hogg, M.A., Abrams, D.: Social identifications: A social psychology of intergroup relations and group processes. Routlegde, London (1988)
27. Pelet, J.-E., Papadopoulou, P.: The Effect Of Colors Of E-commerce Websites On Mood, Memorization And Buying Intention. European Journal of Information Systems 21, 438–467 (2012)
28. Rohde, M.: Find what binds. Building social capital in an Iranian NGO community system. In: Huysman, M., Wulf, V. (eds.) Social Capital and Information Technology, pp. 75–112. MIT Press, Cambridge (2004)

"Atlas 2012" Augmented Reality: A Case Study in the Domain of Fine Arts*

Narvika Bovcon[1], Aleš Vaupotič[2], Bojan Klemenc[1], and Franc Solina[1]

[1] Computer Vision Laboratory,
Faculty of Computer and Information Science,
University of Ljubljana
Tržaška cesta 25, 1000 Ljubljana, Slovenia
[2] Research Centre for Humanities,
University of Nova Gorica,
Vipavska 13, 5000 Nova Gorica, Slovenia
{narvika.bovcon,bojan.klemenc,franc.solina}@fri.uni-lj.si,
ales@vaupotic.com

Abstract. The article presents a case study of artistic use of augmented reality built with the Layar augmented reality application. Members of ArtNetLab, a group of new media artists, have conceptualized a series of projects for geolocated virtual objects (augments), that can be perceived by means of smart-phone or tablet-computer applications in the urban space of a city. The user experience in art is not limited to practical and efficient use of a gadget directed towards a predetermined set of actions, instead it has to involve the user in the art experience, and this opens up a broad field of conceivable contexts. Our case study presents an art project that proposes and tests a concrete solution to the latent question proposed by an existing technology, and we describe how the artists encoded meanings by using a ubiquitous mobile platform for augmented reality.

Keywords: augmented reality, new media art, virtual objects in physical environment, emblem, fine art projects, case study.

1 Introduction

Since the beginnings of the human race there seems to be the need that the man makes sense of his physical environment, usually by leaving some material marks of his existence in the environment. Large stones are, for example, still standing across large parts of Europe as remnants of Megalithic cultures, their true purpose and meaning still disputed. Even if there are no visible features in the landscape ancient peoples such as Australian aborigines overlaid the often featureless and uniform Australian landscape with a symbolic meaning. Bruce Chatwin describes how this symbolic layer can be accessed by following sacred

* This work was supported by the Slovenian Research Agency, research program Computer Vision (P2-0214).

A. Holzinger et al. (Eds.): SouthCHI 2013, LNCS 7946, pp. 477–496, 2013.

pathways or "songlines" which each generation learns from their ancestors [1]. Cultural landscapes as a combined work of nature and of man slowly evolved over time. Cultural landscapes seem to be the true repository of cultural and spiritual revelations of human history where the past is made visible. Deborah Tall's "From Where We Stand" is an eloquent exploration of the connections we have with places—and the loss to us if there are no such connections [2]. The primordial Slovenian landscape, for example, seems to be green hills topped with small churches, interspersed with fertile valleys and villages in between, although this was at least partly a result of medieval colonial settlement and counterreformation movement [3].

The continuous development of cultural landscapes is normally the result of organized effort of the whole society. Individual people, however, also had the urge to leave a mark of their existence in the physical world, be it a paleolithic artist who almost 20.000 years ago left his handprints in the Altamira cave by placing his hand on the cave wall and blowing pigment over it to leave a negative image, be it American landscape artists who created monumental earthworks in the 1970s and 1980s in the American west [4]. Another intriguing example of marking the existence of ordinary individuals in the physical space is the art project "Stolpersteine/Stumbling stones" by the German artist Gunter Demnig [5]. He remembers the victims of National Socialism by installing commemorative brass plaques in the pavement in front of their last address of choice. There are now stumbling stones in over 610 places in Germany as well as in Austria, Hungary, the Netherlands, Belgium, the Czech Republic, Norway and Ukraine. Each "stone" begins with HERE LIVED ... The artist believes that "a person is only forgotten when his or her name is forgotten".

The placement of individual "signs of existence" in the modern urban society is however difficult due to the normative and legislative nature of modern human society that often overly regulates the environment. Graffiti artists are well known for breaking the rules by leaving their signatures in public spaces. Even Gunter Demnig had problems with the implementation of his project "Stolpersteine/Stumbling stones" since several German cities prohibited the placement of these brass plaques in pavements [6].

A possible way of expressing individual initiative by leaving a mark in correlation to a particular physical point without breaking any regulations is to use augmented reality. The Internet and the World Wide Web technology were initially so exciting because they removed all geographical and temporal boundaries for the exchange of information. But due to the enormous amount of information available over the web, one of the filters for limiting the search for information, particularly on hand-held devices, has become again geographical or physical proximity. Since we exist in the physical space and many types of information relate to some location in the physical space, maps and mapping applications soon evolved also on the web. For example, we developed a pilot web application for collaborative georeferencing of Slovenian works of literature based on Google Maps so that the users of the system could cross-reference the imagined locations in literary works with points in the real world [7].

Although the technology for augmented reality has been available for decades, it is only now that it is becoming ubiquitous, when augmented reality browsers (AR browsers) can be run on smart phones, as in the case of the Layar platform [8] that we eventually used in our projects. Any user can easily obtain the application on the Internet and use it. On some smart phones it is even pre-installed. For the average end user no additional coding or payments are required. In the case study that is presented in this article, artists (with no formal training in computer engineering) used the application to communicate their artistic statements. However, in collaboration with computer engineers, this case study became a foundation for interdisciplinary research, where the results of the specific use of a technology were evaluated first "intuitively" from the primary user's, i.e. artist's point of view, and second, by using the concrete findings of the first phase in a broader usability evaluation of a family of similar software and hardware solutions. Of course, while realizing the project the two phases would merge in the dialogue of the disciplines. It is important to keep in mind that when a technology is accessible, it has to be actually used in different ways to find out, how useful it really is and what are its limitations for specific uses. The interdisciplinary effort elucidates the ties of a new way of exchanging meanings with the existing "older" modes of communication.

The artists working under the framework of the ArtNetLab society [9] experimented in a series of projects entitled "Atlas" by placing virtual objects into physical locations and extending printed editions with digital content. In one of their projects they actually succeeded in informally joining an exhibition by superimposing virtual forms on the physical environment where the exhibition was taking place [10].

The article continues in the following way: Section 2 talks about the development of virtual and augmented reality, Section 3 describes the cultural and technological influences that fostered the project series "Atlas", Section 4 talks about artistic use of augmented reality platforms, Section 5 presents the exhibitions from the augmented reality "Atlas" series, Section 6 gives the technical details of our project's implementation, and Section 8 concludes the article.

2 Recent History of Imagining the Transition between Physical Reality and Virtual Reality

Virtual reality and augmented reality have been used by artists many times, even before it actually existed on computers. Illusionistic paintings, for example, can be considered as forerunners of virtual reality since they present an invented image that from a standard viewpoint looks as if it were reality [11]. The best known examples are Baroque ceiling paintings that from a particular viewpoint make a flat ceiling look like extending into imaginary architecture of domes, towers or the heaven itself.

In the 20th century augmented reality was imagined most influentially by film directors, who could create a filmic image of it, which didn't require that the technology would actually work. An important early model of virtual reality in film was "Tron" (1982) by Steven Lisberger, where the image was created using "green-screen" technology, i.e. by compositing a filmed actor and for that time advanced computer graphics that represented the virtual environment. Film "Disclosure" (1994) by Barry Levinson showed the hero of the movie entering the virtual reality by being scanned and his avatar is instantly reconstructed as his 3D mirror image in a virtual cathedral/bank, then he walks through the rooms and almost tumbles into a virtual abyss, because he stepped onto the edge of his highly original interface for walking, a kind of a concave tracking mat. "Johnny Mnemonic" (1995) by Robert Longo, based on a short story with the same title (1981) by the famous cyberpunk writer William Gibson, uses data gloves and helmet, he juggles the data and brakes the code in a predominantly tactile manner.

The materializations of virtual and mixed reality are more limited by the possibilities of technology in the fine arts and the conceptual arts. "EVE" (Extended Virtual Environment, 1993) by Jeffery Show is a colossal interactive computer graphic installation with virtual reality. However, it is much less illusionistic than the augmented reality in the films. An industrial robot with a video projector attached is synchronized to the moves of a user equipped with a helmet and a data-manipulation stick. The robotic arm projects a rectangular video image onto the hemispherical dome that contains the installation. The CAVE (Cave Automatic Virtual Environment) technology was another notable solution since its first implementation in 1992 [12]. It models virtual reality as a synchronized video projection onto the six walls of a cubic room. However, CAVE was expensive financially as well as in terms of spatial requirements so that only few institutions have it. Its fixed spatial position in research institutions and commercial facilities limits the users' possibilities to build content for the CAVE environment.

The full-body immersion of a person into a computer generated virtual reality, as seen in previous examples, has been a rare occasion until the arrival of portable smart screen devices with augmented reality applications. When you look through the camera of a portable screen device, you see your immediate surroundings with no temporal delay as though you had looked through a piece of glass, which means that you can look at your other waving hand or at your colleague with whom you are involved in a conversation. However, your recognizable environment in which you find yourself standing and moving is filled with virtual augments, i.e. images or 3D models. The image of virtual reality is not confined to the frame of a computer screen and thus totally isolated from the environment in which the computer screen is placed, but it is combined with the three-dimensional space that extends around you, holding a smart phone in your palm, and allows you to move freely in the city. In this sense the augmented reality on portable smart screen devices comes as close as it is currently possible to the imagined possibilities of being fully immersed into virtual reality spaces. The focus of this paper are AR projects that are positioned "in" or "over" public spaces. We are not considering a special section of interactive art installations in gallery space that involve the AR connected to some marker and displayed by a video projector. These installations confine the AR to the closed space of art institutions and are not ubiquitous.

3 Artistic Experience: Cultural and Technological Influences That Fostered the Project Series "Atlas"

In London there are several small, although very interesting, contemporary art galleries, which are hidden away in obscure streets. It would be quite impossible to find them, if there was no "London A-Z" [13], a book with extremely accurate maps of all parts of London. The (mostly fictional) anecdote says that once it used to be only a quite unusefull map of London until a lady decided to correct it by herself [14]. On her bicycle she criss-crossed every single street and alley and draw it accurately on the map—now contained in "London A-Z". Her endeavour was not a matter of hours, it was of true Borgesian [15] proportions: a translation of a huge archive into another medium at a 1:1 scale.

"Google Maps" is a similar project, only that it stretches the mapping over the whole world and therefore employs hundreds of people, who drive the streets, record the "Street View" and manually draw the exact street directions into the satellite images of the Earth's surface [16]. Computer vision and other algorithms can undertake a huge part in this project, however only to a certain level of accuracy. For the correct notation of the traffic flow human experience and understanding are still more relevant and reliable. Google's motto that better data is more data combined with the promise that huge collections of data, that cannot be mastered by a single human being, will be sorted and retrieved by computers, still involve people in the process of tagging the data and managing the archive.

A person carries in her body models of spaces that she visited in the past. Memories of a space, of key objects in it with their many details and of the path walked through the space are so strong that in history, and even half way into the modern era, this experience was used as the main mnemotechnic device [17]. Famous rhetors, such as Cicero, distributed in their minds parts of their speeches into memory loci, e.g. rooms, that they built through painstaking exercises of imagining and remembering. While delivering the speech, the rhetor walked in his thoughts through these memory spaces and on his way he met the parts of the speech in correct order and—by means of connecting them to the details of the objects in the space—remembered also the details of the argument. The art of memory, so brilliantly described by Frances Yates [17], was finally replaced by a new technology of printed media. In 18th century the famous "Encyclopedia" of Diderot and d'Alembert arranged knowledge in a new way, into the forms of diagrams [18] and "atlases" of scientific disciplines. The conceptual forerunners of atlases of knowledge were the geographical maps ...of the world sphere that the Titan Atlas carried on his shoulders[1].

Another concept that represents the humanist's point of view on the new media technologies is the "synthetic realism", coined by Lev Manovich [19]. This type of "reality" consists of virtual models and nothing in it exists unless somebody made it. E.g. there is no aerial perspective to soften the image, no filth to add detail to the texture of surfaces. Therefore a conscious decision and effort is needed to realize every single detail of a virtual model. In a similar way allegories and emblems were built, where each detail carries a special meaning. The "Emblemata" collection by Andrea Alciato [20] was used in the 16th and 17th centuries as a collection of practical wisdom and directions about how to live, and in the contemporary society of crisis, a similar reference would be similarly useful.

4   Artistic Use of Augmented Reality Platforms

The giant carrying the globe nowadays is Google, containing the archive of all knowledge, through which anyone can search, and also the map of the world, a photographic image of the world's surface that responds to the user—who is holding a smart mobile networked screen device—with meaningful information about her measurable current geolocation. The archive of Internet-based data and the information about the user's location on the map, which are both the basis for the localized search on the Internet, provide a multi-layered mixed reality. We can have a look into virtual augmentation of reality through the camera of a smart phone or a tablet with an AR browser activated. An AR browser shows—on a "layer" superimposed over the live video stream of the surrounding reality—additional digital information, e.g. images, videos and even virtual 3D models, that are linked to geographical coordinates or to objects that the AR browser can recognize with the help of previously uploaded images.

The virtual 3D models in augmented reality are a new field of spatialized images that still have to be thoroughly explored by artists. The new possibilities are opening up in the wide use of phones-computers. Lori Waxman, an independent art critic, wrote about the guerilla project by ArtNetLab—as part of her official intervention at the "dOCUMENTA (13)"—that the emblematic models of the artists are interesting enough to be interpreted, but that it is far more important to acknowledge the existence of a whole new layer of imagery and artistic projects that inhabit the streets of Kassel and can be viewed with smart phones alongside the official selection of art works made by the director of the exhibition Carolyn Christov-Bakargiev [10].

---

[1] The term atlas is first used for a collection of maps in the 1595 posthumous publication of Gerard Mercator's "Atlas sive Cosmographicæ meditationes de fabrica mvndi et fabricati figvra". The Titan Atlas was tied to maps earlier by Antonio Lafreri in the engraving for his collection "Geografia tavole moderne di geografia de la maggior parte del mondo ...", however, Mercator's title page image referred to Atlas, king of Mauretania, as explained in the preface.

Since 2010 there has been a rapid development in the use of AR on mobile platforms in the fields of art and culture. The artists used AR to put the images of their artworks in renown galleries and museums such as MOMA in New York that was invaded by the international artists collective Manifest.AR in 2010 [21]. The restrictive and highly selective character of art institutions could be relativized by the possibility of exhibiting your works in those galleries, at least in a virtual form that is nevertheless open to anyone. The medium specificities of AR models in contrast to the real material models was explored in the project "the world's biggest interactive sculpture" by Sander Veenhof launched in 2010 [22]. In this case, the artist built the concept on three facts: that the virtual model can be easily multiplied, that the construction of such a simple model as a cube is cost free and that it can be effortlessly spread over the whole world since the access to any geo-location is just one click away. Additionally, the models can be manipulated by anyone, so that a simple change of color of each cube is already a visual sign of a community of users interacting with the project.

Another frequent use of AR is to recreate lost or destroyed buildings from previous historical periods. In this way the twin towers of the WTC in New York were recreated by Brian August in 2011 [23]. The virtual recreation of the Berlin wall by the companies Hoppala and Superimpose in 2010 was a part of a larger AR information system about the history of post war Berlin [24]. Another example, which involves a tourist guide aspect as well as a more playful "treasure hunt" approach is the project "ArchaeoApp Rome" [25].

5   The Exhibitions from the "Atlas" Augmented Reality Series

The current crisis of ideas and morals demands a response, which was reflected in the first exhibition in the "Atlas" series by ArtNetLab entitled "Atlas, 5. 12. 2011", which is the date when Slovenian people were deciding how to tackle the crisis in political terms on the extraordinary parliamentary elections. The project "ΜΗΔΕΝ ΑΝΑΒΑΛΛΟΜΕΝΟΣ/Never Procrastinate" by Narvika Bovcon and Aleš Vaupotič presents a virtual model of an emblem from Alciato's book [20] that speaks about Alexander the Great and his instructions for success, however, the artists' effort was not enough to (magically) help to reform the Slovenian society at that time (in March 2011 when the project started) and thus prevent the regression into an atmosphere similar to the one from the 1930s.

Augmented reality "Atlas" is a group project that consists of individual artistic statements, these however are confronted with each other to form an archive of statements themselves and of the dialogic exchanges among the authors. The archive of the "Atlas" series can be ordered by three categories: by the authors from the ArtNetLab group, by the works or by the concepts that describe the different exhibitions. Five "Atlas" exhibitions were realized so far.

"Atlas, 5. 12. 2011" in Kino Šiška [26] in Ljubljana thematized video installations in urban space. From the Celovška street through the panoramic windows of Kino Šiška building it was possible to view video projections; the videos on the

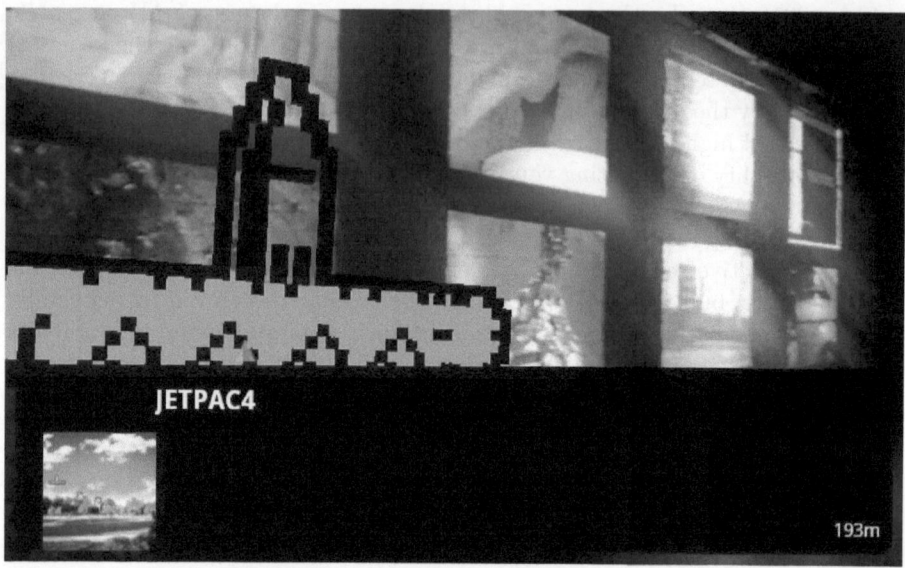

Fig. 1. The Figure shows the video installation of eight video projections at the exhibition "Mnemonic Mirrors" in SC Zagreb. The photo in the Figure was taken with a smart phone with Layar application enabled, hence an augment from the project "JET PAC" by Gorazd Krnc is visible too. The augment is a virtual model representing one of the pieces of the rocket that Jet Man has to assemble to leave the planet.

screens inside the building were integrated as part of the furniture of the bar and of the information system of the institution; one project was exhibited as city light poster near the parking lot; a QR code that led to the exhibition catalogue was attached to the walls and windows. At the entrance a video showed instructions how to use the augmented reality part of the exhibition, which spread over installations in the real space.

The exhibition "Mnemonic Mirrors" in SC Gallery in Zagreb was completely different [27]. Eight videos were projected onto a large gallery wall, ordered as a regular grid of rectangles with two rows of four videos (Fig. 1). The concept of this video installation is based on the sheets from Gerhard Richter's "Atlas" [28]—we have replaced the photographs with video projections. Augmented reality was another layer over the grid of videos, the installation and the perceivable parts of the gallery architecture.

The guerilla intervention at the "dOCUMENTA (13)" showed a possible way of a non-invasive exhibition in augmented reality, non-material, illusional and ambivalently located—at the dOCUMENTA and not an official part of it (Fig. 2). However, "Atlas, dOCUMENTA (13)" will remain a permanent addition to the Karlsaue space.

At the "Month of Design" event in Ljubljana [29], the printed catalogue with augmented pages "Atlas 2012" (Fig. 3) was exhibited at the "Design Expo" (18–19 October 2012) and a signage system for the series of exhibitions "Design in the

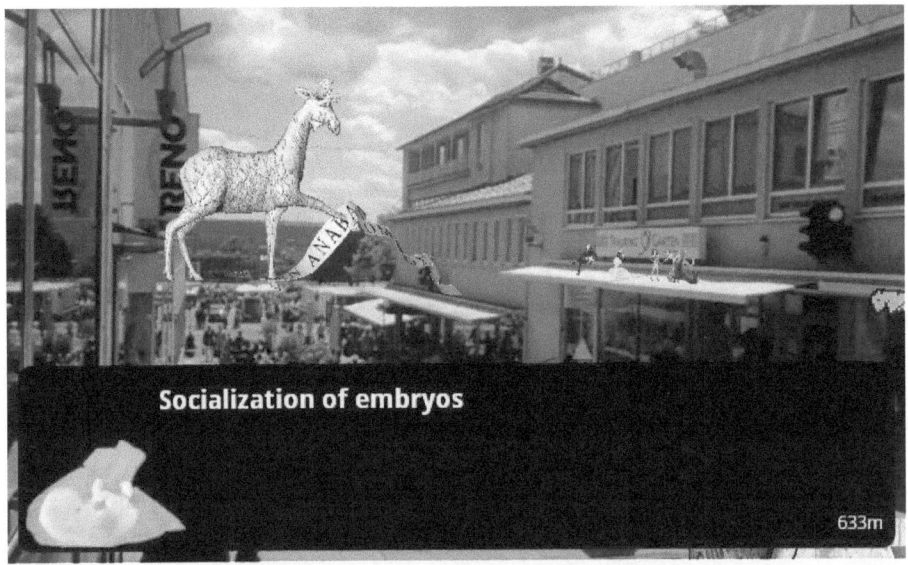

Fig. 2. The photo shows urban sculptures in augmented reality at Kassel. On a projecting roof there are Eva Lucija Kozak's virtual models of active pregnant women from the project "Socialization of Embryos". On the left side of the street there is the elk from the project "MHΔEN ANABAΛΛOMENOΣ/Never Procrastinate" by Narvika Bovcon and Aleš Vaupotič. The interface of Layar application shows an image and a short text, in this case the title of the project, and the distance from the geolocation at which the virtual model is placed to the point from where the photo was taken.

City" (18 Oct.–18 Nov. 2012) was built in Layar and linked to the geolocations in the centre of Ljubljana. The virtual models by the ArtNetLab artists were placed among the signs pointing to exhibition venues as urban augmented-reality sculpturs (Fig. 4).

Another "exhibitional" realization of the "Atlas" augmented reality project is a 4cm × 4cm × 3cm miniature sculpture "Atlas Air Tagging", cast in silver (by Narvika Bovcon and Aleš Vaupotič, 3D print by IB-PROCADD, 2011)— see Fig. 5. The virtual models from the augmented reality were gathered into a compound virtual model, which was printed by using rapid prototyping in paraffin, from which a mould was made that was used for the final casting of this miniature sculpture in silver. Thus the virtual reality was materialized in a metal object and returned to the non-technologically visible reality. The piece was, however, always exhibited in the form of a video document.

5.1 The List of Authors and Their Projects for the "Atlas" Series

From the artistic point of view it is remarkable that the AR system on the mobile screen devices looks and feels surprisingly similar to the "Large Glass" (1915-23) by Marcel Duchamp. You see the ever changing flux of people and the

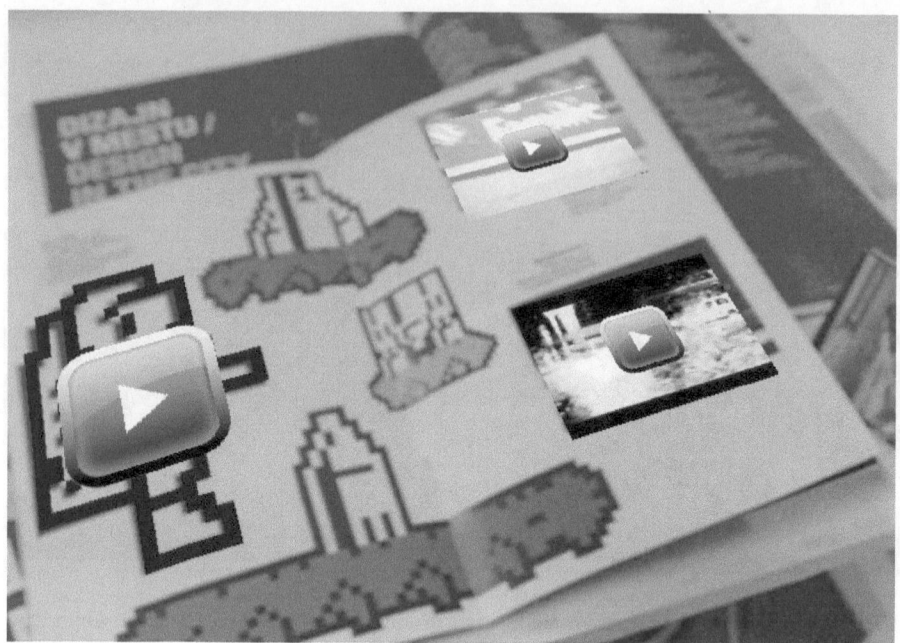

Fig. 3. "Atlas 2012" is an augmented catalogue of the "Atlas" series by ArtNetLab. The photo taken through the camera on mobile device with Layar Vision enabled shows the pages, on which projects by Gorazd Krnc are presented: there are three videos that can be played as video augments connected to the images on the page.

continuous perspective of the surroundings, while the augments float in the air, with sharp contours, flat, like strange stickers on the screen—as the chocolate grinder, the bride and the bachelors in the "The Bride Stripped Bare By Her Bachelors, Even". Isolated as shapes, containing some inexplicable meaning, yet appealing in their form and presence—the 3D models even pore so than the photos. The models look like rendered technical drawings of simple machines by Duchamp, 2.5-dimensional, since they are perceived as flat images. And yet they suggest, they are alive.

The projects used as augments were separate artistic statements encoded into emblematic images. The augments "float" superimposed over the live video stream on a smart screen device, whereas the lower part of the screen is covered with a dark rectangle with an inscription and a small icon linked to the project. The inscription provides a title or a verbal commentary on the project, while the icon is a related image, it shows a blow-up of a significant operational detail of the project or, contrarily, a wider view as a contextual image for the augment.

The artist Gorazd Krnc conceptualized an intervention into the real space by a man in a spacesuit. The viewer recognizes the familiar pixellated image of the spaceman and his disassembled rocket: it is the popular character from an old video game Jet Pac, which brings back the memories of a lost time when the computer technology altogether and we the users were much younger than today.

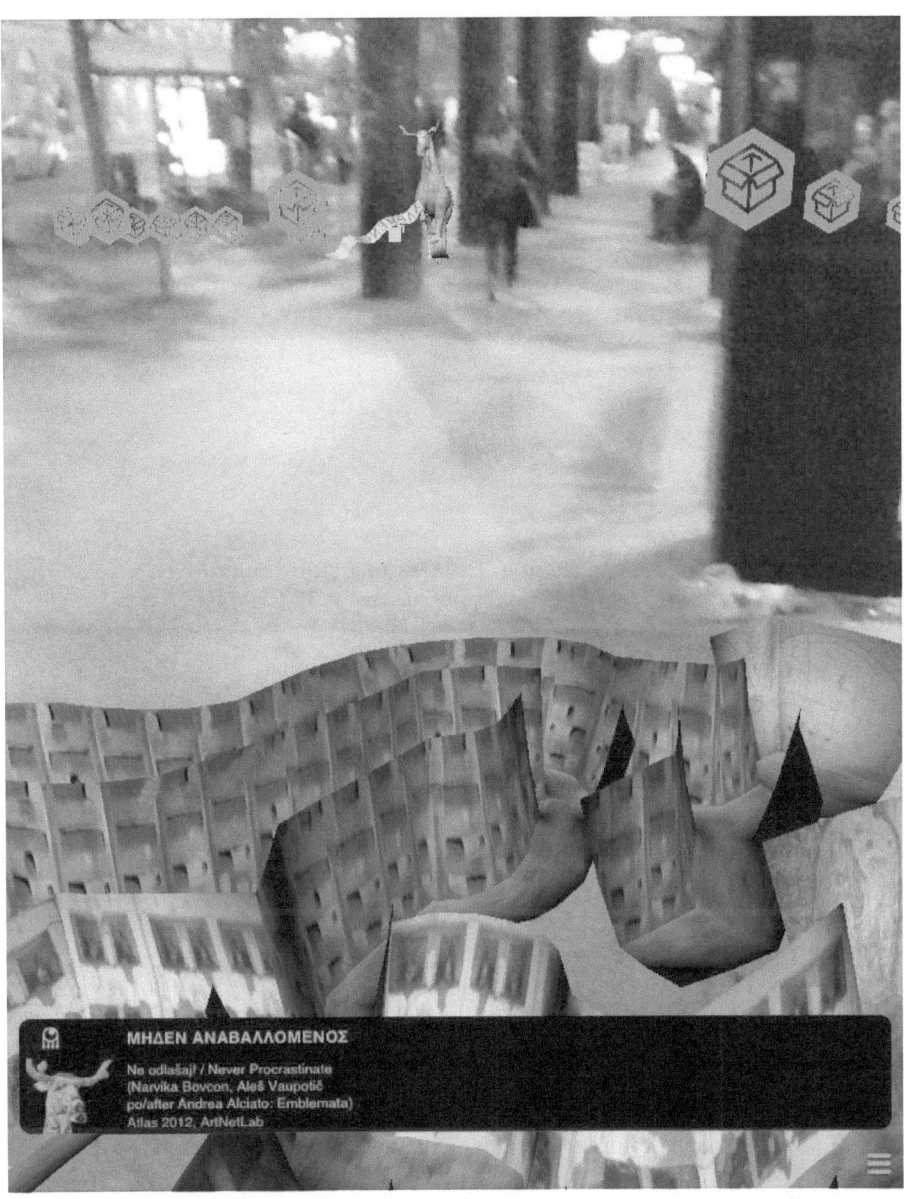

Fig. 4. By looking at the streets in Ljubljana city centre through the camera of a tablet computer, one will find on the "Atlas – Mesec oblikovanja" layer in Layar around fifty signs that guide the user/visitor to the exhibitions of "Design in the City". The signs carry basic information about each exhibition that is displayed in the black rectangle, and by moving towards the location of the exhibition, the sign gets bigger as the perspective in space changes. Among the signage for the design event there are urban sculptures by ArtNetLab artists. The bottom of the screen is covered with Dominik Mahnič's "CATACUMBAE".

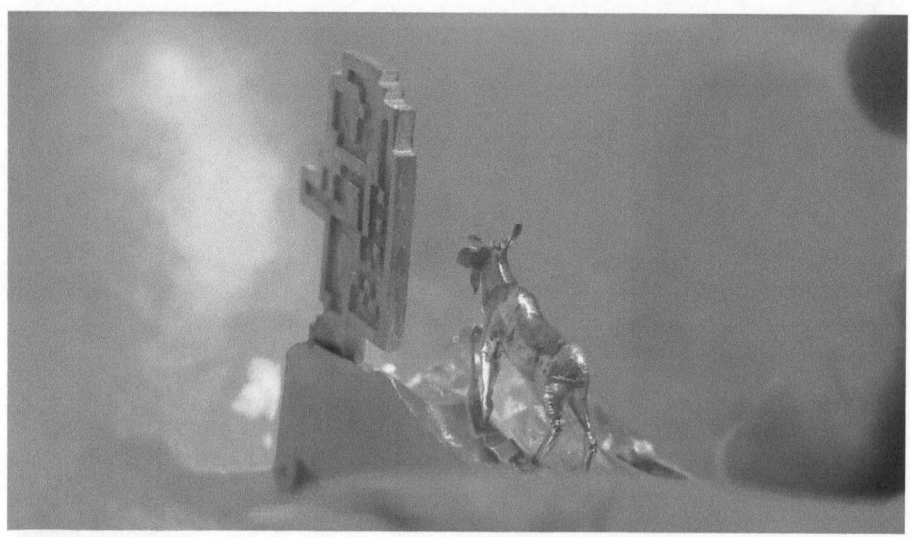

Fig. 5. "Atlas Air Tagging" is the title of a silver miniature sculpture, in which virtual models from the "Atlas" series materialise by means of 3D printing

The political connotation of the project, a quite pessimistic attitude towards our reality, resounds in the enterprise of the Jet Man: he wants to leave the planet, this is why he is combining together the parts of his rocket, to fly away. The icon shows a photo of an idyllic park as the departing point for the Jet Man to fly up into the summer sky.

Eva Lucija Kozak prepared augments in the form of elaborate tiny figurines based on images of pregnant women performing a plethora of activities, which she gathered from mass-media sources. The title of the project "Socialization of Embryos" comments on the fact that nowadays the parents are overwhelmed with the pressure to raise their children actively and responsibly, taking full advantage of each of the multitude of possibilities that are offered to everybody in the civilized world, even to the point when some future mothers start to socialize their not yet born babies by prenatally creating a Facebook page for them. The icon shows an embryo as a commodity item. In her second project "The Walk" Eva Lucija augmented a crossing of a neighborhood road with life-sized images of small children and elderly people, all of them needing assistance to cross.

Dominik Mahnič conceptualized a 3D model of catacombs and placed it beneath the users' feet extending over a vast territory. The project "CATACUM-BAE" reminds us of the city of the dead below ground as a complementary city to the one that we perceive as our reality. For the exhibition "Mnemonic Mirrors" Dominik selected a video titled "Merda d'artista", showing exactly that; on the request of fellow artists, it was not projected in the grid of large video projection on the gallery wall, but was shown (or hidden) more discretely on a virtual "layer" of AR.

Vanja Mervič conceptualized the project "Thinking Colours—Hommage to Rodin" as an intervention that connects the geo-located AR layer with the augmented pages of the printed catalogue. A 3D model of a stylized Rodin's sculpture "The Thinker" was placed at significant spots in the city of Ljubljana. Each virtual sculpture of the thinker sitting on a large cube was colored in a different hue. When you come close to the virtual sculpture, then the cube covers the whole screen of your hand held device, thus you see only the color, not the shape or the surroundings. You start to contemplate—"think"—the colour. In the (duotone) printed catalogue there is a page with the map of Ljubljana with marked spots where the virtual sculptures are located. The colorless spots on the printed page—when scanned with Layar application—appear colored on the screen of the hand held device. When you click on any one of them, an e-mail is automatically generated with the Subject stating e.g. "Thinking blue" if you clicked the blue spot. You can write the e-mail and send it to the author or even to another person. Here the problem of privacy comes to the fore, since the Layar requires the user to disclose her or his identity by using the personal e-mail account.

Due to a space limitation in this article we will not explicate the meanings of the individual art projects by the ArtNetLab artists in the "Atlas" series, however, we shall list them and their projects to indicate the scope of this archive:

- Narvika Bovcon, Aleš Vaupotič: "Atlas Air Tagging", "Car", "Never Procrastinate",
- Jure Fingušt Prebil: "A Pig's Life", "Redefinition of Space",
- Eva Lucija Kozak: "Presence", "Socialization of Embrios", "The Walk",
- Gorazd Krnc: JET PAC, "Roadmovie 1", "Die unbekannte Stadt (Familie Werbung)",
- Dominik Mahnič: CATACUMBAE, "Art Slaves", "Merda d'artista", "Podnanos", "Dark Greenwood",
- Vanja Mervič: "Thinking Colours—Hommage to Rodin", "Blue", "Leaky Tension", "King Midas Room",
- Evelin Stermitz: "ArtFem.TV", "Women in War",
- Tilen Žbona: "Ikko tre", "Light Over", "Hobby AMG 63 outside", "AMG 65".

The projects were placed on different (sometimes simultaneously) levels of the augmented reality installation space: the physical objects in the gallery space, videos on screens and projections, 2D and 3D augments on GPS coordinates, the augmented catalogue pages, websites, and public presentations by the authors and curators[2].

6   Implementation

The main feature of "Atlas 2012" project is a series of virtual objects (models) on various geolocations, which are displayed as augmented reality on user's mobile

---

[2] Curators Narvika Bovcon and Aleš Vaupotič; Layar augmented reality co-curated by Dominik Mahnič; videos of Layar augmented reality by Gorazd Krnc.

device (Fig. 4). We wanted the augmented reality content to be accessible to as many users as possible—users of various backgrounds, with various levels of experience using augmented reality and also users of various mobile platforms. Therefore, it was not feasible to develop a custom AR browser, but we decided to select one of the existing AR browsers.

There are quite a few commercial and open source AR browsers for mobile platforms available, among others: Junaio[3], Layar[4], Wikitude[5], ARViewer[6], Sekai Camera[7], LibreGeo Social[8], Mixare[9], Arlab[10]. At the start of the "Atlas 2012" project we examined different AR browser providers to find a provider whose browser's feature set adequately covers the requirements for our project realisation.

The browser has to support displaying augments on geolocations (location based tracking), however, the accompanying "Atlas 2012" catalogue also uses marker based augments (optical tracking), which also serves as one of the entry points for accessing geolocated augments. Therefore, an AR browser that supports both geolocation and marker-based augments is needed. The virtual objects in our project are 3D models so the AR browser has to support the rendering of 3D objects as well.

Other considerations which were taken into account are: the support for 3D animations, display of video, POI actions (such as sending e-mails and SMS), offline data and caching possibilities, support of at least Android and iOS platforms, open and free publishing model, ease of use for developers and end-users, existing user base and existing web services.

Most browsers support only location based tracking or only optical (marker or markerless) tracking. The only two browsers with location based tracking and optical tracking are Layar and Junaio. They are together with Wikitude the three most used AR browsers according to survey by Grubert et. al [30]. All three AR browsers support 3D models and are open publishing platforms. Layar and Junaio are end-user and developer friendlier [31]. These properties are subject to change and there has been development on many AR browsers since the start of the "Atlas 2012" project. Examining the aforementioned features of different AR browsers at the start of the project, we decided to use Layar.

6.1   Layar AR Browser

Layar uses an architecture with three main components: client, "gateway" server and web services, which is a commonly used architecture in AR browsers [32].

---

[3] http://www.junaio.com
[4] http://www.layar.com/
[5] http://www.wikitude.com/
[6] http://www.libregeosocial.org/node/24
[7] http://sekaicamera.com/
[8] http://www.libregeosocial.org/
[9] http://www.mixare.org/
[10] http://www.arlab.com

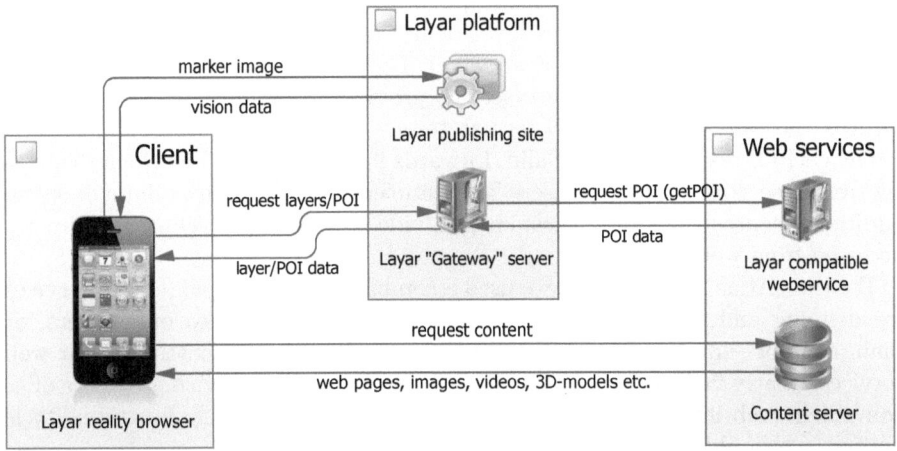

Fig. 6. A schematic view of the Layar architecture, which was used in the project "Atlas 2012"

Fig. 6 shows Layar's architecture [8], which is made up of the following components:

- the Layar reality browser, which is the client (AR browser) on users mobile device,
- the Layar server, which serves as a proxy for external Layar service providers and provides data concerning layers to clients. It also processes image markers sent from clients. Layer data can be managed using the Layar publishing web site.
- The Layar web service providers which provide POI (point of interest) data and content sources which contain the actual content. Service providers serve as interface for general content sources, which usually do not support Layar developer API.

Layar offers two possibilities to retrieve augmented reality content: geolocation and optical tracking. Geolocation based content is displayed on top of the live-camera image. The display coordinates are calculated from POI coordinates relative to user coordinates and users orientation. These are acquired from mobile device's GPS module and compass. When using marker based retrieval, the user photographs a marker image, which was in the case of "Atlas 2012" project printed in the accompanying catalogue. The image is sent to the Layar server for recognition. If the image is recognized, the client receives the corresponding augmented reality content. The content (interactive web page, movie etc.) is than displayed on top of the marker image (Fig. 3).

A typical request and response cycle in case of a geolocation layer display is as follows: the user launches the client AR browser (Layar Reality Browser) on his mobile device. The client sends a request to the Layar server, which returns layer definitions. The layer definitions are previously set through Layar publishing website. When the user receives layer definitions, he can choose a layer and a getPOI request is sent to the Layar server. Layar server than forwards the POI request to the appropriate Layar service provider. The Layar service provider returns the POI data in JSON format to the Layar server, who validates the JSON getPOI response and, if valid, forwards it to the client. The client displays the response content to the user. The returned content can contain links to additional content like web pages, images, videos, 3D-models, which are directly accessed from web services.

For the "Atlas 2012" project we used a combination of Hoppala[11] web services for defining and serving geolocation layer POI in addition to our servers for main content—image, video and webpage data. The use of existing Layar web services greatly facilitates deployment as some Layar web service providers offer convenient web interface for defining POIs. However, if specific functionality is desired, we would have to develop our own services.

The presented architecture offers flexibility, although there are still performance issues and consequently a limit on the number of POIs is needed. However, as hardware capabilities are steadily increasing, these issues will probably become less noticeable in the future. As previously mentioned, the AR browsers are constantly changing and during the course of this project the previously free publishing of vision based layers is now subject to a fee, which may be a deterrent for similar projects in the future.

Another possible issue is the reliability of services. As can be seen on Fig. 6 the architecture depends on multiple servers and if one of the servers goes off-line, a part of the content or the whole content is inaccessible. Compared to physical world artefacts, which tend to be more persistent, the augmented reality content must be monitored if accessible to ensure availability in the future.

To enable the augmented reality content the user has to provide data to the servers. This data includes for example geolocation of the user, device identification data and images taken by camera for optical-based tracking. The images sent to the server may contain personal information (including third party personal information). This issues are usually covered by usage terms and conditions pertaining to privacy policy, which the user accepts before staring to use the service. The terms depend on the service provider, in case of Layar, the user permits the service provider to store and process the personal data to provide their services (pertaining to serving augmented reality content and associated services)[8]. However, the user has to pay attention not to send third party personal information, as submission of third party information would require the consent of the affected third party.

7   User Experience Evaluation

At dOCUMENTA(13) in Kassel the "Atlas" project was very well accepted, which is supported by the fact that one curator considered it to stand out among

---

[11] http://www.hoppala-agency.com/

several artistic projects. Actually, the AR aspect of the project was preferred over the other artistic media: the non-material guerilla exhibition that colonizes the real space on an augmented layer without cluttering the real space, with its versatile, smooth and ubiquitous intervention.

The augments were also very successful in the gallery of SC Zagreb, since the audience connected the images-virtual models with the projected videos in the installation of "Mnemonic Mirrors". The images and stories from the large video projections combined with the non-visible, surprising presences of the augments.

At the "Design Expo" the audiences were less inclined to appreciate the virtual objects, since they came to see the material exhibits from the industrial and fashion design domain. The whole point of design objects is their fetish existence, they are ownable, they adorn you or your living space, you can touch them, feel the textures and materials, feel the shapes in space. These are all categories and aspects that are opposite to the function of augments. Your iPhone is a design object, a fetish, but the data on it are not.

The augmented geo-located signage system for the "Design in the City" proved to be functional, playful and surprising for most users, although the technology itself is not accurate enough to allow for much experimentation. The geo-located points move substantially due to the gyroscope and GPS system limitations, the data are quite slow to load and follow as we point the hand held device in different directions, especially when we approach the limit of 50 items. With a dozen or more of them simultaneously on the screen, it is difficult to click them, particularly when they are very close together or when they become superimposed onto each other, because a certain area is required for the finger tip to touch the screen. The change in perspective, i.e. the distance dependent changeable size of the augments, gives only a vague notion of the distances to the objects, which is corrected by the information in meters displayed in writing in the lower part of the screen when an augment is selected. The above mentioned technological limitations were considered while we designed the signage system and most of the problems were solved with the right solution of the information coding by graphic design strategies. The Layar service addresses this issue by linking AR object to the reliable Google maps platform.

The printed catalogue with augmented pages was well-accepted in the gallery context and with other users that were able to experience it. The catalogue was conceptualized and realized as an artist book, experimentally, it is in fact a book of videos, of moving images. However, the functional, design oriented and educational aspects of augmented printed material soon took us into the direction of future projects of collaboration with museums. Our next step is under way, we are creating an augmented reality flyer that the visitors of a museum, especially younger audiences, can take home. They can see the multimedia documentation of the exhibition again, browse additional information, show the leaflet with videos to friends and parents and thus spread the knowledge of and on the exhibition.

8   Conclusions

We present a case study of using augmented reality in a series of fine art projects. Virtual sculptures and other objects were placed in physical space using location based tracking and a printed catalogue was enhanced with video clips using optical tracking. Augmented reality technology is now most accessible to a wider public due to hand held devices equipped with AR browsers which use built-in cameras and location tracking functions. Setting up augmented reality applications using one of the existing augmented reality systems is also fairly straightforward since it does not require any programming as demonstrated by the artists who initiated their project series using the Layar AR browser. The most serious problem that we encountered is the unstable environment which is due to the intensive development in this area. There are many competing augmented reality applications and the conditions for their use are not stable. Handling of personal information that images sent to Layar may contain is also not clearly defined.

In the future one would hope that augmented reality systems would become more universal. Virtual objects connected to specific physical locations should be accessible with any universal AR browser. In that way, any virtual object connected to a geographical location could be seen by anyone, much like web pages created by anyone can be seen with any web browser by practically anyone else. Physical landscapes as well as particular objects could therefore be overlaid by different layers of information related to history, culture, administration, economics etc. Practically any human intervention related to a particular location or object could be "seen" just by using the proper layer in an universal AR browser. Instead of a lifetime of learning the connections between our environment and its relevant information, these relations would become "evident"[12] with the proper device. First envisioned in fiction, the technical development in this direction is already well on its way[13]. How permanent and stable will these virtual objects remain in the long run is still not clear. Probably in their present form virtual objects will not be as permanent as cave paintings or brass plaques in the physical space turned out to be.

References

1. Chatwin, B.: The Songlines. Viking (1987)
2. Tall, D.: From Where We Stand: Recovering a Sense of Place. Alfred A. Knopf, New York (1993)

---

[12] "evident"—ORIGIN late Middle English: from Old French, or from Latin evidens, evident— "obvious to the eye or mind," from e- (variant of ex-)"out" + videre "to see."

[13] Google Googles
http://en.wikipedia.org/wiki/Google_Goggles,
Project Glass http://en.wikipedia.org/wiki/Project_Glass,
Eye Tap http://en.wikipedia.org/wiki/EyeTap, etc.

3. Urbanc, M.: Kulturne pokrajine v Sloveniji. Založba ZRC, Ljubljana (2002)
4. Hogan, E.: Spiral Jetta: A Road Trip through the Land Art of the American West. The University of Chicago Press (2008)
5. Demnig, G.: Stolpersteine: An Art Project for Europe, http://www.stolpersteine.com (accessed December 12, 2012)
6. Stolpersteine, http://de.wikipedia.org/wiki/Stolpersteine (accessed December 12, 2012)
7. Solina, F., Ravnik, R.: Georeferencing works of literature. In: Proceedings of the ITI 32nd Int. Conf. on Information Technology Interfaces, Cavcat, Croatia, pp. 249–253 (2010)
8. Activate print with digital content, http://www.layar.com (accessed December 12, 2012)
9. ArtNetLab – Drutvo za povezovanje umetnosti in znanosti, http://black.fri.uni-lj.si/ (accessed December 12, 2012)
10. Kunstkritik, L.W.: ArtNetLab – documenta (13) - Nachrichten – HNA Online, http://www.hna.de/documenta-13/objekte/lori-waxmans-kunstkritik-artnetlab-2353568.html (accessed December 12, 2012)
11. Grau, O.: Virtual Art: From Illusion to Immersion. MIT Press (2003)
12. Cruz-Neira, C., Sandin, D.J., DeFanti, T.A., Kenyon, R.V., Hart, J.C.: The CAVE: audio visual experience automatic virtual environment. Commun. ACM 35(6), 64–72 (1992)
13. A-Z Maps - Phone, Pocket PC, Digital & Paper street & road maps, http://www.az.co.uk/ (accessed December 12, 2012)
14. Pearsall, P.: Design/Designer information, http://designmuseum.org/design/phyllis-pearsall
15. Borges, J.L., Hurley, A.: Aleph and other stories. Penguin Books (2000)
16. Madrigal, A.C.: How Google Builds Its Maps—and What It Means for the Future of Everything. The Atlantic, http://www.theatlantic.com/technology/archive/2012/09/how-google-builds-its-maps-and-what-it-means-for-the-future-of-everything/261913/
17. Yates, F.A.: The Art of Memory. Routledge and Kegan Paul (1966)
18. Bender, J., Marrinan, M.: The Culture of Diagram. Stanford University Press (2010)
19. Manovich, L.: The Language of New Media. MIT Press (2001)
20. Alciato at Glasgow: Home, http://www.emblems.arts.gla.ac.uk/alciato/ (accessed 12 December 2012)
21. Manifest, A.R.: http://manifestarblog.wordpress.com/ (accessed March 10, 2013)
22. Biggar—world's biggest interactive sculpture, http://www.sndrv.nl/biggar/ (accessed March 10, 2013)
23. BBC, http://www.bbc.co.uk/news/magazine-16387833 (accessed March 10, 2013)
24. Layar, http://www.layar.com/blog/2010/04/16/the-berlin-wall-is-back/ (accessed March 10, 2013)
25. Holzinger, K., Koiner-Erath, G., Kosec, P., Fassold, M., Holzinger, A.: ArchaeoApp Rome Edition (AARE): Making invisible sites visible—e-business aspects of historic knowledge discovery via mobile devices. In: Proceedings International Conference on e-Business, ICE-B 2012, Rome, pp. 115–122 (2012)

26. Atlas, Razstave in film – Kino Siska (December 5, 2011),
    http://www.kinosiska.si/sl/dogodki/
    razstave-in-film/2011-12-05/atlas_5_12_2011/452/
    (accessed December 12, 2012)
27. Galerija SC Zagreb (May 22-June 2, 2012),
    http://black.fri.uni-lj.si/atlas/GSC_artnetlab_reduced.pdf (accessed December 12, 2012)
28. Richter, G.: Gerhard Richter: Atlas. Köln: Walther König (2006)
29. Mesec oblikovanja, http://www.mesecoblikovanja.com/ (accessed December 12, 2012)
30. Grubert, J., Langlotz, T., Grasset, R.: Augmented reality browser survey. Technical Report 1101, ICG, University of Technology Graz, Austria (2011)
31. Butchart, B.: Augmented reality for smartphones. Technical report, JISC Observatory (March 2011)
32. Butchart, B.: Architectural styles for augmented reality in smartphones, Taichung, Taiwan, Open Geospatial Consortium, pp. 1–7 (2011)

Unfolding – A Library for Interactive Maps

Till Nagel[1,2], Joris Klerkx[2], Andrew Vande Moere[3], and Erik Duval[2]

[1] Interaction Design Lab, FH Potsdam
mail@tillnagel.com
[2] Department of Computer Science, KU Leuven
{joris.klerkx,erik.duval}@cs.kuleuven.be
[3] Department of Architecture, Urbanism and Planning, KU Leuven
andrew.vandemoere@asro.kuleuven.be

Abstract. Visualizing data with geo-spatial properties has become more important and prevalent due to the wide spread dissemination of devices, sensors, databases, and services with references to the physical world. Yet, with existing tools it is often difficult to create interactive geovisualizations tailored for a particular domain or a specific dataset. We present Unfolding, a library for interactive maps and data visualization. Unfolding provides an API for designers to quickly create and customize geo-visualizations. In this paper, we describe the design criteria, the development process, and the functionalities of Unfolding. We demonstrate its versatility in use through a collection of examples. Results from a user survey suggests programmers find the library easy to learn and to use.

Keywords: toolkits, maps, geovisualization, information visualization, interaction design, programming.

1 Introduction

Until the extensive digitalization of geo-spatial data, cartographic products have been nearly exclusively created by cartographers, geographers, and scientists from other disciplines with a spatial context. Nowadays, interactive maps and geo-visualizations are prevalent on the internet, on navigation devices and smart-phones, as well as on large-scale multitouch displays in exhibitions and public spaces. Similarly, interactive or animated maps are used increasingly to communicate facts or stories related to geo-spatial information in various application domains [1].

Areas are ranging from social networks to mobility patterns to data journalism to many more. For example, Dodge et al [2] argue that there is a "spatial turn" in social sciences, and that researchers are exploiting the geo-spatial components of large data to understand spatial relations and interactions. They describe interactive geographic visualization as an essential research tool. MoMA Design curator Antonelli sees visualization as one of the central design disciplines [3], and demonstrates current trends with eight examples of "highest quality of design", of which six use geo-spatial data visualized on maps. Moreover, there is an

A. Holzinger et al. (Eds.): SouthCHI 2013, LNCS 7946, pp. 497–513, 2013.

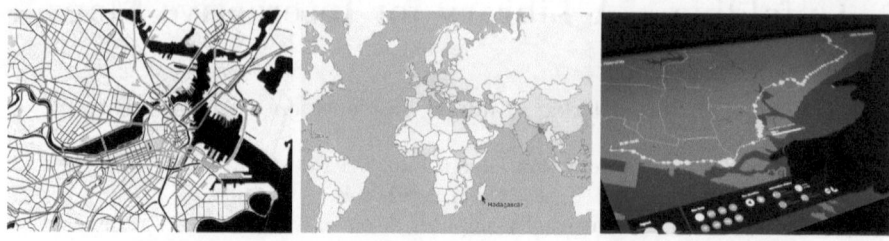

Fig. 1. Three applications created with Unfolding: An animated map showing subways in Boston (left), an interactive choropleth map showing population density (middle), and a visualization showing ridership in Singapore for a multitouch tabletop (right)

increase in the interest of the general public, among others due to the widespread use of location based apps for smartphones. Due to the recent 'creativity boom', in which "novel types of graphic [...] and interaction were being applied to new data and new scenarios" [4], different user groups should be encouraged to experiment in the geovisualization field.

But while interactive geovisualization is useful in a variety of domains, the tools that can be employed to generate the visualizations are either cumbersome to use, or lack the appropriate functionalities. There is an increasing need for interactive maps and geovisualizations, and many amateurs and non-GIS researchers are now creating and customizing geo-spatial data representations. In order to support a democratization of tools and technology we developed the Unfolding library.

With our library we strive to support three different purposes, i.e. (i) having a simple API that is easy to learn and use, (ii) support creating prototypes to quickly visualize data and to rapidly test novel interaction techniques, and (iii) building applications for a broader audience. We chose to implement Unfolding as a Processing library, and are going to introduce Processing and explain our reasoning for choosing it in Section 4.3. Since its inception, Unfolding has been used in course assignments, research projects and commercial products. The iterative development of Unfolding was guided by the needs of, and with constant feedback from the library users.

The remainder of this paper is structured as following: We give an overview on related work (Section 2), and describe our design goals (Section 3). In Section 4 we introduce the Unfolding library, its interaction and visualization features, and our design rationales. We demonstrate its usefulness with exemplary applications for each of the three purposes, and summarize the results of a user survey in Section 5.

2   Related Work

In the following we examine software and tools for the creation of interactive geovisualizations. We describe their different goals, and how they are only partly fitting for the purposes we aim to support. We discuss their advantages and drawbacks, and describe how they differ from Unfolding.

2.1 GIS Software

Standard geographic information systems (GIS) foremost aim is to support analyzing geospatial data, but often do not allow extensive adaptation and simplification for a non-GIS-experts audience. Researchers in the field of geovisual analytics have argued that software "should be lightweight, easily deployable and usable, rather than huge and complex like current GIS." [5]. There is the need for less complex software which encourages interactivity [6], and supports interactions facilitating a knowledge construction process [7].

Thanks to easier tools for creating customized maps since the release of Google Maps and other web mapping services there are more and more interactive maps created by persons who have no expertise in GIS. This kind of map mashups needs little or no programming to visualize information spatially [8]. While such mashups often only include dots on a map or other basic display techniques, the mashup principle of re-using existing technology has been described as a means to rapidly create prototypes for geovisualization [9]. Simpler web-based GIS applications support selected visualization (e.g. IndieMapper [10]) or interaction techniques (e.g. GeoCommons [11]), and customization to a certain degree.

Generalized, GIS software facilitates in-depth analytics, but is complex, has a high learning curve, and is intended for experts. Mashup tools are easy-to-use, suitable for quick data exploration, and intended for non-experts, but only allow employing a fixed set of techniques. An approach to fill this gap is the geoviz toolkit [12], which offers a graphical user interface (GUI) for users without programming expertise, yet it targets an audience of GIS experts.

Effective geo-visualizations employ established techniques, but tailor the visualization to the application domain and to the specific dataset. Thus, custom visualizations have to be created with toolkits or with software libraries.

2.2 Visualization and Map Libraries

The Java GIS library GeoTools provides extensive functionality for geospatial data, and aims to support developing complex spatial data processing applications [13], but is targeted to professional software developers.

In recent years, multiple libraries have been published with the intent to allow designers and web developers to create interactive visualizations. As we are not aware of surveys on modern visualization libraries aimed at these new user groups, we chose an online collection [14], of which 12 out of 43 tools include map or other geo-spatial components. Data visualization libraries such as d3 [15] or Prefuse [16] aim to supporting general purpose visualizations and include a broad spectrum of techniques. With this, however, they tend to not focus on the geospatial area.

Dedicated map libraries such as Leaflet [17] or Polymaps [18] offer functionality to create interactive maps, and display geo-spatial data. These libraries have proven value in practice, which is also why design and functionality of Unfolding were guided by them. However, they are intended exclusively for a web environment, and thus only partially support more advanced interactive applications such as exhibits for large multitouch devices. Furthermore, they are not developed for the Processing environment, which prevents the usage in existing Processing projects, and reduces the applicability for less advanced users (see Section 4.3).

We are aware of three libraries providing basic map functionality for Processing. Their purpose is to provide rudimentary mapping features: all of them offer the display of a geo-referenced map, with conversion methods between geo-locations and Cartesian screen coordinates and vice versa. The geomap library by giCentre [19] provides functionality to load and display Shapefiles, a standard file format for GIS data. It allows interactive feature picking, and color coding, e.g. for choropleth maps (a thematic map with its areas shaded according to a data value). Google Mapper [20] allows downloading a Google map section and storing it as single image. Unlike Unfolding, none of these Processing libraries provide zooming and panning, dynamic map tile handling, an event system, multiple coordinates map views, additional geo data loading, or custom markers. Lastly, ModestMaps [21] is an extensive map and geovisualization JavaScript library for the web, for which a port to Processing was created in 2008. The main JavaScript library has many of the features missing in the other Processing map libraries, but the port for Processing is not actively developed, and only supports some of the basics. However, the tile-handling mechanism was mature and feature rich, which we therefore used as basis for Unfolding's own tile-handling functionality.

3   Design Goals

This section introduces the design goals of Unfolding, and how the library enables developers[1] (i) to easily create simple sketches[2] with interactive maps, (ii) to quickly implement prototypes, and (iii) to create sophisticated visualizations, or even extend Unfolding's functionality.

For these purposes, Unfolding was developed with the main goals of learnability, simplicity, and extensibility. To support the first goal, the library comes with extensive documentation, mostly in the form of tutorials and example code. The documentation can be found both online at unfoldingmaps.org as well as in the downloadable distribution. The library uses a simple programming interface (API) to support the second goal. Library users can create interactive maps in very few lines of code (see Code sample 1). And thirdly, the library provides reusable components, and employs a software architecture allowing to extend its functionality in order to create advanced visualizations.

3.1   Task Areas

We identified design goals and requirements, based on the experience from our own design projects, from our teaching, and collected as feedback from

---

[1] This paper differentiates between *developers* or *library users* for Unfolding library developers, and *end users* for persons using applications created with Unfolding.

[2] This paper uses the term *sketch* as introduced by Reas and Fry [22] where small programs act as software sketchbook allowing to quickly explore different ideas.

external users of the library, and grouped them into three main task areas. These groups partially converge, and are not necessarily strictly disjoint, but are useful nonetheless to refer back to and to describe how we aim to support the dominant tasks of the target audience. We describe the activities, user groups, and typical use cases.

i **Learning** Includes all activities in which developers learn how to display geo-spatial data. Users in this group mostly create simple sketches where they show markers on an interactive map. They use it for experiments and small projects.

ii **Prototyping** Includes all activities in which library users explore and understand geo-spatial data in an iterative data visualization design process. This also includes to quickly prototype sketches to try out new visualization or interaction ideas. Developers include both beginners and advanced users.

iii **Creating** Includes all activities in which library users create larger projects. This can be for design studies by researchers to be able to evaluate novel techniques. This also can be for commercial or art projects where developers create complex geovisualizations.

All library users – that is persons creating visualizations or interactive applications with Unfolding – must have programming skills, ranging from beginner (learning) to intermediate and expert level (prototyping and creating). All of them have in common, that they not necessarily have expert geography or cartography knowledge.

Overall, Unfolding is developed to have a gentle learning curve, i.e. empowering to create standard visualizations in a few lines of code, and to create more complex visualizations when users are accustomed and more experienced with the library.

3.2 Design Process of Unfolding

Since the first version of Unfolding in 2008, we continuously gathered feedback from library users. In the process of designing Unfolding its functionality was based on the lessons learnt from class room usage, and on the requirements of our own case studies in visualization. We follow the argument of Heer et al [16], and see iterative development, an established method for designing HCI, to be also a valuable design process for software libraries. In this vein, we discuss how the utilization of Unfolding in each task group helped the progress of Unfolding, and how the feedback from developers with different expertise levels helped us to balance learnability and functionality.

Learning. Since 2009 Unfolding has been used in six courses at Fachhochschule Potsdam, and two at IUAV University of Venice by the authors. Besides, it has been endorsed in various coursed at international universities (e.g. Carnegie Mellon, ITP, MIT), with departments ranging from interaction design to computer science to urban studies. The use in courses and workshops for teaching basics on geospatial data visualization allowed us to observe how beginners were using the library, and simplify the API and improve the documentation.

Prototyping. In early stages of designing an application, quick visual representations of geo-spatial data help to understand them. While these data loading and visualization methods can be implemented with other software or libraries, Unfolding provides them too in order to support library users all the way from learning up to creating. In addition, users have employed Unfolding to create geovisualizations with the purpose to prototype and evaluate new techniques. Unfolding aims to bridge the gap between traditional and novel visualizations by easing the creation of rapid design experiments.

Creating. Comments and suggestions from advanced users employing Unfolding in research, design, and commercial projects helped us refine existing and add frequently demanded features. Furthermore, successful design projects can act as flagship and inspire new groups of users.

4   The Unfolding Library

This section introduces Unfolding, describes some of the basic interactions and visualizations methods, demonstrate its features and usage by examples, and explains our design rationales.

The code samples in 4.1 are to demonstrate the usage of the library in order to implement some of the fundamental functionality. This is to show how the basics are achievable in just a few lines of code, as stated in one of our design goals. For longer code examples we deem a paper not as the most appropriate form, and refer to the example section on our web page.

4.1   Interaction and Visualization

Unfolding supports basic techniques for interactive maps such as zoom and pan, but also other common but slightly more advanced techniques such as Overview+Detail, i.e. showing a large scale map view while keeping the context by displaying the selected region on a large scale map.

Basic map. In just three lines of code library users can create an interactive map. The map is displayed in a default style with cartographic data from OpenStreetMap [23] and tiles from CloudMade [24].

```
UnfoldingMap map = new UnfoldingMap(this);
MapUtils.createDefaultEventDispatcher(this, map);
map.draw();
```

Code Sample 1. Creating an interactive map in Unfolding

To use another map style, developers can specify a different provider as second parameter when creating an UnfoldingMap. Our library provides eight pre-configured map tile providers for educational purposes. Developers can also create their own map provider to use customized map styles adapted to the requirements of their visualization. For instance, if the objective of the map is to support general spatial recognition while being discreet enough to not hinder the display of the data and interface layers, a minimal style with selected geographical features could be employed.

Basic Interactions. By creating the default event dispatcher (as shown above), end users already can interact with the map. They can pan the map by dragging it with the mouse, or by using the arrow keys on the keyboard. Using the mouse wheel zooms in or out, which also works by pressing + or - keys. Double-clicking on the map centers it around that location, and zooms in one level. These basic interaction patterns were based on studies for map interactions ([25], [26]) and well-established design patterns for navigating and browsing [27].

Basic interactions with markers, i.e. visual representations of geographic features or data entries, are also provided out of the box. These include selecting and highlighting markers by clicking or tapping on them. More sophisticated interactions such as brushing and linking have to be implemented by the developers, but can employ Unfolding's event mechanism.

Multitouch Interactions. Unfolding also provides interaction handling for multitouch devices. To turn on this feature developers have to register Unfolding's multitouch handler, which maps gesture input to map manipulation methods.

We focused on simple navigation patterns (e.g. pinch to zoom, drag to pan, tap to select) to support end users interact with the maps in ways more laymen have experience with, due to the wide-spread dissemination of smartphones and tablet computers with multitouch capabilities.

Visualizing data on a large-scale multi-touch surface allows the application of natural interaction techniques to engage a broad audience. Unfolding supports a high fluidity of the visualizations, with smooth transitions and low responsive times, in order to create enjoyable user experiences. See the project descriptions in Section 4.2 for examples of visualizations on multitouch tables.

Visualization Features. Developers can use Unfolding's built-in marker mechanism to display geo-spatial data on the map. When end users interactively change the map area, or when the map is animated, latitude and longitude of the locations are converted to the correct screen positions, in the background.

```
Location berlinLocation = new Location(52.5, 13.4)
Marker berlinMarker = new SimplePointMarker(berlinLocation);
map.addMarker(berlinMarker);
```

Code Sample 2. Adding a location marker to display

Unfolding provides a default marker style, and has point, line, and polygon markers out of the box. Besides these markers, developers can also create multiple markers consisting of two or more markers of any kind, or use various connections representing some relationship between markers.

```
UnfoldingMap map;
void setup() {
  map = new UnfoldingMap(this);
  MapUtils.createDefaultEventDispatcher(this, map);
  List features = GeoRSSReader.loadData(this, "quakes.xml");
  map.addMarkers(MapUtils.createSimpleMarkers(features));
}
void draw() {
  map.draw();
}
```

Code Sample 3. A Processing sketch loading and displaying earthquakes on an interactive map. The earthquake data comes from the U.S. Geological Survey institution provided in the GeoRSS format

The library also allows reading standard formats for geospatial data, and automatically creating the respective graphical representations. The provided data readers support basic functionality, and do not fully implement the respective specifications. The GeoJSON parser supports most features, while the GeoRSS reader supports only Simple and W3C Geo, but not GML, and the GPX reader only enables reading track points. The aim was not to re-implement functionality developers can use and integrate from more sophisticated GIS libraries, but to enable getting quick results in a rapid prototyping approach. By building upon the Processing framework, developers can easily create own data readers. For example, Fig. 1(left) shows the display of subway lines in Boston, in which the geospatial routes as well as the train schedules comes from General Transit Feed Specification (GTFS) files provided by the transport authority.

The marker style can be customized, or completely implemented anew by the designers. The second option allows using data glyphs such as donut charts or any other data display technique (see Fig. 3). By mapping a value to the brightness value of a polygon marker, one can create simple choropleth maps. The example in Fig. 1(middle) shows an interactive version displaying population density of the world. End users can select single countries by hovering over (one of) the country's polygons, and additional data is display on demand.

4.2   Example Projects

The following two Unfolding projects were selected to represent the spectrum of how the library can be used, and to exemplify various advanced features of Unfolding.

Max-Planck-Research Networks. A visualization of research networks on a multitouch table [28]. It uses three coordinated multiple views: one showing a network with institutions and their connections based on co-published papers, and two maps showing the locations of institutions in Germany and the world (see Fig. 2). Tapping on an institution in any view highlights it in all other

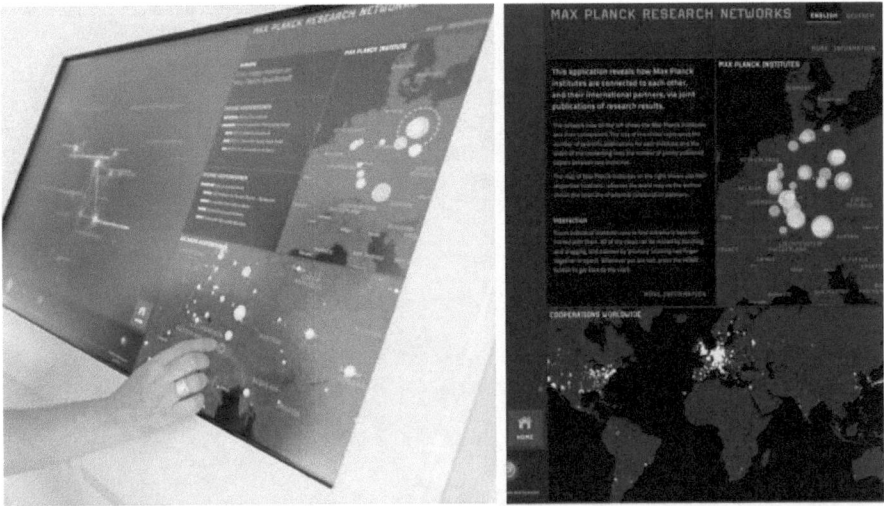

Fig. 2. Visualization of research networks on a multitouch table (left) with two Unfolding maps showing institutions (clipping right)

views. The maps are implemented with Unfolding, and use custom styled map tiles. The application uses Unfolding's multitouch capabilities in order to allow end users to slide for panning and to pinch for zooming the maps. Brushing and linking interactions can be developed with Unfolding's event system to coordinate multiple maps.

Live Singapore. A visualization of public transit ridership in Singapore [29]. It shows bus passenger flows in three coordinated visualizations (map, time chart, arc diagram), and allows users to interactively explore bus lines and areas of interest (see Fig. 3). Unfolding was used for the map view and for the display of the geo-spatial data glyphs. Interactions with the map are restricted to the city state of Singapore, i.e. when an end user pans or zooms outside of that area, the map gently animates back. One of the challenges in developing this visualization was to create a performant data display method in order to keep high responsiveness on every user interaction. End users can slide through the time dynamically which is directly reflected in the geo-spatial markers. Unfolding supports traversing the visualization pipeline in an efficient way, so that after users adapt the time range the data gets newly aggregated and displayed nearly instantaneously.

4.3   Design Rationale

In this section we explain the reasoning for our design decisions in developing Unfolding.

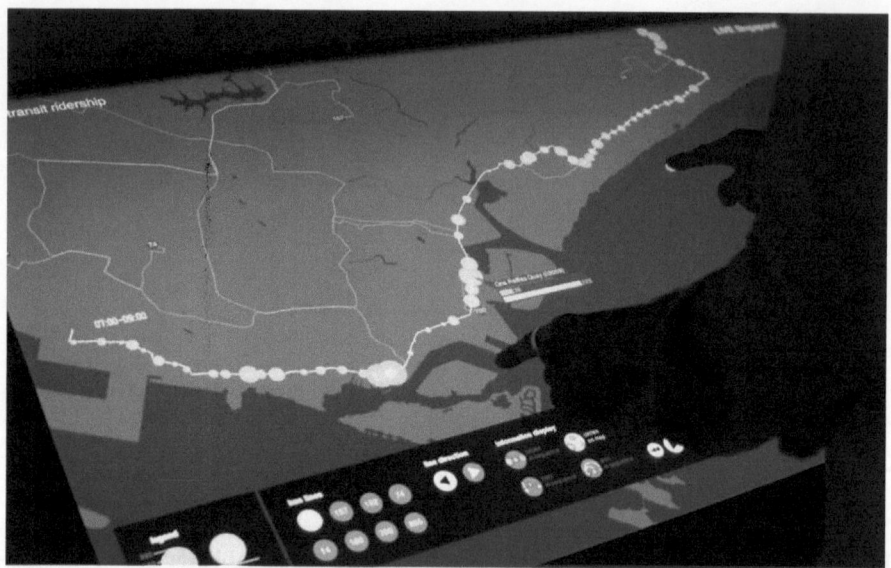

Fig. 3. Visualization of public transit ridership in Singapore, using Unfolding's built-in multitouch interactions for map manipulations

Simplified Java Dialect. Processing is a programming language to create interactive graphics, which is used for learning, prototyping, and production [22], and "targets an audience of computer-savvy individuals who are interested in creating interactive and visual work through writing software but have little or no prior experience" [30]. It has a large and active community, with many libraries providing particular additional functionality if needed. Furthermore, Processing is beneficial for more advanced developers: in comparison to visualization libraries which often use high level programming languages, and an elaborate component structure, Processing provides a low level graphic based environment. The flexibility to investigate and develop new visualization and interaction techniques usually requires relatively low level programming and considerable development time [9]. With Unfolding we aim to support this flexibility while reducing the complexity.

One drawback for more advanced developers is the very simple editor (due to the aim of not overwhelming beginners), with nearly no features of modern Integrated Development Environments (IDE), such as code assistance. To circumvent this, Unfolding provides its library for Processing, as well as for full Java IDEs such as Eclipse.

Tile-Based. Users know and expect the interaction possibilities of online maps. Tile-based maps are a established way of providing zoom and pan functionality. It furthermore enables to select from a huge range of existing map styles, or customize styles with existing tools. The library uses the so-called Slippy Map technique [23], which uses a tile-based algorithm with pre-rendered map tiles for fixed geographical locations in different provided zoom levels. This is used widely for online web map services (e.g. Google Maps), and custom map styling applications (such as CloudMade [24], TileMill [31]). While map tiles technically support other tile sizes or other map projections, typically the same size of 256x256px, and the same Spherical Mercator projection is used. This restricts geovisualizations to a subset, but simplifies the handling. By using such tiles, non-GIS-experts can easily use existing web tiles or custom map styles, and not care about an own map server stack.

Desktop-Based. For creating sophisticated geovisualization applications, i.e. for big sets of data, or creating multitouch interactions for exhibitions, the use of the Java based programming language Processing includes the ability to use OpenGL for high performance visualizations of tens of thousands of visual elements. While web technology such as WebGL more and more includes these abilities, it still needs more advanced programming skills, and extensive knowledge of the newest browser developments at the moment. Another reason for using a desktop based programming language is the ability to employ large-scale interfaces, such as visualizations on interactive multitouch tabletops.

Simple Software Architecture. While one of the principles of Processing and many Processing libraries is to provide most methods in a single class for easier access, this comes with a cost: the API itself becomes unstructured and bloated, and the functionality more complex to extend. Similarly, visualization libraries offer lots of functionality, and while they can be extended it tends to be difficult. This is due to the complex software architecture, where new components need to adhere to the sophisticated class structure. The advantage is that – after learning the deeper parts of the API and implementing new features correctly – an integrated component can profit from existing mechanisms, e.g. interaction or transition patterns. In Unfolding, we intended combining the simplicity of Processing with proven design patterns in software architecture to achieve the extensibility of other libraries. One of our aims was to create a clear Unfolding API enabling beginners to create own sketches showing geo-spatial data, while at the same time allowing more advanced developers to enhance functionality in a reusable way.

Documentation. To support good learnability, the library comes with extensive documentation, mostly in the form of tutorials and example code. The basic API documentation comes in standard JavaDoc format, and describes the methods of Unfolding. We followed Robillard [32], who proposed to use examples, and categorized them in snippets (short code examples), tutorials (code examples with prose), and applications (longer code examples from actual applications). We distribute various examples in the Unfolding library. On the website we additionally publish tutorials and example applications, so beginners can use or copy these code samples directly in their sketches.

4.4 Summary

In summary, Unfolding provides functionality to handle geo-spatial data and display them on interactive tile-based maps by using reusable components in Processing. Unfolding is not just a collection of existing visualizations; it provides the foundation to create interactive maps, and a basic set of reusable components for building customized or novel geovisualizations.

5 Evaluation

In this section we demonstrate the usefulness of Unfolding by presenting selected projects, and describing our user survey and its results. We also give some numbers indicating the library's acceptance.

5.1 Applications

We follow the argument of the authors of the widespread Protovis visualization library that one of the main values of a toolkit is in the design and dissemination of successful visualizations [33]. We collected 40 projects which were publicly accessible on the web and referred to the Unfolding website, or were described in publications. From these, we selected notably successful projects as examples for each of the three task groups.

Learning. Student projects have won student competitions (Tweetography [34] is the Winner of the Harvard Conant Prize for "Best Non-Traditional Project", and Foreign Domestics [35] is one of the winners of the Visualizing Marathon 2012.), or have been featured in design magazines (LiquiData [36] in Weave magazine [37]).

Prototyping. An example of using Unfolding as a prototyping tool to quickly analyze data-sets is an animation of viewers of TED talks [38]. Various research projects have employed Unfolding to create interactive prototypes to be able to develop and evaluate novel visualization and interaction methods (e.g. [39], [29]). In a visualization for exploring geo-spatial networks a new interaction technique for solving the fat-finger problem was introduced. Their user study showed that end users could casually interact with the system and were satisfied with the ease of use of this multitouch visualization [29].

Creating. In the last group, successful design projects were publicly exhibited (e.g. Max-Planck-Research Networks [28], a visualization of research networks on a multitouch table, or The Quiet Walk, a system for sonic exploration of urban space [40]). A commercial project for visually analyzing tax-free sales on an airport [41] has been featured in Cairo's book on visualization [42].

We believe these Unfolding applications demonstrate compelling real-world usage.

5.2   Dissemination

Unfolding was publicly released in August 2011, and the first public version (0.8) was downloaded over 3000 times in the following twelve months. The next version (0.9) was published end of September 2012 and downloaded over 2200 times in the first three months (as per 31st December 2012). While these numbers are just a single measurement, it indicates that Unfolding is widely used, and well accepted. (For instance, the authors of the Prefuse library mention in [16] it had been downloaded 1300 times after the alpha-release.)

5.3   User Survey

We ran a user study as an online survey after the design and implementation of the second release of Unfolding. The purpose of the survey was to gather feedback on library and feature usage, and measure satisfaction on several aspects such as learnability and suitability. A secondary intention was to gather feedback in order to further improve Unfolding.

Survey Design. The questionnaire consisted of sections on the participant's background and prior experience, on the projects they used Unfolding for, and on their satisfaction with the library's features and use.

The survey is partly based on an ISO standard to evaluate software quality [43], and partly on the System Usability Scale (SUS) to collect the subjective rating of the library's usability [44]. We adapted the phrasing in order to have precise yet not overly formal questions. The drawback is that we did not adhere to the standard, and would not be able to compare our results with the usability of other systems. As we have not found other studies on visualization libraries using SUS, we deemed this as acceptable. We mainly tried to keep the survey form brief. We encouraged participants to give comments and constructive criticism, by providing free-form text fields with open questions (e.g. "Do you have any suggestions on how to improve Unfolding?"). All these aspects were based on recommendations to increase response rate in online surveys [45].

We used a 5-point Likert scale for satisfaction (ranging from "Highly satisfied" to "Not at all satisfied"), and for agreement to given statements (ranging from "Strongly agree" to "Strongly disagree"). Overall, the survey contained 12 multiple choice, 7 Likert-scale grid, and 6 open questions. Test participants from our group needed circa 15 minutes to fill out the complete form.

The survey was designed as an online questionnaire[3], was accessible under a public URL, and ran for 10 days in early December 2012. All responses were anonymous.

Participants. As our intention was to gather feedback from persons familiar with Unfolding, we chose library users as potential participants. These persons

---

[3] Find the full survey archived at
http://unfoldingmaps.org/survey-2012-archived.pdf, and the original results at http://unfoldingmaps.org/survey-2012-results.pdf

identified themselves by being active in the Unfolding community, be it on the forum, having published their Unfolding projects online, or having contacted us with questions before. We invited 93 persons via e-mail, from which 32 participated (34% response rate). This of course means we did not collect feedback from developers who decided against Unfolding, which might have biased the satisfaction results. However, we announced the survey on the Unfolding website and in the Processing community forum, via which we received another 5 responses. Overall, this resulted in a total of 37 survey submissions.

Participants were from all age groups (16% under 24, 44% 25-34, 31% 35-44, 9% over 45 years), and nearly half of them students (41%). They stated their expertise mainly in Design (21 participants) and Visualization (18 p.), with Software Development (15 p.), Data (10 p.) and GIS (2 p.) as runner-ups (participants could enter more than one area). They self-assessed their skill level mostly not as novices, with 25% expert, 41% advanced, 25% intermediate, and 9% beginner skills.

Survey Results. In the following, we present how satisfied participants were with Unfolding's usability and features, and discuss some further results.

Participants were mostly highly satisfied or satisfied with Unfolding's learnability, understandability, and suitability (see box plots in Fig. 4). They also

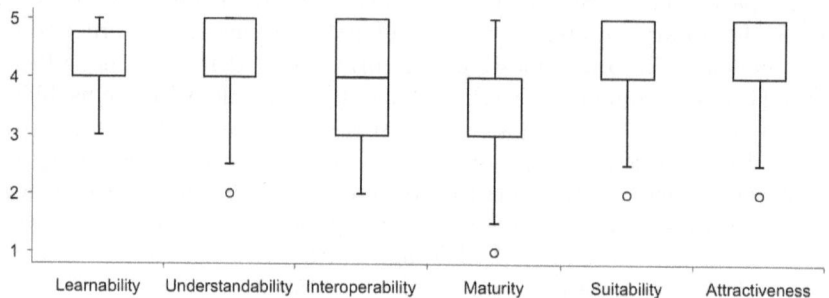

Fig. 4. Satisfaction with Unfolding

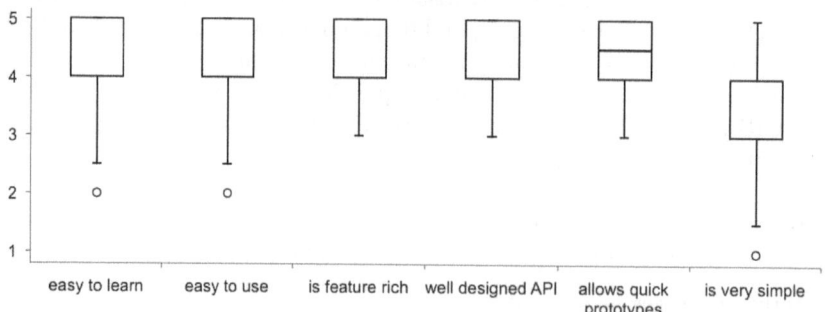

Fig. 5. Agreement with statements

agreed to the statements that Unfolding is feature rich, and has a well designed API (Fig. 5).

Nearly all participants were highly satisfied or satisfied with Unfolding's basic features (such as displaying maps (97%), or enabling zoom and pan interaction (91%)). However, fewer participants were satisfied with more advanced functionality such as displaying labels (51%) or loading geo-spatial data (54%). While these numbers still indicate a majority of users being satisfied, we assume a connection to the documentation of these more advanced features.

Most participants were highly satisfied or satisfied with examples (62%) and tutorials (53%). This reflects our decision of focusing on these sections for learning Unfolding (cf 4.3). However, participants were not fully satisfied with the API documentation (38% highly satisfied or satisfied). This suggests that even though studies have shown developers use examples and tutorials to learn a new API, and re-use existing code snippets to quickly create own prototypes [32], library users expect a complete and well-written interface description, in any case. Three participants suggested improving the documentation in our general free-form comment field.

More than half the participants had some prior experience with GIS software (19% use it often, 19% occasionally, and 22% at least once). Besides the Google Maps API (57%) few have used other map libraries often or occasionally (9% Leaflet, 12% Open Layers, 12% PolyMaps, 15% ModestMaps). However, around one third or more have used these libraries at least once (28% L, 40% OL, 31% PM, 46% MM, respectively). To the question why Unfolding was chosen over other libraries, free-form responses included the Processing environment (e.g. "well integrated with Processing"), and the ability for quick prototyping (e.g. "it's quite easy to get results quickly", "It allowed me to dump geo data directly on a map in less than an hour"). Three participants named the integration with TileMill as reason. We did not expect the latter, as other libraries also allow this. We assume this is due to a tutorial about Unfolding's TileMill functionality which was linked on well-known visualization blogs.

Participants used Unfolding for visualizations ranging from student to research to commercial projects. They achieved what they planned (81% agreed or strongly agreed), and found Unfolding to be helpful in doing so (87%).

Overall, participants were highly satisfied (53%) or satisfied (38%) with the library. Most participants (88%) plan to use Unfolding in the future (with 6% not, and the rest don't know).

6   Conclusion

We presented the Unfolding library to create interactive maps and geovisualizations. Both creating our own applications, as well as collecting feedback from visualization projects by others has helped us to adapt the library, and to repeatedly refine its function range. The results from our user survey prove that Unfolding achieved our design goals. Most participants were highly satisfied or satisfied with our library. We see the use in various courses, in student, research and commercial projects as further indicator for the learnability and usability of the library.

Overall, we have shown that Unfolding is beneficial for learning, prototyping, and creating interactive maps and geovisualizations.

Acknowledgments. We like to thank Felix Lange, and all other library contributors. We also thank the users of Unfolding, especially students from FH Potsdam and from IUAV University of Venice for their feedback, and the participants of the survey. And we like to thank the anonymous reviewers for their helpful feedback.

References

1. Heidmann, F.: Interaktive Karten und Geovisualisierungen. In: Weber, W., Burmester, M., Tille, R. (eds.) Interaktive Infografiken, pp. 43–74. Springer, Heidelberg (2013)
2. Dodge, M., Perkins, C., Kitchin, R.: Mapping modes, methods and moments. In: Dodge, M., Perkins, C., Kitchin, R. (eds.) Rethinking Maps: New Frontiers in Cartographic Theory, pp. 220–243. Routledge, London (2009)
3. Antonelli, P.: States of Design 01: Visualization. Domus 946 (2011)
4. Dykes, J., Andrienko, G., Andrienko, N., Paelke, V., Schiewe, J.: GeoVisualization and the Digital City. Computers, Environment and Urban Systems 34(6), 443–451 (2010)
5. Andrienko, G., Andrienko, N., Demsar, U., Dransch, D., Dykes, J., Fabrikant, S., Jern, M., Kraak, M., Schumann, H., Tominski, C.: Space, time and visual analytics. International Journal of Geographical Information Science 24(10), 1577–1600 (2010)
6. Wisniewski, P., Pala, O., Lipford, H., Wilson, D.: Grounding geovisualization interface design: a study of interactive map use. In: Proceedings of the SIGCHI Conference on Human Factors in Computing Systems Extended Abstracts, pp. 3757–3762. ACM (2009)
7. Jones, C., Haklay, M., Griffiths, S., Vaughan, L.: A less-is-more approach to geovisualization–enhancing knowledge construction across multidisciplinary teams. International Journal of Geographical Information Science 23(8), 1077–1093 (2009)
8. Batty, M., Hudson-Smith, A., Milton, R., Crooks, A.: Map mashups, Web 2.0 and the GIS revolution. Annals of GIS 16(1), 1–13 (2010)
9. Wood, J., Dykes, J., Slingsby, A., Clarke, K.: Interactive visual exploration of a large spatio-temporal dataset: reflections on a geovisualization mashup. IEEE Transactions on Visualization and Computer Graphics 13(6), 1176–1183 (2007)
10. IndieMapper, http://indiemapper.com/
11. GeoCommons, http://geocommons.com/
12. Hardisty, F., Robinson, A.: The geoviz toolkit: using component-oriented coordination methods for geographic visualization and analysis. International Journal of Geographical Information Science 25(2), 191–210 (2011)
13. Turton, I.: Geo Tools. In: Hall, G., Leahy, M. (eds.) Open Source Approaches in Spatial Data Handling. Advances in Geographic Information Science, vol. 2, Springer, Heidelberg (2008)
14. DataVisualization.ch Selected Tools, http://selection.datavisualization.ch
15. Bostock, M., Ogievetsky, V., Heer, J.: D^3 Data-Driven Documents. IEEE Transactions on Visualization and Computer Graphics 17(12), 2301–2309 (2011)

16. Heer, J., Card, S., Landay, J.: Prefuse: a toolkit for interactive information visualization. In: Proceedings of the SIGCHI Conference on Human Factors in Computing Systems, pp. 421–430. ACM (2005)
17. Leaflet, http://leaflet.cloudmade.com/
18. PolyMaps, http://polymaps.org/
19. GeoMap, http://www.gicentre.org/geomap/
20. Google Mapper, http://googlemapper.pt.vu/
21. Modest Maps, http://modestmaps.com/
22. Reas, C., Fry, B.: Processing: programming for the media arts. AI & Society 20(4), 526–538 (2006)
23. Haklay, M., Weber, P.: Openstreetmap: User-generated street maps. IEEE Pervasive Computing 7(4), 12–18 (2008)
24. CloudMade, http://cloudmade.com/
25. Harrower, M., Sheesley, B.: Designing Better Map Interfaces: A Framework for Panning and Zooming. Transactions in GIS 9(2), 77–89 (2005)
26. You, M., Chen, C., Liu, H., Lin, H.: A usability evaluation of web map zoom and pan functions. International Journal of Design 1(1), 15–25 (2007)
27. Tidwell, J.: Designing interfaces. O'Reilly Media (2010)
28. Max Planck Research Networks, http://max-planck-research-networks.net/
29. Nagel, T., Duval, E., Vande Moere, A.: Interactive exploration of geospatial network visualization. In: Proceedings of the SIGCHI Conference on Human Factors in Computing Systems Extended Abstracts, pp. 557–572. ACM (2012)
30. Reas, C., Fry, B.: Processing: a programming handbook for visual designers and artists. MIT Press (2007)
31. TileMill, http://tilemill.com/
32. Robillard, M.: What makes APIs hard to learn? Answers from developers. IEEE Software 26(6), 27–34 (2009)
33. Bostock, M., Heer, J.: Protovis: A graphical toolkit for visualization. IEEE Transactions on Visualization and Computer Graphics 15(6), 1121–1128 (2009)
34. Patel, S., Sun, W.: http://tweetography.herokuapp.com
35. Foreign Domestics, http://visualizing.org/visualizations/foreign-domestics
36. LiquiData, http://liquidata.org/en/
37. Kiefer, C., Nagel, T.: Neue Sichtbarkeit. Weave Magazine (6) (2011)
38. TED Talks - A Visual Map,
    http://blog.ted.com/2012/09/28/
    who-else-is-watching-tedtalks-a-visual-map/
39. Nagel, T., Heidmann, F., Condotta, M., Duval, E.: Venice Unfolding: a tangible user interface for exploring faceted data in a geographical context. In: Proceedings of the 6th Nordic Conference on Human-Computer Interaction: Extending Boundaries, pp. 743–746. ACM (2010)
40. Altavilla, A., Tanaka, A.: The Quiet Walk: Sonic Memories and Mobile Cartography. In: Proceedings of the 9th Sound and Music Computing Conference (2012)
41. Tax Free Retail Analysis Tool,
    http://tulpinteractive.com/projects/tax-free-retail-analysis-tool/
42. Cairo, A.: The Functional Art: An introduction to information graphics and visualization. New Riders (2012)
43. ISO 25010: Systems and Software Quality Requirements and Evaluation (2011)
44. Brooke, J.: SUS-A quick and dirty usability scale. Usability Evaluation in Industry 189, 194 (1996)
45. Nulty, D.: The adequacy of response rates to online and paper surveys: what can be done? Assessment & Evaluation in Higher Education 33(3), 301–314 (2008)

Improving Students' Technical Skills Using Mobile Virtual Laboratory: Pilot Study of Assembly Language Input Methods for Touchscreen Devices

Mihael Kukec[1], Sandi Ljubic[2], and Vlado Glavinic[3]

[1] Medimurje University of Applied Sciences in Cakovec,
Bana Josipa Jelacica 22a, HR-40000 Cakovec, Croatia
mihael.kukec@mev.hr
[2] Faculty of Engineering, University of Rijeka,
Vukovarska 58, HR-51000 Rijeka, Croatia
sandi.ljubic@riteh.hr
[3] Faculty of Electrical Engineering and Computing, University of Zagreb,
Unska 3, HR-10000 Zagreb, Croatia
vlado.glavinic@fer.hr

Abstract. The process of improving technical skills requires students to spend many hours both observing real systems at work and working in laboratories equipped with specially prepared apparatus. Beside personal motivation and discipline, there are objective factors which limit the amount of available laboratory time for students. To deal with the afore mentioned problem for electrical engineering and computer science courses teaching basic concepts of computer architecture at the undergraduate level, we have devised a pocket-size prototyping system which can be controlled from any kind of computer device, here including contemporary mobile phones and tablets. The issue which we tackle in this paper is the efficient use of touchscreen devices to input assembly language code controlling the operation of the main processing unit on the prototyping system. The results of the pilot study performed, which addresses accuracy and time needed to accomplish the task, are rather encouraging, and shows that our special variant of virtual keyboard did not deteriorate students' performance when inputting assembly code.

Keywords: Technology enhanced learning, usability, mobile devices, touchscreen keyboards.

1 Introduction

In the era of mobile ubiquitous computing, mobile devices are becoming preferred tools in many contexts of use, whereat m-learning represents one of the emerging fields. Advanced concepts for learning and training "on the move", such as Mobile Virtual Laboratories (MVLs), were already introduced in the period of feature phones, when mobile application development possibilities were much constrained and limited. Nowadays, improved capabilities of popular touchscreen smartphones and

A. Holzinger et al. (Eds.): SouthCHI 2013, LNCS 7946, pp. 514–533, 2013.

tablets, combined with attractiveness of mobile operating systems such as Android and iOS, lay foundation for many m-learning systems to be implemented at a "full strength". At the same time, the opportunity to introduce new and engaging interaction methods for mobile platforms promises a higher level of both performance and usability of mobile applications.

We elaborated our initial idea of MVL, making it a prototyping hardware tool (PHT) able to be programmed/controlled via Android-based mobile devices. As such, this prototype is entirely suitable for inclusion in several undergraduate courses concerning microcontroller/embedded systems, and can serve as a support for appropriate laboratory exercises. Since mobile devices can be used for programming our remote microcontroller-based system, the main focus of this paper is put on the performance of assembly language input. Three interaction techniques that correspond to one standard keyboard and two originally devised tablet keyboards are presented and thoroughly analyzed via a usability testing experiment. Our main goal is to assess whether special keyboard designs for tablets can help students to improve while working on laboratory tasks involving PHT programming in assembler code.

The paper is structured as follows. Section 2 shortly outlines an overview of related work both on mobile virtual laboratories and customized virtual keyboards. In Section 3 we present the results of a preliminary study concerning (i) students' usage of SW/HW tools during individual learning, (ii) their motivation in existing course(s) setup, and (iii) their opinion about possible PHT involvement into a teaching and training process. Section 4 deals with design principles for two specially developed tablet keyboards, the first of them being similar to the traditional desktop keyboard and adjusted for limited touchscreen size, while the second one being comprised of touch buttons with assembler mnemonics. In Section 5 we describe our user testing setup, by presenting information about participants, apparatus, and protocol of the corresponding experiment. Obtained results are given in Section 6 along with discussion and our considerations, while the last section offers a brief recapitulation.

2   Related Work on Mobile Virtual Laboratories and Customized Virtual Keyboards

Introduction of the Mobile Virtual Laboratory concept is an ongoing effort in the area of mobile learning. In fact, MVL represents a continuation of the Remote Virtual Laboratory paradigm with mobile devices acting as primary client platforms. Proof-of-concept examples can be found in related research for several domains. In [1] authors propose the *M-lab* – the prototype of a virtual chemistry laboratory accessible through a mobile device. Two activities are enabled for mobile clients: video streaming of real experiments, and interacting with GUI objects that represent elements of the chemistry apparatus. However, the proposed prototype is simulation-based and there is no possibility to interact with real remote devices. In [2], a MVL system was developed for executing virtual experiments by controlling real hardware and performing measurements wirelessly. J2ME-enabled devices were used for running simple experiments from the domain of digital design (basic logic gates, combinational and sequential circuits). Target domains in another MVL system, proposed in [3], include factory automation, data acquisition, data management, and manufacturing processes. The respective mobile application was developed as a *LabView PDA Module* able to send commands and receive outputs from real signal generator hardware. Our previous work addresses a MVL implementation for learning and training digital systems design [4][5], whereas current attempts are focused in delivering the MVL for dealing with embedded systems, and particularly for remote microcontroller programming on mobile devices. Within our research, special emphasis is given on mobile software usability, by addressing interaction efficiency of keyboards for assembly language code typing.

Regarding touchscreen keyboards, being software based allows them to be customized and automatically adapted, as well as supported by new interaction methods. Contemporary virtual keyboards are usually provided with full QWERTY layout and integrated dictionary support with related algorithms able to predict the next letter in the word and/or next word in the sentence that is being typed. When it comes to interaction, the dominant technique used for text entry across the most of the available keyboards is comprised of direct touch (*Tap*) and sliding gesture (*Swipe*). While conventional keyboards usually use *Tap* for character entry, and *Swipe* for control features (e.g. character layout change, keyboard settings dialog activation), more sophisticated implementations require combined *Tap-and-Swipe* interaction. This especially applies for zone-based keyboards, where less frequently used letters are entered after tapping into the appropriate zone, and swiping in the proper direction (see Fig.1).

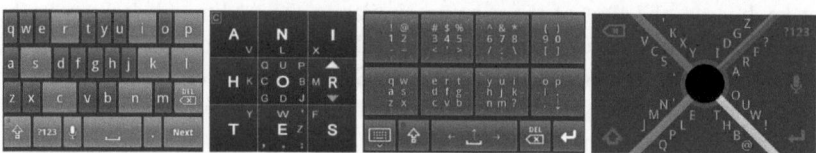

Fig. 1. Examples of non-standard touchscreen keyboards. From left to right: *ThickButtons* – adaptive change of key dimensions [6], *MessagEase* – zone-based keyboard with 9 main zones [7], *Flit Keyboard* – zone-based keyboard with 8 main zones and preserved QWERTY formation [8], *8Pen* – handwriting mimic using *Swipe* only [9].

One of the most popular touchscreen text entry interaction styles is *Swipe-only*, where the user is required to draw a gesture that connects all the letters in the desired word with one continuous finger or stylus motion. Well-known example implementations include *ShapeWriter* [10], *Swype* [11], *SlideIT* [12], and *8Pen* [9]. The *Dasher* project [13] provides a novel text entry method which discards the traditional keyboard concept, and introduces zoom-and-point interaction for selecting "flying letters" in 2D space. It is worth noting that all of the aforementioned keyboards and associated interaction styles are particularly tailored for massive text input (e.g. writing SMSs and e-mails), promising higher entry speed and lower error rate features. However, these solutions are not appropriate for assembly language typing, as dictionary support and prediction algorithms cannot provide the desired benefit. To the best of our knowledge, there exists no virtual keyboard specifically customized for assembler programming.

3   Motivation: Preliminary Study Results

The idea of building an MVL was derived from several years of observation of students in several forms of laboratory training which took place at the respective institutions of the authors. All of the authors of this paper are directly involved in the teaching process of courses related to digital system design, microcontrollers and computer architecture and as such they all had a good perspective on student's achievements, their motivation and satisfaction with the respective curricula. The process of working with students in laboratories and grading their achievements revealed a somewhat noticeable absence of enthusiasm and motivation to work at home. In an attempt to take further positive actions to remedy this situation we have interviewed one study group consisting of 26 students taking *Computer Architecture* classes about their views on the curriculum and especially on the amount of time they spend learning topics outside the official teaching premises and laboratories (Fig. 2).

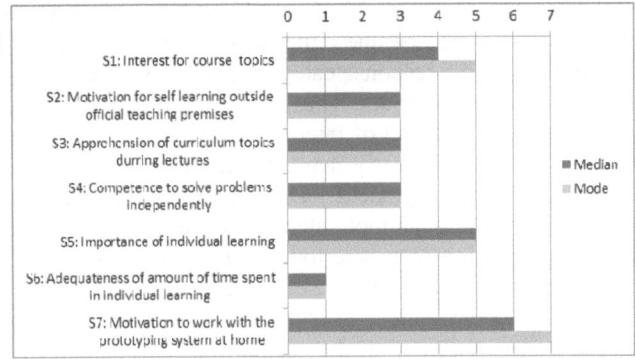

Fig. 2. Results of Likert scale questionnaire concerning student's opinions related to motivation for individual learning

Prior to answering the questionnaire, the MVL prototyping hardware tool was presented to the students. It was explained them that this prototyping hardware tool (PHT) was made in such a way as to be compatible with the curriculum, thus enabling them to gather skills and knowledge needed for the successful fulfillment of their obligations (in this case the homework ones) during the semester. Students were informed that the PHT had been in development and that at some point in future it would be available for their laboratory use. The study group was then asked to grade the questionnaire statements, as given in the following:

- Statement 1 (S1): I am interested in course topics.
- Statement 2 (S2): I am motivated for learning course topics at home.
- Statement 3 (S3): I can grasp new topics and follow lectures with ease.
- Statement 4 (S4): I feel competent to independently solve almost any problem regarding curriculum topics.

- Statement 5 (S5): Individual learning is important for overall apprehension of course topics.
- Statement 6 (S6): The amount of time I spend learning individually is adequate for me to understand almost all course topics.
- Statement 7 (S7): The PHT would motivate me to spend more time working on my homework and other curriculum related assignments.

A seven-point Likert scale [14][15] was used to describe the levels of agreement with the above statements: (1) – *Strongly disagree*, (2) – *Disagree*, (3) – *Disagree somewhat*, (4) – *Neither agree nor disagree*, (5) – *Agree somewhat*, (6) – *Agree*, (7) – *Strongly agree*. Student's opinions regarding statements S1–S7 are represented with median and mode values as depicted on Fig. 2.

Evaluation results for statement S1 show a positive attitude towards the course topics, albeit this is not as prominent as the results for statements S2, S3, and S4. From our personal experience derived both from lecturing and working with students in laboratories, we can assert a students' more than satisfactory response to the course topics, thus a slight disappointment with the evaluation results of S1. We can therefore assume that this results can be due either to the inherent Likert scale weakness (i.e. participants avoid extreme response categories) or it is a matter of isolated view on one course in the whole curriculum. Thus, to have a broader view on the subject, one must take into account the level of interest for the entire curriculum. Evaluation outcomes for statements S2–S4 clearly demonstrate the problem. All of these latter were evaluated slightly negative (grade 3 – *Disagree somewhat*), meaning that (i) the students are not sufficiently enough motivated for self-learning outside official teaching premises; (ii) apprehension of course topics during lectures could be better; (iii) the students do not regard their skills to be sufficient enough for independent problem solving. The most conspicuous indicator for the amount of the effort students put into individual learning is their opinion on the adequateness of amount of time spent in self-learning (Statement S6). Although they realize the importance of individual learning (Statement S5), evidently this does not adequately enough translate into the time actually spent in individual learning.

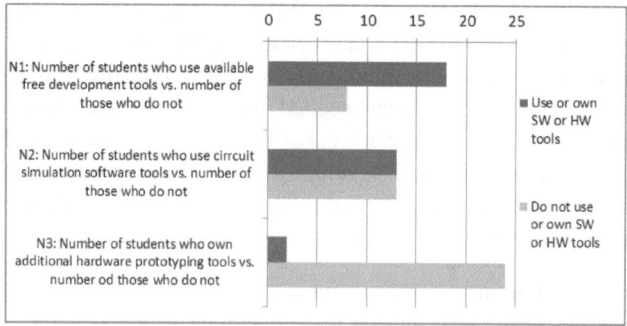

Fig. 3. Number of students who use additional software (SW) and hardware (HW) tools during individual learning: (N1) - number of students who use available free integrated development environments, (N2) - number of students who use microcontroller and circuit simulation software tools, (N3) - number of students who own additional hardware prototyping tools

In addition to the seven items Likert scale questionnaire, we asked students to "digitally" answer (Yes–No) whether during their individual learning time they use: (i) either of the three: freely available software tools, integrated development environments (IDE) or any other combination of freely available source code editor, assembler, compiler, and debugger; (ii) microcontroller and digital circuit simulation software tools; (iii) their own additional hardware prototyping tools. The study group was also asked for additional explanation of negative answers.

As expected, and given the availability of software development tools (which can be freely downloaded from the respective Web pages of microcontroller manufacturers), the majority of students is using such an opportunity (see Fig. 3 – N1). However, the percentage of those than do not use freely available software tools (28%) is somewhat worrisome. Unfortunately, although we specifically required for an explanation of negative answers to be provided, the students provided no feedback.

The number of students using circuit simulation software tools (Fig. 3 – N2) is equal to the number of those who do not use, what is a rather expected result since electronic circuit simulation tools are complex and rather expensive software packages. In fact, the high price of respective licenses is emphasized as the reason for the negative answer to question N2. Students that do use simulation software mostly indicated the use of free and open source software (FOSS) equivalents. The response to the third question (Fig. 3 – N3) was generally negative, as students were not expected to own any such tools.

Most encouraging of all the answers are the results for statement S7, as our study group demonstrated an evident enthusiasm with the PHT (see Fig. 2 – S7). The majority of the students emphasized their agreement or even a strong agreement with the statement, clearly communicating their positive motivation to work with the tool. There is, however, a prominent discrepancy of this finding with the current level of utilization of such tools in the studied group (see Fig. 3 – N3), as only 7% of students currently use such tools. This possibly comes from the fact that many existing prototyping tools are in general not aligned with course assignments, thus causing additional efforts to make them acceptable as a learning tool.

We can comment on the overall quite positive reaction to the introduction of the PHT as an acceptance of a new tool in a wish to improve personal knowledge and skills, while it could certainly be only a facet of the Hawthorne effect [16]. This latter alternative could essentially be caused by the students' knowledge of the primary design goal for the PHT, which is to create a tool that will help students with homework and individual learning.

Although with a limited scope, the study revealed some tendencies concerning students' opinions on the proposed improvements of the teaching process. The initial assumption was proven to be correct: students are indeed not dedicating an adequate amount of time to learning and working on homework assignments and, what is more, they are aware of it (see Fig. 2 – S6). While this awareness is a good starting point towards a possible positive action, it is definitely not enough just to be aware of it. Beside an inefficient utilization of available time, it is apparent that students have limited access to proper tools. Even in situations when they do have access to some sort of simulation tools and/or hardware prototyping systems, these tools are usually not sufficiently aligned with the course curriculum, making it harder for students to make initial steps in using them properly. This result makes the basis for our work in creating a solution to this problem.

4   Design Principles and Implementation of Special Touchscreen Keyboards

The previous section presents issues regarding students' motivation for learning beyond the mandatory time at the teaching premises and laboratories, as required by the curriculum. Motivation for learning, along with students' abilities for meaningful self-regulated learning, are complex issues [17][18]. One potential motivational element revealed by our pilot study is the access to proper tools. Trying to improve students' motivation for individual self-regulated learning we have devised a small pocket-sized PHT which can be used in electrical engineering and computer science courses teaching basic concepts of computer architecture. The primary design principles for the PHT we have set forth are: (i) it must foster the constructivist learning theory [19], (ii) it must be aligned with the main course topics, and (iii) it must leverage mobile learning principles [20][21][22].

The PHT can be regarded as a safe place for experimenting without consequences in the real world, thus establishing a playground for learning and utilizing the acquired knowledge to create new solutions [23]. However, we believe that learning by constructing must be somehow guided, possessing at least some sort of loose structure, thus the PHT must be aligned with the main course topics. The third main design principle is the provision of a truly ubiquitous learning experience without any restrictions. With these goals in mind, the PHT is implemented with the ability to be controlled from any kind of computer device, including contemporary mobile phones and tablets.

Computing power in the form of mobile phones and tablets is a relatively new phenomenon that rapidly gains momentum. Although contemporary mobile phones and tablets have arguably been widely available in the last three to five years, research efforts to create learning systems supported by such devices had begun more than forty years before these events [24]. Today, mobile phones and tablets embody only the hardware part of Alan Kay's Dynabook. Due to the large reduction of dimensions, these devices are both personal, as "in personal ownership of their user", and portable, as the "user can carry additional things", beside the device [24]. Since they are personal and portable, this makes them ideal for the "anyplace and anytime" paradigm supported by mobile learning, but not without some additional cost in the field of human computer interaction (HCI) [23][25]. Standard input devices – keyboard and mouse – have been merged into a primary output device, hence creating a new output-input device (the touchscreen). Although an encouraging new wave of natural user interface (NUI) [26] methods is becoming increasingly prominent, touchscreen devices still suffer from common usability issues.

Overcoming issues like interaction design [27], maximizing screen real-estate [28][29][30], adequate input techniques provision [31][32], and usability in general [33][34], represents a great challenge for mobile applications, resulting in designers and developers of mobile applications having complex tasks of finding the best way to meet user expectations. In our previous work [35] we have detected what we believe are "typical usability issues, common to all touchscreen applications: optimal size of touchscreen objects, visual search-and-selection, edge-positioning, occlusion, dragging gestures, and efficiency of virtual on-screen keyboards". In this paper, we describe our efforts towards performance evaluation of virtual on-screen keyboards for assembly language code input.

4.1 Design of Virtual Keyboard for Assembly Language Input Using Touchscreen

The main intention of our study is to evaluate user performance on virtual on-screen keyboards used in assembly language code input tasks. Hence, we have designed and implemented two variants of virtual keyboards for touchscreen devices: (i) a standard one (SK) and (ii) a mnemonic one (MK). It must be noted that both keyboards are especially tailored for assembly language code input.

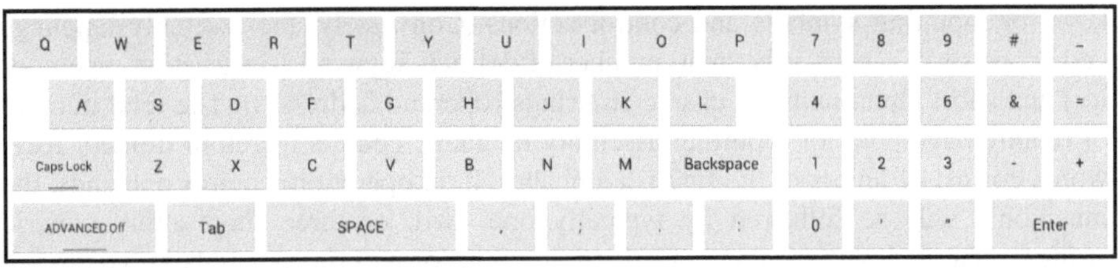

Fig. 4. The layout of the standard keyboard (SK) for assembly language input for touchscreen devices. On the left part of the keyboard is the classic QWERTY key (software buttons) arrangement, which takes approx. 2/3 of the available width. On the right side of the keyboard, taking about 1/3 of the entire width is the numeric part of keyboard.

4.2 Standard Virtual On-Screen Keyboard

The SK layout (see Fig. 4) is similar to a classic desktop personal computer (PC) keyboard, but, in order to save screen space, we have omitted both function and number keys (the two rows of keys usually placed above the "QWERTY" keys row). While function keys have no role in our application, digits can be parts of almost every assembly code line; therefore we had decided to dedicate one (smaller) part of the screen to an additional numeric keyboard. In order to make the arrangement as much similar to the standard PC keyboard, the numeric keyboard is placed to the right of its letter counterpart. Contrary to present day touchscreen solutions, both keyboard parts are simultaneously displayed on the screen. Namely, taking into consideration the importance of numeric keys for assembly language code input, we regarded as not advantageous enough the tradeoff made for general text input keyboards on touchscreen devices. As already known, in these latter applications, a balance between the opposite requirements of trying to place as many keys on screen as possible, and making them as large as possible, is implemented by alternating as needed the on-screen display of the letter and numeric keyboards.

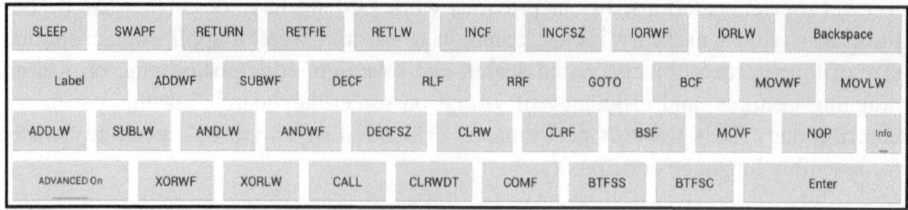

Fig. 5. Mnemonic keyboard (MK) consisting of 35 keys (software buttons), each key representing an assembly language instruction. Beside 35 mnemonic keys, there are also the Backspace, Enter, Label, Info, and Advanced On/Off keys. Each mnemonic key is placed as close as possible to the location of its first letter on the standard keyboard (SK).

4.3   Mnemonic Virtual On-Screen Keyboard

Beside letters and digits, keyboards for arbitrary text input must provide a number of keys for inputting symbols and control actions. Conversely, the assembly language code consists of a relatively small number of defined keywords (instruction mnemonics) and short alpha-numeric character strings (operand addresses). The total number of required symbols for inputting assembly language code is therefore limited. Keywords consist of letters of the English alphabet. If an operation requires operands, the mnemonic will be followed by typically one, two, or three short alpha-numeric strings, separated with the comma. Given the rigid form of the assembly language and the relatively small number of mnemonics, we have devised a keyboard layout which is comprised solely of keys representing mnemonics (see Fig. 5). The rationale behind this approach is rather simple. Take that e.g. to write a CLRWDT mnemonic using the SK one has to tap six keys (or software buttons on the virtual on-screen keyboard) as opposed to tapping only one on the MK. Additionally, if the instruction requires operands, writing the DECFSZ mnemonic using SK will require six key taps for each mnemonic letter plus one key tap for inputting a whitespace character to separate the operands from the mnemonic. Note however that whitespaces are typically space or tab characters which are inserted automatically after a key tap on the MK.

The arrangement of mnemonic keys on the MK is not incidental. In fact, the location of a mnemonic key tries to be as close as possible to the location of the first letter of the mnemonic on the SK. E.g., mnemonic keys SLEEP and SWAPF start with the letter "S" which is placed on the left side of the SK in its second row, thus SLEEP and SWAPF try to mimic the position of the key "S" on the SK. The same applies to the other 33 mnemonic keys. Unfortunately, this rule cannot be enforced for all the mnemonics, as there are more mnemonics starting with the same letter. E.g., there are four keys representing mnemonics starting with the letter "I" and five keys representing mnemonics starting with the letter "C", hence making it difficult to fully follow our rule for placement mnemonic keys.

Nevertheless, we regard that such a keyboard layout can have positive impact on the accuracy and especially on the speed of typing with the MK. Hopefully, instead of visually searching for mnemonic keys, the user will try to instinctively position her/his fingers above the area where (s)he assumes the key should be located. This approach leverages the existing information a user has stored in her/his spatial memory regarding classic keyboards layout. Although it would be very interesting to analyze the impact of different mnemonic keyboard layouts on user performance, this is not the primary consideration of this paper.

Beside 35 mnemonic keys (Fig. 5), the MK has five additional keys: Backspace, Enter, Label, Info, and Advanced On/Off. The Backspace key is used for deletion of previously entered text, while Enter is used to confirm the input of one line of assembly language code and to place the editor cursor in the next line. The Label key is used for inputting labels which can consist of arbitrary strings of characters; this key moves the cursor to the first column in the current line and enables inputting of arbitrary alpha-numeric strings by activating the SK. Advanced On/Off is used for switching between standard and mnemonic keyboards, while Info displays otherwise hidden parts of the screen showing technical documentation for using mnemonics, providing the user needs it.

4.4   Assembly Language Syntax Rules and Keyboard Switching

Our model of the assembly language code input makes interchangeable use of both the SK and the MK. At any given moment the user can switch between them using the Advanced On/Off key located at the lower left corner of both keyboards. Hence, the user has the freedom to choose the keyboard that is most appropriate for her/his purpose. Other than reducing the number of keystrokes per mnemonic, we have designed a slightly different mode of operation for the MK, which we believe can further improve the user performance.

The grammar rules of assembly languages are pretty rudimentary, and can be summed by the following line:

```
[label]      mnemonic      [operand], [operand]
```

Labels are optional; they are used to make a reference to an arbitrary code segment. The mnemonic part of the assembly code line is however mandatory. To be able to distinguish between labels and mnemonics, the general rule of assembly languages dictates that labels should be written in the first column, while mnemonics must be separated from them with at least one white-space character. If the assembler instruction does not have any label, then the mnemonic should be preceded by at least one white-space character, in order not to confuse the mnemonic for a label. Other that conforming to this basic grammar rule, the assembly language code must be legibly written. Legibility of assembly code can be achieved following some simple rules: (i) use the tabulator for separating labels and mnemonics, (ii) if there is no label in the line, use the tabulator to move the mnemonic away from the first column, and (iii) separate the mnemonic from the operands with a tab. Using the tabulator to separate labels, mnemonics and operators produces a legible code formed into three distinct columns.

Taking into account the above rather simple grammar rules, we have additionally slightly enhanced the MK operation by further reducing the number of the required keystrokes when inputting assembler code through the introduction of a number of actions automatically performed by the keyboard. Namely, coding with the MK can benefit from mnemonic "shortcuts", but there is a need for switching the keyboard to the SK layout when operands or labels are required. For this specific context, an automatic switching mechanism is provided according to the syntax rules. The detailed explanation of this action is beyond the scope of this paper and will be skipped.

In the following text, the "SK" annotation refers to the explicit SK-only code input method, while the "MK" addresses mnemonic-based input with keyboard switching.

5   Experiment Setup and Tools Used

To evaluate the efficiency of inputting assembly code on our (MK, SK) keyboards, we have performed an experiment which will be described in this section.

Fifteen male students, with an average age of 20 years, participated in the study. All of them had fulfilled the requirements and had passed the *Computer Architecture* course hence we regarded them as being acquainted with the assembly language for the Microchip 14 bit instruction microcontroller family and associated tools [36]. The students were accommodated in a laboratory equipped with 15 workplaces equipped with a personal computer and a 10" capacitive touchscreen Toshiba AT100-100 Android tablet.

```
L1:   BROJAC    equ     0xC
L2:   GRANICA   equ     0xD
L3:             org     0x0
L4:             bsf     STATUS, RP0
L5:             bcf     TRISB, 0
L6:             bsf     TRISA, 0
L7:             movlw   B'11010011'
L8:             movwf   OPTION_REG
L9:             bcf     STATUS, RP0
L10:            clrf    PORTA
L11:            clrf    PORTB
L12:            movlw   D'195'
L13:            movwf   GRANICA
L14:  poc       nop
L15:  lab1      btfss   PORTA, 0
L16:            goto    lab1
L17:            clrf    TMR0
L18:  lab2      btfsc   PORTA, 0
L19:            goto    lab2
L20:            movf    TMR0, W
L21:            movwf   BROJAC
L22:            movf    BROJAC, W
L23:            call    provjeri
L24:            goto    poc
```

Fig. 6. The assembly language program for Microchip 14-bit instruction microcontrollers used to test the efficiency of the SK and the MK

As the same student group was to be used in testing three keyboards (PC keyboard, SK, MK), in order to avoid the bias caused by gradually learning the assembler code segment to be inputted, we used the standard counterbalancing technique of dividing the student group into three subgroups, each one consisting of five students, to test the different keyboards in three different alternations.

Before the experiment, its purpose was explained to the participating students. They were explained that both speed and accuracy are equally important. Each student was handed a sheet with the printed assembly program segment. They were given a couple of minutes to familiarize themselves with the program segment and to ask possible questions. Concerning errors, we instructed them to correct all of the errors they notice during writing the current line of the assembly code, but never to go back to previous lines even if they noticed errors.

5.1   Tools for Collecting and Analyzing Quantitative Data

During the three experiments performed by the study group, the three different methods were tested, basing on (i) the desktop computer keyboard (DK), (ii) the tablet computer with the SK, and (iii) the tablet computer with the MK. Event logging was performed in the background of the respective operating systems, by recording every user action together with its associated time-stamp into an appropriate log file. Timestamps and event identifiers were fetched using .NET system calls on Windows OS, and Android API system calls on Android. The only technical difference found when fetching event data and the associated timestamps was that the logging software for Windows was implemented as a self-standing executable file while the one for Android was an integral part of our prototype. The log files conformed to the same format on both platforms.

The collected log files were subsequently analyzed with a specially prepared software utility written solely for the purpose of this study. This utility software was written in Java (about 400 lines of code), and extensively used the character string handling capabilities of the *java.lang.String* class. The motivation to create such a utility was twofold. First of all, keystroke logs collected from the three experiments consisted of 45 files (fifteen participants performing three experiments), each one having approximately 250-350 logged keystrokes with associated timestamps. Even data from such small an experiment consisted of a large number of individual units, whose processing would be otherwise very time-consuming even when using general purpose software tools such as LibreOffice Calc or Microsoft Excel. The second reason was the need to process the logs from all three experiments without any bias, completely in the same way, with an identical algorithm.

6   Results and Discussion

The examination of gathered data revealed the issue of establishing the accuracy measurement method. The whole experiment was set to assess accuracy and efficiency of the assembly code input methods, therefore accuracy measurement methods for arbitrary text input could not be applied.

The measurement unit for text input speed is words per minute (wpm), and relies on the smallest element of text that by itself has a meaning, which is a word. On the other hand, morphemes are defined as the smallest units with a meaning, which cannot necessarily stand alone, thus one word can be made from one or more morphemes. Considering the assembly language, a mnemonic can be regarded as a morpheme, while a line of assembly code can be regarded as the elementary unit which by itself has a meaning. However, this analogy is not completely correct. There are assembly language instructions which do not have operands, thus having only one morpheme, i.e. the mnemonic. Furthermore, there are assembly language instructions that require operands, thus they consist of both the mnemonic and operands. Although the mnemonic can be regarded as the morpheme, operands cannot. If separated from the mnemonic, operands do not have any meaning by themselves. Nevertheless, given the analogy with word and morpheme definition in arbitrary text, we will consider one line of assembly code to be the smallest element that by itself has a meaning. From the assembly language point of view, there is no smaller unit of logical meaning than one line of code.

6.1   Accuracy of Typing the Assembly Language Program

Since one line of assembly language program is defined as an elementary unit of logical meaning, the log processing utility was set to seek correct lines in the log files. If such a line was found, the duration of its typing was calculated, otherwise the utility reported a duration of "-1". The total number of assembly code lines the study groups had to copy during the experiment is 360 (15 participants × 24 lines of code). Using the DK, the touchscreen device with the SK, and the touchscreen device with the MK, the study group achieved a total accuracy of 63.1%, 54.7%, and 62.5%, respectively (see Fig. 7). The results show a slight degradation of accuracy when using touchscreen devices with the SK, while there is almost no difference between the DK and touchscreen device with the MK.

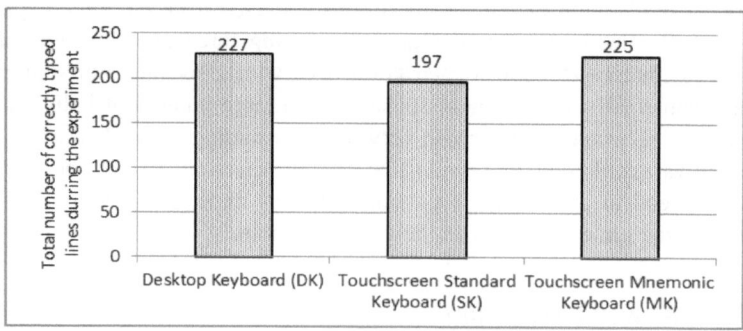

Fig. 7. Total number of correctly typed lines during the experiment for three input methods: (i) desktop computer with attached keyboard (DK), (ii) touchscreen device with standard keyboard (SK), and (iii) touchscreen device with mnemonic keyboard (MK)

A closer inspection of the accuracy test results (see Fig. 8.) reveals a rather similar distribution of data in the case of the DK and the MK, while the SK has a much wider spread of results. The mean values for all the three cases are almost identical (15.130, SD=3.313; 13.133, SD=7.317; and 15.000, SD=3.273 for DK, SK, and MK respectively). Nevertheless, a similar result distribution for the DK and the MK together with a noticeable degradation of performance is evident from the results for SK and cannot be ignored. Due to inherent usability issues of touchscreen devices [31][32], this difference between DK and SK was however anticipated. Moreover, the prominent degradation of performance for the SK of the touchscreen device was not only expected, but was the primary incentive for this study.

A one-way repeated measures ANOVA (RM ANOVA) with a Greenhouse-Geisser correction was used to test for accuracy differences among the three cases. The accuracy of assembly code typing did not differ significantly across three types of input methods, $F(1.223, 17.123)=1.018$, $p=0.344$.

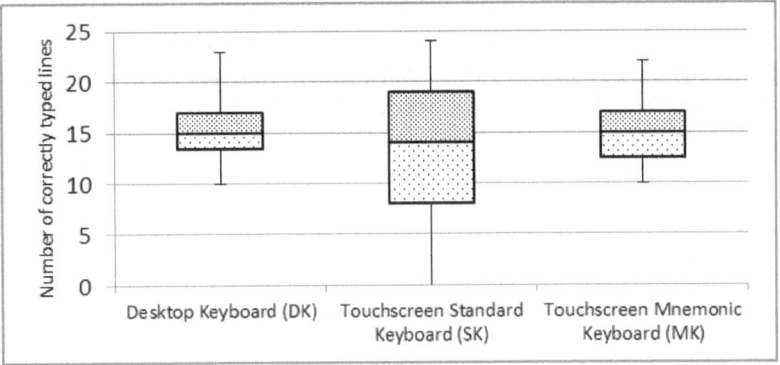

Fig. 8. Box plot with whiskers for correctly typed lines for the three input methods: (i) desktop computer with attached keyboard (DK), (ii) touchscreen device with standard keyboard (SK), and (iii) touchscreen device with mnemonic keyboard (MK)

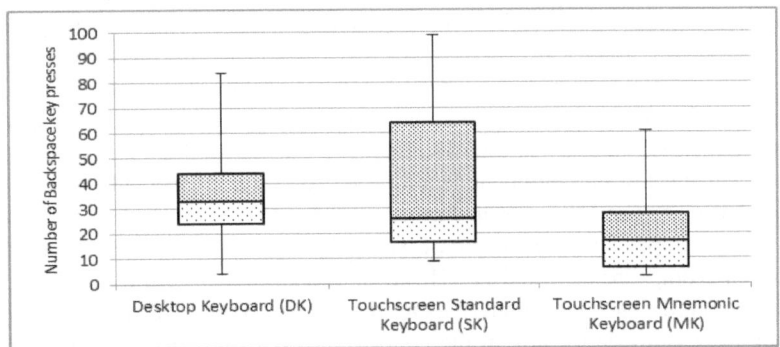

Fig. 9. Number of backspace key presses for three input methods: (i) desktop computer with attached keyboard (DK), (ii) touchscreen device with standard keyboard (SK), and (iii) touchscreen device with mnemonic keyboard (MK)

Regarding the total number of corrections made during code typing, (see Fig. 9), the MK proved to be the least error prone, with a total number of 303 corrections (M=20.20, SD=17.201). The DK follows with a total number of 534 corrections (M=35.60, SD=20.402), while the SK was the most susceptible to errors, with a total number of 604 errors (M=40.27, SD=33.165). A one-way RM ANOVA with a Greenhouse-Geisser correction was used to test for differences among these three cases. The number of corrections did not differ significantly across these three types of input methods, as $F(1.378, 19.292)=3.237$, $p=0.076$. The statistical inference test showed no difference between the three cases regarding the number of backspace key presses at the significance level $\alpha=0.05$ ($p>\alpha$); however, this result is statistically significant at the level $\alpha=0.1$ ($p<\alpha$).

It must be noted that the primary objective of this study was to evaluate whether touchscreen devices deteriorate students' performance when inputting assembly code. To that end, we have shown that there is no significant difference ($\alpha=0.05$) between DK, SK, and MK, hence all of this three types of devices and input methods can be used interchangeably. Nevertheless, at the significance level of $\alpha=0.10$, a post hoc test using Bonferroni correction revealed that the reduction of number of backspace key presses between the DK and the MK is statistically significant ($p=0.018$). Both differences, between the DK and the SK ($p=1.000$), and between the SK and the MK ($p=0.180$), were not statistically significant. Due to the significantly lower number of keystrokes per mnemonic, comparing the DK input method and the MK input method, we can say that the latter reduces the total number of corrections by more than 40%.

6.2   Analysis of Time Needed for Assembly Program Typing

The assembly language program that the participants were asked to type consisted of 24 lines of code, albeit not all of them were taken into consideration when computing the total time needed to type the code. This total number of lines was further reduced to 19, as lines L6, L9, L14, L15, and L18 were discarded because of the following reasoning.

Upon closer inspection, we have noticed that the above mentioned lines of code have been typed correctly by only five or less participants during one of the three experiments. Lines L6 and L9 have been typed only four times using SK, thus they were excluded from further consideration. Lines L15 and L18 have been typed only once using the MK, and, using the MK, line L14 wasn't typed correctly at all. Given the rather small set of measurement data for lines L6, L9 and especially L14, L15, and L18, we have excluded them from further consideration. Unfortunately, there is no sufficient data to provide explanation of why did the study group make so much mistakes when typing lines L6 and L9. However results of typing lines L14, L15, and L18, which were typed inaccurately using the MK by almost all of the participants revealed an obvious deficiency in the course of typing lines of code which include labels.

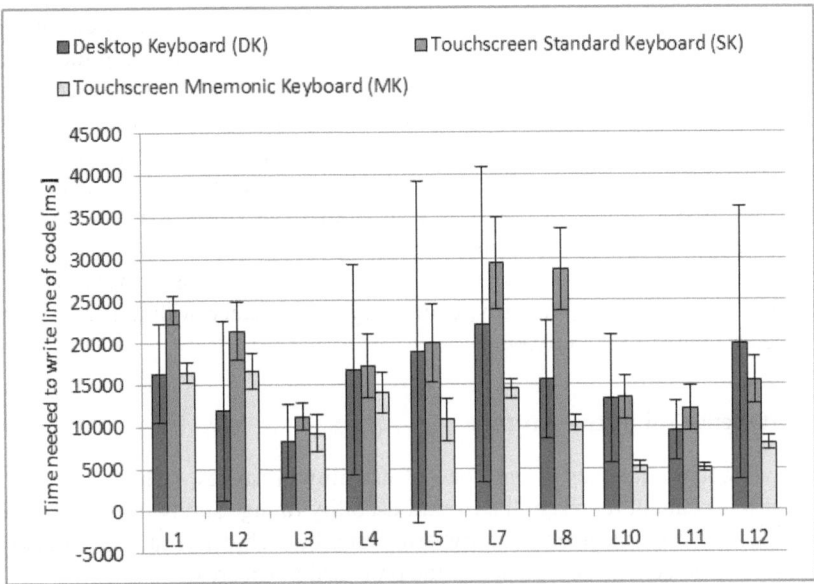

Fig. 10. Analysis of time needed to type lines L1–L12, excluding lines L6 and L9. The graph shows average times needed to type assembly language code lines with error bars depicting the standard error for each line.

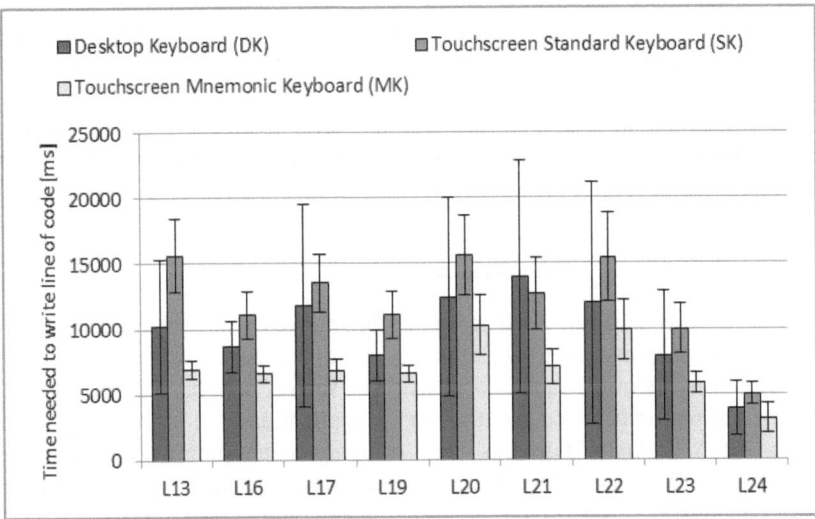

Fig. 11. Analysis of time needed to type lines L13–L24, excluding lines L14, L15, and L18. The graph shows average times needed to type assembly language code lines with error bars depicting the standard error for each line

The total time needed for typing the 19 lines of assembly code is calculated by adding the average times for typing each line. The total time for typing the assembly language program for DK, SK, and MK is 242.04 seconds, 303.52 seconds and 173.96 seconds, respectively. A one-way RM ANOVA was used to test for differences among average times needed to type a correct line using the three methods: DK, SK, and MK. The significant difference was found between these three methods: $F_{(2, 36)}=28.007$, $p<0.01$. Post hoc analysis with Bonferroni correction revealed significantly lower code entry time per line when using MK (M=9155.9 ms, SD=899.6 ms) over DK (M=12739.2 ms, SD=1076.0 ms; p=0.002) and SK (M=15974.7 ms, SD=1451.1 ms; p<0.001). Similarly, code entry performance with the DK is significantly better than the SK (p=0.007).

6.3   Students Subjective Attitude

Since code entry efficiency is only one of usability attributes, task completion time and error rates cannot represent the overall usability rating. Surely, it is very valuable to provide speed enhancement and low error rate, but subjective attitude is also very important for the general acceptance of the proposed keyboards.

In order to qualitatively compare proposed touchscreen keyboards, we sent an e-mail to participants asking them to make a final choice between SK and MK, with a presumption that the selected keyboard and associated interaction technique would become the only available one for our PHT. We suggested that both ease of use and user friendliness experienced in the lab setting should implicate individual response. Furthermore, we explicitly underlined that choosing the SK assumes code typing without mnemonic keys, whilst choosing the MK implies possible keyboard switching.

Users responded with answers favoring the MK, as no less than 11 participants (approx. 73%) picked MK as their first and preferred option to be included in the MVL setting.

6.4   The Tablet/Smartphone Argument

The proposed keyboards are modeled and implemented with tablet screens (approx. 7"–10") being the main target platforms. For our experimental setup, we were able to acquire 15 instances of the same model with 10" screen, and that was the only device model used in research. Of course, the mobile application used in the experiment can be run on different Android devices, here including contemporary touchscreen smartphones (approx. 3.2"–4.8"). However, our research budget limit prevented the possibility of including a 15 smartphone series in the laboratory apparatus.

Surely, different screen sizes may affect the ways users interact with the virtual keyboard. Larger screens usually provide easier text entry, as key buttons and their mutual distance are larger, thus lowering the effect of the "fat finger" syndrome. Thus, one can argue that the SK may benefit from larger screens while the MK may be suitable for smaller ones. However, the experiment results revealed the MK (with larger mnemonic keys) outperforming the SK on a 10" screen, hence we can reasonably assume a similar performance ratio within the smartphone class. Since the particular keyboard layout and functionality are totally equal among various screen sizes, we can additionally expect that the MK would obtain better user experience effects than the SK, even in smartphone applications.

Although comparing the PC desktop keyboard to the SK and the MK in the smartphone setting has no particular significance (because of the considerably different context of use), a smartphone-based SK/MK comparative evaluation deserves a thorough insight. For our future work, we plan to enlarge the experimental research of SK/MK, by assessing various screen sizes, screen orientations (landscape, portrait), and code entry interaction styles (one-hand, and two-hand usage).

7   Conclusion

The primary objective of this pilot study was to evaluate the feasibility of using contemporary mobile phones and tablets in an MVL setting, especially considering a particular aspect of its usage. Fostering the constructivist learning paradigm of our MVL model, we are challenging the ability of tablet computers to be utilized as an input device for assembly code which in turn controls the operation of the primary processing unit of our PHT. To that end, a small scale study was performed which involved fifteen participants in a within-subjects design experiments. Participants were asked to type the assembly language code three times, using a desktop computer with the attached keyboard (DK), a modified version of standard on-screen virtual keyboard of a touchscreen device (SK) and our variant of the on-screen virtual keyboard specially tailored for mnemonic input (MK). While using the SK envisaged assembly code typing without mnemonic keys and without keyboard switching, handling the MK included mnemonic "shortcuts" and keyboard switching for labels and operands. During the experiments, every keystroke with the accompanying timestamp was logged. After analyzing the results thus gathered, we concluded that the initial results were rather encouraging. Regarding typing accuracy there was no statistically significant difference among the used methods ($p>0.1$). Concerning the total number of corrections made, the mnemonic keyboard proved to be the best method for assembly code input, with the smallest number of corrections made. It was even better than the desktop keyboard, reducing by 43% the total number of corrections made. As for the average time, the MK was the fastest method for code typing, as it produced a result that is 28% better than the DK and 42% better than the SK. A simple qualitative comparison revealed that the MK solution is favored with respect to the SK approach.

Taking all results into consideration, we can conclude that touchscreen devices can be efficiently used for assembly code input. Moreover, we have shown that the mnemonic keyboard had positive effects on typing speed and reduces the total number of errors.

Acknowledgments. This paper describes the results of research being carried out within the project 036-0361994-1995, as well as within the program 036-1994, both funded by the Ministry of Science, Education and Sports of the Republic of Croatia.

References

1. Bottentuit Junior, J.B., Coutinho, C.: Virtual Laboratories and M-Learning: learning with mobile devices. In: Proc. Int'l Multi-Conf. Society, Cybernetics and Informatics, pp. 275–278. International Institute of Informatics and Systemics (2007)
2. Alkouz, A., Al-Zoubi, A.Y., Otair, M.: J2ME-Based Mobile Virtual Laboratory for Engineering Education. International Journal of Interactive Mobile Technologies (iJIM) 2(2), 5–10 (2008)
3. Auer, M.E., Al-Zoubi, A.Y., Zutin, D.G.: Implementation of a Mobile Accessible Remote Lab. International Journal of Interactive Mobile Technologies (iJIM) 2(3), 7–11 (2008)
4. Glavinic, V., Kukec, M., Ljubic, S.: Mobile Virtual Laboratory: Learning Digital Design. In: Luzar, S.V., Hljuz, D.V. (eds) Proc. 29th Int'l Conf. Information Technology Interfaces (ITI 2007), pp. 325–410. SRCE University of Zagreb, Zagreb – Croatia (2007)
5. Glavinic, V., Kukec, M., Ljubic, S.: Digital Design Mobile Virtual Laboratory Implementation: A Pragmatic Approach. In: Stephanidis, C. (ed.) Universal Access in HCI, Part I, HCII 2009. LNCS, vol. 5614, pp. 489–498. Springer, Heidelberg (2009)
6. ThickButtons, http://www.thickbuttons.com/
7. Nesbat, S.B.: A System for Fast, Full-Text Entry for Small Electronic Devices. In: Proc. 5th Int'l Conf. Multimodal Interfaces (ICMI 2003), pp. 4–11. ACM Press, New York (2003)
8. Flit Keyboard, https://sites.google.com/site/flitkeyboard/
9. 8Pen, http://www.8pen.com/
10. Zhai, S., et al.: ShapeWriter on the iPhone – From the Laboratory to the Real World. In: Extended Abstracts on Human Factors in Computing Systems (EA CHI 2009), pp. 2667–2670. ACM Press, New York – USA (2009)
11. Swype, http://www.swype.com/
12. SlideIT, http://www.mobiletextinput.com/
13. Inference Group: The Dasher Project,
    http://www.inference.phy.cam.ac.uk/dasher/
14. Likert, R.: A technique for the measurement of attitudes. Archives of Psychology 22, 1–55 (1932)
15. Maurer, T.J., Andrews, K.D.: Traditional, Likert, and Simplified Measures of Self-Efficacy. Educational and Psychological Measurement 60, 965–973 (2000)
16. Franke, R.H., Kaul, J.D.: The Hawthorne Experiments: First Statistical Interpretation. American Sociological Review 43, 623–643 (1978)
17. Dignath, C., Büttner, G.: Components of fostering self-regulated learning among students. A Meta-Analysis on Intervention Studies at Primary and Secondary School Level. Metacognition and Learning 3, 231–264 (2008)
18. Dignath, C., Buettner, G., Langfeldt, H.: How can primary school students learn self-regulated learning strategies most effectively? A meta-analysis on self-regulation training programmes. Educational Research Review 3, 101–129 (2008)
19. Jonassen, D., Mayes, T., McAleese, R.: A Manifesto for a Constructivist Approach to Uses of Technology in Higher Education. In: Duffy, T., Lowyck, J., Jonassen, D., Welsh, T. (eds.) Designing Environments for Constructive Learning, vol. 105, pp. 231–247. Springer, Heidelberg (1993)
20. Gil-Rodríguez, E.P., Rebaque-Rivas, P.: Mobile Learning and Commuting: Contextual Interview and Design of Mobile Scenarios. In: Leitner, G., Hitz, M., Holzinger, A. (eds.) USAB 2010. LNCS, vol. 6389, pp. 266–277. Springer, Heidelberg (2010)

21. Sharples, M.: The design of personal mobile technologies for lifelong learning. Computers & Education 34, 177–193 (2000)
22. Sharples, M., Corlett, D., Westmancott, O.: The Design and Implementation of a Mobile Learning Resource. Personal and Ubiquitous Computing 6, 220–234 (2002)
23. Holzinger, A., Nischelwitzer, A., Meisenberger, M.: Mobile Phones as a Challenge for m-Learning: Examples for Mobile Interactive Learning Objects (MILOs). In: Proc. 3rd IEEE Int'l Conf. Pervasive Computing and Communications (PerCom 2005), pp. 307–311. IEEE Computer Society, Washington, DC (2005)
24. Kay, A.C.: A Personal Computer for Children of All Ages. 1 (1972)
25. Shudong, W., Higgins, M.: Limitations of Mobile Phone Learning. In: Proc. IEEE Int'l Workshop on Wireless and Mobile Technologies in Education (WMTE 2005), pp. 179–181. IEEE Computer Society, Washington, DC (2005)
26. Wigdor, D., Wixon, D.: Brave NUI World: Designing Natural User Interfaces for Touch and Gesture. Morgan Kaufmann Publishers Inc. (2011)
27. Stephanidis, C.: Editorial. International Journal – Universal Access in the Information Society 1, 1–3 (2001)
28. Repokari, L., Saarela, T., Kurki, I.: Visual Search on a Mobile Phone Display. In: Proc. Research Conf. South African Institute of Computer Scientists and Information Technologists on Enablement through Technology (SAICSIT 2002), pp. 253–253. SAICSIT (2002)
29. Baudisch, P., Rosenholtz, R.: Halo: a technique for visualizing off-screen objects. In: Proc. SIGCHI Conf. Human Factors in Computing Systems (CHI 2003), pp. 481–488. ACM, New York (2003)
30. Burigat, S., Chittaro, L., Gabrielli, S.: Visualizing locations of off-screen objects on mobile devices: a comparative evaluation of three approaches. In: Proc. 8th Conf. Human-Computer Interaction with Mobile Devices and Services (MobileHCI 2006), pp. 239–246. ACM, New York (2006)
31. Lee, S., Zhai, S.: The Performance of Touch Screen Soft Buttons. In: Proc. 27th Int'l Conf. Human Factors in Computing Systems (CHI 2009), pp. 309–318. ACM Press, New York (2009)
32. Parhi, P., Karlson, A.K., Bederson, B.B.: Target Size Study for One-Handed Thumb Use on Small Touchscreen Devices. In: Proc. 8th Conf. Human-computer interaction with mobile devices and services (MobileHCI 2006), pp. 203–210. ACM Press, New York (2006)
33. Nielsen, J.: Usability Engineering. Morgan Kaufmann (1993)
34. Holzinger, A.: Usability engineering methods for software developers. Communications of the ACM 48, 71–74 (2005)
35. Glavinic, V., Ljubic, S., Kukec, M.: Supporting universal usability of mobile software: touchscreen usability meta-test. In: Stephanidis, C. (ed.) Universal Access in HCI, Part III, HCII 2011. LNCS, vol. 6767, pp. 26–35. Springer, Heidelberg (2011)
36. Microchip PICmicro x14 Instruction Set, http://techtrain.microchip.com/x14/instruc/

Exploring the Adaptation to Learning Styles: The Case of *AdaptiveLesson* Module for Moodle

Jelena Nakić[1], Sabine Graf[2], and Andrina Granić[1]

[1] University of Split, Faculty of Science, Nikole Tesle 12, 21000 Split, Croatia
[2] Athabasca University, School of Computing & Information Systems, 10011-109 Street, Edmonton, AB T5J-3S8, Canada
{jelena.nakic,andrina.granic}@pmfst.hr,
sabineg@athabascau.ca

Abstract. Understanding learners and acknowledging diversities in their learning behavior is the key to design effective e-learning systems. This paper presents an innovative solution focused on adaptation to learning styles in the context of the learning management system Moodle. A new activity module named *AdaptiveLesson* has been developed as an extension of the *Lesson* module. It simplifies the interface for teachers who are creating lesson content while on the other hand provides students with individually adapted on-line courses in respect to their learning styles. Modifications in adaptive lessons with respect to regular lesson are described and the mechanism for adaptation to learning styles is presented. In order to evaluate the effectiveness of the proposed solution, a pilot evaluation of an on-line course developed by the *AdaptiveLesson* module has been conducted. The experiment is based on the comparison of an adaptive and an equivalent regular course. Results are discussed and guidelines for further research are established.

Keywords: e-learning systems, Moodle lessons, learning styles, adaptive course.

1 Introduction

Research in the academic community confirms that understanding learners and acknowledging diversities in their learning behavior is the key to design effective e-learning systems [3; 12]. The handicap of insufficient presence or even absence of the teacher in modern class needs to be compensated by the capabilities of e-learning systems. A respectable teacher senses the class, knows the capabilities of her/his students and recognizes their current motivational state. Thus she/he can change the approach and adapt the lecture to all these factors trying to engage the most of the students to catch the best of the lecture. A vast number of e-learning systems are developed with the intention to do the same, with more or less success. Among the most widely used systems are Virtual Learning Environments (VLEs) also well known as Learning Management System (LMSs) which support a number of activities for course creation, administration and delivering as well as facilities for

A. Holzinger et al. (Eds.): SouthCHI 2013, LNCS 7946, pp. 534–550, 2013.

communication between participants and sharing information on a course. Besides commercial environments such as Blackboard [1] and Sakai [25], there is a number of open-source systems, for example Moodle [21], Ilias [15], Claroline [6] and others.

It appears that Moodle is one of the most commonly deployed systems as up to February 2013 it has over 66 million of registered users, both teachers and students in 229 countries, using more than 7 million courses [21]. Moodle courses are intended to be learner-centered resources rather than just repositories of documents previously used for face-to-face learning and additionally enriched with on-line tests and communication tools. In addition to existing core facilities (some of them yet poorly exploited, such as the Lesson activity) there is a possibility to develop plugins for supporting a variety of additional resources and activities. For example, a teacher can use the Lesson module to create lessons in form of series of HTML pages which is already a step ahead of the commonly used courses consisting of documents developed elsewhere and imported into Moodle. Another step towards a highly learner-centered course is to enable developing of a new kind of lessons that will be adapted by the LMS to individual characteristics of the students, such as background knowledge, preferences, cognitive abilities, learning styles, preferences, and so on. In this paper one such initiative focused on adaptivity to learning styles is presented along with the first evaluation of an adaptive on-line course.

The paper is structured as follows. The next subsections discuss learning styles definition and description with special attention to the Felder-Silverman learning style model. Section 2 deals with on-line courses in Moodle. Regular lessons designed through the *Lesson* module are introduced followed by the description of the new *AdaptiveLesson* module and lessons that are adapted to learning styles of the students. Modifications in adaptive lessons with respect to regular lessons are described, and the mechanisms for adaptation to learning styles are explained. Section 3 presents the pilot study on effectiveness of the *AdaptiveLesson* module through the first adaptive on-line course implementation. Results are interpreted and discussed in light of related research.

1.1   Learning Styles

A set of attitudes and behaviors which determine an individual's preferred way of learning is considered as a learning style [13]. While there is a number of learning style theories, researchers agree that it is possible to diagnose a student's learning style and that learners with a dominant preference for certain learning style may have difficulties in knowledge acquisition in conditions where their learning styles is not compatible with the teaching strategy [7]. The thesis that incorporation of learning styles in learning environments enables more pleasant learning experience and higher performance of students has inspired development of a number of adaptive educational systems. These implementations employ different learning style models relying on diverse concepts, each proposing distinctive descriptions and classifications of learning types. One of the most popular models of learning styles in adaptive education is Felder-Silverman learning style model, FSLSM [7], implemented for example in CS383 [4], eTeacher [26], INDeLER [16], as well as an add-on for the LMS Moodle [9].

1.2   Felder-Silverman Learning Style Model

FSLSM places student's learning tendencies along four dimensions: sensing/intuitive, visual/verbal, active/reflective and sequential/global.

The sensing/intuitive dimension classifies learners according to the type of information they preferentially perceive: sensing learners prefer concrete information with lots of facts and examples, while intuitive learners learn better from abstract learning material such as theories and principles. As described in Graf *et al.* [11], sensing learners are usually more practically oriented and more patient with details. On the other hand, intuitive learners tend to see relationships between concepts and to discover additional possibilities.

The visual/verbal dimension reflects students' preferred perceptual tendencies: visual learners like to see pictures and graphs while verbal learners learn better what they hear and discuss out loud. Verbal learners also deal better with textual representation of data than visual learners.

The active/reflective dimension considers students' way of processing information, i.e. converting it into knowledge: active learners prefer to be engaged in physical activity, collaborative discussion or any kind of experimentation, while reflective learners benefit from introspection and quiet observation. Active learners learn best by doing any kind of exercise with the learning material, while reflective learners prefer to observe and reflect on the material. Unlike reflective learners who like to learn alone, active learners prefer communication with peers, especially if it includes group work and active discussion.

The sequential/global dimension describes the way learners make progress towards comprehension of the subject: sequential learners proceed through the material in a logical order, usually in the manner the material is presented, while global learners prefer to glance through the whole material and then select the topics to grasp more deeply. Global learners usually master the material by jumping to more complex issues, filling the gaps afterwards. In problem-solving activities, sequential learners usually follow logical steps to find a solution. On the other hand, global learners can solve complex problems using original approaches but they often cannot explain the way they did it.

To assess students' learning style according to FSLSM, the Index of Learning Styles (ILS) is generally used [8]. It contains 44 two choice questions distributed along the four learning style dimensions, where one choice increments and the other decrements the score of the particular dimension. The resulting index of preference for each dimension is expressed by an odd integer, ranging [-11, +11] since 11 questions are posed for each dimensions. The ILS questionnaire provides a very precise quantitative estimation of a learner's preference for each dimension of FSLSM.

Reliability and validity of the ILS questionnaire were confirmed in several studies, as reported in Graf, Liu and Kinshuk [10]. Test-retest reliability studies showed moderate to strong reliability with correlation coefficients between 0.505 and 0.683 for eight-month interval [33] and between 0.60 to 0.78 for a seven-month interval [19].

Regarding internal consistency reliability, literature suggests that Cronbach's alpha coefficient of 0.5 or higher is an acceptable value for attitude-assessing instruments [29]. Several studies showed that the ILS questionnaire met this limit for all dimensions, with Cronbach's alpha values between 0.51 and 0.76 [19; 30; 33], except of one result which showed an alpha value of 0.41 for the sequential/global dimension [30]. Findings of our previous study [23] are in line with those results. Cronbach's alpha coefficient for sequential/global dimension was 0.45. When the weakest item of the instrument is removed, as suggested in Litzinger *et al.* [18] alpha scores 0.48, and after removing two items the alpha value is 0.51. These results confirm that ILS questionnaire can be considered as reliable for sequential/global dimension as well.

Graf, Liu and Kinshuk [10] also reported several studies that support construct validity of the ILS questionnaire and concluded that the ILS questionnaire may be considered as reliable, valid and suitable instrument for measuring learning styles according to FSLSM.

These features of the ILS questionnaire probably led to the fact that FSLSM is one of the most widely used learning style models in adaptive education. Research suggests FSLSM as one of the most appropriate learning style models for application in e-learning systems [4; 17]. In addition to that, Graf *et al.* [11] stressed the advantages of FSLSM over other learning style models. The fact that the model distinguishes between strong and weak preferences for a particular learning style makes it a very suitable theory for application in adaptive systems design and development.

2   Adaptive On-Line Course Design

The Learning Management System (LMS) Moodle enables teachers to create a lesson in form of a series of HTML pages. Lessons are created through the *Lesson* module and consist of content pages and question pages. There are several types of questions available via the *Lesson* module: true/false, multiple choice, numerical, pair matching, short answer, essay, and so on. Teacher can provide a response to a learner's answer and decide what page the learner will see next in case of correct answer, and in case of incorrect answer. After submitting an answer to a question, a student gets appropriate response and follows the path predefined by the teacher.

On the other hand, the content pages can be equipped with several navigation buttons which enable students to choose what page they want to read next. Figure 1 shows a typical content page of a lesson in Moodle. The page content covers the central part of a page; buttons are in beneath of the content, while the map of the lesson is placed on the left. The lesson map contains captions of all content pages as hyperlinks. The question pages are not visible in the map. The teacher decides how many buttons will be on each content page and for each button what is the target page ("jump to"). The "Next page" button allows direct guidance of a student, i.e. he/she will follow the default path determined by the teacher. The other buttons along with map of the lesson allow the students to create their own path through the lesson.

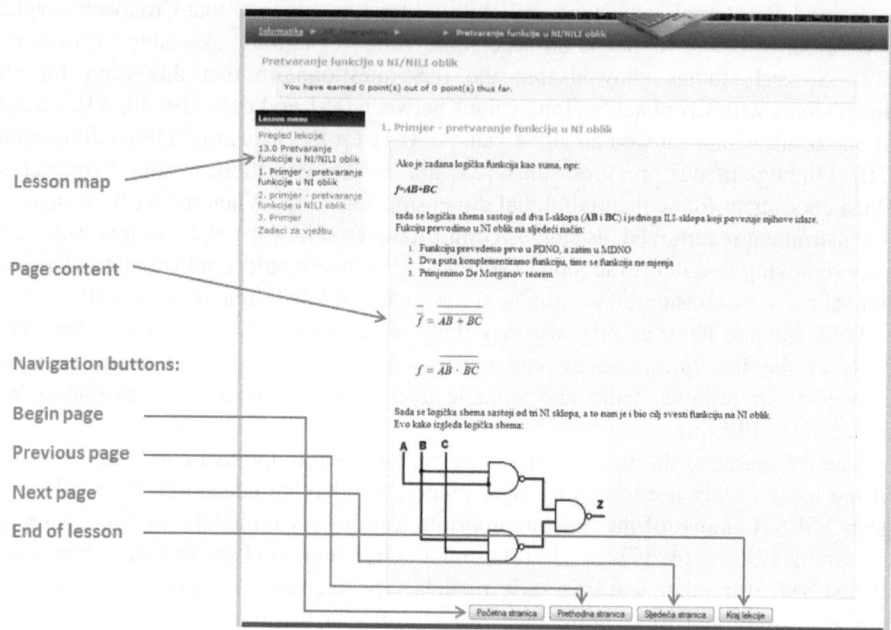

Fig. 1. Interface of a typical content page created by the *Lesson* module

As it allows the students to create a self-directed path through the lesson, the *Lesson* module is often claimed as adaptive [22]. However, in such contexts it could be argued about the claimed "adaptive ability" since this type of adaptivity is quite restricted to learners' knowledge. In order to enable this type of adaptivity teachers are required to do a lot of additional work, besides creating the lesson content, as they have to write captions and target pages for each button on each page and for each question.

The interaction of the teacher and the student with the *Lesson* module is shown in Figure 2a.

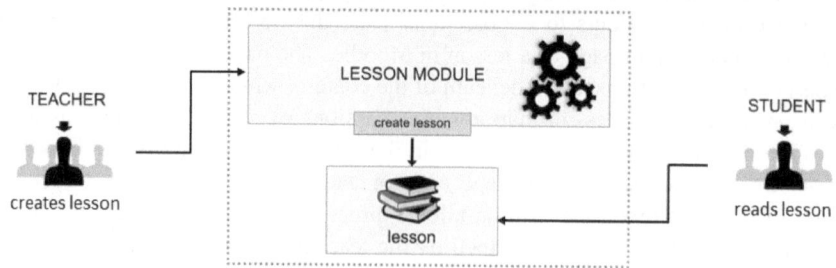

Fig. 2a. Teacher's and student's interaction with the *Lesson* module

To provide advanced adaptive behavior, we have developed a new module called *AdaptiveLesson*, which enables the creation of lessons adapted to the learning styles of students according to FSLSM. Adaptive lessons have several advantages over the regular lessons as the module implements a number of techniques to provide content adaptation as well as adaptive navigation support [2]. At the same time the effort of teachers creating adaptive lessons is reduced in regards to regular lessons. The next subsections bring the *AdaptiveLesson* module description followed by in-depth report on modifications of teacher's and students' interface.

2.1   *AdaptiveLesson* Module Description

The *AdaptiveLesson* module of the LMS Moodle is developed as an extension of the *Lesson* module. In addition, ILS questionnaire, i.e. its translation into Croatian, is integrated in the *AdaptiveLesson* module. A student is required to fill out the questionnaire at his/her first attempt to read an adapted lesson. Once a student fills out the ILS questionnaire, her/his learning style is detected and discrete values of every learning style dimension are stored in the *AdaptiveLesson* module database. Once students have filled out the ILS questionnaire, they can read all the lessons of any adaptive on-line course each time logged in.

Teacher and students have a specific interaction with the module, as shown in Figure 2b. The teacher creates lessons and triggers adaptation. The students fill out the ILS questionnaire, get information about their learning styles and read adaptive lessons.

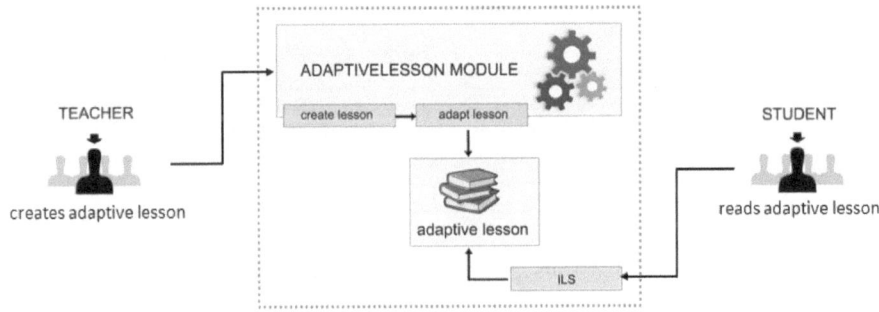

Fig. 2b. Teacher's and student's interaction with *AdaptiveLesson* module

2.2   Modifications for Teachers

In order to unify the interface of all pages, as well as to reduce the effort of teachers, the *AdaptiveLesson* module includes several changes in default settings compared to the *Lesson* module. The number of buttons for each page is set to four, and the text for buttons captions and target pages are filled in by default.

The mechanism for content adaptation is based on different content types. In order to use this mechanism, teachers/course creators are required to annotate a page type as one of the following: example, exercise, outline and theory.

While designing a lesson, the teacher usually determines several examples and exercises that are fundamental for understanding the basics of the lesson. For students who want to learn more, the teacher can prepare a few extra examples as well as additional exercises to be done as a single or group assignment. According to FSLSM, some students prefer more examples while other students prefer more problem-solving activities [7]. Those extra pages are considered for adaptation to learning styles. With that purpose, the teacher's interface for creating a content page is supplied with a checkbox for annotation of a content page as optional. The checkbox is enabled for examples and exercises, but disabled for outline and theory. Figure 3 shows the new items on teacher's interface for creating or editing a content page.

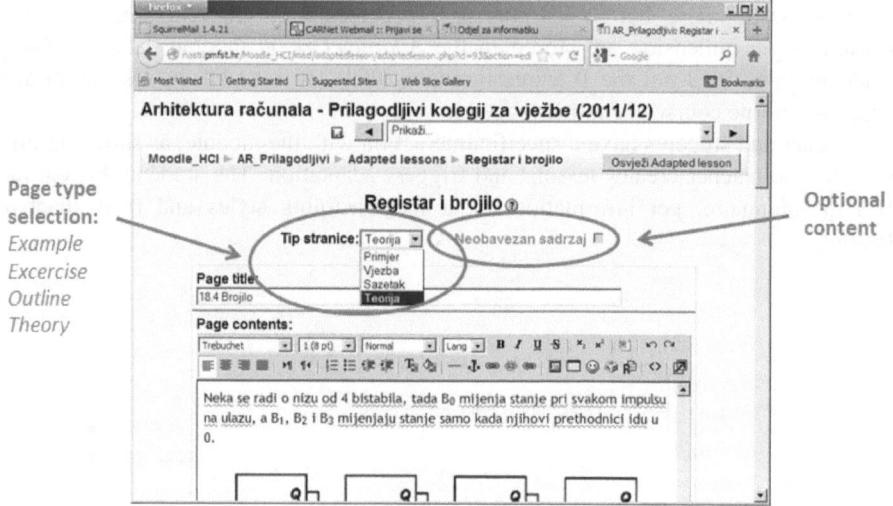

Fig. 3. Interface for creating or editing a content page of an adaptive lesson

The question pages are used occasionally throughout the lesson in order to provide self-assessment for students. In the *AdaptiveLesson* module no changes have been conducted in the interface for creating question pages.

Upon creation of all pages of the lesson, both the content pages and the question pages, the teacher triggers the adaptation algorithm. Figure 4 shows a new "Adapt lesson" tab with a button for triggering the adaptation of the lesson. Adaptation algorithm performs several techniques for adaptive presentation and adaptive navigation support [2] thus creating an adapted course as described in the next subsection.

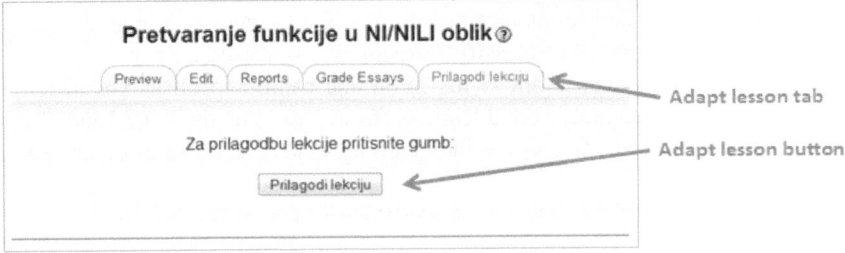

Fig. 4. Interface for triggering the adaptation algorithm

2.3   Modifications for Students

Two types of modifications have been done for the students' interface in the *AdaptiveLesson* module. First, modifications were done in order to provide students with adaptive courses that fit their learning styles, as described in more detail in the next subsection. Second, a few modifications were done for students regardless of their learning styles. Those modifications of students' interface are designed upon results of our previous study on navigation behavior of students while learning from regular Moodle lessons [23]. Those lessons were supplied by several navigation tools, but the study showed that the "Next" button is the most frequently used navigation tool for students, independent of their learning styles. This supports the decision to enlarge the "Next" button on all pages, for each learning style, as shown in Figure 5a. This feature prevents accidentally clicking on other buttons and improves students' navigation through the lesson.

Another improvement of students' interface is made in the *AdaptiveLesson* module. In contrast to the *Lesson* module, all question pages are shown in a lesson map, which improves students' orientation through the lesson, regardless of their learning styles. Visibility of the question pages enables students to reach any question any time they want, thus supporting navigational possibilities. Position of the questions inside the lesson structure depends on students' learning styles, so the next page a student will see after the correct answer is determined by the adaptive path of the lesson for each student.

Adaptivity Mechanisms. This subsection describes the modifications of the students' interface in order to provide them with courses that fit their learning styles. According to the ILS results, students are classified into several categories. For example, for active/reflective dimension, we refer learners who scored from -11 to -5 as active, those who scored from -3 to 3 as balanced between active and reflective, and those who scored from 5 to 11 as reflective learners. In the same way, the learners are categorized along sequential/global dimension as sequential, balanced and global learners.

Adaptation to visual/verbal dimension implies the existence of two different modes of presentation for the same content. Thus we do not consider any learner as balanced between visual and verbal, but classify learners as visual (scored from -11 to -7 on ILS) and moderately visual (from -5 to -1) on one hand, as well as verbal learners (from 7 to 11) and moderately verbal learners (from 1 to 5) on the other hand. Table 1 presents the distribution of ILS scores into learning styles categories as described.

Table 1. The distribution of ILS scores into learning styles categories

active	balanced between active and reflective		reflective
-11 -9 -7 -5 -3	-3 -1 1 3		5 7 9 11
visual	moderately visual	moderately verbal	verbal
-11 -9 -7	-5 -3 -1	1 3 5	7 9 11
sequential	balanced between sequential and global		global
-11 -9 -7 -5	-3 -1 1 3		5 7 9 11

The module does not have any adaptive features for sensing/intuitive dimension. Such adaptation would have additional requirements for teachers creating a lesson (for example to annotate the percentage of facts and concrete data in the page content). We assumed it would be very difficult for teachers and their motivation to make adaptive content could decrease to a great extent if this dimension would be added.

Adaptation to active/reflective dimension. The adaptation algorithm implements adaptive selection of pages for active and reflective learners and ensures pages to display in a corresponding order according to a certain type of learner. These techniques are known as adaptive content selection and adaptive sorting of pages, and they are widely applied in adaptive hypermedia [2; 3].

According to Felder and Silverman (1988), active learners are comfortable with problem-solving activities and group discussions, they prefer answering questions and doing exercises but less theory and examples. In contrary, reflective learners learn by reflecting on the matter and thinking things through. Thus, they are introduced with the theory pages first and examples afterwards. Exercises are following, but the number of exercises is limited and only obligatory exercises are recommended for reflective learners. If there are any optional exercises in the lesson, reflective students will see them at the bottom of the lesson map and annotated as additional pages. Those pages are adaptively annotated by different link color thus improving students' orientation through the lesson. Page layout for an active student is shown on Figure 5a, and for a reflective student on Figure 5b. The differences in page layout for active and reflective learners are shown in terms of selection of recommended pages and page ordering.

A student whose learning style is balanced between active and reflective see the lesson pages in default order as determined by the teacher.

Adaptation to visual/verbal dimension. Content adaptation is enabled by using two different modes of presentation wherever possible, namely text and graphics for the same learning concept. Visual students are presented with parallel modes of presentation, having graphics shown by default while accompanying text is hidden. Students can "stretch out" or "stretch in" the textual explanation by clicking on the link. Visual learners cannot hide graphics. The page layout for visual learning style is shown on Figure 5b. Moderately visual learners have an additional link to hide/show graphics. They can hide graphics if they have too much items on a page after stretching out a lot of text. This option seems to be very convenient for pages rich with content.

Adaptation for verbal and moderately verbal learners works in a similar way. Graphics are hidden by default, while textual explanation is stretched out. Verbal learners see the textual explanation all the time (Figure 5a), while moderately verbal learners have an option to stretch the text in.

Adaptation to sequential/global dimension. According to FSLSM, sequential learners tend to learn in small incremental steps, mastering the learning content in the presented order. They might have difficulties in learning if using learner control tools frequently, as also confirmed in [23]. As the findings of the study suggest, sequential learners who jumped a lot through the lesson achieved lower learning outcomes compared to sequential learners who followed the linear path through the lesson.

To restrict navigation possibilities for sequential learners, the left menu is hidden by default but available via hyperlink on the left side on the lesson page. Once stretched out, the left menu can be hidden again. For students balanced between sequential and global, the left menu is always visible, i.e. without option to be hidden, thus enabling students to browse all the pages of the lesson (Figure 5b). Finally, adaptation for global learners is accomplished by vertically displaying left menus of all lessons of a course theme on each page (Figure 5a). Thus global learners get the "big picture" of the subject and can randomly jump from one lesson to another inside a theme representing a chapter of the course. For global learners all the left menus are always visible.

In addition to that, the enlarged "Next" button is expected to be beneficial to sequential learners. This feature is accepted to encourage sequential learners to follow the path that the *AdaptiveLesson* module has recommended for them with respect to other dimensions of their learning styles.

Flexibility for Students. The module implements soft adaptivity, meaning that all adaptivity features are very flexible. The students can easily ignore some of the features recommended for their learning styles and activate them later. There are two reasons supporting this decision. First, FSLSM is based on tendencies, indicating that even learners with a high preference for a certain behavior can act sometimes differently, enabling the learning style model to consider exceptional behavior. Second, the ILS questionnaire is very sensitive and one wrong answer can classify a student to a different category of a learning style dimension or even to a different learning style (e.g. moderately verbal instead of moderately visual). It is possible that a student

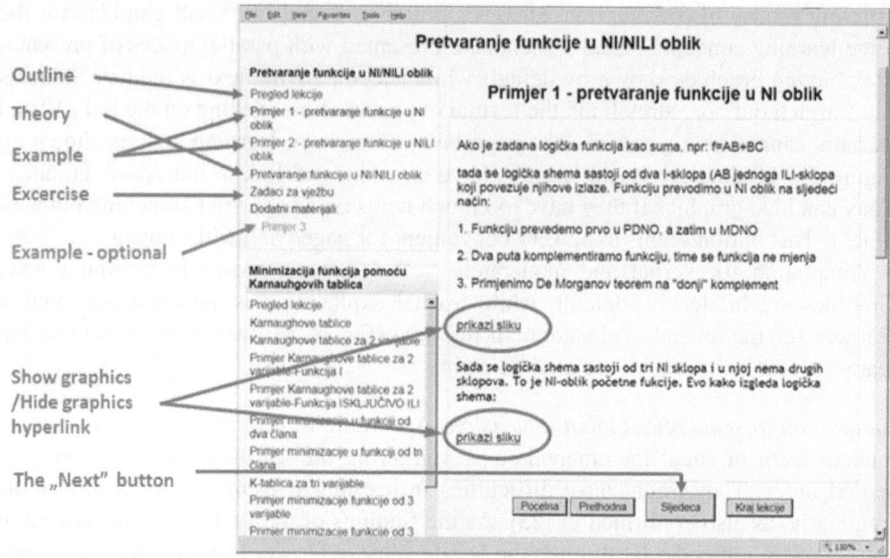

Fig. 5a. Page layout for student with active, verbal and global learning style

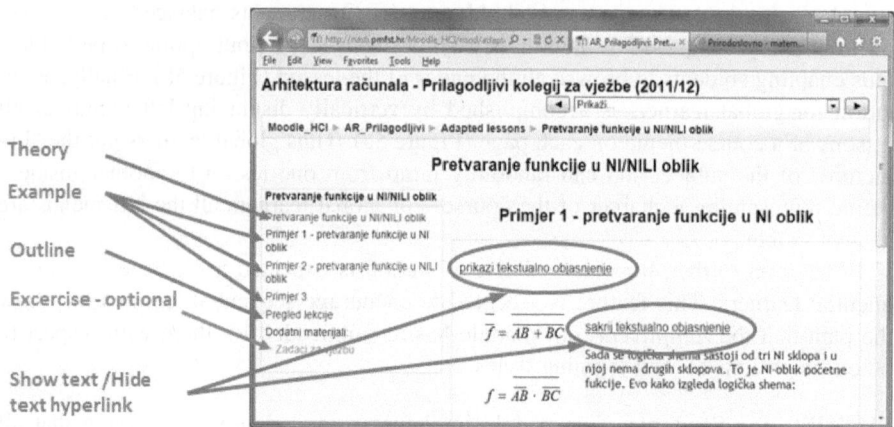

Fig. 5b. Page layout for student with reflective and visual learning style. A student has balanced learning style between sequential and global.

accidentally provides a wrong answer, but on the other hand it is true that some students do not feel like properly fill-out the questionnaire. They simply do not provide answers that are describing them in the best, thus their resulting learning styles are not reliable.

For these reasons, we have offered to the students the freedom not to follow recommended content. This is the option they can use occasionally in some situations or constantly through the whole course.

3   Evaluation of an Adaptive On-Line Course: A Pilot Study

The first evaluation of *AdaptiveLesson* module effectiveness was conducted in the spring semester 2011/12 at University in Split, Croatia, Faculty of Science. The study was carried out in the Computer Architecture class which is supported by two on-line courses developed and delivered via Moodle: a regular course consisted of lessons built by *Lesson* module, and an adaptive course consisted of lessons built by *AdaptiveLesson* module. The study examines the hypothesis that learning in an environment that matches students' learning styles results in higher learning outcomes than learning in an environment that does not match learning styles of the students.

3.1   Experimental Procedure

The class had total enrollment of 83 undergraduate second-year students and 67 of them have taken the class for the first time. These students have been considered as participants of the study and were assigned to one of three groups, controlled by background knowledge calculated from students' grades on five previously passed exams on Computer Science during the first year of their study. Because of the small number of participants, to eliminate the influence of background knowledge to learning outcomes, all of the students were first categorized into three groups according to their background knowledge: novice, intermediate and experts. After that the students from each group were randomly assigned to one of the three groups for the experiment. One group of students was enrolled in the regular course, referred to as standard group, while two groups were enrolled in the adaptive course as follows. The first group of students was enrolled using their actual learning styles (referred to as matched group) and the second group was enrolled using the opposite learning style categories for all dimensions of learning styles (referred to as mismatched group). For example, a student classified as active, visual and global learner was provided with a course for reflective, verbal and sequential learners. The students were not aware of belonging to a particular group while the experiment was carried out.

Participants were learning introductory concepts on both on-line Computer Architecture courses on Moodle, the regular and the adaptive course. The first three out of twenty lessons of the courses were considered as part of the pilot experiment. The content of all respective lessons of two different courses was exactly the same, and this content was not presented to students in any other way or from any other resources outside these courses.

The students' scores from mid-term and final exams were taken as the measures for learning outcomes. Only the answers to the first and the second question of these exams are taken into account since only those questions dealt with content taught in the experiment. The criterion variables were (i) the scores on the first and the second question in mid-term exam and (ii) the scores on the first and the second question in final exam.

3.2   Data Set

Since some of the students did not attend the mid-term and/or the final exam, a total of 61 datasets were completed and analyzed. Data analysis was performed using SPSS 16.0 software statistical package. The number and percentage of students in each category of learning styles is shown in Table 2.

Table 2. The frequencies of learning styles in the sample

active	balanced between active and reflective		reflective
10	47		4
16.4%	77.0%		6.6%
visual	moderately visual	moderately verbal	verbal
21	23	15	2
34.4%	37.7%	24.6%	3.3%
sequential	balanced between sequential and global		global
6	55		0
9.8%	90.2%		0.0%

There were 23 male (38%) and 38 female (62%) students in the sample. The standard group consisted of 18 students, matched group of 23 and mismatched group of 20 students.

3.3   Results

One-way ANOVA is used to compare the means of standard, matched and mismatched group. The significance level of 0.05 was adopted for the study. The results are shown in Table 3.

Analysis showed no statistically significant difference between groups in respect to background knowledge, confirming that the influence of background knowledge to criteria variables is eliminated.

Criteria variables q11 and q12 represents the scores on question 1 and question 2 on mid-term exam, while q21 and q22 represents the scores on question 1 and question 2 on final exam. Sums are calculated as follows: Sum1=q11+q12, Sum2=q21+q22, thus Sum1 is related to mid-term exam as the first students' attempt to answer the questions, and Sum2 refers to final exam as the second attempt to answer related questions. Data analysis has shown no statistically significant differences between standard, matched and mismatched group in respect to all criteria variables.

Table 3. One-way ANOVA by learning styles categories

		Sum of Squares	df	Mean Square	F	Sig.
Background	Between Groups	53,411	2	26,705	,857	,430
	Within Groups	1807,901	58	31,171		
	Total	1861,311	60			
q11	Between Groups	196,332	2	98,166	2,499	,091
	Within Groups	2278,685	58	39,288		
	Total	2475,016	60			
q12	Between Groups	9,663	2	4,832	,098	,906
	Within Groups	2845,189	58	49,055		
	Total	2854,852	60			
q21	Between Groups	27,287	2	13,644	,287	,752
	Within Groups	2756,352	58	47,523		
	Total	2783,639	60			
q22	Between Groups	1,815	2	,908	,017	,983
	Within Groups	3147,267	58	54,263		
	Total	3149,082	60			
Sum1	Between Groups	177,674	2	88,837	,692	,504
	Within Groups	7441,113	58	128,295		
	Total	7618,787	60			
Sum2	Between Groups	38,859	2	19,429	,128	,880
	Within Groups	8778,387	58	151,352		
	Total	8817,246	60			

4   Discussion and Concluding Remarks

There are two limitations of presented research that have to be acknowledged. The limitations are caused by uncontrollable factors of the study which could have affected the obtained results. First, the *AdaptiveLesson* module enables students to not follow recommended content. This flexibility allows the students not to behave as expected according to their ILS scores. Although FSLSM indicates that students can act sometimes differently from their primary tendencies, we can assume that some students have used this possibility more often than the others: first, the students who did not carefully and accurately fill out the ILS questionnaire, and second, the students who have been assigned to mismatched group.

The second limitation of the study is the fact that students' learning achievements on the studied lessons were measured with a significant delay in respect to time of learning. The mid-term exam was four weeks and the final exam ten weeks after the learning sessions included in the study. This additional time enabled students to consult other resources besides the on-line resources that were recommended for them in the course.

Limitations of the study can be addressed as follows. Monitoring student's behavior is suggested to dynamically check the use of adaptivity features and update students' learning styles according to their learning behavior. The flexibility of the system is a desirable feature and should be preserved in order to provide a high level of learner control. Moreover, to support students' learning styles better, the system should be able to recognize the navigation and behavior patterns that are in line with particular learning styles and dynamically compute the new values of learning styles. To address the second limitation, learning outcomes have to be measured immediately after the learning session. A pre-test should also be involved in the study to enable more accurate measuring of learning outcomes on particular lessons. In addition to that, inclusion of the time limit for learning session would probably decrease the influence of flexibility of the system to learning outcomes. If all the students have equal time for learning, we can conclude that students in standard group and even more in mismatched group would spend some time to find the resources that fit to their learning styles. Consequently, these students would have less time for reading those resources which could affect their learning outcomes. We conclude that the *Adaptive-Lesson* module enables teachers to easily create on-line courses that adapt to learning styles of the students. Compared to the *Lesson* module, the effort of teachers creating adaptive lessons is reduced. The teachers can create adaptive lessons without any knowledge about learning styles definition or identification methods. Once the lesson is finished, teacher triggers the adaptation algorithm and the *AdaptiveLesson* module automatically adapts the content presentation as well as navigation options to learning styles according to FSLSM.

Although the adaptation mechanism strictly follows the theory of FSLSM, the pilot evaluation has shown no evidence of higher effectiveness of adaptive over regular Moodle lessons. The findings are in-line with related research where objective standard criteria such as learning outcomes usually fail to find a difference between adaptive and non-adaptive versions of a system [32]. Compared to studies with a similar design such as Graf and Kinshuk [9] we conclude that the lack of significant difference in learning outcomes occurred due to the fact that students had the flexibility to use all resources of the adaptive course in the way that suits for them the best. There is a high probability that students were quite aware of how they prefer to learn and they were using the flexibility that we provided them with. Research on improvements of criteria to find the valid indicators of interaction quality or adaptivity success is on-going and the new criteria are proposed [27; 28]. Acknowledging also a number of subjective criteria, e.g. user perception, motivation and satisfaction, complementary approaches to evaluation of adaptive systems are emerging suggesting the using of usability evaluation methods such as usability testing and heuristic evaluation [20; 24].

The advantage of presented research compared to similar studies is that the comparison of adaptive and non-adaptive lessons is grounded on fair basis as required in literature [14; 31]. The study contributes to the body of knowledge on adaptive education, as well as on methods of evaluation of adaptive systems.

Further research needs to be conducted in controlled conditions that address the lessons learned from the limitations of pilot experiment. A number of qualitative criteria regarding user motivation and satisfaction should be included in future studies.

Acknowledgments. This work has been carried out within project 177-0361994-1998 *Usability and Adaptivity of Interfaces for Intelligent Authoring Shells* funded by the Ministry of Science and Technology of the Republic of Croatia.

References

1. Blackboard, http://www.blackboard.com, (last accessed February 1, 2013)
2. Brusilovsky, P.: Adaptive Hypermedia. User Modeling and User-Adapted Interaction 11(1-2), 87–110 (2001)
3. Brusilovsky, P., Millán, E.: User Models for Adaptive Hypermedia and Adaptive Educational Systems. In: Brusilovsky, P., Kobsa, A., Nejdl, W. (eds.) Adaptive Web 2007. LNCS, vol. 4321, pp. 3–53. Springer, Heidelberg (2007)
4. Carver, C.A., Howard, R.A., Lane, W.D.: Addressing different learning styles through course hypermedia. IEEE Transactions on Education 42, 33–38 (1999)
5. Chin, D.: Empirical evaluation of user models and user-adapted systems. User Modeling and User-Adapted Interaction 11(1-2), 181–194 (2001)
6. Claroline, http://www.claroline.net (last accessed February 1, 2013)
7. Felder, R.M., Silverman, L.K.: Learning and Teaching Styles in Engineering Education. Engineering Education 78(7), 674–681 (1988)
8. Felder, R.M., Soloman, B.A.: Index of learning styles questionnaire (1997), http://www.engr.ncsu.edu/learningstyles/ilsweb.html (retrieved January 11, 2013)
9. Graf, S.: Providing adaptive courses in learning management systems with respect to learning styles. In: Proceedings of the World Conference on E-learning in Corporate, Government, Healthcare, and Higher Education (E-learn), pp. 2576–2583. AACE Press, Chesapeake (2007)
10. Graf, S., Liu, T.C.: Kinshuk: Analysis of learners' navigational behaviour and their learning styles in an online course. Journal of Computer Assisted Learning 26(2), 116–131 (2010)
11. Graf, S., Liu, T.-C., Kinshuk, C.N.-S., Yang, S.J.H.: Learning Styles and Cognitive Traits - Their Relationship and its Benefits in Web-based Educational Systems. Computers in Human Behavior 25(6), 1280–1289 (2009)
12. Granić, A., Nakić, J.: Enhancing the Learning Experience: Preliminary Framework for User Individual Differences. In: Leitner, G., Hitz, M., Holzinger, A. (eds.) USAB 2010. LNCS, vol. 6389, pp. 384–399. Springer, Heidelberg (2010)
13. Honey, P., Mumford, A.: The Manual of Learning Styles. Peter Honey Publications, Maidenhead (1992)
14. Höök, K.: Steps to take before intelligent user interfaces become real. Interacting with Computers 12(4), 409–426 (2000)
15. Ilias, http://www.ilias.de (last accessed February 1, 2013)
16. Jovanović, D., Milošević, D., Žižović, M.: INDeLER: eLearning Personalization by Mapping Student's learning Style and Preference to Metadata. International Journal of Emerging Technologies in Learning 3(4), 41–50 (2008)

17. Kuljis, J., Liu, F.: A comparison of learning style theories on the suitability for elearning. In: Proceedings of the IASTED Conference on Web Technologies, Applicationsand Services (2005)

18. Litzinger, T.A., Lee, S.H., Wise, J.C., Felder, R.M.: A Study of the Reliability and Validity of the Felder-Solomon Index of Learning Styles. In: Proceedings of the 2005 American Society for Engineering Education Annual Conference & Exposition (2005)

19. Livesay, G.A., Dee, K.C., Nauman, E.A., Hites, L.S.: Engineering student learning styles: a statistical analysis using Felder's Index of Learning Styles. Presented at the Annual Conference of the American Society for Engineering Education, Montreal, Canada (June 2002)

20. Magoulas, G.D., Chen, S.Y., Papanikolaou, K.A.: Integrating layered and heuristic evaluation for adaptive learning environments. In: Brusilovsky, P., Corbett, A.T., de Rosis, F. (eds.) UM 2003. LNCS, vol. 2702, pp. 5–14. Springer, Heidelberg (2003)

21. Moodle, http://moodle.org (last accessed February 1, 2013)

22. Moodle Docs, http://docs.moodle.org/24/en/Lesson_module (last accessed February 1, 2013)

23. Nakić, J., Marangunić, N., Granić, A.: Learning Styles and Navigation Patterns in Web-Based Education. In: Stephanidis, C. (ed.) Universal Access in HCI, Part IV, HCII 2011. LNCS, vol. 6768, pp. 587–596. Springer, Heidelberg (2011)

24. Paramythis, A., Weibelzahl, S., Masthoff, J.: Layered Evaluation of Interactive Adaptive Systems: Framework and Formative Methods. User Modeling and User-Adapted Interaction 20(5), 383–453 (2010)

25. Sakai, http://www.sakaiproject.org/portal (last accessed February 1, 2013)

26. Schiaffino, S., Garcia, P., Amandi, A.: eTeacher: providing personalized assistance to e-learning students. Computers & Education 51(4), 1744–1754 (2008)

27. Tarpin-Bernard, F., Marfisi-Schottman, I., Habieb-Mammar, H.: AnAmeter: The first steps to evaluating adaptation. In: 6th Workshop on User-Centred Design and Evaluation of Adaptive Systems at UMAP 2009, pp. 11–20. CEUR, Trento (2009)

28. Tobar, C.M.: Yet Another Evaluation Framework. In: Brusilovsky, P., Corbett, A.T., de Rosis, F. (eds.) UM 2003. LNCS, vol. 2702, pp. 15–24. Springer, Heidelberg (2003)

29. Tuckman, B.W.: Conducting Educational Research, 5th edn. Wadsworth Group (1999)

30. Van Zwanenberg, N., Wilkinson, L.J., Anderson, A.: Felder and Silverman's Index of Learning Styles and Honey and Mumford's Learning Styles Questionnaire: how do they compare and do they predict academic performance? Educational Psychology 20, 365–380 (2000)

31. Weibelzahl, S.: Problems and pitfalls in evaluating adaptive systems. In: 4th Workshop on the Evaluation of Adaptive Systems at UM 2005, Edinburgh, UK, pp. 57–66 (2005)

32. Weibelzahl, S., Lippitsch, S., Weber, G.: Advantages, opportunities, and limits of empirical evaluations: Evaluating adaptive systems. Künstliche Intelligenz 3(2), 17–20 (2002)

33. Zywno, M.S.: A contribution to validation of score meaning for Felder–Soloman's Index of Learning Styles. Presented at the Annual Conference of the American Society for Engineering Education, Nashville, USA (June 2003)

Design and Evaluation of a Learner-Centric Immersive Virtual Learning Environment for Physics Education

Johanna Pirker[1], Christian Gütl[1,2], John Winston Belcher[3], and Philip H. Bailey[3]

[1] Graz University of Technology, Austria
{jpirker,cguelt}@iicm.edu
[2] Curtin University of Technology, Australia
cguelt@iicm.edu
[3] Massachusetts Institute of Technology, United States
{jbelcher,pbailey}@mit.edu

Abstract. There is a growing interest in virtual immersive environments such as virtual worlds for gaming, socialization, and also learning purpose. Frequently three major issues are mentioned, when using 3D worlds for educational scenarios: high technical requirements, low user acceptance and missing technical know-how. The last two issues can be decreased using an elaborate user-centric design with focus on the pedagogical objectives to improve the user experience and enhance the usability. This paper discusses design principles for immersive, three-dimensional environments and in-world tools with focus on pedagogical aspects and presents based on these principles an implementation of a virtual world environment for physics education which integrates the pedagogical model TEAL. A first showcase was built in Open Wonderland and evaluated and tested by student groups and domain experts with focus on usability and pedagogical ambitions. The evaluation shows how the implementation of a learning-centric model focusing on the pedagogical main objectives and designed in-line with the usability guidelines can minimize issues such as user acceptance and missing technical know-how.

Keywords: Virtual World, Open Wonderland, Physics Education, TEALsim, TEAL, Collaborative Learning, Usability Heuristics, Learner-Centric Design.

1 Introduction

While three-dimensional virtual worlds (VW) for games such as Word of Warcraft or for social platforms as Second Life are already widely used, VWs with learning and teaching purpose are seen quite controversially by learners and teachers [1][2]. In particular, interactive activities, such as synchronous collaborations and training, or immersive, three-dimensional experiences, are increasingly attracting features in line with modern, interactive enhanced pedagogical scenarios and advanced requirements.

Physics education, for instance, integrates learning, understanding and application of formulas, concepts and phenomena. The TEAL (Technology-Enabled Active Learning) model, implemented at the Massachusetts Institute of Technology, uses

A. Holzinger et al. (Eds.): SouthCHI 2013, LNCS 7946, pp. 551–561, 2013.

different interactive and collaborative activities and advanced three-dimensional si-mulations and desktop experiments to teach freshmen physics. This approach focuses on two main aspects. First, students are motivated to discuss and solve problems to-gether to develop a common knowledge. Second, it enables students to conduct hands-on experiments and use advanced simulation software to enhance the concep-tual understanding [1]. But not many institutions can afford the resources and physical environments necessary to benefit from this approach. By integrating the entire peda-gogical model with an immersive virtual world environment, not only a cost-effective, but also a remote e-solution can be provided. However, using three-dimensional worlds for education, frequently three major challenges are mentioned in the literature [2]. First, users need modern PCs, with advanced graphics cards and a good internet connection. Second, it is important to motivate the users, so that they like and want to use the system and also see a reason to use it. Third, many users still need to learn how to use a three-dimensional environment. The last two issues can be decreased by improving the user experience and enhancing the usability. Hence, it is necessary to develop an elaborate user-centric design with focus on the pedagogical purposes.

The question rises how can we integrate an entire teaching model into a three-dimensional environment in line with usability-heuristics? How well are TEAL's objectives met in the virtual environment in comparison to the traditional hands-on model? This paper aims to discuss design principles and problems of virtual worlds, assess how a teaching approach, such as TEAL, can be integrated into a VW envi-ronment, sustaining the defined usability requirements and to evaluate the outcomes of a first showcase in the domain of electrodynamics. To this end a model to enable remote, synchronous, collaborative learning activities based on the pedagogical model TEAL in a virtual world environment has been developed. This VW model of TEAL is referred to as Virtual TEAL World (VTW) [3].

The structure of this paper is divided into three parts. First, the design process and according requirements to integrate the TEAL model into a virtual world framework are introduced. The design process focuses on being in line with the pedagogical prin-ciples and usability heuristics, especially defined for virtual world environments and in-world tools. In the second part the VTW model and a first prototype in Open Won-derland are introduced. The third part focuses on the evaluation of this prototype. It was studied by logging activities, conducted surveys and interviews with four student groups, one physicist and one physics instructor. We discuss how the technology of virtual worlds supports the learning process and how the user experience was in line with the designed user heuristics.

2   Background

There is an increasing number of initiatives and research trying to improve today's STEM (science, technology, engineering, and mathematics) education. But designing a pedagogical model, which motivates and helps students, but which also does not frustrate teachers or exceed a moderate budget, is a challenging task. Many modern approaches are using interactive and engaging learning activities to impart the required knowledge. Examples for teaching models are interactive engagement, introduced by Hake [4], Mazur's peer instruction [5] or ranking tasks [6]. A very successful approach in the field physics education is the TEAL model [1]. As a learner-centric approach, it is designed to focus on the needs of the students and supports different learning types and styles [7]. All the different activities and tools used by TEAL, such as the simulation framework TEALsim, were carefully designed and implemented to enable the entire experience [8]. In [9] and [1] advantages and issues of the integration of the single modules of the TEAL approach into a 3D virtual world environment are discussed.

Many studies and research projects provide information about learning environments in 3D virtual worlds [1][2][10] but say little about the design principles or used usability heuristics to integrate a particular teaching model and according necessary tools with the VW. The main research interests in literature are design strategies of 3D virtual learning environments (VLE), strategies to engage the users and implementation of different learning scenarios and application examples. Saleeb and Dafoulas [11], for instance, discuss architectural design aspects, such as room and interior specification of VLEs. Schmeil, Eppler and Freitas [12] provide a high-level framework for the design of avatar-based collaborations, but do not address usability principles.

Muñoz, Barcelos and Chalegre [13] propose 16 usability heuristics with a mapping to Nielsen's 10 heuristics [14]: (1) feedback, (2) clarity, (3) consistency, (4) simplicity, (5) orientation and navigation, (6) control camera and visualization, (7) low memory load, (8) avatar's customization, (9) flexibility and efficiency of use, (10) communication between avatars, (11) sense of ownership, (12) interaction with the VW, (13) support to learning, (14) error prevention, (15) helps users to recover from errors, (16) help and documentation. However, this mapping focuses on heuristics for the entire environment and interactions with the VW, but does not address user interactions with in-world tools and scenarios. Due to the lack of missing usability principles, also guidelines how to evaluate VLEs with focus on the pedagogical models are missing. In particular, quantitative methods, such as logging data, or qualitative evaluations from experts were used in previous studies [15].

3   Design Principles

To design and develop a learner-centric environment addressing human interaction, design principles and requirements were identified and updated following an iterative approach [2]. It is important that already in early iterations the pedagogical design model is in-line with usability principles. Therefore, the requirement definition was conducted in two steps. First, usability-centric design principles were defined, which should apply for the entire environment, but also for the tools within the environment. Second, TEAL's main objectives were identified and design principles were separated and adapted to be in-line with the usability-centric design principles. These requirements and design elements were updated after each iteration step.

Usability Heuristics for 3D Virtual World Environments. Designing a 3D virtual environment is a challenging process, which should not only address technical issues, such as the rendering performance, but should also approach the issues user acceptance and usability failures. User studies show that disorienting navigation, complex user action, and annoying occlusions can slow performance in the real world as well in a three-dimensional environments and interfaces [16].

Based on a literature study, different usability requirements adapted from [2][13][16], which are valid for virtual worlds, but also for in-world tools, were identified and selected and on the basis of Nielson's usability heuristics [14] sorted and adapted. Nielson's usability heuristcs was used as a common basis to combine VW-specific 3D elements with in-world 2D tools. The extended and revised list of Nielson's heuristics, which is based on [3], can be used as guideline for designing three-dimensional virtual world interfaces and environments and the according tools and scenarios:

- *(H1) Feedback and visibility of system status:* The VW system should give users appropriate feedback within reasonable time about what is going on at the moment. Users should be aware of potential in-world activities and interactions with other objects and users [13].
- *(H2) Match between system and the real world:* A common language familiar and easy understandable to the user should be chosen. Following real-world conventions and adapting the VW to familiar systems and environments [2] helps the user in understanding the system. Asynchronous and synchronous remote collaboration should be enabled [16] and should be analogue to real world interactions [13].
- *(H3) User control and freedom:* User actions and interactions should be intuitive and reversible. A history should be provided, so that users are able to record, undo and replay actions. Different actions on object (such as saving, copying, annotating, sharing or sending) should be possible [16]. The navigation must be intuitive and memorable [13]. In particular, three-dimensional objects require adapted manipulations. X-ray vision should be provided to see into or beyond objects. Semantic zooming and movement should be supported to focus on the objects' front and center to reveal more details [16].
- *(H4) Consistency and standards:* The VW system, situations and interactions must be consistent in all aspects [13]. Also, the design and usage of the different in-world tools should be similar constructed.
- *(H5) Error prevention:* A careful design should prevent users from making mistakes in the first place [13].
- *(H6) Recognition rather than recall:* The user's memory load should be minimized by making places, objects, actions, and options visible. Explanatory text should be controllable on demand by users by adding, for instance, pop-up or floating elements. Places inside the VW should be easily accessable using landmark indexes. An overview, such as a map, should be provided to the users, so that they can see the big picture [16] [13].

- *(H7) Flexibility and efficiency of use:* Accelerators and editable interfaces should be provided or definable to enhance the efficiency of the interactions for advanced users [13]. Novel 3D icons to represent concepts that are more recognizable and memorable should be developed. Users should be able to shift the context rapidly. Hence, teleportation should be possible [16].
- *(H8) Aesthetic and minimalist design:* Dialogues should not contain irrelevant information. The VW should not contain objects or actions, which are not or rarely needed. Control panels should be well-arranged and not overloaded [13].
- *(H9) Help users recognize, diagnose, and recover from errors:* Error messages must provide the user relevant information about the problem and how to solve it in plain language [13].
- *(H10) Help and documentation:* Help and documentation must be easily accessible not only online, but also inside the VW [13]. Explanatory pop-ups or floating elements can give such information about specific objects or actions [16].

Design Principles of the TEAL Model. The TEAL approach uses different concepts and teaching methods with the four different pedagogical main concepts (1) collaborative learning, (2) hands-on experiments, (3) media-rich software and simulations, and (4) information. Table 1 gives an overview of the single concepts and the according objectives. Different cycle steps were defined and assigned to the concepts, objectives and pedagogical tools. This step facilitates the in-world implementation. The three main objectives (1) basic knowledge acquisition, (2) enhancement of the conceptual understanding and (3) measurement of the learning progress can be cycled for the different learning concepts. These objectives can be used to build functional requirements, which should be in-line with the defined usability heuristics and form the basis of the pedagogical scenario in the virtual world environment. This scenario consists of different activities and required instruments, which can be construed from the concepts and pedagogical tools. Figure 2 gives an overview of the single conversion processes. Based on this representation three main design objectives of the learning model can be identified [3].

- *Interactivity*: In particular, interactive elements should raise the students' interests and motivation. Simulations of physical phenomena should enhance their conceptual understanding.
- *Collaborative tasks*: Collaborative in-world tasks, such as brainstorming or the joint discussion of concept questions raise the students' understanding and their motivation. Different tools such as collaborative whiteboards should enhance collaboration possibilities and motivation.
- *Assessability*: Instructors should be able to follow the students' activities and answered questions to measure the actual learning progress.

The identified requirements enable the implementation of different physics courses with different learning content based on the TEAL approach in a VW environment.

Table 1. Overview of the single TEAL components, concepts and simplified cycle steps [17][3]

Cycle Step	Objective	Concepts	Pedagogical Tool
Prior class	Preparation	Textbook reading	
1	Basic knowledge acquisition	Instructions	Oral explanation Course notes
2	Enhancement of the conceptual understanding	Experiments, simulations and visualizations, discussion about concept questions and assignments	Collaborative learning (Collaboration) Networked laptops (Hands-on experiments) Media-rich software – TEALsim (Simulations) Concept questions
3	Measurement of learning progress	Quizzes, assignments	Concept questions (PRS) Assessment
After class	Consolidation	Home assignments	

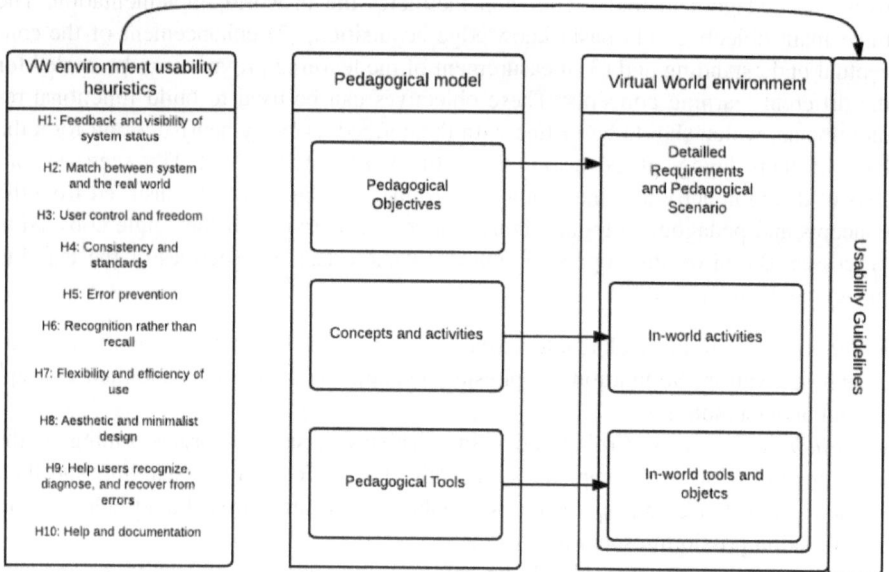

Fig. 1. Conversion process of the pedagogical model into the VW environment

4   The Virtual TEAL World in Open Wonderland

The Virtual TEAL World was implemented in the open source VW environment Open Wonderland (OWL) [18]. OWL already comes with many tools and functionalities required by the TEAL model. Table 2 gives an overview of the integration of the single pedagogical tools used by TEAL in the OWL framework. The first prototype focuses on introducing Faraday's Law. Students meet in groups of 3-4 in the VTW and start a so-called 'learning round-trip'. The single concepts used for this round-trip are based on the three cycle steps (1) basic knowledge acquisition, (2) enhancement of the conceptual understanding and (3) measurement of the learning progress. Hence, it is necessary to provide documents and videos to teach the students the first basic concepts. After that, they can enhance the conceptual understanding based on those concepts by simulating experiments. For this purpose the simulation framework TEALsim, which is also used by TEAL, was integrated into OWL [8]. The simulation was integrated in line with the usability heuristics and the design objectives collaboration, immersion and interactivity. Students are able to watch and use the simulations together. Due to the 3D integration of the single simulations it is possible to provide the feeling of immersion and presence. For assessment objectives a learning module was developed to simulate TEAL's concept questions. Students are motivated to discuss the different concepts. To answer a concept question they are first sent to a separated discussion area, where they should find a consensus before getting back to the main area.

Table 2. Adaption of the pedagogical tools in the virtual world environment [9]

	TEAL Environment	**Virtual TEAL World**
Oral explanation	In class.	Videos and documents in-world.
Collaborative learning	Groups of 3, with 9 students sitting at a round table and discussing electromagnetic phenomena.	A group of 3-4 students conducts a 'learning round-trip' in-world.
Networked laptops	One for each group of 3, with data acquisition links to desktop experiments that students perform and analyze.	Desktop experiments are either simulated in-world using the simulation software or shown via videos.
Multimedia visualization	Media-rich software (TEALsim) delivered via class laptops and the Web.	3D simulations of experiments via the TEALsim module in-world.
Course notes	With links to the visualizations.	In-world documents.
Conceptual questions	Using Personal Response Systems (PRS).	Using a specially designed learning-module with an optional interface to a conventional e-learning tool.

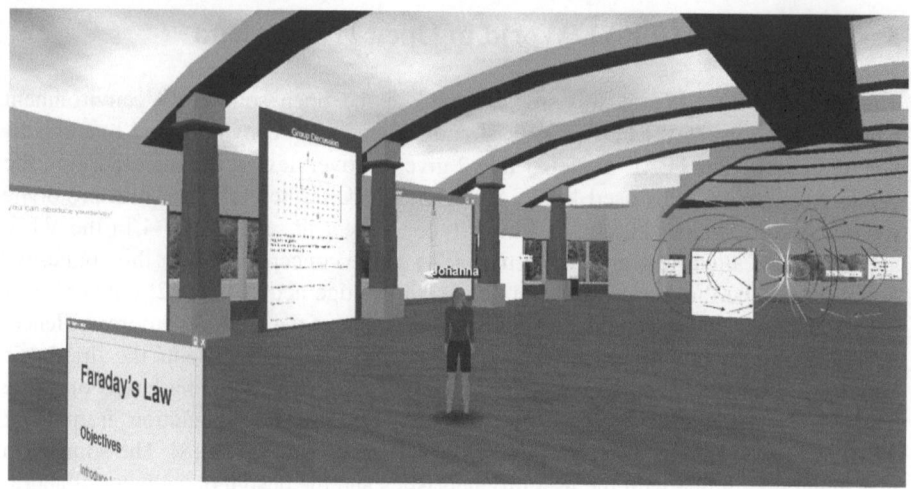

Fig. 2. Overview of the Virtual TEAL World in Open Wonderland [9]

5   Evaluation of the Virtual TEAL World in Open Wonderland

To evaluate the Virtual TEAL World we used quantitative and qualitative methods. The study was developed in the framework of [3] on basis of the usability heuristics and TEAL objectives. We conducted two different studies for the two different stakeholder groups. First, two physics experts with pedagogical background (SG1) evaluated the VTW with focus on usability and teaching objectives. In the second step eight students at university level (SG2) with minor physics knowledge were asked to make a short learning round-trip in the VTW. This study focused on measuring the students' learning progress, usability aspects, and compliance of the learning objectives. Each study took approximately one hour and consisted of three parts. First, they filled out a pre-questionnaire with focus on demographical data and background information, such as computer experience, experience with virtual world environments and stakeholder specific questions. In the second part of the study they explored the world. The first stakeholder group SG1 focused on trying out different tools with focus on subject-specific relevance. The second group SG2 conducted a shortened learning round-trip in the Faraday's law scenario. Therefore, they were grouped into pairs to do a collaborative round-trip and learn a single basic principle about Faraday's law. Their learning progress was measured with the in-world concept question tool. The third part of the study consisted of a post-questionnaire with focus on usability aspects, learning objectives, motivators and common impressions. The questionnaires were a combination of open-ended questions and questions with a Likert scaling between 1 (strongly agree) and 5 (strongly disagree). To measure the usability VW specific questions based on the usability heuristics list for virtual world environments and in-world tools and also the standard questionnaire SUS [19] were used. The next sections briefly describe and summarize the results of the user studies. Further details can be found in [3].

Previous User Experience. In the pre-questionnaire, the majority of SG1 and SG2 stated to be experienced in the use of computer systems, are used to play computer games and 80% of the participants already had experience with VWs. SG1 mentioned collaborative and interactive activities as important learning tools. The majority of SG2 stated to be less experienced in physics (M=4.24; SD=0.83) and only a few already heard about Faraday's law (M=3.25; SD=1.4).

Common Impressions. The participants agreed with a mean score of 1.83 (SD=0.8) that the Virtual TEAL World was a good experience. The majority of the participants would like to use the environment with the appropriate resources (mean score = 2.0; SD=1.0). At the beginning of the round-trip, the students got a question testing their common comprehension of Faraday's law concept. 5/8 students were already able to answer the question, two answered with 'I do not understand the concept' and one student answered the question wrong. After the short course all students were able to answer the question. They agreed that they learned something new, and have a better comprehension about Faraday's law (M=1.625; SD=0.86). All participants agreed in the importance of collaborative, interactive and assessment aspects of the environment and rated also the used methods and in-world tools as useful and important.

Experiencing Collaborative Activities. SG1 emphasized the importance of collaborative activities as part of a teaching model and liked in particular the different in-world discussion possibilities and motivators. "In real learning spaces it would be also very nice to be able to offer students separated discussion areas." SG2 rated collaborative activities as important learning tool as well. The mean rating of all participants of the collaborative ability of the VTW was rated positively with 1.4 (SD=0.49).

Experiencing Interactivity. SG1 was excited about the interactive simulations. Even if the main objective of the integrated simulation of Faraday's law was rather designed for explanatory experiments than for gaming, one of the participants had great fun in using the simulation in a playful way. "I like to try out innovative learning methods. In particular, such a playful animation can motivate also students, which are not really interested in the topic." The mean rating of the interactivity of the system was rated 1.6 (SD=0.66).

Experiencing Assessability. The stakeholder groups evaluated the assessability with a mean of 2.4 (SD=0.92). In particular, the missing possibility to assess the performance of individuals was raised, which is not only an issue of e-learning systems, but also of real courses using group exercises.

Experiencing Usabiliy. The participants were satisfied with the usability of the environment and the related components. Only two participants rated the usability according to the SUS with a score less than 70. The mean SUS score was 73.89 (SD=22.81). They were very satisfied with the different in-world tools and did not rate any in-world element with 'not important' or less. In comparison to previous similar studies [2] it was surprising that the tester determined to be able to use the system immediately without the support of a technical person or a first tutorial.

Problems and Reviews. The overall evaluation of the participants was very good. The participants used pre-setup PC system for the evaluations. Therefore, no severe technical problems occurred. An improvement nearly every user suggested were the increase of the performance and the adoptions of graphics. One participant recommended the use of additional realistic three-dimensional experiment settings instead of videos as complement to the existing simulations. "I really like the system and I am sure people would like to use it, if the performance would be better."

6   Conclusion

This paper presented the design and evaluation process of a virtual world environment for the pedagogical model TEAL with focus on resolving the two major issues of VWs: missing user acceptance and missing technical know-how. To identify the different requirements and design objectives an iterative approach was used. The final objectives for the design were (1) interactivity, (2) collaboration and (3) assessability, which should all be in-line with usability aspects and a user-centric design. Therefore, ten usability guidelines for virtual worlds and in-world tools were defined on basis of Nielson's heuristics.

The first evaluation of the VTW setup was very successful. The results state that the environment supports a high-level of collaborative and interactive activities. The participants were in particular very interested in activities and tools, which they can't access in the real world. This includes the three-dimensional simulation tool and also the discussion area. "It would be nice to have such a system also at our university." "It would be great for our physics course. The setup of real experiments always takes half an hour."

In comparison to previous studies, the participants barely experienced the issue of missing technical know-how or had problems how to access or use different tools or activities. Using usability heuristics especially designed for VW environments, but also supporting in-world tools is an enhancement for the user experience, what can result in an improved user acceptance. Focusing on the main pedagogical objectives, which are already useful and successful in real life, can also enhance the users' motivation and their willingness to use and suggest the system. Also, no major technical problems or lack of understanding occurred. The main issue they addressed was an improvement of the overall performance and an enhanced graphical interface. They also suggest the integration of further experiments and setups. After this first positive evaluation, the VTW will be advanced and extended. Further courses will be implemented and in particular more TEALsim simulations and interactive elements will be integrated.

Acknowledgement. We would like to thank the CECI at MIT for hosting this research. The authors would also like to thank the Open Wonderland team for the valuable knowledge support.

References

1. Gütl, C.: The Support of Virtual 3d Worlds for Enhancing Collaboration in Learning Settings. In: Techniques for Fostering Collaboration in Online Learning Communities: Theoretical and Practical Perspectives, pp. 278–299. IGI Glocal, Hershey (2011)
2. Gütl, C., Pirker, J.: Implementation and evaluation of a collaborative learning, training and networking environment for start-up entrepreneurs in virtual 3D worlds. In: 14th International Conference on Interactive Collaborative Learning 2011 (ICL), pp. 58–66 (2011)
3. Pirker, J.: Master Thesis: The Virtual TEAL World – An Interactive an Collaborative Virtual World Environment for Physics Education, Graz University of Technology (2013)
4. Hake, R.: Interactive-engagement versus traditional methods: A six-thousand-student survey of mechanics test data for introductory physics courses. American Journal of Physics 66(1), 64–74 (1988)
5. Mazur, E.: Peer Interaction, A User's Manual. Prentice Hall (1996)
6. O'Kuma, T.L., Maloney, D.P., Hieggelke, C.J.: Ranking Task Exercises in Physics. Prentice Hall, Upper Saddle River (2000)
7. Brandes, D., Ginnis, P.: A Guide to Student-Centred Learning. Nelson Thornes, Cheltenham (1996)
8. Berger, S.: Master Thesis: Virtual 3D World for Physics Experiments in Higher Education, Graz University of Technology (2012)
9. Pirker, J., Berger, S., Gütl, C., Belcher, J., Bailey, P.H.: Understanding Physical Concepts using an Immersive Virtual Learning Environment. In: Proceedings of the 2nd European Immersive Education Summit, Paris, pp. 183–191 (2012)
10. Thackray, L., Good, L., Howland, K.: Learning and Teaching in Virtual Worlds: Boundaries, Challenges and Opportunities. In: Research and Learning in Virtual Worlds, pp. 139–158. Springer, London (2010)
11. Saleeb, N., Defoulas, G.: Architectural Evolution of E-Learning Virtual Worlds. In: Hinrichs, R., Wankel, C. (eds.) Engaging the Avatar, pp. 49–80 (2012)
12. Schmeil, A., Eppler, M.J., de Freitag, S.: A Framework for the Design of the Avatar-Based Collaboration. In: Hinrichs, R., Wankel, C. (eds.) Engaging the Avatar, pp. 15–48 (2012)
13. Muñoz, R., Barcelos, T., Chalegre, V.: Defining and Validating Virtual Worlds Usability Heuristics. In: Ninth International Conference on Information Technology: New Generations, pp. 690–695 (2012)
14. Nielson, J.: Heuristic evaluation. In: Nielson, J., Mack, R.L. (eds.) Usability Inspection Methods. Wiley & Sons, New York (1994)
15. Erickson, T., Shami, N.S., Kellogg, W.A., Levine, D.W.: Synchronous Interaction Among Hundres: An Evaluation of a Conference in an Avatar-based Virtual Environment. In: CHI 2011, Vancouver, BC, Canada (2011)
16. Shneiderman, B., Plaisant, C.: Designing the User Interface - Strategies for effective human-computer interaction. Pearson Higher Education, Boston (2010)
17. Dori, Y.J., Belcher, J.: How Does Technology-Enabled Active Learning Affect Undergraduate Students' Understanding of Electromagnetism Concepts? The Journal of the Learning Sciences 14(2), 243–279 (2005)
18. Open Wonderland, `http://openwonderland.org/` (retrieved from)
19. Brook, J.: A "quick and dirty" usability scale. In: Usability evaluation in industry. Tayler and Francis, Longon (1996)

Towards Unification for Pointing Task Evaluation in 3D Desktop Virtual Environment

Mathieu Raynal, Emmanuel Dubois, and Bénédicte Schmitt

IRIT – ELIPSE, Université Paul Sabatier,
31062 Toulouse cedex 9, France
{firstname.name}@irit.fr

Abstract. New visualization systems for large and complex datasets are emerging and 3D Virtual Environments turn out to be a relevant solution. Interaction tasks in these 3D VE have been defined, especially to support evaluation of these applications. Nevertheless there is a lack of unified protocol to assess these elementary tasks in this context. Moreover it can be complex to determine the appropriate technique to perform these tasks as there is a lack of reference data. A standard is available for 2D pointing task, but there is no equivalence in 3D. In this paper, we propose an adaptation of this standard to a pointing task in a 3D VE. We detail our protocol and an instrumentation, which aims at assessing performance, comfort of techniques and satisfaction of users. We also present results of a user experimentation conducted according to this standard's adaptation.

Keywords: Pointing task, 3D virtual environment, 3D interaction, usability study.

1 Introduction

3D Virtual Environments (3D VE) are emerging in many different domains ranging from games to industrial applications (Geographic Information System - GIS, Computer-Aided Design - CAD, etc). A 3D VE can be defined as a space where one or more users interact in real time through physical means, and devices, with 3D digital data generated by a computer [1]. Recently new polyvalent technologies, like the Wiimote, successfully appeared in public spaces to offer advanced interaction techniques for using 3D [2]. They are initially intended to be used in game applications, and they should turn out to be satisfying and comfortable. In parallel, dedicated devices (e.g. Rockin'Mouse [3], Cubic Mouse [4]) have been proposed to offer advanced forms of interaction with 3D environments in more professional contexts. But they are uncommon and not yet part of the democratized and the well accepted set of interaction devices for professional activities; classical devices such as mouse or joystick remain the most common and used devices, even if they are not always well adapted to the tasks. Anyway to develop the use of advanced interaction techniques in

A. Holzinger et al. (Eds.): SouthCHI 2013, LNCS 7946, pp. 562–580, 2013.

such professional contexts, these techniques should match several usability requirements: accuracy, execution speed and ease of learning. Moreover satisfaction and level of comfort should also be part of their acceptance due to their daily use. Therefore determining the device that can be efficient and well-accepted is a major need to contribute to the development of these advanced interaction techniques in such context, their evaluation and validation. It is also a complex need that requires appropriate means to measure and to compare techniques for 3D interactions.

So far, studies traditionally deal with one or several of the well established 3D tasks: selection, manipulation and navigation [5]. It results in complex user experiments, attempting to combine 6DOF input devices, 3D tasks, different interaction techniques, etc. And yet, focusing on a 3D pointing task only, which is a prevalent task, would simplify experiments' protocol. The pointing task consists in moving a cursor to a specific location by changing the coordinates of the cursor in translation (tx, ty, tz). A parallel can be drawn with the specification of an object position of the manipulation task and recommendations extracted from the evaluation of the pointing task could be transposed to this part of the manipulation task. Moreover a study of Masliah [6] revealed the interest to break the evaluation of the manipulation task into a separate evaluation of the translation and rotation tasks because users consider them as two different tasks. This reinforces the need to assess a low-level task interaction, such as the pointing task in 3D. However, even in such simplified contexts, facing the growing interest in advanced forms of interaction for 3D VE requires additional considerations: there is a need to support reproducible evaluations, in different application contexts, with a wide variety of advanced forms of interaction techniques; it is also required to support a composite approach, combining quantitative aspects, i.e. performance, and qualitative aspects, i.e. satisfaction.

To create a structured and replicable evaluation method for assessing pointing task in 3D Virtual Environments, we propose an adaptation of the ISO 9241-9 standard. Initially dedicated to pointing in 1D or 2D, this standard gives recommendations for assessing non keyboard technique and combines quantitative and usability measures. Usability here refers essentially to effort and comfort. Our adaptation aims at extending its applicability to a 3D environment and to additional consideration related to the performance and the user satisfaction. After reviewing existing works for evaluating interaction techniques in 3D environments, we describe and justify the required adaptations in the ISO standard. We finally present a software tool used to conduct a user's evaluation of a 3D pointing task and report on the evaluation conducted on the basis of the adaptation and its associated tool to compare and assess two different interaction techniques for pointing in 3D.

2   Evaluation of Input Devices in 3D Environments

Two approaches presented in the literature to assess input devices in 3D environments can be opposed: structured approaches for pointing task evaluation and ad-hoc approaches for 6-DOF interaction techniques evaluation.

2.1   Pointing Task Evaluation Approaches

Fitts' Law and its Extensions. Fitts' Law is originally designed to predict the time (MT) required to move to a target in 1D where a and b are two constants, determined empirically for a device and an interaction context. W is the width of the target and D the distance to the target. The log term is the Index of Difficulty (ID) and is measured in bits.

$$MT = a + b \times ID \text{ with } ID = \log_2(^D/_W + 1) \tag{1}$$

Recently, some models have been proposed to extend Fitts' Law. MacKenzie and Buxton [7] proposed different approaches to compute the index of difficulty in 2D. But Zhai and Accot demonstrated some limitations to those models, especially when target height and target width are not equal, and proposed in reaction a model for bivariate pointing.

Ware and Lowther [8] proposed an extension of the Fitts' Law for 3D. Targets are now defined in 3D with a width, height and depth and the computation of the indexes of difficulty relies on the smallest of these three dimensions. However this extension of the model has the same issues as the reference model. Furthermore according to our knowledge, no experience with explicit 3D targets has already been performed to fully validate this model. Grossman and Balakrishnan [9] adaptation consists in studying physical movements of users in a XZ plane for a volumetric display. They validated their model for a volumetric display but not in a 3D Virtual Environment. Moreover, movements were constrained on one plane (X,Z) with (Y=0), so movements were not evaluated on all axes. So far these alternate models have not overcome the classical Fitts' Law to study and predict pointing performance in a 3D VE. Hence the classical model is used regardless of the dimensions.

Throughput. The throughput (TP) has been introduced by the ISO 9241-9 standard to describe and compare the performance of at least two pointing devices in a given context. It is measured in bits per second and the formula to compute the TP is:

$$TP = \frac{ID_e}{MT} \text{ with } ID_e = \log_2(\frac{D_e}{W_e} + 1) \tag{2}$$

This is an overall performance measure, based on the Fitts' model, and is independent of the speed-accuracy tradeoff contrary to the Index of Performance. MT is the average movement time performed by users over a block of trials and IDe is the effective Index of Difficulty. These terms represent how a user effectively performed rather than what the user can do in theory. Indeed De is the effective travelled distance between two targets covered by users during the evaluation and We is the effective width corresponding to the distribution of users' selections in or around the target during the evaluation. But no throughput measures are currently available for 3D interaction techniques in 3D VE.

ISO 9241-9 Standard. The ISO 9241-9 standard [10] gives requirements about design and evaluation of non keyboard devices such as mouse, joystick, etc. The standard provides recommendations and a set of variables for different kind of tests depending on the task to evaluate: for example tapping and dragging test respectively corresponds to a pointing and a drag-and-drop task. The use of this standard aims at simultaneously measuring the throughput of such devices, to compare the performance of devices, and leading a qualitative study based on a comfort assessment and an effort scale. This standard has been used in recent studies to assess the performance of diverse techniques, e.g. [11]. However these recommendations concern 2-DOF interaction techniques used to perform 1D or 2D tasks. The standard does not give recommendations to assess interaction techniques with 3-DOFs or more and does not address 3D environment. Nevertheless some attempts have been proposed to extend the ISO standard to a 3D environment.

Proposition of Adaptation of the ISO 9241-9 Standard to a 3D Environment. Recent studies of Teather et al. [12,13] deal with pointing task evaluation in a 3D environment based on the ISO standard. In the first study [12], targets are spheres disposed on a 2D circle on a vertical plane. In the second study, the representation used is a 3D scene [13] in which targets are circles placed on cylinders. In both cases, due to the perspective rendering mode, targets representation appears on a plane, either horizontal or vertical: selecting a target thus results of the combination of a 2D pointing on the plane with the use of a ray-casting technique to reach the appropriate depth. In these settings interactions with the device are thus confined to the plane (X,Y): the depth is not processed with one specific DOF but is a software computation. Cursor movements are therefore not considered in all directions. Moreover these studies take place in immersive environments and not desktop environments.

Another recent study [14] evaluates 3D object manipulation using virtual hand techniques. They based their evaluation on the ISO standard and adapted the formula to compute a 3D projection, onto the task axis, of the user's selection, i.e. of the position of the cursor when the user validated the target selection. Nevertheless their evaluation took place in a Tangible Augmented Reality Environment and they did not propose a digital 3D VE to interact with. This work illustrates the interest to base an evaluation on the ISO standard but their results can not be compared with evaluations conducted in 3D Virtual Environment like Teather's works.

Beyond these propositions, we are not aware of any other study based on the ISO standard performed in a 3D VE and involving interaction techniques with 3DOF or more. Therefore results provided by structured approaches do not yet constitute reusable references. More concrete results have been measured through empirical studies. The following section summarizes ad hoc evaluations lead in 3D Virtual Environments.

2.2   Evaluation of 3D Interaction Techniques in 3D Environments

Among existing studies in the domain of 3D interaction techniques evaluation, we here focus on three representative examples: (1) the Airmouse technique [15], (2) a study lead by Berard [16], (3) a study lead by Zhai [17].

These studies differ in terms of task and settings. In terms of settings, the studies (1) and (2) manipulate only 3 axes for translations while the study (3) uses all 6 axes for translations and rotations. In terms of task, study (1) assesses a pointing task: moving a little sphere in a spherical area; study (2) evaluates a placement task: moving a cube as close as possible to a target represented by a cube with a smaller size; study (3) evaluates a docking task: manipulating a tetrahedron in another tetrahedron with the same size. This task consists in putting the object exactly in the same position and orientation than the target. But for each task, users aim at moving a cursor or an object as quickly as possible to a specific location.

Even if all these experiments focus on quantitative results, in particular performance time, each one considers and relies on different variables. Studies (2) and (3) define an error rate. Studies (1) and (2) use the notion of index of difficulties, as defined in Fitts' law to modify task conditions, but only study (1) matches indexes of difficulties and times to perform the task. However traditional parameters a and b of a Fitts' law analysis are not studied. In addition, as opposed to study (2), studies (1) and (3) include qualitative measurements by assessing the fatigue; however the evaluation of the fatigue is not similar among the two studies.

These studies show a lack of formalization for 3D interaction techniques evaluation and highlight limits that are commonly observed in similar users' studies: DOF considered, task, measurements and method. Furthermore the analyzed measures are not identical and there is no overall measure to easily compare these interaction techniques.

To summarize, the first set of approaches gives recommendations to assess the pointing task in a structured way, while the second set of approaches provides concrete results and measures, which are complex to compare. Our goal is thus to take advantage of the structured approach to guide and to standardize the design of such experiments. We also take advantage of the variables and measures promoted in the ad-hoc approaches and denoting relevant aspects of the users' experiment in 3D VE. Our work is based on an extension of the ISO standard.

3   Unification for the Pointing Task in a 3D Desktop VE

Among the type of tests covered by the standard, we focus on the multi-directional tapping test as we intend to evaluate the pointing and selecting tasks. The movement is multidirectional as we consider pointing movements in any direction (x, y and z). The adaptation we propose is explicitly targeted at pointing tasks in 3D context. A first introduction to this adaption has been briefly presented in [18]. In this section, we more clearly refer to the sections of the existing standard for which modifications are proposed. We therefore detail 5 main dimensions addressed by the initial standard, three of them related to the performance (task, targets, and variables) and two related to qualitative aspects (representation and finally, comfort and satisfaction). For each one, we present and justify the adaptation introduced to fit with a 3D pointing context.

3.1   Adaptation from a Performance Point of View

Three major aspects of the standard structure the quantitative assessment: task, targets and variables.

Task. In the ISO standard, the recommended task consists in selecting a fixed target as quickly and accurately as possible (ISO 9241-9 - Annex B.B.3). Selection comprises the pointing of a target by moving a cursor from a starting target to a destination target with the pointing technique. The pointing task ends in the validation of the selection when confirming the selection by pressing a button or key. If the cursor is inside the destination target when the user confirms the selection, the pointing task is successful. If the cursor is outside the target, the validation raises an error. In every case, pressing the button or key is the end of the current task and the beginning of the next pointing task of the protocol. The task difficulty varies according to different IDs as defined in Fitts' Law: targets size and distance between targets are modified over the experiment.

In our adaptation, the task instruction, the existence of a source and destination target and the need for a confirmation has been kept. The adaptation first concerns the validation. Indeed, the 3D cursor does not need to be fully inside the target to consider the validation as a successful selection: when validating, detecting a collision between the target and the cursor is sufficient. In the absence of collision, the validation raises an error.

The ISO standard also describes the use of the task axis (line between the start target and the end target) implied by user's movements during the task and used to measure the throughput: this has been kept in our adaptation.

Targets. Although the form of targets is not explicitly constrained by the standard, circle targets are the most used in evaluations of the literature, because a circle has one width regardless of the user's movement. As a result, our adaptation to 3D recommends that targets become spheres to keep one measure for the width regardless of the 3D movement: the size of the target will thus be given by the diameter of the spheres.

Regarding the arrangement and position of targets, the ISO standard recommends to equally space the targets around the circumference of a support circle (ISO 9241-9 - B.B.6.2.2). In addition, the place of the target on the circle must be defined so that each target has a symmetric with respect to the center of the support circle. This ensures that the distance between two targets is always the same, and equals to the support circle diameter (ISO 9241-9 - B.B.6.2.2).

In our adaptation, the arrangement of the targets must be revisited to fit with 3D: the support circle is thus replaced by a support sphere. Targets are still equally spaced on the circumference of a support sphere. But their position is defined so that each target has a symmetric with respect to the center of the support sphere. And the distance between two targets is still equal to the diameter of the support sphere and constant over the task.

Variables. The ISO standard recommends different independent and dependent variables (ISO 9241-9 - B.B.5). Independent variables inherent to the experiment are input technique, targets size, targets distance and the resulting IDs. Dependent variables mentioned in the ISO standard include the throughput and the mean movement time.

In our adaptation, these variables have been kept. However the calculation of IDs is modified, because the cursor is volumetric. Its computation, as illustrated in the equation below, thus includes the size of the cursor:

$$ID = \log_2\left(^D/_{W_{target}} + W_{cursor} + 1\right)$$

(3)

The calculation of the effective IDs (IDe) is also modified and relies on the coordinates of the point effectively reached by the center of the 3D cursor when the user selects the target. The effective width is then computed by solving a 3D parametric equation to project the effective users' selection point onto the "task axis". The effective distance corresponds to the 3D Euclidean distance computed between the starting users' selection point and the destination users' selection point of the "task axis". The effective width and distance, used in the computation of the TP, are computed as an average over all repetitions for a given condition.

Our adaptation of the standard also recommends considering two additional dependent variables: the error rate and the inefficiency ratio. Very frequently used as a dependent variable in ad-hoc approaches, we recommend considering the error rate because it complements the TP measure. Furthermore the 3D context induces more movements' variability during the task than 2D contexts; a deeper investigation of the users' performance is thus required to qualify this quantitative measure. Masliah [19] suggests the inefficiency ratio, defined by Zhai and Milgram [20], to support the analysis of the performance quality: this ratio compares the user's travelled distance to the optimal distance (cf. Figure 1). This ratio indicates the coordination of users during the task: the closer the ratio is to 0, the better is the coordination as 0 indicates that users navigated the optimal distance. The inefficiency ratio therefore complements the error rate, one aspect of users' performance. We thus recommend considering this variable in the set of dependent variables.

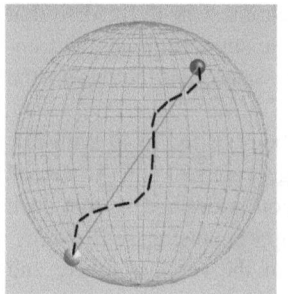

$$Inefficiency\ ratio = {}^{UD - OD}/_{OD}$$

Dashes trajectory : User's travelled distance (UD) = 309px
Straight trajectory: optimal distance (OD) = 150px
IR = (309 − 150) / 150 = 1.06

Fig. 1. Illustration of the coordination for one task

3.2   Adaptation from a Qualitative Point of View

Two elements structure the qualitative assessment: representation with especially 3D indices and, comfort and satisfaction.

Representation and 3D Indices. The ISO standard does not recommend any specific elements of representation. Despite that, the pointer is commonly represented by a cross. In our adaptation, the volumetric representation of the cursor we recommend is a red sphere. In addition its recommended width is about 70% of the littlest target width (10px in our case) to remain visible regardless of its position in the 3D environment. The shape of the cursor is defined in order to ensure that the collision point is captured at a same distance from the cursor center to the target center whatever the 3D movement, which is not possible with a square.

Our adaptation to 3D VE is also facing the traditional problem of depth perception in 3D. Due to the desktop environment and the lack of effective hardware and software solutions, users may not be able to correctly sense the depth of a digital object, thus making the modeling of the 3D pointing relatively difficult. For these reasons, 3D perception requires to define some additional and specific aspects to the representation. Some 3D visual indices are defined to overcome difficulties of depth perception: a color graduation combined with a transparency [21] of the target spheres. This transparency reduces the occlusion with other spheres and allows users to see the cursor behind spheres. A relative size of spheres is due to the perspective of the 3D scene, so spheres placed behind seem to be smaller. Furthermore, the support sphere is represented by a transparent wireframe. These indices have been explored and defined during an iterative design made with the participation of 3D experts. Although shadows are commonly used in 3D scenes, our adaptation does not encourage the use of shadows to avoid overloading the environment. Indeed Hubona et al. [14] showed that user performance for a docking task decrease when increasing shadows number and scene complexity. These recommendations thus constitute a scene of reference for evaluating interaction techniques for pointing tasks in 3D; using this common scene of reference will avoid inserting biases from the depth perception that could jeopardize evaluation results of interaction in 3D spaces.

Comfort and Satisfaction. The ISO standard recommends two complementary rating scales to assess the comfort of interaction techniques: a comfort questionnaire to measure the comfort and fatigue of techniques and an effort scale to measure the effort perceived by users during the task (ISO 9241-9 - Annex C).

In our adaptation, the two rating scales are kept and we reinforce the usability analysis of the comfort questionnaire by adding the SUS questionnaire that covers user's satisfaction and learning. Indeed the comfort questionnaire does not cover aspects of usability, such as user' satisfaction, learning and users' preference. SUS includes 10 items and computes an overall usability score for each technique, useful to easily compare different techniques assessed in a same context. We further enrich the analysis of the satisfaction aspect by inserting the use of 6 SUMI items focusing on the frustration and the stimulation for example. Finally we complete this part of this qualitative aspect by asking users their 3 preferred points and their worst points about each 3D input technique.

In addition to these main adaptations of the ISO standard, we developed an interactive tool to support the use of the resulting adaptation when performing an evaluation. Its main features are presented in the next section.

3.3   Instrumentation

The interactive tool aims at supporting the deployment of the protocol to evaluate 3D input techniques and at collecting logs. The interactive tool is composed of a 3D environment (cf. Figure 2) and a configuration panel. The 3D graphics software is written in C++ using OSG toolkit. The configuration panel is written in C#, and to propose an evolutive software tool, all software elements are linked through a software bus called Ivy. The pointing task is composed of a number of targets that the experimenter can manage with the configuration panel: targets can be placed at specific longitude and latitude. A block is composed of a series of pointing tasks, which have the same Fitts'ID. The experimenter can configure the targets' size (width) and the support's size (distance) to adjust the ID of the block. Running the task on one block is a three-step process: 1) the pointing task begins when the participant selects the starting sphere, colored in blue, without making an error. 2) It then highlights the symmetric destination sphere, colored in yellow. 3) The task ends when the participant selects the destination sphere, even if there is an error (i.e. no collision with the cursor). The target sphere becomes orange when the cursor and the target are in contact.

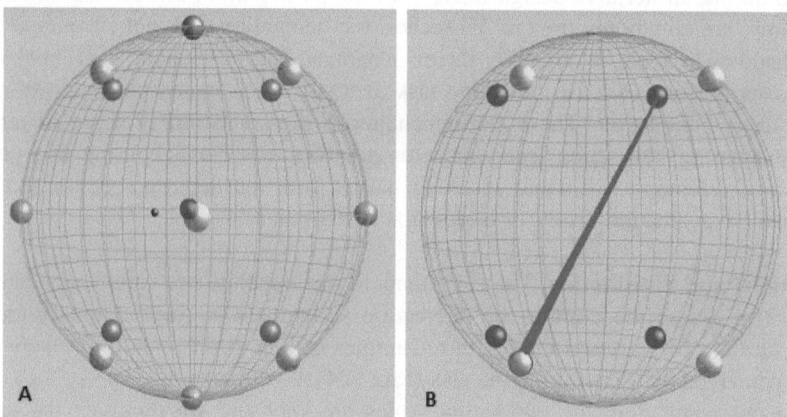

Fig. 2. Illustration of the 3D scene (A), of the depth perception indices and of a task axis (B)

During the task, the software tool records temporal data, such as beginning and end of each pointing task, validation of the selection and execution time. It logs the position of the 3D cursor and errors when the validation was done without collision between the cursor and the target. All experiment events are dated and recorded in a XML format.

In order to concretely show the use of the recommendations of our adaptation, we present a case study, the protocol for the evaluation of two interaction techniques. We then analyze and discuss results of this evaluation.

4   Concrete Use of the Adaptation of the Standard and Evaluation Results

The case study we consider in this section is taken from an industrial context. A partial set of results regarding has already been mentioned in [22, 23].

Nevertheless, instead of just using an ad hoc evaluation protocol as in these previous publications, we here tightly follow the adaptation of the standard presented in this paper to measure and analyse a well identified and justified set of variables and protocol steps.. We first detail the experimental protocol and report on the quantitative and qualitative results of this evaluation.

4.1   Case Study: Aircraft Static Test Design

Our case study is based on a real application proposed to design and manage campaign of static test for aeronautics (cf. Fig. 3). Designers have to manipulate and position sensors on a 3D digital mock-up, which represents a real aircraft, including dimensions and volume. Interactions with these models enable users to perform tasks in 3D as if they were manipulating the real aircraft. Users can apply transparency on parts of the digital mock-up to easily interact with otherwise hidden elements of the 3D structure: techniques like ray-casting are not usable given the digital mock-up complexity, and its multi-layered structure.

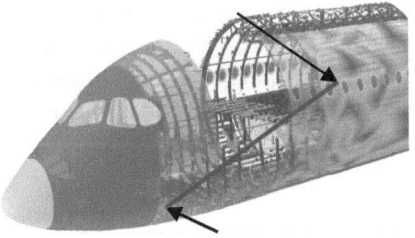

Fig. 3. : View of the 3D model in EasySensorManager application

Task. 3D pointing task is regularly performed to place or manipulate sensors in the 3D aircraft. Designers frequently have to successively select two elements of the digital mock-up to measure a distance for example: this corresponds to the selection task described in the standard between two points of the aircraft placed at different depth in the mockup (cf. Fig. 3 - points A and B).

Targets. Targets are typically elements of the plane structure (e.g. extremities of wings) or sensors. Designers can select sensors placed on the inside or outside surface of the nose plane, the left or right wing and the tail plane. The volume of these elements and the distance between them are variable, and these variations match different task difficulties (ID) of the standard.

Variables. Designers have to accurately position a large number of sensors for one test, so small movement times and error rates are important to reduce the time of the task.

Representation and 3D Indices. To help perceive the 3D in the complex mock-up and to avoid jeopardizing its understandability, no "decorating" elements, such as shadows, are added to the digital mock-up. Conversely objects are represented in different colors and with different transparencies to highlight different depths present in the digital mock-up. This is also in line with the recommendation expressed by the standard.

Comfort and Satisfaction. The sensors positioning is a daily activity for designers and they can spend many hours to realize this activity; it is therefore important that they feel comfortable and satisfied by the techniques they use. SUS score and other fatigue scale will be helpful in this use case.

Two techniques have been designed and implemented to support this activity. Concretely, the first technique is an advanced interaction technique: a physical object is manipulated in a 3D physical space in order to move the digital pointer in the 3D mock-up. The position of the object in the physical space matches with the position of the pointer in the 3D environment. This technique is based on a position-control mode and constitutes an isotonic controller. The second technique is based on the users force applied to an object similar to a joystick in order to move the digital pointer. The input force is transformed into speed to change the position of the pointer in the 3D environment. This technique is based on a rate-control mode and corresponds to an isometric controller. The evaluation of the pointing task with these two interaction techniques will illustrate the use of the standard adaptation.

4.2   Participants

Fourteen non-paid users (3 female and 11 male) were recruited to participate in this study and to test the two techniques. But usable results were only available for 13 users, because logs for one user were corrupted due to an issue with data recording. Participant ages ranged from 22 to 39 (mean: 27.5, SD: 5.26). They were regular computer users but they were not familiar with our 3D interaction techniques. They used their dominant hand (12 right-handed and 1 left-handed participants).

4.3   Hypothesis of the Experimentation

A goal of the evaluation is to assess the speed and the accuracy of techniques, our second hypothesis (H1) is that the isotonic technique is more efficient than the isometric technique and has a better throughput measure. We also hypothesize that users prefer interacting in a 3D environment with the isotonic technique (H2) as the interaction seems more usual than for the isometric technique. The assessment of these hypotheses will rely on the results provided by our adaptation of the standard.

4.4   Apparatus

The experiment was conducted using a HP EliteBook 6930p laptop PC with Windows 7 and a LCD screen with a resolution of 1920*1080. The computer's processor was a 2.4GHz Intel Core Duo CPU with 4GB of RAM and an ATI Mobility Radeon HD 3450 graphics controller of 256Mo. The goal was to compare two interaction techniques presented above: the technique based on a position-control mode and the one based on a rate-control mode were respectively implemented with a Polhemus Patriot, an isotonic tracking system, and the SpaceNavigator, an isometric joystick. In order to implement these interaction techniques, a pre-experiment has been conducted to determine optimal parameters for position-control and rate-control modes.

4.5   Procedure

At the beginning, each participant completed a consent form and a demographic questionnaire. Then participants sat in front of a desk where the LCD screen and both devices were placed. Instructions, in accordance with those specified in the adaptation of the standard, were given to participants and they performed a 15 minutes-training before the experiment. As mentioned in the adaptation, the pointing task began when participants selected the starting sphere. The task ended when participants selected the destination sphere. Participants were allowed to rest whenever they wanted between two pointing tasks. When all pointing tasks were performed with the first technique, they filled out a scale to assess technique comfort and a satisfaction questionnaire to assess technique usability. Participants followed the same procedure for the second technique. At the end of the experiment, participants filled out a questionnaire in order to compare both techniques. Complementary interviews, as recommended in our adaptation, were used to gather users' preferences and to identify the three best and the three worst points of each technique. In this case study, the effort scale was not used as it is generally used to assess large muscle groups (arm, shoulder and neck) but may not be appropriate for smaller muscles, such as those involved in manipulating our two techniques. Assessment of efforts was thus limited to the use of the 5 indices of the comfort scale.

4.6   Design

As recommended in our adaptation, different IDs need to be specified. In our experiment, the IDs were defined as a combination of width and distance. Unlike [23], we chose to present, in this article, indices of difficulty according to the calculation presented in (3). Cursor size is 10 px so target width + cursor width=25px, 40px, 55px and distance=150px, 450px, 750px. IDs were ranged from 1.898 to 4.954. In this instance of the adapted standard, the number of targets to point has been fixed to 14 targets: 6 targets were placed on the extremities of the axes and 8 at longitude and latitude Π/4. Participants were divided into 2 groups and each group tested techniques in a counterbalanced order.

Finally, we collected 3276 pointing times as we had 13 participants * 2 devices * 9 blocks (counterbalanced by a Latin square) * 14 target selections.

4.7   Quantitative Measurements

Based on the logged data, we analyze the quantitative results by use of descriptive statistics and inferential statistics (i.e. One-way RM ANOVA).

Movement Time. The ISO standard includes the mean movement time as a dependent variable based on the Fitts' law. So we analyzed the mean time required to select a target: the mean time measure for the isometric technique (hereafter referred to as the SpaceNavigator) is 10681ms and for the isotonic technique (hereafter referred to as the Patriot) is 6265ms. The analysis shows a significant difference between these techniques ($F(1,12) = 179.05$, $p < 0.0001$). So the Patriot enables users to perform the pointing task significantly faster than the SpaceNavigator. Based on observation and answers during the semi-guided interviews, we believe that this higher efficiency of the Patriot is due to the use of more usual and less constrained arm motions.

Throughput. Among the dependant variables identified in the standard, the throughput is a performance measure to easily compare two techniques. Computing the throughput for each input technique relies on effective widths and effective distances. This computation uses a per-participant and a per-block basis to produce the "grand throughput". Throughputs for the isotonic technique and the isometric technique respectively are 2.1bps and 1.69bps, that is to say the rate of information transfer during the task. So we infer that the Patriot is more efficient than the SpaceNavigator. This confirms our hypothesis (H1) about the higher efficiency of the isotonic technique.

Inefficiency Ratio and Movements Analysis. As a complement to the TP, the measure of the inefficiency ratio is recommended in our adaptation of the variables of the standard. The computation of the inefficiency ratio for both techniques reveals that the translation inefficiency of the isotonic technique (1.06) is lower than the translation inefficiency of the isometric technique (1.56). This means that translation trajectories with the isotonic technique are 106% longer than the optimal distance and translation trajectories with the isometric technique are 156% longer than the optimal distance. The analysis shows a significant difference between these techniques ($F_{(1,12)} = 218.75$, $p<.0001$). We infer that the isotonic technique supports a better coordination than the isometric technique.

In addition to the quantitative measures recommended in the adaptation of the standard, we analyzed users' movements to better understand the impact of the 3D on results of this experiment. Movement required to achieve every pointing task is performed in 3D. We analyzed the difference between movements involving translations realized along one axis (simple movements) and movements involving a combination of translations along the 3 axes (complex movements). A first analysis shows a significant difference between movements in terms of time ($F_{(1,12)}$ = 13.67, p<0.001) and distance ($F_{(1,12)}$ = 16.91, p<0.0001) regardless of the technique (see Fig. 4 and Fig. 5). Users perform the task quicker and with a shorter travelled distance when simple movements are involved than when complex movements are proposed. This means that users have less difficulty to manipulate the pointer during simple movements than during complex movements.

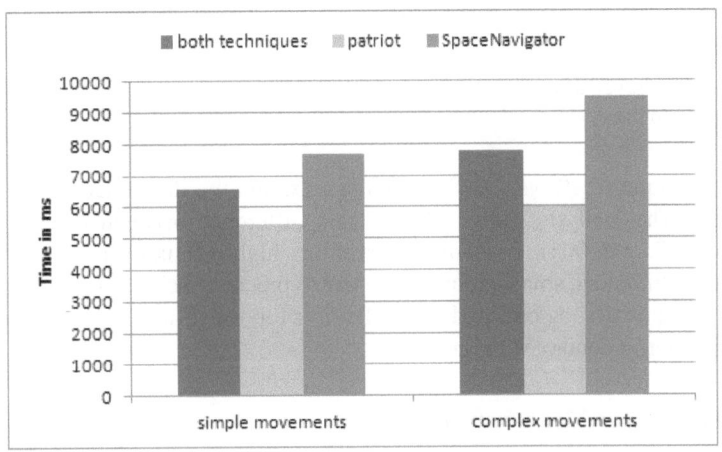

Fig. 4. Time to complete the task according to the difficulty of the movement and to the device

A second analysis shows a significant difference between the two techniques in terms of time ($F_{(1,12)}$=56.74, p<0.0001) and of distance ($F_{(1,12)}$=4.81, p<0.05) with simple movements (see Fig. 4 and Fig. 5). A significant difference also exists between the two techniques for the time ($F_{(1,12)}$=123.86, p<0.0001) and for the distance ($F_{(1,12)}$=47.68, p<0.0001) during complex movements. The *Patriot* enables users to perform the task quicker and with a shorter travelled distance for both kinds of movements. These results confirm the inefficiency ratio and the best performances of the isotonic technique.

Error Rate. Our adaptation of the standard establishes the measure of the error rate as a dependent variable. So we analyzed error rate for both techniques to know how successful the pointing task is and to determine the effectiveness of these techniques. The measured error rate of the isometric technique is lower than the one of the

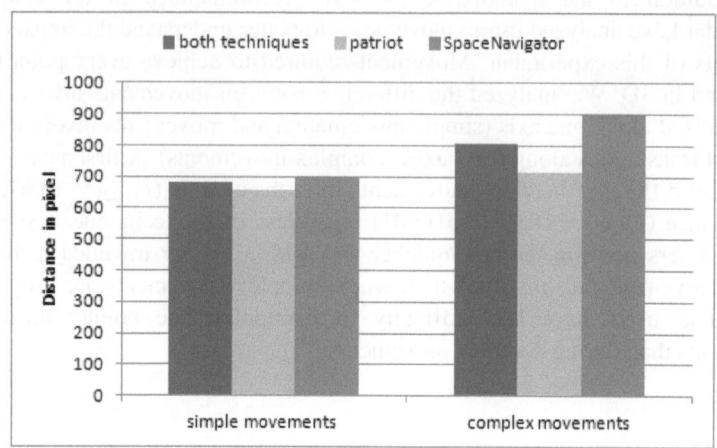

Fig. 5. Distance traveled by the cursor to complete the task according to the difficulty of the movement and to the device

isotonic technique (4.4% vs 7.6%), which can explain the difference of mean movement times. The analysis shows a significant difference between these techniques (F(1,12)=20.77, p<0.005). In-study observations highlight that the SpaceNavigator enables users to realize small motions in order to precisely select targets and to maintain a neutral position as opposed to the Patriot, for which users have difficulties to keep the pointer in contact with targets.

4.8   Qualitative Measurements

Our composite approach also includes qualitative aspects that we analyzed by use of non-parametric statistics.

Comfort Assessment. Participants completed the comfort questionnaire, which includes two indices, general indices and fatigue indices, and based on a five-level Likert scale. As described in the procedure, in a first phase, participants completed a questionnaire after testing the first technique in order to assess the comfort of this first technique. Results of the first questionnaire do not show any major significant results for all indices according to the Mann and Whitney test, except for the arm fatigue. The mean score over all scales of the first phase is 3.41 (SD=0.45) for the isometric technique and 3.54 (SD=0.35) for the isotonic technique: this result shows that users tend to have a better feeling about the comfort of the isotonic technique. After testing the second technique in a second phase, participants filled out a scale to compare both techniques according to the same indices. A sign test shows no significant difference (|Z|=-0.28, p>0.5) between both techniques. But results of the two phases (p=0.091 for the first phase) reveal that the isotonic technique tends to cause more fatigue than the isometric technique for arm or shoulder, so it would be relevant to envision another design for this point of focalization.

Users' Satisfaction. The adaptation of the standard recommends analyzing usability of techniques with a SUS questionnaire in addition to the comfort questionnaire. We computed a SUS score to measure the usability of each technique. The score of the isometric technique (52.5) is marginal at a low level whereas the score of the isotonic technique (76.3) is acceptable, according to [24]. The techniques' usability can be improved, even if the usability of the isotonic technique is good. Both SUS scores establish that the current usability of the techniques does not jeopardize their use for pointing tasks. Besides, answers to the SUMI items questionnaire highlight the isotonic technique is perceived as more stimulating and less frustrated than the isometric technique.

Users' Preferences. As proposed by the adaptation of the standard, we used interviews since users' answers are usually a fair indication of improvements, indicating what could be developed to reach a better usability level. Users mentioned the most frequently a good aestheticism of the device, as the best point of the isometric technique (based on the *SpaceNavigator*) and an inappropriate association between input and output interactions, especially depth interactions, as the worst point of this technique. They mentioned the most frequently the ease of use, as the best point of the isotonic technique (based on the *Patriot*), and the fatigue lead by the technique during the task, as the worst point. Results of the interviews highlight a main difference about these techniques: users did not well perceived the depth by manipulating the isometric technique whereas they could find bearings in space with the isotonic technique to move easily in 3D and it seems to be more "intuitive". Besides, users made no negative comments about the representation and the 3D indices suggested in our standard's adaptation.

With regards to users' preferences, 85% of users like to interact with the isotonic technique and 77% of them estimate this technique is more usable than the isometric technique. This confirms our second hypothesis (H2). Indeed they are 69% to estimate that the isometric technique is more constraining in terms of freedom of movement.

5   Discussion

This paper progressively introduces and justifies the modifications required to adjust a standard for evaluating 2D pointing to the specific context of 3D VE. The adaptation of the standard includes 3 main aspects of enrichment. The first aspect is the addition of the SUS questionnaire to the comfort questionnaire to enable an easy comparison between techniques in terms of usability; it also provides an overall measure, similar to the throughput but related to satisfaction and not to performance. The second aspect is the set of variables of the experiment, which is enriched by a measure of coordination to better understand users' movements in 3D. The third aspect is the adjustments of the task and targets to fit with 3D pointing contexts: forms, arrangements, representations and 3D indices are proposed in order to help users better perceive the depth.

We also propose a software tool to support the execution of experiments in a 3D VE in accordance to the adaptation of the standard.

As a result, our adaptation of the standard presents a generic evaluation method and proposes a structured protocol to lead the evaluation of interaction techniques for pointing task in 3D VE. According to Zhai [25], the usability of 3D input techniques can be defined by 6 criteria: speed, accuracy, fatigue, device persistence and acquisition, coordination and at last, ease of learning. This adaptation offers a composite approach and a set of recommendations, which address all the criteria defined by Zhai. Indeed, in our adaptation, speed and accuracy are measured by the throughput. The fatigue and, persistence and acquisition are evaluated with the comfort questionnaire from the standard and additional semi-directive interviews. The coordination is computed with the inefficiency ratio that we recommend in our adaptation. To measure the ease of learning, we recommend adding an overall score of usability and users' satisfaction measured thanks to the SUS questionnaire.

Furthermore, we show in this paper the use of our adaptation on a concrete case study. It reveals the advantage of having a generic and composite approach. Overall scores of throughput and SUS support a quick and overall comparison of 2 techniques: in our case study, it revealed that the isotonic technique is more efficient and usable than the isometric technique. Moreover, interviews show that users preferred using the isotonic technique to move the pointer as the manipulation seemed more natural, although it may infer more fatigue. This experiment also highlights a tradeoff between the mean movement time and the error rate: the confidence measure of the SUS questionnaire shows that users were more confident using the isotonic technique than the isometric technique and may explain that they paid less attention to the task accuracy. These results enable a complementary analysis to better understand the users' performance and satisfaction for a pointing task in 3D VE.

Using the adaptation of the protocol lead to some already known results (tradeoff between error and speed, preference towards isotonic device, etc), but also provided a framework to explore additional considerations and refine the initial outcomes (inefficiency ratio, impact of ID, complexity of movements, SUS question).

Being an extension of an existing standard, it contributes to the standardization of pointing evaluation in 3D VE. Future uses of the standard by designers will therefore contribute to classify the results according to considerations that are specific to 3D pointing and highlighted in this adapted protocol. Actually this protocol is a guide to set up an experiment and it will contribute to empirically generate recommendations based on these results.

6   Conclusion

In this paper we presented an adaptation of the existing ISO 9241-9 standard to a pointing task in 3D VE. We based our work on an existing standard addressing 2D situations only, because the literature in 3D mentions elements for 3D evaluation that are not present in the ISO 9241-9 standard and does not refer to other standards.

The adaptation of such a standard presents the advantage to propose a structured approach to evaluate a 3D low-level interaction task combining quantitative and qualitative aspects. It offers a unified method to perform pointing task evaluation in 3D VE and constitutes a first step towards 1) a standardization of such procedures and 2) the starting point for the creation of a coherent usability knowledge for pointing in 3D VE.

References

1. Bach, C., Scapin, D.: Ergonomic criteria adapted to human virtual environment interaction. In: 15th French-Speaking Conference on HCI, pp. 24–31. ACM, New York (2003)
2. Gallo, L., de Pietro, G., Marra, I.: 3D interaction with volumetric medical data: experiencing the Wiimote. In: 1st International Conference on Ambient Media and Systems (AmbiSys 2008) (2008)
3. Balakrishnan, R., Baudel, T., Kurtenbach, G., Fitzmaurice, G.: The Rockin'Mouse: integral 3D manipulation on a plane. In: SIGCHI Conference on Human factors in computing systems (CHI 1997), pp. 311–318. ACM, New York (1997)
4. Froehlich, B., Plate, J.: The cubic mouse: a new device for three-dimensional input. In: Conference on Human Factors in Computing Systems (CHI 2000), pp. 526–531. ACM, New York (2000)
5. Bowman, D.A., Kruijff, E., LaViola, J.J., Poupyrev, I.: 3D User Interfaces: Theory and Practice. Addison Wesley Longman Publishing Co., Inc.
6. Masliah, M.: Measuring the allocation of control in 6 degree of freedom human-computer interaction tasks, PhD thesis, University of Toronto (2001)
7. MacKenzie, I.S., Buxton, W.: Extending Fitts' law to two-dimensional tasks. In: Conference on Human Factors in Computing Systems (CHI 1992), pp. 219–226. ACM, New York (1992)
8. Ware, C., Lowther, K.: Selection using a one-eyed cursor in a fish tank VR environment. ACM Trans. Comput.-Hum. Interact. 4(4), 309–322 (1997)
9. Grossman, T., Balakrishnan, R.: Pointing at trivariate targets in 3D environments. In: Conference on Human Factors in Computing Systems (CHI 2004), pp. 447–454. ACM, NY (2004)
10. ISO, 9421-9 Ergonomic requirements for office work with visual display terminals (VDTs)-Part 9: Requirements for non-keyboard input devices. ISO (2000)
11. Natapov, D., Castellucci, S.J., MacKenzie, I.S.: ISO 9241-9 evaluation of video game controllers. In: Graphics Interface 2009 (GI 2009), pp. 223–230 (2009)
12. Teather, R.J., Stuerzlinger, W.: Target Pointing in 3D User Interfaces. In: Poster at Graphics Interface (GI 2010) (2010)
13. Teather, R.J., Stuerzlinger, W.: Pointing at 3D targets in a stereo head-tracked virtual environment. In: IEEE Symposium on 3D User Interfaces (3DUI 2011), pp. 87–94 (2011)
14. Hubona, G.S., Wheeler, P.N., Shirah, G.W., Brandt, M.: The relative contributions of stereo, lighting, and background scenes in promoting 3D depth visualization. ACM Trans. Comput.-Hum. Interact. 6(3), 214–242 (1999)
15. Ortega, M., Nigay, L.: AirMouse: Finger Gesture for 2D and 3D Interaction. In: Gross, T., Gulliksen, J., Kotzé, P., Oestreicher, L., Palanque, P., Prates, R.O., Winckler, M. (eds.) INTERACT 2009. LNCS, vol. 5727, pp. 214–227. Springer, Heidelberg (2009)

16. Bérard, F., Ip, J., Benovoy, M., El-Shimy, D., Blum, J.R., Cooperstock, J.R.: Did "Minority Report" Get it Wrong? Superiority of the Mouse over 3D Input in a 3D Placement Task. In: Gross, T., Gulliksen, J., Kotzé, P., Oestreicher, L., Palanque, P., Prates, R.O., Winckler, M. (eds.) INTERACT 2009. LNCS, vol. 5727, pp. 400–414. Springer, Heidelberg (2009)

17. Zhai, S.: Investigation of feel for 6 DOF inputs: isometric and elastic rate control for manipulation in 3D environments. In: Proc. of The Human Factors and Ergonomics Society 37th Annual Meeting, vol. 37(4), pp. 323–327 (1993)

18. Schmitt, B., Raynal, M., Dubois, E., Bach, C.: Extension de la norme ISO 9241-9 au pointage en 3D. In: 23rd French Speaking Conference on Human-Computer Interaction (IHM 2011), pp. 117–120. ACM, New York (2011)

19. Masliah, M.:
    http://etclab.mie.utoronto.ca/people/moman/timeandspace/timeandspace.html

20. Zhai, S., Milgram, P.: Quantifying coordination in multiple DOF movement and its application to evaluating 6 DOF input devices. In: Karat, C.-M., Lund, A., Coutaz, J., Karat, J. (eds.) Conference on Human Factors in Computing Systems (CHI 1998), pp. 320–327. ACM Press/Addison-Wesley Publishing Co., New York (1998)

21. Zhai, S., Buxton, W., Milgram, P.: The "Silk Cursor": Investigating transparency for 3D target acquisition. In: Adelson, B., Dumais, S., Olson, J. (eds.) Conference on Human Factors in Computing Systems (CHI 1994), pp. 459–464. ACM, New York (1994)

22. Schmitt, B., Dubois, E., Raynal, M., Bach, C., Croenne, D.: Evaluation d'une technique d'interaction ubiquitaire pour le pointage de données complexes et spatialisées. In: Journées Francophones Mobilité et Ubiquité (UBIMOB 2011), pp. 1–8 (2011)

23. Schmitt, B., Raynal, M., Dubois, E.: A composite approach to evaluate two interaction techniques for a 3D pointing task. In: IEEE Symposium on 3D User Interfaces, pp. 159–160 (2012)

24. Bangor, A., Kortum, P.-T., Miller, J.-T.: An empirical evaluation of the System Usability Scale. Journal of Human-Computer Interaction, 574–594 (2008)

25. Zhai, S.: User performance in relation to 3D input device design. SIGGRAPH Comput. Graph. 32(4), 50–54 (1998)

Design Culture for Ageing Well:
Designing for 'Situated Elderliness'

Özge Subasi[1], Geraldine Fitzpatrick[1], Lone Malmborg[2], and Britt Östlund[3]

[1] Vienna University of Technology, HCI-Group
subasi@igw.tuwien ac.at, geraldine.fitzpatrick@tuwien.ac.at
[2] IT University of Copenhagen
malmborg@itu.dk
[3] Rehabilitation Engineering, Design Sciences, Lund University, Sweden
britt.ostlund@design.lth.se

Abstract. The "Design Culture for Ageing Well: Designing for 'Situated Elderliness'" special track focuses on everyday practices and notions of ageing that can be relevant to Human Computer Interaction (HCI). In collaboration with senior associations, designers and theoreticians we elaborate on how newer notions of ageing might inform HCI design. With this track, we concentrate on bottom-up practices of ageing in everyday life, such as used language (visual and verbal) and diverse practices of senior communities (e.g: in different cultures). Our ambition is to go beyond framing support for ageing through a disability-support assistive lens and explore new approaches to designing through ageing well and life experiences as sources for innovations.

1   Background

The topic of designing for ageing well, working with seniors, or assistive technologies have long been discussed in Human Computer Interaction (HCI). In relation to an ageing society, we face a variety of needs and wishes that may or may not be supported with HCI. Existing studies on ageing and technology in e.g: Ambient Assisted Living (AAL) aim to formalize a definition for an "older person" based on biological age, a list for "needs" in the particular technology related context e.g.: see EC Report 12 [2]. Even with a good purpose, this kind of approach usually results in a functional assistance service design for particular deficits (see AAL Project catalogues for project abstracts [2]). Some recent work from Human Computer Interaction discuss an emerging need for distinguishing between this assistive deficit-driven approach and the heterogeneous everyday and situated needs of an ageing community [6, 4]. In a similar topic, recent discussions on healthcare and technology point to the importance of emotional wellbeing and its relevance to emerging technological themes such as social networks, digital storytelling, technologies that provide emotional support and monitoring emotional health [1]. A recent overview on HCI research on the topic of designing for elderly [4] has showed that the simplistic assumptions on what "being old means" do not always hold. For example, loneliness

A. Holzinger et al. (Eds.): SouthCHI 2013, LNCS 7946, pp. 581–584, 2013.
© Springer-Verlag Berlin Heidelberg 2013

and isolation are overplayed, or having a few good close friends may be more important than a larger social network [4].

A situated perspective on 'elderliness' would help us to think beyond the formalized understanding of ageing well. 'Situated elderliness' as a notion aims to define ageing and old age not with biological age, nor with institutional categories, but rather by looking into everyday practices [6]. For example a particular change in an established context (e.g: e-government) can suddenly disable a particular community in their daily practices (accessing governmental services). Situatedness is not only about challenges of ageing. Based on the communities of practice, it is possible to develop an alternative approach by using "elderly's existing everyday practices as frame and starting point"[6]. This approach can help us define specific situations where a community of people has common aims. Looking into everyday practices of elderly in their existing communities can have other benefits. Designers look into different contexts to get inspired for a particular problem in a particular context. By looking into "notions of ageing" through looking into everyday practices of specific senior communities, there might be new lessons to learn for the designer. Taking this as base, we aim to ask some questions on designing for "old age". Some questions here might be: what are the communities out there related to "old age"? How can their practices be brought closer to designers? What is the appropriate language around "notions of ageing" of academia, practitioners and senior organizations? What theories have not yet been considered to explore life experiences? How can modern ageing benefit from innovation research theory and practice [7,8]? We further discuss an early framework on how designers can interpret aging & design, and how they can place themselves in this design research community [9].

1.1 Special Track Outline and Papers

This special track aims to open up interdisciplinary discussions between social scientists, seniors' association members, researchers in human-computer interaction and related fields, healthcare practitioners and other interested persons. The special track brings together people from diverse backgrounds and provides a forum to explore the above introduced issues. Roles of "diversity", "heterogeneity" and "abilities" are core themes, based on an ability-based understanding of aging [5] and situated elderliness [6]). The organizers invited position papers that focussed on topics related to "ageing well", "ambient assisted living" or similar:

- Community based practices in relation to ageing (senior associations, clubs)
- Situated elderliness (practices of "feeling old", "being old")
- Bottom up research on ageing
- Defining heterogeneity in "ageing well"
- Creative space of life-span changes
- Case studies and examples of real-world seniors' related technology designs
- Design process and continuous involvement of senior participants
- Life experiences as sources of innovations

- Broader understanding of ethics, including design ethics, giving-back mechanisms, language and sustainability
- Broader understanding of accessibility and exclusion (e.g: semantic access)

The special track received more than twenty papers. After a double blind peer review process, four papers were selected for full tack presentations to reflect the scope of our understanding. Another 11 papers were selected for a workshop session to showcase interesting studies and to give an impulse to provocative thought around the topic. Further we invited speakers from senior associations to give talks about their communities of everyday practice. Here is an overview of selected papers to illustrate the diversity of approaches. On a theoretical level, Huldgren et. Al. in "Towards community-based co-creation" propose that "the engagement of citizens and stakeholders in their own social and cultural environment, as a natural context for designing and implementing their own solutions would be a key" for future solutions. Similarly, Sustar, Jones and Dearden in Older People as Equal Partners in Creative Design demonstrate the importance of older people's engagement in the creative design process with designers in the design of digital devices. Heimgärtner in „Course and Perception of Ageing in Different Cultures Relevant for Intercultural HCI Design" discusses how the course of perception of ageing in different cultures will be elucidated to derive recommendations for intercultural human-computer interaction (HCI) design. Bagalkot, Green and Lutz in „Designing With Senior Citizens as Mediating Memories: A Retrospective Account" discuss that by looking at 'designing with seniors' as mediating the seniors' rendering of memories is a fruitful stance to take to embrace how seniors and their concerns participate in a design process through three example cases. Ramer in „ A Historical Criticism of Telemedicine as Context to Consider Participatory and Experience-Based Design Applications in Healthcare Service Delivery for Aging Populations" explore the historical origins of telemedicine and reflected back to the importance of participation.

On exploratory papers part, Luckner et. al. discusses a series of design sketches, based on experiences from the field and studying with people, for a playful digital application designed to trigger reminiscence in older adults as a preventive measure against cognitive disabilities such as dementia and Alzheimer's disease. Schulte points to the importance of lack of guidelines for garments for people affected by Dementia. Markovic and Subasi discuss their findings from participant observations and introduce initial design ideas for a particular community. Kouhla et. al. discuss the use of USB-sticks within the context of ageing and health promotion in terms of their visual appearance, functionality, package, implementation and additional services. Arets and Weidema point to the importance of radical design changes in relation to the drastic situation of healthcare in Netherlands. Ehrenstrasser and Spreicer present the analysis of the three years iterative design process of an accessible communication system with tangible user interface to support digital inclusion of elderly people. Güldenpfennig and Fitzpatrick discuss the potential of using rapid prototyping techniques for creating robust, easy to use solutions in long term terchnology probe deployments at home. Culén, Finken and Bratteteig indicate a need for the "smart gym" to be much smarter in order to address the complexities of exercise for an elderly person: as in order to exercise one has to master the gym equipment and its technology. Giorgi et. al. describe an ongoing co-design project of a cooperative distributed space, based on multi-touch technologies, through which older adults engaged in the activities of recreational centers in their everyday contexts could keep in touch with others, for example other recreational centers, and with a general public. Leitner, Mitrea and Fercher reflect upon existing Ambient assisted living related acceptance models and discuss initial results from a project.

Acknowledgements. This special track is 'intellectually' connected to our previous international peer-reviewed workshops such as: AMI Workshop 2008 *DAI-"Capturing AAL Needs"*, in AMI 2008, Nurnberg. CHI Workshop 2009 *"Age matters: bridging the generation gap through technology-mediated interaction"* AMI Workshop 2009 *DAI-"Designing Ambient Interactions for Older People"* in AMI 2009, Salzburg. NordiCHI Workshop 2012 *"Elderly's everyday practices"*, Nordichi 12, Copenhagen. We further thank our international committee members: Marie Ertner (IT University of Copenhagen); Jean Hallewell, University of Applied Sciences Upper Austria; Dave Harley, University of Brighton; Michael Leitner, Northumbria University; Charlotte Magnusson, Lund University; Francisco Nunes, Vienna University of Technology; Kirsten Rassmu-Gröhn, Lund University; Marjo Rauhala, Vienna University of Technology; Tomas Sokoler, IT University of Copenhagen; John Vines, Northumbria University. This special track is partially supported by Ambient Assisted Living Joint Program through STIMULATE Project Sustainable E2 Mobility Services for Elderly People (Austrian Code: 829314).

References

1. Coyle, D., Linehan, C., Tang, K., Lindley, S.: Interaction design and emotional wellbeing. In: Proc of CHI EA 2012, pp. 2775–2778. ACM, New York (2012)
2. European Commission – DG ECFIN. The 2012 Ageing Report (2012), http://ec.europa.eu/information_society/newsroom/cf/itemlongdetail.cfm?item_id=4286 (accessed November 6, 2012)
3. Anon. Catalogue of Projects 2012 (2012), http://www.aal-europe.eu/wpcontent/uploads/2012/08/AALCatalogue2012_V7.pdf (accessed November 6, 2012)
4. Lindley, S.E., Harper, R., Sellen, A.: Designing for elders: exploring the complexity of relationships in later life. In: Proc. of BCS-HCI 2008, vol. 1, pp. 77–86. British Computer Society, Swinton (2008)
5. Wobbrock, J.O., Kane, S.K., Gajos, K.Z., Harada, S., Froehlich, J.: Ability-Based Design: Concept, Principles and Examples. ACM Trans. Access. Comput. 3(3), Article 9, 27 pages (2011)
6. Brandt, E., Binder, T., Malmborg, L., Sokoler, T.: Communities of everyday practice and situated elderliness as an approach to co-design for senior interaction. In: Proc. of OZCHI 2010, pp. 400–403. ACM, New York (2010)
7. Essen, A., Östlund, B.: Laggards as Innovators? Old Users as Designers of New Services & Service Systems. December Issue of the International Journal of Design (2011)
8. Kohlbacher, F., Herstatt, C. (eds.): The Silver Market Phenomenon. Marketing and Innovation in the Aging Society, 2nd edn. Springer, Berlin (2011)
9. Subasi, Ö., Malmborg, L.: Ageing as Design Culture. In: Proc. of Nordes 2013 (2013)

Towards Community-Based Co-creation

Alina Huldtgren, Christian Detweiler, Hani Alers, Siska Fitrianie,
and Nick A. Guldemond

Interactive Intelligence, Delft University of Technology,
Mekelweg 4, 2628CD Delft, The Netherlands
alina@hexgroup.nl,{c.a.detweiler,h.e.b.al-ers,s.fitrianie,
n.a.guldemond}@tudelft.nl

Abstract. Current AAL solutions are often rejected by senior end-users, who do not perceive their benefits or themselves as the target group. This is due to the prevailing technology-driven design process that does not account for human needs. To shift the focus from the technology to the human, involvement of stakeholders in the design process is crucial. In this paper we outline some issues with involvement and continuous engagement of seniors and propose the concept of community-based co-creation as a way forward. Key is the facilitation of long-term collaboration of a community comprised of stakeholders including among others seniors, caregivers and researchers. Their neighborhoods serve as a natural context for designing and implementing their own solutions. We raise several points for consideration and first steps to be discussed.

Keywords: co-creation, co-design, seniors, ambient assisted living.

1 Introduction

Europe's demographic changes are expected to lead to a proportional imbalance of working population to dependent seniors and people with chronic conditions. This will require a shift from public care services to informal community support. Much research and development effort is devoted to technological solutions to solve these issues [1]. Outcomes include assistive technologies, telehealth and telecare systems. Despite these efforts, few systems have been introduced to the market successfully and readily accepted by the targeted user groups [2]. This could be due to the technology-driven development, which accounts little for human needs and values. As a result the proposed systems are often misaligned with the daily lives of end-users, who do not perceive benefit of using the system. In one of our studies of a homecare platform we found that the calendar function was not useful to many of the participants, as a 72-year-old man's quote reflects: *"I don't think it will be used that much. Everyone already has it written down somewhere."* Another problem was that some of the functionality (e.g. a rally round service) required an informal care network around the end-user, which was not in place for some of the seniors. For instance, as one participant said after we presented the system: *"My neighbor does not care about me. And my*

A. Holzinger et al. (Eds.): SouthCHI 2013, LNCS 7946, pp. 585–592, 2013.
© Springer-Verlag Berlin Heidelberg 2013

family lives far away. So, I don't think the system is relevant for me." This
example shows that technical solutions alone are insufficient to innovate the
care system. Greenhalgh's [3] discourse analysis shows that our experiences are
no exceptions; many projects follow a technology-focused, futuristic vision that
is not person-centered and grounded in reality.

In order to shift the focus from the technology to the relevant stakeholders, HCI methodologies such as user-centered design or participatory design are
more appropriate. Building on these methodologies, the concept of co-design
has become popular within HCI. In its broad sense the term refers to any act of
joint creativity in which designers, end-users untrained in design, and perhaps
other stakeholders work together in design processes [4]. It provides a way to
create knowledge by doing, and by that brings tacit knowledge of how people
perform everyday activities and how they may be supported to the foreground
[5]. End-users are treated as experts within their own context [6].

A concept often used synonymously, but stemming from a different field (i.e.
management instead of design) is co-creation. Co-creation, as introduced by [7],
stands for a process of designing with people and not for them. It has become
a popular approach in the public sector to driving innovation. "Co-creation can
[...] lead to radical solutions that overcome the silos, dogmas, and group thinking
that trap much of our current thinking..." [8], which often hampers the creation
of successful solutions. This is relevant and necessary in the care domain, where
traditional silos hinder the communication and collaboration of stakeholders
across disciplines. Nowadays, care is often provided on an informal basis by
spouses, relatives or friends [9]. This can be challenging when social networks
decrease due to retirement, loss of peers and remoteness of family members. The
need for support and care within local communities becomes more prominent.

Co-creating supportive solutions for these new situations is the focus of our
work. A central concept is the engagement of stakeholders, in particular, senior end-users. After highlighting issues that we encountered with regard to
engagement of seniors, we argue for a community-based co-creation approach,
which constitutes a shift from using participatory methods with carefully selected stakeholders in a defined (lab) setting to forming and facilitating local
communities, where stakeholders co-create together over long periods of time. In
South-Holland, and particularly in Delft, we are currently working on building
a local community for co-creation to provide a proof of concept to be applied on
a national level. We raise some of the important questions with regard to the
process of forming and facilitating communities as well as ethical and scientific
considerations. Finally, we provide a description of our first steps.

2   Issues with Senior Engagement

In our research in EU and national projects we commonly employ a human-
centered design methodology. Engaging end-users in all stages of the design
process is central. We collected qualitative data in semi-structured interviews,
participatory design workshops and have run formative evaluations of (early

stage) interactive design mock-ups. Besides design activities, we are in touch with a local community of stakeholders and, in particular, seniors, to whom we regularly present and demo our ideas and prototypes. In the following, we will focus on a number of aspects that we identified in these activities that hindered the collaboration with seniors and technology acceptance. We highlight selected experiences and link them to the literature.

2.1 Stigmatization and Self-image

Similar to the experiences of [10] that "... almost nobody among the group of people between 55 and 75 years old identified themselves as elderly' or senior citizens'", almost all participants (between 70 and 80) in our interviews made references to the usefulness of the envisioned system for older people but not for themselves. This is reflected by the following conversation about sensors in the home with a 76-year-old woman: *"I don't need it myself, but I can imagine that people would need this when they are older."* Importantly, similar thoughts were expressed both by participants who lived active lives without physical and mental challenges as well as by participants that had significant physical handicaps (e.g. paralyzed). The concept of self-image is an interesting point to consider when recruiting participants. A 73-year-old woman's comment reflects her self-image with regard to the system: *"Well you know, I'm still pretty modern. There are many things I wouldn't use right now, but when I'm older and I won't leave home as much, I think there might be some more things I'd want to use then."*

2.2 Language-Related Issues

Within the AAL literature the user group is mainly described as the elderly'. However, in 2009 the Telegraph published an article stating *"Words to describe elderly people such as 'codger', 'fogey' and even 'elderly' itself should be banned from media reporting, ageism campaigners are urging."* A guide was created for journalists saying that *"[i]nstead, people aged over 50 should be referred to as 'older people' or simply 'man' or 'woman' followed by their age, the guide suggests."* Within recent HCI publications, e.g., [11], new labels emerged such as 80-somethings, elders or people of the 3rd age. In a discussion with a project partner representing the end-users, he concluded that seniors' is more acceptable than elderly', as it is comparable it to being a senior in a company reflecting experience and knowledge. An example from our fieldwork shows very clearly that using the right wording is important. When a couple aged over 80, who were active in social volunteering work, received a letter with an invitation to present their work at a local event targeted at senior citizens, they were upset about being addressed as elderly and refused to go.

2.3 Stances of Researchers and Society

We should also consider that our language reflects our perspectives on ageing and could lead others to think in similar ways. The same perspectives are then used to design new solutions. For instance, having the opinion that people over a certain age are fragile and in need of assistance would focus the design process on assistive systems and may lead developers to build a system that assists and monitors people in taking their medication, getting the groceries, sending alarms etc. In a workshop, attended by one author recently, a group of young students presented a design for social inclusion of seniors. Their design entailed that *"elderly, so 65+"* moved into a house where they would have a room equipped with a computer on which they could play an interactive game with other residents. After this presentation an older workshop participant criticized the design heavily claiming that the students had not considered the target group and their current lives appropriately.

2.4   Lack of Continuation of Ideas

When taking part in a study, participants put time and effort giving their ideas on a certain research domain. People take pride in offering such information because it represents their thought, experiences and identity. While executing our activities, we found that participants in user studies were expecting a continued use of their collected ideas. A lack of continuation may hinder the long-term engagement of stakeholders in a research trajectory. Some people were reluctant to participate in consecutive studies, because they did not see the follow-up on ideas and feedback that were collected previously and thus felt exploited or disappointed as shown by the following example.

In a local information evening for seniors, a woman said that sometime ago she and some peers were invited to brainstorm ideas to improve the quality of life and inclusion of seniors in society. In the meeting the idea of adopting a grandmother/father came up, which many seniors liked. However, the city never implemented or followed up on this idea. The woman stated that this was disappointing and it made her doubt whether the seniors' feedback would ever be used. Not every idea can be continued, but as stated in [8], *"what is necessary is to clarify expectations."* He suggests stating clearly that not every idea will be put into practice, but that all input will be taken seriously.

3   Discussion

The issues discussed in the previous section highlight some of the salient difficulties of engaging prospective senior end-users in the design of new technologies. The first three are closely related. Stigmatization and language-related issues stem from researchers' (and society's) preconceptions and assumptions about stakeholders, which often do not align with stakeholders' self-image. Addressing these issues calls for more accurate perspectives on ageing and forming more realistic images of stakeholders. To achieve this, it is important to (1) be in close contact with seniors and other stakeholders to experience their daily lives, (2) give stakeholders the opportunity to present themselves as they see themselves, and (3) understand the assets and capabilities of all stakeholders, not just their problems.

The engagement of researchers with stakeholders in everyday life settings can provide rich insights into the stakeholders' daily life environments and experiences that would be lost in lab settings [12]. In the early stages of co-creation, where the focus lies on a shared understanding of the design space, it is important that all stakeholders get to experience the context first hand. Furthermore, stakeholders may more easily provide tacit knowledge by being observed in their own environments than a lab [6]. In the later stages of co-creation, it is important to test and evaluate solutions in real-life to see the effects of contextual factors on the interaction with the system, which would not be encountered in controlled lab settings [13].

Furthermore, engagement needs to go beyond a single phase of design or a single project. If stakeholders' involvement is short-term, e.g., when they are merely involved in the process of gathering requirements, it is often unclear to them how their input was used. Moreover, if stakeholders' involvement is limited to a particular design phase, there are few opportunities for them to voice their interests or concerns, potentially hindering a sense of influence or ownership. It needs to be transparent how ideas elicited in participatory sessions led to next steps. Additionally, channels of communication and involvement need to remain open beyond elicitation and evaluation, throughout the process of design and deployment. By putting innovation into people's own hands, we can ensure the innovation meet people's essential need (regardless who was the owner of the initial idea) and with the help of local business partners and infrastructure ideas can be implemented quickly.

Bringing together stakeholders and facilitating co-creation is key. We believe it is our role as researchers to initiate and become part of local communities where stakeholders (senior citizens, informal carers, volunteers, care organizations, etc.) meet and collaborate, supported by our knowledge about demographic and technological developments. At the same time, we should take care not to impose fixed processes or methods on the people, but instead promote mutual learning that could lead to a common understanding (and shared language) to reduce stereotypes, e.g. of younger people towards ageing and of older people towards technologies. Each stakeholder's perspective is needed and no perspective should be privileged. To form a methodical approach following our arguments above, we propose a new concept: *community-based co-creation*.

3.1 Community-Based Co-creation

Community-based co-creation refers to active collaboration between stakeholders to build communities and related infrastructure where long-term co-creation will take place. To set co-creation in a relevant context, living-labs can provide a basis for researchers and stakeholders to work together to create, validate and test new products and services in real life contexts [12]. Community-based co-creation aims at mutual learning to reach a shared understanding (and language), long-term engagement, and continuation of ideas.

We define community as a spatially bound group of individuals (e.g. a neighborhood) and their close social network (e.g. family members who frequently visit the neighborhood) that share a common goal (i.e. in our case active and healthy ageing) and common values, and take collaborative action towards achieving the goal. Members of this community can take on different roles (not necessarily fixed) such as giving or receiving support or representing a company or organization (e.g. the municipality, local service providers or knowledge institutes). Our notion of communities differs from communities of (everyday) practice as it includes stakeholders with different professions and skills. However, it relates to communities of action or purpose.

Our role as researcher is to make co-creation more transparent and to build the trust of the stakeholders by (1) creating awareness about the possibilities and the limitation of innovation, and (2) informing stakeholders how contributions are utilized and how designs are adjusted to fit the situation and the stakeholders' need. Community-based co-creation entails the following key features:

- A sustainable community of stakeholders (including researchers, citizens, businesses, etc.) with (technological) infrastructure

- Continuous communication among stakeholders (reducing issue of 2.2)

- Equality of stakeholders (reducing stigmatization as in 2.1)

- Facilitation of mutual learning among stakeholders (addressing issue of 2.3)

- Transparency of processes and outcomes (handling issue of 2.4)

As this approach is more complex than research and development in discrete lab settings it poses new challenges of organizing the process while balancing the researchers' interference into communities and creation of scientific knowledge. We raise the following issues to be discussed with the HCI community:

Identifying, forming and managing communities: Communities may not readily exist and it is therefore a key task to facilitate the forming of communities by identifying relevant stakeholders and providing communication means to them. Key questions are; Who should be engaged? How can we engage all relevant stakeholders, including the people who are normally difficult to involve, to establish a representative community?

Ethical considerations: Community-based co-creation may affect social structures in the chosen neighborhoods. Key questions are; Which social-cultural and ethical aspects should be taken in consideration and incorporated in the process? How can we ensure that stakeholders can voice themselves and that their ideas and interests are considered equally?

Methodological considerations: As a scientific method, generalizability is one of the concerns. Key questions are; What kind of approaches and methods are appropriate for successful co-creation in the community? What are the indicators for co-creation contexts to transfer a developed method to a new context? What are the success criteria of co-creation?

4   Ongoing Actitivies and Future Work

Based on the considerations above we defined these goals for implementing community-based co-creation: (1) identify, build and manage communities where co-creation will take place, (2) create awareness of technological developments within these communities. (3) create an inspiring and comfortable environment for co-creation supporting intergenerational stakeholder interaction and (4) develop co-creation techniques and success criteria. *Stakeholders:* For senior support and care we identified the following stakeholders.

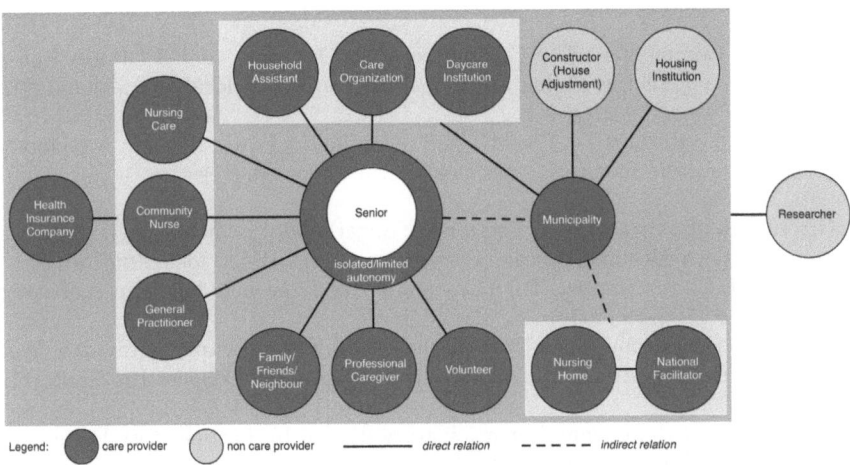

Fig. 1. Stakeholders related to care domain in the Netherlands

Living Lab: A prerequisite to community-based co-creation is an infrastructure with a defined network (e.g. public-private partnership). Our local community setting (highly populated urban neighborhood) comprises relevant stakeholders, facilities and a mixed demographic population. A dedicated ICT-infrastructure and service platform is envisioned and a multidisciplinary team is developing proposals, engaging partners, raising funds and managing the activities. Activities - We have initiated several first activities to facilitate citizens to learn about our work as well as provide their opinion. Two examples are:

– iCare videos contest: Sponsored by the municipality, we organized a video contest for young people about care, technology, and community to collect positive stories about how seniors use technology in their regular activities. We invited young and old to work together and present their stories to other community members (goal 3). Prices were handed over at a public community event (goal 2).

– Active living fair: an event organized by the local volunteer organization aimed at people aged 55+ where more than 30 organizations offered their services. We joined the fair and demonstrated 'easy to use technologies' (e.g. 'Word Lens' that uses augmented reality to translate texts from foreign languages) to raise awareness about new technologies (goal 2). Other activities include, e.g., debates and presentations at local events, think tanks with stakeholders and a stakeholder video documentary that will be used in an online platform for communication between stakeholders. These activities are crucial steps in laying the foundation for a community-based co-creation process.

References

1. European Commission, The Committee of the Regions, AGE Platform Europe: How to promote active ageing in Europe: EU support to local and regional actors (2011)
2. Brownsell, S., Bradley, D., Blackburn, S., Cardinaux, F., Hawley, M.: A systematic review of lifestyle monitoring technologies. J. Telemed. Telecare. 17(4), 185–189 (2011)
3. Greenhalgh, T., Procter, R., Wherton, J., Sugarhood, P., Shaw, S.: The organising vision for telehealth and telecare: discourse analysis. BMJ Open 2012 (2012)
4. Sanders, E.B.-N., Stapper, P.J.: Co-creation and the new landscapes of design. CoDesign 4(1), 5–18 (2008)
5. Nardi, B., Engeström, Y.: A Web on the Wind: The Structure of Invisible Work. In: Nardi, B., Engeström, Y. (eds.) Computer Supported Cooperative Work, vol. 8, pp. 1–2 (1999)
6. Crabtree, A.: Ethnography in participatory design. In: Participatory Design Conference, pp. 93–105. CPSR, Seattle (1998)
7. Prahalad, C.K., Ramaswamy, V.: Co-Creation Experiences: The Next Practice in Value Creation. J. I. M. 18(3), 5–14 (2004)
8. Bason, C.: Leading Public Sector Innovation. Co-creating for a better society. The Policy Press, Bristol (2010)
9. Eurostat: Active ageing and solidarity between generations. A statistical portrait of the European Union, European Commission (2011)
10. Brandt, E., Binder, T., Malmborg, L., Sokoler, T.: Communities of everyday practice and situated elderliness as an approach to co-design for senior interaction. In: OzCHI 2010, pp. 400–403. ACM, New York (2010)
11. Vines, J., Blythe, M., Dunphy, P., Vlachokyriakos, V., Teece, I., Monk, A., Olivier, P.: Cheque mates: participatory design of digital payments with eighty somethings. In: Proceedings of the 2012 ACM Annual Conference on Human Factors in Computing Systems (CHI 2012), pp. 1189–1198. ACM, New York (2012)
12. Følstad, A.: Living Labs for Innovation and Development of Communication Technology: A Literature Review. eJOV 10, 99–131 (2008)
13. Kushniruk, A.W., Borycki, E.M., Kannry, J.: Commercial versus In-Situ Usability Testing of Healthcare Information Systems: Towards Public Usability Testing in Healthcare Organizations. Enabling Health and Healthcare Through Ict: Available, Tailored and Closer, 157 (2013)

Course and Perception of Ageing in Different Cultures Relevant for Intercultural HCI Design

Rüdiger Heimgärtner

Intercultural User Interface Consulting (IUIC)
Lindenstraße 9, 93152 Undorf, Germany
ruediger.heimgaertner@iuic.de

Abstract. The course of perception for ageing in different cultures is elucidated to derive recommendations for intercultural human-computer interaction (HCI) design. How ageing influences the usage and the design of intercultural HCI is analyzed. Software development and usability engineering are perceived quite differently in various parts of the world according to the age of the respective interpreters. The main tasks are discussed which users request depending on their age. The discussion covers how age influences software developers and how UI designers collaborate with respect to different cultural backgrounds.

Keywords: Learning, Challenges, Cross-Cultural, Culture, Communication, Interpretation, HCI, Intercultural, Cultural Studies, HCI Design, Cultural Differences, Understanding, Empathy, Intercultural Communication, Intercultural HCI Design, Age, Ageing, Perception.

1 Course and Perception of Ageing in Different Cultures

Life-span developmental psychology investigates factors that have an influence on adaptation to the challenges of the aging process, mechanisms of developmental regulation and successful aging. This includes experimental as well as questionnaire-based studies with focus on different topics, such as context specific age stereotypes and subjective well-being (cf. [1]), age discrimination, depression in later life, adaptive changes in goals and values (cf. [2]), control beliefs in later life as well as coping with age-related deficits and losses (cf. [3]).

Changing lifestyle, sensory and cognitive changes as well as reducing mobility and increasing illness are the characteristics of older adult users (cf. [4]). In detail, there are physical changes in vision, hearing, and motor; cognitive changes in memory and attention; as well as psychological and social changes (cf. [5]). Older adult users usually have high life experience. They had the chance to enjoy education and gain fundamental soft skills applied in several contexts over long time.

Functional ageing relates to the way in which a user's cognitive, perceptual and physiological capabilities may degrade at a rate that is faster than might otherwise be expected for their age (cf. [6]). This form of ageing can be a particular problem for certain industries. For example, some commercial aviation pilots suffer significant

A. Holzinger et al. (Eds.): SouthCHI 2013, LNCS 7946, pp. 593–600, 2013.

sinus problems that ultimately may lead to hearing loss. According to [6], there are three different ways in which 'functional ageing' can affect interface development:

- it can affect an entire workforce and so additional cues and prompts may be introduced for all users who suffer from this problem;
- it may only affect certain individuals within a population and so studies will have to be conducted to determine whether initial assumptions about user capabilities hold for the entire group;
- the rate of functional aging may vary from individual to individual and so further studies may be needed to determine the extent of the additional support that may be necessary. Ultimately, it may not be possible for some people to use the system even with significant enhancements to the interface, for example in safety-critical applications.

Moreover, based on ageing, there are changes in methodologies for involving older adults in the design process (cf. [7]). Ageing in general influences the usage of 'user interfaces' and the design of them. In addition, only by assuming the perspective of a user by the HCI designer to grasp their needs depending on world view, general knowledge, context, and purpose of usage can lead to good user interfaces of high usability, thereby evoking excellent user experience also from an ageing point of view also in the cultural context.

Therefore, the aim is to research the basic cultural differences in ageing while discussing and adapting well-known methods for their usage in intercultural HCI design, i.e., the culture-oriented design of interactive systems and products by taking into account the cultural context of the user depending on product usage and required tasks (cf. [8]), and related areas such as intercultural user experience (UX) design and intercultural usability engineering.

2   Effects of Ageing on Using and Designing Intercultural HCI

Influences of social structures of the age on the thoughts and actions of individuals – and in this respect anticipated changes – are mediated by age norms, age stereotypes and personal age images (cf. [9]). These age-related notions are pre-conditions for first conceptions of personal future self-images of their own age. In a second step, these personalized age images are internalized in the self-image of older people (cf. [10] and [11]). For different areas of life there exist different and independent age images that strongly differ in their valence and their age limits (cf. [12]).

[13] found inflated self-views across the lifespan and around the world present investigation examined associations among narcissism, age, ethnicity, world region, and gender, using a large sample of participants (n=3445) representing several different world regions and ethnicities. The results suggest that (1) reported narcissism declines in older participants, (2) consistent with previous findings, males report being more narcissistic than females, (3) that ethnic differences in reported narcissism are generally comparable to those found in the self-esteem literature, and (4) that world region appears to exert influence on narcissism, with participants from more individualistic

societies reporting more narcissism. The results are discussed in terms of how age and culture might impact narcissism. The aging experiences gathered by [13] describe the diversities and commonalities across several cultures. In an attempt to understand the meaning of ageing and the treatment of the aged in different cultures seven anthropologists have made studies of 10 communities on four continents. The authors used both qualitative and statistical data to examine such issues as: health and well-being, perceptions of the life course, material resources, and functionality of elders. This resource provides a detailed comparative analysis of ageing worldwide. The intercultural comparison of the images of old age, including Germany, the United States and Hong Kong showed a systematically enlarged view and yielded characteristics and correlations between individual age images, time and life in old age and personal preventive action (cf. [13]). The approach adopted in the study comparing the findings to the German case of old age, usage of time and maintenance and preventive action in the United States and Hong Kong is scientifically highly relevant. The case selection leads to three sophisticated late-or post-industrial societies to be considered for structural analogue (although the extent of different) affected by demographic change exhibiting significant differences with regard to the socialization of the (higher) age, the cultural patterns of age-specific life management, the individual action time as well as social structures of time. So, for example, [14] showed how the pace of social time, depending on socio-structural and socio-cultural framework conditions vary and is subject to specific modes of change. Stability and change social experience of time and social time horizons in turn affect the individual ways of dealing with time and temporality. [15] showed that compared to Chinese respondents for the U.S. and Europe the experience of time result in different patterns. [16] showed that negative expectations about the future can have positive consequences for the well-being of older Chinese. At the same time social upheavals such as had the return of Hong Kong to China or the SARS epidemic on their own experience of time and shaping their own development (cf. [17]). Corresponding differences are assumed in the face of structurally divergent norms of ageing, age transitions and age stereotypes in the three societies, also with regard to issues of age perception and self-perception as well as to their impact on personal age-related action orientations (cf. [18, 19]). [10] demonstrated that in China hardly prejudices regarding age-related cognitive deficits prevail, so that activation of the category "old" in elderly subjects without self-stereotyping effects in terms of a poorer truncation of older people could be detected during memory tasks. Background of these differences are often deeply rooted differences with regard to cultural adjustment pattern about individualism and collectivism (or familism), the idea of self-determined life or the normative place occupied by short-or long-term nature of action orientation (e.g., [20]). [1] initiated two successive interdisciplinary research projects on transitions in adulthood and perceptions of aging and older persons which are funded by the Volkswagen Foundation until 2015. There are first indications that the internalization of general age images regarding the personal age and the personal self-image is context-specific (cf. [12]), which implicates that cultural contexts influence the perception of aging. Finally, it is stated that there are no affective priming effects in a valent/neutral-categorization task (cf. [21]) and that the activation of specific facets of age stereotypes depend on individuating information (cf. also [1]). [22] researched the adjustment and age through the eyes of Portuguese and English community-dwelling older adults. The most prevalent response of the interviewed participants for contributors was 'sense of limit and exis-tential issues' and 'with congruence'. Portuguese elderly were explained by a three-factor model: 'integrated', 'involved' and 'young at heart'. A three-dimension model formed by 'attentive', 'driven' and 'connected' was indicated as a best-fit solution for English elderly. There are also influences of ageing on action and cognition. Goal orientations and processes of action regulation influence – and are in turn influenced by – micro mechanisms of cognition and information processing (cf. [23]). Informa-tion processing is tuned to what is relevant for action regulation and goal pursuit. As long as action resources are available for active goal pursuit (i.e., in an assimilative mode of action regulation), information processing is focused on the current goals and the means towards achieving the goals. When action resources become scarce and attempts to reach a goal are chronically frustrated (i.e., in an accommodative mode of action regulation), cognitive resources are withdrawn from blocked goals and redi-rected towards other, more promising goals and projects. Experiments examined the relation between assimilative and accommodative modes of coping and cognitive processes relating to selective attention (cf. [11] and [3]), perception (cf. [23]), and motivated reasoning (cf. [24]).

In overall, the results of all these studies are highly relevant for intercultural user interface design from an ageing point of view regarding ageing images, time usage and preventing actions at least according to its influences on the values of cultural dimensions such as individualism and collectivism (cf. [25]).

3   Discussion: Challenges and Recommendations

3.1   Challenges

Successful usage and adaptation of methods depends crucially on the capability for empathy of the people involved (cf. [26], [27], [28, 29], e.g. to avoid quarrel by gen-eration conflicts, i.e. "critical incidents" in the cultural context, cf. [30]). In this sense, "same age groups" or "ageing groups" can be regarded as different cultural groups processed with the same methods used for handling culture groups ("cultures"). Communication without empathy does not deliver the desired results (cf. [26]). This in turn assumes a certain level of confidence and trust (e.g. Principle of Charity, cf. [27]) and includes the knowledge of how to read between the lines of the counter-part's communication depending on culturally different rules. This includes the usage of linguistic rules, for example, Austin's felicity conditions or Gricean maxims (cf. [28, 29]). Therefore any literal translation of a conversation is prone to misinterpreta-tion since the extension of the concepts can be different in different cultures ("linguistic relativity", cf. [31]). As context must also be taken into consideration, it is important to consider these aspects in communicating and focus on the intellectual horizon of the communication partner as widely as possible. This can occur in par-ticular through personal and on-site communication and is particularly difficult over the phone due to the absence of mimical and gestical signals. Even more problems arise for ageing in intercultural communication compared to intra-cultural communication due to differing world views and the context in which clarification occurs. For this reason, the empathic capability to put oneself in someone else's situation is particularly important. The application of empathy in the end contributes to a successful communication supporting a mutual linguistic code. In particular, intercultural user experience designers must be able to put themselves in the position of the user in order to know and understand his or her intentions and needs, to ideally experience them, and to implement them in the product. However, empathy also presupposes the capability to separate oneself from other persons to get the chance to recognize the differences to them and then to put oneself in their position. Within the intercultural ageing context, this requires being aware of one's own cultural standards before it is possible to compare and recognize differences to other cultures (cf. [30]).

In addition, global user interfaces, which would suit all culture domains, users and contexts, do not yet exist, at least for technical if not for more fundamental reasons. Computers do not yet possess empathy (cf. the so-called „hard problems of AI" (cf. [32])). At the moment computers lack environmental data (through sensors), the complex processing patterns and the respective knowledge of the world needed to develop empathy. Furthermore, the cultural differences involved in the interaction of the user with the system must be integrated in such knowledge of the world so that the system can adjust for it respectively. Finally, even if these challenges were met the so-called 'bootstrapping' problem of adaptive systems would remain. Because the system is not yet acquainted with the user on his first encounter, the system cannot adapt to him. It is a matter of time until the system gets acquainted with the user and can adapt itself to him. At least the following areas must be considered in HCI, i.e. Human-Computer-Interaction: task, context/situation and tools used (cf. [33]). In this case the cognitive processes of the user differ from the results of studies or discrete situations due to his cultural and environmental conditioning and personal experience. The concept of the task intended (as well as the task itself) is no longer congruent. That requires the system (computer / machine / tool) to adapt as perfectly as possible to many different aspects, which however has not yet been possible to implement because of the multitude of aspects and the resultant complexity.

3.2   Recommendations

A detailed model for intercultural HCI design has been worked out by the author (cf. [25]), which is used as inspiration for thinking things through in this area and helps to elucidate the complex entanglement of the huge amount of data and information pieces forced by the number of aspects to consider for ageing in cultural context (like current situation, ambience, mood, cognitive style, cognitive state, context, use case, perspective, role, status, profession, experience, education, ability to be empathic, personal character, use of language). In addition, a compiled list of examples of HCI problems resulting from ageing have been analyzed according to the aspects mentioned just now and the results are stored in a matrix representing the ageing and cultural differences related to examples of HCI. From this matrix in conjunction with the model, rules must be derived to adjust the methods for intercultural HCI design concerning ageing such that the results and the design recommendations from applying the methods can be compared according to different cultures as well as applied for adequate use cases in the right situation and context. To show the applicability of this model as a basis for further studies, the influence of age images in different cultures must be investigated and connected to intercultural HCI design.

However, even if some evidence and rules have been obtained to narrow the challenges in analyzing ageing perspectives relevant for HCI design using the mentioned matrix and model, the final analysis of the intercultural HCI design process and it's relating cultural differences is still outstanding.

As long as the problems of automatically adapting the user interfaces to the users have not been completely solved, human beings must accordingly attune HCI to the intended cultural domain, user group and context (cf. [34]). To do so, the HCI designer must be able to immerse himself in these cultural domains, user groups and contexts in order to extract the relevant requirements for the HCI design.

In order to build up not only understanding but also the ability to put oneself in someone else's position, it is initially necessary to be on the same wavelength to find a connection to the other person. This requires the alignment of communication coding (vocabulary and grammar) and to achieve a situation where the other person wants to communicate including taking into account different mental models, cognition, and metaphysics. Thereby a relationship is built up in such a way that future communication remains possible. If this connection is given, it is important to preserve access to the other person's knowledge base ("Web Of Belief", cf. [35]) using a mutual topic of conversation in order to examine the knowledge base of the counterpart in regard to extent, type, and quality. Only then it is possible to find the right "hook" in further conversations and consequently "fetch up" the other person's web of belief at the most relevant point to quickly pick up the same wavelength again. The web of belief contains beliefs and desires derived from premises, assumptions and facts using logical rules and are recursively formed by experience from birth. Through training intercultural competency, approaching the web of belief of a member of other cultures is possible. Thereby, exchange of experiences is very effective, trust can be conferred from one person to another by introducing the persons and critical interaction situations (cf. [30]) because of ageing can be weakened. This works, if it is clear how the other person thinks (i.e. what world view he or she holds i.e. which premises and assumptions about the world he or she has). This is necessary in order to make choices which are relevant to the job at hand and correct for successful communication with a continually expanding set of extra information.

This is particularly the case in intercultural ageing contexts. The ability to assess and understand the person's thinking patterns enables an adequate reaction to the people involved. In the same way, the leading and guiding of conversation, e.g., as facilitator or investigator is successfully supported especially in the cultural context.

4   Conclusions

This paper just touches the problems in intercultural HCI design arising from ageing, which should be investigated in detail in further studies. The design rules for ageing differ from culture to culture because of different expectations (by experiences, education, and context) of the members of the respective cultures. The final analysis of the challenges by ageing in intercultural HCI design is still outstanding. Nevertheless, this paper should be a first step to come closer to a scientific understanding and to apply adequate methods considering ageing in intercultural HCI design.

References

1. Casper, C., Rothermund, K., Wentura, D.: The activation of specific facets of age stereotypes depends on individuating information. Social Cognition 29, 393–414 (2011)
2. Brandtstädter, J., Rothermund, K., Kranz, D., Kühn, W.: Final Decentrations. European Psychologist 15, 152–163 (2010)
3. Rothermund, K., Brandstädter, J.: Coping with deficits and losses in later life: from compensatory action to accommodation. Psychology and Aging 18, 896 (2003)
4. Dickinson, A., Arnott, J., Prior, S.: Methods for human-computer interaction research with older people. Behav. Inf. Technol. 26, 343–352 (2007)
5. Nunes, F., Silva, P.A., Abrantes, F.: Human-computer interaction and the older adult: an example using user research and personas. In: Proceedings of the 3rd International Conference on PErvasive Technologies Related to Assistive Environments, pp. 1–8. ACM, Samos (2010)
6. Johnson, C.A., Adams, A.J., Twelker, J.D., Quigg, J.M.: Age-related changes in the central visual field for short-wavelength-sensitive pathways. J. Opt. Soc. Am. A 5, 2131–2139 (1988)
7. Newell, A.F., Arnott, J., Carmichael, A., Morgan, M.: Methodologies for Involving Older Adults in the Design Process. In: Stephanidis, C. (ed.) HCI 2007. LNCS, vol. 4554, pp. 982–989. Springer, Heidelberg (2007)
8. Röse, K., Zühlke, D.: Culture-Oriented Design: Developers' Knowledge Gaps in this Area. In: 8th IFAC/IFIPS/IFORS/IEA Symposium on Analysis, Design, and Evaluation of Human-Machine Systems, September 18-20, pp. 11–16. Pergamon (2001)
9. Kotter-Grühn, D., Hess, T.M.: The impact of age stereotypes on self-perceptions of aging across the adult lifespan. The Journals of Gerontology Series B: Psychological Sciences and Social Sciences 67, 563–571 (2012)
10. Levy, B., Langer, E.: Aging free from negative stereotypes: Successful memory in China among the American deaf. Journal of Personality and Social Psychology 66, 989 (1994)
11. Rothermund, K., Brandtstädter, J.: Age stereotypes and self-views in later life: Evaluating rival assumptions. International Journal of Behavioral Development 27, 549–554 (2003)
12. Kornadt, A.E., Rothermund, K.: Contexts of aging: assessing evaluative age stereotypes in different life domains. The Journals of Gerontology Series B: Psychological Sciences and Social Sciences 66, 547–556 (2011)
13. Keith, J., Fry, C., Glascock, A., Ikels, C., Dickerson-Putman, J., Harpending, H.: The aging experience. Sage Pub. (1994)
14. Levine, R.V., Norenzayan, A.: The pace of life in 31 countries. Journal of Cross-Cultural Psychology 30, 178–205 (1999)
15. Fung, H.H., Stoeber, F.S., Yeung, D.Y.-I., Lang, F.R.: Cultural specificity of socioemotional selectivity: Age differences in social network composition among Germans and Hong Kong Chinese. The Journals of Gerontology Series B: Psychological Sciences and Social Sciences 63, 156–164 (2008)

16. Cowling, B.J., Chan, K.-H., Fang, V.J., Cheng, C.K., Fung, R.O., Wai, W., Sin, J., Seto, W.H., Yung, R., Chu, D.W.: Facemasks and Hand Hygiene to Prevent Influenza Transmission in Households A Cluster Randomized Trial. Annals of Internal Medicine 151, 437–446 (2009)
17. Carstensen, L.L., Mikels, J.A., Mather, M.: Aging and the intersection of cognition, motivation, and emotion. Handbook of the Psychology of Aging 6, 343–362 (2006)
18. Westerhof, G.J., Whitbourne, S.K., Freeman, G.P.: The aging self in a cultural context: the relation of conceptions of aging to identity processes and self-esteem in the United States and the Netherlands. J. Gerontol. B. Psychol. Sci. Soc. Sci. 67, 52–60 (2012)
19. Westerhof, G.J., Whitbourne, S.K., Freeman, G.P.: The Aging Self in a Cultural Context: The Relation of Conceptions of Aging to Identity Processes and Self-Esteem in the United States and the Netherlands. The Journals of Gerontology Series B: Psychological Sciences and Social Sciences (2011)
20. Cross, S.E., Hardin, E.E., Gercek-Swing, B.: The what, how, why, and where of self-construal. Pers. Soc. Psychol. Rev. 15, 142–179 (2011)
21. Werner, B., Rothermund, K.: Attention please: No affective priming effects in a valent/neutral-categorisation task. Cognition & Emotion 1-14 (2012)
22. Humboldt, S.V., Leal, I., Pimenta, F.: Adjustment and Age Through the Eyes of Portuguese and English Community-Dwelling Older Adults. Studies in Sociology of Science 3, 1–9 (2012)
23. Brandtstädter, J., Rothermund, K.: The life-course dynamics of goal pursuit and goal adjustment: A two-process framework. Developmental Review 22, 117–150 (2002)
24. Rothermund, K., Bak, P.M., Brandtstädter, J.: Biases in self - evaluation: moderating effects of attribute controllability. European Journal of Social Psychology 35, 281–290 (2005)
25. Heimgärtner, R.: Cultural Differences in Human-Computer Interaction. Oldenbourg Verlag (2012)
26. Stueber, K.R.: Rediscovering empathy: agency, folk psychology, and the human sciences. MIT Press, Cambridge (2010)
27. Dennett, D.C.: The intentional stance. MIT Press, Cambridge (1998)
28. Austin, J.L., Savigny, E.V.: Zur Theorie der Sprechakte = (How to do things with words). Reclam, Stuttgart (2010)
29. Grice, P.: Studies in the way of words. Harvard Univ. Press, Cambridge (1993)
30. Thomas, A., Kinast, E.-U., Schroll-Machl, S.: Handbook of intercultural communication and cooperation. Basics and areas of application. Vandenhoeck & Ruprecht, Göttingen (2010)
31. Whorf, B.L.: Sprache - Denken - Wirklichkeit Beiträge zur Metalinguistik und Sprachphilosophie. Rowohlt, Reinbek bei Hamburg (2008)
32. Winograd, T., Flores, F.: Understanding computers and cognition: A new foundation for design. Addison-Wesley, Boston (2004)
33. Herczeg, M.: Software-Ergonomie: Grundlagen der Mensch-Computer-Kommunikation. Oldenbourg, München (2005)
34. Van Kleek, M., Shrobe, H.E.: A practical activity capture framework for personal, lifetime user modeling. In: Conati, C., McCoy, K., Paliouras, G. (eds.) UM 2007. LNCS (LNAI), vol. 4511, pp. 298–302. Springer, Heidelberg (2007)
35. Quine, W.V.O.: Word and object. MIT Press, Cambridge (2004)

Memoryscape: Designing with Senior Citizens as Memory Meditation

Naveen L. Bagalkot[1], William Green[2], and Peter Lutz[3]

[1] Srishti School of Art, Design and Technology, India
naveen@srishti.ac.in
[2] Leicester University, UK
wg32@leicester.ac.uk
[3] IT University of Copenhagen, Denmark
plutz@itu.dk

Abstract. Supporting senior citizens with tools to recollect past experiences about everyday life is gaining ground within HCI research. In this paper, we focus on how seniors reminiscing can be a resource for designers to uncover the situated aspects. In particular, we argue that an analytical focus on seniors' memories is a fruitful stance for tracing how design practice situates issues of senior wellbeing. We employ the case of designing with senior citizens to design ICT for supporting adherence to physical therapy at home and discuss two retrospective examples. These examples highlight how seniors' physical wellbeing was situated in, memories of a musically rich and mobile life, and memories of youthful male body. Through retrospection, we offer the preliminary notion of *memoryscape* as a conceptual term for orienting how a design process can mediate seniors' memories as a way of accounting for situated elderliness in design.

1 Introduction

Literature from gerontology and geriatric care strongly suggests that a care-plan needs to include reminiscence sessions, where the seniors are facilitated to come together and share their memories and experiences about various aspects of their life, which can help them deal with and overcome age related psychological disorders [4,8].

Case in point is the reminiscence sessions organized by a local senior citizen group, aptly titled as "Then and Now"[1]. Here a set of senior citizens meets once a month to share their experiences and thoughts about a particular topic through recollecting how things were then, when they were young, as compared to now, when they are old. The author attended one of the sessions that focused on 'care for elderly: then and now'. Participating seniors recollected how care back then was mostly taken for granted and was a reciprocal affair between seniors, their children and grand children who mostly lived together: the seniors took care of the grandchildren by inculcating the traditional values through stories, etc., the children and grandchildren

---

[1] http://nightingaleseldercare.com/programs/enrich

A. Holzinger et al. (Eds.): SouthCHI 2013, LNCS 7946, pp. 601–608, 2013.

were always there to cater to the various needs of the seniors. They also shared how it has changed now, where they live alone or with their spouse and their children living in cities and abroad. While they mentioned that it is understandable due to the changing economic opportunities, which are mostly focused in the urban areas, they felt that it is a problem if they fall ill living alone. However, even as everyone shared this concern, by the end of the one-hour session, they moved towards finding solutions for this concern: "Let's Google and make a list of (privately funded) senior care home in and around the city!" They decided to make such a list, visit the facilities in a group, and then decide together which ones suit their needs and budgets.

This snippet from the field suggests that supporting seniors to recollect and reminisce on the issues in a group would help seniors to find solutions to their problems. This strand of thought is already being explored by works that focus on designing and developing Information and Communication Technology (ICT) for supporting senior citizens to collect and recollect about various aspects of their life [9,10].

However, in this paper, we posit that designers can consider the seniors' acts of recollecting memories as fruitful resources for uncovering the situated aspects of senior wellbeing [5] while designing ICT in participation with the senior citizens. Specifically we argue that an analytical focus on seniors' memories is a fruitful stance for tracing how a design practice situates issues of senior wellbeing. While the above snippet highlights explicit framing of recollection, in this paper we argue through bringing forward examples of how seniors recollect during a design process in a subtler manner and hence require a particular orientation to uncover.

To support our argument, we make a retrospective glance at our experiences in engaging with a participatory design of ICT to support senior citizens adhere to prescribed physical therapy at home. The aim of the project was to explore the design of digital technological tools that can support the seniors to self-monitor how they perform the physical exercises at home, reflect on the collected data, and share them with their therapists and friends [1,2]. The project through the help of senior citizen groups recruited senior participants to inform the design process. The process involved a series of semi-structure interviews with the participants in their homes, and collaboratively sketching [3] and experiencing early forms of the possible digital tools.

Through retrospection on two explorations within the project, we demonstrate how recollecting memories was the dominant way through which the senior participants asserted to the designers the situated aspects of their physical wellbeing. In particular, the two examples highlight how adhering to physical therapy was situated in, a) memories of a musically rich and mobile life, and b) memories of youthful male body. For both the examples we highlight how designing meant mediating seniors' memories of the past and the designers' aspirations of a technological tool to support adherence to therapy, and how this mediation was shaped by the social and material settings of the design situation at hand.

Through this retrospection we offer the beginnings of a *memoryscape*, a conceptual term for orienting how a design process can mediate seniors' memories as a way of accounting for situated elderliness in design. We consider memoryscape as a series of examples that nuance how the seniors render memories to shape the design process, and how a design process can mediate these memories and move towards exploring a range of new possibilities that were previously unforeseen.

2   Designing as Mediating Memories

Drawing from Latour [7] we position mediating as transforming matters of concern. In this case, the concern of the design was to understand how do seniors adhere to physical therapy and at the same time, to explore the design of possible digital technological tools to support and enhance this adherence. However, the senior participants had their own concerns, which they expressed and articulated through recollecting and reminiscing. These recollections opened the door for the designers towards how adhering to physical therapy was shaped not only by the social and physical settings of the present but also by the memories of past. To consider these situated aspects the designing a digital technological tool had to open up to a range of new possibilities that were unforeseen at the beginning of the process.

In the following sub-sections we reflect on the two examples to highlight this process of mediating memories; of transforming not only the design concerns but also of memories of aging and wellbeing.

2.1   Mediating Memories of a Musically Rich and Mobile Life

The first example concerns the situation of Gita. Gita is a 74-year-old lady who has had her knee joints replaced five years ago from a hospital in Pune, after which she underwent two months of physiotherapy to be mobile and reduce the pain. Her doctor prescribed her an exercise regime to continue at home so that she remains mobile and not experience much pain. Back at home she has integrated these exercises into her everyday routine. One standout example is the way she has integrated some of her knee exercises with the swing in her garden (figure 1). Everyday she swings back and forth by pressing her feet on the ground, thereby exercising her knees, while listening to a musical broadcast on her radio.

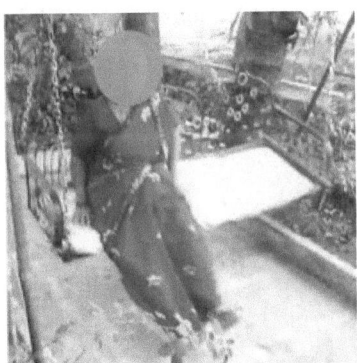

Fig. 1. Gita exercising on the swing

Our concern here, following up from an early exploration [1], was to explore a possibility of a device that can help Gita to time and pace her activity on the swing everyday, so that she can have quantitative data about the time she spends on the swing and how that helps in reducing pain. When we suggested this possibility, Gita rejected it smiling, "I do not need to time my exercise, I listen to this music program everyday and when it gets over, I stop and come in the home."

Gita made apparent her attachment with music in other ways too. She recollected how before the surgery she was the leader of a 'bhajan mandal', a group of musicians who perform devotional songs. She used to go around nearby towns and villages to perform, and has collected a fair amount of awards and trophies congratulating her effort, which she had displayed in her living room where we held the interviews (figure 2). Even now she plays the music with the group when the performance is in the same town, but as she cannot travel, she is not a leader anymore.

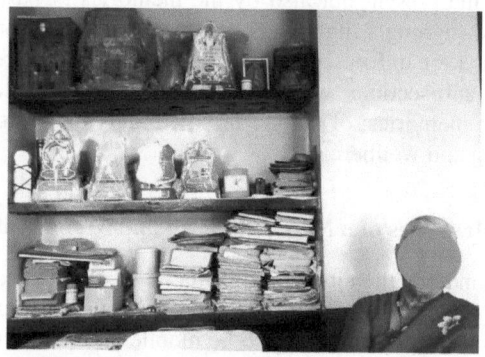

Fig. 2. Gita recollecting memories of a musical life

This recollection opened up a possibility for us to explore if Gita can record her swing exercise movements as a memorabilia that she can employ as a resource to share her rehabilitation story of five years. We sketched a simple electronic ensemble that detected the swing movements and lit up two LED lights on a trophy that had congratulated Gita and her husband Kumar for successful rehabilitation (see figure 3 and refer [2] for more details).

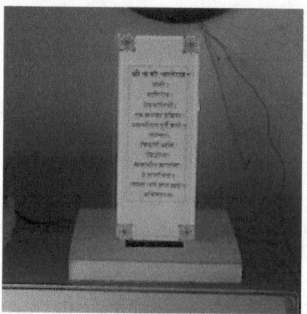

Fig. 3. The sketch of the rehabilitation trophy

We left the sketch with the couple and asked them to try it out. When we returned after a week, it was Kumar who engaged the trophy as a resource to tell stories about his role in Gita's rehabilitation, "thank you for mentioning my name there. I have done a lot of work to get her on her feet... close friends and family knew about my efforts, but now you have given me something to make it permanent." He further recounted the details about his active role in the rehabilitation of his wife, telling stories about him staying in the hospital in Pune during Gita's surgery, encouraging Gita to keep exercising everyday, and modifying her exercises to suit their home environment.

2.2   Mediating Memories of Youthful Male Body

This was of a situation of Madhav, a 69-year-old man and a secretary of the neighborhood senior citizens group, which runs a physiotherapy center, an activity center, and a gym. Due to the nature of his activities he suffers from weak knees, and according to Ravi, his physiotherapist at the physiotherapy center, he is couple of years away from a knee replacement. Ravi has prescribed him an exercise regime to push the surgery further. Madhav has to keep a soft pillow or a rolled towel under his knee while lying down, apply pressure on the towel and count till 10. He has to repeat this 10 times each, while lying down and while sitting everyday. However as he admitted in the interview, he does not consistently perform these exercises. Furthermore, Madhav is supposed to visit the therapist once every week to discuss his progress, but he drops in sporadically as he is busy. And as the secretary of the senior citizen group that runs the therapy center, Ravi cannot help much to enforce the periodicity of his visits, but remind him of his weakening knees.

Initially we envisioned a basic self-monitoring technology that consisted of a force-measuring sensor fixed on the soft pillow he keeps under his knees. The sensor counts the number of times he presses his knees and sends this count to his mobile device as text messages for him to keep a record and to negotiate his treatment with Ravi.

However, during our interactions with Madhav he performed a memory of a person who is not reaching 70 years of age, and but of a body-builder who has a strong and able body. He mentioned how he is actively engaged in exercising at the nearby gym that he built and now oversees. He goes to the gym everyday at 4 am, performs a series of upper body exercises, lifts weights, and is back home by 5 am. He and his wife, who is a yoga enthusiast, then do a series of yogic breathing exercises. Madhav is proud of his 'fit' body, recollecting only his gym exercises and the yogic breathing whenever we asked about his exercise regime at home; we had to specifically ask him to talk about his knee exercises to know more about his weak knees.

Hence, we came to an understanding that we need to move away from the simple measure, record and display kind of a technological tool, and to explore the possibility where Madhav engages with technology as a resource to merge his favorable activities of yogic breathing and weight lifting with the knee exercises. We sketched this possibility by using Madhav's weight-lifting support belt and Wizard-of-Oz technique.

We envisioned that Madhav will wear this belt on his chest, which detects his breathing patterns and hence can perform his knee exercises while doing the yogic breathing, using the yogic breathing as a means to count his knee exercise repetitions. For about five minutes, and as we now think mostly for the sake of the camera, Madhav wore the belt and enacted both the breathing and performing the knee exercises at the same time (see figure 4). Soon after he went on demonstrating how he can use this belt to monitor his breathing patterns while he is weight-lifting, going back to an energetic male body (see figure 5).

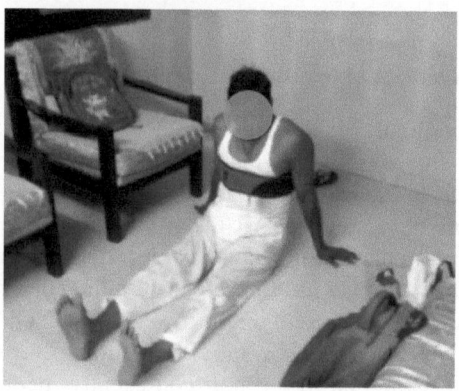

Fig. 4. Madhav wearing the support belt to use his breathing to count the repetitions of knee exercises

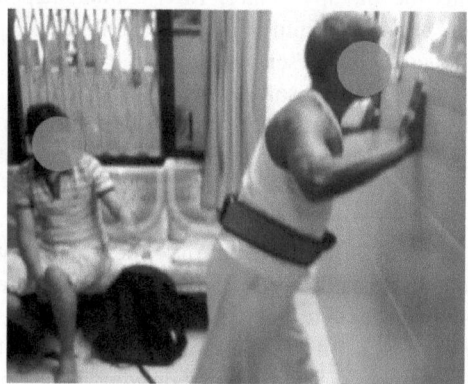

Fig. 5. Madhav wearing the support belt to use his breathing to count his vertical push-ups

3   Discussion: Constructing a Memoryscape through Design

The two examples described a process of design that was inherently speculative and hence open to being informed and shaped by the situated aspects of senior wellbeing: The aim was to explore the possibilities without an a-priori typology of such possibilities. At the same time, because of the speculative foundations, the process led us to uncover the aspects of situated elderliness. The examples highlighted how the speculative design process and situated elderliness together charted an unfolding landscape of possibilities for the design of digital technological tools.

For orienting the designers towards the relation between design process and situated elderliness, we suggest that the unfolding landscape be termed as a *memoryscape*. Memoryscape is a series of emerging examples that nuance how the seniors render memories to shape the design process, and how a design process can mediate these memories and move towards exploring a range of new possibilities that were previously unforeseen.

The examples presented here being to chart out such a memoryscape. While Gita demonstrated how her association with music over the years shaped her physical wellbeing, and vice versa, the design outcome demonstrates a possibility for Gita to make this association explicit in a material form and a part of her living room. Meanwhile, Kumar's recollection of his role in supporting Gita renders another possibility where a spouse engages with the digital technology to care for their partners. Similarly, while Madhav demonstrated how he is more of a strong and able body builder, rather than an aging 70-year-old with knee problems, the design outcome demonstrates a possibility for him to engage with both kinds of memories. Madhav's exploration of the sketch further produced a range of other possibilities where he can engage with the technology to monitor how he performs his muscle-building exercises.

In sketching the notion of memoryscape, we draw from Ingold [6] who mentions how exploring a landscape is a process of learning to spot the clues of information held in the environment to unearth issues. In our case we were led to uncovering aspects of situated elderliness through the ways in which the senior participants recollected how their wellbeing is situated by the memories of past and present.

For Ingold the landscape is already there waiting to be uncovered through an expert cartographer. However, while memoryscape does contain already existing pockets (the situated aspects of wellbeing) that are to be uncovered, a large part of it is constructed through the mediation of design aspirations and senior memories. As the examples demonstrated, this mediation leads to construction of a range of possibilities that were previously unforeseen. In this way the memoryscape is rather a creation of a series of possibilities for design through mediating the matters of concern.

4   Conclusion

In this paper we reflected on our experiences of designing digital technological tools to enhance adherence to physical therapy at home to argue that considering designing as mediating memories is a fruitful stance to take to account for the situated aspects of senior wellbeing. We discussed two examples of seniors recollecting memories of past and present that highlighted how their adherence to therapy was entangled with these memories. Positioning design as a speculative engagement moved the process towards exploring a range of unforeseen possibilities of digital technology. We further positioned this process a creating a memoryscape.

We offer this notion of memoryscape as a conceptual term for orienting how a design process can mediate seniors' memories as a way of accounting for situated elderliness in design. While we presented and discussed two of such memories, the paper is an open invitation for the researchers in the field to add and contest these memories and their mediation through design, and thereby further unfold the memoryscape of designing of senior wellbeing.

References

1. Bagalkot, N.L., Sokoler, T., Shaikh, R.: Integrating physiotherapy with everyday life: exploring the space of possibilities through ReHandles. In: Proceedings of the Sixth International Conference on Tangible, Embedded and Embodied Interaction, pp. 91–98. ACM (2012)
2. Bagalkot, N., Sokoler, T.: ReHandle: towards integrating physical rehabilitation in everyday life. In: Proceedings of the 2011 Annual Conference Extended Abstracts on Human Factors in Computing Systems, pp. 1795–1800. ACM (2011)
3. Buxton, B.: Sketching User Experiences: Getting the Design Right and the Right Design. Morgan Kaufmann Publishers Inc. (2007)
4. Coleman, P.G.: Uses of reminiscence: Functions and benefits. Aging & Mental Health 9(4), 291–294 (2005)
5. Brandt, E., Binder, T., Malmborg, L., Sokoler, T.: Communities of everyday practice and situated elderliness as an approach to co-design for senior interaction. In: Proceedings of the 22nd Conference of the Computer-Human Interaction Special Interest Group of Australia on Computer-Human Interaction (OZCHI 2010), pp. 400–403. ACM, New York (2010)
6. Ingold, T.: The Temporality of the Landscape. World Archaeology 25(2), 152–174 (1993)
7. Latour, B.: Reassembling the social-an introduction to actor-network-theory. Oxford University Press (2005)
8. Merriam, S.B.: The Uses of Reminiscence in Older Adulthood. Educational Gerontology 19(5), 441–450 (1993)
9. Pavel, D., Callaghan, V., Dey, A.K.: Looking Back in Wonder: How Self-Monitoring Technologies Can Help Us Better Understand Ourselves. In: 2010 Sixth International Conference on Intelligent Environments (IE), pp. 289–294. IEEE (2010)
10. Staahl, A., Höök, K., Svensson, M., Taylor, A.S., Combetto, M.: Experiencing the Affective Diary. Personal and Ubiquitous Computing 13, 365–378 (2009)

Design and Interaction in a Smart Gym: Cognitive and Bodily Mastering

Alma Leora Culén, Sisse Finken, and Tone Bratteteig

Department of Informatics, University of Oslo, Oslo, Norway
{almira,finken,tone}@ifi.uio.no

Abstract. Being physically active is perhaps the most important factor influencing the health of elderly people. As a consequence, technologies that support and encourage physical activity have been developed. In this paper, we study a "smart gym" in a residential care building. Our findings indicate that the "smart gym" does not address the complexities of exercise for an elderly person: in order to exercise one has to master the gym equipment and its technology, cognitively as well as bodily. Both the equipment and the smart technology turn out to be difficult to master by its elderly users. Our study reports these difficulties and suggests a more nuanced concept of mastery as a way to address the challenges in designing for elderly users. We unfold physical and bodily dimensions of mastery and consider how these differ between individuals, and within the context and situation.

Keywords: situated elderliness, cognitive mastery, bodily mastery, smart gym technology.

1   Introduction

The changing demographic development with an increasing elderly population has spurred technological development aimed at technical support for elderly people living independently at home longer [1, 2, 3]. Smart home technologies have become robust enough to be used in practice [4], and in this paper we report from fieldwork following the introduction and use of smart home technologies in a residential care building in Oslo, Norway. The smart house, and the smart gym, opened in September 2012. The 91 flats in the smart house are equipped with sensors responding to fire, water flooding, light, and temperature changes. In addition to sensor technology, each flat comes with a tablet. The tablet may be used to order food from the local in-house cantina and keep track of appointments using the calendar functionality [5, 6]. The smart house is certified as a Care+ unit, implying that safety, security, wellbeing, quality of life, and independence are central concerns for the municipality. Within such policy older people are encouraged, through different health caring and social means, to preserve their current state of self-sufficiency and, accordingly, their capabilities of continuing to live as independently at home, as their resources allow and make possible [6]. The smart house is open for rent to citizens aged 67+, having

A. Holzinger et al. (Eds.): SouthCHI 2013, LNCS 7946, pp. 609–616, 2013.

impairments such as e.g. chronic illnesses, rheumatism, allergy, and/or disabilities with hearing, walking, seeing, or orienting [6].

Physical activity is an important factor influencing the health and wellbeing of elderly people [1]. Thus, much research has focus on supporting and encouraging physical activity. Solutions include diverse approaches, from pedometers to exercise games with gesture-based interaction [7]. The Care+ smart house includes a "smart gym" equipped with smart cards and touch screens. In this paper, we talk about how the gym works in practice, and how technology is part of the gym experience. We focus on mastery and report on challenges encountered during a gym hour. We suggest a more nuanced concept of mastery as a way to address the challenges in designing smart solutions for ageing.

The paper is structured as follows: in the next section we enter the smart gym and report from an evening with smart gym hour where we observed interactions between the residents and the technology, including exercising machines, while working out. We then discuss our observations and relate them to cognitive and bodily mastery.

2   Using the Smart Gym

This section describes the use of the smart gym in the smart house Care+ building, observed by the first two authors on a quiet Sunday afternoon. We arrived at the building at 16:55, and went with a caretaker to the gym to take some pictures without residents, see Fig. 1a). At first sight, the gym did not appear very different than many commercial ones. After taking the pictures we joined the tea and coffee chat in the common room, attended by seven residents and one caretaker. At 17:30, six residents made their way to the smart gym, Fig. 1b).

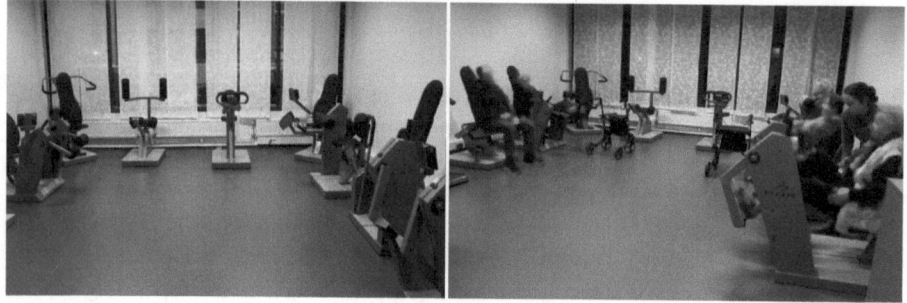

Fig. 1. a) The gym before the exercise hour. b) Gym with elderly, exercising.

The building is new and not all routines are fully in place yet. While the residents know that there are training sessions, the training hours are not yet firmly established. However, each apartment is equipped with a tablet, on which information about activities is available. This information is also posted daily in the reception/entrance area (printed and digital). Furthermore, a pamphlet is printed quarterly describing different social and cultural activities such as crafts, gym, walks and trips, cinema, live music, reading club, resident meetings etc.

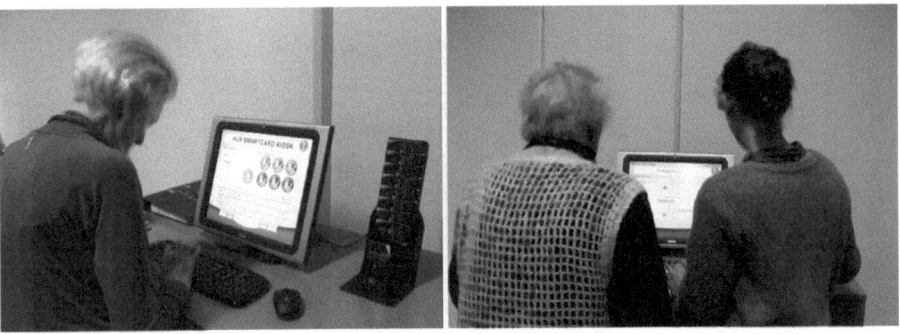

Fig. 2. Residents registering for the session; activating their cards by themselves, or with help

Our experience of the smart gym starts with observing how the residents get registered for the gym hour on a desktop computer. One registers with a name. After successful registration, a smart card is inserted, and personal data such as weight, gender and height are transferred to the card. Every exercise machine in the room has a touch unit that allows for the insertion of a smart card. However, the cards are not personal, and a registration at each visit is necessary. Some of the elderly can carry out the registration process on their own; some need help, see Fig. 2. Fig. 3 shows the stack of the cards to use for registration; a nonregistered card inserted into the touch unit and position of the touch units at various exercise machines. The positioning of touch units throughout the room is not consistent.

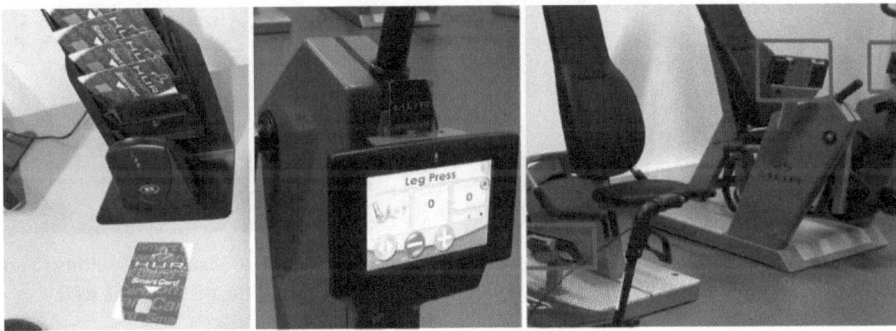

Fig. 3. a) The smart card with a microchip b) the non-registered card inserted into the touch unit c) the positioning of touch screens is not consistent

When the card is registered for the given user, and then inserted into the touch unit, the screen shows the user's settings for the particular machine, i.e. the weight and the number of repetitions. The machine keeps the count of repetitions. However, interacting with screens is not easy. Part of the difficulty is due to different possible interpretations of the icons, Fig. 4a), or the icons having different meanings, Fig 4b).

Further, changing the settings for the next exercise is not easy, Fig. 5a). For the time being the caretaker takes care of such interactions, as well as adjustments of the training machines, for those who need help, see Fig. 5b).

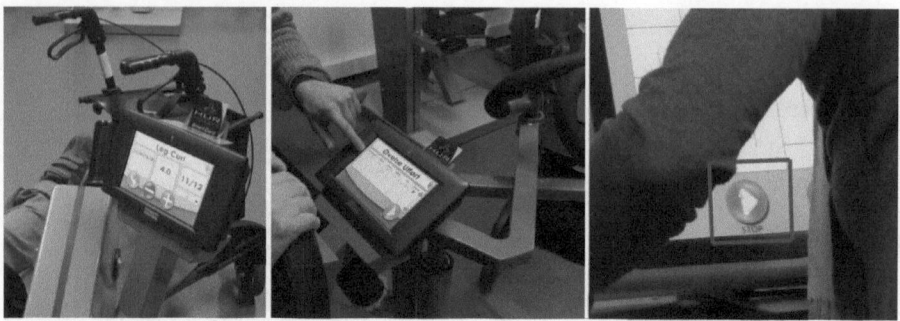

Fig. 4. a) The meaning of the + and the – buttons is not clear at once b) the green arrow takes the user to the next exercise c) the same green arrow stops the exercise on another machine

While the caretaker spends time with one person adjusting their equipment (regulating the seat height, strapping the legs etc.) or adjusting their body position so that they can receive the best effect of the exercise, the other residents have a light chat while waiting for their turn. Most of them do need help, either because they are physically incapable to adjust the equipment, or they do not know how to do it. The later is true for some residents, even after repeated visits to the gym.

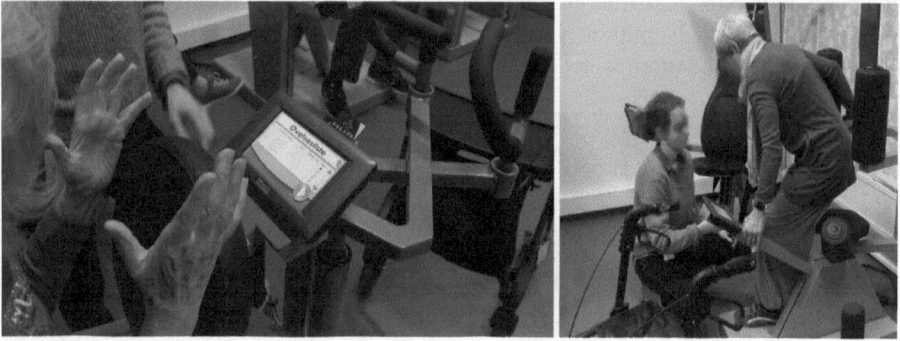

Fig. 5. a) A resident using her smart card. It is difficult to see how to change the settings and perform more repetitions. b) The caretaker helps with adjustments of the machines as well.

At 18:30, people start leaving. We chat with one resident a bit longer and then leave. Observing this "smart gym hour" provoked many thoughts about situated elderliness [8] and what it means for this community of practice. One particular aspect, or rather the lack of it, connected to the experience we just had, stood out: mastery – both bodily and cognitive mastery.

3   Cognitive and Bodily Mastery

The elderly living in the smart house experience decline in abilities as described over; it is a condition that gives the possibility to apply for renting the flat. Some have physical, some cognitive limitations, and some have both, to a various degree and in a multitude of ways.

The elderly living in the building may be considered a community of practice as defined in [8, p. 3]: *... one could talk about communities of everyday practice, where senior citizens similarly are skillfully enacting everyday practices as seniors. Gradually as they get older they enact what we would call situated elderliness. With situated elderliness, we refer to practices that include activities that for some reason or another has become more challenging or perhaps even impossible to carry out by himself or herself.* In what follows, we discuss situated elderliness in the smart gym, through the lens of mastery.

In Collins Thesaurus of the English Language mastery (noun) is defined (with our emphasis italicized) as:

1. *understanding, knowledge, comprehension, ability,* skill, *know-how, command,* grip, grasp, expertise, prowess, familiarity, attainment, finesse, proficiency, virtuosity, dexterity, cleverness, deftness, acquirement 2. *control,* authority, command, rule, victory, triumph, sway, domination, superiority, conquest, supremacy, dominion, upper hand, ascendancy...

The definitions emphasize being able, knowing – both understanding and knowing how, and control. However, ageing comes with a decline of abilities including cognitive skills, hence losing know-how and control. It is then reasonable to ask if the mastery is possible? Is mastery of technology possible? Mastery of the body? If so, how to retain it for as long as possible, given the progressive reduction in abilities due to the ageing process. Are there different kinds of mastery involved?

In psychology and learning, researchers often use self-efficacy [9] as a measure of one's ability to perform tasks and reach specific goals. Psychologist Bandura defined self-efficacy as a belief in one's ability to be successful in reaching a goal or in a specific situation in life [10]. Thus, self-efficacy is an important factor motivating the work, practice, persistence, etc. that may lead towards mastery.

The field of gerontechnology includes two areas of concern: studying elderly and ubiquitous and pervasive technology [11]. For the case presented above, a study by Alvseike and Brønnick [12] is relevant. The authors report the results of a feasibility study involving the iPad as a hub for smart house technology. They found that the age of the participants in their study was not correlated to how successfully they used the technology. However, cognitive impairments and self-efficacy were detrimental factors. Those with severe impairments and low self-efficacy were unable to use the technology. Further, Malinowsky, Almkvist, Kottorp and Nygård have shown that persons with cognitive impairments, such as mild dementia, are likely to have decreased ability to manage everyday technology [13]. Thus, retaining, or even slightly increasing this ability to master interaction with technology is necessary in order to use the technology as means for improving health and wellbeing. To achieve the mastery, self-efficacy is a vital factor, often absent with elderly. During the observation at the smart gym, we noticed a lack of understanding related to the technology and the machines. Everyone in the group had, to a varying degree, need for *cognitive mastery* of technology: tablets in the apartment to see the information about the smart gym timetable, desktop computer to transfer data onto a smart card and last, but not least, touch interface at every machine in the gym. Cognitive mastery was also a factor in knowing how to use the exercise machines.

Another important factor for the cognitive mastery is a cultural familiarity with commonly used visual language in today´s computing. Elderly are often not familiar with the most common icons and symbols used in everyday technology for younger people. This lack of familiarity may lead to insecurity, less self-efficacy and in some cases a denial to use the technology at all. A simple experiment was conducted in another elderly center by our students who designed a communication platform for elderly. They made a heat map to see what elderly touch given the task to start a conference call, which simply implied touching the green phone icon. Fig. 6a) shows the result for 5 elderly [14, 15]). The results in Fig. 6a) may also be due both to non-familiarity with icons and physical problems, such as tremors. However, some of these are clearly due to non-familiarity, for example, trying to initiate the call by touching the image of the person to be called instead of the phone icon. We could not use the heat map on touch units in the gym, but we observed that elderly had problems with screen interactions.

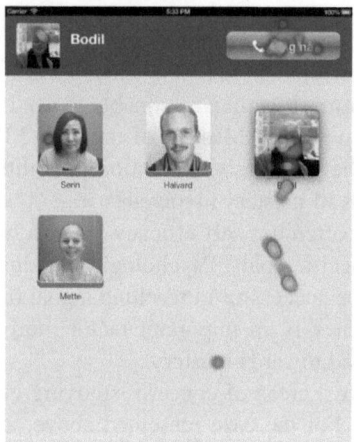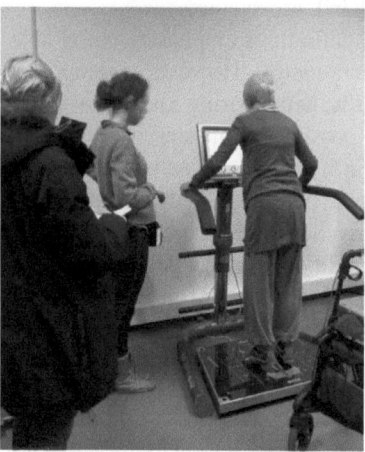

Fig. 6. a) Cultural language of modern computing is a hindrance for elderly. b) Physical disability as a hindrance to completing the task.

During the gym hour we observed an example of problems with bodily mastery when a resident had difficulties finalizing a task on a machine training the body balance, due to the lack of bodily strength, Fig. 6b). When performing her task on the exercise machine the resident had to lean her body forward to make a figure on the screen move towards a certain destination. This seemed to be a difficult task for her to perform and the caretaker helped her by re-locating her feet on the bottom of the machine to see if that would help. Ultimately, the resident decided to move onto another task on the same machine. We read this experience as an example where cognitive and bodily mastery become equally important in order to complete a task, both in terms of understanding how to navigate the screen and in terms of being able to engage physically with the exercise machine in order to complete a task. Thus, in defining *bodily mastery* we put emphasis on strengths and capabilities of moving the body or a specific body part in order to perform a specific task.

A second example related to the importance of bodily mastery came forth when one of the residents was asked about previous experience with exercising in a gym. The reply was that she had none. She added that she liked going to the smart gym to move her body as the long winter had kept her indoors.

In terms of bodily mastery and command of technology, there has been much focus on assistive technology such as gloves for people with callous fingers, large icons for those with tremors and reduced vision, multimodal interactions etc., see [14]. However, the assistive technology does not solve the problem of self-efficacy related to bodily mastery, rather it assumes that such solutions are needed and welcome.

With the above examples from the gym, we want to highlight that mastery has several dimensions, which need to be accounted for in design efforts for situated elderliness. This is not to say that we follow a line of Cartesian reasoning aiming at dichotomizing body and mind. Philosophers have long done beautiful work debunking this divide e.g. [16]. Such philosophical orientation has also made its way into HCI (e.g. Larssen et al. [17], who draw on the work of phenomenologist Merleau-Ponty in order to describe bodily interaction in relation to technology). We aim at opening up an analytical space in design work that includes both the cognitive and the bodily, and, which brings them into focus on equal terms while still accounting for their differences. These differences are significant in that they have real effects in terms of what can and cannot be accomplished. The examples from the gym show that both dimensions of mastery came into play as instantiations of a heterogeneity that affects the possibilities of interaction/engagement in and with the world. Taking into consideration these dimensions of mastery becomes important in other everyday situations where technology moves into the homes of elderly in an effort to support their independent everyday living. This is to say that when moving within a perspective of interaction design we find it productive to make an analytical distinction between the two dimensions in order to account for the very heterogeneity of elderly's mastery.

4   Conclusion

When designing spaces for elderly, considering the process of ageing and diversity of abilities that elderly people have, we find mastery of tasks and goals to be decisive in the use of those spaces by elderly. We have discussed self-efficacy and ability to understand cultural symbols as important factors contributing to the mastery. In order to address the complexities of exercise for an elderly person we have considered what they need to master, both in terms of the equipment and the smart technology. We conclude that facilitation of both bodily and cognitive mastery together need to be considered by designers when working with elderly.

Acknowledgements. We are grateful to all the participants in the study: thank you! This research is part of the project *Autonomy and Automation in an IT society for All*, funded by The Norwegian Research Council, grant number 193172.

References

1. Velferdsteknologi. Fagrapport om implementering av velferdsteknologi i de kommunale helse- og omsorgstjenestene 2013–2030. Report IS-1990, Helsedirektoratet (2012)
2. Finken, S., Mörtberg, C.: The Thinking House: on Configuring of an Infrastructure of Care. In: 3rd International Workshop on Infrastructures for Healthcare: Global Healthcare, IT-University Copenhagen, pp. 44–47 (2011)
3. Stefano, D.H., Bien, Z., Bang, W.C.: The Smart House for Older Persons and Persons With Physical Disabilities: Structure, Technology Arrangements, and Perspectives. IEEE Transactions on Neural Systems and Rehabilitation Engineering 12(2), 228–250 (2004)
4. Smarthusteknologi. Planlegging og drift i kommunale tjenester. Report IS-1216,Sosialoghelsedirektoratet, Deltasenteret, Oslo (2004)
5. Jansson, M., Mörtberg, C.: A Cup of Coffee: Users' Needs and Experiences of ICT in Homecare. In: Ziefle, M., Röcker, C. (eds.) Human-Centered Design of E-Health Technologies: Concepts, Methods and Applications, pp. 253–271. IGI Global, Hershey (2010)
6. Finken, S.: Case Description – When Technologies Move to the Home. In: Bratteteig, T., Finken, S., van der Velden, M., Verne, G. (eds.) Chapter to appear in a book based on the A3-project "Autonomy and Automation in an IT Society for all" (forthcoming)
7. Cornejo, R., Hernández, D., Favela, J., Tentori, M., Ochoa, S.F.: Persuading older adults to socialize and exercise through ambient games. In: Pervasive Computing Technologies for Healthcare (PervasiveHealth), pp. 215–218. IEEE (2012)
8. Brandt, E., Binder, T., Malmborg, L., Sokoler, T.: Communities of everyday practice and situated elderliness as an approach to co-design for senior interaction. In: Proceedings of the 22nd Conference of the Computer-Human Interaction Special Interest Group of Australia on Computer-Human Interaction, pp. 400–403. ACM, New York (2010)
9. Ormrod, J.E.: Educational Psychology: Developing Learners, Merrill (2006)
10. Bandura, A.: Self-Efficacy: The Exercise of Control. Worth Publishers (1997)
11. Bouma, H., Fozard, J.L., Bouwhuis, D.G., Taipale, V.T.: Gerontechnology in perspective. Gerontechnology 6(4), 190–216 (2007)
12. Alvseike, H., Brønnick, K.: Feasibility of the iPad as a hub for smart house technology in the elderly; effects of cognition, self-efficacy, and technology experience. Journal of Multidisciplinary Healthcare 5, 299–306 (2012)
13. Malinowsky, C., Almkvist, O., Kottorp, A., Nygård, L.: Ability to manage everyday technology: a comparison of persons with dementia or mild cognitive impairment and older adults without cognitive impairment. Disability and rehabilitation: Assistive technology 5(6), 462–469 (2010)
14. Culén, A., Bratteteig, T.: Touch-Screens and Elderly users: A Perfect Match? In: Proceedings of the Sixth International Conference on Advances in Computer-Human Interactions, pp. 460–465 (2013)
15. Åmdal, V.S., Klette, K., Simonsen, H.L., Selskap, A.S.: http://www.uio.no/studier/emner/matnat/ifi/INF2260/h12/projects/elderly/Elderlyaidapp/
16. Foucault, M.: The Care of the Self. The History of Sexuality, vol. 3. Vintage (1988)
17. Larssen, A.T., Robertson, T., Edwards, J.: How it Feels, not Just How it Looks: When Bodies Interact with Technology. In: OZCHI 2006 Proceedings, pp. 329–332. ACM, New York (2006)

From Research to Design - Sketching a Game to Trigger Reminiscence in Older Adults

Naemi Luckner[1], Fares Kayali[1], Oliver Hödl[1], Peter Purgathofer[1],
Geraldine Fitzpatrick[1], Erika Mosor[2], Daniela Schlager-Jaschky[2], and Tanja Stamm[3]

[1] Vienna University of Technology, Institute of Design and Assessment of Technology, Austria
{naemi,fares,oliver}@igw.tuwien.ac.at,
{peter.purgathofer,geraldine.fitzpatrick}@tuwien.ac.at
[2] FH Campus Wien, Department of Health, Vienna, Austria
erika.mosor@aon.at, danhar@drei.at
[3] FH Campus Wien, Department of Health / Medical University of Vienna,
Department of Rheumatology, Vienna, Austria
tanja.stamm@meduniwien.ac.at

Abstract. This contribution describes a series of design sketches for a playful digital application designed to trigger reminiscence in older adults. The goal of the intervention is to be a preventive measure against cognitive disabilities such as dementia and Alzheimer's disease. Research shows that reminiscence and cognitive activities are beneficial in this area. The presented sketches have been developed as part of a design workshop and are based upon the results of a focus group study which involved older adults, their families, experts and care personnel. The ideas are all rooted within the context of the project which revolves around the playful use of media such as photos, video clips and audio recordings. These personal media artifacts shall trigger reminiscence and engage players cognitively.

Keywords: reminiscence, dementia, older adults, play, serious games.

1   About Us

The Human-Computer Interaction (HCI) group seeks to merge relevant technical-al/engineering and social sciences research with a practical contribution to the design of technology particularly mobile, tangible and sensor-based technologies. The group combines multiple disciplines like informatics, engineering, psychology, sociology, medical-informatics, game studies, design and media arts. The HCI group at the Vienna University of Technology is part of the Institute for Design and Assessment of Technology. The authors of this contribution combine experiences in game design, serious games and HCI-related projects. Their professional backgrounds bridge academic research with actual design practice.

2   Introduction

Today's (western) society benefits from continuous advances in the prevention and treatment of diseases. This also leads to a steadily growing demographic of older

A. Holzinger et al. (Eds.): SouthCHI 2013, LNCS 7946, pp. 617–624, 2013.

adults. As people get older the prevalence of cognitive disabilities such as dementia or Alzheimer's disease increases. This puts a heavy burden not only on people suffering from these diseases but also on their relatives and on care institutions. Presently there is no medication or cure for these diseases but it has been shown that an increase in cognitive, physical and social activities can prevent the aforementioned diseases or slow down their progress [1-4]. To further engagement across these areas, technological solutions can help by building a framework which embeds them with everyday routine, and which helps to sustain motivation.

The main focus of the designs presented here, reminiscence, is the cognitive process of remembering and reliving events from the past. This process can be caused by triggers. Memories can be sparked in conversations through words, clues or other stories. Triggers can be smells, objects or familiar impressions. Reminiscence happens interpersonally, meaning that it can be told and heard by others, or interpersonally within the person reminiscing [5]. Reminiscence serves various functions described by [6] as the social, directive and self functions. The social function of reminiscence facilitates engaging and interacting with other people. The directive function serves for problem-solving or predicting an outcome by comparing situations with the past. The self function boosts one's self-esteem, and helps to create and preserve a sense of self.

Reminiscence can be used in a therapeutic setting, also for older adults who suffer from dementia. Some memories create positive feelings, some negative. A therapist can help to reframe negative memories, so that it is easier for the patient to cope with them. Adults with dementia suffer from short time memory loss but can often remember events from their past. Reminiscence can help them train their cognitive functions and generates a feeling of accomplishment, self-worth and facilitates a reintegration into society [7].

Recent research in games designed for older people shows a tendency to positively impact their well-being [8-11]. A detailed review of literature on reminiscence and games to encourage social, cognitive and physical activities is given by [12].

This paper presents insights on research-to-design practice in the context of games for older adults. The core focus is a presentation of design sketches for a game about reminiscence intended to prevent or slow cognitive decline. The sketches were conceived in a workshop with experts from the fields of computer science, ergo therapy and game research as well as professionals in health care, game development and project management.

3   The "Lebensnetz" Project

This contribution is made in context with a particular project called 'Lebensnetz' (which could be roughly translated to the term 'life network'). The project's goal is the user-centered development of a gesture-based application using the Microsoft Kinect sensor, which is meant to activate patients in a physical, mental and social way. The topic of the game-like application is that the users collect memories and map their life using photos as well as other auto-biographical information. The project started with a phase of investigating demands and needs of the target audience through a focus group study. The implementation takes place within an iterative design process to get permanent user feedback on the prototype. The iterative process includes two test periods and features observation and a survey. The learnings are to be looped back into game development. The result of the project will be an interactive prototype.

4   Focus Group Study

The design sketches presented here were informed by insights gathered in four focus groups. The focus groups were held separately with experts, the target audience (people 60+), caring relatives, and professional health care staff during November and December 2012. Each group was made up of 8-12 participants and two moderators and lasted for 90 minutes.

The focus group study has not yet been fully evaluated but preliminary insights indicate that the primary motivation to play is to be together with others, to have fun, to tackle challenges and to hone one's skills. There were also mentions of playing to relive or exchange memories. It seems that the understanding of play varies greatly with many differentiating strictly between work and play, cognitive training being seen as work activity. It was a common understanding that an intervention would suffer from lower acceptance if training / treatment aspects are disguised as play activities. In general there was a strong demand for the intervention to primarily be fun and playful. An emphasis was also put on the need of the system to be easily accessible, to remove technological barriers and to have as much guidance as possible. Specific game ideas included board games, musical play, puzzles, and physical play. We think that one of the biggest challenges in this context is the great age range and heterogeneity of the target audience.

5   From Research to Design

The next step of the project and core focus of this contribution was to turn the results of the focus groups into practical sketches, which then serve as basis for the iterative development of interactive software prototypes. Each of the following four sketches was produced by a group of experts with one game designer per group to facilitate the design process. The experts were comprised of researches from the fields of computer science, ergo therapy and game research as well as professionals in (health) care, game development and project management.

The goal of the sketches was to describe an idea how biographical content like songs, pictures, photos, postcards, geographical data and more can be collected in one place and presented in a way that individuals can easily interact with them.

The workshop was structured as follows:

- Preliminary focus group results were presented and discussed
- A joint brainstorming session was held to come up with terms to base game ideas on (see table 1). The terms were supposed to relate to the previous discussion of focus group results.

- The group split into diverse teams of four. Each team included a game designer, researchers and practitioners.
- Each team chose a term from the below table and came up with a game idea.
- The whole group reconvened and each team's ideas were presented and a sketch for each idea was made collaboratively.

Table 1. Terms resulting from of a group brainstorming session during the workshop

competition	board games
self expression	musical play
virtual worlds	home(land)
tangible interface	social play
autobiographical play	media
role play	triggering memories

5.1   Sketch 1

Every user can create a timeline, which they fill with personal media contents. The timeline can represent a person's life, but can also be used to create a fictitious life story, for example a story they would have liked to live. Users can interact with other users by overlaying and comparing their timelines to talk about similarities and differences (Fig. 1). The application can be used by all generations to bring young and old together, create a safe surrounding to talk about the past and provide new topics based on the personalized content. Quizzes about one's own past can be generated in order to support people with dementia to train their cognitive abilities or to induce a reminiscence session.

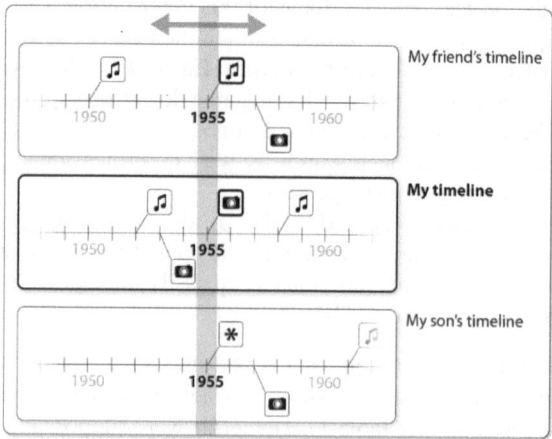

Fig. 1. Three timelines navigated together

5.2   Sketch 2

Users create a slideshow with personal content. The interface should be as simple as possible and support only creating, inserting and deleting entries (Fig. 2.). The games are played by older people and their children or grandchildren and revolve around navigating through the slideshow. Possible games are a really slow jump'n'run in which the grandchild needs to navigate through the diashow and stop and balance on one of the entries if their grandparent wants to take a closer look at it. Another game could be a quiz where three possible next entries are shown at the same time and the grandchild has to guess which of the entries their grandparent chose next.

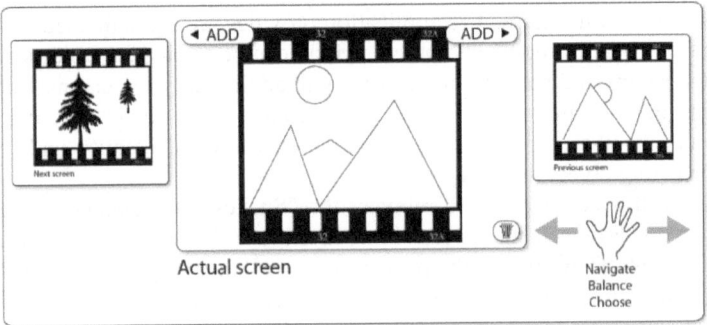

Fig. 2. A slideshow with navigation and the possibility to add contents

5.3   Sketch 3

Every user chooses an avatar and can decorate it with various objects. Each object is connected to a story that the user tells while placing the object on the avatar. The story is audio-recorded and can be replayed at any time. Avatars can be themed, for example each resident of a retirement home can choose a tree and visitors can "walk" through the forest of tree avatars (Fig. 3). Users can play mini games together. For

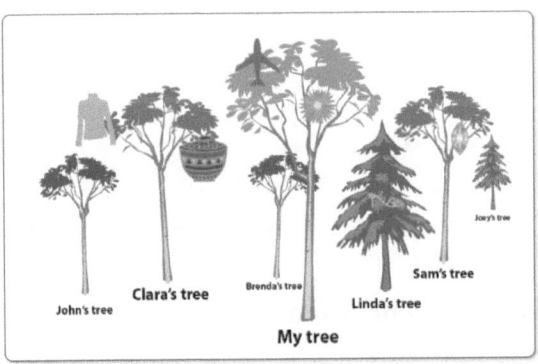

Fig. 3. Tree avatars with attached memory objects

example players see an object and try to figure out which of three possible stories it stands for. The avatars have to be kept alive which happens by interacting with them, looking at connected stories, and answering questions about their content. Users don't only interact with their own trees, but also with others. That way they get to know their peers better while at the same time also dealing with their own past. Also avatars of deceased users are kept alive by others who interact with them.

5.4   Sketch 4

Users create "memory rooms". Each room can have a different topic, for example "my highschool years". Rooms are filled with objects from that time, for example an old gramophone or old furniture. The application provides pre filled themed rooms, like a "20s room", a "beatles room" and others, which can be looked at. Objects can be taken from the rooms and put into one's own room additionally to personal content. The content can be used in game contexts. Grandchildren can "hide" memories of their grandparents in other rooms and the grandparents have to identify and replace the missing or wrong object in the room.

An idea in this context was to reinvent the "Snakes and Ladders" board game to use the players' arranged memories. The players use the same board but are shown different content. They start in the present and work their way "back" over the board to arrive at their time and place of birth (Fig. 4). They can choose to answer questions to different categories to advance further on the board. If they just want to watch and listen to entries, they advance in their normal speed. The game could also be used to get more information for a certain time period and acts as an educational tool.

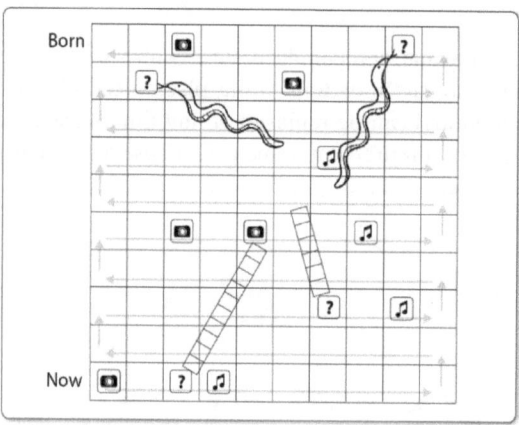

Fig. 4. A Snakes & Ladders board with memory objects

6   Discussion and Conclusion

So far we managed to transform the findings from the focus groups and our literature review into the four presented designs. The general idea was to create a biographical game and all sketches are based on a personalized database of video clips, pictures, music and similar objects. We found that the main difference between the sketches is the way data is collected and presented and the proposed gameful approaches can mostly be used in any given setting. The sketches took similar approaches in trying to present data in a way older people might find comfortable. The look and feel of the sketches was often described as old-fashioned or customizable. Metaphors like dia-shows as picture timelines or old radios as music players were often proposed. As mentioned before, this approach might be appropriate for parts of the target audience, but leaves out those, who are comfortable with new technologies.

Our contribution to the workshop will be to describe our particular research and design approach towards a game-like application for older adults. We will discuss how focus groups helped us build a solid basis for brainstorming and shaping several designs.

We expect to learn about related example practices in designing technology for older adults and how others involve senior participants in their design and development processes.

Acknowledgements. The project Lebensnetz is funded by Austrian funding agency FFG. The design sketches presented here were conceived collaboratively by all of the project's partners, Ovos media, Vienna University of Technology, Plansinn, University of Applied Science Campus Vienna, Caritas Vienna, and the Austrian Interdisciplinary Platform on Ageing as well as two game design experts, Sabine Harrer and Lev Ledit.

References

1. Zunzunegui, M.V., Alvarado, B.E., Del Ser, T., Otero, A.: Social Networks, Social Integration, and Social Engagement Determine Cognitive Decline in Community-Dwelling Spanish Older Adults. The Journals of Gerontology Series B: Psychological Sciences and Social Sciences 58(2), 93–100 (2003)
2. Voelcker-Rehage, C., Godde, B., Staudinger, U.M.: Cardiovascular and coordination training differentially improve cognitive performance and neural processing in older adults. Frontiers in Human Neuroscience 5(26), 17–26 (2011)
3. Brassington, G.S., Atienza, A.A., Perczek, R.E., DiLorenzo, T.M., King, A.C.: Intervention-related cognitive versus social mediators of exercise adherence in the elderly. AJPM 23(2), 80–86 (2002)
4. Rolland, Y., Abellan van Kan, G., Vellas, B.: Physical activity and Alzheimer's disease: from prevention to therapeutic perspectives. Journal of the American Medical Directors Association 9(6), 390–405 (2008)
5. Webster, J.D., Bohlmeijer, E.T., Westerhof, G.J.: Mapping the Future of Reminiscence: A Conceptual Guide for Research and Practice. Research on Aging 32(4), 527–564 (2010)
6. Bluck, S., Alea, N., Habermas, T., Rubin, D.C.: A Tale Of Three Functions: The Self-Reported Uses Of Autobiographic Memory. Social Cognition 23(1), 91–117 (2005)
7. Alm, N., Dye, R., Gowans, G., Campbell, J., Astell, A., Ellis, M.: A Communication Support System for Older People with Dementia. Computer, 35–41 (2007)

8. Grosinger, J., Vetere, F., Fitzpatrick, G.: Agile Life: addressing knowledge and social motivations for active aging. In: Proceedings of OzCHI 2012 (2012)

9. Gerling, K.M., Schulte, F.P., Masuch, M.: Designing and evaluating digital games for frail elderly persons. In: Proceedings of the 8th International Conference on Advances in Computer Entertainment Technology - ACE 2011, pp. 62:1–62:8. ACM Press, New York (2011)

10. Tanaka, K., Parker, J., Baradoy, G., Sheehan, D., Holash, J., Katz, L.: A Comparison of Exergaming Interfaces for Use in Rehabilitation Programs and Research. Canadian Game Studies Association 6(9), 69–81 (2012)

11. Nouchi, R., Taki, Y., Takeuchi, H., Hashizume, H., Akitsuki, Y., Shigemune, Y., Sekiguchi, A., Kotozaki, Y., Tsukiura, T., Yomogida, Y.: Brain training game improves executive functions and processing speed in the elderly: A randomized controlled trial. PloS one 7(1), e29676 (2012)

12. Kayali, F., Luckner, N., Hödl, O., Fitzpatrick, G., Purgathofer, P., Stamm, T., Schlager-Jaschky, D., Mosor, E.: Elements of play for cognitive, physical and social health in older adults. In: Holzinger, A., Ziefle, M., Hitz, M., Debevc, M. (eds.) SouthCHI 2013. LNCS, vol. 7946, pp. 296–313. Springer, Heidelberg (2013)

kommTUi – A Design Process for a Tangible Communication Technology with Seniors

Lisa Ehrenstrasser[1] and Wolfgang Spreicer[2]

[1] iDr-inklusiv Design & Research
design@lisaehren.net
[2] Vienna University of Technology
wolfgang.spreicer@tuwien.ac.at

Abstract. In this paper we present the analysis of the three years iterative design process of the research project *kommTUi*. In *kommTUi*, the goal was to design and develop an accessible communication system with tangible user interface to support digital inclusion of elderly people. We propose our qualitative approach for user involvement and identify the atmosphere as key factor for successful research outcome when working with older adults. Therefore, we introduce a graphical analysis tool for comparing the conducted workshops by means of different trigger elements like tangible input, location, participants and communication.

Keywords: user centered design, tangible user interface, design process, AAL.

1 Introduction

Efforts to support elderly people staying in their homes or in supported housing through assistive technologies (Ambient Assisted Living – AAL) have grown into a big research field with a lot of technological innovations in recent years. A large number of AAL research projects deal with topics like fall detection, health monitoring or smart homes, but also digital inclusion. A key requirement for all these technologies is accessibility, which means that they should be equally available to as many people as possible coming from diverse backgrounds with different technology knowledge. A lot of research has been done regarding user involvement and participation in this field [1-7]. However, there is little research on designing tangible user interfaces for and with elderly people. We describe our design approach for user involvement in the development process of a tangible communication tool. To achieve the goal of an accessible and senior-friendly system, our research project *kommTUi* focuses on a very high level of user integration and scrutinizes the possibilities of tangible user interfaces for user interaction. The integration of potential future users throughout the whole design process ensures early feedback on the interaction- and system design and therefore avoids possible design flaws from the very beginning of the development. We aim for an accessible information and communication technology (ICT) which is not only functional but is also accepted by elderly users and enables them to take an active part in the digital society [8]. In order to achieve this objective,

A. Holzinger et al. (Eds.): SouthCHI 2013, LNCS 7946, pp. 625–632, 2013.

we had to carefully plan our user-centered design process, with special focus on creating a respectful and pleasant atmosphere when working with elderly people.

2   Tangible Interfaces

Tangible User Interfaces combine digital data with physical objects. Through interacting with tangible elements it is possible to access or manipulate data linked to these elements. Unlike in Graphical User Interfaces there is not necessarily a clear separation between systems' input and output - it is also possible to have direct feedback at the input elements (Fig. 1) [9].

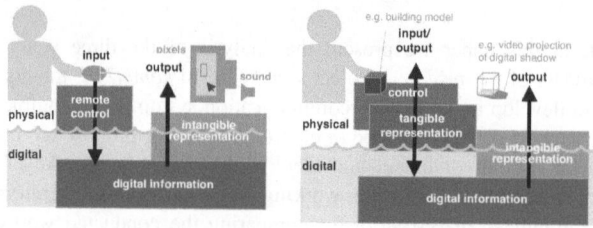

Fig. 1. Comparison of Graphical User Interface (left) and Tangible User Interface (right) [9]

In *kommTUi* we examine the possibilities of tangible interfaces to improve accessibility of ICTs. Accessible communication technologies can help elderly people to use applications and services of digital society and thereby avoid being confronted with (what Brandt et al. call) situated elderliness. Mainly we focus on the design of generic- and personal objects for user interaction. Well-known and often cited examples for tangible user interfaces, like the Marble Answering Machine [10] and the reacTable [11], are using generic objects with geometric shapes as interface elements i.e. marbles or cubes. The usage of generic objects like cubes supports users in the interaction through the natural affordances [12] of their shapes. There are several affordances of cubes, which are already learned in early childhood, i.e. rotate, roll, twist, turn, etc. [13]. They can also be easily included in a token+constraint setup to trigger well-known chains of actions and shape patterns [10]. While generic objects support the user through triggering simple interactions, personal objects can enrich user interfaces on a very individual and emotional level. Personal objects "can be everyday or self-made objects, representing physical, autobiographical objects of memory, reminding the owner of special moments or friends" [14]. They inhere an emotional linkage to the user, turning them into keys, which can only be decoded by the owner of the object. The MEMODULES project uses these relations to create "tangible shortcuts". Personal objects are recognized through a mixture of RFID tagging and image recognition, triggering special functionalities [15]. More recently, Samsung has released the Samsung TecTiles, attachable to every object and usable with every NFC-enabled Smartphone [16]. In kommTUi we scrutinize how tangible interfaces can be used by elderly people and could further improve accessibility of new communication. This has been realized in a user-centered design process, which will be introduced in the next section.

3   kommTUi Approach

From the very beginning of *kommTUi* we focused on the integration of elderly people in the design process. As previous research shows, user involvement has to be carefully composed and well-organized. This has been identified as especially important when working with elderly users: To overcome a potential lack of knowledge of and confidence in (new) technologies [1,4], to raise their motivation to engage in the design process although the benefit isn't immediately clear to them [2], to consider and react to age-related physiological impairments [5], to provide them a pleasant and welcome surrounding not reminding them on a "testing situation" [6], to support an inspiring collaboration in a very heterogeneous group of people [4] or to focus them on the given tasks in a respectful way [3].

Existing participatory user involvement strategies, like the *Future Workshop* format or the *say-do-make* framework, share the challenge of enabling unfamiliar people in an unfamiliar surroundings to produce a creative and successful outcome [17]. Therefore, it is crucial to put maximum effort in providing a respectful and pleasant atmosphere for successful user involvement. As we were confronted with very limited resources (3 team members: project leader, designer, computer scientist, cf. [18]), we had to carefully plan the design process. We defined three iterations for the development of our prototype, each containing user workshops, evaluation and redesign. The structure of the workshops was a mixture of qualitative methods for user-centered design [19]: design sessions, interviews, focus groups, usability testing and feedback rounds. For evaluation, we introduced multimodal analysis frames, a tool for qualitative content analysis with focus on multimodal interaction [20]. This formed the basis for the redesign phase, which completed the iteration. For an overall analysis of the workshops of all three iterations, we designed a graphical analysis tool (Fig. 2) to better compare and understand the similarities and diversities of the conducted workshops. The figure below is the basis of the analysis. As we developed a tangible

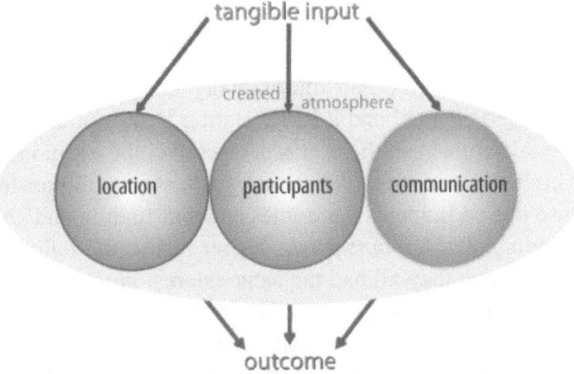

Fig. 2. Basic graphic as analysis tool for *kommTUi*

interface, the role of tangible objects and physicality was high. Therefore, "tangible input" stands for our core variable defined by the research team for each workshop year, influencing communication, interaction, design sessions, location and participants.

The graphic shows the structure of our analysis and enables direct comparison of the three workshops series conducted in 2010, 2011 and 2012. *location l* stands for the location of the conducted workshops and its relation to the participants. *l* can be supportive for the atmosphere when participants know the physical environment or challenging when they are unfamiliar with it [17, 21]. *Participants p* represents the invited participants for each workshop setting and their relation to each other. This trigger element can be modified by inviting participants, who share commonalities or are unfamiliar with each other, thus influencing group dynamic [21]. *Communication c* signifies the whole communication including initial contact, pre-information, pre-talks, interaction and the interactive design sessions. *c* changes through workshop design (exploratory or more focused on technology) and whether including a contact person known by the participants into the communication process [1]. These three elements form the basis to create a specific atmosphere, which we defined as playful, engaging and inviting from the start of *kommTUi* in 2010. More specific, the atmosphere has to enable openness for exchange, interaction and creativity and reduce barriers towards new technologies, especially when working with elderlies. Knowing the atmosphere we wanted to achieve for each workshop, we had to identify the trigger elements facilitating us to reduce or enhance them as needed. This was essential as we had fixed resources in time and person month for the project and wanted to realize similar quality in the workshops each year. Hence, the analysis technique consists of *l*, *p* and *c* as trigger elements and the overall tangible input, which formulated the header of the development. For the workshop comparison we chose the perspective of our participants (user´s perspective), to scrutinize the effects of the conducted events and better understand user involvement and inclusion. In this way we visualize the impacts on planning and designing the *kommTUi* process to reach the specific inviting and playful atmosphere: our basis for successful workshops and research outcome.

3.1   Workshop Series in 2010

The focus of the workshops in 2010 was on exploration of communication habits of elderly people. Therefore, we provided several workshop stations with different kinds of playful user interaction. We had multisensory board game, an interactive board game played via video channel and a RFID station to try out tangible interaction. As we analyze the workshops from the user's perspective, the location in 2010 was totally new for our invited participants: *location l* was just a small part for the atmosphere to create, because our participants were uneasy about finding and getting along in the unknown surrounding. *Participants p* was bigger than *l*: the fellow participants were familiar in the sense, that they all had the same interest group as background, but they did not know each other directly. As a consequence, *communication c* was important and had to be great, to balance the atmosphere to be achieved. In 2010 we invested a lot of time and resources to meet the interest group in one of their events, we wrote

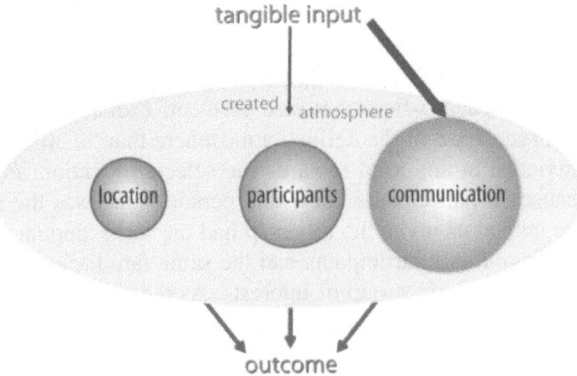

Fig. 3. Analysis of workshops in 2010

emails, designed and gave away cultural probes to each participant and phoned them to explain and getting to know each other. Before and after the workshops itself we conducted discussions and feedback rounds, during the workshops we interviewed each participant with the help of objects (like flyers, flowers, photos, lucky charms etc.,) as mediator to find out more about communication partners and content. Participants brought own flyers, photos etc. to explain topics of communication. *Effects: tangible input was only possible and defined for **c**, due to the early project phase. By having **c** as a mayor player, **l** and **p** could be less to create our specific atmosphere.*

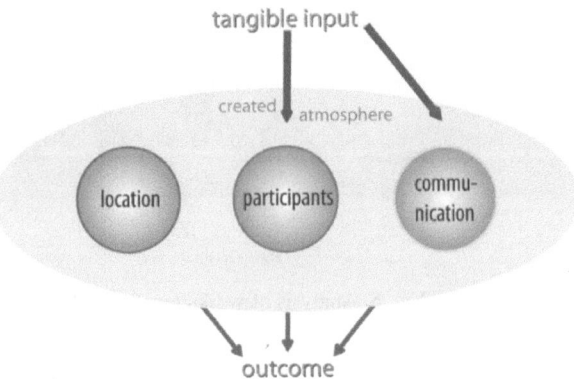

Fig. 4. Analysis of workshops in 2011

3.2   Workshop Series in 2011

In the workshops series of 2011, we focused on the interaction design. Based on the findings of the workshops in 2010, we developed different technology probes to examine basic tangible interactions with elderly people. For that reason, we introduced pre-produced, specially shaped objects made of wood, which we called "generic objects" [13]. Additionally, we asked the participants to bring a personal object to the workshop, reminding them on a special communication partner. This "personal to-ken" was equipped with an RFID-chip during the design session and immediately used for user interaction. In 2011 the participants knew the location well. We were allowed to adopt the space, where they use to meet, exchange and arrange events, therefore *l* had a larger share of the defined atmosphere than in 2010: participants had no barriers or anxieties in any kind towards the selected location. *Participants* *p* in-creased too, because all participants knew one person – she was the initial person of the group and she helped us invite the others. *p* had the same amount of impact for the atmosphere as *location l*. All participants had the same familiarity towards the others, as they were part of an elderly group of interests. As the two trigger elements *l* and *p* were more significant, this meant reducing *communication c* by achieving a similar atmosphere to 2010 was possible. For *c* we had a personal meeting with the initial person, we emailed and phoned again in advance to the workshops and gave away an information leaflets explaining our project and the workshop agenda. Tangible input was raised as we introduced personal objects into the interaction. Additionally the workshops started with a design session, where each participant equipped and de-signed the pre-produced generic tokens and described their personal object and the special relation it represents. *Effects: tangible input was increased by fostering partic-ipant's involvement in c and increasing it in p. By enhancing l and p, the effort for c could be reduced – l, p and c were equal in achieving the pre-defined atmosphere.*

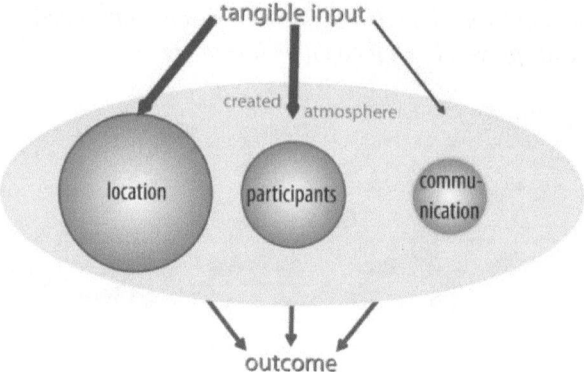

Fig. 5. Analysis of workshops in 2012

3.3 Workshop Series in 2012

The focus of the workshops in 2012 lied on evaluating the usability of the *kommTUi* prototype, which has been developed on the basis of the findings of the workshops in 2010 and 2011. The interaction design stayed basically the same, we had pre-produced generic tokens, which have been equipped and designed by participants, and personal tokens contributed by the participants. The *kommTUi* prototype has been extended to a USB pluggable device, to use it with a standard notebook or PC system. By placing the generic and personal tokens on the *kommTUi* device, the participants were able to use distinct functionalities like starting a Skype call or opening a website. In 2012 the location came to be the major player for the created atmosphere:

Each participant was visited at home - we moved the workshop in the domestic surrounding. From the user's perspective *location l* had a great influence in creating the defined atmosphere. *Participants p* stayed similar to 2011: They knew one person accompanying the research stuff. We had 2 different initial persons, hence one always was very well-known and liked by each participant. *Communication c* could be even smaller than in 2011, besides phone calls directly with the initial persons, we just fixed dates for the visits and talked to each participant shortly about what they had to expect. In 2012 we succeeded in introducing tangible input also in *l* and experienced once more the importance of involving known objects for interaction. The possibility of looking around in one's own home during personal objects selection was experienced as very homey and created an openness for telling relations and meanings of the selected objects. *Effects: tangible input was enabled in l, p and c. Participants got involved even stronger by enhancing the tangible input in p and l. The relation of l, p and c totally reversed compared to 2010: l was the major and c the minor player then.*

4   Conclusions

Our contribution lies in the specific analysis of our design process and our goal to achieve a respectful and pleasant atmosphere by relating specific components like location, participants and communication. Reflecting our analysis and the results, we were amazed by the fact, how clear the analysis tool showed insights in the relation of *tangible input, location, participants* and *communication* creating a successful workshop atmosphere. We set up the workshops in a way to create for each a similar atmosphere, realized how to increase or decrease each trigger element and how they relate. This was essential, since we had the same time and personal resources throughout all three years and could not increase certain parameters, without reducing others. We had to understand how we could reduce our input in time and effort in one trigger element, if the other was getting bigger in consequence of the chosen workshop structure. A good example for keeping this balance is the fact that the relation of *location* (*l*), *participants* (*p*) and *communication* (*c*) reversed from 2010 to 2012 (Fig. 2, 3, 4). We used different methods throughout the design process to keep *p* as an important factor for the atmosphere. This allowed us to increase/decrease *l* and *c* and still reach the desired atmosphere. The importance of *p* is also underscored by the constant *tangible input* throughout the whole design process. By integrating personal objects, the user involvement was getting even more intimate. This highly individualized interaction as part of our overall *tangible input* (Fig. 2) is able to reduce emotional barriers towards the interface and therefore increases the accessibility of the technology – a revelation for design and development of future communication products and an issue we found essential to scrutinize more. However, the high degree of personalization demands for a very sensible and respectful dealing with the elderly people, which underlines the importance of atmosphere for user involvement.

References

1. Eisma, R., Dickinson, A., Goodman, J., Syme, A., Tiwari, L., Newell, F.: Early user involvement in the development of information technology-related products for older people. Univers. Access Inf. Soc. 3(2), 131–140 (2004)

2. Hawthorn, D.: Interface design and engagement with older people. Behaviour & Information Technology 26(4), 333–341 (2007)
3. Zajicek, M.: Aspects of HCI research for older people. Univers. Access Inf. Soc. 5(3), 279–286 (2006)
4. Lindsay, S., Jackson, D., Schofield, G., Olivier, P.: Engaging older people using participatory design. In: Proceedings of the SIGCHI Conference on Human Factors in Computing Systems, pp. 1199–1208. ACM, New York (2012)
5. Fisk, A., Rogers, W., Charness, N., Czaja, S., Sharit, J.: Designing for Older Adults. In: Principles and Creative Human Factors Approaches, 2nd edn., CRC Press (2009)
6. Newell, A., Arnott, J., Carmichael, A., Morgan, M.: Methodologies for involving older adults in the design process. In: Stephanidis, C. (ed.) HCI 2007. LNCS, vol. 4554, pp. 982–989. Springer, Heidelberg (2007)
7. Brandt, E., Binder, T., Malmborg, L., Sokoler, T.: Communities of everyday practice and situated elderliness as an approach to co-design for senior interaction. In: Proc. of the 22nd Conf. of the Australian Computer-Human Interaction, pp. 400–403. ACM, USA (2010)
8. Shinohara, K., Wobbrock, J.: In the shadow of misperception: assistive technology use and social interactions. In: Proceedings of the SIGCHI Conference on Human Factors in Computing Systems, pp. 705–714. ACM, New York (2011)
9. Ishii, H.: Tangible bits: beyond pixels. In: Proc. of the 2nd Int. Conf. on Tangible and Embedded Interaction, pp. xv-xxv. ACM, New York (2008)
10. Ullmer, B., Ishii, H., Jacob, R.: Token+constraint systems for tangible interaction with digital information. ACM Trans. Comput.-Hum. Interact. 12(1), 81–118 (2005)
11. Jordá, S., Geiger, G., Alonso, M., Kaltenbrunner, M.: The reacTable: exploring the synergy between live music performance and tabletop tangible interfaces. In: Proc. of the 1st Int. Conf. on Tangible and Embedded Interaction, pp. 139–146. ACM, NY (2007)
12. Norman, D.: Psychology of Everyday Things. Basic Books, New York (1988)
13. Sheridan, J., Short, B., Van Laerhoven, K., Villar, N., Kortuem, G.: Exploring cube affordances: towards a classification of non-verbal dynamics of physical interfaces for wearable computing. In: Proceedings of the IEE Eurowearable 2003, pp. 113–118. IEE (2003)
14. Ehrenstrasser, L., Spreicer, W.: Personal Interaction through Individual Artifacts. In: Workshop-Proc. Mensch & Computer 2012, Konstanz, September 9-12, pp. 129–134 (2012)
15. Mugellini, E., et al.: MEMODULES as Tangible Shortcuts to Multimedia Information. In: Lalanne, D., Kohlas, J. (eds.) Human Machine Interaction. LNCS, vol. 5440, pp. 103–132. Springer, Heidelberg (2009)
16. Samsung TecTiles (2013),
   http://www.samsung.com/us/microsite/tectile/
17. Muller, M., Druin, A.: Participatory design: the third space in HCI. In: Jacko, J., Sears, A. (eds.) The Human-Computer Interaction Handbook, pp. 1051–1068. L. Erlbaum Associates Inc., Hillsdale (2002)
18. Mao, J., Vredenburg, K., Smith, P., Carey, T.: The state of user-centered design practice. Commun. ACM 48(3), 105–109 (2005)
19. Vredenburg, K., Mao, J., Smith, P., Carey, T.: A survey of user-centered design practice. In: Proceedings of the SIGCHI Conference on Human Factors in Computing Systems, pp. 471–478. ACM, USA (2002)
20. Ehrenstrasser, L., Spreicer, W.: Defining Multimodality for Tangible Interaction. In: Workshop-Proceedings NordiCHI, Copenhagen, October 14-17, pp. 27–29 (2012)
21. Hultcrantz, J., Ibrahim, A.: Contextual workshops: User participationin the evaluation of future concepts. In: Proceedings of PDC 2002. CPSR, Malmö (2002)

Keeping "InTOUCH": An Ongoing Co-design Project to Share Memories, Skills and Demands through an Interactive Table

Sabina Giorgi, Miguel Ceriani, Paolo Bottoni, Alessandra Talamo, and Silvia Ruggiero

Università di Roma "Sapienza" (Italy)
{bottoni,ceriani}@di.uniroma1.it,
{sabina.giorgi,alessandra.talamo}@uniroma1.it, silviaruggiero5@gmail.com

Abstract. We describe the first phases of an ongoing co-design project for a cooperative distributed space, based on multi-touch technologies, through which older adults engaged in the activities of recreational centres in their everyday contexts could keep in touch with others, for example other recreational centres, and with a general public. The project's main goal is to foster the active participation of older people as producers of resources related to their experience and know-how and to the activities carried out in the centres, to be shared in a community context. The project aims to fulfill some seniors' needs and wishes as "always learning new things", "being with others" and "not staying at home".

Keywords: co-design, older people, memories, skills, interactive table.

1 Ageing and ICT

In 2002, the World Health Organization adopted the expression "Active Ageing" to express the concept of ageing in connection with concepts of social participation and safety, with the aim of improving older people's quality of life [15]. The United Nations identifies specific psychological dimensions behind the concept of Active Ageing that are: dignity, independence, participation, care, self-fulfillment. Even though most of these dimensions rely on the emotional aspects of ageing, many research projects in the domain of Ageing and Information and Communication Technologies (ICT) primarily focus on the design of assistive technologies and monitoring systems, offering a representation of older persons mainly characterized by their weaknesses, passiveness and failings [8,9].

More recently, a growing number of research studies have focused on the design of ICT systems which aim to foster social interactions for older adults in peer-to-peer communicative contexts [2], in intergenerational communities [3,16], also through the development of virtual game platforms [4].

From a technological point of view, the last years have witnessed considerable advances in the possibily of interaction with ICT systems. The advent of mobile computing devices as smartphones and tablets quickly widened the access to multi-touch technologies and multimedia integration. These technologies

A. Holzinger et al. (Eds.): SouthCHI 2013, LNCS 7946, pp. 633–640, 2013.

have proved to be effective in lowering the digital divide between different generations [1]. A standing research challenge is to use them in forms that can be inclusive and supporting of older adults and of their needs and wishes.

The ongoing co-design process we present here, called InTOUCH, aims at creating a service that is rewarding from the emotional and social point of view. It provides older people with the chance of maintaining already existing meaningful personal connections and building new relationships inside a community in which experience and competences they gained through life are shared with others, in order to support their active participation in their life environments.

At the same time, also the other users of the service, with a special regard to younger adults, can benefit from the contents and information produced within the system and the interactions shared.

We propose, as a "community tool", an interactive table, i.e. a horizontal multi-touch screen designed to digitally support collective activities in their usual meeting space (a recreational centre) without losing the communicative posibilities of "around the table" meetings. This technology is proposed integrated with standard tablet technology (to be used outside of the centre or in the centre for special purposes like recording).

Paper Organisation. In Section 2 we discuss the methodology of the InTouch project and in Section 3 we report on findings from a previous study. Section 4 presents the ICT service, while Section 5 sketches interaction with them through a multi-touch tabletop. Finally, conclusions are given in Section 6.

2   The "InTOUCH" Co-design Project: Methodology

A co-design project is based on some main assumptions, first of all the definition of "users" as unique experts of their own experience [12] and not only the "prototype" of users who will evaluate and test the new service/product [11]. Recently, many research projects focused on ageing and ICT adopted a co-design perspective in order to better include seniors in the design process [2,6,16]. The InTOUCH project follows the same approach, involving as co-designers a group of 14 older adults (13 females and 1 male) aged between 76 years old and 86, who are members of two daily recreational centres for frail older adults in the X Municipality of Rome. Both centres are part of a local social co-operative.

Since the start of the project, the design team recognised that a co-design process with the group of older adults required the active participation and involvement of two main groups of stakeholders: the management of the cooperative and the group of caregivers who work every day with seniors, in order to better stimulate them during the work sessions and to avoid frustrating experiences due to requests for skills they could not support.

The InTOUCH project has started in June 2011 and is running for three years. It is a long-term design process undertaken by an interdisciplinary research team, organized around some main phases. In the first phase seniors participated in an in-depth user experience (UX) research, whose main activities were:

- a first "user forum", during which the project, its phases, goals and methodology were described;
- co-construction of the seniors' life stories and interviews on their everyday activities, a crucial activity for better knowing seniors' past and present lives, their competences and know-how;
- co-realization of guided video tours in the seniors' homes, to "situate" their narrations about daily activities and life events in their everyday spaces;
- two workshops on specific subjects: the first focused on the interactions of seniors with modern technologies; the second on the experience of sharing memories related to their own "objects of affection" within a group;
- a workshop of "needs prioritization", in which the most important older participants' needs (and wishes) were better identified (see Figure 1).

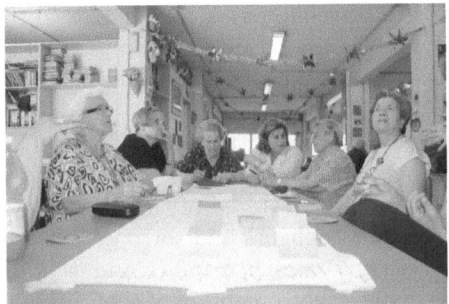

Fig. 1. The workshop of "needs prioritization" in the recreational centre

The second phase of the project, still ongoing, focuses on the development of the concept of the ICT service through the use of some service design tools as personas, narrative scenarios and user journey. Caregivers and managers have played a crucial role in generating the service concept.

Currently, the research team is designing the interaction system and the service interfaces involving seniors and caregivers in workshops with low-fidelity prototypes, also taking into account the critical points related to their use with this specific group of participants [7], as discussed in the next Section.

3   Main Findings from the Co-constructed UX Research

From the UX research some main needs emerged. We describe them in order of importance from the senior participants' point of view:

- *Always learning new things.* Learning is described as what allows self development and synchronicity with the present time. It supports the perception of the life progression. The main learning wishes expressed by seniors are to be able to use computers (especially in order to gather from the Web information about practical aspects of their lives), to cook, to better know the city where they live. Many older participants recognize their know-how and expertise (typically cooking and sewing, as participants were mostly women) as "gifts" they have and they would like to share with others. Other seniors, however, have difficulties in identifying their skills or abilities.

– *Being with others.* The need to be in touch with people, to share activities within a group is quite important for senior participants. The time spent with others is mostly dedicated to informal communication and storytelling. The most gratifying communication is with friends or people close to them in everyday life (e.g. young volunteers met in the recreational centre). Beside chatting, older participants like to share activities like cooking or sewing, already carried out in the recreational centers. Other activities they would like to do together are traveling and strolling around the neighborhood and the city, as they did in the past. But they complain of the growing difficulty to meet other people due to their health problems and to the lack of a large and supportive social network.

– *Do not stay at home.* The home time, spent in loneliness, on the edge of recreational centers activities, is mostly described by seniors with an emotional tiredness. The home, scattered of tangible memories and emptied of real presences, remember "delights and sorrows", as a participant said.

– *Helping others* (or *feeling oneself helpful*) and *being helped.* The need of helping others, to enhance the perception of their usefulness, emerged during the user forum with the older adults. But during the final workshop of "needs prioritization", terms changed in favor of the need of being helped. "Who can we help? We need to be helped", an older participant says. Helping others seems to be something done in the past when their abilities and agency were better recognized than now.

3.1   The Experience of Storytelling

The life story activity presents an emotional ambiguity between the opposite needs to forget and to remember through storytelling. The experience of narrating their own stories is most positive when it is possible to choose and select what to tell, e.g. in workshops focused on objects of affections, in which objects are selected and stories are told about them. The shared dimension of storytelling within the group adds value to the experience. Seniors' narrations are also characterized by their strong localization in the places where events happened.

3.2   Representations of Technology

In the course of the UX research, older adults have also expressed some specific representations of the "modern technologies". Technology is useful and comfortable if it answers specific needs otherwise unsatisfied (see also [5]), as in the case of the cellular phone. Technology is also "intriguing", especially for some familiar features seniors already know as the visual functionalities of digital technologies, for example watching films, documentaries, photos of cherished persons and "to talk with others", as a participant says. The written dimension is perceived as too tiring and not appealing. Digital technology enters older people's everyday life trough the mediation of meaningful others: children, grandchildren or caregivers of the recreational center.

4   The InTOUCH Service and Its Objectives

On the basis of our findings, we created a concept for an ICT service that responds to the cognitive, emotional and social needs of the older participants.

InTOUCH is an ICT service that allows older adults who participate in activities of recreational centres to become part of a community in which a specific pool of resources is created and shared, in order to build meaningful relationships among users.

The members of the community interact with each other in an interactive map where the resources are localized. The choice of the map as metaphor of the service is due to the will of enhancing the seniors' wishes to learn new things about places where they live, not to stay home, and to be with others for traveling and strolling around. The InTOUCH service is a journey within geographical places, known and unknown, and the resources associated with them. These consist in: 1) TALES, short stories of events, biographical or not, linked to places; 2) KNOWLEDGE IN ACTION, video tutorials for learning specific activities; 3) TOURS, guided tours of places; 4) QUESTIONS, requests coming from the members of the community for specific competences or know-how they want to learn and to know. Resources will be produced and enjoyed under the form of short clips, taking advantage of the seniors' interest towards the visual functionalities of digital technologies. They will be localized in the map and visualized according to categories described above.

Older adults of the two recreational centres, with the support of caregivers, will be the first active members of the service, by creating a first pool of resources to share, that are related to the activities usually carried out in the recreational centres. In short, the InTOUCH service allows:

- *to foster the learning* of the digital technologies by using them as tools for creating new knowledge on that domains most quoted by seniors, among them the knowledge of places;
- *to enhance the sharing* of seniors competences and expertises, also by empowering the awareness of their abilities and skills;
- *to keep in touch with others* by carrying out practical activities together;
- *to empower the usefulness perception* of older adults and their ability to help others, and to answer for others' requests, as something not only related to their past life experiences but also to their present time;
- *to foster the storytelling* as positive experience, by activating the selectivity of reminiscence and improving the normal attitude of older tellers to link their narrations to their life places (past and present);

- *to enhance the representation of digital technology as useful* and comfortable since it answers for specific needs otherwise unsatisfied;
- *to make use of the mediation of meaningful others* for the introduction of the InTOUCH service in older adults' everyday environments. In particular the recreational centre will be the first touch-point of the service for older adults, taking into account its role in their everyday lives.

The InTOUCH service also aims at becoming a tool for creating new relationships between older adults and other people that could become vis-à-vis relationships. Caregivers have to be able to use the service to fulfill their role of guiding activities and facilitating comprehension and access to technologies. People close to seniors will support them when using the service outside of the recreational centre and will also access and request contents as a way to share knowledge and interact with older people. Other persons using the system will access and request contents to share knowledge and build social relationships.

5   Devices

We defined some requirements for the devices to be used by the older adults and caregivers: 1) Audio/Video Recording Capability; 2) Portability (for ease of recording and transportation between centre and home/outside); 3) Graphical and Natural User Interface; 4) Possibility of exploring/organizing contents in a map based view; 5) Possibility of playing contents; 6) Support for group activities in the recreational centre. The first three requirements are met by the use of tablets. To support collective activities we propose an interactive table. The service will be available also to the general public as a web application in order to provide the desidered openness.

5.1   An Interactive Table

The interactive table consists of a table whose upper surface accommodates a multi-touch display (see Figure 2). The table is designed to support collective activities of a small group, up to four active users at a time, centred on the research and exploration of the available resources (see Section 4).

To provide comfort and support interpersonal interaction [14] we opted for a basic rectangular table with space for legs below and some free space near the edges of the tabletop (to rest arms or to put objects). At each side there will be an earphone plug to be used in case of independent content fruition.

The layered interface has the Interactive Map at the bottom. On the map lay the Points of Interest (POIs), that are the locations which are related to some content. When a POI is tapped or dragged it exposes its content throught the appearance of a Floating Content Thumbnail (FCT) that can be arbitrarily dragged and reoriented to support natural collaboration roles [10].

To support and suggest personal areas of action [13] Personal Panels can be summoned from each side and dragged to allow different arrangement of users.

In each Personal Panel, among the other commands, there is a clearly designated Personal View Area in which a FCT can be dragged to be viewed. The content on display can then be also enlarged, becoming a Resizable Content View that can reach the most comfortable size depending on user and group needs [1].

The interface is multidirectional, the map being the only graphic component with global orientation, which can, however, be changed to favour another user through the "Navigate the Map" command. The favoured user is the only one who can change the map view searching for a location or filtering visible POIs.

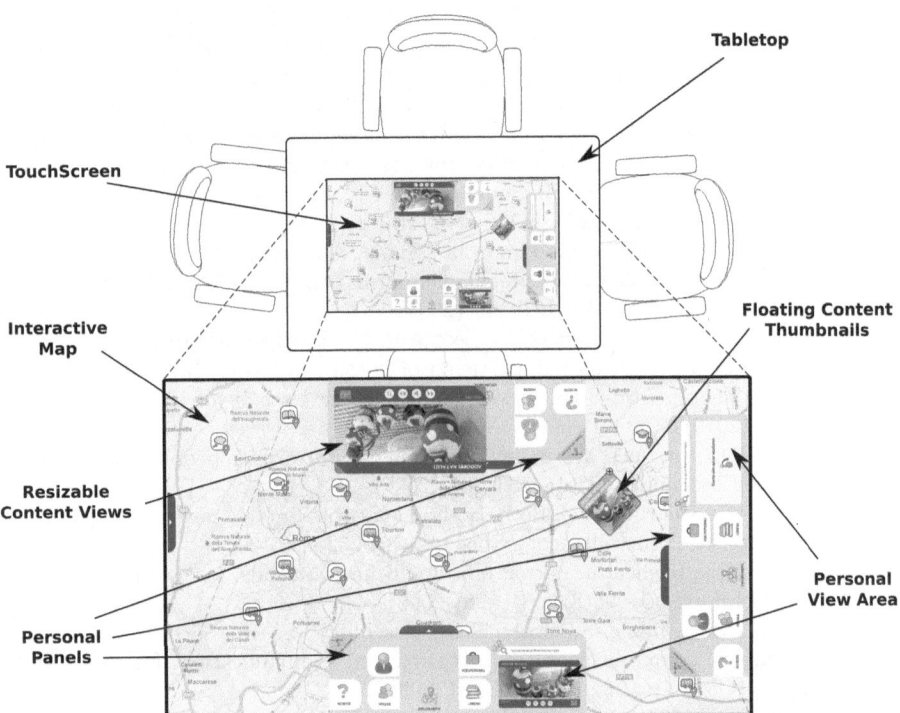

Fig. 2. The interactive tabletop. A view from above with the active area enlarged.

6   Conclusions

We described the methodology and experience of co-design with a community of older adults participating in activities of a recreational centre, in order to realize an ICT service fostering "active ageing" and participation in their cultural and social life contexts. We studied their needs and wishes, their relationships with memories and storytelling and their representations of technology. From the findings of our study we designed a service to reach social engagement by sharing of knowledge and life experiences, both in digital form and vis-à-vis.

We chose to use a digital tabletop system as main access point to the system and sketched the design of the device and the interface. Currently, we are carrying on the proccess of co-design of the interfaces of the InTOUCH service. In the meanwhile we plan to carry out some UX research aimed to reach a general public, especially young people, through the service.

References

1. Apted, T., Kay, J., Quigley, A.: Tabletop sharing of digital photographs for the elderly. In: Proc. 24th HFCS, pp. 781–790. ACM (2006)
2. Brandt, E., Binder, T., Malmborg, L., Sokoler, T.: Communities of everyday practice and situated elderliness as an approach to co-design for senior interaction. In: Proc. 22nd Australia CHI, pp. 400–403. ACM (2010)
3. Budweg, S., Müller, C., Lewkowicz, M.: Designing for Inter/Generational Communities. International Reports on Socio-Informatics 9 (2012)
4. Dewsbury, G., Rouncefield, M., Sommerville, I., Onditi, V., Bagnall, P.: Designing technology with older people. UAIS 6(2), 207–217 (2007)
5. Eisma, R., Dickinson, A., Goodman, J., Syme, A., Tiwari, L., Newell, A.: Early user involvement in the development of information technology-related products for older people. UAIS 3(2), 131–140 (2004)
6. Grönvall, E., Conci, M., Giusti, L., Leonardi, C.: The intrinsic fragility of elderly care networks: five challenges in participatory design practices. In: Proc. NordiCHI workshop: Therapeutic Strategies-a Challenge for User Involvement in Design, pp. 20–24 (2010)
7. Hawthorn, D.: Interface design and engagement with older people. Behaviour & Information Technology 26(4), 333–341 (2007)
8. Kenner, A.M.: Securing the Elderly Body: Dementia, Surveillance, and the Politics of Aging in Place. Surveillance & Society 5(3), 252–269 (2008)
9. Koch, S.: Home telehealth. current state and future trends. International Journal of Medical Informatics 75(8), 565–576 (2006)
10. Kruger, R., Carpendale, S., Scott, S.D., Greenberg, S.: How people use orientation on tables: comprehension, coordination and communication. In: Proc. ACM SIGGROUP 2003, pp. 369–378. ACM (2003)
11. Marti, P., Bannon, L.: Exploring User-Centred Design in Practice: Some Caveats. Knowledge, Technology & Policy 22, 7–15 (2009)
12. Rizzo, F.: Strategie di co-design. Teorie, metodi e strumenti per progettare con gli utenti. Franco Angeli, Roma (2009)
13. Scott, S.D., Carpendale, M.S.T., Inkpen, K.M.: Territoriality in collaborative tabletop workspaces. In: Proc. CSCW 2004, pp. 294–303. ACM Press (2004)
14. Scott, S.D., Grant, K.D., Mandryk, R.L.: System guidelines for co-located, collaborative work on a tabletop display. In: Proc. 8th ECSCW, pp. 159–178 (2003)
15. WHO. WHO Active Ageing - A Policy Framework (2010), http://whqlibdoc.who.int/hq/2002/WHO_NMH_NPH_02.8.pdf
16. Xie, B., Druin, A., Fails, J., Massey, S., Golub, E., Franckel, S., Schneider, K.: Connecting generations: developing co-design methods for older adults and children. Behaviour & Information Technology 31(4), 413–423 (2012)

Assisting Lifestyles: "Laughing, Living and Learning"

Boris Markovic and Özge Subasi

Vienna University of Technology, HCI Group, Austria
e0625198@student.tuwien.ac.at
subasi@igw.tuwien.ac.at

Abstract. This paper reports on practices of a senior community based on the findings from three participatory observation sessions, a short survey and wrap-up interviews. Our findings suggest that both the lifestyle of individuals and the constraints of the specific community settings play a role for designing for senior communities. We introduce our insights from our studies on the setting, the artifacts used in the sessions and on senior individuals. Further we introduce our initial design ideas and discuss their relations to the presented design space.

1 Introduction

Ageing is an important personal and demographic change. Without a clear starting point when somebody is considered old, many issues that are related to the quality of life of a person can also be related to the process of ageing. As an understanding a homogenous ageing society based on the sum of their deficits is losing popularity [3][1][8]. As designers, we feel a need for a better understanding of particular practices of a group of ageing people in relation to those situations, in order to think an inclusive perspective together [8][6]. In this paper, we concentrate on a case of senior individuals that weekly meet in a group called LIMA (Lebensqualität im Alter - „quality of life in age") for training their body and mind, based on interviews and participatory observations. To strengthen social networks and interaction among seniors, one has to pay attention to their everyday practices [2] as a well-designed system is useless without a community that accepts its use [9]. In our particular locality (in Vienna), Senior Offices and Senior Federation centrally organize senior clubs and communities for a lively senior culture and the Association of Seniors are also a part of the organization culture (http://www.wien.gv.at/menschen/senioren/). Vienna has 166 Senior Clubs, which are mostly intended for entertainment, offering excursions, travel possibilities, holidays and theater visits, and they also support living alone at home, providing mobility training and help in a household (http://www.kwp.at/). In addition to senior clubs, there are other support groups e.g. for supporting the mental and physical health. LIMA is an organization of the Catholic Church that is founded more than 10 years ago (http://www. bildungswerk.at/content/lima/0/articles/2010/09/30/a4340/). It's aimed at senior people, who want to stay mentally fit, healthy and mobile. The LIMA program is

A. Holzinger et al. (Eds.): SouthCHI 2013, LNCS 7946, pp. 641–648, 2013.
© Springer-Verlag Berlin Heidelberg 2013

based on a study from the University of Erlangen, Institute of Gerontopsychology from 1991, called SIMA (Selbstständigkeit im höheren Lebensalter – "autonomy in age") [7]. The study established, that repeating cognitive and motoric training on a regular basis, results in a higher autonomy of people. That's why the LIMA-program today consists of memory and movement training. In addition, questions of meaning and faith were a part of it too. Participants are also discussing every day habits and capabilities to find solutions, how to make life easier. Recently, since 2012, The Association of Seniors (main organization for all issues around senior society in Vienna), started to offer LIMA. This made us think about the existing structure of LIMA and its fit to new understandings on aging. In addition to standard support for mental fitness, both emotional values and everyday rituals are also interesting for engaging solutions [8]. For example theoretical debates around ageing and design [8][1] and new perspectives from HCI such as philosophy of slow technology (e.g: [6]), related solutions such as designing paychecks for "eighty somethings" [9] or a materialistic photobox that prints flickr pictures [6] motivate us on how design and creation of new technology must take into account the material, shape and meaning of an object for seniors and how such examples fit into the texture of the everyday. Our main aim is letting people feel less old, by letting them being able to handle things, even if they are newly introduced [2].

2   LIMA Study and Findings

Our initial goal was to understand the existing LIMA course better in order to see some potentials of improvement and a possible fit of technology and design to this everyday texture. For this study we interviewed one expert on how LIMA groups are organized, what the topics and motivations are and what practices they have, we conducted a short survey on level of technology access of the individuals and observed three LIMA sessions. We attended two sessions from Monday meetings (with same participants, N_{G1}=12, 11F, 1M) and one session from Thursday meeting (N_{G2}=13, 10F, 3M), all meetings having the same structure and procedures. Each session took around 1,5 hours, taking place only on Mondays and Thursdays. Participants pay around 6.50 Euro per LIMA session (not for our study) for practicing mental training. LIMA sessions are planned in 10 units a year and most of the participants were attending LIMA for years. We observed the groups and audio-recorded the sessions, took photos of activities, participants and environment. Initially, we applied thematic analysis [1] by two researchers. On the next section of the paper we give a short overview on our observations, themes and design ideas. To make it easy for mapping to design ideas, we initially categorized our LIMA observations according to the following points: (a) LIMA people: practices, motivations (b) LIMA topics and structure (c) LIMA utensils & environment. We found three important themes related to LIMA everyday by saturating them from around fifty different issues we detected. These three themes are "LIMA as lifestyle", "LIMA as fun" and "LIMA as family, social contacts". An overall theme of "life balance as lifestyle" was chosen to define the umbrella term for LIMA participants and their motivations around LIMA. We then documented sets of constraints and issues for each theme in relation to given LIMA structures. This means, each theme was once more evaluated in relation to LIMA people, practices, motivations, topics, structure, utensils and environment (via line-by-line coding). Our results pointed to "learning" and "socializing" as opposite sides in LIMA and "using existing topics" and "defining new topics" are constraints that we cannot overcome due to strict structure of LIMA sessions. We created a Cartesian coordinate system (CCS) [5] based on these two themes and constraints. CCS is a design technique that is used for defining a spectrum of possibilities (with x- and y-axes) and mapping design ideas on this spectrum, to find the most attractive idea [5]. In the next part, we discuss insights from our observations and how we interpreted them for the created ideas and CCS. We discuss 5 ideas and their value on CCS at the end of this paper.

2.1   LIMA People

LIMA people as a community have various characteristics. To name a few, although people are attending LIMA for mental training and exercises they usually have broader motivations such as looking for companionship, contact with other like-minded persons and fun. As a participant explains what LIMA means for them: *"Mental, cognitive and physical recreation, running, laughing, living and learning is the program for me."* (George, 75, Thursday group). The atmosphere in the group is very personal and they take care of each other, as seen in Fig. 1. As another example of this, when Martha was not in the session on that day, her LIMA colleague Dora said: *"Please give me an exercise sheet for Martha, ... should I also keep exercise sheets for you? ... Where is Martha, is she fine?"* (Dora, 68, Monday group). This type of 'caring' and 'companionship' is manifested in many different facets in the sessions. Furthermore, family is a very important mechanism to motivate a person visiting LIMA.

In some cases LIMA also functions like a network for distributing news, e.g. when there is a new event –not related to LIMA-, the information is passed on by mouth: *"May I allowed to say something, ... there is a book flea at our parish, upcoming Monday and everybody is invited to come..."*(Ruth, 77, Monday group). Family, society and sharing events are major themes for participants, however communication between different groups of LIMA (e.g: between Monday and Thursday groups) is not available at the moment. We thought an asynchronous communication with other LIMA groups concerning LIMA topics could motivate people, without adding the initial burden of extending their networks, as new friendships are usually not sought by seniors [8]. One design idea we had was the following: Different groups are scanning self-made LIMA-relevant material and sharing with each other through a mobile scanner and tablet solution shown in Fig. 2, called *My Life, in Paper-Form.*

Taking the prototype to each class by the LIMA leader, every group member can use it during, before or after lessons. This way an asynchronous communication on LIMA related issues could be managed. After putting a paper in the scanner slot of the prototype, the "share with"-screen is called and participants can choose groups to share with. Clicking on the mailbox keyhole, participants can view their scanned pictures and explore what kind of mail arrived from different groups.

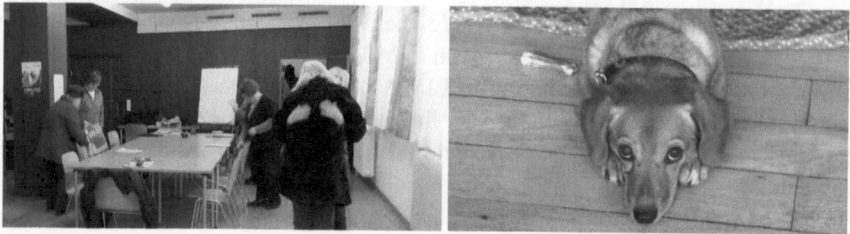

Fig. 1. Although there is little or no contact between LIMA sessions, each group atmosphere is very personal, participants are also bringing their dogs to the group

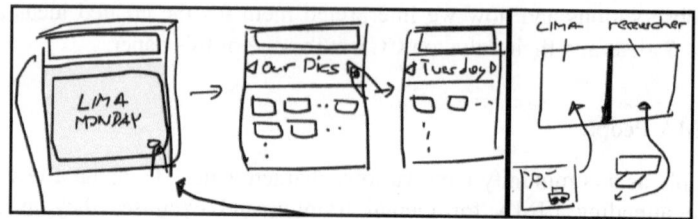

Fig. 2. (Left) "My Life, in Paper-Form", (right) "My week"

LIMA is a heterogeneous group concerning the psychological and physical state and personalities (e.g: introverts and extroverts). Regarding new people attending to LIMA sessions, LIMA-members appreciate the engagement of external people a lot and like it when somebody new is interested in working with them. This brought us to the idea of keeping our connections to them via sharing weekly activities between LIMA members and design researchers using the prototype *My Week*:

At the beginning of a LIMA session, people are talking with each other, about their week, homework and other topics. We thought a book of impressions could be placed in the LIMA room, bound with a mobile printer and smartphone for internet connection, printing a researchers week and splicing it in the book as shown in Fig. 2. Motivated by the researchers week, LIMA people can create their own impressions (activities and daily routines) and feedback them to the researchers. Writing with a digital pen, both notes and audio can be transmitted to the researcher. This can help researchers learn about seniors' life out of LIMA and improve products and services on this direction. It can also be an unobtrusive way for seniors to share their concerns on designs with researchers.

We found that people are motivated to use technology for staying in contact: "I'm very impressed of Facebook and proud that I'm using it. I need it because of my grandchildren living abroad, knowing what is going on in their lives is very important for me." (Marie, 77, Monday group). So they would see some value in using technology: "If you are looking for companionship, Facebook is a good option … My grandchild is continuously on Facebook … (George, 80, Monday group). But this interest and appreciation is not without doubts: "If there's something happening on my computer, I call my grandchild to help me, unfortunately he can't always explain how he solved the problem… (George, 80, Monday group).

Creating *Emotion-Tech-Cards* by family members (via text and pictures) and explaining technology usage to LIMA group in every LIMA session by printing the cards, can motivate seniors to write about their technology usage on these cards and send it back to corresponding people by using a scanner. The heterogeneity of LIMA people and their openness are very important components for our work. There were a couple of issues, where conflicts came along due to heterogeneity of people in contrast with the homogeneity of LIMA training structure. In the following parts we tried to categorize both homogenous LIMA practices and diversity of people.

2.2   LIMA Topics and Structure

At the beginning of each LIMA session, people are showing their homework from last week. The range of subjects is based on cognitive and balance training (each taking 1/3 and ¼ of session time), so they are reading, counting, doing short balance exercises and memory work, dancing to music and other cognitive exercises as seen in Fig. 3. They are also doing handicrafts, but mostly at home. The aim is to get away from every day habits. It is important that the fluid intelligence is trained, that means the concentration and logic of each individual in order to think faster. The background theory behind that is taught in approximately 10 minutes per lesson.

But problems in managing the subject area occurs, so it is not always clear, which topics have been presented to each group: *I thought we did crossfoots, or was it with another group? May we have done it once, but just in oral form?* (LIMA-leader, 62).

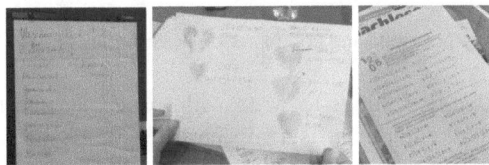

Fig. 3. Themes like "What two household appliances do I like the most?" as memory work, the homework topic "My heart" and concentration exercises are parts of LIMA

People, who are psychologically or physically in a bad mood (due to family problems or not having family any more), often won't cooperate and are negatively affecting the group. *They just feel very bad and are thinking in a negative way, producing aggression to everything new, even on things that I do, they are shouting at me, it's like a valve for them, ... then, the whole group is shouting too ...* (LIMA-leader, 62). The LIMA-leader plays an important role in these cases, as the group must be led, to avoid not LIMA related discussions, although they're well-liked by participants. As individuals, some participants are playing the piano or organ, are sewing or reading at public book sessions and this is a conflict that LIMA is sometimes too simple as Gerti puts it: *Our pastor wants us just accompanying church songs; ... this is so boring ...* (Gerti, 78, Thursday group).

Our concept here was letting participants introduce their own old objects, pictures, pieces of clothes or paperwork to the group by telling stories and making notes, as to increase the sense of self-worth as described in [8]. With the idea *That's Me - Memory Recollection*, this data is saved in order to recollect memories later on, finding out who told a story or what the meaning of a particular picture is, by showing the material on a display or playing it on the speakers.

2.3   LIMA –Utensils and Environment

LIMA takes place in a medium-sized room in medical practices, rectories or clubs. Both the seating position of participants and the room size can differ from group to group. For example the Monday group was sitting mostly in a row and the group on Thursday around a round table, which is shown in Fig. 5.

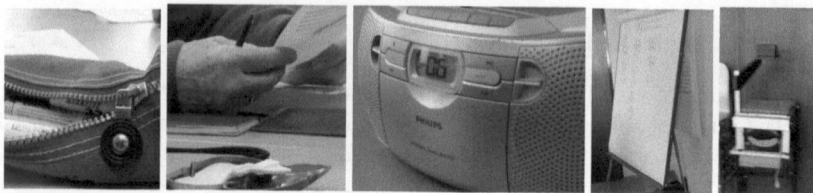

Fig. 4. LIMA Utensils: felt tip pens, exercise sheets, a portable CD player, flipchart and a projector are parts of the standard equipment in the classroom

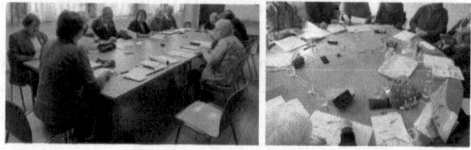

Fig. 5. Seating positions and collaboration possibilities of LIMA-members

Every participant carries things to write with, paper and mostly reading glasses. The classroom standard equipment is a flipchart, felt tip pens, exercise sheets and a portable radio with a CD-player, showed in Fig. 4. There are no records of a LIMA session. Both the sitting positions and the utensils emphasized a "fix structure" for a particular aim of "mental training". However we realized that most of the informal communication was taking place during small breaks around a water corner, gathering together around a table. Therefore, a bottle of water is always a part of LIMA-utensils which brought us to the following idea: Some of the times, when lifting the bottle, a picture-card is printed for each senior over a hidden printer in a box as seen in Fig. 6, explaining on what project the researcher is currently working on. Seniors can give feedback by scanning paper about topics they are elaborating at this time or writing feedback on the back of the card using the prototype *We are drinking. And You?.*

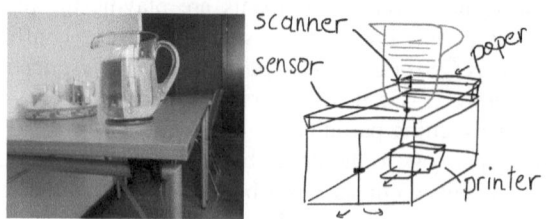

Fig. 6. (Left) "Water corner", (right) "We are drinking. And You?" - prototype

3   Conclusions and Future Work

During our observation we noted down several issues that are interesting to follow up with. Still being a group with a community character, the individual wishes for how LIMA should be in the future were diverse. Most people enjoyed company and participation of new people. Some people didn't much appreciate the monotonous structure of lessons. The administrative load for organization of all things, even they are monotonously designed, was high for the leaders. In general people indicated a lack of interest for any new technology, saying that "*I became so old without knowing this exercise, therefore I do not need to learn it now*". The utensils used in a LIMA session are things to write, exercise sheets, flipcharts and a radio player. Another issue was, that people in LIMA don't get informed concerning external events and many people don't know about LIMA. Sharing the fun experience from LIMA was interesting for some members.

Based on these insights we defined themes and created a model from three main themes and their relations to around fifty subthemes (not reported in detail in this paper). We then created a Cartesian coordinate system (CCS) [5] for the most important conflicting themes and sketched 5 ideas from the design space to tackle with the issues with a design technology perspective. "I1: *My Life, in Paper-Form*", "I2: *We are drinking. And you?*", "I3: *Emotion-Tech-Cards*", "I4: *That's Me – Memory Recollection*" and "I5: *My Week*". Two design researchers using CCS as described in Fig. 7, evaluated these ideas.

We found that concerning our main issues ("learning" and "socializing") and their constraints ("using existing topics" and "defining new topics"), all listed ideas are possible to implement in a LIMA-setting. Ideas I2-I5 however, generate new topics either by family, design researcher or LIMA-leader and a more asymmetric way of communication (one peer knows more than the other), causing a feeling of assistance for the senior, described in [8]. The idea "I1: *My Life, in Paper-Form*" presents the most compelling case, building on most common practices (writing, reading, discussing), is easy to integrate by offering a design space for seniors and also easy to manage by both seniors and facilitator. It is mainly an idea that strengthens communication between elderly people, more than assisting them. For future work we want to follow this idea, in an out of LIMA class context, allowing participants to share topics, thoughts and opinions with each other, observing what kind of data they will share, when they are no or fewer constraints, if they will meet each other more often and if the external LIMA class opens new possibilities in senior community building and working with design researchers teams as peers.

In this paper we showed some insights from our studies with LIMA-community and discussed our initial design proposals, in relation to the design space for LIMA. Our work showed a way of dealing with emerging themes from bottom-up research and their connections to design ideas. By using design as a 'communication tool', we aimed to overcome some of the conflicts from the existing LIMA structure, and to open up LIMA to a broader understanding on positive aspects of aging.

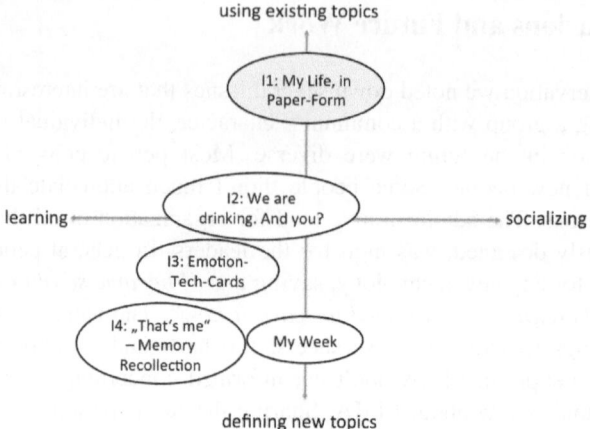

using existing topics

I1: My Life, in Paper-Form

I2: We are drinking. And you?

learning   socializing

I3: Emotion-Tech-Cards

I4: „That's me" – Memory Recollection

My Week

defining new topics

Fig. 7. By mapping ideas (generated by LIMA observations) on the CCS and defining issues ("learning", "socializing") and constraints ("using existing topics", "defining new topics"), we found the most compelling case for the LIMA framework: I1: *My Life, in Paper-Form*

References

1. Bødker, M., Nielsen, J.: Vision labs: seeing UCD as a relational practice. In: Proceedings of the 20th Australasian Conference on Computer-Human Interaction: Designing for Habitus and Habitat, pp. 283–286. ACM, Cairns (2008)
2. Brandt, E., Binder, T., Malmborg, L., Sokoler, T.: Communities of everyday practice and situated elderliness as an approach to co-design for senior interaction. In: Proceedings of the 22nd Conference of the Computer-Human Interaction Special Interest Group of Australia on Computer-Human Interaction, pp. 400–403. ACM, Brisbane (2010)
3. Essén, A., Östlund, B.: Laggards as innovators? Old users as designers of new services & service systems. International Journal of Design 5(3), 89–98 (2011)
4. Leonardi, C., Mennecozzi, C., Not, E., Pianesi, F., Zancanaro, M., Gennai, F., Cristoforetti, A.: Knocking on elders' door: investigating the functional and emotional geography of their domestic space. In: Proc. CHI 2009, Boston, pp. 1703–1711 (2009)
5. Odom, W., Jung, H., Hazlewood, W.R.: Reflective inquires: a multi-dimensional approach to designing for domestic elderly life. In: Proceedings of Design and Emotion, D&E (2010)
6. Odom, W., Selby, M., Sellen, A., Kirk, D., Banks, R., Regan, T.: Photobox: on the design of a slow technology. In: Proceedings of the Designing Interactive Systems Conference, pp. 665–668. ACM, Newcastle (2012)
7. Oswald, W.D., Rupprecht, R., Hagen, B.: SimA-50 in Stichworten. Universität Erlangen-Nürnberg. SimA-Akademie, Erlangen (2012)
8. Sian, E.L., Richard, H., Abigail, S.: Designing for elders: exploring the complexity of relationships in later life. In: Proc. of BCS-HCI 2008, vol. 1, pp. 77–86. British Computer Society, Swinton (2008)
9. Vines, J., Blythe, M., Dunphy, P., Vlachokyriakos, V., Teece, I., Monk, A., Olivier, P.: Cheque mates: participatory design of digital payments with eighty somethings. In: Proc. of CHI 2012, pp. 1189–1198. ACM, Austin (2012)

Older People as Equal Partners in Creative Design

Helena Sustar[1,*], Sara Jones[2], and Andy Dearden[1]

[1] User Centred Healthcare Design, Sheffield Hallam University, Sheffield, Great Britain
{h.sustar,a.m.dearden}@shu.ac.uk
[2] Centre for Human Computer Interaction Design, City University London, Great Britain
s.v.jones@soi.city.ac.uk

Abstract. Active older people want to be actively engaged by contributing their experiences to design better services and products. This paper demonstrates the importance of older peoples engagement in the creative design process in a small study where older people were engaged together with designers in the design of digital devices. Three creative workshops were conducted: the first with designers, the second with designers and older people, and the third with older people only. During the illumination stage of the creative process flexibility and flow were measured with topics and turns. Results show that when older people were working with designers more topics and a higher total number of turns were developed than by older people or designers working on their own, which indicates that they had the highest flexibility of ideas and possibly also the greatest flow.

Keywords: Older People, Creative process, Creativity, Flexibility, Flow.

1 Introduction

Active older people (from 55 to 74 years) desire to be part of society, they have fewer disabilities and shorter periods of illness than very old people (from 75 to 90 years); they care for their children, and they are financially independent [1]. Active older people are *"everyday people"*, who do not want to be just consumers, but also *'creators'* [2]. Older people want to be actively engaged in their own healthcare services, as well as wanting to know how services will be part of their life [3]. They have to cope with the various ageing and technological challenges that life brings. Interfaces, systems, services and digital products are designed for a broad market [4] and designed by designers, who know the technology, but are not familiar with older people's lifestyles [5]. Older people's influence on design is minimal and their attraction to services and products is low [5]. They are rarely engaged in the design process, and if they are, this is at the beginning in focus groups [6] or at the end as part of usability tests [7].

This paper describes a study that demonstrates, by measuring two components of creativity in the creative process (flexibility and flow), the importance of engaging

---

* Corresponding author.

A. Holzinger et al. (Eds.): SouthCHI 2013, LNCS 7946, pp. 649–656, 2013.

older people in the design process. The literature review introduces everyday creativity and different levels of older people's engagement in creative design. Components of the creative process are then presented, and following that, the case study. Our approach is described in section 5, following results, discussion and conclusions.

2   Literature Review

People use *everyday creativity* to find creative solutions to everyday problems [8]. Everyday creativity helps people to cope with daily life, increases physical and psychological health, well being, self-actualization and contribution to the world [9]. Ordinary peoples' creativity is not very innovative [9], and these people *"never produce anything that is publicly acknowledged or acclaimed"* [10]. However, the *"production of novelty can be fostered in everybody not just the chosen few"* [11]. For people who do not apply creativity in a daily routine, creative ability is likely to be latent, and therefore it is necessary to stimulate it, with the use of appropriate methods [6].

Researchers have involved older people in their studies with different levels of engagement from the more passive (e.g. to give feedback on the system), to more active e.g. as creative partners in co-design processes. Gaver et al [12] were the first to engage older people as creative participants, adopting Cultural Probes to collect their experiences, feelings and memories through diaries to identify their presence in local communities. Human Computer Interaction (HCI) studies involve older people as subjects providing opinions on design through participation in focus groups, for example in redesigning interactive systems [13]. Participatory design (PD) studies involved older people as inspiration for designers in designing various future prototypes, for example, in transforming mobile phones into specially-designed memory aids [14]. Another PD method used in Healthcare Service design adopted for gathering patients experience is Experience Based Design (EBD) [15] which [10] and [16] implemented with older patients to improve an outpatient health service in the UK. Finally, older workers were engaged in the preparation stage of the co-design process to investigate their lifestyle and values using Design Probes and Make Tools [17]. Our case study was building among others on apporach [12] and research [17].

3   Components of the Creative Process

Some of the most important work on the nature of creative processes has been carried out by [18] and [19] among others. The four characteristics of creative processes: fluency, flexibility, originality and elaboration were identified by [18]. Understanding of flow by [19] has become central to our understanding of creativity.

The first to identify flexibility as one of the components of divergent thinking was by Guilford [18] who stated that *"creative thinkers are flexible thinkers"* and distinguished between two types of flexible thinking: i.) spontaneous flexibility that is the ability to produce *"a great variety of ideas"* and ii.) adaptive flexibility which facilitates the solution to a problem. Also interested in the idea of flexibility as a characteristic of creative thinking, describing it as *"the number of categories of ideas that were generated"* was [21]. Building further on this definition, [22] view flexibility as *"the number of different approaches or categories of ideas produced"*.

Perhaps the best known for defining flow during the creative process was Csikszentmihalyi [19], who described it as *"the optimal state of experience that yields novelty and discovery"*. Experience of flow occurs for every activity or people, gender, age or cultural background; sportsmen, artists, scientists and ordinary people [19]. The concept of flow includes among others the following elements: clear goals for every step of the way, immediate feedback given to one's action, action and awareness are merged, distractions are excluded from consciousness, there are no worries of failure, sense of time becomes distorted, and activity becomes autotelic [19]. The importance of flow was also recognised by Cropley [8], as well as Kerne et al [23], who state that results from the creative process include direct products (for example innovation) and experiential by-products, one of which is flow. The definition of flow by [23] is as follows:

> *"Flow is an intrinsically rewarding motivational and behavioural state in which one's experiences are optimal. Flow activities facilitate concentration and involvement. They enable people to achieve peak performance, by generating feedback that sustains engagement. ... Flow states are highest when one is successfully engaging in challenging activities. Flow occurs in activities with clear goals and unambiguous feedback. .... The experience of flow has been correlated with the production of creative products."*

4   The Case Study

Participants in the study included 9 designers (HCI design researchers and HCI postgraduates) and 9 older people (recruited from an organisation which provides IT training for older people). The designers were aged between 27 and 48 years of age and older participants were aged between 57 and 78. These participants took part in three separate workshops: the first workshop ('designers' workshop') involved 6 designers, working together in two groups of 3 (referred to as 'yellow group' and 'red group'). The second workshop, the 'mixed workshop', involved 3 designers and 3 older people. These participants also worked together in two groups of 3, where the 'yellow group' included one older person and two designers, and the 'red group' included two older people and one designer. Finally, the third workshop ('older people's workshop') involved 6 older people, also working in two groups of 3 and referred to as 'yellow group' and 'red group' [24].

The design process followed the Wallas-Poincare four stage model of the creative process including preparation, incubation, illumination and verification [25]. The first part, intended as preparation, involved the use of Cultural Probes and was conducted individually. The second part of the process involved different group creative activities in the creative workshops to support the three remaining stages of incubation, illumination and verification.

In the preparation stage, participants worked individually on a package of Cultural Probes for a period of one week. The main aim of Cultural Probes was to mentally prepare participants for activities in the creative workshop by thinking how, where and when they used a computer.

During the 5-hour long creative workshop participants were asked to design a digital device for the older population. The incubation stage, among other activities also included brainstorming exploring questions *'what will the device do?'* and *'when, where and how will the device be used?'*, stimulated by use of *'Creative cards'*, containing a concept (e.g. 'connection') and a visual image relating to one of the key questions. At the end of this session participants had a chance to vote for the *'golden idea'*, which was then developed further in the next illumination stage. At this stage participants were asked to develop their ideas in three different ways: visually, using storyboarding techniques - *'Draw it'*; as a concrete prototype, using materials from a *'Magic box'* – *'Make it'*; or verbally, by recording an oral description or written concept definition - *'Tell me'*. The session finished with presentations where participants presented their ideas. Finally, in the verification stage, participants were asked to evaluate their own and the other group's ideas in terms of novelty and appropriateness using a questionnaire (for information see [24]).

5   Approach

All workshops were video recorded in order to allow later analysis of the creative process. Based on experiences from the pilot study we decided to analyse data from the illumination stage, which lasted approximately 45 minutes. For this analysis, we chose to use *'topics'* and *'turns'* as our main units of analysis, and as indicators of flexibility and flow, as described above. A topic was defined as *'discussion, or exchanging of ideas, among members of the group about a certain theme'* and typically lasted from one to ten minutes. A new topic was judged to start when a person in a group asked a question or started a conversation about a different theme from the previous one. The topic finished when the discussion was interrupted for some reason, for example when someone started a conversation on a new theme or asked a question, which was not related to the previous theme. Topics were, for example, discussions about the design of the device (illustrated below) [24]. A turn was defined, according to [27] as *"sentences spoken by a participant until his or her partner next spoke"*, and speech by one participant that contained a significant pause was segmented into two turns. The following example of a discussion between two designers (D1 and D2) and an older person (OP1) about a personal safety alarm illustrates the way in which a conversation was broken down into turns. Each turn is shown starting on a new line [24]:

> D1: *And it should have one big button.*
> D2: *Maybe one big one in the middle.*
> D1: *Yes. It is some kind of release button - you press it again and it will pop out.*
> OP1: *I'm a bit worried. If you fall and if you panic, I don't think that you will remember to press it once or twice or three times. But, I don't know.*

D2: You can have green.
OP1: Oh, you can have a colour. When you press the button a colour comes.
D1: It could light up; the whole button could light up.

Based on the definition of flexibility as *"the number of categories of ideas that were generated"*, it was possible to use the number of topics discussed by a group as an indicator of the variety of ideas they considered, and hence their flexibility [21]. Thus, a group who covered a wide range of topics could be said to exhibit high flexibility, and therefore be collaborating more creatively than a group that covered only a low number of topics.

Flow was defined as being characterised by many factors, including obtaining immediate feedback on one's actions [19] and also defined flow in individuals: *"flow occurs in activities with ... unambiguous feedback"* [23]. Building on these definitions, we used turns, or responses of one group member to another, as indicators of feedback, and hence flow in a group context. Thus, a group with a high number of turns could be said to exhibit good *'group flow'* [24].

Alongside measuring different parameters during the design process also a small study – an on-line survey with two independent external experts was conducted. Experts evaluated final outputs by watching videos where groups presented their work and evaluated them in terms of their appropriateness and novelty for the older population. Definition for appropriateness was stated as *"Artefacts need to have some potential value, it must be useful or appropriate"* by [28] and novelty was defined as situated creativity *(S-creativity)* which occurs when *"a designer or reasoned has an idea for a specific task, which was novel in that particular situation"* [29].

6   Results

According to our analysis (Fig. 1), the mixed groups covered the highest numbers of topics (20 and 25), suggesting that they demonstrated the greatest flexibility (Chart 1, left). The mixed groups also had high numbers of turns (491 and 604), as did the older people's red group (513), which indicates high levels of flow (Chart 2, right) [24]. Fig. 2 shows a prototypical example of a section of the conversation for the mixed red group, where there was good flow. In this example, there is a high number of turns in the topic (62), and approximately 16 turns per minute during this exchange. We can see a high number of exchanges between the designer (D1) and the two older people (OP1 and OP2). Closer examination of the notes in column 6 reveals that all three participants were engaged in a discussion about design options for a new device based on existing technology (TV and touch screens), and the photograph shows a sketch of the design idea that was generated during the conversation. There were some examples of poor flow, especially in groups of older people only, where participants spent a minute or more with no productive conversation [24].

In summary, more topics and a higher total number of turns were developed by mixed groups than by older people or designers working on their own, which means that they had the highest flexibility of ideas [18] and possibly also the greatest flow

[23]. A review of the workshop outputs by external experts also suggested that when older people and designers work together they may design more appropriate products for the older population than designers or older people working alone.

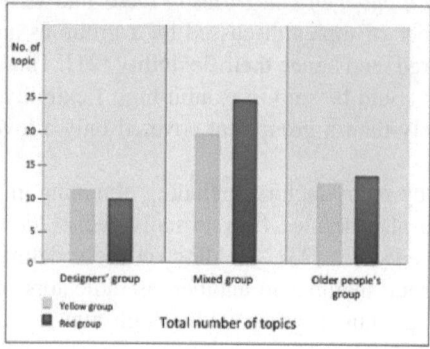 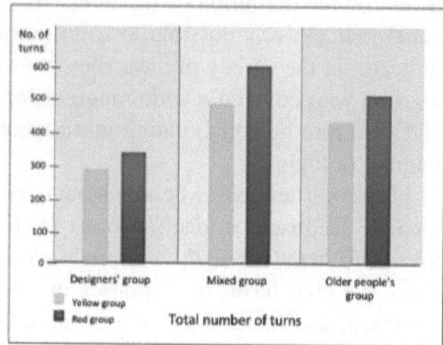

Fig. 1. The Chart 1 illustrates the higher number of topics and therefore high flexibility in the mixed groups, in comparison to both the designers' and older people's groups (left) (Source: Sustar, 2010, vol.1 p. 231). The Chart 2 presents the total number of turns and high levels of flow in the mixed groups (Source: Sustar, 2010, vol.1 p. 232).

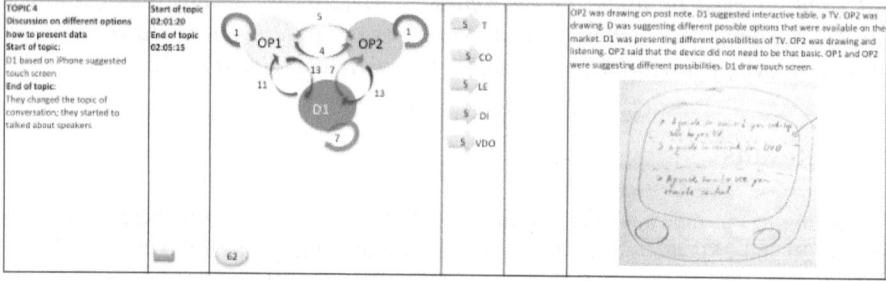

Fig. 2. This figure represents a good group flow (Source: Sustar, 2010, vol. 2, p. 115)

7   Discussion

The evidence shows that while older people make different contributions to designers in the design process their contributions are equally important when designing digital devices for the older population. While designers contribute knowledge of what is possible, older people contribute their life experiences and an understanding of what would be appropriate for the older population. In the mixed groups designers were challenged by the older people's views on what would be usable by other older people. Also mixed groups developed the most positive conflict, discussing more different options and had a lively information exchange which was leading to more complex ideas.

8   Conclusion

According to several of the measures used in our study, it appears that the most effective way of including older people in creative workshops aimed at the design of digital devices may be to include them as members of teams in which they can collaborate directly with designers. Perhaps the least effective approach is to have older people working in teams where they can collaborate only with other older people. These findings obviously need to be treated with caution, since they are based only on an initial lightweight analysis of the data, and a relatively small sample of participants. However, they suggest interesting avenues for further research.

Acknowledgments. This paper presents independent research by the National Institute for Health Research Collaboration for Leadership in Applied Health Research and Care for South Yorkshire (NIHR CLAHRC SY). The views and opinions expressed are those of the authors, and not necessarily those of the NHS, the NIHR or the Department of Health. CLAHRC SY would also like to acknowledge the participation and resources of our partner organisations. Further details can be found at www.clahrc-sy.nihr.ac.uk.

References

1. Bjerre, A., Mogensen, K.Æ., Rasmussen, B.N., Dons, J.L., Schüle, H., Kruse, M.: Young Seniors Will Shape Society,
   http://www.cifs.dk/scripts/artikel.asp?id=1767&lng=2
   (last accessed December 12, 2008)
2. Sanders, E.B.N.: Information, Inspiration and Co-creation. In: Conference of the European Academy of Design, University of the Arts, Bremen, p. 5 (2005)
3. Dearden, A., Wright, P., Bowen, S., Cobb, M., Wolstenholme, D.: User Centred Design and Pervasive Health Position paper for workshop on User Centred Design of Pervasive Healthcare Applications. In: Pervasive Health Conference 2010, Munich (2010)
4. Gregor, P., Newell, F.A., Zajicek, M.: Designing for Dynamic Diversity Interfaces for Older People. In: ACM SIGACCESS Conference on Assistive Technologies, Edinburgh, p. 781. ACM Press, New York (2002)
5. Healy, F.: Towards a Usability Research Methodology for Use with the Older Population. Amberlight Partners Ltd., London (2003)
6. Sanders, N.E.B.: Collective Creativity. LOOP: AIGA Jnl. Int. Design Education 3, 1–6 (2001),
   http://www.maketools.com/pdfs/CollectiveCreativity_Sanders_
7. Engdahl, K., Leclerc, K., Loring, B.: Conducting Field Studies with Older Adults. User Experience 8(1), 14–16 (2009)
8. Cropley, A.J.: Definitions of Creativity. In: Runco, A.M., Pritzker, R.S. (eds.) Encyclopedia of Creativity, p. 11, 115. Academic Press, California (1999)
9. Richards, R.: Everyday Creativity. In: Runco, A., Mark, P.R.S. (eds.) Encyclopedia of Creativity, pp. 683–687. Academic press, San Diego (1999)

10. Milgram, R.M.: Creativity: An Idea Whose Time Has Come and Gone? In: Runco, A.M., Albert, R.S. (eds.) Theories of Creativity, pp. 215–233. SAGE Publishing, Newbury Park (1990)
11. Cropley, A.J.: Creativity in Education and Learning: A Guide for Teachers and Educators, p. 27. Kogan Page Limited (2003)
12. Gaver, B., Dunne, T., Pacenti, E.: Design: Cultural Probes. Interactions 6(1), 21–29 (1999)
13. Hawthorn, D.: Interface Design and Engagement with Older People. Behaviour and Information Technology 26(4), 333–341 (2007)
14. Massimo, M., Baecker, R.: Participatory Design Process with Older Users. In: Proceedings Ubicomp Workshop (2006)
15. Bate, S.P., Robert, G.: Experience-based design: From redesigning the system around the patient to co-designing services with the patient. Quality and Safety in Health Care 15, 307–310 (2006)
16. Bowen, S., Dearden, A., Wolstenholme, D., Cobb, M., Wright, P.: Different Views: Including Others in Participatory Health Service Innovation. In: Proceedings of PINC 2011, Sønderborg (2011)
17. Vaajakallio, K., Mattelmäki, T.: Collaborative Design Exploration: Envisioning Future Practices with Make Tools. In: Designing Pleasurable Products and Interfaces, DPPI 2007, Helsinki, pp. 223–238. ACM Press, New York (2007)
18. Guilford, J.P.: Traits of Creativity, in Vernon, P.E. (Ed.) Creativity. Harmondsworth, pp. 167-234. Penguin Education (1959)
19. Csikszentmihalyi, M.: Creativity: Flow and the Psychology of Discovery and Invention, pp. 110–113. Harper Perennial, New York (1996)
20. Runco, A.M.: Divergent Thinking. In: Runco, A.M., Pritzker, R.S. (eds.) Encyclopedia of Creativity, pp. 577–582. California Academic Press, San Diego (1999)
21. Torrance, E.P.: The Torrance Tests of Creative Thinking: Norms-Technical Manual. Personal Press, Princeton (1966); Warr, A., O'Neill, E.: The Effect of Operational Mechanisms on Creativity in Design. In: Interact 2005: Human Computer Interaction, pp. 629–642. Springer, Rome (2005)
22. Warr, A., O'Neill, E.: The Effect of Group Composition on Divergent Thinking in an Interaction Design Activity. In: Proceedings of the 6th Conference on Designing Interactive systems, University Park, pp. 122–131. ACM Press, New York (2006)
23. Kerne, A., Smith, S.M., Mistrot, J.M., Sundaram, V., Khandelwal, M., Wang, J.: Mapping Interest and Design to Facilitate Creative Process During Mixed-Initiative Information Composition. In: Creativity & Cognition, p. 14. Studios Press, Sydney (2004)
24. Sustar, H.: Older People as Equal Partners in the Creative Design of Digital Devices. PhD thesis, City University London, vol. 1, pp. 231–232, vol. 2, 115 (2010)
25. Wallas, G.: The Art of Thought. Harcourt Brace, New York (1926)
26. Sustar, H., Jones, D., Maiden, N.: Creativity in Older People Designing Digital Devices. In: Create 2010, London (2010)
27. Kulesza, T., Weng-Keen, W., Stumpf, S., Perona, S., White, R., Burnett, M.M., Oberst, I., Ko, A.J.: Fixing the Program My Computer Learned: Barriers for End Users. In: Challenges for the Machine, IUI 2009, pp. 187–196. ACM, Sanibel Island (2009)
28. Suwa, M., Gero, J., Purcell, T.: Unexpected Discoveries and S-invention of design requirements: Important Vehicles for a Design Process. Design Studies 21, 539–567 (2000)
29. WordNet: Version 2.1, http://www.cogsci.princeton.edu/wn/ (last accessed January 15, 2005)

Designing Guiding Garments for People Affected by Dementias

Britta Friederike Schulte

Nottingham Trent University, Nottingham, England
Britta.schulte2009@my.ntu.ac.uk

Abstract. Our society relies heavily on written or verbal instructions to collate and share information. Cognitive impairments such as dementias decrease the ability to process information on an intellectual level, even though sensory information might still be appreciated. This paper supports the view that aesthetic design can not only make garments more appealing to the target group, but can also enhance the ease of use and ease of understanding of objects. Design can be made functional as well as aesthetically pleasing by encouraging correct use through sensual pleasure and discouraging incorrect use through disagreeable stimuli. This paper focuses on an ongoing short-term research and design project based on literature survey and design proposals with the aim to develop a collection appealing to and easy to use by elderly people with cognitive impairments.

Keywords: information design, craft, interaction design, garment design, aging, dementia.

1   Introduction

Interest in this topic was stimulated by the personal experience of caring for a family member with dementia. As the illness progressed, everyday tasks became more and more complicated so that the need for care and support increased. Dressing has been one of the tasks that took up a lot of time due to the complexity of the process. Even though it is an everyday task, dressing is an intricate matter. To understand when to get dressed, which garments are appropriate, where to put the garments on the body, how the garments function are just a few examples of the decisions to be made. (compare e.g. Moore, 1988) While aging it becomes increasingly important for many people to keep up a tidy appearance as "any lapses in dress can be interpreted as signaling mental and physical decline and might communicate an impending dependency." (Day; Hitchings, 2011, 889) Very practical garments have been developed, which facilitate easy dressing. But they focus on care, i.e. through easy care fabrics, use of Velcro and stain hiding fabric prints. As stated by Julia Twigg in her article about clothing and dementia: "Clothes are central to identity" (2010, 227), and therefore an assumed identity focusing on the need for care should be avoided.

This paper focuses on the research for the Final Year project "No place like home – a conceptual collection appealing to and easy to use by people affected by

A. Holzinger et al. (Eds.): SouthCHI 2013, LNCS 7946, pp. 657–663, 2013.

dementias using visual, tactile, and olfactory stimuli to create a feeling of home, identity, and belonging in the wearer", for the course BA (Hons) Fashion Knitwear Design and Knitted Textiles at Nottingham Trent University. The project started in September 2012 and will end in May 2013 with an exhibition of the resulting prototypes and information about the research. Four design guidelines have been developed from the initial research and the resulting prototyping.

The main aim of this project was to create a range of garments in which the aesthetic appeal is as important as the functional approach. The aesthetic and personal preferences of the people concerned are often neglected in research when considering dress for the elderly, as has been observed by Twigg in her article regarding clothing, age and the body:

> "This has produced an emphasis on the recourses of the public and semi-public sectors rather than the world of private consumption, and on the themes of need, functioning and deficiency rather than expressivity, identity and choice." (Twigg, 2007, 286)

After an extensive research on the requirements of elderly people including literature about the changes of the body when aging, inclusive design and architecture projects aimed at elderly people, the focus was set on developing a range of garments for people with cognitive impairments such as dementia. This area is neglected in garment design, even though research indicates the importance of enabling people with cognitive impairments to keep up their way of dressing to maintain their feeling of identity: "Identity is thus present in habitual gestures and actions, and is retained by an individual even in circumstances of considerable cognitive damage." (Twigg, 2010, 224)

All elements of the garments are chosen to enhance interaction between wearer and object, facilitating understanding and handling of the garments to enable independent dressing for longer, while supporting the feeling of comfort in the wearer. In addition interactive elements are incorporated which provide guidance beyond the act of dressing.

2   Research and Project Development

On first glance the connection between garment design and interface design is not an obvious one. But not only in the development of wearable technologies do those two cross over. Although mostly considered from an aesthetic viewpoint, the study of dress and dressing can reveal information about the interaction of the wearer of the garment with the outside world, which in turn might lead to a more intuitive usable design, due to the inclusion of all senses:

> "While the two-dimensional painted bits of GUI link the handling of information almost inclusively to the sense of vision, leading to passive physical behaviour, multi-dimensional tangible bits are intended to allow inclusion of all other sense and activation of the body's motor system. In this manner, they provide access to a whole series of new approaches based in spatial and everyday experiences, and therefore inherently more intuitively."(Klooster, 2009, 136)

The focus of this project is on the ability of garments to create homely and welcoming feelings in the wearer. All features are chosen to create positive sensation, either by facilitating easy understanding of the garments or by evoking positive memories.

Bodily changes taken into consideration for the design of the garments are: reduced grip of fingers, overall reduced strength, decreased range of upper and lower limbs, increased incontinence, yellowing of the lenses and blurred vision.

Other practical considerations such as garments cuts that allow the caregiver to support the dressing without the need to touch the genital area or garment shape that can facilitate incontinence pads have been incorporated, but are not the main focus for these garments.

Cognitive changes taken into consideration for the design of the garments are: decreased ability of recalling information, problems with making decisions, problems to communicate discomfort, decreased concentration, and loss of initiative.

If a decision had to be made between functionalities that enable either physical handling or understanding of the garments the focus was laid on enabling understanding of the garments, following Bucheggers advice: "Ease of learning is more important for seniors than ease of use." (Buchegger; in Calori, 2007, 32f)

The garments are developed following guidelines to communicate with people affected by Alzheimer's disease such as stated by Brawley: "People with Alzheimer's disease respond on a sensory level rather than on an intellectual level." (2006, 30) From this it has been established that information about the garments should be provided through the garments themselves to decrease the need for verbal instructions as much as possible. By reducing the level of frustration while dressing, overall well-being might improve and agitation or depression might be decreased. Being able to understand ones surroundings is a trait inherent in humans:

> "When we are uncertain we actively seek information. Certainty is enhanced by similarities, and minimized by differences. That of which we are uncertain becomes less favourable." (Calori, 2007,88)

Seen in this context enabling understanding of garments might motivate independent dressing for longer and as such help to maintain autonomy.

To achieve a better understanding and easier handling of the garments the following considerations are made:

Fabrics are manipulated in a way that the inside of the garments is more appealing next to the skin, to promote putting them on in the correct way without encouraging from the caregiver. The inside is treated differently from the outside either by colour or structure or both, so that they are recognisable faster, which will enable an easier handling of the garments: e.g. parts have been covered with latex on the outside, which appears to be cold, while the inside is made from a warm, soft brushed wool.

Fig. 1. Different structures surfaces to facilitate orientation, Fabric swatches (Source: own photography)

All edges and trims of the garments are highlighted through structure as well as changes in colour, so that they can be easily recognized and the handling of the garments is made easier.

A special colour palette was developed which features motivating, bright colours. The colours for the garments worn on the lower part of the body are darker than the ones which are worn on the top half of the body. This idea has been generated from the assumption that this is a natural occurrence in nature which might enable intuitive handling. As a motivator colours with a high saturation have been chosen. Hues have been carefully selected that do not blur much when seen through yellow lenses, to ascertain that they will appeal to their target group.

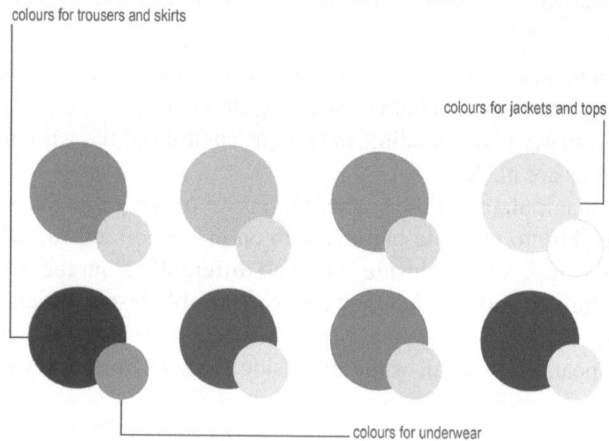

Fig. 2. Colour palette (Source: own illustration)

The fasteners of the garments are either magnets, which can be opened and closed easily or specialised ergonomic toggles. These fasteners are all placed on the front, in plain view of the wearer, so that "users see and recognize their options rather than having to recall them" (Johnson, 2010, 166); a guideline taken from UI design. The male and female parts of all fasteners have the same colour, to facilitate the assumption that they belong together and to discourage confusion.

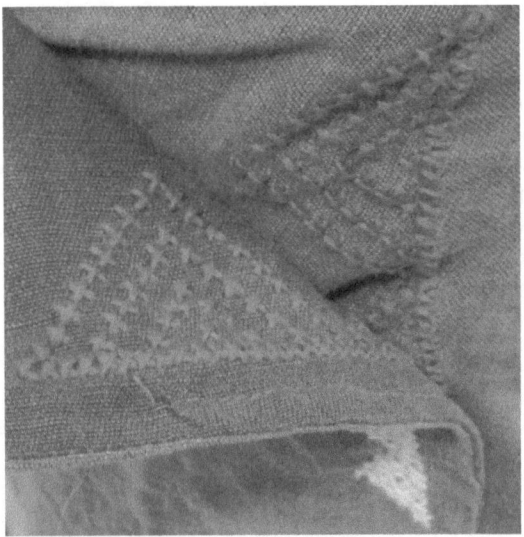

Fig. 3. Highlighting matching fasteners, Detail of skirt (Source: own photography)

The buttons can be treated with essential oils, providing positively connoted olfactory stimuli, which according to some care workers might decrease agitation, although this practice is controversial. (compare Nguyen; Paton, 2008)

Where it has not been able to facilitate easier decision making, the garments are designed and constructed in a way that making a decision is not needed, which means that the garments can be worn inside out without any difference in handling or recognition of this.

As patterns have been proven to be confusing for people with dementia, all fabrics are kept monochrome with the exception of highlighted trims or fasteners.

To make the handling of the garments easier, mere decoration has been eliminated, as not to create distractions or confusions, following advice to "reduce the number of information chunks that need to be kept in mind at any given time ...." (Clarkson, 2007, 4-94) Nonetheless all guiding elements inherent in the garments are designed aesthetically, to keep the garments interesting and to increase the motivational value of the garments.

Dress it is a very sensual experience. Bradley Quinn observes: "Because many of our earliest haptic experiences are fibre-based, a single textile can evoke a lifetime of memories and sensations." (2010, 10) This is taken into consideration while choosing the fibres to work with. In a care environment garments need to be able to be washable at 65 ° for 10 min, so that they can be sterilized. Therefore garments for people in care are quite often made from polyester, polyacrylics or other man-made fibres that are easy care, even though those do often not make up the fibres mature people are used to or would buy themselves. While man-made fibers have considerate practical properties, they are considered more uncomfortable to the skin than natural fibers and as a result natural fibers have been chosen for this project. Linen and wool change their appearance when washed at such a high temperature, but the fabrics created can be pre-washed and manipulated to avoid disappointment by the consumer. This choice of materials does not only enhance comfort of the garments, but circumvents social notions of easy care fabrics.

The sleeve was chosen as the place for detachable gadgets which offer orientation and allow communication with the wearer of the garments. Three devices are developed which can be chosen according to the personal preference of the wearer: a note pad, a photo frame, or a recordable audio device. The note pad can be used for short, simple information or personal notes. Based on the idea of the memory book, the photo frame allows the wearer to carry a photo which might provide a topic for conversation or consolation. The audio device plays back pre-recorded messages which again might be used to provide information or personal notes.

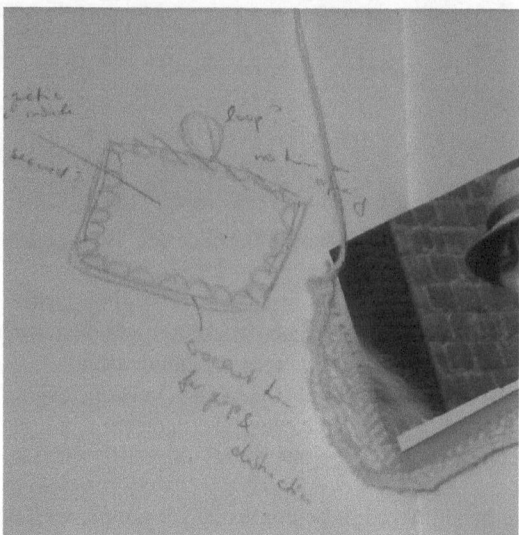

Fig. 4. Development of the photo frame (Source: own photography)

3   Outlook

Based on literary review and design proposals four guidelines are introduced as a result of this research and design project:

- Simple: All functions on the garments should be easily perceived, rather than having to be recalled
- Guiding: All information should be provided as sensory, i.e. visual or tactile clues, rather than relying on verbal instructions by caretakers

- Motivating: All items should be easy to handle, regarding use of fasteners, weight of the garments and understanding of the functions
- Homely: All items should appear familiar and should trigger memories

To test the assumptions on which the project is based, a survey between health care workers and between medical students focusing on dementia is in planning, but has not been executed. The results of these will help to make to garments even more functional for their target group.

But even though the practical outcome of the project is important to illustrate the underlying guidelines to a wider audience, the project has further implications. Because of our everyday familiarity and experience with the act of dressing and the social connotations of clothing, it might have the ability to spark a discussion about design for an aging population. By providing an alternative to the care garments available, this collection can question the focus on need and facilitation of care inherent in many objects marketed at the elderly.

Due to time limitations and the focus on domesticity all gadgets have been developed analogously. But the research undergone for this project indicates much scope for development of interactive items, which might benefit people affected by dementia by providing guidance, support or enhance general well-being, e.g. via wayfinding support, unobtrusive medical monitoring or interactive garments that respond to the wearers mood.

References

Brawley, E.C.: Design Innovations for Ageing and Alzheimer´s – creating caring environment. John Wiley & Sons, Hoboken (2006)

Calori, C.: Signage and wayfinding design. John Wiley & Sons, Hoboken (2007)

Clarkson, J., et al.: Inclusive design toolkit. University of Cambridge, Cambridge (2007)

Day, R., Hitchins, R.: Only old ladies would do that: Age stigma and older people's strategies for dealing with winter cold. Health and Place 17, 885–894 (2011)

Johnson, J.: Designing with the mind in mind – Simple guide to under-standing user interface design rules. Elsevier, Online (2010)

Klooster, T.: Smart surfaces – and their application in architecture and design. Birkhäuser, Basel (2009)

Leibrock, C., Harris, D.: Design details for health – making the most of design´s healing potential, 2nd edn. John Wiley & Sons, Hoboken (2011)

Moore, P.: Dressing matters – a handbook to help people with learning difficulties to dress themselves. The Disabled Living Foundation, London (1988)

Nguyen, Q., Paton, C.: The use of aromatherapy to treat beha-vioural problems in dementia. International Journal of Geriatric Psychiatry (23), 337–346 (2008)

Quinn, B.: Textile futures – fashion, design and technology. Berg, Oxford (2010)

Twigg, J.: Clothing, age and the body: a critical review. Ageing and Society 27(02), 285–305 (2007)

Twigg, J.: Clothing and dementia – a neglected dimension? Journal of Aging Studies 24, 223–230 (2010)

Towards Rapid Technology Probes for Senior People

Florian Güldenpfennig and Geraldine Fitzpatrick

Institute for Design & Assessment of Technology, Vienna University of Technology,
Argentinierstraße 8, 1040 Vienna, Austria
{florian.gueldenpfennig,geraldine.fitzpatrick}@tuwien.ac.at

Abstract. In HCI, there is much interest in exploring novel technology-mediated communication that can empower older users who don't have easy access to regular computers. In this paper we exploit the potential of smart phones and tablet computers to create a series of technology probes that we deploy long-term making use of close family members. By this means participants can gain experiences with robust and fully implemented devices at a very early stage of design. We lay out four prototypes of communication technologies with different forms and functions for older adults. We describe the features of these devices including some indicative feedback from our informal deployment study. We thereby suggest that mobile phones are a suitable means for the rapid prototyping of communication technologies for senior people and can possibly provide useful input to later participatory or co-design activities. The overall work is still ongoing hence the main contribution of the paper is about the potential of rapid technology probes as a design technique and in less detail about the potential of the prototypes as AAL communication devices.

Keywords: AAL, Communication, Empowerment, Mobile phones, Older adults, Research Through Design, Tangible Computing, Technology Probes.

1   Introduction

Special need groups such as senior people often times get disconnected from their peers due to decreased mobility. To tackle this and related problems, researchers in HCI develop and explore technologies to reconnect those senior users and to grant them access to information over the Internet or cellular networks, e.g. in [1, 2]. User-centered design approaches and Participatory Design (PD) [3] or Co-Design [4] are common methods for creating such systems. In this paper we take yet another approach to this problem space and use a technology probe approach [5] that exploits the potential of new smart phones and tablet computers to enable the designer to test ideas at a very early stage of design. This means that we give various completely developed and robust prototypes to participants in order to provoke reactions and to gather feedback from the prospective users. This approach is also loosely related to Research through Design (RtD) [6] where artifacts are used to study segments of reality that would not exist and hence couldn't be examined without the artifact.

A key characteristic of the research endeavors in this paper, as compared to more bespoke and complex probe systems as in [5], is that we were able to develop the

A. Holzinger et al. (Eds.): SouthCHI 2013, LNCS 7946, pp. 664–671, 2013.

prototypes rapidly and with low resources due to the affordances of modern smart phones. To emphasize this, we introduce the concept of *rapid technology probes (RTP)* and argue, that mobile phone or tablet computer powered technology probes are an adequate and timely technique for the design process of AAL systems due to the opportunities offered by such 'off-the-shelf' devices. Technology probes based on mobiles provide the designers with quick feedback from the participants and allow them to quickly iterate their products. At the same time, the user experience of a working system is made accessible to the participants and potentially empowers them to be more educated participants in any later participatory or co-design process.

As such, we propose that RTP can complement established design methods such as PD and Co-Design. They can be employed after the initial understanding of the design context or user requirements gathering in order to probe experiences and receive meaningful feedback. Hence, RTP allows additional iterations with high-fidelity prototypes in the course of the advanced design process. Moreover, we argue that RTP can also be employed right in the beginning of the design process, as in this paper, for testing of ideas and receiving initial feedback or inspiration for further design concepts.

In the following, we describe a project for empowering senior users by means of Internet technology featuring four different prototypes. It is supposed to function as a case study or showcase for illustrating what kind of devices can be created relatively quickly, facilitated by modern smart phones and tablets. In this case the four prototypes presented are not direct iterations of one particular product. Rather they are different flavors of similar ideas and were deployed roughly simultaneously for the purposes of informally gathering user experiences with the probes. We conclude the paper with some exemplary insights gathered by means of the rapid technology probes and with discussing those qualities that all four probes have in common, which make mobile devices appropriate for rapid prototyping in AAL.

2   Related Works and Design Inspirations

Besides assistive technologies that have explicitly been designed for older users, there are a number of research projects where regular mobile phones are equipped with extra software to make the devices more accessible. For instance, Olwal and colleagues developed a software toolkit for customizing the user interfaces of phones according to accessibility needs [7]. Besides this kind of 'software-hacking' there are also efforts of hardware-modification where 'envelopes' mask or enhance certain buttons and functions. Panasonic's *Pixi* camera glove is a commercial example for this kind of 'hacking' and turns a regular phone into a camera for social networking.

Coleman et al. [1] investigated reasons for older adults not being interested in digital technologies. According to them older adults would accept technology when they can see a direct benefit. This can be easy access to information or getting in touch with family and friends. They also found that older users often show fear for technology, however they accept "invisible computers", that is computers that are not perceived as a classical computing machine [1].

An example for a suitable and more "invisible" technology is depicted in [8]. In this paper Spreicer describes the potential of tangible computing technologies for engaging older adults [8].

Focusing on the task of communication instead of tangible computing, Lindley et al. investigated the desire of older adults to stay in touch with their loved ones employing focus groups and prototyped technologies. They summarize that their participants accepted the idea of communication supported by technology, however, there was a strong desire of the older adults to have two-way communication, since they wanted to be able to contribute and not only consume passively [2]. We go on now to introduce our prototypes.

3   Rapid Technology Probes with Mobile Devices

In our project for empowering older users through Internet technology, we draw on features of the cited work from above to develop four related prototypes based on Android powered mobile devices: *TwoButtonCamera, Wired TabletCompanion, Wireless TabletCompanion* and *Integrated TabletCompanion*. Those devices function as the computer since they feature a decent performance and also give easy access to the Internet via a LAN or a telephony network provider. In addition, we employ Arduino microcontroller boards for the quick extension of the Android phones by, e.g., physical buttons or RFID readers and corresponding RFID reader antennas. *TwoButtonCamera* is a device for low effort and uncomplicated taking of digital photos and publishing them to a *photo-blog. Wired TabletCompanion, Wireless TabletCompanion* and *Integrated TabletCompanion* are designed to provide older users with no prior computer experience with an easy to operate computer and Internet.

Table 1. Approx. time spent working on different prototypes for an experienced developer

Prototype	Time spent on hardware	Time spent on softw.
TwoButtonCamera	8 hrs	10 hrs
Wired TC	10 hrs	20 hrs
Wireless TC	10 hrs	20 hrs
Integrated TC	10 hrs	20 hrs

As mentioned before, an important characteristic of the prototypes is that they can be created rapidly in relation to the complex tasks that they can handle. Table 1 gives workload estimations for an experienced developer. In contrast to a classic user-centered design approach with subsequent iterations, we can run several test studies with different advanced prototypes in parallel and thus explore different directions at a time. This has the potential to quickly gather feedback from participants or co-designers that have been provided with 'real' user experiences and enables us to explore the design space together with users. Later, this feedback can be considered in further iterations by the designers. Also, possible follow-up workshops might benefit from the fact, that the participants have already been exposed to the experience of high-fidelity prototypes. We leave these high-fidelity prototypes with the participants for a longer period of time as is common practice in various RtD projects. Thus, by denoting the devices as *rapid* technology probes, we do not necessarily mean that we also take them away quickly but rather that they were quick to prototype. In our case, we were interested more in informal feedback from long-term use. The work presented is still ongoing.

3.1   Motivation and Method

More specifically, our motivation was to use the potential opened by Android smart phones in combination with tangible computing components to explore easy to use communication technologies for older users. One principle that we employed was putting the Android devices into customized boxes, thereby covering some of the technical appearance of the phones as well as hiding interaction complexity (unnecessary buttons etc.). We also aimed at giving the prototypes a friendly tone by using wood as a material or painting the box. Besides being built into a cover, the phones were very suitable for attaching customized hardware buttons and shortcuts for hiding even more complexity.

In these ways the prototypes modify the appearance of regular smart phones in terms of their looks and software. The motivation for this was to reduce the fears of inexperienced users, to encourage them to interact with the devices and to ease their operation of the computers in general. This puts a different emphasis on 'accessible' computing compared for example to the efforts of the World Wide Web Consortium (W3C), which focuses on the interactions accessible by standardization guidelines. We want to not only ensure that there are the 'big buttons' to make it easier to operate but that the devices are also inviting to use, so that people can find their own value in it. For this they also need access to the devices over a longer period of time to undertake this exploration.

We have collected this informal, but long-term user feedback by exposing two of the designer's family members to the artifacts, since one of the driving motivations behind this project was to later provide those individuals with the finished devices. Both participants are female, have no prior experience with computers and are aged 65 (P1) and 86 (P2) years. Total amount of experience with the probe systems is more than a year for each person. Data has been collected by informal participant observation during visits with the family members and informal interviews. In addition, we have access to the photos and browsing history produced by the participants.

4   Probes and Informal Feedback

We go on now to describe each of the probes and point to some of the feedback from the informal long-term deployments.

4.1   TwoButtonCamera

TwoButtonCamera is the most straightforward device in terms of functions (photo-sharing). From a technical standpoint *TwoButtonCamera* (see Fig. 1) is an Android phone in a wooden casing with our custom software installed. However, to the user it is presented as an 'online photo camera' with the possibility to audio-annotate the pictures. Its purpose is to take photos, optionally attach an audio recording and imme-diately upload it to a web photo-blog, which has been implemented as part of the system. Family members and friends get automatically pushed email notifications as soon as a new photo is available on the blog. The interaction is designed to be as sim-ple as possible and demands only 2-3 button touches. Hence, it is a technology that enables user groups that don't have easy access to online photo sharing to document their life, capture functional photos (e.g. an image of an important newspaper article to be send to friends) or to simply enjoy themselves by taking creative or appealing pictures. It lets them contribute digital photos and stories actively, which is an activity usually performed by younger adults.

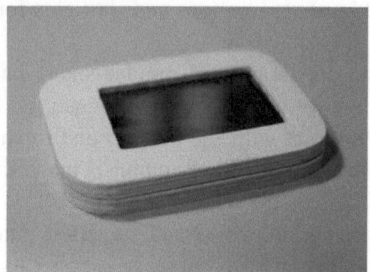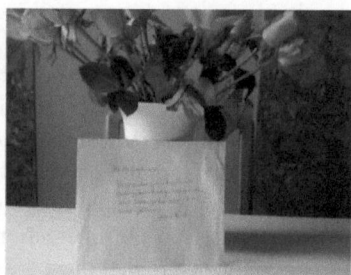

Fig. 1. *TwoButtonCamera* prototype (left) and birthday greeting note including a vase with flowers captured by P2 and sent to a relative (right)

TwoButtonCamera – Feedback. Each participant (P) was provided with a TwoBut-tonCamera and has been using it for approximately half a year. P1 captured 44 photos and 7 audio annotations. P2 took 40 images, 6 with accompanying audios. The feed-back about the device was very positive and usage frequency was constant over time since they did not lose interest but continued using it at special occasions. However, both participants decided most of the time not to use the audio annotation to skip that extra effort and because they "liked providing pure visual messages" (P1). Common triggers for use as shown across the collected images were *sharing of experiences*, virtually *giving presents* in a somewhat tangible way (see Fig. 1, right), *documenting visits* of friends/family and *sharing messages* such as photos of newspaper articles.

4.2   TabletCompanion

The *TabletCompanion* (TC) is a product- or prototype-line for exploring how Internet computers could be designed to be understandable and convenient to use for senior or inexperienced users. Currently three devices are in use: *Wireless TabletCompanion* (Wireless TC, Fig. 2 left), *Wired TabletCompanion* (Wired TC, Fig. 2 right) and

Integrated TabletCompanion (Integrated TC, Fig. 3). Overall the *TabletCompanion* series of probes has different form factors and different levels of assistance (help buttons, video tutorials). Still, all versions of TC have the same set of supported programs (writing and reading e-mails, reading newspapers, watching videos, reading the weather, watching photo-blogs of family and friends, etc.).

Wireless TC (Fig. 2 left) is a peripheral radio module with a build in RFID reader. Switching the device on will pair it with an Android tablet. Placing RFID tokens on the device will trigger various actions on the Android tablet, for instance starting the e-mail client. Of course, the Android device can still be operated conventionally. It is not mandatory to pair the devices, the Wireless TC is meant to be of help when the users get stuck. Accordingly, there are also RFID tokens that will start short tutorial videos or audio guidance for the user-intended actions to be performed on the tablet. In this regard, it is important to note, that a certain kind of context awareness can be implemented easily on the Android devices: it can be learnt from the operation system what kind of task is being performed by the user at the moment, e.g. writing an email to uncle Tom. As a consequence, we can explicitly offer guidance on how to write a message to that uncle. Wired TC (Fig. 2 right) is very similar to Wireless TC (Fig. 2 left), but it is connected to an Android tablet by a USB cable. It features additionally quick access buttons for common tasks such as opening a text field for triggering a web search. *Integrated TabletCompanion* (see Fig. 3) integrates a tablet into the companion. It has a bigger form factor with space on it for taking notes.

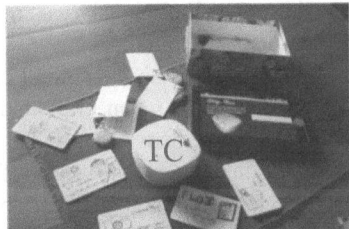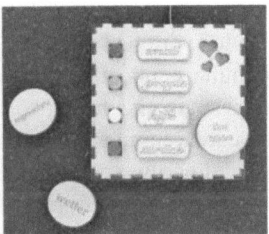

Fig. 2. Black, 7-inch tablet computer with *Wireless TabletCompanion* and various RFID tokens (left). *Wired TabletCompanion* with four quick access buttons and three RFID tokens (right).

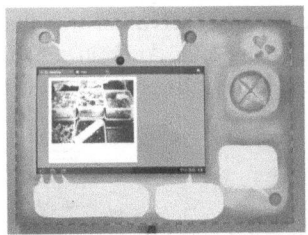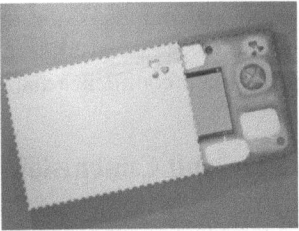

Fig. 3. Integrated *TabletCompanion* with 10-inch display (left and right). The device features several quick access buttons and space for notes by the users. It comes with a wooden casing (right) for easy and appealing storage.

TabletCompanion Feedback. Both participants were equipped with a *Wireless TabletCompanion* for permanent use about a year ago. Five months and four months ago P1 was provided with an additional Integrated TC and P2 with a Wired TC. However, after about two months they were asked to switch devices to provide them with the experience of both flavors of the *TabletCompanion*. All are still in use.

In general the devices were perceived as nice, not frightening and useful. In particular, the Wireless TC was appreciated for its small form factor and the possibility to more easily store or hide it away. This was important to both participants because of their desire to "not have too many things lying around" (P1). However, its drawback compared to the Wired TC was that it was used less frequently due to a small but still existing pairing effort. They also tended to forget about it lying in the drawer and, as a consequence, operated the Android tablet less often. This seemed not to be the case with the Wired TC that always sat next to the Android tablet or phone.

Integrated TC is the complete merging of *TabletCompanion* and the tablet computer, i.e. with it the user only has to mentally deal with one artifact. According to our participants they benefited from having to learn and work with 'only one' single new device. Also, the extra space around the screen was appreciated where they could attach their own notes for explaining the functionalities of the system. P1 and P2 both preferred taking their own notes in contrast to having predefined explanations (e.g. "Google search", "push when lost"). Surprisingly, P2 preferred to use the Wireless TC (often times even without the RFID) module, despite her appraisal of the improved usability of Integrated TC. In this case having the device stored away and setup up again quickly (in order to have a "tidy room") obviously was more important than a larger device with improved functionalities and guidance.

The most popular applications of the TC series comprised the email client, visiting photo-blogs of friends and trying to find information e.g. on craftsmen services by means of web search engines. Both participants made heavy use of the RFID tokens and the customized hardware buttons especially during the first weeks of employment when they haven't had a lot of practice yet. E.g., "I like having a real object for starting programs, because this makes the program more like a real thing, it gives it a face" P1 said. They both reported that the design of the prototypes helped them lose their over-exaggerated respect towards computing devices and the fear of breaking the system, because it didn't look like conventional technology and enabled them to have an impartial go on the computers. An interesting observation was that both participants treated the TC increasingly like a conventional Android tablet (ignoring TC helper functions) as their confidence and computer skills grew over the time.

5   Discussion and Conclusion

In summary we introduced four examples of rapid technology probes for establishing digital communication channels for senior users. What the prototypes have in common is that they could be developed relatively quickly. This was due to the capabilities of modern Android devices and easy to program microcontroller boards such as the Arduino. The wooden casings also gave the technologies a 'solid' non-threatening appearance that made them more appealing to the participants than traditional computers, and made them robust enough for long-term deployments. In addition, two more features accounted for that robustness: While the mobile Android devices provided a stable technological backbone, the tangible computing components assured robust or intuitive interactions and hence made the user experiences accessible. As a consequence of the relatively low-cost development process, we were also able to quickly incorporate user feedback into the later prototypes (e.g. quick access buttons) and deploy these new versions in a real life setting where the participants again could fit these devices into their everyday practices.

Having family members as participants turned out to have the advantage that they were not shy about giving unmasked opinions. To date we have also had several demands to fix some broken (minor) features of our prototypes. We see this as an indicator for their true demand and interest to ensure that they still operate.

Reflecting our observations of this ongoing field study so far, one of the most striking insights is that both P1 and P2 were very eager of not only consuming digital content, but rather to also actively generate emails and photo messages. For future work we will therefore consider this by supporting these user needs even more directly. As there was also great desire for revisiting photos, it might be interesting to explore more interactions around going back to created content and around digitally supported creative engagement for senior people more generally (e.g. extending the photo taking device and study). Such insights can also complement other approaches such as PD or Co-Design and serve as initial experiences to seed these processes. As mentioned before, the work in this paper is still ongoing and the focus here is on RTP as a design technique. Hence, studying the proposed prototypes with regards to their potential as an AAL communication device in more detail also is for future work.

References

1. Coleman, G.W., et al.: Engaging the disengaged: How do we design technology for digitally excluded older adults? In: Proc. DIS 2010, pp. 175–178. ACM (2010)
2. Lindley, S.E., et al.: Desiring to be in touch in a changing communications landscape: Attitudes of older adults. In: Proc. CHI 2009, pp. 1693–1702. ACM (2009)
3. Schuler, D., Namioka, A.: Participatory Design: Principles and practice. Lawrence Erlbaum, New Jersey (1993)
4. Sanders, E.B.-N., Stappers, P.J.: Co-creation and the new landscapes of design. CoDesign 4(1), 5–18 (2008)
5. Hutchinson, H., et al.: Technology probes: Inspiring design for and with families. In: Proc. CHI 2003, pp. 17–24. ACM (2003)
6. Zimmerman, J., et al.: Research through design as a method for interaction design research in HCI. In: Proc. CHI 2007, pp. 493–502. ACM (2007)
7. Olwal, A., Lachanas, D., Zacharouli, E.O.: Mobile phone personalization for older adults. In: Proc. CHI 2011, pp. 3393–3396. ACM (2011)
8. Spreicer, W.: Tangible interfaces as a chance for higher technology acceptance by the elderly. In: Proc. CompSysTech 2011, pp. 311–316. ACM (2011)

Towards an Acceptance Model for AAL

Gerhard Leitner[1], Oana Mitrea[2], and Anton J. Fercher[1]

[1] Institute of Informatics-Systems
Alpen-Adria Universität Klagenfurt
Universitätsstrasse 65-67, 9020 Klagenfurt, Austria
{gerhard.leitner,antonjosef.fercher}@aau.at
[2] Institute for Smart System Technologies
Alpen-Adria Universität Klagenfurt
Universitätsstrasse 65-67, 9020 Klagenfurt, Austria
oana.mitrea@aau.at

Abstract. As one of the major goals in the ambient assisted living
project Casa Vecchia (performed in 20 real world household installations) we want to thoroughly evaluate the life circumstances of elderly
people in order to be able to establish a basic ontology including all
relevant factors that are actually or potentially influencing the acceptance of AAL technology. A prototype system enabling the participants
to observe automated features of an AAL system as well as to perform
basic interaction and communication tasks was installed. Periodic evaluation cycles that were accompanying the project which were based on
a customized mix of methods and concepts frequently discussed and applied in the context of AAL research. The main concepts used are the
technology acceptance model (TAM), contextual design and the analysis
of social networks. The project is still up and running, but first results
could already be achieved which show a different access to technology
between men and women.

Keywords: Ambient Assisted Living, Technology Acceptance, Gender
Differences.

1 Introduction

An extensive body of AAL research is existing which constitutes a solid basis to face the challenges of population overageing. One of the most important
questions in aging research is, however, what efforts it will take to make basic technology accessible to large sections of elderly. Population overageing is a
global phenomenon, but although a large number of AAL solutions have been developed in the recent years, a large scale real world deployment still constitutes,
to quote Neil Armstrong as saying, *"a giant leap for mankind"*, because the ecological validity of a significant proportion of research results is questionable. Two
statements illustrate the basic problems pointedly, [1] contemptuously refers to
usability studies as *one night stands* based on expensive and fragile technology
not comparable to a long-term relationship the interaction with technology in

A. Holzinger et al. (Eds.): SouthCHI 2013, LNCS 7946, pp. 672–679, 2013.

a home can be seen as. Another problem emphasized by [2] is that *people often take a deontological stance when artificially probed.* Everyday behavior probably differs from needs expressed within questionnaire investigations as well as from behavior observed under artificial or experimental conditions. Although AAL technology can - on the technical level - be considered as mature enough to provide the required functionality there is still an unknown number of variables which are potentially influencing the access to technology, in the context of ICT oftentimes subsumed under the term technology acceptance. The identification of dimensions of technology acceptance potentially influencing the widespread deployability of AAL technology was one of the major challenges of the Casa Vecchia project presented in this paper. The dimensions are ranging from technological over sociological to psychological ones. In order to identify and evaluate them a completely as possible, a mixed-method approach based on concepts frequently discussed and used in the related literature was followed.

The remainder of the paper is structured as follows. In section 2 the theories, concepts and models serving as a basis for developing a customized set of evaluation methods is presented. Section 3 describes the methodological approach in detail. The paper finishes with a presentation of results and a discussion section.

2   Related Work

On the basis of psychological theories on product usage and/or buying behavior such as the theory of reasoned action (TRA) or the theory of planned behavior (TPB) [3], the technology acceptance model (TAM) [4] introduced in the 1980es was the pioneer concept to evaluate the acceptance of technical systems on different dimensions. Although competitive models and approaches with comparable dimensions are existing (e.g. Iso 9241-11, User Experience) the TAM builds the basis of numerous scientific studies focused on the evaluation of access to technology, specifically when the behavioral aspect, i.e. to determine the likelihood of the usage (or purchase) of a technological product, service or system, has been in the focus of interest. Since its first publication the TAM has been further developed and enhanced, for example as TAM2, UTAUT and TAM3 [5], the latter building one of the basic components of the approach described in this paper.

However, in regard to the goal of the project the TAM has some limitations which made necessary to combine it with other concepts and methods. As emphasized by the statements *methodological one night stand* and *taking an deontological stance* it is of high importance to ensure the ecological validity of the collected data and achieved results. The preceeding psychological theories of TAM (cf, e.g. [3]) were often critizised for the low correlation between the expressed intention to use or buy a product and actually doing it. A pure questionnaire based approach asking participants about their opinion on AAL and the probability of purchasing such systems would not be adequate to identify the entire set of relevant dimensions. The TAM model is therefore combined with a method focusing on the observation of the use of ICT under real world conditions, concretely the concept of contextual design introduced by [6]. This concept is based on an iterative user centered design approach and was originally designed for work-related contexts. Therefore it had to be adapted to the domain of the project which is living environments. The steps of the original concept and the adaption to the project's domain are enumerated below:

- Talk to specific customers while they work
  ("work" was exchanged by "are at home")
- Interpret the data in a cross functional team
  (the project team consists of computer scientists, psychologists, sociologists)
- Consolidate data across multiple customers
  (commonalities in our participant sample were identified)
- Invent solutions grounded in user work practice
  ("work practice" was exchanged by "activities of daily living (ADL)")
- Structure the system to support this new work practice
  (the prototype was customized to fit into daily living activities)
- Iteration with customer through mockups
  (instead of mockups a high fidelity prototype was serving as illustrative example)
- Design an implementation object model or code structure
  (the implementation was an adaptation and customization to specific needs)

A second addition to the TAM model is the consideration of social relationships. In contrast to shortterm usage under artificial circumstances, the usage of technology at home can also have a social relevance. In order to evaluate this aspect a method based on sketching a circular representation of the social network was taken from [7]. Within the contextual inquiries[6] participants are asked to draw their own social network. This was done in order to evaluate the possibilities of enhancing the existing social network with ICT functionality as well as the potential influence of technology on social relationships.

3   Method

The technological basis of our approach built a high fidelity prototype system which enabled the participants to evaluate whether an AAL solution would fit in their current or future life circumstances. The system at hand constitutes a state-of-the-art, OSGi based multilayer system [8] with a radio operated off-the-shelf smarthome subsystem customized to the project requirements. By providing basic AAL functionality it supports real world prototyping as described in [2]. Twenty households were equipped with our system, about half of them inhabited by elderly singles, the other half inhabited by couples. Within the three years of project duration periodic evaluations based on the methods described in the previous section were performed. The first evaluation cycle was focused on a status quo survey including questions of current life circumstances, relevant aspects of personal history and the expectations with regard to the project. In parallel to the first contextual inquiries [6] the basic AAL system was initially installed and customized step-by-step to the environmental conditions of the households

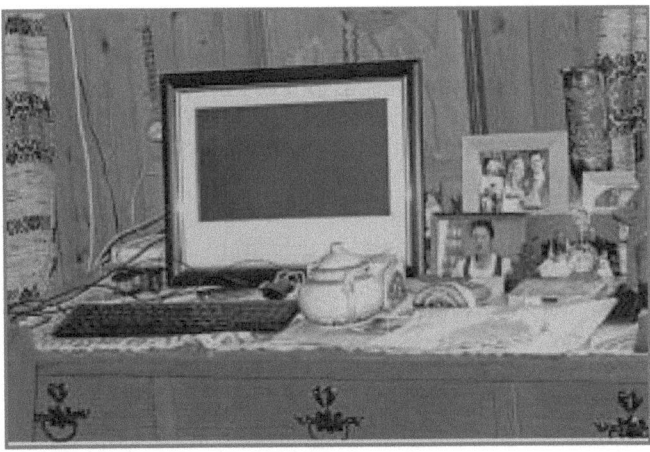

Fig. 1. The central unit is designed to smoothly integrate into the environment. As shown in the example its shape is similar to a digital picture frame and therefore fits into the collection of family photographs.

as well as to the needs and requirements expressed by the participants. Fig. 3 shows an example placement of the central unit of our system.

Because of the fact that the project takes place in real world setting an important prerequisite was to deploy the system as unobtrusively as possible. Therefore only components which could be integrated into the environment but no body worn sensors or cameras were used. Moreover, the installation was done in a way that the participants could use their present devices as usual without, for example, the need of pressing additional buttons or using remote controls. The AAL features provided were focused on security and safety functions. One function ensured that somebody outside the household would be informed (in our case a trusted person) if something extraordinary happened. The identification of extraordinary events was realized by the observation of activities of daily living. In the course of the initial contextual inquiries the participants were asked about their activities and routines and components were installed on neuralgic points connected to those activities. For example, in the household of one participant who stated: *"When I don't drink coffee in the morning, I'm most probably dead"* we equipped the coffee maker with a sensor observing the status (on/off). Most participants cook frequently throughout the day, so we equipped their stoves with sensors. The TV news in the region our project is taking place is viewed by the vast majority of seniors and therefore by our participants, too. Thus the TV set was also connected to our system. Following this approach we installed between five and ten components in each household and were able to observe events over the entire day in a frequency between one or two hours on average. Another feature of security were automated functions, for example, to switch off potentially dangerous devices, such as the kitchen stove or the iron by connecting them via our system with smoke detectors. If the smoke detector is triggered, the devices are switched of and the trusted person is alerted.

Additionally, comfort functions were provided. For example, if a room such as the vestibule is crossed frequently at night a motion sensor was placed there to switch lights automatically. The central unit of the system shown in Fig. 3 served two purposes. The first was to act as a local server coordinating the specific AAL functions provided by the off-the-shelf smart home subsystem and processing, locally buffering and periodically transferring all the collected data to a server at our university. The second purpose was to provide additional functionality and features to the participants they could benefit from. For example, participants in remote locations were provided with RSS feeds of major media providers, they can access weather forecast services and write e-mails to their relatives in an easy way. We expected that these features combined with the possibility to try out the system in the familiar environment for a sufficient period of time (up to 3 years) should generate meaningful results building the basis of a comprehensive ontology including the most relevant dimensions influencing the acceptance of AAL.

Each of the 20 participants nominated a trusted person (a relative, a good friend or a neighbor) who was also involved in the project. Depending on the relevance of an actual topic of the evaluation (e.g. focused on singles or couples, on technological or sociological aspects), the number of participants within a certain evaluation loop differed. Altogether three evaluation cycles have been performed involving the participants in different constellations as well the trusted persons. Some dimensions (such as the social networks) were discussed repeatedly to identify whether the presence of the AAL system changed, for example, the access to technology of the participants or the relationships in the social network. Another point of interest were the different viewpoints of participants and trusted persons on AAL.

4   Results

Due to the fact that the project is still up and running only preliminary and qualitative results are available. On the technical level a huge amount of data (2 million datasets) has been collected which is currently analysed in depth. It turns out that the observation of daily activities based on environmental sensors works satisfactorily. Deviations in activities can be identified on a reasonable quality and significance level and the system would be able to react and alert trusted persons or professional emergency services in case of a problem. However, because of ethical reasons and the fact that our system constitutes a prototype we explicitly did not promise never-known-to-fail security features. Potential participants suffering from severe health problems or chronic diseases were not considered for the project. The alerting functions are therefore only used for simulation and testing purposes and to enable the the participants to give feedback on a higher level of detail (e.g. on the frequency of correct and false alarms).

Based on the outcome of the periodic interviews an initial acceptance ontology for AAL systems could be sketched, however, it is far from being complete and meaningful at the moment. Future work on the completion of the ontology as well as on the interpretation of the result achieved so far is planned for the remaining period of the project.

5   Discussion and Conclusion

What we want to discuss in more detail is the preliminary result that the men participating in the project seem to confirm a *"toys for boys"* cliche. They frequently provide ideas for additional devices, for enhanced functionality and show an intrinsic interest in the data processing and on features of the central unit's interface. In contrast to that the women in the sample are more conservative in regard to the number and combination of components installed in their households and more critically reflecting the benefits of the system (the utility) and the costs (e.g. power consumption, electrical smog, complexity of interaction, fault probability). In the nomenclature of TAM the men seem to have a higher level of computer self-efficacy, playfulness and enjoyment in interaction, or as the concept of user experience [9] describes it, focus on the experiental aspect of technology, whereas the women are more focused on the instrumental aspects.

However, this result seems to show that elderly in our sample are not shying away from technology in general, which would be a positive signal. But this aspect has to be evaluated carefully, because as, for example, [10] illustrates, the access to computing technology is influenced by many aspects. In the context of Casa Vecchia it has to be considered that from the potential target group of around 50.000 elderly in the region only about one per mill has indicated interest in the project, although we used target-group-specific channels such as daily newspapers or local radio for project promotion. So some sort of technology-avoidance is probable, but cannot be seriously evaluated based on the small sample.

Despite the small size of our sample, the observed differences between men and women seem to point to an important aspect to be considered in the final ontology. When taking into account the current population statistics as well as the estimations for future demographic development, the majority of elderly is currently and will remain women. The group of women therefore constitutes the biggest target group of future AAL systems. Therefore it is necessary to investigate the reasons for gender differences as well as possibilities to overcome the eventual problems associated with them.

The differentiation or ambivalence hypothesis [11] stresses the existence of differences between distinct categories of women as well as between men and women and tries to give explanations. Women are characterized as technically behaving and technology using persons who have to work and live - in the technological sense - in *"a men's world"* and have to assert themselves there, a fact that results in ambivalent feelings towards both working and living conditions and their own perceptions about the attributions on women and technology. In our study the abovementioned ambivalence can be observed on the contrast between the overall positive attitudes towards technology of women and the involvement with technology during previous employment on one hand but the feeling that they don't fit in a present world filled with complex and inscrutable ICTs, for which they don't have the necessary comprehension clues (mainly ICT knowledge, skills) on the other. The difficulties of women to deal with technology can be observed, for example shown, on a comment of a women about user manuals: One has to study this in order to understand it everything is so complicated, I ve red everything and did not understand, these settings there I did not understand them without help. Female participants tend to be more critical then the men about the characteristics of (advanced) technology such as perceived opacity (black box), the (sometimes for them not necessary) complexity, the necessity to continuously learn about technological changes and updates. The necessity for a straight and easy technology usage is clearly highlighted by a female respondent: I don't want to think how to use technology, I just want to use it. However, the diversity and ambivalence in female positions is confirmed by the active acquisition of ICT competencies by another female respondent: I really enjoy trying this I had my first computer without hard disk ..I taught myself without help. In contrast to this diversity the men in our sample seem to feel at home in technology and show a higher similarity in regard to their access to technology. Most of them have stressed their general openness towards technical things, their existing competencies going even to extreme (technology freak)and their joy of technology usage (joy and readiness to acquire, use and even construct gadgets), in other words, they like to try out and explore technology. The findings show parallels to the work of [12]. Whereas elderly in general [13] and women in particular typically access technology in a step-by-step, reflective way, men in general as well as in our sample seem to have less problems to explore technology with a trial-and-error approach. According to [12] this constitutes also an approach male software designers find adequate for themselves and they therefore rather design systems to support this approach which again privileges male users. That gender-based differences in the principal access to technology are not genetically determined is illustrated by an example given by [11] which emphazises that in the 1940s and the 1950s as many women as men did programming tasks, since women experts had the necessary mathematical competencies and education and many men were fighting in war. After the second world war the profession had been gradually establishing and had become financially and socially attractive, with the consequence that the returning men edged their female colleagues out. The working on and with computers had turned to be a "male thing" with male connotations. Computing technology so turned into a technology constructed predominantly by males for males [11]. Such lesson from history of computer technology should be considered in the future evolution of AAL systems in a sense that their development should carefully examine and avoid the dangers of both power/dominance and development perspective asymmetries that may put female consumers and users at disadvantage.

We believe that the declared objective of going into field with a prototype system, to talk to users in their very living environment, to collect and interpret user requirements reduces the problem of a limited viewpoint from the perspective of male, young and technophile programmers eliciting their requirements on (as [12] terms it) I-Methodology is constantly being scrutinised by the continuous adaptation and customization of the system to the users needs. The customization has already introduced a variety of changes in the lives of the participants which may have a significant impact on the initial attributions of men and women, for example, increased technical knowledge and competencies, experiencing of various interactivity forms, new functionalities. An important task for our future work in progress is to investigate the dynamics of the seemingly different modes of technology access/usage and the extent to which they do represent consolidated real world behavior.

Acknowledgements. We thank the reviewers for their valuable comments. This paper is originated in the context of *Casa Vecchia* funded by the Austrian research promotion agency within the benefit program (Project.Nr. 825889).

References

1. Rode, J.A., Toye, E.F., Blackwell, A.F.: The fuzzy felt ethnography? Understanding the programming patterns of domestic appliances. Personal Ubiq. Computi. 8(3-4), 161–176 (2004)
2. Iachello, G., Truong, K.N., Abowd, G.D., Hayes, G.R., Stevens, M.: Experience prototyping and sampling to evaluate ubicomp privacy in the real world. In: Proceedings of CHI 2006, pp. 1009–1018 (2006)
3. Armitage, C.J., Conner, M.: Efficacy of the theory of planned behavior: a meta-analytic reivew. Br. J. Soc. Psychol. 40, 471–499 (2001)
4. Davis, F.D.: Perceived usefulness, perceived ease of use, and user acceptance of information technology. MIS Quarterly 13, 319–340 (1989)
5. Venkatesh, V., Bala, H.: Technology acceptance model 3 and a research agenda on interventions. Decision Sciences 39(2), 273–315 (2008)
6. Beyer, H., Holtzblatt, K.: Contextual Design. Interactions 6(1), 32–42 (1999)
7. Scott, J.: Social Network Analysis: A Handbook, 2nd edn. Sage, London (2000)
8. BMBF/VDE Innovationspartnerschaft AAL: Interoperabilität von AAL- Systemkomponenten. Teil 1: Stand der Technik. VDE Verlag, Berlin (2010)
9. Hassenzahl, M., Tractinsky, N.: User Experience - a research agenda. Behavior & Information Technology 25(2), 91–97 (2006)
10. Wandke, H., Sengpiel, M., Sönksen, M.: Myths about older people's use of information and communication technology. Gerontology 58(6), 564–570 (2012)
11. Degele, N.: Einführung in die Techniksoziologie. Fink/UTB, München (2002)
12. Oudshoorn, N., Rommes, E., Stienstra, M.: Configuring the user as everybody: Gender and design cultures in information and communication technologies. Science, Technology & Human Values 29(1), 30–63 (2004)
13. Nap, H.H., Kort, Y.D., IJsselsteijn, W.A.: Senior gamers: preferences, motivations and needs. Gerontechnology 8(4), 247–262 (2009)

Gestyboard 2.0: A Gesture-Based Text Entry Concept for High Performance Ten-Finger Touch-Typing and Blind Typing on Touchscreens

Tayfur Coskun, Christian Wiesner, Eva Artinger, Amal Benzina, Patrick Maier,
Manuel Huber, Claudia Grill, Philip Schmitt, and Gudrun Klinker

Technische Universität München, 85748 Garching bei München, Germany
{coskun,wiesner,artinger,benzina,maierp,huberma,schmittp,
klinker}@in.tum.de, claudia.grill@yahoo.de
http://campar.in.tum.de/Main/TayfurCoskun

Abstract. This paper presents the second version of the **Gestyboard**, which is an innovative approach of text entry on multi-touch devices like tabletops or tablets. To overcome the lack of tactile feedback, we use unique gesture-to-key mappings for each finger according to the ten-finger touch-typing method. As a key feature, the Gestyboard only accepts keystrokes when they are performed with the finger corresponding to the ten-finger touch-typing method. This way, missing a keystroke is not possible, and therefore blind typing is naturally supported by the concept. The first version of the Gestyboard was optimized according to the qualitative and quantitative results of our first formal evaluation. This paper presents two new evaluations which give new insights on the comparative performance and conceptual improvements of the Gestyboard. In the second evaluation, our participants reached a speed of 108 cpm (characters per minute [21.6wpm]) and an error rate of 4% which is close to the performance of standard users on classic touchscreen keyboards. The third evaluation additionally revealed that our participants increased their typing speed with the Gestyboard by 44% and decreased their error rate by 48% in just 3 trial sessions. This steep learning curve is mostly due to the familiarity to the QWERTY layout.

Keywords: Gestyboard, Iterative UI Development, Text input, Gestures, ten-Finger-System, UI Evaluation, User-Centered Design.

1 Introduction

Besides the well-known advantages of touchscreens there are also disadvantages compared to the classical WIMP-based interaction with mouse and keyboard. One important disadvantage is the lack of tactile feedback. Many studies have focused on solving this challenge by either introducing new touchscreen technologies that offer some kind of tactile or haptic feedback or by developing new, suitable touchscreen-based keyboard concepts. This paper presents the second iteration of a novel text input concept, called **Gestyboard**, designed for touchscreens. The name is derived from the fact that unique finger-based **gestures** (taps and slidings) are used to activate keystrokes. The intention of this core characteristic is to tightly link the Gestyboard text input mechanism to the

A. Holzinger et al. (Eds.): SouthCHI 2013, LNCS 7946, pp. 680–691, 2013.

10-finger-system[1]. For example if the user performs a tap gesture with the left pinky finger, the system will always interpret this as the letter 'a', immaterial of where the tap is executed. On sliding the pinky finger up, the letter 'q' will be typed. This way, it is impossible to miss-type the intended key or to accidentally hit an adjacent key while performing the gesture with the correct finger. However, errors still can occur by using the wrong finger or more than one finger simultaneously for a single intended gesture. The goal of this concept is to enable high performance and blind typing without the need for tactile feedback. This can be achieved by abiding with well-known concepts like the QWERTY layout and the 10-finger-system.

2   Related Work

With mobile computing becoming more and more ubiquitous the development of new keyboard concepts have also rapidly evolved. Inspite of this, the performance of touch-screen-based keyboard concepts still suffers, primarily due to the lack of tactile feed-back [1]. Goldberg et al. [2] developed a text input concept called Unistrokes based on simple gestures. These gestures were designed to satisfy three major criteria: simplicity in learning, simplicity in execution and uniqueness. The execution of the gestures does not rely on tactile feedback, this makes blind typing possible. However, learning of those gestures is neccessary. Another text input concept developed for mobile use is called Swype[3]. This concept is based on a dictionary and the QWERTY layout. Here, the user strokes through the letters of the desired word. By combining this approach with error-correction, words can be recognized correctly even if the swipe is not precise.

2.1   Stationary Text Input Concepts

Attempts have also been made to increase the performance of text input for larger touch-screen devices like multi-touch monitors or tabletops. In 2008, Patrick Bader developed a touchscreen keyboard that ergonomically adapts to the users hand [4]. Figure 1 shows the layout of this keyboard which is based on the QWERTY layout. The fingers rest on the home row keys and a keystroke is performed by tapping the keys. One year later, in 2009, Microsoft published the US patent 2009/0237361 A1 which is a QWERTY key-board split into two halves. On placing the hands on the touchscreen, the left half of the keyboard appears below the left hand while the right half below the right hand. Additionally, the two halves follow the hands of the user while moving or rotating. Sax et al. improved this concept by dividing the keyboard into ten parts – one for each finger[5]. Each part follows the corresponding finger and keystrokes are performed with taps.

2.2   Text Entry Evaluation

Typing-speed is usually measured in words per minute (wpm). One word is defined as a sequence of 5 characters inclusive of spaces and signs [6] ($5cpm = 1wpm$). Another important parameter characterizing the performance of the text input is the error

---

[1] This is also called touch typing in literature. However, to avoid confusion in the context of touchscreens, the term 10-finger-system will be used here.

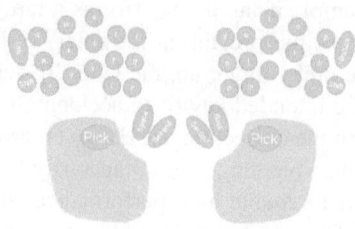

Fig. 1. The layout of the touchscreen keyboard from Patrick Bader

rate. Apart from these performance oriented factors there are other equally important aspects to consider when comparing different text input concepts. These include the acceptance, the learnability, the accessibility, the scalability, and the size needed for the visual representation. Different approaches for evaluating text input methods have been presented in literature. One such method is to let the participants type freely any text that comes to their mind [7]. The advantage is that time is not spent in looking at the predefined text in order to follow it. However, using this method makes it impossible to differentiate between mistakes and intended words. It is also not possible to ensure that the distribution of the letters matches the natural distribution found in the corresponding language. For those reasons, we chose to use another technique: The participants see the text they should type either on a sheet of paper or on a screen. Since each participant types the same text under these controlled circumstances, the individual results can also be better compared. We used the phrase set of MacKenzie and Soukoreff to ensure that the frequency of the letters are similar to their frequency in the English language[7]. To further ensure that each letter appears at least once in our text, a pangram was part of each subset.

3   Requirements

We believe that the classical keyboard can only be replaced by a text input mechanism if the same requirements are fulfilled that are already met by the classical keyboard. Based on this assumption, we collected the following requirements. These are also the requirements which form the foundation of the **Gestyboard** concept.

(R1) No additional hardware: Additional hardware slows down the distribution, and therefore decreases the acceptance of the concept.

(R2) No dictionary: While a language model can improve the performance of a text entry technique, it can also reduce the power of the technique.

(R3) Comparable performance to the classic keyboard: Any new concept needs to be at least as fast and robust as the classical input. Otherwise the new concept can not compete.

(R4) Avoid missing the intended keys: The main reason for the worse performance of a standard touchscreen keyboard is hitting accidentally the wrong keys because of the lack of tactile feedback.

(R5) Enabling blind typing: Blind typing increases the performance of the user because the attention can be focused on the text instead of searching for keys.

Table 1 shows a small survey of touchscreen-based text input concepts developed in the
last decade and whether they fulfill R1 to R5 or not.

Table 1. Several text input concepts and their relation to our requirements. In this table a requirement is fulfilled if we found an evidence for it.

Concept	Year	R1	R2	R3	R4	R5
TCube [8]	1994	no	yes	no	no	no
Quikwriting [9]	1998	no	yes	no	no	no
Dasher [10]	2000	yes	yes	yes	no	no
EdgeWriting [11]	2003	no	yes	no	yes	yes
Graffiti [12]	2008	no	yes	no	no	yes
Bader keyboard [4]	2008	yes	yes	no	no	no
Microsoft Split [13]	2009	yes	yes	no	no	no
Fitaly [14]	2010	yes	yes	no	no	no
LiquidKeyboard [5]	2011	yes	yes	no	no	no
Swype [3]	2011	yes	no	no	no	no

4   Concept

The Gestyboard is activated when the user touches the screen with all ten fingers. A
visual representation of the Gestyboard is then displayed showing the QWERTY layout
as illustrated in Figure 2 a). The home row key letters 'a','s', 'd', 'f', 'j', 'k', 'l' and
';' appear directly below the fingers of the user (see Fig. 2 a). Each finger is associated
with a group of keys, with the home row key as the center key (see Fig. 2 b).

4.1   Gestures

The Tap Gesture: To type one of the home row letters simply a tap with the appropriate
finger is required. Each finger is only allowed to type letters according to the ten-finger-
system. For instance, if the user wants to type an 'a', the left pinky finger is used.
Even if the graphical representation of another letter is hit an 'a' appears. This feature
eliminates the requirement of the user to physically look at the graphical representation
of the Gestyboard. This enables blind typing, hence meeting one of the most challenging
of the requirements listed (R5, see section *"Requirements"*). Moreover, the group of
keys which are linked to the pinky finger is re-centered at the position where the tap
was performed.

The Sliding Gesture: The keys positioned directly below or above the home row keys
are typed by sliding the appropriate finger down or up, respectively. However, in the

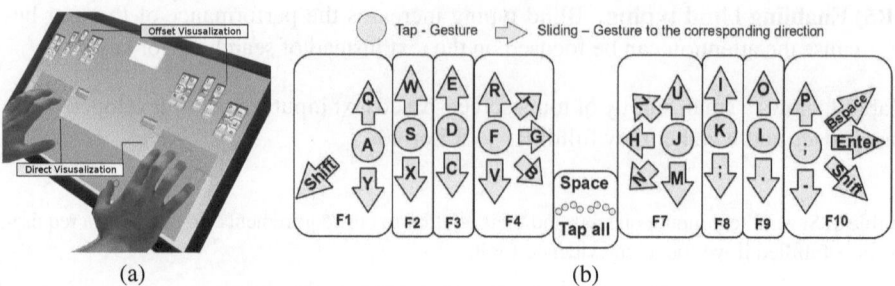

(a)   (b)

Fig. 2. a) The graphical representation of the Gestyboard b) The gesture overview. Fx = Finger x.

case of the pinky and index fingers additional sliding gestures have to be defined, due to additional keys located horizontally and diagonally adjacent to those home row keys. For example if the user desires to execute the enter key, then the right pinky finger must be slided to the right. An overview of all gestures for each finger is given in Figure 2 b).

Space Activation Gesture: To conform to the the rules of the ten-finger-system, the Space key was activated by tapping with either the left or the right thumb in the first version of the Gestyboard. However, we discovered in our first evaluation that space keystrokes were executed accidentally. The reason for this was that due to their larger size, thumbs sometimes were recognized not as one, but two touch points. This was interpreted as a rapid alternation between two corresponding touch points by the software. To overcome this source of errors a new Space key activation metaphor was implemented. To input a space, a simultaneous tap with all ten fingers has to be performed. As a positive side effect, each time a space is typed, all keys are re-centered according to the positions of the user's fingers.

4.2   Challenges

This section describes the most important challenges and the proposed solutions.

Move Fingers Independently: One basic challenge can be attributed to human anatomy. Without further training people are usually not able to move their fingers completely independent from each other. According to the feedback of our first test users, the separate movement of the ring fingers is even more challenging than that of the other fingers.

Hit Wrong Keys: Another result of the first evaluation was that users were accidentally hitting additional keys as they tried to perform the more challenging diagonal sliding gestures. The reason for this can be seen in Figure 3. On the left side the less error-prone approach is shown. A keystroke is only performed when the user re-centers the finger after the visual representation of the letter was reached. That way it is guaranteed that the finger of the user always returns to its appropriate home row letter. However, to support more advanced users the second a option was implemented, which is illustrated on the right side of Figure 3. The user is still able to re-center the finger, but for some words there might be a gain of speed by following the second alternative. However, this was one of the main sources for errors in our first version of the Gestyboard.

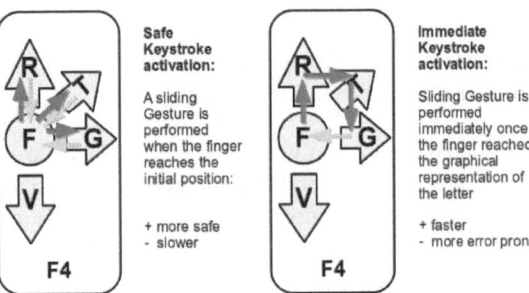

Fig. 3. Two alternatives to type the letters "RTG". Left side: The finger always has to be re-centered to activate a keystroke. Right side: A keystroke is activated when the key is reached by the finger.

Learning Curve: One goal of the evaluation is to determine if our solutions for the mentioned challenges improved the Gestyboard's performance. Another goal is to find out how fast people adapt to this input method over the course of multiple sessions. To be able to compare the performance of a new text input concept with the performance of the classic keyboard, the users need a lot of training. An evaluation over three sessions typing 1000 characters each was performed to gain an initial insight on the associated learning behavior.

5   Evaluation

The results of the first formal evaluation (Pilot Study) with 42 pupils trained in ten-finger touch-typing described in [15] showed a lot of enthusiasm for the concept among the users. The second (Proof of Concept) study is described in the first part of this section while the third (long-term) evaluation is described in the second part of this section.

5.1   Second Evaluation: Proof of Concept

Participants. Two developers having limited experience with the Gestyboard were chosen as the participants for this evaluation. Due to their experience in this field and their prior exposure to the concept they could provide valuable insights on how the technique could be improved.

Procedure. In order to detect some learning effects, each participant had to complete eleven sessions. 1371 characters were typed in session eight and eleven while in each of the remaining sessions, 248 characters were typed. There was a time interval of one to two day between the sessions. For each session we chose a different subset from MacKenzies phrase sets for evaluating text entry techniques [7].

5.2   Third Formal Evaluation: Learning Effect

We conducted yet another study involving unbiased test subjects. The principles of the third formal evaluation are described in the following:

Participants: We evaluated the system with 12 students (11 male 1 female). All were between the ages of 21 and 32 years and have had no prior experience with the Gestyboard. Moreover, none of the participants were accustomed to the ten-finger-system.

Procedure: The evaluation was a within-subject design and consisted of three individual sessions, conducted on separate days with a time period of two to three days. For each session a different subset of MacKenzies phrase sets[7] was used. The participants were asked to enter a text with 1000 characters per session. In the first session our participants typed the phrase set using the Gestyboard, the classical touchscreen keyboard and the classical hardware keyboard (3 stations). There was a ten minute break granted between each station. During this break the participants filled out the System Usability Scale (SUS) questionnaire [16]for each station. The second and third session had exactly the same setup except the classical hardware keyboard was excluded, as it was not necessary to collect learning effects on the already well known classical hardware keyboard. After the third session, the participants were interviewed to get qualitative feedback. On an average it took the participants 70, 52, and 47 minutes to complete the first, second, and third sessions, respectively.

5.3   Apparatus for both Evaluations

The Gestyboard was shown on a 3M Multitouch Monitor with a size of 22". We decided to use Tipp10[2] for our evaluation purposes because of its configurability and capabilities. Tipp10 is an open source typing tutor. Tipp10 presents the text to type in a continuous text ticker. The speed of the ticker is controlled by the user through typing. The ticker stops when a wrong character is pressed and proceeds again by pressing the correct letter. There is no acoustic feedback when a wrong letter is pressed. Thus, the users have to notice mistakes themselves. We measured the following data with Tipp10: duration to type the sentences, overall number of errors and the number of errors per character in each session.

6   Results

This section presents the results of the conducted evaluations.

6.1   Second Formal Evaluation: Proof of Concept Results

The two participants of the proof of concept study were familiar with the Gestyboard. As expected, the speed increased while the error rate decreased throughout the sessions. Figure 4 a) shows the results of the two participants individually. The measured typing speed was 108 cpm (21.6 wpm) and the lowest error rate was 4% in average.

---

[2] http://www.tipp10.com/

6.2   Third Formal Evaluation: Learning Effect Results

Learning Effect: Figure 4 b) shows the cpm, the number of errors and the time needed to type 1000 characters for each session. Average speed increased from session one to session three from 42 to 63 which is an increase of 44%. Simultaneously, the error rate decreased from session one to session three from 25 to 14 errors (-48%).

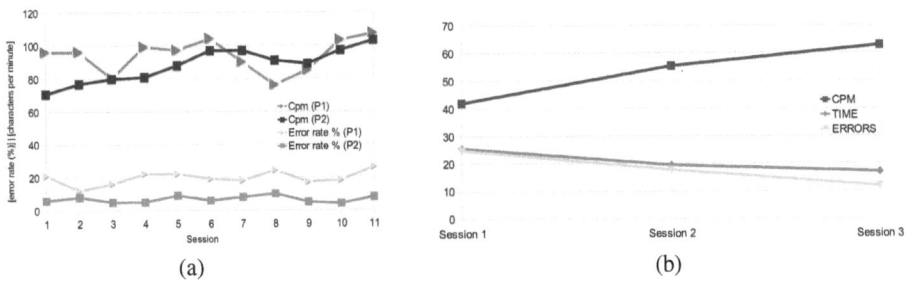

(a)   (b)

Fig. 4. a) Proof of Concept: Performance of two developers during eleven sessions with 276 characters per session. b) Mean values for cpm, errors and the time needed to type 1000 characters for each session.

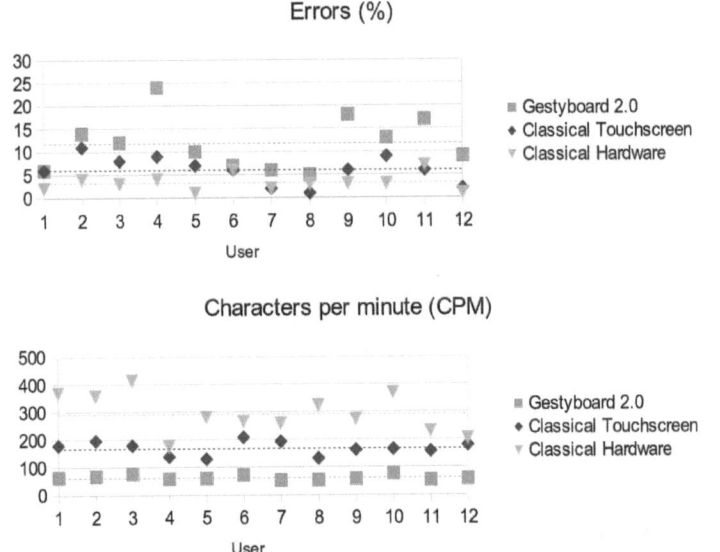

Fig. 5. Comparison between the Gestyboard, the classical touchscreen keyboard and the classical hardware keyboard for each user (Last session). The lines represents the mean values.

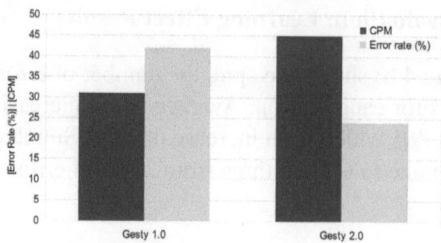

Fig. 6. Comparison between Gestyboard 1.0 and Gestyboard 2.0

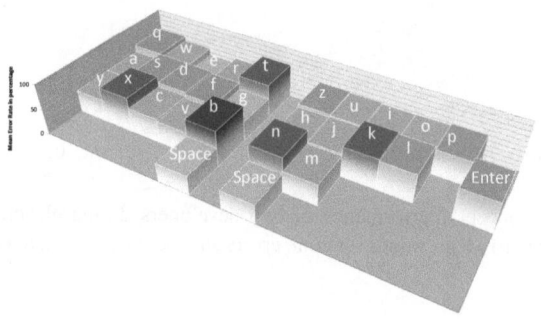

Fig. 7. Errors per character for the first version of the Gestyboard (1.0)

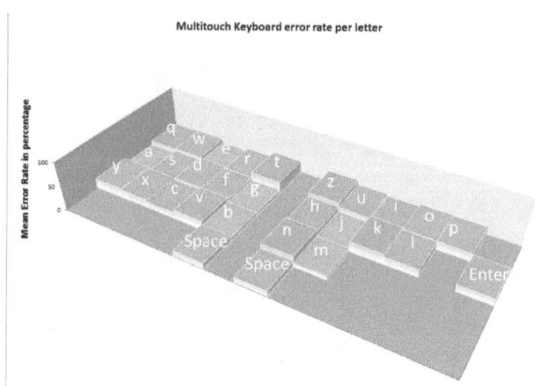

Fig. 8. Errors per character for the current version of the Gestyboard (2.0)

Comparison to the Classic Touchscreen and Hardware Keyboard: Figure 5 shows the comparative results of the characters per minute and the absolute error value for each participant. Overall, the Gestyboard still does not perform as good as the classic virtual touchscreen keyboard and the classic hardware keyboard (both in speed and error rate).

Comparison between Gestyboard 1.0 and Gestyboard 2.0. Figure 6 compares the first version of the Gestyboard with the current version. While the average cpm was 31 for the previous version of the Gestyboard, it increased to 45 for the current version, which is an improvement of 45%. The number of errors decreased from 42 to 24, which is a decrease of 42%.

Figure 7 shows the mean error rate in percentage for each character of Gestyboard 1.0 and Figure 8 shows the same for the current version of the Gestyboard. By comparing these two figures it is noticeable that the number of errors made for each character on version 2.0 of the Gestyboard diminished significantly compared to its predecessor. This is especially the case for the letters 'x', 'b', 't','n', and 'k'.

7   Conclusion and Discussion

In the second formal evaluation the participants reached a typing speed of 108 cpm (21.6 wpm). According to Sax et al. [5] this is already a competitive result when compared to the classical virtual touch-screen keyboards. Sax et al. argued through the work of Lopez et al. [17] that the mean typing speed of classical touchscreen keyboards is 92.5 cpm (18.5 wpm). However, our evaluation of the classical touchscreen based keyboard resulted in a mean typing speed (in our third session) of 168 cpm (33.6 wpm). This difference to the results given in [5] can be attributed mainly to two factors: First, our participants also improved their typing speed for the classical touchscreen keyboard during our sessions. Second, and even more important, the evaluation in [17] was performed on an Apple iPhone which is a small screen device and therefore not as ergonomic as a keyboard used on a large screen. Consequently, the results of our second formal evaluation prove that the Gestyboard can compete with touchscreens on small screen devices but not yet on standard touch-screen keyboards. The participants in our third formal evaluation could not yet reach the performance of the classic touchscreen keyboard (62.8 cpm and 11.75%error rate), but it nevertheless revealed that there is a fast learning behavior. Our participants improved their typing speed by 44% with an average of 63 cpm in just three sessions, and reducing their errors by 48%. The performance can increase dramatically once a user familiarizes with the keyboard layout and the movements on the Gestyboard. A potential benefit from the ten-finger touch-typing method is also evident. Additionally, some of our participants reported that they also became habituated to the finger movements required for a whole sequence of gestures. This was more apparent for words which they typed frequently. This not only improves the typing speed, it also enables the user to blind type without any haptic feedback. Additionally, the participants reported errors made due to moving of the wrong finger. A large amount of time being spent in search of the correct letters. However, this was more the case at the beginning of each session, where the participants required time to re-acquaint themselves with the gestures. The space key gesture was another source of error. When users remove their hands for a short period of time and then position their hands back on the screen, the system detects the entry of a space key. However, a space key was often initiated even when the users just wanted to relax their fingers or recenter them. It also occurred when they wanted to abort an action.

8   Future Work

Our qualitative interviews with our participants revealed some flaws in the current implementation and the concept itself. To remove one such flaw, we decided to change the gesture for the space key from tapping with all ten fingers to merely tapping with the five fingers of the left hand. The same gesture performed with the right hand would then be used for the backspace key. This way, people can remove both hands without the risk of performing the space gesture. We are also investigating algorithms to keep the group of keys following the individual fingers when the movement of the finger is not intended by the user, as fingers tend to drift on the screen over time. For this, the speed of the finger might be an indicator. To eliminate another source of errors, the tap gesture will be optimized. To enable the user to cancel a tap, the tap gesture will be aborted when the user immediately slides the finger a certain amount after the finger touches the screen again. By eliminating those weak points, the performance of the Gestyboard itself can be further improved. In addition to these improvements, we plan to conduct an extended long term evaluation. This way, the performance of the Gestyboard can be better compared with the performance of the classical keyboard. We will then choose those participants who claim to be already proficient in blind typing to conduct another evaluation in which the visualization of the Gestyboard is hidden. We will do the same with the classical touchscreen keyboard (providing some visual or haptic feedback to know where the keyboard is) and compare the results with each other.

References

1. Luk, J., Pasquero, J., Little, S., MacLean, K., Levesque, V., Hayward, V.: A role for haptics in mobile interaction: initial design using a handheld tactile display prototype. In: Proceedings of the SIGCHI Conference on Human Factors in Computing Systems, pp. 171–180. ACM (2006)
2. Goldberg, D., Richardson, C.: Touch-typing with a stylus. In: Proceedings of the INTERACT 1993 and CHI 1993 Conference on Human Factors in Computing Systems, pp. 80–87. ACM (1993)
3. Swype: Swype (April 02, 2012), http://www.swypeinc.com
4. Bader, P.: Entwicklung eines virtuellen Eingabegeräts für Multitouch Screens. Bachelor's thesis, Hochschule der Medien, Stuttgart, Germany, GE (August 2008)
5. Sax, C., Lau, H., Lawrence, E.: Liquidkeyboard: An ergonomic, adaptive qwerty keyboard for touchscreens and surfaces. In: The Fifth International Conference on Digital Society, ICDS 2011, pp. 117–122 (2011)
6. Arif, A.S., Stuerzlinger, W.: Analysis of text entry performance metrics. In: 2009 IEEE Toronto International Conference on Science and Technology for Humanity (TIC-STH), pp. 100–105. IEEE (2009)
7. MacKenzie, I.S., Soukoreff, R.W.: Phrase sets for evaluating text entry techniques. In: CHI 2003 Extended Abstracts on Human Factors in Computing Systems, CHI EA 2003, pp. 754–755. ACM, New York (2003)
8. Venolia, D., Neiberg, F.: T-cube: a fast, self-disclosing pen-based alphabet. In: Proceedings of the SIGCHI Conference on Human Factors in Computing Systems: Celebrating Interdependence, pp. 265–270. ACM (1994)

9. Perlin, K.: Quikwriting: continuous stylus-based text entry. In: Proceedings of the 11th Annual ACM Symposium on User Interface Software and Technology, pp. 215–216. ACM (1998)
10. Ward, D., Blackwell, A., MacKay, D.: Dashera data entry interface using continuous gestures and language models. In: Proceedings of the 13th Annual ACM Symposium on User Interface Software and Technology, pp. 129–137. ACM (2000)
11. Wobbrock, J.O., Myers, B.A., Kembel, J.A.: Edgewrite: a stylus-based text entry method designed for high accuracy and stability of motion. In: Proceedings of the 16th Annual ACM Symposium on User Interface Software and Technology, pp. 61–70. ACM (2003)
12. Castellucci, S.J., MacKenzie, I.S.: Graffiti vs. unistrokes: an empirical comparison. In: Proceedings of the Twenty-Sixth Annual SIGCHI Conference on Human Factors in Computing Systems, pp. 305–308. ACM (2008)
13. Mosby, T.J., Wiswell, C.N.: Virtual keyboard based activation and dismissal. US-Patent 2009/0237361 (September 2009)
14. Fitaly: Fitaly, http://www.fitaly.com/fitaly/fitaly.htm (April 02, 2012)
15. Coskun, T., Artinger, E., Pirritano, L., Korhammer, D., Benzina, A., Grill, C., Dippon, A., Klinker, G.: Gestyboard: A 10-finger-system and gesture based text input system for multi-touchscreens w ith no need for tactile. techreport (2011)
16. Brooke, J.: SUS: a 'quick and dirty' usability scale. Usability evaluation in industry (1996)
17. Lopez, M., Castelluci, S., MacKenzie, I.: Text entry with the apple iphone and the nintendo wii (2009)

On-Screen Marker Fields
for Reliable Screen-to-Screen Task Migration

Rudolf Kajan, István Szentandrási, Adam Herout, and Michal Zachariáš

Graph@FIT, Brno University of Technology
{ikajanr,iszent,herout,izacharias}@fit.vutbr.cz

Abstract. Our goal is to deliver unobtrusive task migration, typically between a desktop computer and a mobile device. We propose to overlay an aesthetically acceptable marker field across (a part of) the monitor screen. This marker field must be easily detectable even by a low-end ultramobile device, unobtrusive to the user, and easy to mix in the natural screen image. We show that Uniform Marker Fields are a good choice for this task and propose a methodology for inserting them into the screen image. The experimental results show that our solution provides reliable task migration on a video stream in interactive frame rates ($\sim 30\,\mathrm{FPS}$ marker detection, $340\,\mathrm{ms}$ whole processing time including wireless communication, HTC Desire from 2010). This substantially outperforms the existing solutions based on natural keypoints ($\sim 7\,\mathrm{sec}$ processing). Our user tests also led to selection and design of appropriate marker fields and their mixing parameters.

Keywords: Task Migration, Uniform Marker Fields, Document Reaccess, Fast Localization, Visual Codes, Multi-Device Interaction.

1 Introduction

Although file sharing services (SkyDrive, Google Drive, Dropbox, etc.) and cloud-based systems (e.g., cloud based solutions for synchronization of bookmarks) are on the rise and found their way to millions of users and devices, work state reconstruction is still a fairly unexplored area. A recent study by Bales et al. [1] focused on methods and content of web information reaccess among personal devices. It showed that cross-device reaccess is often very spontaneous and unplanned and that currently native applications play an important role in how users reaccess content. Unfortunately, contemporary solutions for content sharing and information reaccess are mainly document-centric and rely on complicated infrastructure, thus creating barriers for users trying to perform tasks on mobile devices and continue tasks on other platforms [2].

Dearman et al. [3] state that for most users, the migration from PC to a mobile platform is more frustrating than any other means of follow-up. The main source of this frustration is the fact that users are often forced to use many creative, although very time-consuming, methods to enable content and task migration among their devices, because of lack of support from software. Among most commonly observed means of content reaccess were [3]:

A. Holzinger et al. (Eds.): SouthCHI 2013, LNCS 7946, pp. 692–710, 2013.
© Springer-Verlag Berlin Heidelberg 2013

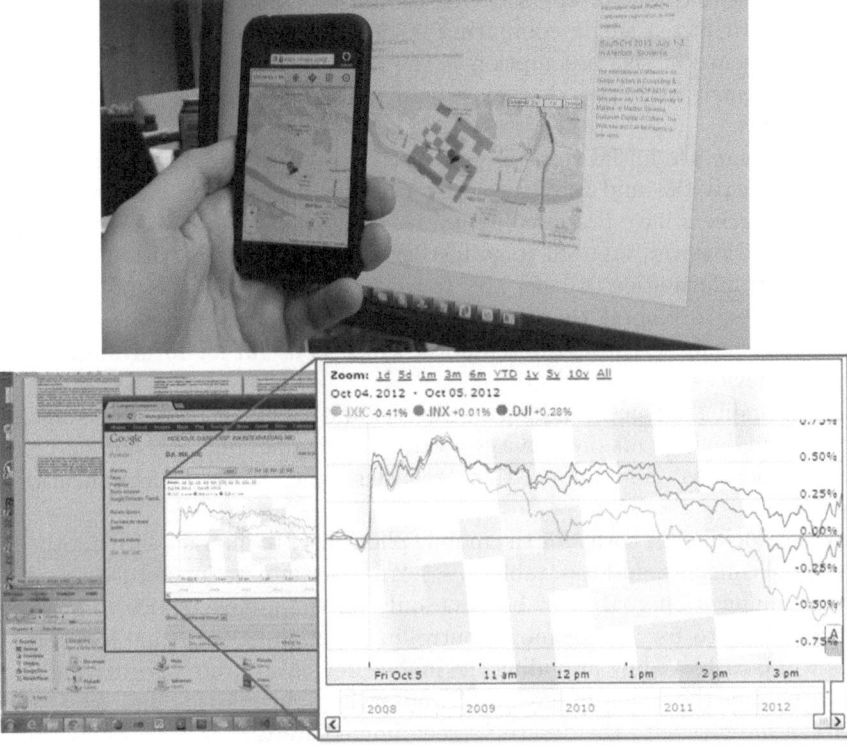

Fig. 1. The goal of our work is to insert a subtle piece of information into the monitor screen that would be reliably detectable and could accurately establish the location within the screen observed by an ultramobile device

- Leaving browser tabs open on the mobile device as a reminder to reaccess them on another device.
- Using handwritten or printed information, carried between the devices, and inputted on the second device.
- Utilizing shared bookmark systems access data between devices. Using these systems users save a bookmark on one device and have it available on their other device automatically.
- Unplanned reaccesses are frequently executed by entering search queries into another device.

As Bales at al. [1] state, users would often use features that were made for different purposes as methods to find information later. Many tools, such as Context Clipboard, Evernote, and Dropbox, have attempted to address this problem by enabling easy capture and reaccess, such as saving a link to find later [4]. Although these tools are seamless and easy to use, they still require planning on the part of the user.

For a vast majority of applications, the initial assumption is still that users interact with just a single computing device throughout the day. The practical consequence of this assumption is the lack of collaboration among devices and user-centric activities that may span multiple devices as well as multiple applications.

While there are initial steps in this direction [5], they must support a wider variety of activities and fully recognize the members of a user's device collection. Researchers have proposed supporting activities that span multiple applications [6]. However, we need to go farther and provide users with a lightweight solution for information transfer able to work with different types of information and contexts, to respect the need for privacy support and supports additional metadata generated through interaction which is useful for future interactions on other devices.

These findings suggest focusing on the user and his intent rather than on applications and devices, making devices aware of their roles and focusing on lighter-weight methods for information transfer and task synchronization / migration.

We are looking for a way for the mobile phone user to interact with another device (public display, desktop, tablet, ...). The user interaction needed to achieve the communication goal must be done only on the mobile device to spare the user the need to use two or more controlling appliances at a time (See Fig. 1). This will be achieved by providing the mobile device accurate information about which part of the monitor screen it is observing. Having this information, the user can interact with the desktop screen immediately.

Pierce et al. [7] introduced an infrastructure based on instant messaging which provides mechanisms for applications to send information, events and commands among devices. A system for document redirection based on SIFT features which uses a mobile camera to achieve document drag and drop functionality in a physical environment was presented by Liu et al. [8]. Shoot & Copy [9] is an interaction technique for transferring information from a public display onto a personal mobile phone with its built-in camera.

Chang and Li proposed DeepShot [10] – a framework for capturing work state which uses natural visual features (SURF, [11]) and tracks them. Their approach is a simplified sibling of PTAM (Parallel Tracking and Mapping, [12]). However, despite various techniques to balance the features' density in the camera view, it is impossible to ensure presence of the visual features in the whole camera view. In the case of observing a computer screen the problem is even more difficult because unlike the real world, the monitor screen tends to contain surfaces of exactly constant color, backlit by the monitor lamp and thus avoiding any external lighting which would help distinguish unique places.

A recent step towards direct information transfer from a desktop screen to an ultramobile device are the VR Codes by Woo et al. [13]. In this solution, a digital payload is encoded into solid gray surfaces on the screen by a time multiplex. The encoding requires a significant computational effort on the desktop monitor side, and assumes a particular design of the camera on the mobile side.

This method could be more promising for the desired purpose of task migration if it allowed encoding the information into arbitrary images.

In this paper we build upon the work of Szentandrási et al. on planar marker fields (Binary Uniform Marker Fields, [14]). Uniform marker field is a two-dimensional planar grid of squares (binary, but possibly colored or greyscale) that can be easily and robustly recognized in a camera image, even when disturbed by occlusion, blur, uneven lighting, etc. We are showing that such a marker field is a good choice for imagery pattern to be inserted into the screen image in order to be detected and recognized by a smartphone camera. The detection of the marker fields is very efficient (milliseconds on a contemporary smartphone) thanks to low computational complexity and low memory footprint. The latter is especially important due to the slow memory access on contemporary ultra-mobile processors. The insertion of the marker field into the desktop image is relatively straightforward and also computationally very cheap.

We propose here a system which uses the mixed-in marker field in order to identify an exact spot on the screen in space and time. This identification happens without any need for interaction on the "desktop" side; instead, it is fully controlled from the ultramobile device. It is based on the very intuitive and common metaphor of shooting a video clip with the smartphone. This technique is employed to achieve an easy, human-friendly inter-device task migration. The optical localization part of the solution is designed so that it is computationally as inexpensive as possible. The ease of detection is ensured by using the marker field which is designed for robust and cheap detection. Low computational demands allow for common-man devices to use the technology, sparing battery life, memory resources, etc.

Our article provides an empirical evaluation of the task migration design: reliability of detection and computational demands. Besides that, a preliminary user testing was carried out to determine which way of inserting/blending the marker field into the screen image is best accepted by the users and what level of obtrusiveness they are sensitive to.

2   Overall Structural Design of the Proposed System

The main objective for the design and implementation of our task migration system was to transfer tasks and information among large variety of devices while minimizing configuration time and being as intuitive as possible.

An inspiration and the leading metaphor was video recording on mobile platforms and augmented reality applications in general, where users just point their device's camera at the object of interest and immediately begin to record (capture) it or interact with it. This means that besides transferring a simple document or URL to another device, also complete application state and related metadata are migrated to the requester device.

We have designed our system with the following goals in mind:

1. Fast deployment without changes to existing network infrastructure.
2. Avoid requirements for a shared server or other central hub.

3. Users do not have to manually configure network settings or configure mobile devices.
4. Support of variety of interaction scenarios in both online and offline environments.
5. Because communication protocols and ways in which messages are delivered are always changing, the system must be flexible enough to support these changes and allow easy modification of the existing protocols and addition of new protocols.
6. Implemented security must ensure that users have only access to certain parts of the system and do not access restricted parts of system and applications.
7. Integration of available standard computing components to support effective collaboration by combining the most suitable set of existing resources available on nearby devices.

2.1 Targeted Real-Life Scenarios

There are four basic scenarios where we consider content and task migration:

- *Resuming task on an (ultra)mobile device* which is one of the most desired and at the same time most frustrating scenarios. Very often "going mobile" means significant reduction of comfort, pace of work and accuracy in the favour of accomplishing tasks on the go. Usually this scenario involves explicit planning and preparation, for example synchronization of documents through specialized tools and services, which is time consuming.
- *Resuming task on desktop computer.* Besides consuming information (reading books, content from web pages, games), users also often generate multimedia content on the go – they take photos, record video sequences, create notes and bookmarks. As in previous scenario, specialized synchronization services are commonly used, even though they are document-centric and are not able to capture and work with the application state.
- *Sharing content between (ultra)mobile devices.* Only few solutions exist that allow for sharing of content among (ultra)mobile device. The most commonly seen scenario is a content exchange between devices belonging to different users, and content and state transfer between mobile devices of one user (e.g. task migration from a smartphone to a tablet) is rare [10].
- *Sharing content between desktop computers through an (ultra)mobile device.* Despite wide availability of cloud-based (SkyDrive, Dropbox, ...) and traditional (FTP, email) file sharing solutions, people still tend to rely on USB drives [3] to transfer content from one desktop computer to another.

2.2 High-Level Overview of the Task Migration System

Our system supports two main roles for devices (see Fig. 2) – the *content provider* role and the *content requesters* role. The device in the role of *content provider* is able to share the state of its applications with authenticated clients – *content requesters*. This device handles incoming connections, maintains context and streams requested content. The *content provider* device provides the state of its applications by either querying individual applications for their current work state (URL and internal settings for web applications, document along with current page number for document viewers, streamed multimedia content) or provides general services, e.g. providing high quality screenshots of a selected screen area or text from a selected area, possibly via optical character recognition. A typical *content provider* is expected to be a plugin into existing widely-used software: common web browsers, mail clients, office applications, possibly even integrated development environments. *Content requesters* are responsible for communication initiation with the target provider device, selection of screen region or application and selection of requested/offered content based on the user's intent. In a typical scenario, *content requesters* are mobile or ultra–mobile devices (mobile phone, smart phone, tablet, PDA). The communication between devices is realized through a WiFi connection. Messages which are exchanged among system components are structured key-value pairs based on Javascript Object Notation (JSON). Binary data in messages are encoded in Base64. Using standardized and open protocols ensures portability of provider / requester implementations.

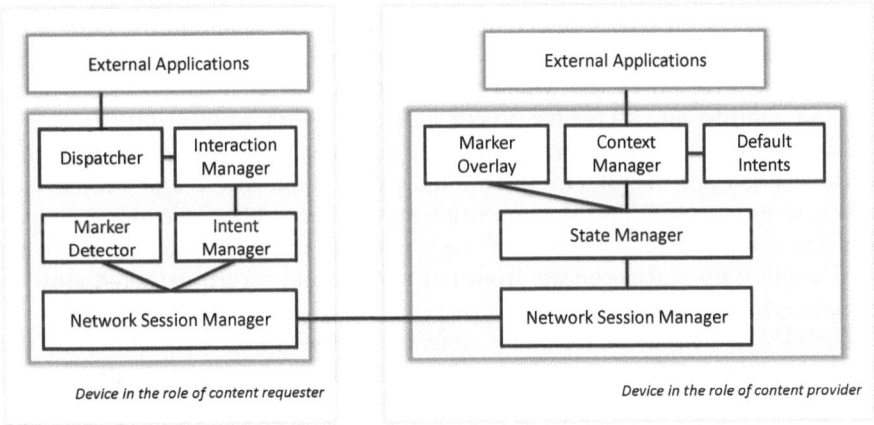

Fig. 2. System overview. Content requester communicates wirelessly with a content provider. The system on both sides consists of a stack of functional blocks (blue rectangle) whose purpose is to ensure information sharing between the built-in or third-party applications (red rectangles). The system thus provides infrastructure for general communication between different devices' applications.

2.3   System Components and Their Functionality in Detail

The content requester's network session manager is responsible for network connection initiation to a remote content provider (e.g., public display, laptop).

At the moment, the communication is implemented through the WiFi connection, due to its availability on a broad range of devices. The target device is located either via network discovery, by manually entering an IP address (or selecting IP address from history) or the user scans a specific code associated with target device (e.g. on-screen or printed visual marker / matrix code). Afterwards, the *content provider's network session manager* accepts the incoming connection and asks for authorization and device capabilities (e.g., camera resolution and internal camera parameters). The target device uses this information to visually adjust the marker field (e.g., change its opacity, color contrast and/or brightness).

When the connection is successfully established, the *content provider* device uses the *marker overlay* (Section 3) to create an unobtrusive on-screen localization marker adjusted for the given *requester* in its current state. After the connection is accepted, the marker overlay covers a larger part of the screen, until the camera's position is detected for the first time (less than a second). Afterwards, the overlay is automatically adjusted, so that it covers just the area captured by the camera. The part of the marker which is observable is defined by the camera's position and by the distance from the *content provider* device.

The *marker field detector* on the *requester* device is used for fast and accurate client-side on-screen marker decoding and sending of within-screen localization information to the target device via the *network session manager*. This approach minimizes the amount of transferred data between the devices because only the unique ID of the currently detected part of the marker field and the homograph data is sent back to the *content provider* (unlike feature-based solutions where either feature vectors or the whole camera stream are sent to the target device or to an intermediate server for processing and camera localization).

Based on the obtained camera-localization information, the *context manager* on the *content provider* device queries individual applications and gathers their status. In order to obtain the application status from web applications, we have implemented an extension for the Google Chrome browser which is able to forward application state requests from our system and return gathered state information for further processing.

The Google Chrome extension is implemented as a persistent Chrome background page, which runs on the *content provider* device even when main browsers windows are closed. The extension communicates with the *context manager* via websocket – full-duplex single socket connection. After receiving a request, the extension finds the active browser window and the tab with a web page and through code injection inserts javascript script into the page. This script is able to extract required parts of the web page - blocks of text, images, videos or links to other web-based resources and send them back to the *content provider*, which forwards them to the *requester device* (See Fig. 3).

If the selected application is unable to provide its state and metadata, only general intents are available. General intents include high-quality screenshots, text and phone numbers recognitions for the selected part of the screen.

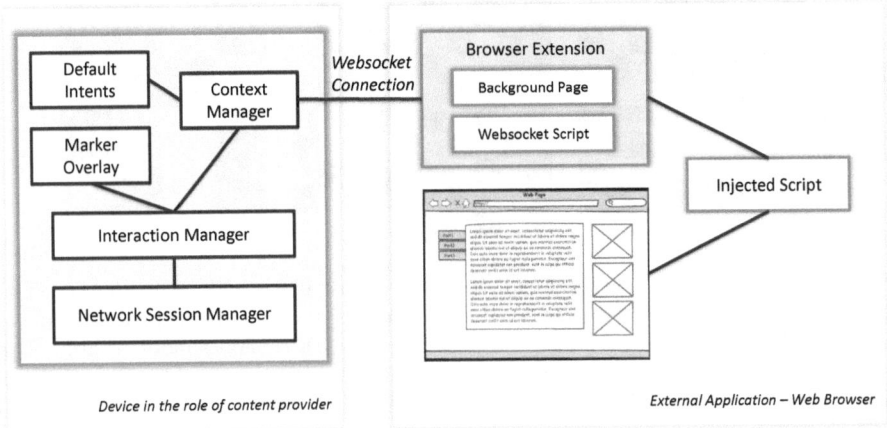

Fig. 3. Example of communication with external application – web browser via browser extension. The implemented browser extension is able to extract state of web application through javascript code injected into the opened web page.

The acquired application state is sent to the *intent manager* on the *requester device* which translates these JSON-encoded messages to intents directly usable on the requester platform (e.g., on the Android platform creates Android intents from JSON messages).

Afterwards, the *state manager* provides the user with a visual feedback and updates the GUI, based on available actions for the selected content. The options include resuming work with web application on current device, editing text in available text editor, manipulation and viewing of images or audio/video playback.

If the user decides to continue the task with a selected application (e.g. web browser or media player), the *application dispatcher* sends the intent along with context to the appropriate application on the *requester device*.

3   Marker Fields Design and Detection

In order to minimize the data transfer between the client and the data provider, we used easily identifiable marker field proposed by Szentandrási et al. [14], the Uniform Marker Fields (See Fig. 5). An advanced version of the detection algorithm, evaluation and comparison with other alternative camera localization markers was described in our latest work [15]. In order for the paper to be self-contained, we give a brief description of the marker field design and the detection algorithm.

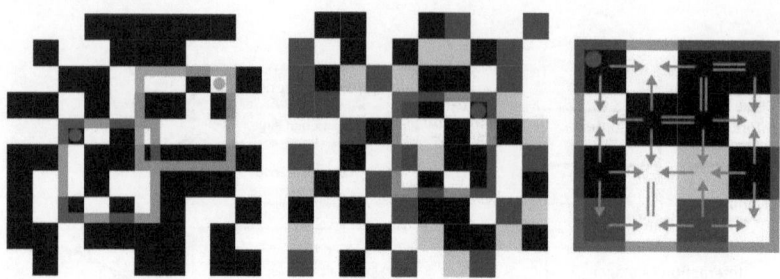

Fig. 4. The use of our Marker Field. **left:** The basic black and white marker. The highlighted green and brown windows are unique in the marker field, just as all other sub-windows in every rotation. **right:** The marker with several shades of grey. The highlighted blue sub-window is unique in the map considering the edge directions as seen on the extracted region.

The Uniform Marker Fields were first introduced as a checkerboard structure, where the black and white fields are mixed up so that every n^2 tile for a given n is unique in the field in every rotation (Fig. 4). The synthesis of such fields is highly time consuming and the size is also limited by the size of the uniquely identifiable sub-windows (n^2). (For $n = 4$ the theoretical upper bound of the field dimensions is 127×127 [14]). In [15], the limitation of using only black and white colors was relaxed, so that different colors or shades of gray could be used to form the marker field. In this case, instead of the intensity of each field, the gradient between them was used to determine the unique location inside a marker. This modification not only helped the detection performance and the robustness of the detection algorithm against occlusion, but also much larger maps could be generated with smaller n. In this work we used binary markers with localization based on the edge gradient orientations.

The detection algorithm supposes that the grid of squares is planar and distorted by a perspective projection. This assumption is always fulfilled by markers displayed on monitors and projections on flat surfaces. Thanks to this

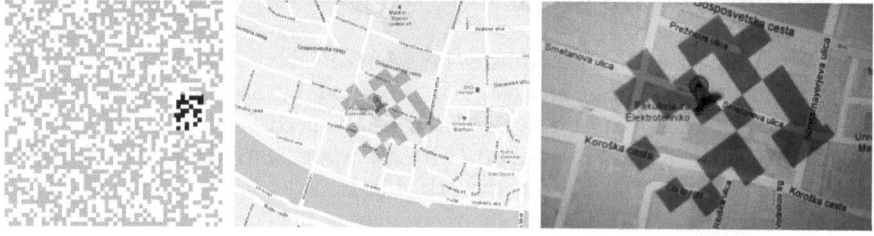

Fig. 5. The use of our Marker Field. **left:** Highlighted region in the Marker Field used for mixing. **center:** Marker Field mixed into the displayed content. **right:** The same Marker Field, as seen by a mobile phone camera.

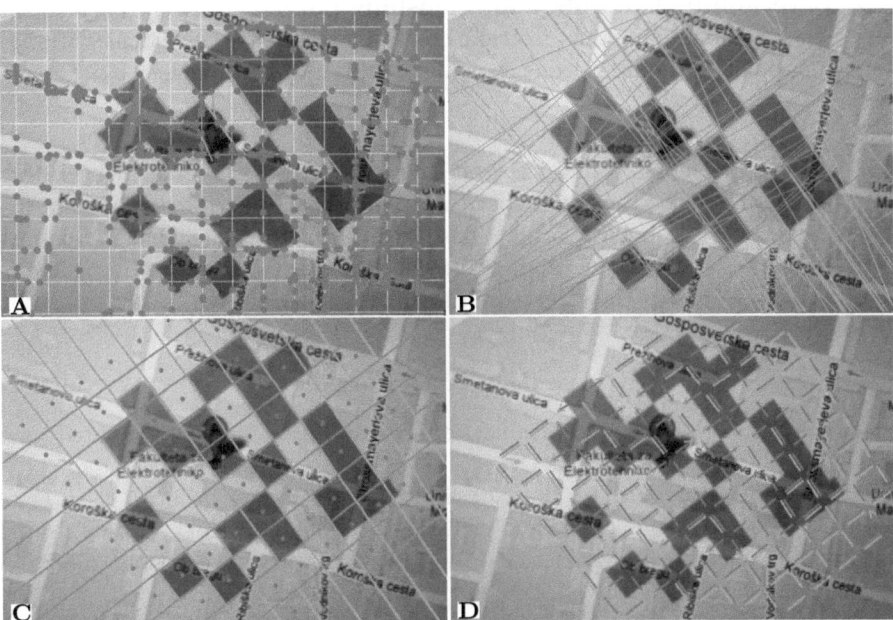

Fig. 6. Detection of the greyscale grid of squares from the image acquired by the mobile phone camera (Fig. 5). **A:** The image is processed in sparse scanlines. On each scanline, edges are detected (Red) and extended to edgels (Green). The edgels are filtered roughly based on the phone's orientations sensors. **B:** The edgels are grouped into two dominant groups using RANSAC; two vanishing points are computed by hyperplane fitting. **C:** Based on the vanishing points, the optimal grid is fitted to the set of the edgels. **D:** Edges between the modules are classified.

assumption, the algorithm is very efficient: the fraction of visited pixels (the algorithm's "pixel footprint") within an average input image is very small ($\sim$ 5 %, [15]).

The grid detection algorithm performs the following three main steps (Fig. 6):

1. Extraction of edgels (edge element or edge pixel) – typically, the algorithm extracts around one hundred straight edge fragments in the whole image. The image is processed only in sparse horizontal and vertical scanlines (Fig. 6A) and edges detected along these scanlines are used as seeds for the edgel detection. For onscreen markers we added one more assumption. The marker will always be roughly in the center of the camera view. This is mostly true thanks to the communication flow between the client and the content provider, which only displays the marker at a given part of the screen. Another improvement in this step compared to the basic algorithm is that we have the information from the gyroscope or accelerometer from the mobile device. This can be used to filter out directions for the marker orientation.

2. Determining two dominant vanishing points among the edgels (Fig. 6B). Lines in one dominant direction are supposed to be coincident with the vanishing point. In homogeneous coordinates this can be expressed by:

$$\forall i : \mathbf{v} \cdot \mathbf{l}_i = 0, \tag{1}$$

for the vanishing point $\mathbf{v}$ and the pencil of lines $\mathbf{l}_i$. Lines $\mathbf{l}_i$ coincident with a vanishing point in the projected space in homogeneous coordinates lie on a hyperplane passing through the origin. The hyperplane's normal vector in this case corresponds to the vanishing point $\mathbf{v}$ in the projective space. The hyperplane's normal can be found as the direction of the least variance by eigendecomposition of the correlation matrix.

$$C = (\mathbf{l}_0 \ldots \mathbf{l}_N)(\mathbf{l}_0 \ldots \mathbf{l}_N)^T. \tag{2}$$

Since matrix C is 3×3 and symmetric, decomposition can be computed very efficiently.

3. Finding the grid of marker field edges as two groups (*pencils*) of regularly repeated lines coincident with each vanishing point. Two vanishing points $\mathbf{v}_1, \mathbf{v}_2$ define the horizon ($\mathbf{h} = \mathbf{v}_1 \times \mathbf{v}_2$). Marker edges of one direction can be computed using the horizon as ($\hat{\mathbf{x}}$ denotes normalized vector)

$$\mathbf{l}_i = \hat{\mathbf{l}}_{base} + (ki + q)\,\hat{\mathbf{h}}, \tag{3}$$

where $\mathbf{l}_{base}$ is an arbitrarily chosen base line through the vanishing point, different from the horizon [16]. The parameter k controls the line density and q determines the position of the first line. A good simple choice for $\mathbf{l}_{base}$ is a line through the center of the image (and through the vanishing point).

In order to find k and q, the value of $(ki + q)$ is calculated for every line (extended edgel) of the input group. These values are clustered, each cluster is assigned an i and then the overall optimal k and q are found by linear regression (Fig. 6C, blue and green lines).

When only a small fraction of the marker field is visible without any noise or distortions, it is crucial that the edge gradients (Fig. 4 right) are recognized correctly. Their recognition can be challenging due to motion blur, uneven lighting conditions, real content displayed on the monitor, etc. (Fig. 7).

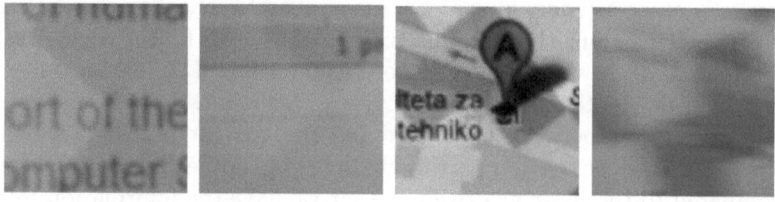

Fig. 7. Examples of problematic edges within the pictures of the marker field. The edges are classified by deterministically sampling a varying number of pixels within the neighboring modules. Wald's SPRT is used to discern the edge by using a minimal number of such samples.

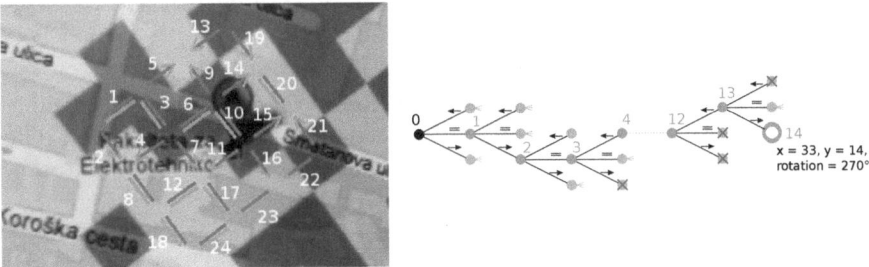

Fig. 8. The use of our Marker Field. **left:** The order in which the edges are visited. **right:** The decision tree. Leaves are either invalid or contain a location and orientation to the marker field.

In order to correctly classify an edge given the locations of the neighboring marker field modules, our algorithm samples pixels from the edge's vicinity. If a small number of samples suffices to decide an edge either way, the decision is made, otherwise more pixels are sampled. If an edge cannot be confirmed, the location between the modules is treated as a place without an edge (Fig. 8 left).

The directions of the horizontal $(e_{ij}^{\rightarrow})$ and vertical $(e_{ij}^{\downarrow})$ edges inside a single unique n^2 subwindow can be used to construct a **decision tree** (Fig. 8). The maximal depth of the decision tree is given by the unique sub-window size n^2, hence the decision is made in constant time for arbitrary sized marker with the given unique sub-window size.

When a compact piece of the marker field is detected in the input image, the edges are classified and used for traversing the tree. The edges in the subwindows are selected in a predefined order (Fig. 8). Any cluster of neighboring edges is recognized by the tree – the leaf node would either define the cluster's location and orientation within the marker field or reject the cluster of edges as invalid (due to misdetection). By using a larger number of deciding edges, the tree can also be constructed **fault-tolerant** – the tree nodes can tolerate one or more falsely classified edges.

From the correctly identified sub-windows we calculate the location of the camera image center in the maker field. This information is sent to the content provider. The content provider then maps the position to display coordinates and updates the mixing mask and size for the marker field.

The complexity of the detection algorithm is dependent on the number of detected edges in the image. For given n edges the edgel search is done in $O(n)$ time, since from every detected edge point on the scanlines we take a finite number of steps to find edgels. The grid detection algorithm has $O(n \log n)$ complexity due to the need to sort the computed $(ki + q)$ parameters for the clustering. The rest of the detection algorithm (edge orientation extraction, sub-window identification and position extraction) requires constant time. More importantly the memory footprint of the algorithm is very low visiting only $\sim 5\%$, [15] of the image pixels. This is crucial for mobile processors.

4 Results: User Testing and Technical Evaluation

We performed a user test to find out the most acceptable shape of the marker field and the parameters of mixing it into the desktop screen image. The technical evaluation involves tests of reliability of detection of the marker field on different screen contents and under different viewing poses. Finally, computational performance is evaluated.

4.1 Marker Unobtrusiveness

We conducted an initial user study to observe how people would use our prototype. Our main goal was to find out how obtrusive was the usage of marker fields for task migration for participants and whether this approach is feasible also for inexperienced users.

The study we conducted consisted of 11 participants (8 male, 3 female). All attendees use at least one ultra-mobile device (mobile phone, smart phone, tablet, PDA) and one desktop computer or laptop on a daily basis. The average device count per participant was 2.9.

18% of our participants use their built-in photo camera on a daily basis, 54% several times in a week and 28% at least once in a month. 54% of participants use multiple devices for content reaccess on a daily basis. Their average age was 29 years, the youngest participant was 21 and the oldest was 46. Seven participants were from non-technical professions.

In the beginning, participants had to fill in a questionnaire. This questionnaire asked them about their technical expertise, their knowledge regarding mobile phones, as well as some demographic statements. Subsequently we introduced our system and three basic task migration scenarios – map state transfer, acquisition of short textual information from a web page and acquisition of an image from a long online article with a photo gallery.

In order to be able to compare feedback from participants, we have created ten marker presets divided into four categories (Fig. 9):

1. Marker with constant opacity (20%, 40% or 60%), without blurred background.
2. Marker with constant opacity (20%, 40% or 60%), with blurred background (gaussian blur with four pixel radius).
3. Marker with variable opacity, pulsing between 20% – 40% or 20% – 60%, without blurred background.
4. Marker with variable opacity, pulsing between 20% – 40% or 20% – 60%, with blurred background (gaussian blur with four pixel radius).

We provided the participants with an Android smartphone and a laptop with our system; the laptop also contained an application which allowed fast change of marker parameters from presets. Participants were asked to rate marker presets based on perceived obtrusiveness on a five point Likert scale (1–least obtrusive, 5–most obtrusive).

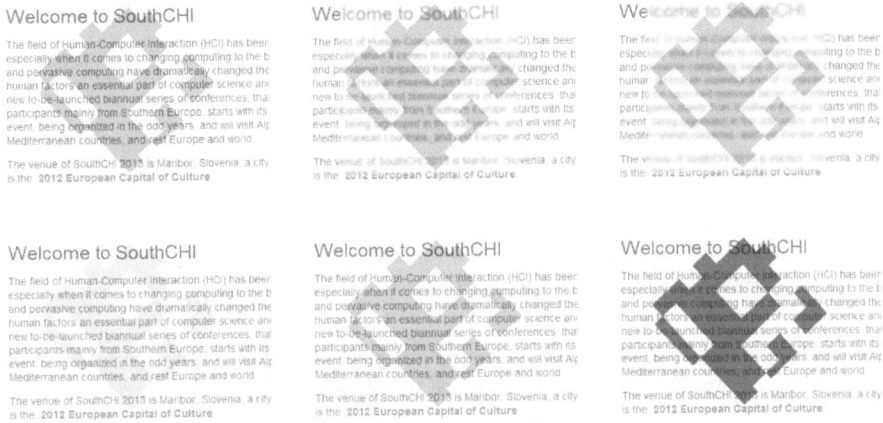

Fig. 9. Examples of mixed-in marker field with varying presets. **top row:** different background blur radii. **bottom row:** varying opacity levels (20, 40, 60 %).

Fig. 10 shows the user-reported average obtrusiveness for marker presets. The average rating across all presets was 2.47. Markers with high opacity were perceived as most obtrusive (average rating 3.76), while markers with 20% and 40% opacity had similar, significantly lower, average rating (1.67 and 2.12). Among our participants, the presence of blurred background or periodic changes in marker opacity had only minimal influence on perceived obtrusiveness. Application of blur on the background decreases the amount of natural edges present in the image and allows for the marker field edges to prevail. Similarly, the pulsing intensity of the marker allows for periodic appearances of highly opaque form of the marker field, which can be tracked afterwards or at least can provide localization information in discrete time frames. The fact that the users tend to tolerate these modes of mixing, offers truly reliable on-screen localization with acceptable levels of obtrusiveness.

We also conducted a test of our system with simulated network latency, in order to find out the maximum time the system should need until a content is returned to the user's device. The average time after which participants perceived system as poorly responding (obtrusiveness rating 3-5 on a 5-point Likert scale) was 4.5 seconds. This slightly contradicts the findings of Boring et al. [9], where a ten seconds response time was acceptable by most users.

In general, our system was perceived very positively, with 81% of participants stating that it would definitely help them with content reaccess. 63% of participants would use it to obtain information from public displays. In this case, the biggest concern were privacy issues – fear that a publicly available system could access private information stored in mobile devices due to security flaws.

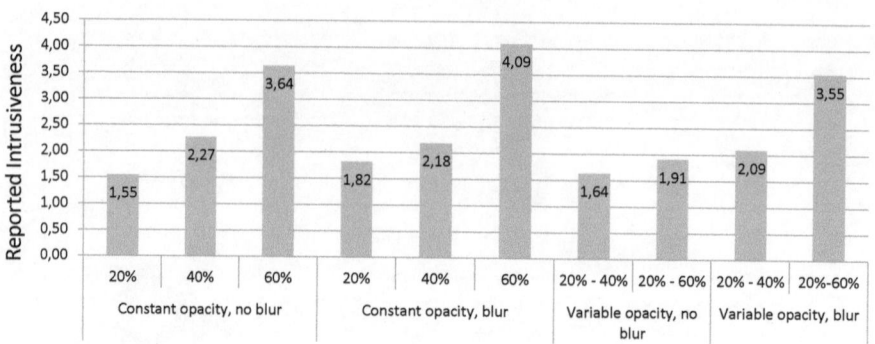

Fig. 10. Reported average obtrusiveness for marker presets. Percents under each bar are the marker opacity; percental ranges are the extremes of pulsing opacity.

4.2 Marker Detection Reliability

We tested the accuracy and reliability of our marker detection algorithm, with the marker mixed into natural screen contents. We created a setup consisting of one device in the role of content provider and one device in the role of content requester. As a content provider device we used a laptop computer with a high-resolution (1920 × 1080) display, and an Android 4.0.4 smartphone HTC Incredible S for the role of information requester device. The requester device was attached to a base perpendicular to the floor, in a fixed height, focused

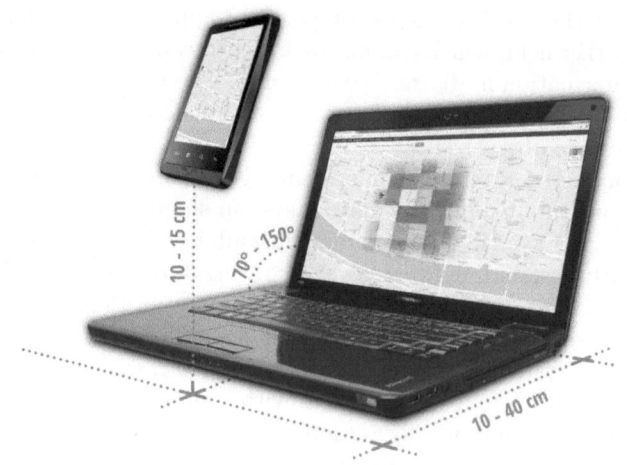

Fig. 11. Parameters of marker detection reliability setup – distance between mobile device and laptop, range of screen angles used during tests and height range of a mobile device in order to be focused on the same point on screen

at a chosen part of the screen (see Fig. 11). The experiment was conducted in a room with artificial (fluorescent) lighting. Devices were connected through a WiFi connection. The requester device was held at a distance of 10 (on graphs shown as near), 20 and 40 cm (on graphs shown as far) and a pitch angle of 70°, 90°, 110°, 130°, and 150°. On the content provider device a fullscreen webpage containing text, several smaller images, and a map was displayed during the experiment. The pulsing period for the pulsing marker was set to 1.5 seconds. The frame rate of the camera was 25 FPS.

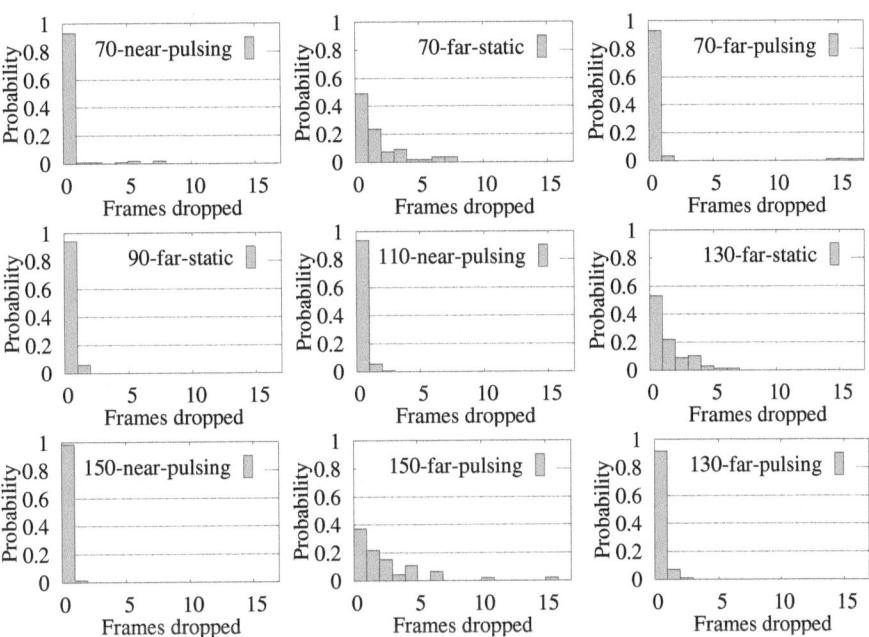

Fig. 12. Selected results of the reliability test. The histograms show the probability distribution of the time (in frame count) between consecutive successful position identifications. The name of the histogram corresponds to the pitch angle, distance from the content provider plane and whether the marker was pulsing (the pulsing period calculated in frames was 37.5 frames).

Fig. 12 shows some of the reliability tests based on the display tilt and the distance between the camera and the display. For the static (non-pulsing) marker mixing we used the average transparency used in the case of the pulsing marker. We chose from each set with different pitch at least one histogram. Between 90° and 110° the results were consistent with the data presented in Fig. 12 and thus they are omitted. The results show that even for 150° pitch angle (which was outside the viewing angles for the monitor) and from a large distance the pulsing marker was still reliably detectable within 5 frames (0.2 seconds) with 90 % probability.

The results indicate that the pulsing marker gave consistently better results then the static marker, especially at the extreme pitch angles (150°, 70°). This is mainly due to the fact that it is tricky to calibrate the correct transparency level for the static marker that is unobtrusive but still detectable by the smartphone camera for all the possible display pitch angles. Notice that histograms for the pulsing markers show two main peaks (Fig. 12 – 70-near-pulsing, 150-far-pulsing). The first one is near zero, since while the marker transparency is lower, the marker is detected in each frame. The second peak marks the interval, where the marker is too transparent during the pulsing period for the algorithm to be able to detect it (in the 70-near-pulsing histogram it is at 15 dropped frames which is about the third of the pulsing period).

Another observation concerning the detection reliability is that the results get better with a larger area of the visible marker in the camera view. This follows from the continuous marker design lacking localization patterns and relying only on regular structure detection. However, since the user during real-world usage would usually want to get the client closer to the content provider for more precise region selection, we do not see this as a limitation. In the near future, the framework will also be extended so that the visible marker region on the content provider would be resized dynamically based on the feedback from the client.

4.3   Speed Performance

In order to be able to compare our solution to other frameworks (primarily DeepShot [10]), we have tested four target applications: maps from Google Maps, photos from Picasa, long articles with images from CNN.com and short textual information from Twitter. For each application, ten information requests were sent and processed. The setup for this experiment was identical to the previous test.

The average time for all forty requests was 336 milliseconds (Standard Deviation 67 milliseconds). Table 1 summarizes an approximate breakdown of the time consumed in different phases of the processing. The marker field decoding (the "computational part" of the process) takes around one third of the time, whereas the rest is spent in network communication and related activities. From the marker field decoding part the edgel extraction and edge classification required on average ~60 % of the time on an older single core smartphone (HTC Desire with 1GHz ARM v7 processor released in 2010) even with the very low

Table 1. Timing breakdown of the mobile client

activity	% time spent
connection initialization	28 %
marker field detect & decode	34 %
network transfers	13 %
information retrieval	25 %

"pixel footprint" of the detection algorithm. The overall average time required by our naive implementation for mobile platforms excluding the system overhead to acquire the image was $34\,ms$ ($\sim$30 FPS) for 800×480 resolution extracting on average $\sim$120 edgels. We used standard web-site content as the background during these evaluations with the marker constantly visible in the field-of-view. Results might differ considerably for different smartphones or display content.

The results show a significant speed increase when compared to task migration solutions based on visual features. When compared to the DeepShot [10] task migration framework, our solution is on average $20.3\times$ faster (authors of the DeepShot report 7.7 seconds (Standard Deviation 0.3 seconds) for processing the frame) and allows for real-time information feedback for a selected screen area. At the same time, our solution operates on a video stream with all the benefits: if one camera frame fails for any reason, the mobile client program determines the location from a subsequent valid one, etc.

5   Conclusions

We presented a technical solution for reliable and unobtrusive interaction between a ultramobile device and another (typically desktop) monitor screen. We proposed a system architecture harnessing this communication in order to achieve task migration between the devices. This task migration procedure is designed to impose minimalistic requirements on the system setup and at the same time to be straightforward and intuitive to the user.

We measured the performance of the system and the results show that it substantially outperforms the existing solutions: the detection and recognition of the marker field is done in real time on a mid-level cellphone on a video stream; the recognition is reliable even for different observation angles and for cluttered screen content. We conducted a user study to select an as unobtrusive as possible variant of the marker field and the mixing parameters.

Our system allows for direct task migration, without any direct interaction with the desktop system – straight from the mobile device. Thanks to the usage of the marker field, the detection is reliable, because the system ensures reliable and easily detectable keypoints in the monitor screen. At the same time, the marker field proves to be unobtrusive and aesthetically tolerable by the user.

In the near future we intend to employ newly developed versions of the marker field design and detector: using colors, various shapes of the modules (not just squares), non-uniform module color/intensity, etc. Then, after implementing the plugins for a selected set of popular desktop and mobile applications, we intend to perform user testing of the whole system and report the users' perception of the practical use of this approach. The tests will focus on the obtrusiveness of the marker field inserted into real-life desktop content. Also, the speed and ease of task migration and reaccess will be evaluated.

Acknowledgments. This research was supported by the research CEZMSMT project IT4I - CZ 1.05/1.1.00/02.0070, by project V3C, TE01020415, and by project D-NOTAM TA02030835.

References

1. Bales, E., Sohn, T., Setlur, V.: Planning, apps, and the high-end smartphone: exploring the landscape of modern cross-device reaccess. In: Lyons, K., Hightower, J., Huang, E.M. (eds.) Pervasive 2011. LNCS, vol. 6696, pp. 1–18. Springer, Heidelberg (2011)
2. Karlson, A.K., Iqbal, S.T., Meyers, B., Ramos, G., Lee, K., Tang, J.C.: Mobile taskflow in context: a screenshot study of smartphone usage. In: Proceedings of the SIGCHI Conference on Human Factors in Computing Systems. CHI 2010, pp. 2009–2018. ACM, New York (2010)
3. Dearman, D., Pierce, J.S.: It's on my other computer!: computing with multiple devices. In: Proceedings of the SIGCHI Conference on Human Factors in Computing Systems, CHI 2008, pp. 767–776. ACM, New York (2008)
4. Harding, M., Storz, O., Davies, N., Friday, A.: Planning ahead: techniques for simplifying mobile service use. In: Proceedings of the 10th Workshop on Mobile Computing Systems and Applications, HotMobile 2009, pp. 1–13. ACM, New York (2009)
5. Bardram, E.: Activity-based computing: support for mobility and collaboration in ubiquitous computing. Personal Ubiquitous Comput. 9(5), 312–322 (2005)
6. Church, K., Smyth, B.: Understanding mobile information needs. In: Proceedings of the 10th International Conference on Human Computer Interaction with Mobile Devices and Services, MobileHCI 2008, pp. 493–494. ACM, New York (2008)
7. Pierce, J.S., Nichols, J.: An infrastructure for extending applications' user experiences across multiple personal devices. In: Proceedings of the 21st Annual ACM Symposium on User Interface Software and Technology, UIST 2008, pp. 101–110. ACM, New York (2008)
8. Liu, Q., McEvoy, P., Lai, C.-J.: Mobile camera supported document redirection. In: Proceedings of the 14th Annual ACM International Conference on Multimedia, MULTIMEDIA 2006, pp. 791–792. ACM, New York (2006)
9. Boring, S., Altendorfer, M., Broll, G., Hilliges, O., Butz, A.: Shoot & copy: phonecam-based information transfer from public displays onto mobile phones. In: Chong, P.H.J., Cheok, A.D. (eds.) Mobility Conference, pp. 24–31. ACM (2007)
10. Chang, T.H., Li, Y.: Deep shot: a framework for migrating tasks across devices using mobile phone cameras. In: Proceedings of the SIGCHI Conference on Human Factors in Computing Systems, CHI 2011, pp. 2163–2172. ACM, New York (2011)
11. Bay, H., Ess, A., Tuytelaars, T., Van Gool, L.: Speeded-up robust features (surf). Comput. Vis. Image Underst. 110(3), 346–359 (2008)
12. Klein, G., Murray, D.: Parallel tracking and mapping for small ar workspaces. In: Proceedings of the 2007 6th IEEE and ACM International Symposium on Mixed and Augmented Reality, ISMAR 2007, pp. 1–10. IEEE Computer Society, Washington, DC (2007)
13. Woo, G., Lippman, A., Raskar, R.: Vrcodes: Unobtrusive and active visual codes for interaction by exploiting rolling shutter. In: 2012 IEEE International Symposium on Mixed and Augmented Reality (ISMAR), pp. 59–64 (2012)
14. Szentandrasi, I., Zacharias, M., Havel, J., Herout, A., Dubska, M., Kajan, R.: Uniform marker fields: Camera localization by orientable de bruijn tori. In: 2012 IEEE International Symposium on Mixed and Augmented Reality (ISMAR), pp. 319–320 (2012)
15. Herout, A., Szentandrási, I., Zachariáš, M., Dubská, M., Kajan, R.: Five shades of grey for fast and reliable camera pose estimation. In: Proceedings of CVPR (2013)
16. Schaffalitzky, F., Zisserman, A.: Planar grouping for automatic detection of vanishing lines and points. Image and Vision Computing 18, 647–658 (2000)

Reading on eInk and Backlit LED – The Influence of Positive and Negative Contrast on Eye Movements

Yves Etienne Bochud and Marc Garbely

Swiss Distance University of Applied Sciences, Institute for Research in Open,
Distance- and eLearning, Brig, Switzerland
{yves.bochud,marc.garbely}@ffhs.ch

Abstract. This preliminary study aims at identifying possible differences in eye movements while reading either dark text on light background or light text on dark background on-screen. To this end, eye movements during reading with two different screen technologies which are dominant in the domain of mobile e-reading devices (i.e. eInk and backlit LED), have been examined for both negative and positive contrast. Results show that for reading on electronic displays, direction of contrast (negative/positive) has no significant influence on central eye movements involved in reading. Therefore, both positive and negative contrasts can be recommended when presenting text to users on-screen and provide good readability. This goes for either eInk or LED screens, however, a tendency for longer fixations was observed when reading with negative contrast on the LED screen. This may be due to the higher contrast on the LED screen, compared to the lower contrast of the eInk screen.

Keywords: readability, legibility, contrast, polarity effect, LED, eInk.

1   Introduction

In the last few years, reading on visual display units (VDU) has changed significantly and with the appearance of light and mobile e-reading devices, reading on-screen gained much popularity. The classic paper-book that formed our reading habits at least since the invention of modern print by Johannes Gutenberg back in the middle of the 15th century now seems to be confronted with serious competition, since studies showed [1] that there is no significant difference in eye-movements involved in reading when comparing paper, liquid crystal display (LCD) and eInk. eInk is a paper-like screen technology especially promoted for reading. The essential difference compared to LCD and LED (light-emitting diode) is the fact that the screen isn't backlit. Furthermore, the shown page is static on eInk, rather than being refreshed at a given frequency. Beside the better mobility due to large storage capacity of such e-reading devices compared to classic paper-books, they offer the possibility to adjust for fontsize, illumination and contrast. Compared to the convention to read on paper, these new possibilities in adjusting the text to personal preferences could have positive effects on reading, for example in terms of visual strain and fatigue.

A. Holzinger et al. (Eds.): SouthCHI 2013, LNCS 7946, pp. 711–720, 2013.

Especially the direction of contrast and its influence on readability are debated in internet-forums and blogs, most of them related to topics like e-reading or web design. The majority of people seems to think that a negative contrast (that is, dark text on light background) is suited best for reading, while others claim that reading light text on dark background (positive contrast) is more relaxing for the eyes and is less fatiguing. There is some experimental proof for such a polarity effect (i.e. light text on dark background is harder to process by our visual system): Studies found that text is less readable and letter identification is decreased [2], [3] text is more difficult to read [4], error rates for character recognition and detection-of-discrepancy tasks are increased [5] and error-detection rates when proof-reading are lowered [6]. Other studies found small differences or very similar results for the two contrast conditions, for example for reading rates [7]. Contrary, other researchers did not find differences in readability but nevertheless showed that the traditional dark-on-light color scheme was preferred by the readers [8]. Research on reading text with impaired vision revealed that for people with low vision, the presentation of light text on dark background leads to a faster reading [9].

However, these studies date back to the mid-eighties and screen technologies have notably improved since then. It is therefore questionable if those results will hold for newer screen-technologies, as well as for newer methods to measure readability of text (i.e. by analyzing eye movements involved in reading). So far, most results concerning those questions are mainly based on user ratings or performance measures, rather than objective data directly related to visual processes involved in reading. Especially the specific eye movements involved in reading have not – to the best of our knowledge – been researched systematically to determine the effect of negative/positive contrast on the reading on-screen.

As of today, dark font on light background seems to be the standard for reading on digital devices. Nevertheless, it has not been prooven that this way of presenting textual information is best in order to be processed by our visual system when reading on-screen. The pilot study at hand therefore investigates eye movements involved in reading light-on-dark vs. dark-on-light text on two different e-reading devices, one using eInk and one LED. Since prior studies revealed no differing effects while reading on eInk vs. LCD in terms of eye-movements or experienced fatigue and eye-strain [1], [10], it is hypothesized that screen technology will have no influence on eye-movements while reading. Based on the results of the studies mentioned above, we expect patterns of eye-movements for the different contrast conditions to vary as follows: For people with normal vision, negative contrast leads to lower readability (in terms of more regressive saccades and longer fixation durations).

2   Methods

2.1   Participants

The six subjects (3 female; mean age = 28.67, SD = 1.97) all reported normal or corrected-to-normal vision. All subjects voluntarily participated in the experiment.

Lowest level of education was tertiary school level. The study was performed according to the latest declaration of Helsinki and participants gave written informed consent before participation.

2.2   Apparatus

For the recording of eye movements, a remote infrared eye tracking device was used (RED500, Sensumotoric Instruments, Teltow, Germany). The device has a sampling rate of 500Hz and a gaze position accuracy of 0.4 degrees of visual angle. The viewing distance was fixed at a distance of approximately 50 cm. The system compensates for minor head movements with a head tracking range of 40 x 20 cm at 70 cm distance. Therefore, no headrest was used to ensure comfortable reading.

2.3   Stimuli

We used two different e-reading devices for the presentation of the text material: one device supporting the eInk-technology (Kindle DX) and the other one with a backlit LED screen (Apple iPad 2). Technical specifications of the devices used in this study are summarized in table 1. Contrasts of both devices were measured with a luminance meter (Minolta LS-110) and computed by means of Weber contrasts ($CW = (I_F-I_B)/I_B$), where I_F is the luminance of the Font and I_B is the luminance of the background (both measured in cd/m^2). Negative contrast indicates dark text on light background, whereas a positive contrast indicates light text on dark background.

We carried out the experiment under an indirect artificial lighting condition (halogen spot light) in order to avoid differential effects related to reflections on the screens of the reading devices used in this study, since the high-gloss display of the LED device used leads – in contrast to the matt display of the eInk device – to irritating reflections on the screen if illuminated directly. The luminance was measured at 535 lux with a Roline digital lux meter (RO-1332) five centimeters above the plane in which the text material was presented.

Table 1. Technical specifications of the e-reading devices used in this study

Device	Screen Technology	Screen Size (Inches)	Screen Resolution	Pixels per Inch (ppi)	Contrast $CW=(I_F-I_B)/I_B$
Kindle DX	eInk	9.7	1022 x 744	150	-0.80 / 0.80
iPad 2	LED-backlit	9.7	1024 x 768	132	-26.53 / 26.53

The text material used was the first two chapters of the novel *Treasure Island* by Robert Louis Stevenson (German translation). Capital letters covered 0.28 to 0.38 degrees of visual angle vertically, depending on head position and optimal viewing distance. The amount of words read in each of the four experimental conditions was equal (600 words). Figure 1 gives an impression of the two contrast conditions (positive vs. negative) used in this pilot study.

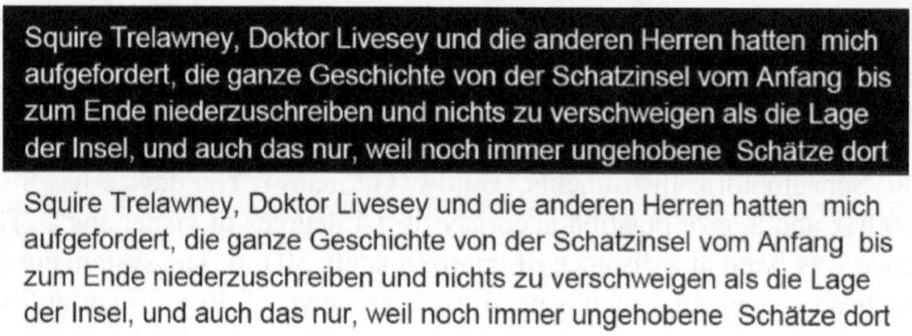

Squire Trelawney, Doktor Livesey und die anderen Herren hatten mich aufgefordert, die ganze Geschichte von der Schatzinsel vom Anfang bis zum Ende niederzuschreiben und nichts zu verschweigen als die Lage der Insel, und auch das nur, weil noch immer ungehobene Schätze dort

Squire Trelawney, Doktor Livesey und die anderen Herren hatten mich aufgefordert, die ganze Geschichte von der Schatzinsel vom Anfang bis zum Ende niederzuschreiben und nichts zu verschweigen als die Lage der Insel, und auch das nur, weil noch immer ungehobene Schätze dort

Fig. 1. Examples of modified text material with positive (top) and negative contrast (bottom) used in the pilot study at hand

2.4   Procedure

The participants were introduced to the experimental procedure by the experimenter. After this short introduction, they filled in a questionnaire which collected demographical data as well as other characteristics relevant to this pilot study (reading experience, education, etc.). Participants were told that they will have to read four different passages of text on two different reading devices. This results in four different experimental conditions: eInk light-on-dark, eInk dark-on-light, LED light-on-dark, and LED dark-on-light. Therefore, the design of the experiment was 2 x 2 whithin-subjects and the order in which the experimental conditions were presented to the participants was randomized. Before starting to read in each condition, the eye tracking-system was calibrated in order to ensure best possible tracking quality. After each experimental condition, participants were asked to indicate the experienced readability of the Text on a 5-point Likert-scale, ranging from "very poor" to "very good". After reading under each of the four experimental conditions, which took approximately 25 minutes in total, the experimenter thanked the participants and released them from the experiment.

3   Results

Legibility influences reading. This fact has been shown for different aspects of readability of text, e.g. [11] for font legibility or [1] and [12] for legibility of text presented on different screen-technologies or media. Generally speaking, the readability of a text is influenced by two factors: First, how easy the text is to understand (= difficulty of the text-material) and second, how easy the text is to process visually (= visual "processability" of the text-material). In this short paper, we will focus on the second factor by manipulating the contrast of the text material and the screen technology used to present the text material to the subjects. All analyses (if not mentioned otherwise) have been carried out deploying a general linear model with repeated measures.

3.1   Fixations

Longer fixation times indicate difficulties in extracting information [13] and a smaller amount of fixations indicates a better visual processability of the text material read, for example due to sub-optimal layout of the materials presented [13].

Fixation Duration
For the analysis of data, only fixations with durations of a range from 80ms up to 2000ms were entered as fixations in the final analysis. Table 2 gives an overview of the mean number of fixations made in each experimental condition. The statistical analysis did not yield any significant differences for the fixation durations under the four experimental conditions ($F = 2.16$, $df = 3$, $p = 0.136$).

Table 2. Fixation durations for the four experimental conditions. $N = 6$.

Experimental Condition	Mean Fixation Duration (in ms)	Standard Deviation
eInk dark-on-light	221.79	62.23
eInk light-on-dark	329.51	125.92
LED dark-on-light	283.79	82.55
LED light-on-dark	247.51	57.06

Number of Fixations
With regard to the number of fixations made under the four experimental conditions, no significant differences have been found ($F = 0.02$, $df = 3$, $p = .996$). Table 3 gives an overview on the mean number of fixations and corresponding standard deviations.

Table 3. Mean number of fixations for both contrast conditions on the two e-reading devices. $N = 6$.

Experimental Condition	Number of Fixations (mean)	Standard Deviation
eInk dark-on-light	314.17	132.84
eInk light-on-dark	325.17	92.05
LED dark-on-light	305.83	76.46
LED light-on-dark	315.67	219.59

Letters per Fixation
In terms of letters per fixation, the manipulation of the screen technology used and the direction of contrast did not have a significant influence on this metric either ($F = 0.50$, $df = 3$, $p = .668$). Table 4 summarizes these results.

Table 4. Letters per fixation for the four experimental conditions. $N = 6$.

Experimental Condition	Letters per Fixation (mean)	Standard Deviation
eInk dark-on-light	3.59	2.19
eInk light-on-dark	3.01	1.13
LED dark-on-light	3.09	0.69
LED light-on-dark	4.41	3.46

3.2   Saccades

Regressive saccades (a saccade against the reading direction) indicate difficulties in reading text and serve to re-examine text passages that were difficult to process or understand [14]. Regressive saccades with amplitudes higher than 70% of line length were classified as line sweeps and excluded from data analysis.

Proportion of Regressive and Progressive Saccades
Table 5 shows the proportion of regressive and progressive saccades under the four experimental conditions. No significant differences between the conditions have been detected ($F = 0.80$, $df = 3$, $p = .516$).

Table 5. Percent of regressive and progressive saccades (*SD* for regressive saccades in brackets, line sweeps excluded). $N = 6$.

Experimental Condition	Porgressive Saccades (%)	Regressive Saccades (%)
eInk dark-on-light	68.88	31.12 (0.13)
eInk light-on-dark	61.61	38.39 (0.09)
LED dark-on-light	62.51	37.49 (0.12)
LED light-on-dark	58.95	41.05 (0.12)

Number of Regressive Saccades
The analysis of the regressive saccades made in each experimental condition didn't indicate significant differences between the two contrast and screen technology conditions ($F = 0.92$, $df = 3$, $p = .455$). Results are shown in table 6.

Table 6. Number of regressive saccades for the four experimental conditions. $N = 6$.

Experimental Condition	Number of Regressive Saccades	Standard Deviation
eInk dark-on-light	84.17	16.28
eInk light-on-dark	122.67	40.96
LED dark-on-light	115.33	46.96
LED light-on-dark	117.50	63.17

3.3   Subjective Measures

Next to the central eye-movement data, we collected data on subjective readability measures after each reading block as well. Table 7 shows the results for each of the four experimental conditions. A simple t-test for repeated measures showed a significant difference in the subjective ratings for the four experimental conditions ($F = 14.61$, $df = 3$, $p = .000$).

Table 7. Subjective readability ratings for the four experimental conditions (Likert-scale ranging from 1 = «very poor readability» to 5 = «very high readability»). $N = 6$.

Condition	Contrast (CW)	Mean Rating	Standard Deviation	Post-hoc: Significant Difference to
1. eInk (dark-on-light)	-0.80	4.33	0.82	2 and 4
2. eInk (light-on-dark)	0.80	2.33	0.52	1 and 3
3. LED (dark-on-light)	-26.53	3.83	0.98	2 and 4
4. LED (light-on-dark)	26.53	1.67	0.52	1 and 3

4   Discussion

The results of this study are preliminary in nature, and therefore more research is needed on this topic to validate the results found in the experiment described. On one hand, more subjects have to be tested in order to get more reliable data. On the other hand, the degree of contrast should be varied, since the highest contrast condition led to longer fixation durations. As [7] already stated when discussing their results on differing contrast conditions, *"this raises the possibility that a contrast polarity effect may be found for low-contrast reading even when it is not evident at high contrasts"*. Furthermore, the kind of task (scanning, reading, proof-reading, etc.) that has to be carried out will presumably have an impact on the results found for differing contrast conditions, especially for positive vs. negative contrast. In addition, despite the fact that there are no significant objective differences for reading on paper vs. reading on LCD or eInk [1], [15] except for the subjective preference of the former by users [15], a control condition where people read on classic paper should be introduced for experimentation check purposes. Finally, it seems likely that reading over a longer period of time could as well be different from reading for short sequences (subjects in this study read for approximately 3 minutes in each of the four conditions).

Another point to consider is the fact that human beings are used to read with negative contrast. Vision is a constructional process and depends on learning processes related to eye movements [16]. Therefore, a learning-effect cannot yet be ruled out in the explanation of the subjective results found in this preliminary study concerning reading with positive and negative contrast. As shown by neuro-psychologists [17], the ability to perceive objects and characters can be increased or decreased by means of long-term potentiation or long-term depression, respectively. In that light, it is likely that earlier experience of the subjects has an influence on their reading performance, as well as on eye movements during reading tasks. It would therefore be advisable to conduct an experiment with tasks where a polarity effect has been found by previous studies and to conduct a second series with participants that were specially trained in positive contrast reading. It could be hypothesized that for trained subjects the polarity effect will be reduced or even removed completely compared to untrained subjects. This consideration is further strengthened by the fact that the objective measures didn't show significant differences between the four reading conditions, whereas the subjective ratings showed a clear preference for the classic dark-on-light color scheme.

One possible explanation for the subjectively bad legibility of light text on dark background could as well be based on lateral inhibition, a neural principle describing how information is processed by bipolar neurons in the upper layers of the retina. The term lateral inhibition refers the fact that a neuron's activity can be inhibited by the activation of its adjacent neurons. If confronted with contrast changes (as for example in reading), this effect leads to the subjective impression of a higher or lower brightness near the edges [18]. This effect of a subjectively increased or decreased brightness perception in edge-detection is illustrated in figure 2.

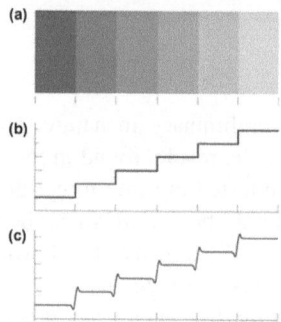

Fig. 2. Schematic illustration of the measured (B) and perceived brightness (C) on the example of Mach bands with increasing brightness intensity (A). Source: [19].

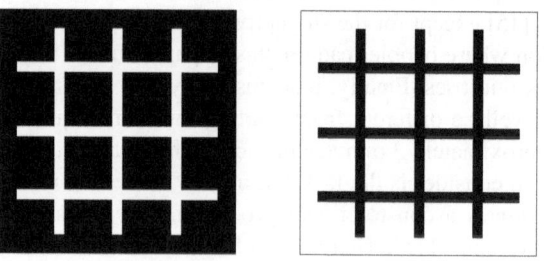

Fig. 3. Example of two Hermann grids for negative and positive contrast

Another example of an optical illusion explained by lateral inhibition is the Hermann grids in figure 3. When not focusing an intersection directly in the examples below, we have the impression of a gray dot appearing right in the middle of the intersections. When focusing the intersections directly, the illusion disappears.

Since we are used to read dark-on-light, the illusion of black shades on the white „text" (left example in figure 3 with positive contrast) is likely to be perceived as more disturbing than in the right example in figure 3. When we think of a conventional and natural reading-setup, then the majority of people will most likely prefer to read black text on white paper, and not black text on a white display or with inverted contrast. The brightness of the background is therefore more similar to the surrounding in most everyday settings (in terms of brightness-differences) than the text material printed on it. If we now read light-on-dark, then the brightness of text is closer to the surrounding and appears to be „framed" by the black background, just as if the text would be a plane behind the background. In Gestalt Psychology this visual discrimination problem is called figure-ground perception. This or the aforementioned lateral inhibition effect could contribute to an explanation as to why subjects tend to feel uncomfortable with the positive contrast condition. In this light, it is possible that participants did not read long enough under the same contrast condition to reveal differing effects. This means that further research has to be carried out, investigating the effect of contrast on eye movements during longer reading. If the effect is in fact dominant and irritating for the visual processing system and thus influences reading, that will as well be further clarified by conducting a follow-up study where subjects read for a longer period of time.

It is obvious that more studies with objective (i.e. eye movements) rather than subjective data (i.e. perceived readability) are required in order to disentangle the mixed results concerning a polarity effect when reading on digital media. The aim of this study was to contribute to the discussion on a polarity effect when reading on e-reading devices, with respect that it raised questions about the influence of positive and negative contrast for text-presentation on screen. Further research is needed to clarify the influence of contrast strength – particularly high contrasts – on the eye movements involved in reading.

This preliminary study suggests for people with normal vision that, especially for low contrast (eInk), the valence of contrast plays only a minor role for readability in terms of subjective preferences, since the objective measures show no significant differences in terms of objective eye movements.

Acknowledgments. We would like to thank all the subjects who participated voluntarily in this preliminary study. Moreover, we would like to thank Prof. Dr. Réne Müri from the Perception and Eye Movement Laboratory at the University Hospital in Bern for the provision of the luminance meter used in this study. The study was supported by the Swiss Distance University of Applied Sciences.

References

1. Siegenthaler, E., Wurtz, P., Bergamin, P., Groner, R.: Comparing reading processes on e-ink displays and print. Displays 32(5), 268–273 (2011)

2. Scharff, L.F.V., Ahumada Jr., A.J.: Predicting the readability of transparent text. Journal of Vision 2(9), 653–666 (2002)
3. Scharff, L.F.V., Ahumada Jr., A.J.: Contrast measures for predicting text readability. In: Rogowitz, B.E., Pappas, T.N. (eds.) Human Vision and Electronic Imaging VII. SPIE Proc, vol. 5007, Paper 46 (2003)
4. Zuffi, S., Brambilla, C., Beretta, G., Scala, P.: Human Computer Interaction: Legibility and contrast. In: 14th International Conference on Image Analysis and Processing, ICIAP (2007)
5. Bauer, D., Cavonius, C.R.: Improving the legibility of video display unitsthrough contrast reversal. In: Grandjean, E., Vigliani, E. (eds.) Ergonomic Aspects of Video Display Terminals, pp. 137–142. Taylor & Francis, London (1980)
6. Buchner, A., Mayr, S., Brandt, M.: The advantage of positive text-background Polarity is due to high display luminance. Ergonomics 52(7), 882–886 (2009)
7. Legge, G.E., Rubin, G.S., Luebker, A.: Psychophysics of reading: V. The role of contrast in normal vision. Vision Res. 27(7), 1165–1177 (1987)
8. Hall, R.H., Hanna, P.: The impact of web page text-background colour combinations on readability, retention, aesthetics and behavioural intention. Behaviour & Information Technology 23(3), 183–195 (2004)
9. Rubin, G.S., Legge, G.E.: Psychophysics of reading: V. The role of contrast in low vision. Vision Res. 29(1), 79–91 (1989)
10. Siegenthaler, E., Bochud, Y., Bergamin, P., Wurtz, P.: Reading on LCD vs. e-Ink displays: effects on fatigue and visual strain. Ophthalmic and Physiological Optics 32(5), 367–374 (2012)
11. Mansfield, J.S., Legge, G.E., Bane, M.C.: Psychophysics of reading: XV. Font effects in normal and low vision. Invest. Opthalmol. Vis. Sci. 37, 1492–1501 (1996)
12. Van de Velde, C., Grünau, M.: Tracking eye movements while reading: Printing press versus the cathode ray tube. Abstract Supplement (2003)
13. Poole, A., Ball, L.J.: Eye Tracking in Human-Computer Research: Current status and future prospects. In: Ghaoui, C. (ed.) Encyclopedia of Human Computer Interaction, pp. 211–219. Idea Group Reference (2006)
14. Morrison, R.E., Inhoff, A.W.: Visual factors and eye movement in reading. Visible Language 15(2), 129–146 (1981)
15. Holzinger, A., Baernthaler, M., Pammer, W., Katz, H., Bjelic-Radisic, V., Ziefle, M.: Investigating paper vs. screen in real-life hospital workflows: Performance contradicts perceived superiority of paper in the user experience. International Journal of Human-Computer Studies 69(9), 563–570 (2011)
16. Hayhoe, M.M., Ballard, D.H.: Mechanisms of gaze control in natural vision. In: Liversedge, S.P., Gilchrist, I.D., Everling, S. (eds.) The Oxford Handbook of EyeMovements, Oxford University Press, Oxford (2011)
17. Beste, C., Wascher, E., Güntürkün, O., Dinse, H.R.: Improvement and impairment of visually guided behavior through LTP- and LTD-like exposure-based visual learning. Curr. Biol. 21, 876–882 (2011)
18. Goldstein, E.B.: Sensation and Perception, 6th edn. Wadsworth, Belmont (2002)
19. Faria, A.W.C., Menotti, D., Pappa, G.L., Lara, D.S.D., Araujo, A.: A methodology for photometric validation in vehicles visual interactive systems. Expert Systems with Applications: An International Journal 39(4), 4122–4134 (2012)

Exploring Hand Posture for Smart Mobile Devices

Ionuţ-Alexandru Zaiţi, Radu-Daniel Vatavu, and Ştefan-Gheorghe Pentiuc

University Ştefan cel Mare of Suceava, 13, Universitatii, Suceava, 720229, Romania
ionutzaiti@yahoo.com, {vatavu,pentiuc}@eed.usv.ro
www.eed.usv.ro/~vatavu

Abstract. In the context of increasing complexity of mobile applications, by not exploring the hands' many degrees of freedom the touch-screen interaction can appear as limited. Current computer interfaces have begun to take gestures into consideration more and more to provide a better user experience. Given that most of the interaction we have with our environment is accomplished through our hands, hand gestures make an ideal candidate for human computer interaction input. In this paper we present a glove based interface to provide additional input data based on hand postures on top of multi-touch gestures in applications for smart mobile devices with touchscreens. We describe application opportunities for employing hand posture for mobile devices. Using hand postures as shortcuts simplifies interactions and interfaces.

Keywords: human computer interaction, gesture recognition, gestural interface, mobile device, smartphone, touchscreen, touch gestures.

1 Introduction

Interactions with mobile devices are achieved using our hands but through gestures that are designed and not naturally occurring. Meanwhile, computer interfaces have begun to take advantage and integrate natural hand gestures in order to provide a more efficient and more pleasant experience. We consider that using hand posture information in smart mobile devices interfaces can lead to the next step in the evolution of mobile interaction. Given the range of gestures and gesture complexity that the human hand is capable of performing [1] we consider that natural hand gestures supporting the interaction with touchscreens would greatly increase the quality of the user experience.

We implemented several applications for smartphones in which the interaction is performed through combinations of hand postures and touch gestures. The information on the hand postures has been collected using a data glove. The posture of a hand is given by the flexion and aperture values of fingers at a point in time. We consider dynamic hand gestures (in which the hand goes through various successive postures such as moving the fingers) as well as static gestures (in which the hand maintains a relatively stable posture for a period of time, such as holding a closed fist).

A. Holzinger et al. (Eds.): SouthCHI 2013, LNCS 7946, pp. 721–731, 2013.
© Springer-Verlag Berlin Heidelberg 2013

2   Interacting with Smart Mobile Devices

Smart mobile devices have had an impressive evolution in both the employed technology and the popularity they have benefited among users. In 2011 the sales of smartphones reached the quota of 472 million units as opposed to the 139.29 million units in 2008[1]. These devices present multiple features such as high resolution cameras, ambient light sensors, proximity sensors, GPS, accelerometer, compass, gyros, pressure, temperature and humidity sensors which combined with a continuously increasing processing power create the opportunity for enriched interfaces.

A large contribution to the popularity of smart mobile devices has been made by the touchscreen, an "electronic visual display that can detect the presence and location of a touch within the display area." [2]. The simple interaction model which allows the direct manipulation of displayed entities leads to one of the easiest to use interfaces [3].

The simplicity of the touchscreen comes with disadvantages as well cause of a single way of interacting with objects on the screen. Any step up in the complexity of the application could potentially bring difficulties in the interaction such as navigating through intricate menus, selecting and combining various actions (a simple example is an image editing application). Simple touch gestures have been introduced to act as shortcuts for various actions such as swipe to browse a page, drag to move an object or double touch to zoom [4]. A further improvement was multi-touch which allowed the detection of multiple touch points on the surface of the screen. This permitted the use of more complex gestures such as pinch open or pinch close for zooming in and out. Based on simple and multi touch gestures various other techniques were designed meant to ease the interaction such as gesture search [5] or avatar gestures [6].

Ultimately, the touchscreen has remained basically unchanged while the processing power and other features of smartphones have significantly evolved. One of the main focus of research is the technology behind it in order to obtain a good physical material for greater durability and resistance to scratches or liquids while maintaining a high image quality, low response times, error rates and power consumption.

2.1   Touchscreen Technology

There are multiple approaches to building touchscreens such as electrical, acoustic and optical [2]. Electrical touchscreens are based on either capacitive sensors [7] or resistive and conductive layers [8]. These two types are currently the most widely spread types of touchscreens due to their low cost [9] but they also present disadvantages. Resistive touchscreens have a lower clarity and resistance to damages while capacitive touchscreens, though offering a higher clarity, have to be engaged with a conductive object which means they cannot be used with most styluses or gloved hands.

---

[1] www.statista.com/statistics/12856/
number-of-smartphones-sold-to-end-users-worldwide-since-2007

The optical technology is based on detecting whenever there is an interruption in the infrared light transmitted across the screen allowing the user to interact with it using any object or gloved hands offering at the same time a very good image quality [2,9]. However, these touchscreens do present the problem of a higher error rate because the sensing technology is outside the screen itself. That can cause a response from the screen even when the user is only hovering a finger or stylus over it without intention to touch.

The most advanced technology used for touchscreens is acoustics in which sound is used to identify the coordinates of screen touches. The surface acoustic wave (SAW) technology [2,9] provides a high image clarity and durability (due to the fact that the technology is not embedded in the glass itself) but it is relatively expensive. The point of touch is determined through the absorption of the waves caused by the touch using a soft tip object (bare or gloved hands, soft tip stylus), which are then intercepted by sensors and translated into coordinates.

Another acoustic technology used in touchscreens is bending waves which is unpowered signal sources, less affected by contaminants as opposed to SAW [10].

2.2 Touchscreen Drawbacks and Solutions

Ultimately, the technology behind touchscreens is set to provide a higher accuracy and response time in returning the touch point coordinates but the interaction remains the same and so do the problems which have been noticed early on in the touchscreen evolution [11,12]. One difficult problem is represented by selecting and manipulating a target on the screen, given that the resolution of the human finger is low. This is even more troublesome in the case of mobile devices with small screen real estate.

Fitts' law [13] gives us a measure of the time needed to select a target on a device using a cursor, which is directly proportionate to the distance to the target over its width. Sears et al. [12] argued a revised version of Fitts' law is required in the case of touchscreens as there is no need to locate the cursor position since the cursor follows the point of the touch. They suggested that the time it takes to reach and touch the screen (using either a finger or a stylus) should be considered combined with the time needed to reach the target from the original touch point (which depends on the target width).

Using either Fitts' law or a revised version could improve touchscreen interaction. The most accessible factor is the width of the target which when increased makes the target much easier to both track and interact with. This however could prove to be troublesome especially in the case of small mobile devices for which the onscreen space is already limited.

Various techniques were introduced for managing the selection and handling problems in touchscreens such as the take-off, first-contact or land-on [11,12,14]. These techniques were designed for technologies that provide a continuous stream of data (take-off, first-contact) as well as for those that do not (land-on). A successful technique is the take-off, in which a cursor is placed at an offset from the touch point in order for it to be visible and easier to control.

Some of the more recent attempts at improving touchscreen interaction take advantage of single and multi-touch gestures to select targets [6,15,16]. The Shift technique [16] considers that targets smaller than the finger tip are harder to control (or visualize once touched) so the area that is being hidden behind the finger is displayed to the user in a small window above the finger. This allows a precision similar to a pen based input using a finger-based input without accommodation on switching between the two. Another approach is Gesture Avatar [6], which allows the user to associate smaller targets with a larger, easier to control avatar.

2.3 Touchscreen Innovations and Improvements Brought on by Other Technologies

Besides the continuous work to provide a better touchscreen technology using the basic quality criteria [2] there have also been improvements from modifications of the actual technology itself to add new features as in the case of Tactus [17]. The Tactus technology provides a touchscreen whose surface is deformable and allows the action of buttons and shapes rising up from the tactile surface and then falling back in when no longer needed. A much more interactive experience is thus provided through the joint actions of using a keyboard and a touchscreen.

Other improvements brought to the interaction with mobile devices are based on using other technologies, either standalone or combined with touchscreens. A very popular approach is based on the motion sensors (accelerometers, gyroscopes, magnetometers) of a mobile device [18,19], an approach used even for text entry methods as in the case of TiltText [20] (text entry using a keypad and aided by the tilt of the device) or GesText [21] (accelerometer only text entry). One of the drawbacks of using motion gestures as an input is the high potential of false positives since the gestures may be similar to many involuntary actions done throughout our daily activity (tilting the device or even any random movement). One solution is using gesture delimiters such as the double flip [22] in order to separate involuntary actions from the deliberate interaction.

Using a technology which is external to the smart mobile device [23,24] is another option to provide an additional input. This presents the advantage that it may also be used to control and communicate with other technologies offering consistency in human computer interaction in an environment quickly evolving towards ubiquitous computing.

3   Merging Hand Posture and Multi-touch

The evolution of the mobile device interfaces has been lead by the requirements of users. A keypad mobile phone still satisfies the condition of making a phone call in an efficient manner. However, today's technology conscious user has a constant need for complex applications and implicitly, the need for an efficient way to interact. The touchscreen itself is a display of the continuous increase in requirements. The simple touch interface for mobile devices has been improved considerably over a relatively short period of time to support touch gestures. Multi-touch followed as well as various other techniques and additions, either software [5,6] or hardware [17,25], overcoming the shortcomings of touchscreens, but up to a point.

Our day to day life can be described by the interaction we have with our environment and with people around us, activities which are heavily supported by hand gestures [1]. The human hand is capable of both simple and complex gestures which makes it a valuable source of information and can be used as an input modality human computer interaction. Even though today's interfaces are based more and more on gestures[2] we consider that the potential of the human hand as an input device has still to be reached [26,27].

We propose the perspective of using hand posture data in order to enrich touchscreen interaction, working with a 5DT Data Glove[3] which offers 14 highly accurate sensors measuring finger flexion (two sensors per finger) as well as the proximity between each pair of successive fingers. Furthermore we consider that using natural hand gestures could benefit the user's experience, providing valuable additional information to the multi-touch interfaces. We implemented several applications to illustrate the improvements in the degree of freedom that can be gained by the use of natural hand gestures. For these applications we used the 5DT Ultra Glove with a regular laptop as an intermediary between the data glove and the smartphone, a Motorola Defy running Android 2.1.

4   Interactive Opportunities

Applications connect to a server application (in our case running on the laptop, to which the data glove is connected, collecting and interpreting hand posture data). When a touch event takes place on the screen of the smartphone the mobile application retrieves the necessary information from the laptop server application. The communication between the two applications running on the laptop and the smartphone is based on network sockets for which a simple exchange protocol was implemented. While not practical in a real life scenario, this implementation allowed us to rapidly prototype gesture based interfaces for mobile devices while being able to replace the gesture acquisition equipment with others that may prove to be more suitable [28,29].

4.1   Drawing with Different Fingers

An application for painting can be extremely difficult using only touch gestures. The various possible colors and actions would be selected individually by going through a menu either hidden or displayed on the screen. In the case of a hidden

---

[2] Video game sensors: Nintendo Wii (http://www.wii.com/), PlayStation MoveMe (http://us.playstation.com/ps3/playstation-move/move-me/),   Microsoft Kinect (http://www.xbox.com/en-GB/kinect), Motion and touch gestures for mobile devices [18,21,5,6,19,20].

[3] http://www.5dt.com/products/pdataglove14.html

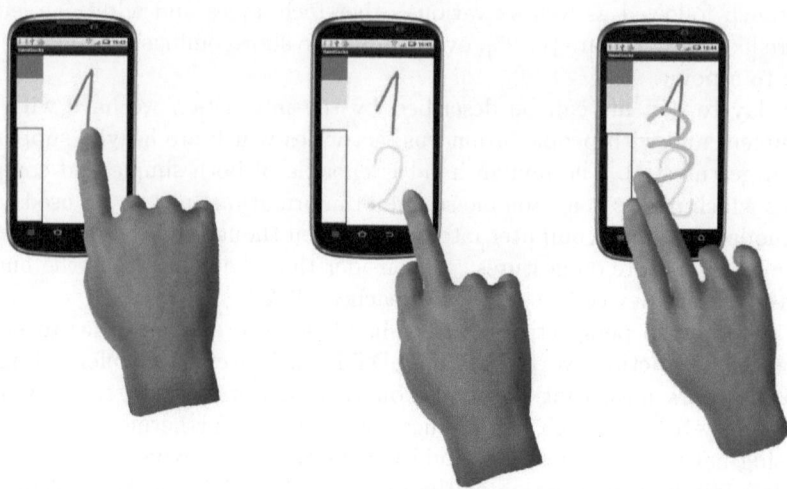

Fig. 1. Paint application using hand postures: (a) Drawing using the index finger which is associated to a color selected by the user. (b) Drawing using the middle finger in a similar manner to the index finger. (c) Drawing using index and middle fingers stuck together which results in a larger mark for which the color is the combination of the colors associated to the two fingers.

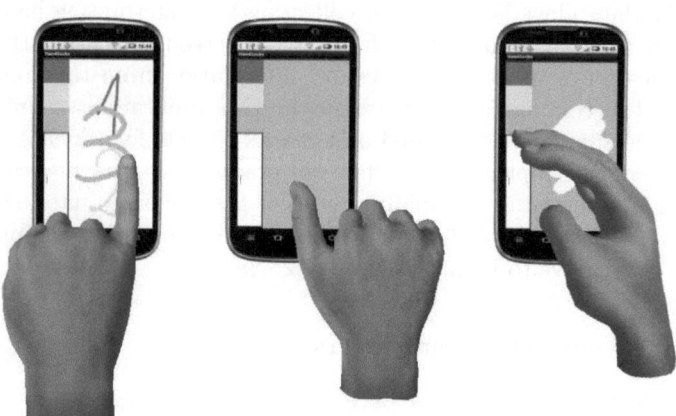

Fig. 2. Paint application for smartphones using hand postures as inputs from left to right: (a) Using the little finger to identify the color obtained in the last step. (b) Filling the screen with that color using the thumb. (c) Erasing by rubbing the screen with the side of the hand.

menu, the process could be tedious to the user, even the simplest of actions requires opening the menu and then navigating to the wanted item (possibly through submenus). A menu which is displayed on the screen could turn out to be inefficient considering it takes space from the relatively small display of smart mobile devices.

Using hand postures we designed a few shortcuts when interacting with the Paint application:

a. **Color fingers** - we explored the opportunity of assigning data to specific postures; more specifically in our case the gestures which have the index, middle or the thumb finger stretched are associated with colors which can be changed by the user at any point (Fig. 1a,b)

b. **Painting** - the index and middle fingers can be used similarly to a brush by touching the screen and leaving a mark of the currently associated color; touching the screen with the index and middle fingers stuck together produces a larger mark using the color which results from combining those currently associated with the two index and middle fingers (Fig. 1c)

c. **Color picker** - through various combinations of colors by using the index and middle fingers stuck together unknown colors may be obtained; touching the screen with the little finger identifies and retrieves for the user the color from the point of the touch (Fig. 2a)

d. **Fill** - as seen the thumb can have an associated color and when touching the screen with the thumb it will be filled with that color(Fig. 2b)

e. **Erase** - rubbing the screen with the side of your hand as if you would brush something off produces the similar effect in the application of erasing the area where the action took place (Fig. 2c)

4.2 PDF Viewer[4]

The PDF Viewer (Fig. 3) presents a simple solution to working with large pdf files on a smartphone. The application allows browsing through the document using swipe gestures (to advance or go back in the document) as any application for viewing a PDF file would but minor improvements have been added. If the swiping gesture is executed with the index and middle fingers stuck together then several pages will be skipped in the document thus allowing a faster browsing. Another improvement is the ability to go directly to the start or the end of the document by either touching the screen with the thumb or with the little finger.

4.3 Missile Intercept[5]

The third application we implemented is a game in which towns displayed at the bottom of the screen have to be protected from missiles coming from the

---

[4] For the implementation of this application we re-used the Vudroid source code available at http://code.google.com/p/vudroid

[5] For the implementation of this application we re-used the source code available at http://www.kirit.com/Missileintercept

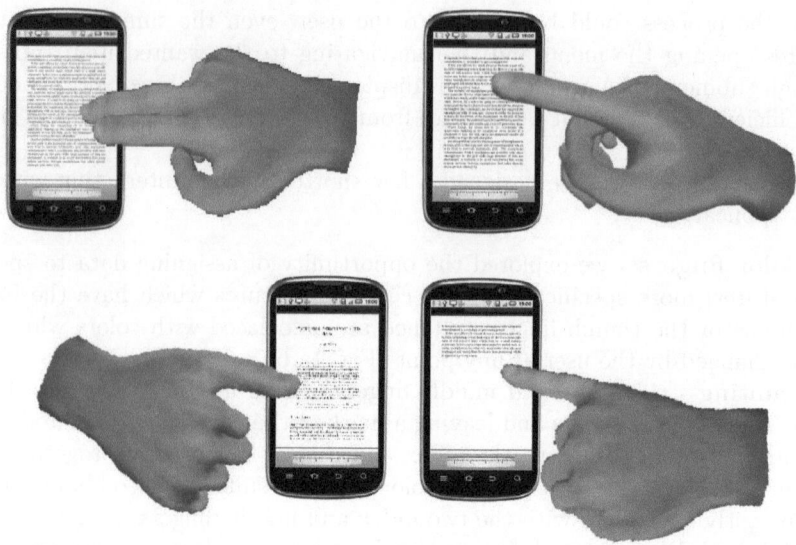

Fig. 3. Browsing documents using hand postures: (a) Swiping the screen using two fingers will result in a fast browsing. (b) Using a single finger for normal speed browsing. (c) Using the thumb finger will browse to the first page of the document. (d) Using the little finger will browse to the last page of the document.

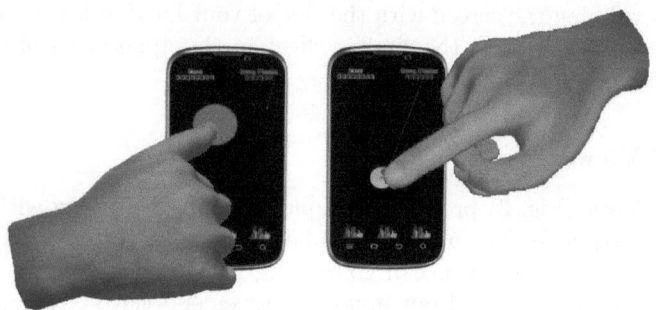

Fig. 4. Missile Intercept for smartphones using hand gestures: (a) Touching the screen with the thumb results in a large explosion. (b) Touching the screen with the index finger results in a smaller explosion.

top of the screen in various directions (Fig. 4). This is usually performed by touching the screen at which point an explosion will take place and hopefully destroy incoming missiles. An addition was implemented in the game in the form of explosions of different sizes. This was achieved by touching the screen with different fingers which had various explosion sizes associated to them.

5   Conclusion

As previously stated the communication between the smartphone and the data glove has been mediated by use of a laptop which allows us to easily replace the technology for hand posture acquisition. The main advantage of a data glove is the relative mobility it confers, a feature essential to the end user who can be found to develop various habits involving unusual positions in the interaction with his smartphone [30]. Vision based technologies such as Microsoft Kinect[6] are popular in gesture acquisition but the hands are required to be in the visual range of the camera at all times. That imposes a restriction for the user to follow and thus negatively influences his experience, an obviously unwanted event. On the other hand, while a data glove confers mobility it can also become cumbersome and uncomfortable. Other technologies are also being considered such as muscle sensing [31] in order to provide highly accurate gesture data with no restriction on the user's mobility and no intrusion in the user's comfort.

We illustrated in this paper the opportunity of the hand posture data as measurements of finger flexure to provide another input dimension for smart mobile devices. By working with just a few easily reproductible postures we managed simplified the interaction for three common applications. These hand postures fulfill three main purposes, retrieving or holding information, such as the little finger identifying and holding a color in the Paint application, carrying out predetermined actions, such as the erase action in the Paint application or carrying out custom actions based on associated data, such as the index and middle fingers painting in the colors which were associated to them by the user. The need for extra menus or buttons either onscreen or hidden has been reduced through use of shortcut gestures. As future work we are considering using hand posture data in more complex applications including other devices and smart environments.

Acknowledgments. This paper was supported by the project InteractEdu (Interactive gesture-based system for the educational development of school-age children: applications in education, tourism and discovery of patrimony) 588/2012, co-funded by UEFISCDI, Romania and WBI, Belgium.

References

1. Jones, L.A., Lederman, S.J.: Human Hand Function. Oxford University Press, Inc., New York (2006)
2. Bhalla, M.R., Bhalla, A.V.: Comparative Study of Various Touchscreen Technologies. International Journal of Computer Applications (0975, 8887) 6(8) (September 2010)
3. Holzinger, A.: Finger instead of mouse: Touch screens as a means of enhancing universal access. In: Carbonell, N., Stephanidis, C. (eds.) UI4ALL 2002. LNCS, vol. 2615, pp. 387–397. Springer, Heidelberg (2003)
4. Android Developers, Gestures,
   http://developer.android.com/design/patterns/gestures.html

---

[6] Microsoft Kinect (http://www.xbox.com/en-GB/kinect)

5. Li, Y.: Gesture search: a tool for fast mobile data access. In: Proceedings of the 23nd Annual ACM Symposium on User Interface Software and Technology (UIST 2010), pp. 87–96. ACM, New York (1866),
http://doi.acm.org/10.1145/1866029.1866044, doi:10.1145/1866029.1866044

6. Lu, H., Li, Y.: Gesture Avatar: A Technique for Operating Mobile User Interfaces Using Gestures. In: CHI 2011 Proceedings of the 2011 Annual Conference on Human Factors in Computing Systems, pp. 207–216. ACM, New York (2011)

7. Baxter, L.K.: Capacitive Sensors Design and Applications. IEEE Press Series on Electronics Technology, NJ (1997)

8. Downs, R.: Using resistive touch screens for human/machine interface. Texas Instruments (2005)

9. Barrett, G.L.: Choose the Right Touch Technology for Your Display. White Paper, Touch International (2012)

10. North, K.D., Souza, H.: Acoustic Pulse Recognition Enters Touch-Screen Market, Information Display. SID Society for Information Display 22(12), 22–25 (2006)

11. Potter, R.L., Weldon, L.J., Shneiderman, B.: Improving the accuracy of touch screens: an experimental evaluation of three strategies. In: O'Hare, J.J. (ed.) Proceedings of the SIGCHI Conference on Human Factors in Computing Systems (CHI 1988), pp. 27–32. ACM, New York (1988),
http://doi.acm.org/10.1145/57167.57171, doi:10.1145/57167.57171

12. Sears, A., Shneiderman, B.: High precision touchscreens: design strategies and comparisons with a mouse. Int. J. Man-Mach. Stud. 34(4), 593–613 (1991), http://dx.doi.org/10.1016/0020-7373(91)90037-8, doi:10.1016/0020-7373(91)90037-8

13. Fitts, P.M., Peterson, J.R.: Information capacity of discrete motor responses. Journal of Experimental Psychology 67(2), 103–112 (1964)

14. Albinsson, P.-A., Zhai, S.: High precision touch screen interaction. In: Proceedings of the SIGCHI Conference on Human Factors in Computing Systems (CHI 2003), pp. 105–112. ACM, New York (2003),
http://doi.acm.org/10.1145/642611.642631, doi:10.1145/642611.642631

15. Benko, H., Wilson, A.D., Baudisch, P.: Precise selection techniques for multi-touch screens. In: Grinter, R., Rodden, T., Aoki, P., Cutrell, E., Jeffries, R., Olson, G. (eds.) Proceedings of the SIGCHI Conference on Human Factors in Computing Systems (CHI 2006), pp. 1263–1272. ACM, New York (2006),
http://doi.acm.org/10.1145/1124772.1124963, doi:10.1145/1124772.1124963

16. Vogel, D., Baudisch, P.: Shift: a technique for operating pen-based interfaces using touch. In: Proc. CHI 2007, pp. 657–666. ACM Press (2007)

17. Tactus Technology, Inc. Taking touch screen interfaces into a new dimension, A tactus technology white paper (2012)

18. Hinckley, K., Song, H.: Sensor synaesthesia: touch in motion, and motion in touch. In: Proceedings of the SIGCHI Conference on Human Factors in Computing Systems (CHI 2011), pp. 801–810. ACM, New York (2011),
http://doi.acm.org/10.1145/1978942.1979059, doi:10.1145/1978942.1979059

19. Ruiz, J., Li, Y., Lank, E.: User-defined motion gestures for mobile interaction. In: Proceedings of the SIGCHI Conference on Human Factors in Computing Systems (CHI 2011), pp. 197–206. ACM, New York (1978),
http://doi.acm.org/10.1145/1978942.1978971, doi:10.1145/1978942.1978971

20. Wigdor, D., Balakrishnan, R.: TiltText: using tilt for text input to mobile phones. In: Proceedings of the 16th Annual ACM Symposium on User Interface Software and Technology (UIST 2003), pp. 81–90. ACM, New York (2003),
http://doi.acm.org/10.1145/964696.964705, doi:10.1145/964696.964705

21. Jones, E., Alexander, J., Andreou, A., Irani, P., Subramanian, S.: GesText: accelerometer-based gestural text-entry systems. In: Proceedings of the SIGCHI Conference on Human Factors in Computing Systems (CHI 2010), pp. 2173–2182. ACM, New York (2010), http://doi.acm.org/10.1145/1753326.1753655, doi:10.1145/1753326.1753655

22. Ruiz, J., Li, Y.: DoubleFlip: a motion gesture delimiter for mobile interaction. In: Proceedings of the SIGCHI Conference on Human Factors in Computing Systems (CHI 2011), pp. 2717–2720. ACM, New York (2011), http://doi.acm.org/10.1145/1978942.1979341, doi:10.1145/1978942.1979341

23. Keir, P., Payne, J., Elgoyhen, J., Horner, M., Naef, M., Anderson, P.: Gesture-recognition with Non-referenced Tracking. In: Proceedings of the IEEE Conference on Virtual Reality (VR 2006), p. 137. IEEE Computer Society, Washington, DC (2006), http://dx.doi.org/10.1109/VR.2006.64, doi:10.1109/VR.2006.64

24. Tsukada, K., Yasumura, M.: Ubi-Finger: Gesture Input device for Mobile Use. Transactions of Information Processing Society of Japan, 3675–3684

25. Harrison, C., Schwarz, J., Hudson, S.E.: TapSense: Enhancing Finger Interaction on Touch Surfaces. In: Proceedings of the 24th Annual ACM Symposium on User Interface Software and Technology (UIST 2011), pp. 627–636. ACM, New York (2047), http://doi.acm.org/10.1145/2047196.2047279, doi:10.1145/2047196.2047279

26. Vatavu, R.-D., Zaiţi, I.-A.: An Investigation of Extrinsic-Oriented Ambient Exploration for Gaming Applications. In: Wichert, R., Van Laerhoven, K., Gelissen, J. (eds.) AmI 2011. CCIS, vol. 277, pp. 245–248. Springer, Heidelberg (2012)

27. Vatavu, R.-D., Zaiti, I.-A.: Automatic recognition of object size and shape via User-dependent measurements of the grasping hand. International Journal of Human-Computer Studies (2013), doi:10.1016/j.ijhcs.2013.01.002

28. Harrison, C., Tan, D., Morris, D.: Skinput: appropriating the body as an input surface. In: Proceedings of the SIGCHI Conference on Human Factors in Computing Systems (CHI 2010), pp. 453–462. ACM, New York (2010), http://doi.acm.org/10.1145/1753326.1753394, doi:10.1145/1753326.1753394

29. Kim, D., Hilliges, O., Izadi, S., Butler, A.D., Chen, J., Oikonomidis, I., Olivier, P.: Digits: freehand 3D interactions anywhere using a wrist-worn gloveless sensor. In: Proceedings of the 25th Annual ACM Symposium on User Interface Software and Technology (UIST 2012), pp. 167–176. ACM, New York (2012), http://doi.acm.org/10.1145/2380116.2380139, doi:10.1145/2380116.2380139

30. Nova, N., Miyake, K., Chiu, W., Kwon, N.: Curious Rituals: Gestural Interaction in the Digital Everyday. Near future laboratory (2012), http://books.google.ro/books?id=XWbelwEACAAJ

31. Benko, H., Saponas, T.S., Morris, D., Tan, D.: Enhancing input on and above the interactive surface with muscle sensing. In: Proceedings of the ACM International Conference on Interactive Tabletops and Surfaces (ITS 2009), pp. 93–100. ACM, New York (1924), http://doi.acm.org/10.1145/1731903.1731924, doi:10.1145/1731903.1731924

Pointing in the Air: Measuring the Effect of Hand Selection Strategies on Performance and Effort

Matthias Schwaller and Denis Lalanne

Department of Informatics, University of Fribourg,
Boulevard de Pérolles 90, 1700 Fribourg, Switzerland
{matthias.schwaller,denis.lalanne}@unifr.ch

Abstract. The research presented in this paper aims at measuring the effect of selection strategies on free-hand pointing performance and effort.

Different evaluations are presented which shows that the selection strategies and the feedback do influence the pointing performance. In the main evaluation presented in this paper, three selection strategies, namely dwell, thumb and pinching, are compared. There was no winning selection strategy, although there was a significant effect of the selection strategies on the pointing performance. Further, the paper shows that it is not enough to compare only the performance of the user, but also the effort, comfort and the selection errors must be taken into account.

Keywords: Deictic gestures, Gestural User Interfaces, Pointing performance, Fitts' Law.

1   Introduction

In recent years, gestural user interfaces have become very popular, mostly because they are fun (in games) and very adapted for teamwork in collaborative settings such as working around interactive walls. Since the launch of gestural consoles like the Wii, PlayStation Move and Microsoft Kinect, gestural interfaces have become accessible to everyone.

Nevertheless, free-hand deictic gestures (pointing and selection) still rely on basic strategies. Microsoft Kinect proposes a selection method based on a temporal threshold, i.e. you must stay on the target for a certain time (about a second) in order to select it. While it works and is reliable with a good visual feedback, we believe it is not an optimal strategy because of the time used for a selection.

This was the major motivation for the work presented in this article: to develop novel hand pointing and selection strategies that do not require holding a device or markers, nor calibration. We implemented three different selection strategies: using depth, temporal thresholding (dwell) and using the thumb. In the article, we focus our presentation on the selection strategies. Further, in order to augment the usability and precision of our deictic gestures, different kinds of visual feedback were implemented. The feedback not only indicates to users whether hands are detected or not,

A. Holzinger et al. (Eds.): SouthCHI 2013, LNCS 7946, pp. 732–747, 2013.

and if not why (too far, out of pointing range, etc.), it also shows how the system actually works.

Another contribution of our paper is the consideration of a general metric that combines comfort, accuracy and perceived quality as complementary factors, in addition to the index of performance.

The remainder of this paper is structured as follows: First, we give an overview of some related work. Next, we present two preliminary evaluations, one about selection strategies and one about selection feedback. Furthermore, the pointing and selection gestures with their recognition algorithms, as well as the feedback are illustrated. Finally, evaluations are presented along with their results, followed by conclusions and future work.

2 Related Work

Concerning the recognition of pointing gestures, known as deictic gestures, research has been done in the past on which we based our implementation. Haker et al. [1] used a time-of-flight camera to acquire and recognize pointing gestures. Their first step for the gesture recognition was the segmentation of the person from the background. For this purpose, they used the intensity data which is similar to the depth map which we use. For the tracking of the hand they used a Kalman filter to do temporal smoothing to avoid jiggling. We also used a Kalman filter. The main difference is that they used the direction from the head to the hand as the pointing direction, while we consider only the hand for the pointing.

Harrison et al. [2] proposed an efficient algorithm for free-hand pointing gesture recognition using a depth camera. In their method, they first looked for fingers and then detected touching for selection. The finger detection started by computing the depth derivate using a sliding window and then looked for vertical slices of cylinder-like objects. However, the method is very sensitive to acquisition conditions (device/user positions) so that with their method the angle can neither be too steep nor too shallow.

Frati & Prattichizzo [3] proposed another approach in which they first calculated the convex hull of the overall hand and then searched for convexity defects to detect the fingertips. For the pinching selection strategy we also use the convex hull. We use the same polynomial approach to detect the thumb in the thumb selection strategy as Klompmaker et al. use in their dSensingNI framework [4] for detecting fingers.

Concerning selection strategies, various approaches have been proposed in recent research, taking into account or not ergonomic and physiological issues. Vogel et al. [5] interestingly noted that "since the hand is also pointing, the click or clutch action should be designed to minimize hand movement side effects, which can be tricky due to the interconnectedness of tendons and ligaments in the hand". They implemented a thumbTrigger method on which preliminary tests led to the conclusion that this method is uncomfortable and tiring. Their thumbTrigger method was initially inspired by the trigger gesture of Grossman et al. [6]. As presented later in this article (section 4.3), in our adaptation of the selection strategy (S2), only the index finger is outstretched and the rest of the fingers (except for the thumb) are folded. The thumb can touch the middle finger or simply be partly hidden behind the palm. This requires only a little movement, and less effort than the thumbTrigger, and is thus less tiring. Such a thumb selection strategy is also presented by Moeslund et al. [7] although their system is wearable and has a head-mounted camera which make it intrusive. A thumb selection strategy was also presented by Gallo & Ciapi [8]. In their implementation, where they used Wiimotes and a data glove with IR LEDs, the thumb is bent for the pointing and outstretched for the selection which is the inverse of our implementation of the thumb selection. Banerjee et al. [9] adapted the thumbTrigger selection strategy of Grossman et al. (where the thumb can touch the middle finger) and instead the thumb has to be leaned towards the index finger, like in our implementation. They used this gesture to reach out-of-reach targets on a tabletop.

Wilson [10] and Gustafson et al. [11] both presented a detection of pinch gestures, but in different settings. Wilson used the pinch gesture over the keyboard in front of the screen. Gustafson et al. used the pinch gesture for drawing in the air detected through a wearable webcam. Benko & Wilson have extended the pinch gesture of [10] and used it in a dome [12]. Foehrenback et al. [13] also presented a pinching gesture, but which required the use of sensors on the fingers, which made it intrusive. In those four versions of the pinching gesture the fingers other than the thumb and index are outstretched. A modified version of the pinch gesture presented by Wilson was presented by Fukuchi et al. [14]. Their adaptation was that the pinch gesture can be done either with thumb and index, thumb and any finger or by thumb and all fingers. This system was used with a tabletop system. The advantage of the pinch gesture is that there is a non-ambiguous state, so either the thumb is touching the index or not and thus has an implicit feedback.

Finally, concerning visual feedback, Grossman et al. [15] presented the Bubble Cursor which is an area cursor which changes its size depending on the proximity of the targets. The bubble cursor does always "point" at a target. We do not have an area cursor but a part of our cursor changes its size according to a threshold (distance or time) the user has to reach to trigger a selection. The property, that a bubble cursor does always point to a target is not implemented in our research in order to compare the pointing performance of the user.

3   Evaluations 1 & 2: Preliminary Tests of the Effect of Selections and Feedback

We started by doing two preliminary evaluations to check whether (1) the selection strategy, and (2) the visual feedback might influence the pointing performance of the user. For this preliminary evaluation we used a time-of-flight (TOF) camera. We have chosen the TOF camera Swiss Ranger 4000, since this camera has a frame rate of about 50 frames per second. We thought to detect a movement it is better to have a higher frame rate than having a big resolution. To evaluate the impact of selection strategies and visual feedback, we first performed a user evaluation with 6 users. For this purpose we developed TargetCatching, an application that allows measuring the performance of pointing and selection gestures. In this application, the user had to click on several round targets of different sizes, located at different positions. The application then calculates, with the help of Fitts' Law, the index of performance (also called throughput) which is measured in bits per second (bps) $IP = ID/MT$, where ID is the index of difficulty $= \log 2(D/W + 1)$, D is the distance from the initial point to the target, W the diameter of the target, and MT is the total time taken to select targets. In the final evaluation presented in section 6, we modified this application to be compliant with part 9 of the ISO 9241 standard for non-keyboard input devices, both in terms of target positioning and index of performance calculation.

3.1   Varying Selection Strategies

In this first evaluation we compared 3 different selection strategies: dwell, distance and thumb selection.

For a selection with the dwell selection strategy, the user has to keep the pointer (controlled with his hand) over the region she or he would like to select for approximately one second (similar to the one presented in section 4.3).

The distance strategy, as the name says, uses distance to perform a selection. The selection is performed when the user passes a certain distance (fixed distance towards the sensor). It is quite similar to a button press or a click in the air. In order to prevent a flickering effect the user has to augment the distance from the hand to the camera in order to make the next selection. The advantage of this distance selection is that the user can use any hand posture which helps to reduce fatigue.

The third selection strategy used in this evaluation was the thumb selection strategy. For this selection strategy the user deploys his thumb for pointing and hides it (or leans it to the middle finger) for selecting (similar to the one presented in section 4.3).

As pointing location we use the topmost point cloud of the contour of the detected hand (see Fig. 1).

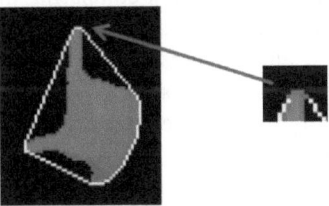

Fig. 1. Pointing with topmost location

The outcome of this evaluation is presented in Table 1 (mean of all users). For each selection strategy, users had to select 20 targets, with varied target sizes and positions. The same set of 20 targets was used 3 times, but only the last 15 were used to compute the index of performance, leaving aside the first 5 selections due to the potential learning effect.

Table 1. Pointing efficiency with different selection strategies

Selection strategy	Errors / selection		Index of performance	
	M	SD	M	SD
Dwell	-	-	1.30 bps	.07
Distance	0.62	.34	0.75 bps	.18
Thumb	0.49	.39	1.57 bps	.26

M = Mean, SD = standard deviation.

There was a significant effect of the selection strategy on the index of performance $F(2, 10) = 310.286$, $p < .001$ (one-way repeated measures ANOVA). Three paired samples t-tests (Bonferroni corrected) were used to make post-hoc comparisons. Significance was found for the two pairs: distance vs. dwell; $t(5) = 8.96$, $p < .001$ and for distance vs. thumb $t(5) = 10.26$, $p < .001$. Between the thumb and dwell ($t(5) = 2.58$, $p = .049$), there was no significant difference when using the Bonferroni correction.

This evaluation measured the effect of selection strategies on the index of performance. With the evaluation, we found that the distance strategy is worse than the dwell strategy. Therefore we put the distance strategy aside and add another one for the final evaluation, the pinching strategy which is often used (see section 4.3). The errors were not measured for the dwell selection strategy since we detected a "pointer over" event (detection if the cursor is over a target) and ran a timer to detect a click. So if the cursor is next to the target, nothing will happen. Therefore we adapted the dwell strategy for the final evaluation to be able to detect false clicks. Further, the selection for the distance strategy was quite difficult since the pointing was also influenced by a movement in depth which made it difficult to "stay" on a target for a selection.

3.2   Visual Feedback

The second preliminary evaluation aimed at comparing the pointing/selection performance using different visual feedback strategies. This permitted us to select a good visual feedback for the user evaluation presented in section 4.4.

In the experiment, the thumb selection strategy was used with three different types of visual feedback: using only the overview (Fig. 2 on the left), using the overview together with a varying size circle cursor illustrating the distance between the thumb and index finger (Fig. 2 on the right), and using the overview with an image of the detected and zoomed hand following the cursor (Fig. 2 in the middle).

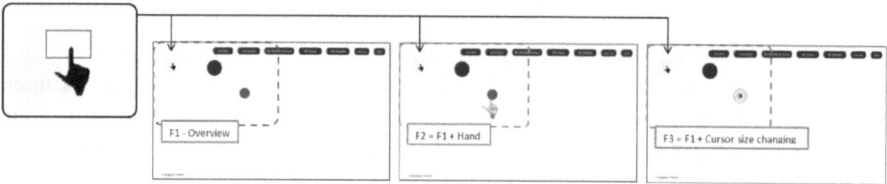

Fig. 2. Feedback: overview, hand and cursor

We found that it makes no sense to use the application without feedback at all. Without the overview it is hard to start because the user will not see where to place their hand so that it is in the camera range and if the hand is too far or too close. Further, if there would be no overview and the user goes sometimes out of the camera range and thus the system would not correctly recognize the movements; the system would probably not be well accepted by the user. The setup for this evaluation was the same as for the first preliminary evaluation.   For this evaluation, 6 users (different from the first preliminary experiment) had to select 20 targets (5 training and 15 to measure the index of performance). This preliminary evaluation was done using the thumb selection strategy. The outcome of this evaluation is presented in Table 2 (mean of all users).

Table 2. Pointing efficiency with different types of feedback

Feedback	Errors / selection		Index of performance	
	M	SD	M	SD
Only Overview	0.21	.20	1.41 bps	.16
Overview with cursor	0.17	.14	1.51 bps	.16
Overview with hand	0.20	.17	1.33 bps	.15

M = Mean, SD = standard deviation.

There was a significant effect of the visual feedback on the index of performance $F(2, 10) = 4.85$, $p = .034$ (one-way repeated measures ANOVA). Post-hoc analysis (Bonferroni corrected) showed a statistically significant difference between the hand feedback and the cursor feedback: $t(5) = 4.84$, $p = .0047$ (between the other two conditions there was no statistically significant difference. For this reason we decided in the subsequent evaluation to use the cursor feedback, which we improved with an arrow indicating the center of the selection more precisely.

This user evaluation permitted us to evaluate that the feedback influences the pointing performance. Normally, one would think that a selection feedback in addition to the overview feedback would improve the performance, but in this evaluation we found out that this is not always the case. If a feedback attracts the user's attention too much, as it is the case with the hand feedback (significant effect on the pointing performance), the performance seems to decrease. For the final evaluation we decided to take the best feedback of this preliminary evaluation and adapted it a bit (see section 4.4).

4   Evaluation 3: Effect of Selection Strategies on User Performance

4.1   Setup and Recognition

In our setting, the user sits on a chair with armrests, in front of a big screen (52 inches). The gestures are recognized through a Kinect for Windows sensor from Microsoft® which is placed in front of the user below the screen (see Fig. 3). The user can put the elbow on the armrest; the forearm has to point towards the top of the screen. The wrist has to be moved slightly up in order that the palm points towards the Kinect. We used in this experiment a Kinect instead of the time-of-flight camera in the preliminary evaluations, because we remarked that 30 frames per second are enough and with the Kinect we have the higher resolution (640x480 pixels versus 176x144 pixels). The distance between the users hand and the screen is about 1.8 m. The Kinect stands on a box of 0.78 m and at a distance of about 1.05 m.

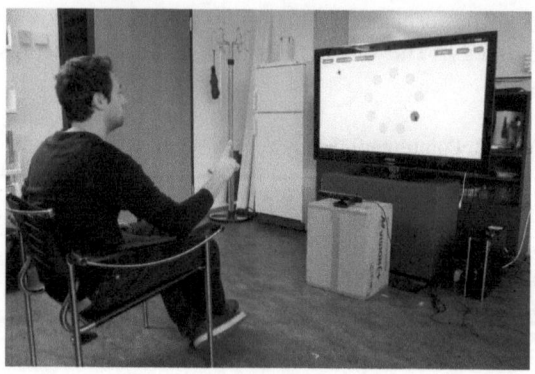

Fig. 3. Setup

The recognition of deictic gestures (pointing and selection) is done through several steps in our implementation: first pre-processing, then pointing and then selection. Next, there is a small tracking algorithm which considers the last 4 states. As state we consider the pointing location and if a selection occurred or not. Finally a Kalman filter is used to make the cursor movement smoother.

Concerning the pre-processing, we filter out the image using the distance. We assume the user's hand to be the closest object in front of the Kinect and take a predefined distance (10 cm) after the closest pixel to the sensor. The current restriction is that nothing can be closer to the sensor than the pointing hand. We then apply a blurring over the image. Next we use erosion and dilatation to prepare the image for the contour detection, which uses canny edge detection.

4.2   Pointing

In our current implementation we use the right hand for pointing, due to our selection methods. In the beginning, we used the highest point of the detected hand (contour) as the pointing position.

This obviously only works for selection strategies where the highest point of the hand does not move during the selection action. For the selection strategy S3 - pinching click - the pointing with the topmost position provokes a pointer moving when just a click is done. Thus, the user would have to move his or her hand up while clicking, which is not comfortable at all. Therefore, we had to find a pointing implementation which works for all the selection strategies in the same way, to be able to compare them equally. Therefore, we now use the center of mass of the detected hand. This works with any hand postures, which reduces fatigue.

To be able to detect the full hand in any position, we reduced the pointing window in which the user points. As a second advantage, this also reduces the movement which the user has to do to go from one side of the screen to the other side. We then directly map the pointing position in this window to the cursor on the screen. We will see later in the article how the visual feedback helps users position their hand in this pointing window.

Furthermore, since the resolution of the sensor is much smaller than the resolution of the screen in our setting, the cursor would have a flickering effect. Therefore, we used a Kalman filter which allow a fluid pointer movement and predict the location in case of a missing frame.

4.3   Selection

Pointing recognition and tracking permits to move a pointer on the screen. Still, a selection must be performed to "click" on a target. An important aspect for a reliable selection is that the movement which is necessary for selecting should not influence the pointing. For the selection, we implemented several strategies, for this research they were only implemented for the right hand with the palm towards the sensor (but of course, the thumb and pinch could be mirrored also be implemented for the left hand):

S1 – Dwell Strategy. The user has to keep the pointer (controlled with his hand) over the region she or he would like to select for one second, which is approximately the time which is used in most Kinect games for Xbox at the time of writing.

The time for a click is a trade-off between speed and accuracy (minimal false clicks). We are currently using 5/6 of a second, which empirically gave the best results. The region in which the cursor has to stay for a click is 60 pixels, which represents the radius of the biggest targets used for the evaluation. Our hypothesis is that since this strategy does not require any additional movement for the selection, it requires less effort and is less tiring than other selection strategies but requires more time for a selection. For instance, we suppose that such a selection strategy is not well adapted for a menu with submenus. Furthermore, no drag-and-drop can be done with such a selection strategy.

S2 - Thumb Click. The user deploys his thumb for pointing and hides it for a selection. In order to hide it, it is enough to lean the thumb to the middle finger. The posture of the thumb selection strategy can be seen in Fig. 4 a.

The hand segmentation for the thumb click starts by detecting a polynomial approximation over the contour (green lines in Fig. 4 c-d). The topology of the edges of this polygon permits to detect if the thumb is present. Therefore, we need to take the left most point and search for the two following points in clockwise order on the polynomial approximation. If the green triangle (left most point), blue cross and the yellow rectangle are in a clockwise order, it means that the thumb is present and if they are in a counterclockwise order, the thumb is hidden or leaned towards the middle finger.

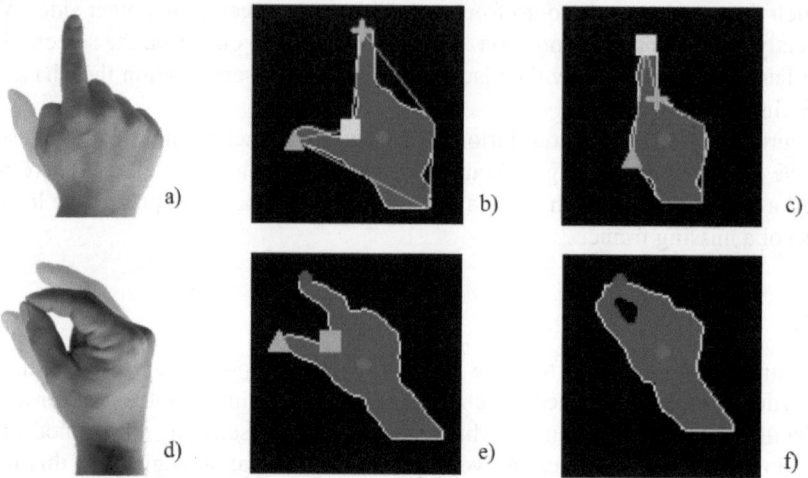

Fig. 4. a) thumb gesture, b) thumb detection with important points, c) Thumb detection with thumb leaned towards the middle finger, d) Pinching gesture, e) Pinch open detection with important points and f) Pinch closed detection with important points.

S3 - Pinching Click. The user performs a gesture like a zoom out on a smartphone. This gesture, where the thumb touches the index finger (Fig. 4 d), is very similar to taking something small from a table. We decided to define that the three other fingers have to be retracted because we found in our tests that this is slightly less tiring than to have them outstretched as in [10–14].

The detection of a pinching gesture starts by detecting convexity defects in the contour of the hand. If the depth of such a defect is above a certain threshold (image width / 45) it means that the thumb does not touch the index. Additionally, the depth point (the farthest point from the convex hull point within the defect, see green rectangle in Fig. 4 e-f) has to be over a certain height (midpoint plus 1/5 of the height of the detected contour).

Tracking. The images of the Kinect sensor may contain noise. Therefore, it is possible that in a frame the contour cannot be detected or that the pointing locations are wrongly detected or selections falsely detected. For this reason, we implemented a simple history queue which tracks the four last locations and four last selections. With the help of the history information, missing locations can be predicted. In order to be able to configure and also change the selection strategy and feedback, a configuration frame was implemented.

4.4   Feedback

The visual feedback shows the user how the system works, meaning that it highlighted the detected hand and the feedback shows if the hand is within the camera range or not. This is important at the beginning until the user has some experience with the system. This facilitates the acceptance of the system by the user. The feedback is composed of three steps. First, there is the overview feedback. This feedback permits the user to see the scene overview in the top left corner. In the overview the user can see the depth image of the detected hand highlighted in black. Furthermore, there is a surrounding frame which shows the pointing zone to the user. The user can only point within this zone, which helps to reduce the size of the movement the user has to do, to go from one side of the screen to the other side. The goal of this overview is to help the user to understand what is detected and what not. This feedback is especially helpful at the beginning to place the hand at the right place or when the user puts the hand outside of the pointing range. This feedback is shown in Fig. 5.

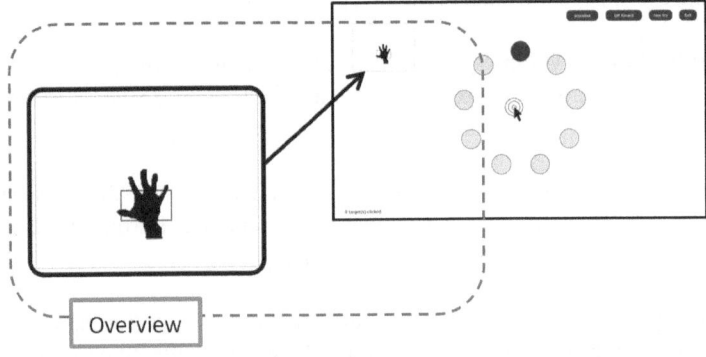

Fig. 5. Feedback

The second feedback provides users with additional information for the selection. The circle around the cursor (see Fig. 6) can have two different colors. If the circle is green, it means that a click occurred and in this case the circle is small. When the cursor is red, its size changes automatically depending on the distance to a click. For the dwell selection strategy the distance represents the time that the user has to wait for the click. At the beginning it is big and if the user stays on the target, its size reduces for 1 second. For the thumb selection strategy it represents the distance from the thumb tip to the index (see green triangle and blue cross in Fig. 4 b). As the user approaches the thumb to the index, the circle gets smaller and smaller. For the pinching selection strategy the size of the cursor represents the distance between the tips of the thumb and the index finger (see the two left most points in Fig. 4 e). Additionally, a sound is played when a selection is made.

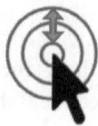

Fig. 6. Cursor changing size for the selection feedback

4.5   Evaluation and Results

We have changed our application (TargetCatching see Fig. 5) to measure the performance so that the evaluations are based on part 9 of the ISO 9241standard for the non-keyboard input devices multi-directional tapping test. So, now the user has to click on circular targets of the same size arranged in a circle on the screen. The size of the circular targets, as well as the circle on the screen, varies. The advantage of this arrangement in a circle is that movements in all directions are equally tested. If the user clicks next to a target, we consider this as an error and the target is not validated and thus the user has to click again on the current target.

Participants. Twelve volunteers, 2 female and 10 male, participated in this evaluation. The range in age of the participants was from 21 to 35 years. All were daily computer users.

Apparatus. For this evaluation we used a 52 inch TV with a 1920 x 1080 resolution as the screen. The user sat in a chair with arm rests about 2 m from of the screen. The Microsoft Kinect sensor was placed below the TV.

Task. The application now calculates the effective index of performance (or throughput), still based on Fitts' Law: $IP = IDe/MT$, where IDe = effective index of difficulty = $\log2((D + We) / We)$, D = radius of the circle, $We = 4.133\ Sx$, Sx = standard deviation of the selection coordinates, MT = total time taken to select targets. This way, the evaluation can be compared to other evaluations based on part 9 of the ISO 9241 standard for non-keyboard input devices.

Procedure. To compare the three different selection strategies (S1: dwell, S2: thumb and S3: pinching) presented above, we conducted a within-subject design user evaluation with 12 users, in which all the users tested all the selection strategies. The selection strategies were counter-balanced to reduce carry over effects (mainly fatigue and learning). For each selection strategy there were 4 circles with 9 circular targets which the user had to click. The target circle used for practice had an ID of 2.807 (using D=600, W=100), the other three target circles had an ID of 3.285 (using D=700, W=80), 3.322 (using D=900, W=100), and 2.585 (using D=600, W=120). The topmost circular target had to be clicked at the beginning and at the end. The first circle was used only as training due to the potential learning effect. As radii of the circles we used 300, 350, 450, and only 300 pixels for training. The target sizes (diameters) were 80, 100, 120, and only 100 pixels for training. The effective index of performance was calculated per circle and we took the average of the second, third and fourth circle. The same set was used 3 times.

Results. The results obtained are presented in Table 3 (mean of all users). There was a significant effect of the selection strategy on the effective index of performance F(2, 22) = 4.98, p = .016 (one-way repeated measures ANOVA). Three paired samples t-tests were used to make post-hoc comparisons. We did not found any statistical significance with the t-tests when using the Bonferroni correction (dwell vs. thumb p = .027, dwell vs. pinching p = .026 and thumb vs. pinching p = .68). The pinching selection strategy gave the best result (IP = 1.38 bps).

Table 3. Pointing efficiency with different selection strategies

Selection strategy	Errors / selection		Eff. index of performance		Mean
	M	SD	M	SD	sel. time
Dwell	0.22	.14	1.19 bps	.14	2.67 s
Thumb	0.38	.18	1.36 bps	.21	2.37 s
Pinching	0.30	.15	1.38 bps	.21	2.29 s

M = Mean, SD = standard deviation.

Concerning the training, we noticed that the index of performance was stabilized after the first of the four circles (with a logarithmic trend line). We remarked during the preliminary evaluations (through the comments of the users), that the users are less stressed if the evaluation starts with training.

Beside the index of performance there was also a significant effect of the selection strategy on the errors per selection F(2, 22) = 4.71, p = .020 (one-way repeated measures ANOVA, values were normally distributed). For the post-hoc comparisons we used three samples t-tests. We did not found any statistical significance with the t-tests when using the Bonferroni correction (dwell vs. thumb p = .017, dwell vs. pinching p = .14 and thumb vs. pinching p = .12).

Furthermore, we used the questionnaire proposed in ISO 9241 part 9 annex C. Each question has a Likert scale from 1 to 7, where 7 is the best and 1 the worst. Also for the force, effort, and fatigue does a higher value mean that it is better (0 means very tiring and 7 means not tiring at all, for the fatigue questions for instance). This is because we followed the ISO. The results (median) of the questionnaire are presented in with a box plot in Fig. 7. Note that for our questions the higher the score, the better it is.

To compare the results we used the Friedman test (used for non-parametric one way repeated measures) since the results of the questionnaire were not normally distributed. There was a statistically significant difference of the selection strategy on the force required for actuation X2(2) = 10.65, p = .0049. Three Wilcoxon signed rank tests were conducted to make post-hoc comparisons. A significant difference was found for dwell (M = 5.08, SD = 1.38) vs. thumb (M = 3.75, SD = 1.54); Z = 49.5, p = .011 and significant effect for dwell vs. pinching (M = 4, SD = 1.48); Z = 39, p = .023. Furthermore, we found significant effect of the selection strategy on finger fatigue X2(2) = 14.8, p = .0006 (Friedman test). Three paired samples Wilcoxon signed rank tests were conducted to make post-hoc comparisons. We also found significance for the two pairs dwell (M = 6.67, SD = 0.65) vs. thumb (M = 4, SD = 1.91); Z = 55, p = .002 and dwell vs. pinching (M = 4.5, SD = 1.78); Z = 36, p = .006.

Our hypothesis, that the dwell strategy is less tiring but needs more time for a selection was accepted since there is a significant effect on the pointing performance as well as on the finger fatigue.

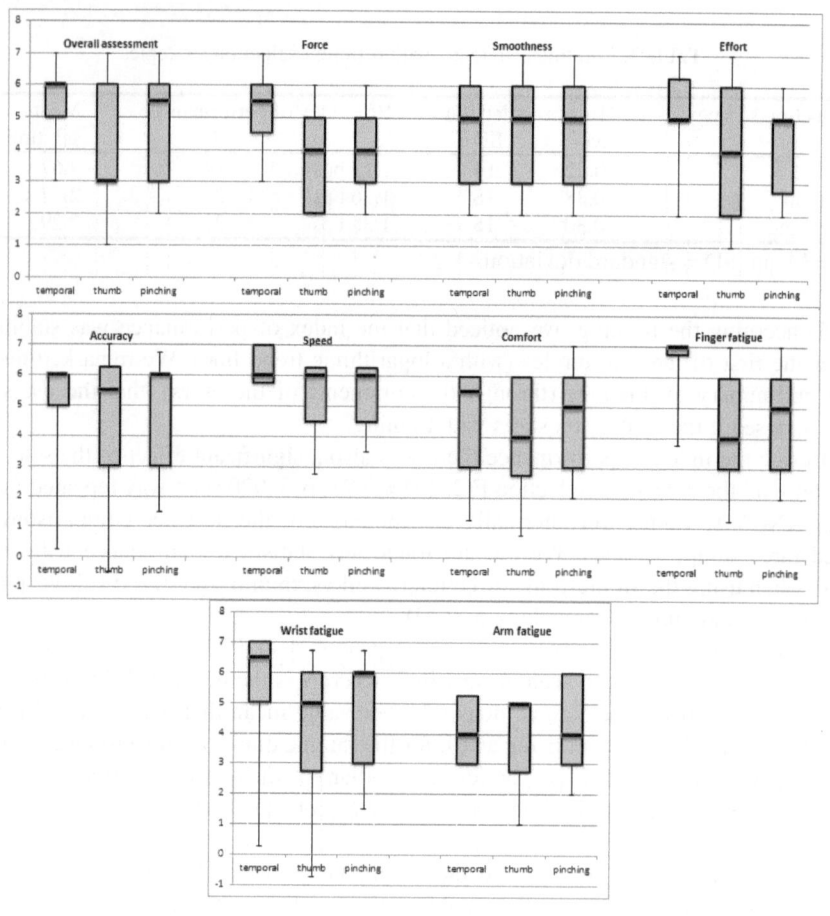

Fig. 7. Box plot summarizing answers to the questions

5   Discussion

To compare the three selection strategies presented in the third evaluation in this paper an overall performance graph was prepared as shown in Fig. 8. Each parameter (perceived quality, overall comfort, accuracy and performance) has a value between 0 and 1. The overall comfort is calculated by averaging the force, effort, finger, wrist and arm fatigue from the questionnaire. The higher the overall score the better the selection strategy. The performance (effective index of performance) of pinching is much better than the one of the dwell selection strategy, but the perceived quality by the user and the accuracy of pinching are worse than those of the dwell strategy. Overall, the pinching strategy is only slightly better than the dwell one. For the future it is clear that we have to work on the accuracy and try to get a better performance and fewer errors for the selection strategies for the users.

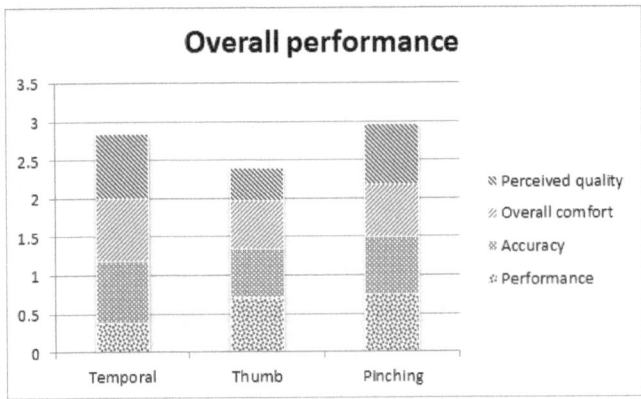

Fig. 8. Overall performance

6   Conclusion

This article presented various recognizers for hand pointing and selection which do not require any calibration or markers. It further presented the design and implementation of three selection strategies and of various visual feedback to support pointing and selection.

Secondly, the paper presented a user evaluation that showed that selection strategies influence the effective index of performance for selecting targets on a screen. Further, it describes two short user evaluations which helped to determine the best selection strategies and visual feedback mechanism for the later user evaluation. No winning selection strategy was found, and we argued that such selection strategy cannot be measure only with the index of performance. The errors, the perceived quality and the fatigue have also to be taken into account, in addition to the index of performance. By comparing the overall performance (see Fig. 8) we remark that the dwell selection strategy has almost the same performance as the pinching selection strategy.

At the performance level, the selection strategy which gave the best index of performance, i.e. pinching, is far from being effective since the effective index of performance is not comparable with the performance of a Wiimote for instance (2.7 bps) [16], there are still numerous false clicks, and the perceived quality for the user is not good enough. More work is thus necessary to improve selection strategies.

In the experiments described in this article, gestures have to be performed towards the camera. For instance, when performing a pinching gesture, the hand has to be turned slightly to the left so that the system is able to recognize it. In order to improve the comfort of gestures we plan to use a second depth sensor on the side of the user to avoid occlusions and also to improve performance. We also plan to continue developing our gesture recognizer in order to enrich the gestural vocabulary with more than only pointing and selection. Our plan is to use the dominant hand for pointing and the non-dominant hand for gestural commands such as selection, zoom, rotation, etc.

Finally, using longitudinal studies, we plan to measure the ergonomics of the chosen gestures, meaning not only whether they support a high effective index of performance for pointing and selection, but also how tiring and usable they are when used in a long period of time.

Acknowledgment. Grateful acknowledgement for proofreading and correcting the English goes to Agnes Lisowska Masson.

References

1. Haker, M., Böhme, M., Martinetz, T., Barth, E.: Deictic Gestures with a Time-of-Flight Camera. In: Kopp, S., Wachsmuth, I. (eds.) GW 2009. LNCS, vol. 5934, pp. 110–121. Springer, Heidelberg (2010)
2. Harrison, C., Benko, H., Wilson, A.D.: OmniTouch. In: Proceedings of the 24th Annual ACM Symposium on User Interface Software and Technology - UIST 2011, pp. 441–450. ACM Press, New York (2011)
3. Frati, V., Prattichizzo, D.: Using Kinect for hand tracking and rendering in wearable haptics. In: 2011 IEEE World Haptics Conference, pp. 317–321. IEEE (2011)
4. Klompmaker, F., Nebe, K., Fast, A.: dSensingNI. In: Proceedings of the Sixth International Conference on Tangible, Embedded and Embodied Interaction - TEI 2012, p. 217. ACM Press, New York (2012)
5. Vogel, D., Balakrishnan, R.: Distant freehand pointing and clicking on very large, high resolution displays. In: Proceedings of the 18th Annual ACM Symposium on User Interface Software and Technology - UIST 2005, pp. 33–42. ACM Press, New York (2005)
6. Grossman, T., Wigdor, D., Balakrishnan, R.: Multi-finger gestural interaction with 3d volumetric displays. In: Proceedings of the 17th Annual ACM Symposium on User Interface Software and Technology - UIST 2004, pp. 61–70. ACM Press, New York (2004)
7. Moeslund, T., Nørgaard, L.: Recognition of deictic gestures for wearable computing. Gesture in Human-Computer Interaction and Simulation, 112–123 (2006)
8. Gallo, L., Ciampi, M.: Wii Remote-enhanced Hand-Computer interaction for 3D medical image analysis. In: 2009 International Conference on the Current Trends in Information Technology (CTIT), pp. 1–6 (2009)

9. Banerjee, A., Burstyn, J., Girouard, A., Vertegaal, R.: Pointable: An In-Air Pointing Technique to Manipulate Out-of-Reach Targets on Tabletops. In: Proceedings of the ACM International Conference on Interactive Tabletops and Surfaces - ITS 2011, p. 11. ACM Press, New York (2011)
10. Wilson, A.D.: Robust computer vision-based detection of pinching for one and two-handed gesture input. In: Proceedings of the 19th Annual ACM Symposium on User Interface Software and Technology - UIST 2006, vol. 255 (2006)
11. Gustafson, S., Bierwirth, D., Baudisch, P.: Imaginary Interfaces: Spatial Interaction with Empty Hands and without Visual Feedback. In: Proceedings of the 23nd Annual ACM Symposium on User Interface Software and Technology - UIST 2010, p. 3. ACM Press, New York (2010)
12. Benko, H., Wilson, A.D.: Multi-point interactions with immersive omnidirectional visualizations in a dome. In: ACM International Conference on Interactive Tabletops and Surfaces - ITS 2010, vol. 19 (2010)
13. Foehrenbach, S., König, W.A., Gerken, J., Reiterer, H.: Tactile feedback enhanced hand gesture interaction at large, high-resolution displays. Journal of Visual Languages & Computing 20, 341–351 (2009)
14. Fukuchi, K., Sato, T., Mamiya, H., Koike, H.: PAC-PAC: Pinching Gesture Recognition for Tabletop Entertainment System. In: Proceedings of the International Conference on Advanced Visual Interfaces - AVI 2010, p. 267. ACM Press, New York (2010)
15. Grossman, T., Balakrishnan, R.: The bubble cursor: enhancing target acquisition by dynamic resizing of the cursor's activation area. In: Proceedings of the SIGCHI Conference on Human Factors in Computing Systems, pp. 281–290 (2005)
16. McArthur, V., Castellucci, S.J., MacKenzie, I.S.: An empirical comparison of "wiimote" gun attachments for pointing tasks. In: Proceedings of the 1st ACM SIGCHI Symposium on Engineering Interactive Computing Systems - EICS 2009, p. 203. ACM Press, New York (2009)

The Influence of Proactivity on Interactive Help Agents

Helmut Lang[1], Melina Klepsch[2], Florian Nothdurft[1], Tina Seufert[2],
and Wolfgang Minker[1]

[1] Ulm University, Institute of Communications Engineering
{helmut.lang,florian.nothdurft,wolfgang.minker}@uni-ulm.de
[2] Ulm University, Institute of Psychology and Education
{melina.klepsch,tina.seufert}@uni-ulm.de

Abstract. The present study examined the effects of proactivity on users' perception of an anthropomorphic user interface agent. The focus was on assessing subjective differences in agent perception between proactive and reactive conditions. Participants of the study were assisted by an interactive agent during seven tasks in a simulation controlling a nuclear power plant. In the reactive condition users had to activate the agent manually in case they needed help. In the proactive condition the agent offered help at a well defined time in the interaction process. Namely when users had confirmed that they were done reading the current task description. The complexity of the simulation ensured that solving the tasks without consulting the agent was virtually impossible. While both conditions performed similarly on objective performance criteria, the reactive agent was perceived more positively than the proactive agent. Especially the reactive agent was rated to be less distracting and less dominant.

Keywords: User Interface Agent, Pedagogical Agent, Help-System, Computer Assisted Learning.

1 Introduction and Theoretical Background

Interaction between computers and their users is not always straightforward. Potential difficulties and problems in dealing with computer systems could be avoided employing effective measures of assistance.

Why the quest for a suitable help system for computer programs is such an important research field has been shown by the results attained by Lazar, Jones, Hackley, and Shneiderman [1]. They describe the negative consequences like frustration or even somatic discomfort (based on prior conducted surveys [2, 3]), including raised muscle tension or anger (e.g. mentioned by [4]) that could be triggered for example by poor interface design. In general four distinct sources of frustration can be identified, namely Internet problems, problems with the application, problems based on the operating system, and problems with hardware [2]. These problems can either be caused by technical failures or could

A. Holzinger et al. (Eds.): SouthCHI 2013, LNCS 7946, pp. 748–767, 2013.

be triggered by erroneous user operations. For problems from the latter category software help systems integrated into applications or operating systems could be sources of assistance. However, in an evaluation with 45 subjects conducted shortly before this study most participants answered for Internet search engines to be their preferred resource when they were in need for assistance [5]. Only nine participants mentioned to use the internal help systems of the software when problems arise. One reason for this neglect might be the fact that help systems have changed little over time and usually consist of a number of indexed and hyperlinked text files that are arranged in sections and subsections and provide some kind of search capability [6].

A change in help request interaction paradigms demands for a changed and adequate assistance in an intelligent manner. The most famous attempt to introduce a new system for user assistance was surely "Clippy the paper clip" an interactive animated character that was part of the Microsoft office suite. Analogous to assistance in human-human interaction the most promising way seemed to be to include a personalized anthropomorphic agent which should try to solve problems in collaborative dialog with the user.

However, Clippy was widely reviewed negatively by users [7]. This is also congruent to findings in the study mentioned earlier. While only two from 45 participants could not remember Clippy when a picture of him was shown, more than 70 percent characterized him as annoying [5].

1.1   Related Work

Up to now the reasons for users' negative perception of Clippy are still unclear.

Taking the importance of the given subject into account we were surprised of the lack of empirical research investigating possible reasons for Clippy's failure. Thus, while a typical assumption for Clippy's failure, is its inappropriate timing of proactive behavior [8], we could not find any empirical evidence confirming this hypothesis.

Rickenberg & Reeves [9] report on anxiety and reduced task performance when an animated character is present in the interface. The idle animations of Clippy along with its proactive behavior might have caused a similar effect as the agent used in their experiment.

Xiao, Catrambone and Stasko [10] evaluated the effects of proactivity in the context of animated agents in a text editing domain. However, their results show that proactivity for an animated agent using spoken output was appreciated by users. Accordingly they also could not find evidence for a substantial difference in users' perception of the agent between the proactive and the reactive group. They concluded that proactive behavior is not problematic in general as long as the information conveyed is actually valuable and presented at the right time.

Kim and Yanghee [11] stated that proactive agents can have a positive impact on recall compared to reactive ones. In their opinion this is due to the fact, that not all information theoretically provided by the agent is requested by the user in reality. However, in terms of subjective evaluation results no differences between a proactive and a reactive version of the agent could be found.

The main differences between Clippy and the two systems used for the evaluations above is that while Clippy uses text based output the other systems rely on speech output.

An agent providing textual help might be perceived to be more disturbing than the agent employed by [10, 11] using spoken output as modality. Conforming to Baddeley's model of working memory [12] spoken output seems to be the preferable choice for agents assisting with graphical user interfaces anyway. Nevertheless computer users are often forced to use systems without auditive output. Especially in open-plan offices auditory output may be distracting.

Another aspect of the agent of Xiao et al. [10] is that its representation is separated from the actual content of the user interface and does not interfere with it. This was definitely not true for Clippy that regularly popped up even in the middle of typing and thus breaking the user's flow of thought [8]. Hence we formulated the following hypotheses.

1.2 Hypotheses

On the one hand we expect a reactive agent using text as output modality, that is presented along with the actual content to be subjectively rated better in terms of intrusiveness potential of distraction and perceived dominance than a proactive one with the same functionalities. On the other hand we expect no differences between the two experimental conditions in terms of help behavior, impact on user, optimism, tolerance, humanity and competence. Variables we consider not to be affected by proactivity.

Also through objective data we expect no differences in users' performance solving the given tasks interacting with the reactive or the proactive agent. Also we expect no differences in erroneous entries and number of restarts of tasks between the two conditions.

To verify our hypotheses we have conducted a study that will be elucidated within the next sections. Firstly the employed methods will be described. Afterwards, the attained results will be presented and subsequently discussed.

2   Method

2.1   Participants

In the experimental study 42 subjects were randomly assigned to one of two treatment groups (proactive agent/reactive agent). Five participants were excluded from the final analysis, as they either stopped interaction after two of the planned seven tasks or their assessed data was incomplete. Hence 37 subjects remained for the analysis. The average age was 22.96 years ($SD = 4.89$). 19 subjects were male and 18 subjects female. Male and female subjects have been evenly distributed among the groups. There were 19 participants in the reactive agent group and 18 participants in the proactive agent group. Participants were mostly students from a variety of majors.

For their participation subjects were compensated with a chocolate bar and had a chance of 1:4 to win a voucher for a cinema ticket. Alternatively psychology students could get a confirmation of participation as needed for their academic studies.

2.2 Material

Scenario. The system employed for the study was Dr. Nick [13] a web-based, interactive and anthropomorphic assistant. Dr. Nick was developed in the context of the bwGRiD portal project[1], where it is used to assist scientists with accessing grid computing resources. Due to various security restrictions it was not possible to use this original grid computing version of Dr. Nick in a public evaluation. Thus an alternative scenario was implemented for this study.

The chosen setting was a nuclear power plant that had to be controlled by the subjects. The nuclear power plant scenario was chosen, as it allows to employ a rather complex model and thus ensures that users heavily rely on assistance.

In the user interface of the system, different controls were distributed among various tabs reflecting the structure of a nuclear power plant (see Fig. 1). There was for example a page to control the water flow in the primary circuit and one to adjust the status of the control rod elements.

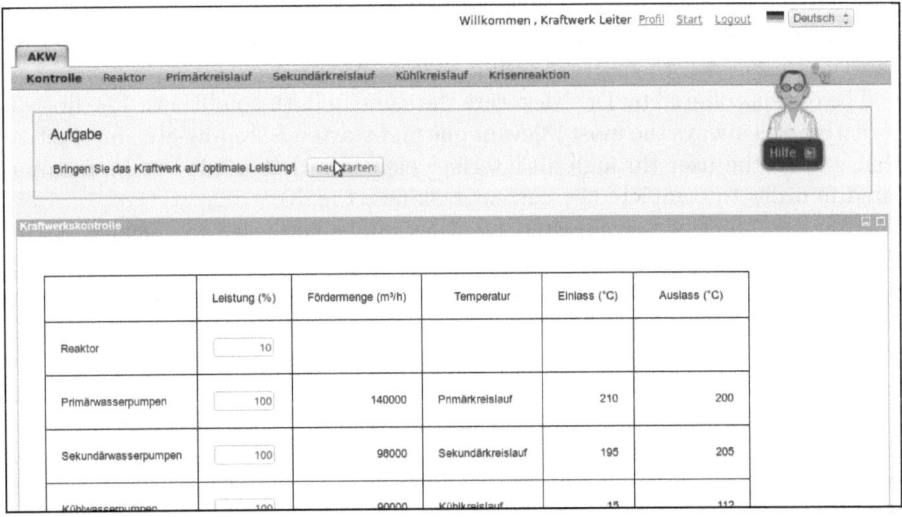

Fig. 1. The main page of the interface for the power plant simulation, with the agent in idle state (The study was conducted in Germany, thus the language used for interface elements was German)

---

[1] http://www.bw-grid.de/portal/

The scenario consisted of seven tasks. For example, the user was instructed to reduce the performance of the power plant to a certain value. Solving the tasks involved navigating to relevant pages, entering values into various input fields and hitting buttons. During three of the tasks subjects were interrupted by warning messages informing them of irregular incidents, like the breakdown of a variable water pump in the primary circuit that made intervention necessary. There was a button allowing participants to restart the current task, in case they felt they made an error and messed something up.

A text with the task description was displayed in a light red box below the navigational area of the page (see Fig. 1). At the beginning of each task only the box containing the task description was displayed and participants had to press a button to confirm that they were finished reading the text and to activate the controls. Warning messages were superimposed on top of the user interface and featured the same button.

After successfully mastering all seven tasks each participant was instructed by the system to log out and was congratulated for mastering all tasks.

Features Dr. Nick. Dr. Nick offered various possibilities for assistance during task completion. In idle state it was displayed as a small icon along with a button (see Fig. 1). To avoid a possibly negative influence of idle animations, as reported by [9], Dr. Nick did not exhibit any idle animation.

In the reactive condition users had to click the button below Dr. Nick in order to activate the agent. In the proactive condition the agent was activated automatically as soon as the user confirmed that he was finished reading the task or error description. When Dr. Nick was activated he offered different options to assist the user with the current task (see Fig. 2).

The options offered by Dr. Nick were the same in both conditions. The first alternative was always the most relevant one and started a step-by-step instruction that guided the user through all interface elements that needed to be manipulated in order to complete the current task (see Fig. 3).

After the guide was completed Dr. Nick could be closed by clicking one of two options in the area below the agent. The first one was a simple "Thank you!" (positive option) and the second one was a rather depreciative statement telling Dr. Nick not to think too great a deal of himself now (negative option). Regardless of the option chosen by the subject, the agent just flipped back into his idle state, to be displayed as a small icon.

As the list of options the agent offered for each task was compiled manually, the best option was always the first one presented. Hence the system was kind of ideal with respect to predicting the user's current goal and perfectly identified users' needs for assistance. Only in 1.4 percent of cases users selected the wrong guide from the list, either by accident or on purpose in order to see what would happen.

The remaining options referred to less relevant information. Dr. Nick was for example also able to explain the structure of a nuclear power plant and make remarks on how the different components interact (see Fig. 4). About 51 percent of the participants opened this explanation at least once. The average time

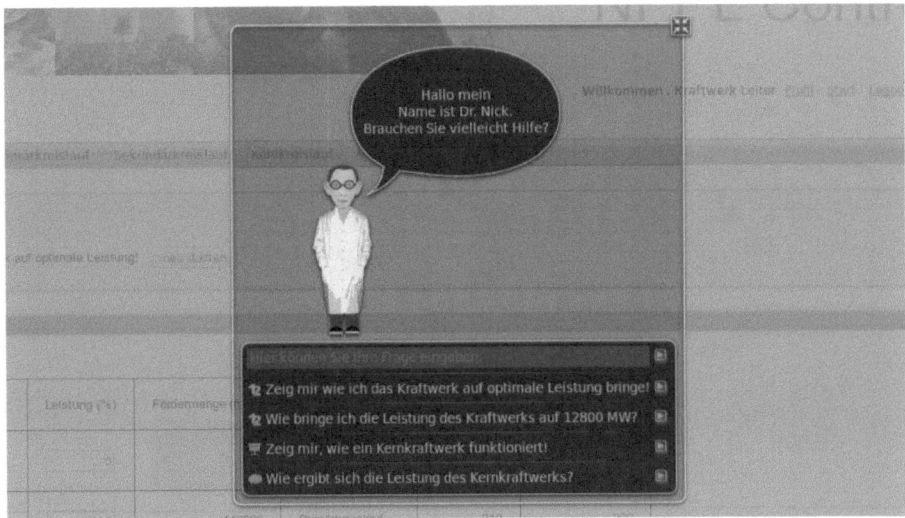

Fig. 2. The agent proposing different options for assistance to the user

users read the information provided was about one minute and the maximum time three minutes. Typically subjects just had a quick glance and then started something else.

In addition to this Dr. Nick was able to provide information on how the correct input values for different states of the power plant were computed. Hence the values that needed to be entered could have been figured out by the subjects manually. However, since the calculus involved was not trivial only one subject, a physics student, opened up a calculator in an attempt to calculate the input values. Overall about 41 percent of subjects opened an explanation of this kind at least once and only six users spent more than one minute reading the explanation.

Thus it may be stated that subjects were not particularly interested in the concepts behind the simulation and rather focused on finishing the given tasks. This was an intention behind the experimental setup, since we wanted users to be completely dependent on Dr. Nick and thus maximize the interaction time with the agent in order to get informative data for the evaluation output even though subjects only had to complete seven tasks. From all subjects only one user was able to complete a single task without referring to Dr. Nick at least once, by following a try and error approach. While it was practically impossible to do a complete task without assistance there were certain sub tasks that were repeated. The plant for example had to be brought to its optimal capacity three times. Users had to remember four numbers to complete this sub task. In 2.2 percent of cases participants were able to complete a given sub task without assistance.

Hence from an objective point of view it may be stated that the design goal of the experiment – to maximize users' dependency on the help system – was met and users definitely needed help. Subjective differences in the rating of the

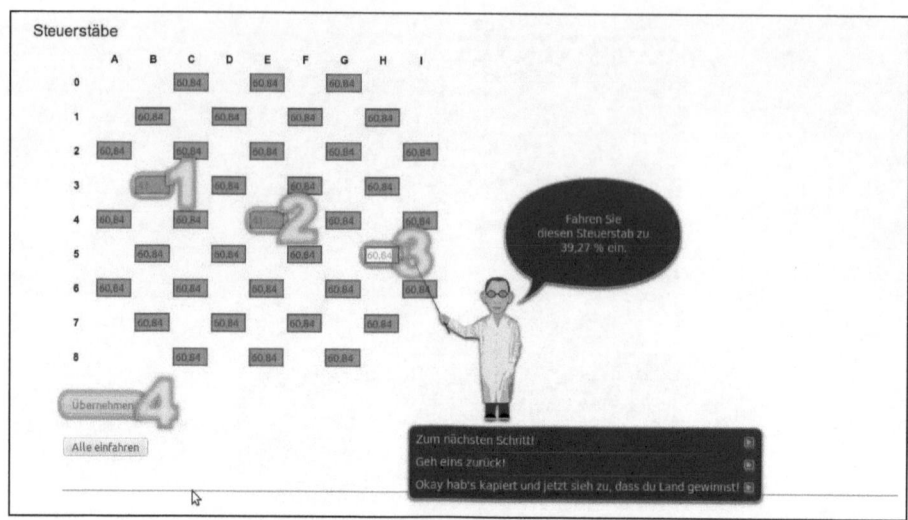

Fig. 3. Dr. Nick pointing at an input field and advising the user about the correct value to enter. Elements that need to be manipulated for task completion are highlighted and sequentially numbered.

agent between conditions are consequently not caused by the fact that the agent did not offer valuable help in the proactive condition.

Subjective Evaluation Questionnaire. As already mentioned previous studies [10, 11] could not find substantial differences in the subjective ratings between proactive and reactive agents. A reason for this might be that the items used in the subjective questionnaires for these studies might not have been elaborated enough or were just inadequate to find possible differences. That is why we decided to develop a new questionnaire containing 41 items especially for this study. Each item had to be answered on a 7-point Likert scale ranging from very high disagreement to very high agreement. The 41 items represent the following nine scales:

help behavior. (3 items, Cronbach's $\alpha=.98$)
   The scale assesses the perceived help behavior of the interactive agent. A sample item is: "The agent is helping in a proper way." High values on this scale show that Dr. Nick's help behavior ist good.

impact on user. (3 items, Cronbach's $\alpha=.63$)
   A sample item says "The presence of the agent appeases me." High values show a positive impact on the user, which means the user feels comfortable with the presence of the agent.

optimism. (3 items, Cronbach's $\alpha=.79$)
   To get an impression on how users assess the personality of Dr. Nick, we developed this scale to evaluate if users ranked the agent to be an optimist

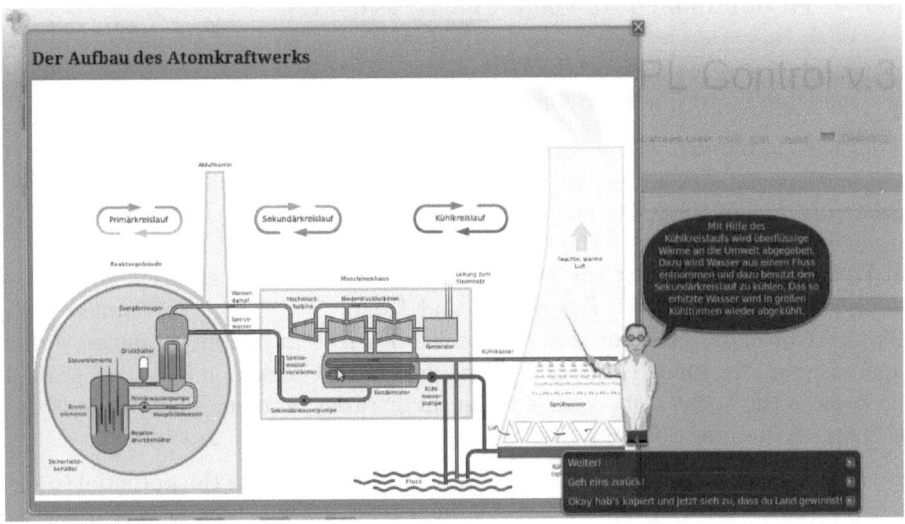

Fig. 4. Dr. Nick explaining the functional units of a nuclear power plant

or pessimist. Again high values reflect a positive evaluation of the interactive agent. A sample item is: "The agent does not lose his courage, even in case of problems."

tolerance. (3 items, Cronbach's α=.82)
An example for an item making up this scale is "The agent is well-disposed towards me." This scale is assessing how users feel to be accepted by the agent and high values are a positive evaluation.

humanity. (6 items, Cronbach's α=.82)
A sample items is "The agent appears lively to me." Within this scale high values are positive and show that the user attests the agent to be human in some sort of way.

competence. (9 items, Cronbach's α=.81)
This scale was used to find out if the agent is experienced as capable. High values are a positive evaluation. A sample item says "The agents seems to be adept and knowing in the area of nuclear physics."

intrusiveness. (3 items, Cronbach's α=.69)
This scale measures the perceived intrusiveness of the agent during task solving. High values for intrusiveness reflect a negative evaluation of Dr. Nick. "The agent likes to be in the center of attention" is a sample item.

potential of distraction. (6 items, Cronbach's α=.82)
As a sample item shows, also high values on this scale are interpreted as negative: "The presence of the agent distracts me from my tasks." The scale was developed to find out how distracting the behavior of the agent is.

perceived dominance. (5 items, Cronbach's $\alpha=.72$)

   With this scale we try to assess the impact of perceived dominance of the agent. A sample item reads: "I think the agent is arrogant and bigheaded", therefore high values are a negative evaluation.

The scales *intrusiveness, potential of distraction, help behavior, impact on user,* and *competence* are assessing the agents actions and behavior. The remaining items are trying to assess how users perceive the agents "personality". These items are loosely based on the German version of the NEO-FFI [14].

For the second part of the evaluation we used the AttrakDiff-questionnaire developed by Hassenzahl, Burmester, and Koller [14]. This questionnaire has 28 items belonging to four different scales. Each item contains bipolar verbal anchors (e.g. "technical – human"). The user has to decide on a 7-point scale if he regards the agent to be rather technical or rather human. The four scales of the AttrakDiff-questionnaire are:

perceived pragmatic quality (PQ). This scale measures the potential to support users' need to achieve behavioral goals. A sample biploar verbal anchor is "confusing – clear".

hedonic quality – stimulation (HQS). The HQS scale measures perceived novelty and potential to grab attention. A sample items says "standard – creative".

hedonic quality – identification (HQI). A sample biploar verbal anchor is "cheap – valuable". This scale assesses potential of identification with the product, which means in our study identification with the agent.

perceived attractiveness (ATT). This scale assesses potential of attractiveness. A sample item is "ugly – beautiful".

In addition to this personality traits of the subjects have been measured with different standardized questionnaires:

self-efficacy. Self-efficacy was measured with a questionnaire by Schwarzer & Jerusalem [15]. It consists of 10 items designed to assess optimistic self-belief. A sample item says I can always manage to solve difficult problems if I try hard enough."

Big 5. To assess the five factors of personality we used a German version of the NEO-FFI [16]. It assesses openness, conscientiousness, extraversion, agreeableness and neuroticism.

Finally demographic informations like age, sex and highest educational achievement of each participant have been recorded. This information along with the assessed personality traits was used as control variables to check for differences in our experimental groups.

Objective Data. To collect objective data screencasts were recorded during interaction. The resulting video material was extensively labeled to gather objective data characterizing the interaction process. Therefore the videos were annotated using ANVIL [17]. Overall more than 10 000 labels were added to about 30 hours of video material. These labels were compiled into the following objective measures:

time on task. Measures the time needed for each of the seven tasks as well as for all tasks combined. Also time on task for login and logout have been measured.

time of interaction. Time of interaction reflects how long participants interacted directly with Dr. Nick on task relevant information. There are again time measures for each task as well as for all tasks together.

wrong parameter input. For each task and also for all tasks combined the number of wrong parameters entered into input fields has been counted.

restarts. Each task could be restarted from the beginning. This value reflects how often this function was used for each participant.

shut down agent. As already mentioned there were two options to close down the agent after completing one of the tasks. This label measures how often each of them was used.

For analysis of the video material the five subjects with incomplete data have also been removed.

2.3 Procedure

The study was carried out during lunchtime and students as well as employees were pointed out to participate in the study by leaflets displayed at the canteen. Before the actual study took place each participant filled out a letter of agreement explaining the intended use of the collected data and that informed about data privacy protection. In the next step the interaction with the nuclear power plant control system and Dr. Nick took place. Therefore, participants were randomly assigned to either the proactive- or reactive-agent group. During the login process users were required to ask Dr. Nick for help for the first time, in order to find out about the correct user name and password. This was monitored by the test conductor in order to avoid problems during testing-time. As already mentioned seven tasks needed to be completed. Participants had a mean time of interaction of about 25 minutes (SD=9 minutes). At the end participants were complimented to their success by the system and asked to logout and quit interaction. After this the evaluation questionnaires and the forms assessing demographic information were filled out. At the end a chocolate bar was handed out and participants could specify an email-address in order to participate in the lottery for cinema ticket vouchers.

3 Results

First of all, no differences in the assessed control variables between our experimental groups could be found. Therefore to test our hypothesis, t-tests were applicable.

In case a Levene-test [18] indicated a possible difference in variances for variables between groups a Welch's t-test [19] was performed. Since this includes computing a corrected value for the degrees of freedom these cases can usually be identified by non integer values for degrees of freedom. For the results reported in this paper the degrees of freedom are different to *35*.

The *d*-values reported specify the effect size according to Cohen [20]. Since reporting effect sizes only makes sense for items that show at least marginal significant effects those values are omitted for not significant results.

3.1 Performance Measures

Means and standard deviations of *time on task, time of interaction, wrong parameter input* and *restarts* can be found in Table 1.

Table 1. Means and standard deviations of objective measures

	reactive agent		proactive agent	
	M	**SD**	**M**	**SD**
time on task [sec]	933.53	534.49	698.60	278.91
time of interaction [sec]	451.19	149.35	446.20	104.67
wrong parameter input [#]	20.11	40.47	9.00	16.91
restarts [#]	1.05	1.96	0.95	1.39

Similar to [10] the time in seconds to complete tasks did not significantly differ as a function of condition (t(23.20)=1.54, n.s.). Despite the relative large absolute difference the time to complete the tasks did not differ significantly due to the high within-group variability.

As we did not limit time for the subjects to finish each task we also measured time of interaction with the agent. We could not find any difference in time of interaction (t(35)=0.12, n.s.).

From the two options that could be used to close the agent after finishing a step-by-step tutorial in only 8.4 percent of cases the negative one was chosen.

Also the values for wrong parameter input did not differ as a function of condition (t(24.38)=1.08, n.s.). There was a high within group variability and we could identify two subjects with more than 100 wrong inputs. Those participants were using the agent to get information on just some correct input variables and figured out the remaining ones with a try and error approach. Both subjects have been in the reactive-agent group.

For restarts we could not find any disparities between conditions (t(35)=0.19, n.s.). The overall number of restarts needed was quite low.

3.2 Self-developed Questionnaire

This section describes the results attained with the self-developed questionnaires. Means and standard deviations are summarized in Table 2, Fig. 5, and Fig. 6.

Table 2. Means and standard deviations of self-developed scales

| | reactive agent | | proactive agent | |
	M	SD	M	SD
help behavior	6.08	1.18	5.63	1.52
impact on user	4.97	1.25	4.75	0.90
optimism	4.87	1.55	4.22	0.89
tolerance	5.55	1.35	4.92	1.05
humanity	2.34	1.02	2.89	0.93
competence	5.62	1.15	5.19	0.97
intrusiveness	2.66	1.35	3.13	1.11
potential of distraction	2.57	1.34	3.65	1.54
perceived dominance	2.24	0.80	3.07	0.87

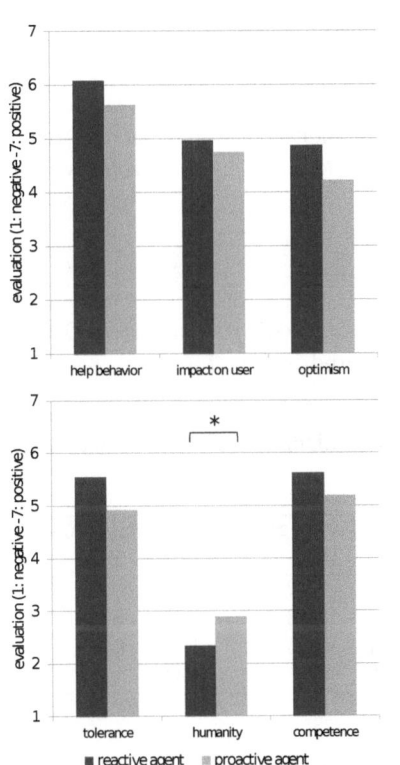

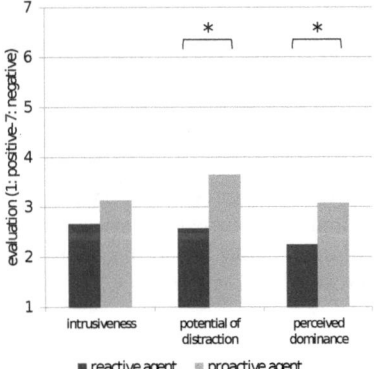

Fig. 5. Means for evaluations scales, where high values are positive. * $p_1 < .05$.

Fig. 6. Means for evaluation scales, where high values are negative. * $p_1 < .05$.

There were no significant differences in the perceived *help behavior* of the agent (t(35)=1.02, n.s.) and the *impact on users* (t(35)=.62, n.s.).

The *optimism* scale revealed a marginal difference between both groups (t(35)=1.54, p₁=.07, d=0.53): The reactive agent group reported Dr. Nick to be more optimistic than the proactive agent group. We found a similar marginal effect for the *tolerance* scale (t(35)=1.59, p₁=.06, d=0.53): Dr. Nick was perceived to be more tolerant by the reactive agent group than by the proactive agent group. *Humanity* of Dr. Nick was rated significantly different by the two experimental groups (t(35)=1.70, p₁<.05, d=0.56): The proactive agent group reported Dr. Nick to be more human than the reactive agent group.

The scale on *competence* of Dr. Nick, which is the last one, where high values reflect a positive rating, showed no significant group differences (t(35)=1.24, n.s.)

The perceived *intrusiveness* of Dr. Nick was rated similar in the proactive- and the reactive-agent-group (t(35)=1.15, n.s.).

For the *potential of distraction* scale we could find a difference between our experimental groups (t(35)=2.29, p₁<.05, d=0.75): The proactive-agent group was more distracted by Dr. Nick than the reactive-agent group. Remember that within this scale high values mean a negative evaluation.

The last scale on *perceived dominance*, where high values again reflect a negative evaluation, also showed that the experimental group with the reactive agent found Dr. Nick less dominant than participants in the proactive group (t(35)=3.04, p₁<.01, d=0.99).

3.3   AttrakDiff Questionnaire

Means and standard deviations for the results attained with the AttrakDiff questionnaire are summarized in Table 3 and depicted in Fig. 7.

Table 3. Means and standard deviations of AttrakDiff-scales for both experimental groups

	reactive agent		proactive agent	
	M	SD	M	SD
perceived pragmatic quality (PQ)	5.40	0.72	4.90	0.70
hedonic quality - stimulation (HQS)	4.25	0.58	3.51	0.98
hedonic quality - identification (HQI)	4.81	0.73	4.44	0.83
perceived attractiveness (AT)	4.87	0.58	4.41	0.78

For *pragmatic quality* we could show that the agent's support of target achievement was significantly better in the reactive agent group than in the proactive agent group (t(35)=2.15, p₁<.05, d=0.70).

Regarding novelty and potential to grab attention (*hedonic quality – stimulation*) a significant difference could be found (t(27.30)=2.81, p₁<.01, d=0.95): hedonic stimulation was higher in the reactive agent group.

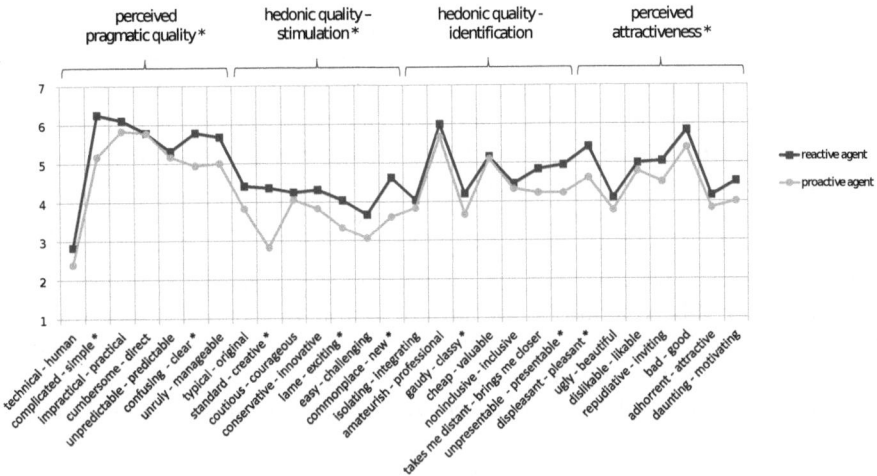

Fig. 7. Means of all AttrakDiff-questionnaire items * p₁<.05

Assessment of potential of identification (*hedonic quality – identification*) showed a marginal significant difference between the two experimental groups $(t(35)=1.46, p_1=.08, d=0.47)$: hedonic identification was slightly lower in the reactive agent group.

According to the *attractiveness (ATT)* scale the agent was rated to be more attractive in the reactive agent group $(t(35)=2.04, p_1<.05, d=0.68)$.

4   Discussion

This study evaluated the effects of proactivity on users' perception of an interactive, anthropomorphic, and assisting agent. We were interested in objective, as well as in subjective measures. On the one hand our hypotheses stated, that we might find differences in subjective measures (e.g. potential of distraction) as a proactive agent might be perceived differently than a reactive agent. On the other hand, we supposed that there would be no differences regarding objective measures. As we assumed that for example time on task or amount of wrong parameter inputs were not different due to Dr. Nick offering the same kind of help in both conditions.

4.1   Subjective Measures – Evaluation Questionnaire

Overall there was a clear tendency to rate the proactive agent worse than the reactive one. For most scales of the self-developed questionnaire we could not find significant differences between the two conditions. However, for scales where high ratings are positive, means showed that the reactive agent was rated better than the proactive version (except for one scale). Whereas for scales where low ratings are positive, the reactive agent was rated lower, which means better.

Most times standard deviation was rather high within each experimental group. This could be an explanation for not finding more significant effects.

For perceived help behavior, our subjects rated Dr. Nick very high in the proactive-agent group as well as in the reactive-agent group. As our subjects had to complete predefined tasks, and our agent was always offering help in a semantic way, which means he only offered help that was related to the task, we might have provoked a ceiling effect.

Also the impact on the user did not differ between our experimental groups. As Cronbach's alpha for this scale was lower than .70, we assume that the developed items for this scale were not optimal to measure the impact of the agent on the user. Therefore this scale might not have been able to differentiate between the two groups. Another explanation could be that Dr. Nick in his reactive and his proactive version is not affecting users in a different way. For further studies the items for this scale need to be reviewed. It might be possible to adapt them in order to improve internal reliability.

The scales for optimism and tolerance of Dr. Nick only revealed marginal differences, where the agent was rated better in the reactive group than in the proactive one. The text output of the agent was the same for both conditions, kind of neutral and not reflecting optimism or tolerance. During interaction Dr. Nick was for example not using emotional speech and he was also not trying to be motivating or anything similar. Thus this marginal effects might be artifacts of differences in intrusiveness, potential of distraction and perceived dominance reflecting differences in proactivity.

While the humanity rating was rather low in both conditions, the proactive version was rated to be significantly more human than the reactive one. This is an indicator that proactive behavior is perceived to be more human like. A similar item appeared in the scale on perceived pragmatic quality. It contained a biploar verbal anchor saying *technical – human*. Compared to our scale on humanity the bipolar verbal anchor *technical – human* did not show significant differences between the experimental conditions. Therefore we argue that our scale on humanity is not measuring human behavior in comparison to technical behavior. Another interesting aspect concerning the amount of humanity the subjects attributed to the agent was found in an objective measurement. Even if users in general rather neglected the human aspects of the agent with rather low ratings on humanity, we found that conforming to Nass, Steuer & Tauber [21] participants nevertheless tended to behave polite towards Dr. Nick. This was expressed by thanking him for his help after finishing a step by step guide and not using the negative option in 91.6 percent of cases.

According to the perceived competence of Dr. Nick no differences could be found between our experimental groups. As the agent did not provide different information in both groups and did not give any wrong information this result is not surprising. Competence on Dr. Nick also correlates high with results in the scale for help behavior ($r=.75$, $p<.001$). This scale also attained very high ratings in both conditions and the lack of significant difference could be due to another ceiling effect.

Within the scales intrusiveness, potential of distraction and perceived dominance we expected significant differences between our experimental conditions. According to peoples' negative responses when they were asked about Clippy [7], the proactive agent was expected to be rated more intrusive, more distractive and more dominant than the reactive agent. While the scale on intrusiveness did not reveal any significant differences, the scales measuring potential of distraction and perceived dominance did. The results on intrusiveness are similar to findings by Xiao et al. [10], they also could not show differences in intrusiveness between proactive and reactive agents. A reason for similar ratings in both conditions could be that in the proactive condition the agent was always activated at a well defined point in time, namely when the user had finished reading the task or error description. Thus users were never interrupted by the agent in the middle of something.

Even though users did not judge the proactive agent to be more intrusive, they nevertheless judged it to be more disturbing. This could be induced by the proactive agent being activated right after the user had finished reading the task description. During task description the actual content of the user interface was not displayed and after the click Dr. Nick popped up and required users' attention, while new elements became visible. Thus users might have appreciated having some time to take a look at the new content, before the agent popped up. Nevertheless, only in 11.2 percent of cases the agent was closed right after it was proactively opened by the system, indicating that due to the high task complexity users appreciated the help and preferred finishing the task quickly over having a closer look at the power plant interface themselves. Perceived dominance is correlating high with potential of distraction (r=.58, p<.001). This indicates that a proactive agent is not only experienced to be distracting but also very dominant. As people usually consider dominance and distraction to be bad characteristics, they rated the proactive agent worse.

4.2   Subjective Measures – AttrakDiff Questionnaire

As expected, we found differences between our two conditions for the AttrakDiff-scales.

We found a significant difference in *perceived pragmatic quality*, which means potential to support users' goals. By looking closely at each item, it can be observed that the significance of the overall scale results in differences in two items (see Fig. 7). As expected the reactive agent was perceived to be less complicated and less confusing under pragmatical aspects. The remaining pragmatical aspects do not differ significantly, but means show that the reactive agent nevertheless is consistently rated better or at least as good as the proactive one. Therefore a reactive agent seems to be the better choice, as it better supports users' goals.

The scale on *hedonic quality – stimulation* also showed significant differences between the two conditions. Again only a few items can be seen as reason for the overall significant difference. Namely *standard – creative, lame – exciting,* and *commonplace – new.* These findings are very difficult to interpret and we think there are some further studies needed to explain them in a proper way. Especially differences in creativity are surprising. Perhaps the proactive agent, that was always performing the same action (user indicated by clicking a button that he had read the instruction, proactive agent popped up), was rated to be rather uncreative and therefore acting very standardized, and lame. This would also make him quite commonplace.

Hedonic quality – identification showed no significant differences for the experimental groups but also within this scale some items showed significant differences. Especially the item *unpresentable – presentable* showed that the reactive agent is rated to be more presentable. This can be seen as confirmation for the result attained with the scales for potential of distraction and perceived dominance.

Last but not least we found differences in perceived attractiveness, which measures, in our case, how attractive the agent appears to the user. Only one item of the whole scale showed significant differences, but for each item the rating for the reactive agent was better than for the proactive agent. Therefore a reactive agent is more attractive to the user than a proactive agent. According to findings by Xiao et al. [10] on Clippy we expected the reactive agent to be more attractive.

4.3 Objective Measures

Similar to Xiao and colleagues [10] and according to our hypothesis we could not find any differences in objective measures. Users amount of time needed for task completion was similar for both groups, as well as time on task and interaction time with Dr. Nick. Both groups had a similar amount of wrong inputs and restarts. As users were forced to accept help from Dr. Nick and tasks were designed not to be solved without Dr. Nick the lack of differences is not surprising.

5 Conclusion and Future Work

In contrast to previous studies we were able to show that proactive behavior has an influence on the subjective rating of animated interface agents.

The reactive agent was especially perceived to be less dominant and less distracting. Additionally, the reactive agent performed significantly better in three of the four different scales of the AttrakDiff questionnaire [14].

Even though the observed effects were rather small, this is a hint that proactivity might have played an important role in building up the resentments towards Clippy. A reason for the effects to be rather small might be that the agent in this study was kind of "well-behaved". It only offered help at a well defined point in the interaction process (at the beginning of each task) and for tasks, users could not accomplish otherwise; it only offered relevant alternatives and it did not exhibit idle animations. Those four points are definitely not true for Clippy. Hence the fact that we nevertheless attained significant results, confirms our point of view.

The key differences between the present study and previously published work, investigating the proactivity of animated interface agents – especially [10] – was the way the agent was presented and the output modality. While the agent in the present study was displayed along with the actual content of the user interface, the agent of Xiao et al. was presented in a separate area. This might not be a problem, if the agent uses spoken language to communicate with the user, but if text based output is required a proactive agent making suggestions might just be overlooked. Another aspect of separating the agent from the interface is the problem that interface assisting agents should be able to interact with the content in order to provide adequate help at the interface level. Consider for example the task, participants had to solve in Fig. 3. Three different numbers had to be entered into three input fields. For an agent with text output as modality that is not able to interact with the content, an instruction for this task would have read something like "First enter 41 into input field B3, then enter 36.8 . . . " This would force the user to remember three times at least two numbers and one letter in order to identify the correct input field and enter the correct value. That is why a typical answer of users, after they have utilized Dr. Nick for the first time and are asked to stress something positive about him, is: "I actually liked that he pointed at things". This ability to point out relevant elements to the user is surely one of the reasons, why in a test in the grid computing domain novice users assisted by Dr. Nick were significantly faster submitting their first grid job than users employing a traditional approach based on help texts. [22].

Thus separating the agent from the interface seems not to be an option. Hence we are planning to focus on changing the output modality of the agent to remedy the negative effects of proactivity pointed out in the present study. Accordingly for our next study we are planning Dr. Nick to proactively offer help using spoken output. Even if spoken output is not very practical in certain environments, we would nevertheless like to verify our hypothesis that the output modality has an influence on the negative effects of proactivity in the context of interactive help agents.

Acknowledgments. This work was supported by the bwGRiD portal project that was funded by the Ministry of Science, Research and the Arts Baden-Wuerttemberg. We would like to thank Maria-Magdalena Attenberger, Luise Knecht, Nelli Maucher, Melanie Partsch, Franziska Perner, Manuela Rappel, and Franziska Rück for helping to conduct this study by recruiting participants and performing part of the data collection.

References

[1] Lazar, J., Jones, A., Hackley, M., Shneiderman, B.: Severity and impact of computer user frustration: A comparison of student and workplace users. Interacting with Computers 18(2), 187–207 (2006)

[2] Ceaparu, I., Lazar, J., Bessiere, K.: Determining causes and severity of end-user frustration. International Journal of Human-Computer Interaction 17(3), 333–356 (2004)

[3] Lazar, J., Jones, A., Shneiderman, B.: Workplace user frustration with computers: an exploratory investigation of the causes and severity. Behaviour & Information Technology 25(3), 239–251 (2006)

[4] Smith, M.J., Conway, F.T., Karsh, B.T.: Occupational stress in human computer interaction. Industrial Health 37(2), 157–173 (1999)

[5] Lang, H., Dolpp, T., Minker, W.: Evaluation of methods to acquire help with computer problems. Unpublished Raw Data (2012)

[6] Nauman, M., Khan, S., Khan, S.: Helplets: A common sense-based collaborative help collection and retrieval architecture for web-enabled systems. In: Web-based Support Systems, pp. 43–63. Springer, Heidelberg (2010)

[7] Xiao, J., Stasko, J., Catrambone, R.: An empirical study of the effect of agent competence on user performance and perception. In: Proceedings of the Third International Joint Conference on Autonomous Agents and Multiagent Systems, AAMAS 2004, vol. 1, pp. 178–185. IEEE Computer Society, Washington, DC (2004)

[8] Dix, A., Lepouras, G., Katifori, A., Vassilakis, C., Catarci, T., Poggi, A., Ioannidis, Y., Mora, M., Daradimos, I., Akim, N.M., Humayoun, S.R., Terella, F.: From the web of data to a world of action. Web Semantics: Science, Services and Agents on the World Wide Web 8(4), 394–408 (2010)

[9] Rickenberg, R., Reeves, B.: The effects of animated characters on anxiety, task performance, and evaluations of user interfaces. In: Proceedings of the SIGCHI Conference on Human Factors in Computing Systems, CHI 2000, pp. 49–56. ACM, New York (2000)

[10] Xiao, J., Catrambone, R., Stasko, J.: Be quiet? evaluating proactive and reactive user interface assistants. In: Proceedings of INTERACT 2003, pp. 383–390 (2003)

[11] Kim, Y., Baylor, A.L.: Pedagogical Agents as Learning Companions: The Role of Agent Competency and Type of Interaction. Educational Technology Research and Development 54(3), 223–243 (2006)

[12] Baddeley, A.: Working memory. Science 255(5044), 556–559 (1992)

[13] Lang, H., Mosch, C., Boegel, B., Benoit, D.M., Minker, W.: An Avatar-Based Help System for Web-Portals. In: Jacko, J.A. (ed.) Human-Computer Interaction, Part II, HCII 2011. LNCS, vol. 6762, pp. 537–546. Springer, Heidelberg (2011)

[14] Hassenzahl, M., Burmester, M., Koller, F.: AttrakDiff: Ein Fragebogen zur Messung wahrgenommener hedonischer und pragmatischer Qualität. In: Szwillus, G., Ziegler, J. (eds.) Mensch & Computer 2003: Interaktion in Bewegung, Teubner, pp. 187–196 (2003)

[15] Schwarzer, R., Jerusalem, M.: Skalen zur Erfassung von Lehrer- und Schülermerkmalen. Dokumentation der psychometrischen Verfahren im Rahmen der Wissenschaftlichen Begleitung des Modellversuchs Selbstwirksame Schulen, Berlin (1999)

[16] Borkenau, P., Ostendorf, F.: Neo-Fünf-Faktoren Inventar. Hogrefe, Verlag f. Psychologie (1993)

[17] Kipp, M.: Anvil-a generic annotation tool for multimodal dialogue. In: Proceedings of the 7th European Conference on Speech Communication and Technology (Eurospeech), pp. 1367–1370 (2001)

[18] Levene, H.: Robust tests for equality of variances. Contributions to probability and statistics: Essays in Honor of Harold Hotelling 2, 278–292 (1960)

[19] Welch, B.L.: The generalization of student's' problem when several different population variances are involved. Biometrika, 28–35 (1947)

[20] Cohen, J.: Statistical power analysis for the behavioral sciences. Lawrence Erlbaum (1988)

[21] Nass, C., Moon, Y.: Machines and Mindlessness: Social Responses to Computers. Journal of Social Issues 56(1), 81–103 (2000)

[22] Lang, H., Minker, W.: A collaborative web-based help-system. In: Proceedings of the 2nd International Conference on Web Intelligence, Mining and Semantics - WIMS 2012, pp. 60:1–60:5. ACM Press, New York (2012)

Platform-Aware Rich-Form Generation for Adaptive Systems through Code-Inspection

Miroslav Macik, Tomas Cerny, Jindrich Basek, and Pavel Slavik

Czech Technical University in Prague,
Faculty of Electrical Engineering,
Department of Computer Graphics and Interaction,
Karlovo nam. 13, 131 25, Praha 2, Czech Republic
{macikmir,cernyto3,basekjin,slavik}@fel.cvut.cz

Abstract. This paper introduces a framework for adaptive user interface (UI) development. Our framework facilitates development and maintenance efforts through code inspection. Information already captured elsewhere is reused in the UI rather than restated. In our approach, inspected information is transformed in multiple stages through an aspect-oriented approach. As each stage may be influenced at runtime, our approach allows systems to be built with context-aware adaptive UIs. In addition, the selection of UI elements and their layout is generated using optimal metrics. The output of our approach can be influenced by the target platform. Our approach to UI is shown in detail in a case study.

Keywords: automatic UI generation, aspect-oriented, adaptive design, context-aware.

1 Introduction

From the user's point of view, the quality of a user interface (UI) is perceived as the quality of the application itself. A UI mediates communication between the user and the rest of the application. The development of application UIs with a conventional approach typically requires significant implementation efforts. Accordingly to [1], about one half of an application code is related to its UI, mostly due to restated information from the data model and duplication in UI fragments that contain tangled code. The development and maintenance costs of interactive applications are therefore greatly affected by the effort invested in their UIs.

For applications where different user roles are taken into the account [2], the problem is even more serious. These applications usually contain a significant amount of code that is related to UIs for individual user roles. A typical problem here is code-replication, which makes application development and maintenance even harder. These efforts become even more complex when clients need the support of various platforms, e.g. Windows, Mac, iOS, Android or HTML 5. The target devices differ, e.g. in form (desktop PC, table PC, smartphone etc.)

A. Holzinger et al. (Eds.): SouthCHI 2013, LNCS 7946, pp. 768–784, 2013.

or in interaction modality (keyboard+mouse, touch, voice, or combinations). It is necessary to implement the UI and the corresponding application logic for each individual platform. The cost of developing and maintaining the UI therefore forms a major part of the total application development costs.

Recent advances in the accessibility of interactive systems suggest that these systems should anticipate users' specific needs and adapt to the usage context. An interesting approach to this problem is through ability-based design [3]. Usage context adaptation is a key feature of ability-based systems. A basic context model [4] consists of a user model, a device model and an environment model. According to [3], a good interactive system should adapt dynamically to context properties expressed by these sub-models at runtime. It is very complicated to implement each possible combination of properties in these models, so an automated solution is necessary. A possible solution to the problems indicated above is to generate a UI automatically, as described in [5] or [6].

This paper aims to address problems related to the development of UIs that adapt to their usage context, i.e. adaptive UIs. First, in section 3.1 we address problems of conventional approaches that need to restate information that is already present in order to extend it. We propose that captured information should be received by automated data persistence model [7] code analysis (code inspection). This information is thus captured only once, which reduces the development and maintenance efforts.

Significant portion of information restated in the UI comes from application persistence model. Rather than to reference the model directly from the UI we apply code-inspection of an extended model. The inspected information are transformed in multiple steps into the UI. Inspecting the persistence model information and transforming into the UI, rather than to restating it, defines a single focal point of information. Application developer needs to address only one location to access or modify the information. Furthermore, the information stated in persistence models are enforced in the UI and no inconsistency or error introduced from restatement may occur.

As the next step, in section 3.2 we introduce a model-based approach for automatic context-sensitive UI generation. Information captured by persistence-model analysis is transformed at runtime into concrete UIs. These UIs can be

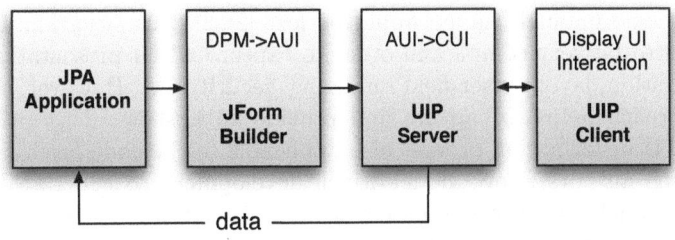

Fig. 1. Architecture overview

displayed on a number of different platforms, including a desktop PC, a tablet PC and a Smartphone. In addition, adaptations for a context model are performed to reflect specific user properties and needs and the actual environment.

The high-level life-cycle of our approach is shown in Fig. 1. Based on data persistence model (DPM) analysis, AspectFaces library generates an abstract user interface (AUI) that is later transformed by context-aware UI generation into a concrete user interface (CUI). CUIs generated at runtime can be displayed on a number of UIP clients. In this paper, we focus on the following platforms: desktop PCs, tablet PCs and smartphones, but other platforms, e.g. smart TV and multi-touch terminals are already being added. One of the key advantages of the proposed approach is that it is not necessary to restate any application code when another user interface platform is added to the system. The proposed framework was evaluated from the perspective of target user audience (section 4.1) and from the perspective of development costs (section 4.2).

2   Related Work

The idea of automating or at least simplifying the process of user interface generation is not novel. Various approaches have addressed this issue, including generation approaches, model-based approaches, inspection-based approaches and aspect-based approaches. Each approach has its own benefits, and a combination of these approaches is usually used. For example, the natural idea of model-driven development [2] suggests itself, as the information source exists in one location and thus code replication will not exist in the UI. This assumption is correct, but there is a problem with context-awareness and adaptivity, because the model-driven approach fails to capture various concerns independent of each other. This results in code-duplication, and as a consequence it makes development and maintenance harder.

Aspect-oriented design [8,9] can be used to deal with cross-cutting concerns. Aspect-oriented design and model-driven development can be combined, but this approach will not be applicable to existing systems where no models exist. Let us consider a case when a model is used to generate an application UI, but a small change to the UI must later be applied. This change often takes place in the UI part, and not in the model, as the model captures only a subset of properties. This pretty much disallows further use of the model to generate the UI, because the manual change would be lost [2]. In this situation, the model would need to be very complex in order to capture all UI presentation details, e.g. presentation, layout, user-field rendering, security, etc. However, the model-driven approach helps to capture and provide an abstract description of the generalised transformation process also applicable to the code level.

In [2], the authors apply model-driven development to generate rich-forms from class models. They apply object-relational mapping stereotypes and validation stereotypes to the model, and further extend it with stereotypes for the UI part and security. This approach allows the generation of variations of UI forms that reflect multiple situations. The properties that are not addressed in this research are its applicability for adaptive UI, and also for a changing environment that may have multiple further concerns to consider. For example, consider that an adaptive UI may have various form presentations. The forms may apply in a different layout, or the UI should adapt to the user context and make adjustments based on it. In this case, additional concerns would have to be captured in the class model, but this kind of extension has a limitation on readability, and not all concerns can be solved on this level (e.g. multiple layouts).

Next, we consider an alternative approach to model-driven development. Code inspection [1,10] uses the existing code base and provides properties similar to model-driven approaches. It allows information to be harvested from the system and re-applied it in multiple places in the UI, or extended according to the user context. In this process, a meta-model is built and then transformed through templates to the UI. The transformation may consider different concerns arising at runtime. The advantage over the model-driven approach is its natural use with common development frameworks. In [10] the authors suggest the use of templates and mapping rules to apply minor changes in the UI, and also configuration by exception, when the mainstream transformation follows general rules and edge cases have special mapping rules and templates.

There are a few tools that apply code inspection and transformation. Aspect-Faces [10] is a standalone tool for Java-based applications. It has the ability to inspect data models and to understand their extension marks, e.g. Java Persistence Architecture (JPA) [11], and has features to support additional user-defined extensions. The MetaWidget tool [1] has a similar aim, but fails to provide the mapping to custom components, and is not able to switch among different presentation and layouts, which is especially needed for adaptive systems. In AspectFaces, the code-inspected information about the data model is composed into a metamodel. This metamodel is then queried in the transformation process through aspect approach to determine the appropriate template to apply for the transformation. Each template has a textual form, and describes a component of the target platform through the domain specific language (DSL). The transformation uses the selected template to inject the relevant meta-model properties related to the data instance. However, AspectFaces does not address native support for UI for different platforms, and it also does not provide global optimisation to derive optimal UI component selection and layout.

There are many types of interactive devices with the ability to display UIs. These devices have various form factors and are based on various platforms. Technologies that allow a single UI to be delivered to various platforms are already available. The most widely-used are (X)HTML+CSS and HTML 5. The problem is to adapt the UIs to particular device properties, e.g. screen resolution, size, interaction modality, etc. There are web frameworks that help to solve this problem to some extent, e.g. [12], but currently there is no general solution. UIP (User Interface Platform) [6] can deliver UIs to various heterogeneous UI clients. UIProtocol handles both the UI description and the communication.

Unlike HTML, UIProtocol UIs are displayed using native UI components of individual client platforms. Each supported platform comes with an implementation of UIProtocol client.

Modifications of UIs are necessary not only in order to adapt UIs to individual platforms, but also to adapt UIs to the specific needs of users with disabilities. Regarding user capabilities and preferences, most solutions currently strive to fit people with disabilities to standard systems, using various assistive technologies. This can stigmatise users with disabilities, and force them to use expensive assistive technologies even when a similar effect can be achieved by adapting the systems. In addition, some expensive assistive technologies are hard to use, and there is a high abandonment rate [13]. Ability-based design [3] has been proposed in response to this problem. It uses context-awareness to provide adaptations to user-specific abilities, instead of forcing users to use a specific assistive technology.

Ability-based systems can be customised to suit the needs and the performance of particular users. They can adapt automatically in response to user behaviour, or they can be customised by a user. In order to provide context-aware adaptations, a context model must be present. There is a context model [4] that builds on the requirements of ability-based design. The main goal of its design is to provide a complex context model that is easy to maintain and powerful enough to describe user abilities and preferences as well as the properties of interaction devices and the actual environment.

UIP [blinded] uses combinatoric optimisation and a context model to generate UIs for various UI platforms and types of users. It allows the generation of UIs optimised to require low interaction effort from their users. For automatic UI generation, UIP requires an abstract UI (AUI) as an input. AUI is a model that is described in domain-specific language – UIProtocol. This language can be harder to understand for newcomers than standard notions like JPA. In this paper we describe the benefits of integrating AspectFaces and UIP Platform to both developers and target users.

3   Proposed Framework

This section describes the proposed framework. Individual components and their input/output are described in detail. Fig. 2 depicts an abstract view on the architecture of the framework. We apply code-inspection of persistence models in order to avoid restatement of information in models that use a markup language with weak type safety. The inspection and transformation derives an AUI model and data model in runtime. In this approach, both models transfer to the user interface platform (UIP) server. In the next phase, the UiGE UI generator derives a context-aware CUI. Finally, this CUI transfers to the target client platform and renders as the final UI.

Dynamic fields of CUI are initialised by values from the data model, using model-wind binding. The application logic that corresponds to user actions is implemented in the UIP Server in the form of event handlers. There are event

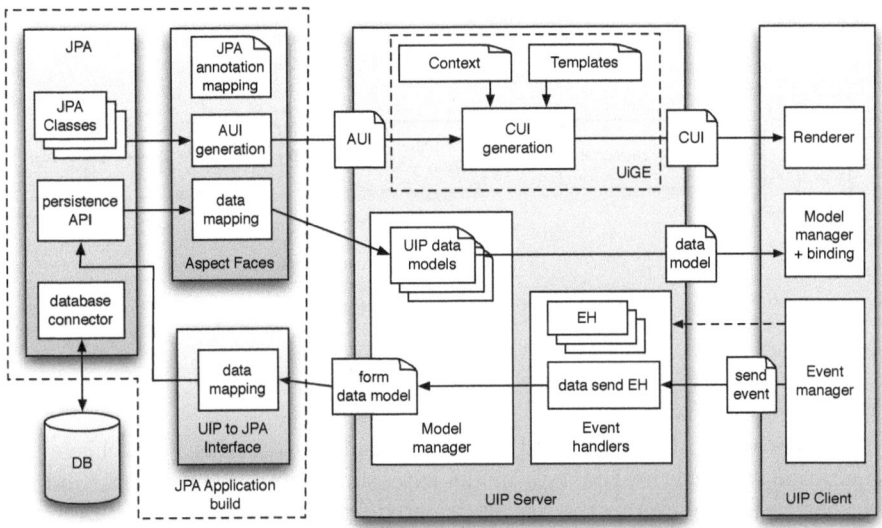

Fig. 2. Framework architecture

handlers for handling events such as navigation in the CUI, validation and injecting the final data back into the corresponding JPA application. In the further text will be presented a detailed description of each phase.

3.1 Code Inspection

Code inspection is based on a code base that must be implemented in any case, for example JPA classes. Information already stated in this existing code base can be reused in order to avoid code duplication, and consequently to achieve improved development and maintenance. In our approach, we assume that an application backend exists. The persistence part most likely consists of a data model represented by classes. Similarly, the persistent state of these classes will most likely be stored in a relational database. In most cases, the persistence process uses object-relational mapping (ORM). In [14], a profile providing an extension to the class model is suggested in order to simplify the mapping. This profile is based on existing Java standards for ORM. Later, in [2] this profile is further extended for input validation and also for presentation. In addition, similar extensions are often used by the annotation driver participant pattern (ADPP)[15] for security purposes. These profiles are represented by stereotypes in UML, and in the source code an equivalent to a stereotype can be seen as an annotation. We mention data model extensions because they can be used to derive fragments of UIs [2].

Since the application data model already uses ORM, it may also consider data field validation and security presentation constraints [2]. As shown in Fig. 3, this information is captured by the data model, the concerns are not necessarily

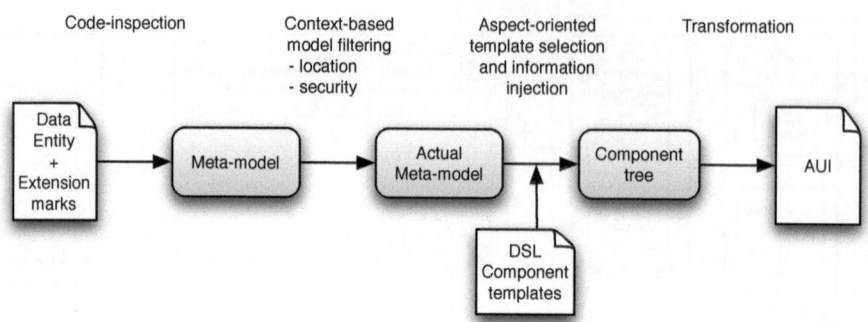

Fig. 3. Code inspection

mixed, because this information is often considered together. To achieve good separation of concerns, the data-model extensions should be minimal, and they can act as join points in the aspect-oriented approach (AO). An inspection of this kind of data model can capture all information that may be needed later in the UI.

This AO code inspection approach is adapted in AspectFaces library. The library inspects a given data instance considering its extensions. All inspected information is captured in a metamodel. This metamodel can be modified or filtered based on the contextual information, or can be extended with separately captured aspects. The context can consider properties such as user preferences, user access rights, or even a target location, and thus all of these may influence the transformation. In the next stage, the library transforms the metamodel to the UI through pre-prepared fragments related to the target language. The library uses generalised transformation rules that match the field information (types, constraints, extensions) via point cuts [8], to select an advice which links to a template that is used by the transformation of a given field to the UI presentation. The transformer selects a given template for each data field and injects there the context from the meta-model and the application. In our case, the target language used for the transformation is the AUI specification, so the product of the transformation is not a UI fragment but an intermediate step towards it. The products are data-specific AUI fragments.

A benefit of the inspection is that the correlation between the persistence model and AUI does not need to be developed and maintained manually. Considering that the data model and its properties are often non-trivial, the manual mapping process is tedious and error-prone. Next, the AUI uses a language without type safety, and it is not easy to notice an inconsistency, unless a careful revision is made. All future changes to the data model are implicitly applied to the AUI fragments by the life cycle process.

3.2   User Interface Generation

The input for the automatic CUI generation process is an AUI. The goal of the process is to generate UIs that require minimal user effort for interaction in a particular situation (usage context). To make this possible, the UiGE UI generator requires an additional input – the context model. The AUI is a hierarchical structure that describes the UI in platform-independent manner. Basically, this structure specifies what the interface should consist of (input, output and action triggers), but there is no specification about the actual representation of the individual elements and the layout. Relationships between AUI elements and parts of the CUI (that can be rendered on a particular client device) are specified by mappings. Each mapping has its cost, which corresponds to the estimated user effort required for interaction using a particular mapped element. These cost values are later used for optimisation during the UI generation process.

UIs generated using this approach respect the usage context constraints. Each platform supported by the UIP can render any AUI. An example of such an interface generated for iOS operating system is presented in Fig. 5. A problem can arise when there is a specific platform element that should be applied in the UI. An example of such a component is an iOS table (UITableView [16]). This structure provides a very good user experience, but it is a specific component of the iOS platform. It can be mapped only when the AUI contains a specific structure (a subset of AUI). The implementation of a mapping that provides the relationship between the AUI elements and such specific structures will make the UiGE generator too complicated and too hard to maintain. In order to solve this problem, the UiGE is extended to support UI templates. In this case, a template is basically a complex mapping that provides the relationship between a subset of an AUI and a platform specific structure. In can be implemented either programatically using UiGE API, or using the XSLT transformation [17]. An example of a UI generated using a template is presented in Fig. 6.

Next, we provide a description of the UI generation process (see Fig. 4). At the beginning, a set of all possible mappings is reduced according to the current context model to a set of feasible mappings. From the point of view of UiGE, the templates are a special case of a mapping. Similarly to mappings, a set templates is reduced to a set of feasible templates using the context model. Both mappings and templates have their particular cost function value that corresponds to the estimated effort required from the user while interacting with a particular UI component.

In the next phase, mappings and templates are ordered according their cost value. The next phase is the optimisation process, which finds the optimal mapping for all AUI elements with respect to the context model. This is a computationally hard problem (for more details, see [5]). Our optimisation process uses a variant of the branches and bounds algorithm [18,19], and for typical instances provides a solution within a few seconds. The product of the UI generation process is a CUI, which is immediately transferred to the particular UIP client and displayed.

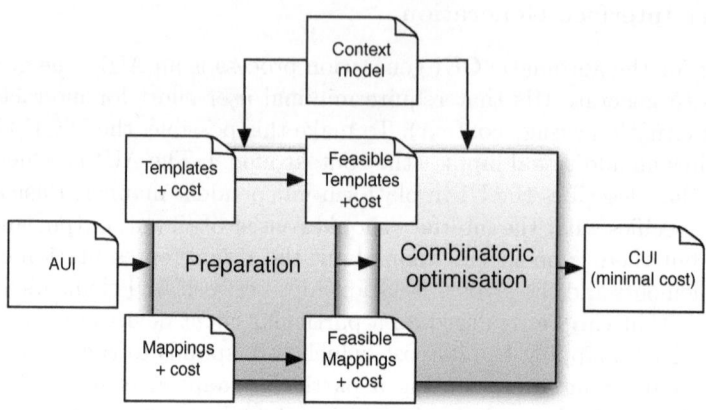

Fig. 4. Simplified scheme of the UI generation process

3.3   Example of a Development Use

This section describes the use of our framework from the developer's point of view. We presume that the context model is already defined in the framework. Context-sensitive UIs for all supported platforms are generated automatically in runtime. The only action that the developer needs to take is to reference Aspect-Faces library and extend the JPA class by a set of corresponding annotations (or add an XML configuration). The code example in Listing 1.1 shows a part of the code used in our proof of concept application. Various UIs that do not need templates can be generated from the amount of code shown in the listing. Examples of such UIs are shown in Figs. 5 and 8.

Additional action is necessary when there is a demand for UIs with platform-specific look and feel, which use specific components. Examples of such UIs are shown in Figs. 6 and 7. In this case, it is necessary to specify a template for each specific component. In our example, only one template is necessary. This template maps the part of the AUI onto an iOS table component. Templates can be specified either in the code or using an XSLT transformation [17].

4   Proof of Concept

In order to verify the correctness of the proposed approach, the framework was tested on the ACM-ICPC registration system, which is a Java EE [20] applica-tion. The aim of this system is to acquire the information necessary for register-ing a new member. Using our approach, the registration form was generated at runtime. The individual steps of the generation process are depicted in Fig. 2. First, the application code is inspected in order to derive an AUI. A subset of the inspected code is presented in Listing 1.1. This phase is provided by Aspect-Faces. In the next phase, the AUI is transferred to the UIProtocol server. The AUI describes UIs on the abstract level, but it does not contain any information about the concrete representation of UI elements and their layout. The CUI is generated from the AUI as soon as a client contacts the UIP server. The CUI is therefore generated on demand for a concrete context (client, user, environment, etc.) Finally, the CUI is transferred to a client platform and rendered. Data is handled separately in so-called data models. These data models are transferred to a client platform on demand, and their updates can later be pushed from the server side.

Fig. 6 depicts a part of the UI generated for the iOS platform (iPhone). Similarly, the proposed framework generates UIs for iPad (Fig. 7) or Windows desktop (Fig. 8). Note that different UI elements are used on different platforms (iOS vs. Windows desktop). A template that enables the use of a platform-specific iOS table component was used for iPhone and iPad UIs. UI properties such as font-size, element-spacing and size of target area (e.g. button or checkbox) are determined according the context model, as proposed in section 3.2. In edge cases, certain UI components mapped by templates prevent the application of given context model properties. If the difference between an actual UI property value and a value specified by the context model (e.g. required font size) is bigger than a specified threshold, the template cannot be applied and a simple mapping is used instead.

4.1   User Study

The aim of this user study was to compare UIs generated by our framework with manually implemented simple web-based UIs. A user study with 12 participants (10 male, 2 female, aged 22 - 48, mean = 30 years) was conducted to evaluate the quality of the UIs generated by our framework. Three platforms were used

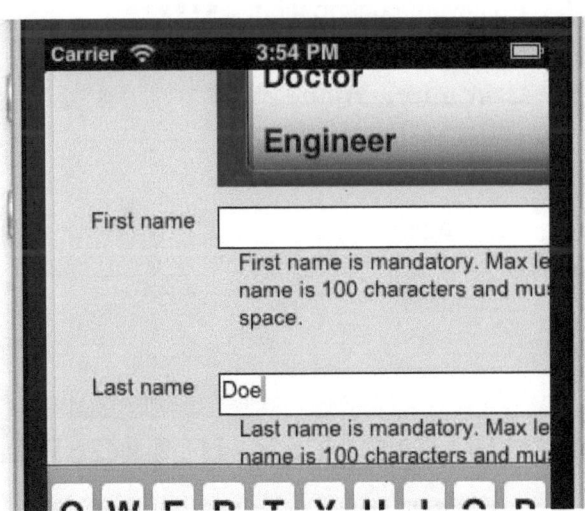

Fig. 5. Example – UI generated without templates

```
class PersonInfo extends EntityObject {

    /*fields*/

    @Column(name = "first_name", nullable = false)
    @Length(max=100) @NotNull
    @Pattern(regexp="^[^\\s].*")
    public String getFirstName() {return this.firstName;}

    @Column(name = "last_name")
    @Length(max=100) @NotNull
    @Pattern(regexp="^[^\\s].*")
    public String getLastName() {return this.lastName;}

    @Email @NotNull
    @Length(max=255)
    public String getEmail() {return this.email;}
}
```

Listing 1.1. Example data entity used for generation of forms in Figs. 6 and 7

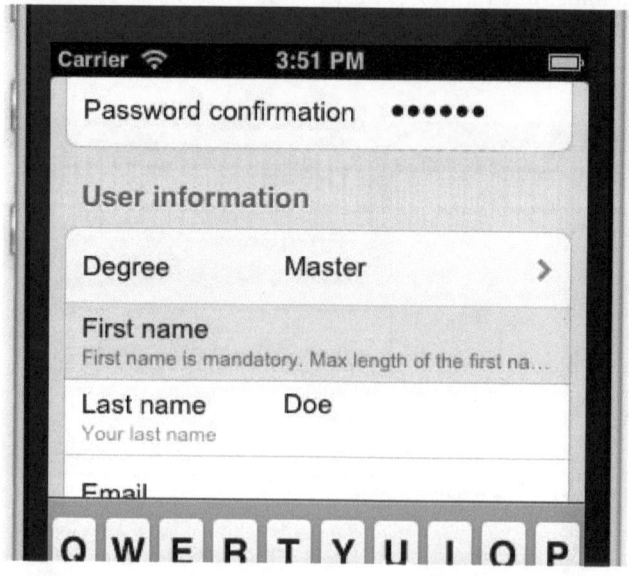

Fig. 6. Example – iOS Client - iPhone

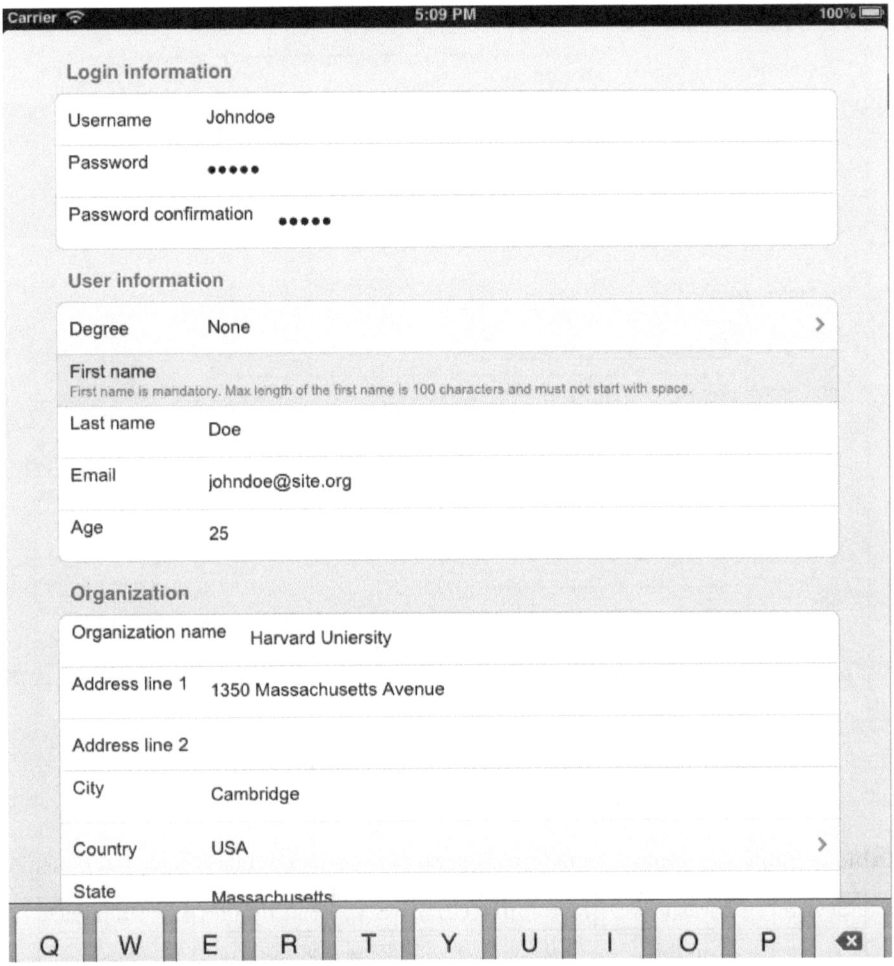

Fig. 7. Example – iOS Client - iPad

during the study – desktop PC, tablet PC and smartphone. At each platform, the participants in the study were presented with UIs generated by our framework and a web UI with a similar functionality. The UIs were assessed subjectively in terms of comfort, efficiency and aesthetic quality. The participants in the study were skilled ICT users who use a computer as their primary work tool. With one exception, all users have a university degree. Each participant was asked to fill in an ACM-ICPC registration form, using both a web browser and UIP client on each platform. The order of the tests was scrambled to avoid possible bias.

Afterwards, the participants were asked to evaluate the six presented UIs for comfort, efficiency and aesthetic quality, on the Likert scale [21] (1 to 5, where 1 is the best score). The Wilcoxon rank-sum test [22] was used to compare the effect of each UI on comfort, efficiency and aesthetic quality. The Wilcoxon rank-sum test is a statistical test that compares two samples and assesses whether

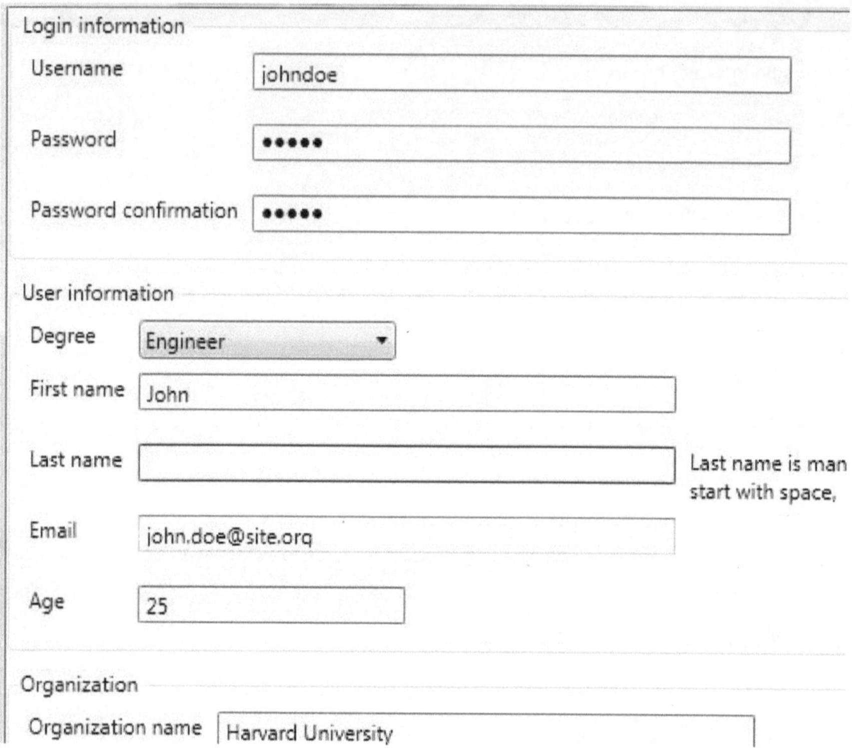

Fig. 8. Example – Windows desktop

Table 1. Subjective evaluation of form UIs. M(x) is median of Likert scale assessments.

Device	UI aspect	M(web)	M(UIP)	Statistical result	Sig. difference
Desktop	comfort	2	1	W = 108, p<0.05	yes
	efficiency	2	1	W = 100, p>0.05	no
	aesthetic quality	4	2	W = 115.5, p<0.05	yes
iPhone	comfort	4	2	W = 121, p<0.005	yes
	efficiency	4	2	W = 114, p<0.05	yes
	aesthetic quality	4	2	W = 134.5, p<0.001	yes
iPad	comfort	3	2	W = 109, p<0.05	yes
	efficiency	3	2	W = 110, p<0.05	yes
	aesthetic quality	4	2	W = 126, p<0.005	yes

their population mean ranks differ. It is used as an alternative to the paired Student t-test in cases when the population cannot be assumed to be normally distributed [23]. The results of the statistical evaluation are presented in Table 1.

The user study proved that the generated UIs provide a better subjective user experience for comfort, efficiency and aesthetic quality. On the desktop

Table 2. Comparison of manual and code-inspected approach regards the size of code

Component	Manual approach (LOC)	AF approach (LOC)
Persistence model	370	370
Extension to the persistence model	-	96
Text label properties	-	108
UIP XML forms	703	-
JavaScript library	300	300
JavaScript in view	446	-

PC, the usage comfort was evaluated as better for the UIP client ($M = 1$), though both UIs provide good results. There is a non-significant difference in efficiency between UIP client ($M = 1$) and web UI ($M = 2$), so their performance can be evaluated as comparably good. The aesthetic quality was evaluated as significantly better for the UIP client ($M = 2$) than for the desktop web UI ($M = 4$).

Using the iPhone smart phone, all three metrics were evaluated as significantly better for the UIP client. For all three metrics, the medians of the Likert scale values were 2 for the UIP client and 4 for the respective web UI. For the iPad tablet, all three metrics were also evaluated as significantly better for the UIP client. For the web UI, the medians for comfort and efficiency metrics were 3, and for aesthetic quality the median was 4. The UIP client provided better results with median $= 2$ for all evaluated metrics.

Generally, our framework provided UIs that were more highly rated in the user study. The biggest advantage over the web UI was on iPhone. In this case, the UI generated by our framework was based on easy-to-navigate iOS Table View. By contrast, the web page required a lot of scrolling and zooming, which worsened its usability.

4.2 Development and Maintenance Efforts

The study is further evaluated from the perspective of development and maintenance. We consider a manually developed system and compare it with a system built using our approach. The persistence model of the considered application consists of 7 entities. For both applications considered here, the model consists of 370 physical lines of code (LOC). With the manual approach, it is necessary to implement XML forms for the UIP, and it consists of JavaScript (JS) references and a JS library. The XML forms have 703 LOC, while the JS references and library have 300 and 446 LOC.

With our approach, the persistence model is extended with additional marks, resulting in 96 additional LOC for the persistence model. Generic UIP configuration, templates and UI handler are designed for AspectFaces library, and all these are applicable to different UIP projects. The UI part is generated through persistence model inspection and transformation. To deal with text labels, we apply them in the text property file rather than in forms (108 LOC). Table 2 summarises the efforts. In order to develop the project manually, we need to implement 370 LOC of the persistence model, 703 LOC of XML with weak type safety, and 746 LOC of JS. With our approach, we only need to implement 466 LOC of the persistence model, define text properties (108 LOC) and use 300 LOC of the JS library.

It must be considered that when we develop the UIP project manually, the entire presentation source code in addition to JavaScript library, must be developed. Especially in the XML part, with forms, there is a burden of restated information in a weak type safety, so future changes to the persistence model must also be manually applied in the XML part. By contrast, with our approach the changes take place only in a single location, the persistence model. We must consider that there is a reduction not only in the source code, but also in the coupling among different subsystems. In addition, the time devoted to both development and maintenance is reduced, because the UI part adjusts to the information already captured in the persistence part, and no manual restating takes place.

4.3   Discussion

We have presented a system that uses code inspection for automatic context-sensitive UI generation. We used an example application, the ACM-ICPC registration system, to prove the concept. A user study was conducted to assess the quality of the UIs generated on three different platforms. The UIs ware compared against web-based UIs with similar functionality. The user study proved that the generated UIs are in most cases better in terms of comfort, efficiency and aesthetic quality. The UIs were assessed subjectively by each participant, using the Likert scale. The user study provides promising results for the population of users that have no disabilities. It is necessary to conduct another specifically focused user study to assess the quality of context-sensitive adaptation for users with specific needs.

One of the main goals of the proposed system is to reduce the development and maintenance effort. We conducted a study to assess the extent to which the solution fulfills this goal. A manually developed UIP application was compared with a system built using the proposed approach. The study proved that much less application-specific code needs to be implemented when our approach is used. There are also other benefits – the amount of restated information is reduced, and the information is specified using a rich persistence model instead of type-unsafe domain-specific language.

5   Conclusion

There were two important objectives for the framework introduced in this paper. The first was to reduce the development and maintenance effort required to generate rich UIs for applications that use data persistence. The second objective was to generate context-sensitive rich UIs that can be delivered on a number of heterogeneous client platforms. As a result, the framework consists of two main components – AspectFaces and UIP.

AspectFaces uses code inspection to effectively capture information already contained in the application code to generate a platform-independent abstract user interface (AUI). In this way the first objective – to reduce the development and maintenance effort – is achieved. UIP uses AUI as an input for context-sensitive generation of platform-specific personalised UIs. The proposed solution uses a context model based on the requirements of ability-based design [3]. Using this context model, the UIs that are generated are adapted to the properties of the interaction device, user, environment and assistive technologies that can be used during the interaction. In this way, the second objective is achieved.

Both main components of our framework can be used as standalone solutions, but in this case, each of them has an important disadvantage. AspectFaces is a very effective tool for code inspection, but it has an important limitation in UI generation. Firstly, it lacks a simple mechanism for delivering the generated UIs to multiple heterogeneous platforms. Secondly, the generation process is based on a set of static rules, and therefore fails to generate UIs that are optimised by global metrics. On the other hand, UIP can deliver context-sensitive optimised UIs to a number of heterogeneous platforms, but it requires a specific input model, which can be hard to understand and maintain separately from an application backend. By putting these two components together, we gained a powerful tool without the disadvantages mentioned here.

As a proof of concept of our approach, we used an existing Java EE application, the ACM-ICPC registration system, to derive context-aware UIs for three different devices. A user study proved that the generated UIs provide better usability than a simple web UI in terms of comfort, efficiency and aesthetic quality.

It is a subject for future work to integrate the proposed solution into a framework that can be used easily by 3rd party organisations. Using a context model, the proposed framework can be used to generate accessible UIs. A special client that uses a Braille script keyboard on touchscreen devices is under development, and will be integrated into the framework. An extensive user study will be performed to reveal the accessibility of the UIs generated using the framework proposed here.

Acknowledgments. This research has been supported by Technology Agency of the Czech Republic, funded by grant no. TA01010784 (Form Cloud). Furthermore, our research was partially supported by the Technology Agency of the Czech Republic under the research program TE01020415 (V3C - Visual Computing Competence Center).

References

1. Kennard, R., Leaney, J.: Towards a general purpose architecture for ui generation. Journal of Systems and Software 83, 1896–1906 (2010)

2. Cerny, T., Song, E.: Model-driven rich form generation. INFORMATION: An International Interdisciplinary Journal 15, 2695–2714 (2012)
3. Wobbrock, J., Kane, S., Gajos, K., Harada, S., Froehlich, J.: Ability-based design: Concept, principles and examples. ACM Transactions on Accessible Computing (TACCESS) 3, 9 (2011)
4. Macik, M.: Context model for ability-based automatic ui generation. In: Proceedings of the 3rd IEEE Interational Conference on Cognitive Infocommunications (CogInfoCom 2012), pp. 727–732. IEEE (2012)
5. Gajos, K., Weld, D., Wobbrock, J.: Automatically generating personalized user interfaces with supple. Artificial Intelligence 174, 910–950 (2010)
6. Macik, M., Klima, M., Slavik, P.: Ui generation for data visualisation in heterogenous environment. Advances in Visual Computing, 647–658 (2011)
7. O'Neil, E.J.: Object/relational mapping 2008: hibernate and the entity data model (edm). In: Proceedings of the 2008 ACM SIGMOD International Conference on Management of Data, pp. 1351–1356. ACM (2008)
8. Kiczales, G., Lamping, J., Mendhekar, A., Maeda, C., Lopes, C., Loingtier, J.M., Irwin, J.: Aspect-oriented programming. In: Akşit, M., Matsuoka, S. (eds.) ECOOP 1997. LNCS, vol. 1241, pp. 220–242. Springer, Heidelberg (1997)
9. Laddad, R.: Aspectj in action: enterprise AOP with spring applications. Manning Publications Co. (2009)
10. Cerny, T., Chalupa, V., Donahoo, M.J.: Towards smart user interface design. In: 2012 International Conference on Information Science and Applications (ICISA), pp. 1–6 (2012) (accepted for publication)
11. Biswas, R., Ort, E.: The java persistence api-a simpler programming model for entity persistence. Sun Microsystems, Inc. (May 2006)
12. Bryant, J., Jones, M.: Responsive web design. In: Pro. HTML5 Performance, pp. 37–49. Springer (2012)
13. Dawe, M.: Complexity, cost and customization: Uncovering barriers to adoption of assistive technology. In: Refereed Poster at ASSETS 2004 (2004)
14. Torres, A., Galante, R., Pimenta, M.: Towards a uml profile for model-driven object-relational mapping. In: XXIII Brazilian Symposium on Software Engineering, SBES 2009, pp. 94–103. IEEE (2009)
15. Laddad, R.: AspectJ in Action: Enterprise AOP with Spring Applications, 2nd edn. Manning Publications Co., Greenwich (2009)
16. Bondo, J., Barnard, D., Burcaw, D., Novikoff, T., Kemper, C., Parrish, C., Peters, K., Siebert, J., Wilson, E.: IPhone User Interface Design Projects. Apress (2009)
17. Transformation, X.: (Version 1.0, w3c recommendation) (November 16, 1999)
18. Land, A., Doig, A.: An automatic method of solving discrete programming problems. Econometrica: Journal of the Econometric Society, 497–520 (1960)
19. Yeoh, W., Felner, A., Koenig, S.: Bnb-adopt: An asynchronous branch-and-bound dcop algorithm. Journal of Artificial Intelligence Research 38, 85–133 (2010)
20. Singh, I., Johnson, M., Stearns, B.: Designing enterprise applications with the J2EE platform. Addison-Wesley Professional (2002)
21. Nielsen, J., Hackos, J.: Usability engineering, vol. 125184069. Academic Press, San Diego (1993)
22. Lam, F., Longnecker, M.: A modified wilcoxon rank sum test for paired data. Biometrika 70, 510–513 (1983)
23. Graziano, A.M., Raulin, M.L.: Research methods: A process of inquiry. HarperCollins College Publishers (1993)

Kinect Web Kiosk Framework

Ciril Bohak and Matija Marolt

Univerity of Ljubljana,
Faculty of Computer and Information Science,
Slovenia
{ciril.bohak,matija.marolt}@fri.uni-lj.si

Abstract. In this paper we present a web kiosk framework based on Kinect sensor. The main idea is to use the framework for creation of simple interactive presentations for informing, advertising and presenting knowledge to the public. The use of such a framework simplifies adaptation of existing web materials for presentation with the kiosk. We can also make use of touchless interaction for browsing through the interactive content, to animate the user and encourage her to spend more time browsing the presented content. We present the structure of the framework and a simple case study on using the framework as an interactive presentation platform and as an education resource. The developed framework has been used for presenting information on educational programs at Faculty of Computer and Information Science, University of Ljubljana.

Keywords: HCI, Kinect, interactive kiosk presentation, interactivity, interaction framework.

1 Introduction

In recent years, several novel approaches to human-computer interaction became popular. Examples include mobile and large touch screens, as well as motion sensors such as Microsoft Kinect[1], Nintendo Wii[2] and Sony PlayStation Move[3] which are mostly used for gaming. While the former two systems still rely on the physical act of touching an appropriate surface, some of the touchless interfaces are able to support the interaction without the need of additional controllers.

To bring the digital content closer to the target audience, it is necessary to attract users attention with interactivity. This kind of presentation is not just suitable for advertising, but also for educational and work purposes. Later on we present a case study of using a touchless system for presentation and education purposes. The system uses the presented kiosk framework for easier preparation of content.

In the following section we present related work, where we point out the important contributions that drive the idea of a touchless kiosk system. In section

---

[1] http://www.microsoft.com/en-us/kinectforwindows/
[2] http://www.nintendo.com/wii
[3] http://us.playstation.com/ps3/playstation-move/

A. Holzinger et al. (Eds.): SouthCHI 2013, LNCS 7946, pp. 785–790, 2013.
© Springer-Verlag Berlin Heidelberg 2013

3 we present our implementation of a web kiosk framework and a touchless kiosk system. The case study is presented in section 4. In the last section we present future work and conclusions.

2   Related Work

While touch interfaces are replacing all other forms of interaction on mobile devices, several authors [1,5,7] have presented examples where touchless interfaces could play an important role. Such scenarios are 3D puppetring or interacting with devices in operating rooms, where doctors usually can not interact by touching due to sterile environment limitations. While the idea of the touchless interfaces is not really new, greater attention for such devices as well as their usage was stimulated when Microsoft has released its Kinect sensor. Some of the methods incorporated in the sensor presented in article [10].

Several authors presented their own implementations of touchless frameworks [3,6,8,9,11]. Some of these approaches use the Kinect sensor as an input device, but several are using their own implementation of touchless interfaces for detecting the user input. Recently, some interest was also given to evaluation of touchless interfaces [4] as well as to the introduction of new challenges and opportunities [1].

In our previous work [2] we have already implemented a simple kiosk system for use with an ordinary web camera. The system supported only simple switching between different web sites and its robustness was quite low due to its basic gesture recognition system.

3   Method

To develop a touchless kiosk system, we first developed a web kiosk framework. We aimed for simple definition of content and possibility of creating content independently of the framework. This feature is very important when we want to use same the system for several different tasks, as it is not feasible to adapt the whole system each time the content changes. In contrast to the previously mentioned works our approach has a strict separation of content and functionality, which means faster adaptation of content for different end use scenarios.

3.1   Web Kiosk Framework

The web platform has been proven as a widespread and very adaptive platform for defining the content in many scenarios such as business and mobile applications, as well as online education platforms. This is also the main reason why we selected the web platform as the basis of our Web Kiosk Framework. The structure of the Web Kiosk Framework is shown in Figure 1, which also displays its relation to the Kinect Kiosk System.

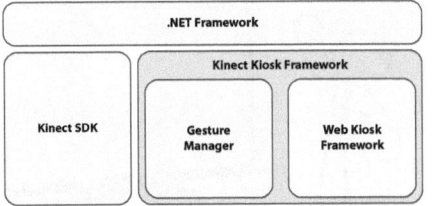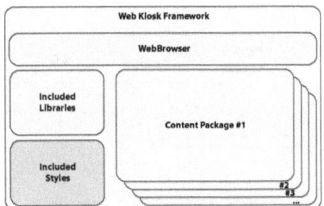

Fig. 1. Structure of the system is presented in the left image. Structure of the Web Kiosk Framework is presented in the right image.

The Implementation of the Framework is done in C# with the .NET Framework[4]. We use the `WebBrowser` class from .NET Framework for displaying the content of our packages. Javascript support in the browser component is used to augment the content with interactive components and for achieving a more attractive look and feel. We leave the support for additional Javascript libraries to content creators, but provide the general interaction functions and support in the framework. Extensive use of libraries such as jQuery[5], Impress.js[6] and similar are supported and encouraged to create a pleasant and appealing content.

The Functionalities of Framework are available through methods implemented in the framework. We can split functionalities into two distinct groups. The first group consists of methods for loading, displaying and transitioning the content and the second group includes methods for interacting with the content such as *clicking, dragging* and responding to gestures. While some frameworks also provide the predefined user interface, this is not the case with our framework. The navigational functionalities are part of the framework, however the navigational GUI is considered as a part of the provided content and must be defined as such.

3.2 Kinect Kiosk System

The presented framework was used in a demonstration system. The structure of the system is shown in Figure 2. It consists of a Kinect sensor, PC and display. Kinect is used for capturing the user input. On PC, the Kinect SDK takes care of tracking the motion of joints, while the Gesture Manager (see Figure 1) performs hand tracking and gesture recognition and sends the interaction data to the Web Kiosk Framework. The Web Kiosk Framework changes the displayed content according to incoming gesture messages and displays the requested content. The user gets immediate feedback of his actions on the display.

---

[4] http://www.microsoft.com/net
[5] http://jquery.com/
[6] https://github.com/bartaz/impress.js/

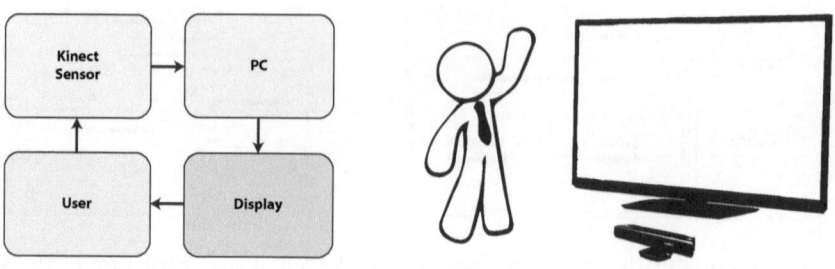

Fig. 2. Interaction cycle of the system is presented in the left image. The hardware setup of the system is presented in the right image.

4   Case Study

During our research we have completed a case study and planned another one that will be done in near future. The first case study addressed the scenario of using the developed system as a presentation kiosk, while the second case study will involve educational use of the system.

In this study we have prepared a kiosk presentation of our laboratory. The presentation consists of several parts such as: personnel introduction, information on their contact hours and locations, information on available diplomas, current projects in the laboratory, information on special events such as summer schools and information on the courses held by our members.

Subjects in our case study were future first year students at our faculty. We have displayed our system in the main hall to get a feedback from end users. Users did not have many problems using the system if they were the only one interacting with it. The system worked well and users could browse through the content without problems. However, if there were more users in the detectable area, users had more problems with the system, as it did not always recognise the user that wanted to interact with the system. In the future development of the system we have to make the selection of the active user more robust. The case study was open for anyone and was conducted only for testing the proof of concept in the real-life environment.

As feedback we got suggestions that the system should pick the closest user for interaction and that it should give some visual feedback to see which user is currently the one that the system has selected. Another suggestion was that we should mark the area where the system detects users and limit it to a certain distance from the system. The system should not detect users that are too far away or at least ignore them when there is an user that is already interacting with the system.

5   Conclusions and Future Work

In this paper we have presented our work on developing the Web Kiosk Framework as a framework for defining content packages and defining the modes of interaction, as well as the Kinect Kiosk system, which is a touchless kiosk system that uses the Kinect sensor for interaction with the user.

Case study shows that the system allows an interesting and engaging way for users to actively browse the presentation and interact with the content. Furthermore we will assess the use of the system for educational purposes. We do not think that the presented system could be used for education in classes, however it could be used in self learning environments such as museums or "hands-on" science centers. We believe that it could also be used in schools, not as the main resource of knowledge but rather as an additional knowledge resource for children and youngsters whose curiosity exceeds the formally established curriculum.

Future work will include a case study conducted on a group of high school teachers at the international conference on using Information technologies in education (SIRikt[7]). We will present a knowledge kiosk at the conference and study the possible usages of our system for education purposes.

In the future we also plan to extend the Web Kiosk Framework for improved interaction with both hands and the entire body. We plan to incorporate the possibility of spawning actions when users enter a certain pose (sitting, standing, etc.). We also plan to extend the framework with a library for easier creation of interactive content. To further evaluate the system, we plan to use the system and create content for a "hands-on" science center as an example of interactive knowledge kiosk.

References

1. de la Barré, R., Chojecki, P., Leiner, U., Mühlbach, L., Ruschin, D.: Touchless interaction-novel chances and challenges. In: Jacko, J.A. (ed.) HCI International 2009, Part II. LNCS, vol. 5611, pp. 161–169. Springer, Heidelberg (2009)
2. Bohak, C.: Gesture based user interface (2007)
3. Burnar, S.: Computer interaction using kinect sensor (2012)
4. Fikkert, W., van der Vet, P., Nijholt, A.: User-evaluated gestures for touchless interactions from a distance. In: 12th IEEE International Symposium on Multimedia, ISM 2010, Taichung, Taiwan, December 13-15, pp. 153–160. IEEE Computer Society (2010)
5. Held, R., Gupta, A., Curless, B., Agrawala, M.: 3d puppetry: a kinect-based interface for 3d animation. In: Miller, R., Benko, H., Latulipe, C. (eds.) UIST, pp. 423–434. ACM (2012)
6. Hirte, S., Seifert, A., Baumann, S., Klan, D., Sattler, K.U.: Data3 – a kinect interface for olap using complex event processing. In: Proceedings of the 2012 IEEE 28th International Conference on Data Engineering, pp. 1297–1300. IEEE Computer Society, Washington, DC (2012)
7. Johnson, R., O'Hara, K., Sellen, A., Cousins, C., Criminisi, A.: Exploring the potential for touchless interaction in image-guided interventional radiology. In: Proceedings of the SIGCHI Conference on Human Factors in Computing Systems, CHI 2011, pp. 3323–3332. ACM, New York (2011)

---

[7] http://www.sirikt.si/

8. Papadopoulos, C., Sugarman, D., Kaufmant, A.: Nunav3d: A touch-less, body-driven interface for 3d navigation. In: Virtual Reality Short Papers and Posters (VRW), pp. 67–68. IEEE (March 2012)

9. Ryu, D., Um, D., Tanofsky, P., Koh, D.H., Ryu, Y.S., Kang, S.: T-less: A novel touchless human-machine interface based on infrared proximity sensing. In: 2010 IEEE/RSJ International Conference on Intelligent Robots and Systems (IROS), pp. 5220–5225 (October 2010)

10. Shotton, J., Fitzgibbon, A., Cook, M., Sharp, T., Finocchio, M., Moore, R., Kipman, A., Blake, A.: Real-time human pose recognition in parts from single depth images. In: Proceedings of the 2011 IEEE Conference on Computer Vision and Pattern Recognition, pp. 1297–1304. IEEE Computer Society, Washington, DC (2011)

11. Spano, L.D.: Developing touchless interfaces with gestIT. In: Paternò, F., de Ruyter, B., Markopoulos, P., Santoro, C., van Loenen, E., Luyten, K. (eds.) AmI 2012. LNCS, vol. 7683, pp. 433–438. Springer, Heidelberg (2012)

Enhancement of Web Application Design of the Open Platform for Clinical Nutrition

Peter Novak, Franc Novak, and Barbara Koroušić Seljak

Jozef Stefan Institute, Ljubljana, Slovenia
{peter.novak,franc.novak,barbara.korousic}@ijs.si

Abstract. In this paper, an enhancement of a web application design is presented. The aim was to modify the visual quality of the application in order to make it simple and visually more easy to understand, which consequently leads to improved user experience. The process of enhancement of user interface of the web application home page and subsequent web pages is based on different methods for establishing clear visual hierarchy of presented information, among them the methods of reduction, regularization and leverage. The web application to which the above principles were applied is Open Platform for Clinical Nutrition, which offers to users effective means for identifying their nutritional state and adjusting diet plans to their way of life and clinical state. Currently, the application has about 3000 active users.

Keywords: web design, visual perception, visual hierarchy.

1 Introduction

This paper reports the initial results of an ongoing work of enhancement of user interface of the Open Platform for Clinical Nutrition (OPEN) i.e., a web-based application (http://www.opkp.si/, accessible in February 2013) aimed for the assessment of nutrient intake and food consumption among adults and children as well as for the personalized diet planning [1]. OPEN has been developed by the Computer Systems Department, Jožef Stefan Institute, in cooperation with the University Children's Hospital Ljubljana, the Oncology Institute Ljubljana, and the international non-profit association EuroFIR AISBL (http://www.eurofir.net/, accessible in February 2013).

The application can apply any food composition database (FCDB) complying with EuroFIR procedures that facilitate access to and exchange of comparable, high quality food composition data for industry, regulators and researchers across Europe. It considers nutrition recommendations from the German (DGE), Austrian (ÖGE) and Swiss (SGE and SVE) Societies for Nutrition as well as guidelines from the European Society for Clinical Nutrition and Metabolism (ESPEN) and the European Society for Paediatric Gastroenterology, Hepatology and Nutrition (ESPGHAN).

In cooperation with the Slovenian Society for Clinical Nutrition, a mobile application that integrates different tools for dietary screening of malnourished patients of different ages and health conditions has been developed. The mobile application is an upgrade of OPEN and allows easy transition to the web application, where patients

A. Holzinger et al. (Eds.): SouthCHI 2013, LNCS 7946, pp. 791–802, 2013.

facing malnutrition can find more information and tools for planning an appropriate diet. By using tablets and mobile application, selected clinical dietitians carried out dietary screening at the Institute of Oncology Ljubljana; Clinical Gastroenterology Department of the Internal Clinic of the University Medical Centre Ljubljana; and the Hospital Dr. Petra Držaja, Ljubljana.

From the above it becomes apparent that OPEN serves a wide range of users, ranging from individuals with relatively low-level computer literacy of all ages to experienced dietitians and nutritionists. Furthermore, the number of active users already exceeds 3000 and is still growing. In order to provide a quality service to the satisfaction of clients, web application design should be focused and allow the user an easy way to find information and/or enter his personal data. Over the years, the web application has grown significantly including new materials, tools and functionalities, which calls for progressive enhancement of website design. In our recent attempt, reported in this paper, we performed an in-depth analysis of visual information of the target web subpages and the corresponding modification of website design in order to provide better comprehensiveness and make the web application more easy to use. Enhancement of visual organization of information of individual subpages aims at improving the experience of current and prospective users of OPEN. Attention has been paid to keep the overall web application organization intact not to disturb the users that are regularly accessing the application and already got accustomed to it. In our work we followed the basic principles of establishing visual contrasts by manipulating visual variables [2]. We also applied simplification techniques such as reduction, regularization and leverage [3] and followed the guidelines for webpage elements and layout design based on eye tracking web usability study [4].

2   Background of the Applied Approach

As stated in [3], effective design respects the capabilities and limitations of visual language, which, at its most basic level, concerns the primitive visual distinctions that are available in human vision. In this respect we refer to the visual variables (Fig. 1) and the rules governing their use [2].

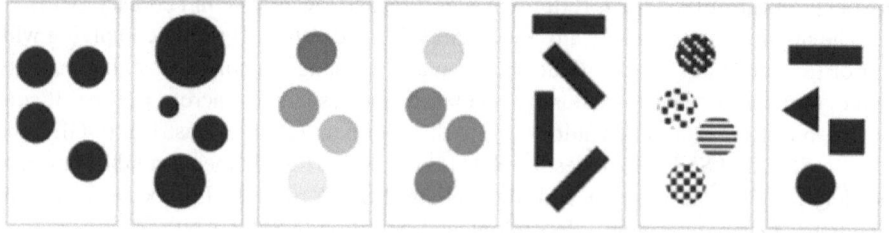

Fig. 1. Visual variables: position, size, value, hue, orientation, texture, shape

We followed the established guidelines by selecting appropriate visual variable for encoding data such that the desired distinctions between visual elements were achieved. Employed visual variables should be chosen such that they match the required communication in the best possible way. For this purpose, the two characteristics of a visual variable: scale (e.g., nominal, ordered, quantitative) and its length (e.g., the number of possible values) are considered. A nominal scale is just a list of categories and the values have no ordering relationship. By using a nominal scale, associative and selective perception can be used to communicate the desired information to the user.

According to [2], a visual variable is *associative* if it permits the immediate grouping of all the correspondences differentiated by this variable. In other words, it does not diminish the visibility of other dimensions applied to the same elements., Position, hue, orientation, texture and shape are associative, while size and value are not. One can, for example, recognize the hue of an object regardless of its position or orientation (which are associative variables). On the other hand, it may be difficult to deter-mine the hue of an object if it is of a very small size or of a light value of color (size and value are not associative).

A visual variable is *selective* if it allows immediate identification of all elements to which it is applied. From the above stated visual variables, only shape is not selective. An illustrative example is given in Fig. 2.

One can recognize at the first glance all the letters b in this paragraph since they are colored red (hue variable is selective), but cannot easily identify all the letters e in the paragraph because they distinguish from the others only by shape (shape variable is not selective).

Fig. 2. An example of selective visual variable

For an ordered visual variable, the user can easily determine the relative ordering of its values along its perceptual dimension. Position, size and value are ordered visual variables. Ranking of elements described by such visual variable is immediately obvious. Furthermore, a visual variable is quantitative if it is possible to determine the amount of difference between two ordered values. From the above mentioned visual variables, only position and size are quantitative.

As mentioned in the introduction, we also applied simplification techniques such as reduction, regularization and leverage [3]. Reduction technique aims at removing non-essential elements from the design. In our case, the information content of individual web page was analyzed and the main design elements were identified. Next, we checked to what extent they support the mission of the web page and removed those which do not make enough contribution. Regularization of the website was performed by unifying color, shape, texture, size, value and orientation of the existing similar visual elements. Visual design can be leveraged if the employed visual elements take over multiple roles. For example, previous paragraph played a double role: it explained the property of a selective visual variable and served at the same time as an illustrative example. In our case, we identified the functionality of each visual element of a web page and thought over if we could possibly combine some of them in a single object.

As regards page layout, organization of pages, navigation, related to the user viewing behaviors on the web, we mainly followed the guidelines derived from the eye-tracking web usability study of Nielsen and Pernice [4] and papers referenced in the next section.

3   Recent Related Work

Extensive work has been published on human perception of visual variables and its application in HCI. In this section we briefly summarize those papers which mostly influenced our work by reported experimental evidence and gave confidence to the decisions we made in the enhancement process of OPEN web application.

Wolfe and Horowitz have made an extensive study [5] which of the visual variables can be used to control the deployment of attention. On the basis of several decades of research, they proposed a list of guiding attributes. They showed that color, size and orientation definitely draw attention of users, value and shape are also probable candidates, whereas others, such as threat, are probably not.

In [6] an empirical evaluation approach to assess the effectiveness (how accurate) and efficiency (how fast) of visual variables size, color value, color hue and orientation is reported. In their experimental study, traditional performance measures (accuracy and speed) were combined with eye movement recordings. They have shown that the visual variable size performs most effectively and most efficiently under flicker conditions, whereas the visual variable orientation proved to be least effective and efficient. No clear results could be derived for the visual variables color hue and color value.

Although not explicitly referred in the previous section, we also considered the principles of the Gestalt theory. For example, in [7] Chang et al. studied how individuals use the sense of touch to group display elements using the Gestalt principles of similarity and proximity. They show that people use touch to group display elements in the same way they group elements visually. A useful observance for our work was that people used texture or color to group the elements when there was an equal spacing between the elements. In the case of an unequal spacing between the elements they used spatial position to determine groupings.

Cognitive strategies and eye movements that people use to search for a known item in a hierarchical computer display are elaborated in [8]. Specific design recommendations are derived from the patterns of visual search behavior obtained from the eye tracking data. The described approach demonstrates how cognitive modeling can be used for predicting, explaining, and interpreting eye movement data. Adopted search strategies, the way how people anticipate visual locations and other experiences discussed in the paper offer useful guidelines for visual page organization.

Another study of predicting the eye movements of a typical user and consequently proposing guidelines for webpage organization was conducted by Johansen and Hansen [9]. Their experimental evidence suggests that the predictions of web designers are generally less reliable than asking the users themselves. Lesson learned for a web designer: besides trusting professional intuition one should also rely on the feedback from the users how they actually look at the interface, and organize the layout accordingly.

Sutcliffe and Namoune investigated the relation between user attention and design quality in websites [10]. A questionnaire was used to assess whether the areas of interest that users attended to were also remembered and rated well in terms of aesthetic design and usability. Based on the analysis, design guidelines for directing user attention are proposed. As stated in the paper, aesthetics proved to be the more important determinant for overall attractiveness; whereas content, brand and usability were more important for overall preference.

4   Enhancement of the Web Application Design

The first step in the enhancement of OPEN web application comprised an in-depth analysis of its functionality. Existing elements of the web application were identified and their roles were studied and discussed in order to determine the corresponding hierarchical dependences. Then, individual visual elements were modified with the appropriate use of visual variables, as shown in the following.

In order to help user to quickly comprehend the information of a web page it is possible to use different ways of grouping the elements that carry data with specific information content. If, for example, the links in a paragraph to other information items are indicated in cursive font (i.e., difference in shape, which is not a selective variable) the user would need more effort to search for the required information than in the case where the links were indicated in a different color (i.e., hue is a selective variable). Consequently, we colored all the links with blue.

Some elements of a web page may play multiple roles (i.e., correspond to different functionalities). For their presentation, associative variables should be employed. In the previous example, some words serve as a part of the overall text message and also as links to some other information content. If those words were shown by a different value (i.e., non-associative variable) instead of a different hue (i.e., associative variable) the user could identify them as links but it would be difficult to read the text.

The OPEN application contains many items that the user may need to compare in quantity. The appropriate use of quantitative visual variables can make the comparison intuitive which subsequently decreases cognitive effort. For example, comparison of the actual energy value of a meal and the daily recommended intake value could look like (400,00 kcal/2000 kcal). In such a case the user may spend some time to make comparisons of different meals. Visually, the above data in brackets can be regarded as elements of different shapes (i.e., shape is not a quantitative variable). On the other hand, comparison becomes immediate if pie charts (i.e., size is a quantitative variable) are used for data presentation.

Buttons placed directly into dialog boxes and pages are a common way of implementing control. They are usually grouped semantically. Many different variants of buttons in the current version of the OPEN web application hampered the user experience and called for regularization. This has been done by unifying the shape and background color and by providing icon cohesiveness as shown in Fig. 3. Similarly, other items like forms, links, etc. also have required some modifications.

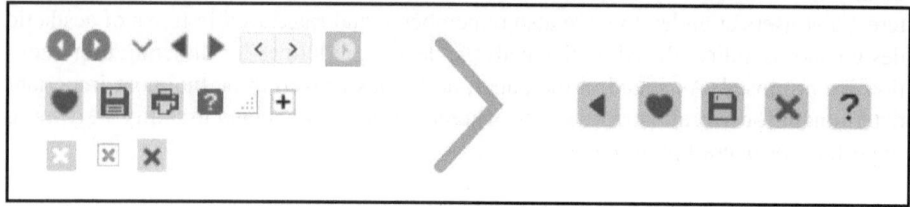

Fig. 3. Regularization of buttons

Some modifications of captions of different data fields were also done (Fig. 4). In the original version, both captions of data fields and actual data values of given items were displayed in bold. In the enhanced version, only captions of data fields remain bold, while data are displayed using normal weight. In this way, the user gaze is directed first to the main categories. Once the desired data field is selected, the user proceeds to the given data values.

Kol.		Kol.	
Skupne beljakovine	9,49 g	Skupne beljakovine	9,49 g
Skupne maščobe	3,18 g	Skupne maščobe	3,18 g
Skupni ogljikovi h...	20,04 g	Skupni ogl. hidrati	20,04 g

Fig. 4. Modification of displaying data in data fields

A considerable part of the OPEN web page space is occupied by a text which appears on different pages in different font weights and colors. In the first step of regularization process, a single font size of the body text was selected. All static text parts were colored black while interactive elements (hyperlinks) were colored blue. Next, the font size of titles was determined. Text of less important information was colored grey. By reducing the number of variants while increasing the contrast between the existing, previous visual clutter was diminished and a clear visual hierarchy among individual text parts was established (Fig. 5).

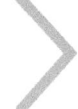

BELEŽITE - ANA
Razmerje med makrohranili
Odprta platforma za klinično prehrar
Tortni graf podaja razmerje med ener
Načrtovanje prehrane
S klikom na razrez se izpiše informacija o vredni
Potrebe po beljakovinah med boleznijo in rekon
Kadar običajno telesno aktivnost toliko poveča

Pomoč pri delu

Kako pravilno načrtovati in beležiti
Odprta platforma za klinično prehranc
odkrijete svoje prehranske navade, tal
in svojemu življenjskemu slogu primeri
Orodje je namenjeno predvsem razisk
organizacij (Onkološkega inštituta in F
datki in izračuni zgolj informativne nai

Fig. 5. Regularization of static text

The remaining work was focused on the enhancement of individual web pages. For illustration we give the following examples of selected web pages: home page, meal plan page and the page presenting the main features of OPEN.

The home page of OPEN serves two purposes. It introduces the main features of the OPEN web application to the new users and enables them to create their account. As for the existing users, it provides an easy way to login. Notice that OPEN is not a commercial publicity based web page, most of its users are accessing it under doctor's recommendation. Consequently, the home page should primarily be designed for easy use rather than attracting possible newcomers.

The initial version of the home page (Fig. 6) comprised many different styles of Arial type-face. In order to reduce the distraction we considerably limit the number styles (for the major part of the text we use a single weight) and consequently unify the text, decrease the number of contrasts, which, on the other hand, increases the impact of the remaining visual variables. The title is moved upwards and switched to minuscule, which retains user attention and adds relaxation. It also allows more natural way of scanning the page (from top down). Individual parts of the title semantically correspond with the figures, so we can remove the former figure captions. Repeated but-tons "Prijava" (login), "več o" (more about) links and other non-unified items are replaced by short and expressive hypertext which directs the user to the corresponding web pages. The line length of the main text is also reduced in order to increase its readability. Furthermore, the second paragraph, which is less essential, is displayed in a lighter font. The login is moved to the upper right position where it is normally expected. In its former place a visually strong blue text box is placed informing the user that the registration is mandatory. The web page is also enhanced by using a more unifying grid. In this respect, the width of the text fits the two upper parts, while the blue text box fits the remaining third upper part. Likewise, the height of the employed elements is also unified.

The new version of the home web page (Fig. 7) is simplified and more user friendly. During the refinement process we used squint test [3] for assessing the performed modifications. The squint test of the resulting web page clearly shows the three visually emphasized main functional parts and the blue box supporting user registration. Web page organization also conforms to the eye gaze pattern (left to right) allowing the user first to identify the main contents and afterwards offering the way to login or register.

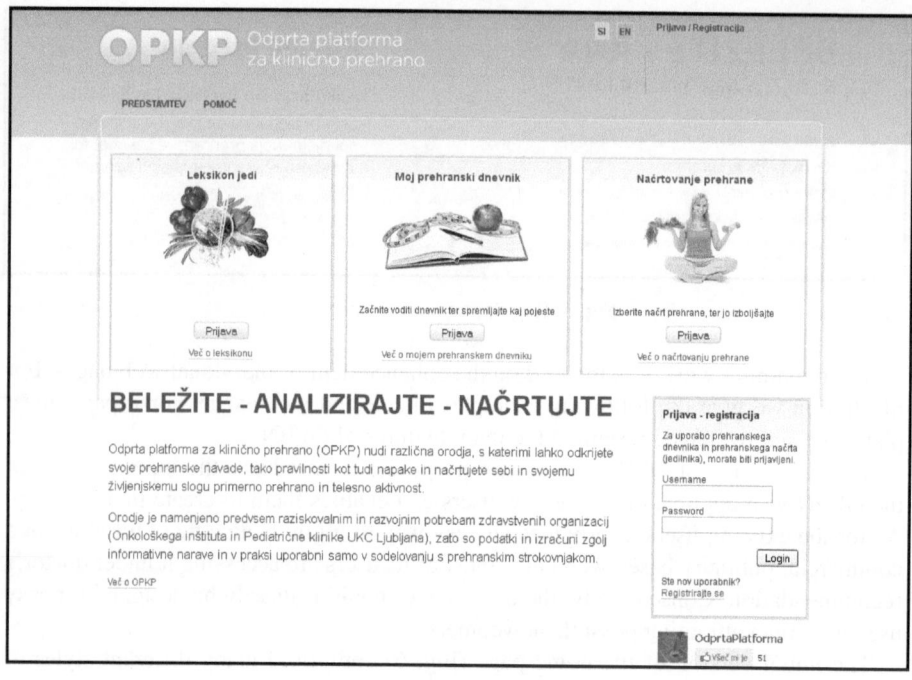

Fig. 6. Original home page

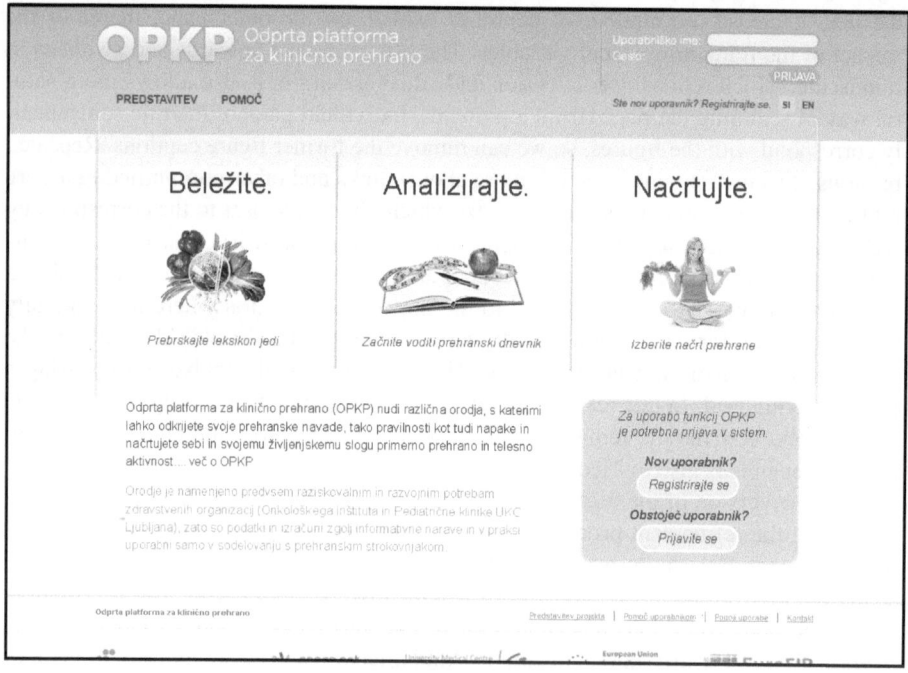

Fig. 7. Enhanced home page

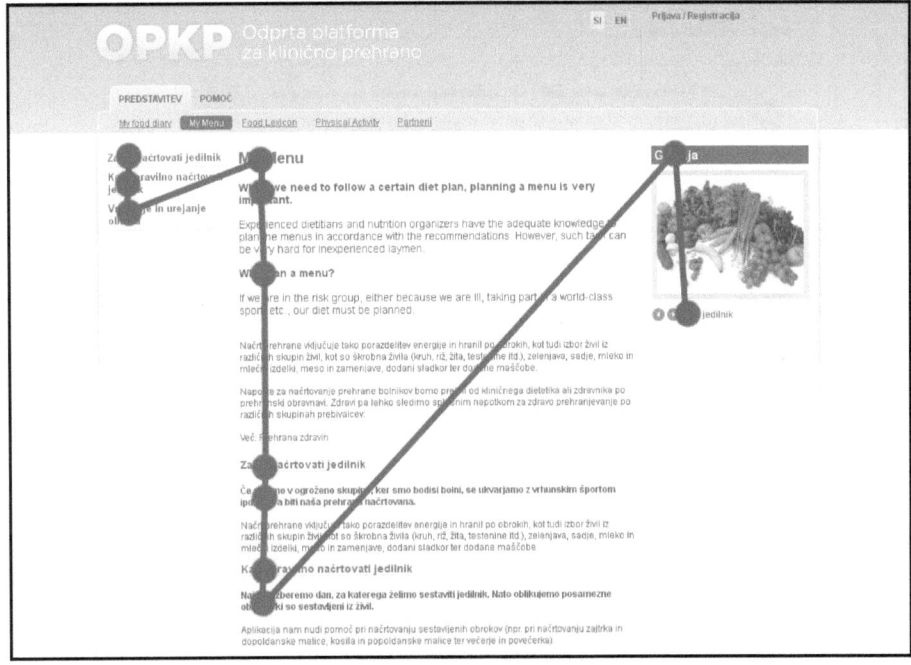

Fig. 8. Original meal plan page

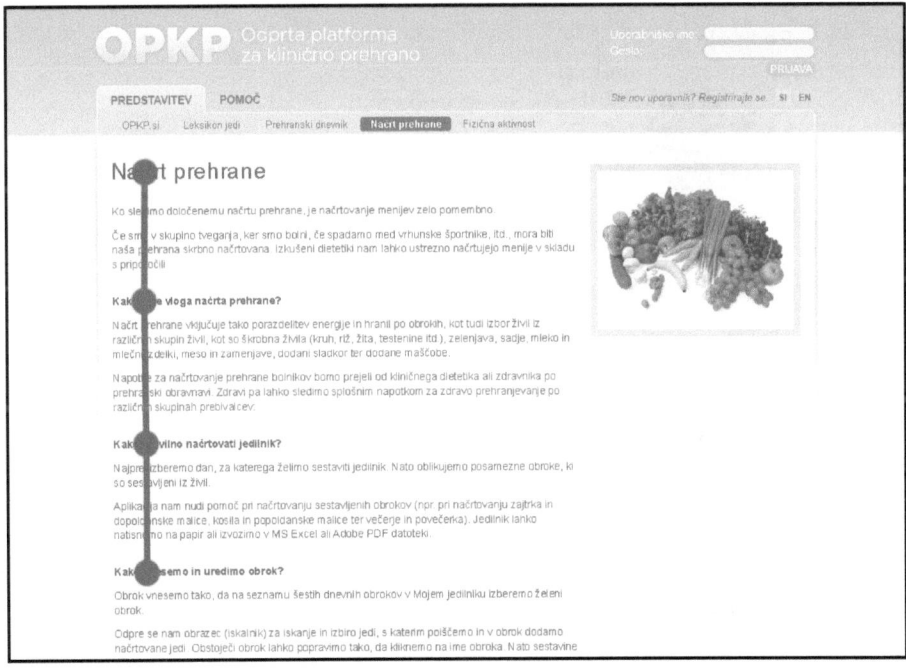

Fig. 9. Enhanced meal plan page

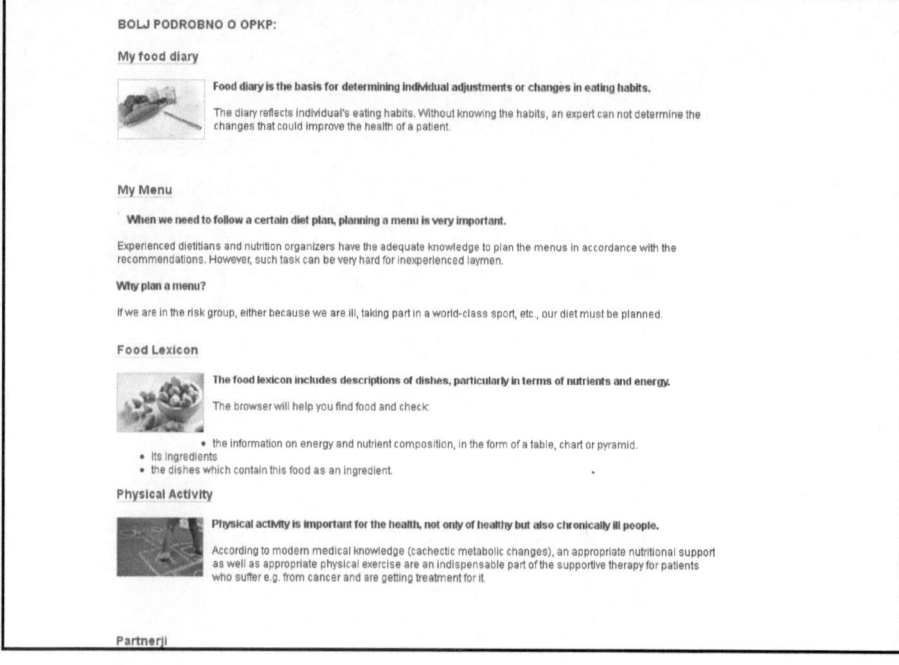

Fig. 10. Original lower part of the web page presenting the main features of OPEN

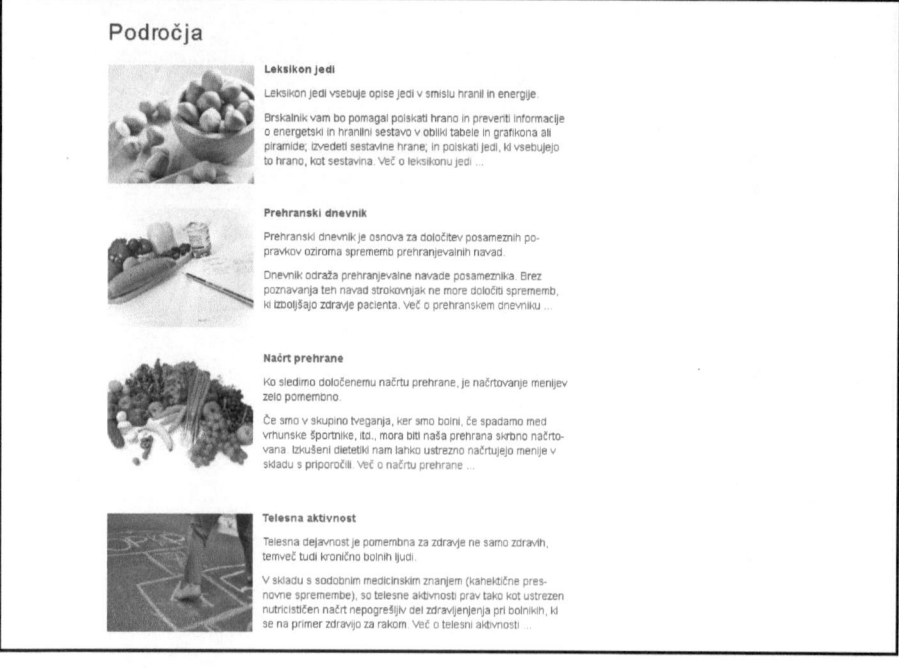

Fig. 11. Enhanced lower part of the web page presenting the main features of OPEN

The second example deals with the meal plan web page. In the original web page shown in Fig. 8 one can notice excessive use of font weights which increases the effort of scanning the page. It is difficult to comprehend the main contents at a glance. The page layout consists of three columns. The simulated gaze plot of user scanning the page is shown in red. The number of fixations is 12. The layout of the enhanced page shown in Fig. 9 is reduced to a single column. The overview is simplified by offering the user only the main (four) items clearly identified by titles with font weights indicating the corresponding hierarchical level. The font weight of the text bodies is unified. The simulated gaze plot of the enhanced page is a single straight line with four fixations. It should be noted that we did not perform actual eye tracking experiments. However, we followed the recommendations and conclusions on this technique presented in [4] and the indicated plots on Fig. 8 and Fig. 9 illustrate the assumed user behavior.

The third example presents the enhancement of the web page which gives the main features of the OPEN application. On the original page, the text was represented in five different styles of Arial typeface. The visual impact of the web page was further degraded by non-uniform and long titles. The length of the page requires vertical scrolling. In the enhanced version, the number of styles of the typeface was reduced. The length of the titles was reduced to one third of the page width which allows faster and easier scanning of the displayed information. Recognition of each of the four entities was improved by introducing one more figure and increasing figure sizes to match the corresponding text boxes. The lower part of the original and of the enhanced web page are shown in Fig. 10 and Fig. 11, respectively.

5   Conclusion

Enhancement od the OPEN web application design is a continuous process. In this paper, the main issues performed in the initial step are described. As the web application expands by including new features, visual appearance and aesthetic quality become even more important factors for its usability. In our future work we plan to perform usability tests with target audiences to improve the efficiency, effectiveness and satisfaction of users. For example, the OPEN has been used at the University Children's Hospital Ljubljana to support clinical dieticians in nutrition care process of dystrophic children and cystic fibrosis patients. The OPEN has also been applied to support research work in a clinical study "The Role of Human Milk in Development of Breast Fed Child's Intestinal Microbiota", in which 230 healthy pregnant and breastfeeding women track and analyze their nutrition (http://www.moje-mleko.si/en/, accessible in November 2011). Since a considerable part of OPEN are also people with disabilities, emphasis will be paid on accessibility of web design.

References

1. Korousic Seljak, B.: Computer-based dietary menu planning. Journal of Food Composition and Analysis 22(5), 414–420 (2009)
2. Bertin, J.: Semiology of Graphic: Diagrams, Networks, Maps. University of Wisconsin Press (1983)

3. Mullet, K., Sano, D.: Designing Visual Interfaces. SunSoft Press (1995)
4. Nielsen, J., Pernice, K.: Eyetracking Web Usability. New Riders (2010)
5. Wolfe, J.M., Horowitz, T.S.: What attributes guide the deployment of visual attention and how do they do it? Nature Reviews Neuroscience 5, 1–7 (2004)
6. Garlandini, S., Fabrikant, S.I.: Evaluating the Effectiveness and Efficiency of Visual Variables for Geographic Information Visualization. In: Hornsby, K.S., Claramunt, C., Denis, M., Ligozat, G. (eds.) COSIT 2009. LNCS, vol. 5756, pp. 195–211. Springer, Heidelberg (2009)
7. Chang, D., Nesbitt, K.V., Wilkins, K.: The Gestalt Principles of Similarity and Proximity Apply to Both the Haptic and Visual Grouping of Elements. In: Conferences in Research and Practice in Information Technology (CRPIT), pp. 79–86 (2007)
8. Hornof, A.J., Halverson, T.: Cognitive strategies and eye movements for searching hierarchical computer displays. In: CHI, pp. 249–256 (2003)
9. Johansen, S.A., Hansen, J.P.: Do we need eye trackers to tell where people look? In: CHI (2006) (extended)
10. Sutcliffe, A.G., Namoune, A.: Getting the message across: visual attention, aesthetic design and what users remember. In: Conference on Designing Interactive Systems, pp. 11–20 (2008)

HDCMD: A Clustering Algorithm to Support Hand Detection on Multitouch Displays

Bojan Blažica[1,2], Daniel Vladušič[1], and Dunja Mladenić[2]

[1] XLAB Research, Pot za Brdom 100, SI-1000 Ljubljana, Slovenia
{bojan.blazica,daniel.vladusic}@xlab.si
[2] Jožef Stefan International Postgraduate School, Jamova 39, SI-1000 Ljubljana, Slovenia
dunja.mladenic@ijs.si

Abstract. This paper describes our approach to hand detection on a multitouch surface i.e. detecting how many hands are currently on the surface and associating each touch point to its corresponding hand. Our goal was to find a general software-based solution to this problem applicable to all multitouch surfaces regardless of their construction. We therefore approached hand detection with a limited amount of information: the position of each touch point. We propose HDCMD (Hand Detection with Clustering on Multitouch Displays), a simple clustering algorithm based on heuristics that exploit the knowledge of the anatomy of the human hand. The proposed hand detection algorithm's accuracy evaluated on synthetic data (97%) significantly outperformed XMeans (21%) and DBScan (67%).

Keywords: Hand Detection, Multitouch, Clustering, Co-located Groupware.

1 Introduction

Intuitiveness and directness - properties associated with multitouch interaction since the advent of the first multitouch displays in the early 80s [1]. Intuitive, because they allow us to interact with digital objects similarly to the way we interact with physical objects in our everyday life. Direct, because the display represents the input and the output of the computer thus enabling us to manipulate directly with what we see. Furthermore, multitouch displays greatly increase the possibilities of interaction between humans and computers. Whereas the ubiquitous WIMP paradigm (windows, icons, menus, pointer) only offers to the user one cursor that moves in two dimensions, multitouch extends this to up to ten cursors per user. Moreover, by detecting an unlimited number of fingers, support for multiple users working simultaneously on the same surface is implied. A recent survey [2] conducted among multitouch interaction researchers showed that multiuser support is one of the top features of multitouch displays. According to their survey, Benko et al. defined an interactive tabletop as "a large surface that affords direct, multi-touch, multi-user interaction". However, despite the ability of sensing multiple touchpoints, a multitouch display cannot be regarded as a multiuser device per se, as it does not distinguish between different users, nor is it capable of assuming how many users are operating with it or even how many

A. Holzinger et al. (Eds.): SouthCHI 2013, LNCS 7946, pp. 803–814, 2013.
© Springer-Verlag Berlin Heidelberg 2013

hands are currently on the screen. We can thus say that multitouch displays are only finger-aware but not hand-aware or user-aware. To overcome this, we need a way to group touches (fingers) into hands and to associate hands with users. This higher-level information broadens the possibilities of interaction with a multitouch display and transforms it into a multiuser device. Even when the display is used by a single user, hand detection could improve interaction by complying to design guidelines that stem from the nature of bimanual interaction [3, 4].

In this paper we present an incremental clustering algorithm, which makes any multitouch display hand-aware. In Section 2, we motivate our work with a review of literature related to hand-aware interaction on multitouch displays followed by an overview of hand detection methods and related work in Section 3. We continue in Section 4 with a description of general characteristics of clustering for hand detection and the definition of our clustering algorithm. Section 5 presents the methods and results of the evaluation on synthetic data, which is then discussed in Section 6. We conclude with a concise definition of the contribution of our work.

2   Motivation

The need for and the positive effects of multiuser support in multitouch displays have been examined by various studies. Researchers have been concerned with the impact of multitouch interaction on group behavior. On the other hand, investigations about the nature of tabletop interaction in the physical world have been conducted to gain valuable insight on how to design digital tabletop interaction with a multitouch display. In this section we present some of these studies that motivated us in our work.

Ringel Morris et. al. [5] explored the potential of collaborative gestures for co-located groupware. They formalized the notion of cooperative gestures as "interactions where the system interprets the gestures of multiple group members collectively in order to invoke a single command". Their conclusion was that the "use of cooperative gestures can add value to applications as a means of increasing participation, drawing attention to important commands, enforcing implicit access control, facilitating reach on large surfaces, and/or enhancing social aspects of an interactive experience." In such a scenario, hand detection is a crucial requirement for the development of groupware interaction.

When designing natural user interfaces (e.g. multitouch interaction, freehand gestures) the underlying paradigm is that interaction with digital objects should resemble interaction with physical objects as much as possible. Terrenghi et al. [6] observed that given a task, participants divided it in the same subtask when performing it in the physical, as well as in the digital domain, although they eventually performed these subtasks differently - most of the bimanual interaction present in the physical domain was lost. The authors conclude that instead of blindly copying real world interaction, we should always think about how a certain task can optimally be performed in the digital domain. Furthermore, this suggests that in the digital world there may be another kind of bimanual interaction, which must not only be supported but also stimulated by an application. Hand detection could thus represent a valuable tool to achieve this.

Rogers et al. [7] performed an experiment where groups of three people were asked to complete a garden planning task under three different conditions: using a laptop, using a tabletop or in a physical-digital setup (by manipulating physical objects on a tabletop). One key finding was that tangibility and accessibility stimulate more participation from those who find it hard to talk or are incapable of verbal communication (e.g. non-native speakers, shy people, and children with learning difficulties). Furthermore, the study showed that the tabletop and physical-digital conditions resulted in a more equitable participation which led the authors to the conclusion that "where creativity and democracy are valued, then having tangible and easily accessible entry points within information and physical spaces can be an effective way of facilitating collaboration." On the other hand, collaborative tasks involving command and control systems require constraints, so that not everything is accessible to everyone, thus facilitating division of work and assumption of roles. In the first case hand and user detection can be applied to stimulate non-verbal communication between users, while in the second it is required to allow the adoption of roles.

If the previously reviewed scenarios, in which hand detection is beneficial, are of a more general nature, the interaction techniques described in [8, 9] are more specific. The first presents a vision-based hand tracking system showcased by a set of one and two-handed gestures in a picture manipulation application, while the second explores multitouch interactions within a room planning scenario. Another specific scenario that implicitly requires hand detection is presented in [10], where Peltonen et al. explore the dynamics of interactions around a public multitouch display installation. They conclude that "design should support performative acts and facilitate asymmetric and ad hoc role-taking, thus letting users learn the opportunities for interaction from their peers."

In this section we explained what motivated our work and why hand awareness is a sought-after feature in multitouch interaction; in the next sections we will overview existing methods for hand detection and show how it can be achieved on every multitouch display.

3   Related Work

The problem of hand detection for multitouch displays can be tackled from a hardware and/or software point of view. Existing solutions mostly rely on additional hardware, while ours is completely software-based. Here we briefly review the existing solutions.

DiamondTouch [11] can distinguish between four users by exploiting an array of antennas, where each antenna transmits a unique signal, embedded in the touch surface and special seats that work as receivers. When a user touches the surface, a small signal is coupled from the antennas near the touch through his body to the receiver. This technology supports two-handed interaction and distinguishes between users. In [12], Schmidt discusses the benefits of hand detection and user identification for multitouch interaction. He also presents a prototype display augmented with an over-head camera. The camera tracks hands and identifies users based on the hand's contours [13]. Instead of hand contours, Dohse et al. [14] use skin color segmentation to distinguish and identify users with an overhead camera. Another similar approach was adopted by Echtler et al. [15]; with an additional light source placed on the ceiling above the display and a dedicated circuit to control the lights and the camera, they were able to detect shadows cast by the users hand's with the camera already present in the display. Besides hand detection, this enabled the authors to implement mouse-like 'hover' functionality. Another hardware based hand detection solution are the fiduciary-tagged gloves presented by Marquardt et al. in [16]. The gloves are equipped with fiducials that enable recognition of various parts of the hand like fingertips, palms, sides etc. Hand and user detection is achieved in a similar fashion.

The methods described are all capable of distinguishing between hands and also between users. Their common drawback is the need for additional hardware, which makes these methods cumbersome and inapplicable to existing multitouch displays.

To the best of our knowledge, the only software-based method for hand detection is the one presented by Dang et. al. in [17]. They adopt "a simple heuristic for mapping fingers to hands that makes use of constraints applied to the touch position combined with the finger orientation." For two touchpoints, this technique first checks if they are within a certain distance. If so, their intersection is checked next. The intersection of two touchpoints is the intersection of the lines described with the fingers' positions and orientations. If this intersection is behind the touchpoints, the touchpoints can be associated to the same hand. This decision is not yet final as other conditions are applied for further disambiguation; we wish to point out this condition because it relies on the definition of what is 'behind' and what 'in front' on the display. This implies that all the users approach the display from the same side, which is plausible in a single user environment as envisioned in the paper, but restricts the possible multiuser expansion of the method to horizontally mounted displays. In other words, the method cannot be applied in a multiuser tabletop scenario. On the other hand, the method's strengths are the fact that it can be implemented on every display that provides information about finger orientation and its reported 97.5% ($\sigma = 0.48$) overall accuracy in distinguishing a single user's left and right hand.

4   Clustering for Hand Detection

This section is divided as follows: in subsection 4.1 we overview the general characteristics of clustering for hand detection on multitouch displays, subsection 4.2 explains why we chose DBScan and XMeans for baseline comparison and finally subsection 4.3 describes our proposed clustering algorithm.

4.1   General Characteristics of Clustering for Hand Detection on Multitouch Displays

Generally speaking, a multitouch display is a touchscreen capable of detecting an unlimited number of touches. Depending on the underlying sensing technology, some constraints may apply. Technology also determines what data we get from the screen. Optical, computer-vision based technologies (e.g. FTIR [18], diffused illumination; see [19] for a full list) are unrestricted in terms of the number of detected touchpoints and provide a rich description of touches. For example, a possible set of data provided by an optical multitouch display is described by the TUIO protocol [20]; each touchpoint is described by a session ID, class ID, position, angle, dimension, area, velocity vector, rotation velocity vector, motion acceleration, rotation acceleration and a free parameter. Besides fingers, some optical displays are also capable of detecting objects placed on the display. On the other hand, non-optical sensing technologies (e.g. capacitive, resistive[19]) can detect only a limited number of touchpoints (e.g. PQ Labs G3 Basic, up to 6 touchpoints[1]) and provide a limited set of information, usually only the coordinates of the touches.

The lowest common denominator of all multitouch displays is the description of touchpoints with x, y coordinates. Therefore, if a hand detection technique is to be generally applicable to all multitouch displays, it must rely only on these data. This is what shaped our goal as 'the development of a method/technique for hand-detection based on the coordinates of the touchpoints.' The goal, as we put it, is similar to the definition of clustering: to determine the intrinsic grouping in a set of unlabeled data.

Furthermore, clustering for hand detection on a multitouch display is characterized by the following properties: a small and highly variable number of instances (touchpoints), the human hand's anatomy, unknown number of clusters and the continuous nature of interaction. These properties must be taken into account when choosing an appropriate clustering algorithm or when developing one. On the one hand, the small number of instances causes problems to most clustering algorithms; on the other hand, heuristics derived from the hand's anatomy can fruitfully be exploited when developing an algorithm from scratch as we will show later.

4.2 Suitable Clustering Algorithms for Hand Detection: DBScan and XMeans

First, we wanted to evaluate the performance of existing clustering algorithms. According to [21], they can be divided as follows: partitioning, hierarchical, density-based, grid-based, model-based, and ensembles of different algorithms. Our choice was dictated by the nature of our problem: assessing the correct number of hands on the screen means that we needed an algorithm capable of automatically detecting the number of clusters in the data. Furthermore, the algorithm should be adept to work in an incremental fashion as fingers come and leave the screen. This led us to the choice of two algorithms: XMeans and DBScan. The first is an extension of the k-means algorithm capable of determining the number of clusters (k) automatically [22], while the second is a clustering algorithm "relying on a density-based notion of clusters which is designed to discover clusters of arbitrary shape [23]." The notion of density of clusters used by DBScan is defined with two parameters: the neighborhood size Eps and minimal number of points minPts. Basically, for a point to be part of a cluster it must satisfy the condition that at least minP points are present in its Eps

---

[1] http://multi-touch-screen.com/store.html

neighborhood. This is only partly true as points on the border of a cluster are an exception to this condition (see [23] for details). Our domain of hand detection determines the choice for both parameters; minPts must be set to 1, so that hands with only one finger can be detected and a hand span seems a sound choice for Eps - 15.9 cm resulted in the highest accuracy (parameters were fine-tuned for performance, data not shown).

4.3   HDCDM: Hand Detection with Clustering on Multitouch Displays

We propose an algorithm HDCMD (Hand Detection with Clustering on Multitouch Displays) that builds upon two premises: the size of the hand span and the fact that a human hand has five fingers. HDCMD maintains a list of hands and each hand in this list maintains a list of fingers associated with it. The algorithm works as follows: when a finger touches the screen, if there is no other already identified hand within maxDistance (approximately half a hand span distance), a new hand is added to the hands list and the finger is associated with it. If one or more hands are within maxDistance, the finger is added to the nearest hand that has less than 5 fingers associated with it. If only hands with five fingers are near, a new hand is created. We achieved the best results with maxDistance set to 10 cm (the parameter was experimentally fine-tuned, data not shown).

5   Accuracy of Hand Detection

The main goal of our evaluation was to determine the accuracy of hand detection for XMeans, DBScan and HDCMD.

To evaluate the performance of clustering for hand detection, a substantial amount of data is needed, therefore we implemented a 'touchpoints data generator' (TDG)[2] to create a suitable database. Besides the amount of data needed, another argument in favor of our simulation approach is the fact that real interaction is highly dependable on the application used while gathering the data and can therefore influence test results. TDG is an algorithm that, given the number of hands, the number of fingers on them and the size of the display, returns randomly generated pairs of coordinates for each touchpoint. It works as follows: for each hand TDG generates a center point that represents the center of the palm. Then it generates touchpoints that are no more than 8 cm away (we empirically determined 8 cm as approximately half of an average hand span) around the palm's center. This center point must be at least a hand span away from all previously generated center points so that hands do not overlap completely thus leading to a better resemblance of real multitouch interaction. In contrast to the dynamic nature of multitouch interaction, the data generated in this way is static and represents a still frame or a snapshot of what is on the screen at a given point in

---

[2] A similar approach was adopted in the development of Microsoft Kinect sensor's skeletal tracking. (C. Bishop, Microsoft Research Cambridge, http://techtalks.tv/talks/54443/, last accessed 25.1.2013).

time. With TDG we created a dataset of 26946 snapshots, 499 for each combination of hands and fingers, where the number of hands ranged from 1 to 8 and the number of fingers from 1 to 5. We also created snapshots with a random number of hands and fingers from the intervals [1,8] and [1,5] for hands and fingers respectively. Snapshots with a fixed number of hands and fingers are useful for analysis, while those with a random number of hands and fingers give a better approximation of real interaction. The size of our virtual table was 200 cm x 200 cm. The combinations of fingers and hands and the size of the table was chosen so that the dataset can represent up to four users interacting with the screen with both hands or 8 users interacting with only one hand.

Table 1. Accuracy [% out of 499 runs] of hand detection with XMeans on synthetic data. Overall accuracy is 21% (5709/26946).

Hands\Fingers	Random 1-5	1	2	3	4	5
random 1-8	22	13	29	27	23	25
1	99	100	100	96	98	99
2	67	0	85	84	87	88
3	0	0	0	0	0	0
4	0	0	0	0	0	0
5	0	0	0	0	0	0
5	0	0	0	0	0	0
7	0	0	0	0	0	0
8	0	0	0	0	0	0

Table 2. Accuracy [% out of 499 runs] of hand detection with DBScan on synthetic data. Overall accuracy is 67% (18185/26946).

Hands\Fingers	Random 1-5	1	2	3	4	5
random 1-8	68	98	58	57	64	60
1	25	100	0	0	0	0
2	46	100	29	31	33	40
3	75	100	59	67	72	73
4	83	98	77	77	83	83
5	85	96	83	81	85	84
5	83	95	80	81	81	74
7	79	90	76	75	76	71
8	70	84	69	65	65	63

We tested all three algorithms on the same dataset. Our algorithm was implemented in Java with the MT4j framework [24], while for DBScan and XMeans we used Weka's implementations [25].

The goal of these algorithms is hand detection, which in turn has two goals: assessment of the number of hands on the screen and mapping fingers to hands. A correct detection happens when both goals are met; the number of hands is assessed correctly and all fingers are correctly mapped to the hands. Tables 1-3 show the accuracy (in %) of the algorithms on the same dataset for XMeans, DBScan and HDCMD respectively. Table 4 shows the results for HDCMD on a different dataset, where hands were allowed to completely overlap one another without any restrictions.

Table 3. Accuracy [% out of 499 runs] of hand detection with HDCMD on synthetic data. Overall accuracy is 97% (26121/26946).

Hands\Fingers	Random 1-5	1	2	3	4	5
random 1-8	100	100	100	100	100	100
1	100	100	100	99	100	100
2	99	99	99	99	98	100
3	98	97	98	98	98	100
4	96	97	97	95	97	100
5	95	97	95	94	95	100
5	95	94	92	92	90	100
7	90	88	89	91	92	100
8	100	100	100	100	100	100

Table 4. Accuracy [% out of 499 runs] of hand detection with HDCMD on synthetic data with completely overlapping hands. Overall accuracy is 93% (25150/26946).

Hands\Fingers	Random 1-5	1	2	3	4	5
random 1-8	100	100	100	100	100	100
1	99	99	99	99	99	100
2	98	98	97	98	97	100
3	96	95	96	96	95	100
4	93	96	93	92	90	100
5	89	89	87	87	85	100
5	88	84	83	86	86	100
7	85	82	78	77	78	99
8	100	100	100	100	100	100

6   Discussion

The goal of this research was to establish whether clustering can be used as a means for hand detection on multitouch displays. We found out that available clustering algorithms suitable for the task fail to provide sufficient accuracy, while the algorithm presented in this paper performs significantly better.

6.1   Hand Detection Accuracy

Table 1 shows that XMeans proved useless in terms of hand detection. The main factor for the poor overall accuracy of the algorithm (21%) is that XMeans tends to underestimate the number of clusters due to the Bayesian information criterion used in determining the number of clusters [22]. This also explains why it only performs well, when there are only one or two hands on the screen as there is a smaller chance for underestimating the number of clusters. When the number of hands (i.e. actual clusters) increases, XMeans always detects less hands than are actually present.

DBScan performs considerably better than XMeans, but still not satisfactorily. Although we are reporting results with the chosen parameters that yield the best overall accuracy (67%), this accuracy is not high enough for the algorithm to be useful in hand detection for multitouch interaction. The main problem is that this choice of minP and Eps results in the algorithm detecting more hands, when there is actually only one hand with more fingers on the screen. Table 2 also shows that DBScan works better when the number of touchpoints on the screen is such that the differences in densities are more distinctive.

To find the best possible results, we experimented with different DBScan and XMeans parameters (in the interest of space, the data is not shown here). Despite this, the aforementioned algorithms performed significantly worse than our human-anatomy inspired algorithm. Due to their poor overall accuracy DBScan and XMeans both proved unsuitable for hand detection for multitouch interaction. In contrast, HDCMD boasts an overall accuracy of 97%. This makes it a suitable means for hand detection. Table 3 shows that, in case all hands are touching the screen with 5 fingers, the accuracy rises to 100%. This can be attributed to the incremental nature of the algorithm that implicitly transforms a snapshot of contemporary touchpoints to a series of touchpoints. This reduces the errors caused by two hands that are close together. For example, consider a combination of 2 hands represented with 4 fingers each. The algorithm correctly maps the four fingers of the first hand and can then make a mistake when mapping the first finger of the second hand by mapping it to the first hand. In the case of hands represented with five fingers this could not happen, because the first hand would already have 5 fingers mapped to it.

6.2   HDCMD's Limitations

Another point observable from Table 3 is that the accuracy of hand detection is consistent across various combinations of hands and fingers; the only noticeable trend is the decrease of accuracy with the increasing number of hands on the screen. Clearly, a lower number of hands on the display and/or a larger display have a positive effect on the accuracy of hand detection. In other words, HDCMD compromises between the maximum number of hands we can detect and the accuracy of the detection. This is due to HDCMD's simplistic nature.

Our algorithm makes errors, when hands are close together. Figure 1 shows these errors; we can see that the errors can be classified in two types. The first type of error is when fingers from two different hands are detected as fingers from a single hand and the second type of error is when fingers of two hands are incorrectly mapped to two separate hands. In the first case both the number of hands detected as well as the mapping of fingers to hands are incorrect, while in the second case only the mapping of fingers to hands is incorrect.

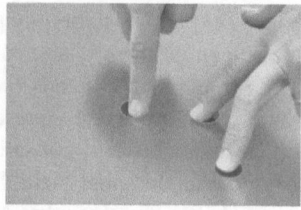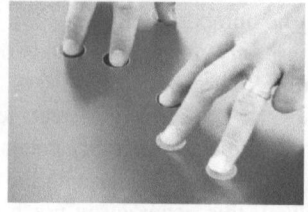

Fig. 1. HDCMD's errors: fingers from different hands are detected as if they were all from the same hand (left) and fingers from hands close together are incorrectly mapped (right). For illustrative purposes we desaturated all the colors in the pictures except blues and greens.

6.3   Use Cases and Future Directions

The aforementioned limitations of HDCMD influence its possible use cases and the directions for future work. In the limited information context we are exploring (x and y coordinates of touchpoints) there is no way of knowing if two hands belong to the same user. This poses a limit to HDCMD - it can only detect hands, but not users. In other words, HDCMD can be used to build applications that are hands-aware, but not user-aware. Nevertheless, in Section 2 we mentioned a valid use-case for hands-aware applications, namely "cooperative gestures for co-located groupware [5]." In these applications, some commands can only be invoked by gestures performed collectively by multiple group members. As a result, in this scenario, the system is only interested in knowing that all users have taken part (hand detection) in the collaborative hand gesture rather than with the identities of the users. Another possible use-case is connected to the notion of territoriality described in [26], where Scott et al. "conducted two observational studies of traditional tabletop collaboration in both casual and formal settings" and found out that "collaborators use three types of tabletop territories to help coordinate their interactions within the shared tabletop workspace: personal, group, and storage territories." Personal territories belong to a specific user and all interaction that occurs in them can be attributed to that user. Within personal territories, HDCMD can be used to support the implementation of bimanual interaction of a single user.

User studies of applications using HDCMD in the abovementioned and other scenarios are one possible direction for future research. Another option originates from the fact that clustering on snapshots is a more difficult problem than clustering dynamic data, because the dynamics of interaction can also be an aid in determining which hand the finger belongs to. For example, the speed of a touchpoint can discriminate it from touchpoints from a nearby hand. As speed is a feature calculated from touchpoint coordinates it does not reduce the general applicability of HDCMD.

7   Contribution and Conclusion

Our work shows that, in contrast to some assumptions, clustering can successfully be exploited for hand detection on multitouch surfaces. Our main contribution is showing how and to what extent this can be achieved. We present an incremental clustering algorithm based on simple heuristics stemming from the anatomy of the human hand. The algorithm determines the number of hands on the screen and maps each finger to its hand with an accuracy of 97%, tested on synthetic data. The features used for clustering are the x and y coordinates of the touchpoints on the screen, which means that the algorithm can be used on all multitouch displays regardless their construction.

Acknowledgements. This research was funded in part by the European Union, European Social Fund, Operational Program for Human Resources, Development for the Period 2007-2013 and by the Slovenian Research Agency.

References

1. Buxton, W.: Multi-Touch Systems That I Have Known and Loved, `http://www.billbuxton.com/multitouchOverview.html` (last accessed January 25, 2013)
2. Benko, H., Morris, M.R., Brush, A.J.B., Wilson, A.D.: Insights on Interactive Tabletops: A Survey of Researchers and Developers (2009), `http://research.microsoft.com`
3. Leganchuk, A., Zhai, S., Buxton, W.: Manual and cognitive benefits of two-handed input: an experimental study. ACM Transactions on Computer-Human Interaction (TOCHI) 5(4), 326–359 (1998)
4. Kin, K., Agrawala, M., DeRose, T.: Determining the benefits of direct-touch, bimanual, and multifinger input on a multitouch workstation. In: Proceedings of Graphics Interface, pp. 119–124. Canadian Information Processing Society, Ontario (2009)
5. Ringel Morris, M., Huang, A., Paepcke, A., Winograd, T.: Cooperative Gestures: Multi-User Gestural Interactions For Co-Located Groupware. In: Proceedings of the ACM Chi Conference on Human Factors in Computing Systems, pp. 1201–1210. ACM (2006)
6. Terrenghi, L., Kirk, D., Sellen, A., Izadi, S.: Affordances For Manipulation of Physical Versus Digital Media on Interactive Surfaces. In: Proceedings of the Sigchi Conference on Human Factors in Computing Systems, Chi 2007, pp. 1157–1166. ACM (2007)
7. Rogers, Y., Lim, Y.K., Hazlewood, W.R., Marshall, P.: Equal Opportunities: Do Shareable Interfaces Promote More Group Participation Than Single Users Displays? In: Human-Computer Interaction, vol. 24(1-2), pp. 79–116. Taylor & Francis (2009)
8. Malik, S., Laszlo, J.: Visual Touchpad: A Two-Handed Gestural Input Device. In: Icmi 2004: Proceedings of the 6th International Conference On Multimodal Interfaces, pp. 289–296. ACM, New York (2004)
9. Wu, M., Balakrishnan, R.: Multi-Finger and Whole Hand Gestural Interaction Techniques For Multi-User Tabletop Displays. In: Proceedings of the 16th Annual ACM Symposium on User Interface Software and Technology, Uist 2003, pp. 193–202. ACM, New York (2003)
10. Peltonen, P., Kurvinen, E., Salovaara, A., Jacucci, G., Ilmonen, T., Evans, J., Oulasvirta, A., Saarikko, P.: It's Mine, Don't Touch!: Interactions At A Large Multi-Touch Display in A City Centre. In: Proceeding of the Twenty-Sixth Annual Sigchi Conference on Human Factors in Computing Systems, Chi 2008, pp. 1285–1294. ACM, New York (2008)
11. Dietz, P., Leigh, D.: DiamondTouch: a multi-user touch technology. In: Proceedings of the 14th Annual ACM Symposium on User Interface Software and Technology, pp. 219–226. ACM (2001)

12. Schmidt, D.: Know Thy Toucher. In: CHI 2009 Workshop Multitouch and Surface Computing, Boston (2009)
13. Schmidt, D., Chong, M.K., Gellersen, H.: Handsdown: Hand-Contour-Based User Identification For Interactive Surfaces. In: Proceedings of the 6th Nordic Conference on Human-Computer Interaction: Extending Boundaries, Nordichi 2010, pp. 432–441. ACM, New York (2010)
14. Dohse, K.C., Dohse, T., Still, J.D., Parkhurst, D.J.: Enhancing multi-user interaction with multi-touch tabletop displays using hand tracking. In: 2008 First International Conference on Advances in Computer-Human Interaction, pp. 297–302. IEEE (2008)
15. Echtler, F., Huber, M., Klinker, G.: Shadow Tracking on Multi-Touch Tables. In: Proceedings of the Working Conference on Advanced Visual Interfaces, Avi 2008, pp. 388–391. ACM, New York (2008)
16. Marquardt, N., Kiemer, J., Greenberg, D.: What Caused That Touch?: Expressive Interaction With A Surface Through Fiduciary-Tagged Gloves. In: ACM International Conference on Interactive Tabletops and Surfaces, Its 2010, pp. 139–142. ACM, New York (2010)
17. Ringel Morris, M., Huang, A., Paepcke, A., Winograd, T.: Cooperative Gestures: Multi-User Gestural Interactions For Co-Located Groupware. In: Proceedings of the ACM Chi Conference on Human Factors in Computing Systems, pp. 1201–1210. ACM (2006)
18. Han, J.Y.: Low-Cost Multi-Touch Sensing Through Frustrated Total Internal Reflection. In: Proceedings of the 18th Annual ACM Symposium on User Interface Software and Technology, Uist 2005, pp. 115–118. ACM, New York (2005)
19. Çetin, G., Bedi, R., Sandler, S.: Multi-touch Technologies, 1st edn. (2009)
20. Kaltenbrunner, M., Bovermann, T., Bencina, R., Costanza, E.: Tuio: a Protocol for Table-Top Tangible User Interfaces. In: Proceedings of the 6th International Workshop on Gesture in Human Computer Interaction and Simulation GW, pp. 1–5 (2005)
21. Kotsiantis, S., Pintelas, P.: Recent advances in clustering: A brief survey. WSEAS Transactions on Information Science and Applications 1(1), 73–81 (2004)
22. Schmidt, D., Chong, M.K., Gellersen, H.: Handsdown: Hand-Contour-Based User Identification For Interactive Surfaces. In: Proceedings of the 6th Nordic Conference on Human-Computer Interaction: Extending Boundaries, Nordichi 2010, pp. 432–441. ACM, New York (2010)
23. Ester, M., Kriegel, H.P., Jörg, S., Xu, X.: A Density-Based Algorithm for Discovering Clusters in Large Spatial Databases With Noise. In: Proceedings of The ACM Sigkdd International Conference on Knowledge Discovery And Data Mining, pp. 226–231. AAAI Press (1996)
24. Laufs, U., Ruff, C., Zibuschka, J.: Mt4j – A Cross-Platform Multi-Touch Development Framework. In: Engineering Patterns for Multi-Touch Interfaces, Workshop of the ACM Sigchi Symposium on Engineering Interactive Computing Systems (2010)
25. Hall, M., Frank, E., Holmes, G., Pfahringer, B., Reutemann, P., Witten, I.: The Weka Data Mining Software: an Update. Special Interest Group on Knowledge Discovery and Data Mining Explorer Newsletter 11(1), 10–18 (2009)
26. Scott, S.D., Sheelagh, M., Carpendale, T., Inkpen, K.M.: Territoriality in Collaborative Tabletop Workspaces. In: Proceedings of Cscw 2004, pp. 294–303. ACM (2004)

Augmentative Requirements Engineering for Trustworthy and Usable ICT-Based Services

Hrvoje Belani

University of Zagreb, Faculty of EE and Computing, Unska 3, Zagreb, Croatia
hrvoje.belani@racunarstvo.hr

Abstract. For people who face certain difficulties to communicate in a conventional manner and participate actively in everyday life, from work engagement to personal settings, a clinical practice called augmentative and alternative communication has been established to improve effectiveness of their communication by using symbols. By enforcing the usage of ICT to help solve these issues, users' needs and wants have to be analyzed carefully, by learning from educational, psychological and rehabilitation methods from other fields already deeply involved with life-care for these people. This paper proposes new paradigm of so-called augmentative requirements engineering that would allow holistic view on ICT service requirements engineering to help these user groups.

Keywords: requirements engineering, complex communication needs, augmentative and alternative communication, usability, trustworthiness, eAccessibility.

1 Introduction

New information and communication technology (ICT) services and emerging digital content being provided for users daily represent an extraordinary enabler for business opportunities, education and infotainment. However, a significant number of users face particular difficulties in benefiting fully from them, and they need enhanced skills to tackle that digital barrier. Their complex communication needs (CCNs) may be associated with developmental (e.g. cerebral palsy, Down syndrome) or acquired disabilities (e.g. stroke, multiple sclerosis), and they can manifest temporarily or permanently. In order to cope with these issues and support CCNs, the area of clinical practice called augmentative and alternative communication (AAC) has been established to improve effectiveness of communication by using symbols, aids, techniques and strategies [1]. When supported by ICT services, the field of AAC suitably falls into human-computer interaction (HCI), a mature research discipline that offers numerous approaches for development of efficient user interfaces and means of people interacting with technology. In order to develop such services that support and enhance AAC, principles of requirements engineering (RE) have to be applied. But, RE techniques have to be carefully considered for users that are not typically considered during the ICT service design process, such as persons with disabilities and special needs [2]. Moreover, such users have to find these services usable and trustworthy.

A. Holzinger et al. (Eds.): SouthCHI 2013, LNCS 7946, pp. 815–818, 2013.

2   Problem Statement: From Requirements to Design for AAC

Bridging the gap from requirements to design and implementation of proper software solutions is often a challenge dealt with methods and tools that tend to trace the status of requirements throughout the development cycle, but these approaches do not help when requirements are gotten wrong in the first place. Considering specificity of target user groups and required service features, it is necessary to make a thorough analysis and define potentials of adequate requirements elicitation techniques that would properly incorporate multidisciplinary approach to the development process.

It seems that ICT has the potential both for enhancing access to different services for people with disabilities and for creating more division and new forms of exclusion. So, it seems crucial to continuously address the issues of accessibility and usability as technology continues to develop and spread and as new technologies emerge [3]. Some usability studies [4] show that even though a product or its features are considered "accessible", users with disabilities may still have difficulty using it easily and efficiently. It is recommended that accessibility and usability should both be measured in tests that include people with a broad range of disabilities, some using assistive technology. Therefore, user centered design (UCD) in this case has to be planned carefully, accepting common approaches from other involved fields and experts, including educators, rehabilitators and caregivers, which are often not well-skilled with advanced AAC services or ICT services at all. Properly developed AAC services can pose economic benefits for disabled people towards their assisted living (AL) practices, and even social benefits for users living by the independent living (IL) principles, in terms of equal opportunities and self-determination.

The three main research questions addressed in this PhD thesis can be formulated:

1. How to make a proper model for engineering software requirements, traceable to the specification that conceives and maintains usability and accessibility of and trust to ICT-based AAC services?
2. Is it possible (and how) to model AAC service requirements using one of widely known formal methods, in order to be able to automatically check the specification for consistency, when reaching for requirements reusability?
3. How do UCD principles, even more user experience design (UED) apply, regarding the dynamics of person's experience, and the specificities of AAC user groups?

3   Proposed Solution: Augmentative Requirements Engineering

We propose new paradigm of so-called augmentative requirements engineering (ARE) that would allow holistic view on service requirements concerning users abilities and needs, service domain (communication, education, entertainment) and associated user supporters (rehabilitators, educators, family). Directions should strive towards fulfillment of principles like: simple and intuitive ICT services providing perceptible information, being tolerant for errors, equitable and flexible for use, with the size and space for approaching and usage with a low physical effort.

Usual requirements gathering methods, such as interviewing or role playing, cannot be universally applied. The crucial fact for people with CCNs is that every person has his/her special needs and specific abilities, not allowing for them to be treated the same way as other AAC service users. Some directions can be driven from experiences of educational, psychological and rehabilitation methods from other fields already deeply involved with life-care for these people.

Although it seems reasonable to assume that the users, regarding their limited abilities, need "as simple as possible" set of functional requirements (FRs) in order to use some AAC service, this does not mean simply reducing already existing set of functions for non-disabled people using the same service. This RE method aims for establishing full understanding which functions are necessary for them, what is the order of function usage, their possible combinations allowed and/or disallowed, etc. Also, non-functional requirements (NFRs), such as those regarding usability, accessibility, security and trust, have to be carefully considered and analyzed, first separately and then in combination with the set of FRs, in order to provide a robust and yet usable AAC service.

Furthermore, some other influential factors for building proper requirements specification for e.g. a mobile AAC service planned to be developed for a person with CCNs have to be properly addressed: (1) contexts of use, such as home, school, or other social places; (2) users and user relations, explaining is the interaction between the user and a service directed or intermediated (supported by parents, caregivers, etc.); (3) using of low-tech and add-on principles to gain a valuable insight to the users' needs; and (4) applying trustworthiness principle to gain user's trust in the service [5]. This PhD thesis proposes building and validating a proper requirements engineering model for specification of FRs and NFRs for ICT-based AAC services, which can be:

- Modeled with certain mathematical rigor, primarily when dealing with usability,
- Instantiated into real, implementable usability and accessibility requirements,
- Checked for consistency, while being reused, by applying automatic tools, and
- Traceable to the other, later phases of AAC service development process.

4   Expected Contributions

A list of the expected contributions from this PhD thesis is given here:

- Broad analysis of RE field of research, with a great emphasis on user groups with special needs, and how the issues relate to software engineering and HCI domains;
- Broad analysis of applicability of known formal methods and according tools to the topic of formal specification of usability and accessibility requirements;
- Proposal of RE model (named: ARE) for lightweight formal specification and modeling of usability, accessibility and trust aspects of ICT-based AAC services;
- Validation of the proposed model on a real-life field studies, by taking into account user experience (UX) aspects, in order to verify the approach from RE to UED. Prototypes will be developed as tablet applications suitable for testing with users.

5   Conclusion

As ICT play an essential role in supporting daily life in today's digital society, European e-inclusion policy aims to achieve that "no one is left behind" in enjoying the benefits of ICT, focusing on participation of all individuals and communities in all aspects of the information society. eAccessibility is a strategy undertaken to identify and overcome barriers that may inhibit or prevent people with specific access needs from being able to successfully use the resource as intended, and participate fully in society. It is also one of the major activities of European Commission's Digital Agenda for Europe, aiming to enhance digital literacy, skills and inclusion.

Regarding this PhD research, preliminary work has already been done outlining the usability requirements taxonomy for mobile AAC services. Also, the statistics regarding people with disabilities in Croatia have been analyzed, along with the causes and types of their impairments, in order to properly recognize the needs and requirements of various potential AAC users. Matching of some types of impairments with common aided, mobile AAC systems have been proposed, along with their typical input and output features suitable for AAC users. In order to show that the work presented in this PhD proposal does indeed solve the targeted challenges, field studies, employing methods like surveys, interviews and observations, have to be conducted and technical soundness have to be proved, along with the model limitations and threats to validity. Field work should be in line with ethnographic methods proven useful for observation of AAC users' cultural practices. Finally, the outputs of this work have to be aligned to the enforced inclusion policies.

Future work plans involve establishing proper requirements management processes for platform-based ICT service development, in terms of efficiency and effectiveness.

References

1. Justice, L.M.: Communication Sciences and Disorders: A Contemporary Perspective. Pearson Education (2008) ISBN-13: 978-0135022801
2. Sears, A., Jacko, J.A. (eds.): The Human-Computer Interaction Handbook: Fundamentals, Evolving Technologies and Emerging Applications, 2nd edn. Taylor & Francis Group, New York (2008)
3. Simpson, J.: Inclusive Information and Communication Technologies for People with Disabilities. Disability Studies Quarterly, vol. 29(1). The Society for Disability Studies, Washington (Winter 2009), http://dsq-sds.org/article/view/167/167 (accessed on March 1, 2013)
4. Burgstahler, S., Jirikowic, T., Kolko, B., Eliot, M.: Software accessibility, usability testing and individuals with disabilities. Information Technology and Disabilities, vol. X(1-2). EASI (2013), http://people.rit.edu/easi/itd/itdv10n2/burghsta.htm (accessed on March 1, 2013)
5. Cranor, L.F., Garfinkel, S.: Security and Usability – Designing Secure Systems that People Can Use. O'Reilly Media, Sebastopol (2005) ISBN 978-0-596-00827-7

Research Goals for Evolving the 'Form' User Interface Metaphor towards More Interactivity

Johannes Harms

INSO Research Group, Vienna Univ. of Technology, Austria
johannes.harms@inso.tuwien.ac.at

Abstract. Forms have been static, document-like user interfaces (UIs) for centuries. This work proposes to evolve the 'form' UI metaphor towards more interactivity. Related work has proposed interactive form elements such as autocompleting or otherwise assistive input fields. But a unified concept and scientific reflection on the topic are missing. Methodologically, this work first provides a deeper understanding of forms as UI metaphor. It then presents relevant research goals for improved usability, including collaborative form filling, easier navigation in long forms, and combined input fields for comfortable data entry. Taken together, the contributions of this work are to provide a deeper understanding of forms, systematically highlight relevant research topics, and hopefully foster a scientific discussion in form design.

Keywords: Form Design, Web Forms, HCI, Usability, User Interaction.

1 Introduction

Electronic forms are embedded in many of todays user interfaces (UIs), enabling users to engage in online communities, e-commerce, and productivity software [1]. These applications may involve multiple concurrent users, large amounts of (semi-)structured data, complex validation and business logic. In contrast to this complexity, the original concept behind forms is very simple: Pre-defined labels and placeholders prompt for information that conforms to the form's structure, diction and intent. As a result, forms do not always cope with the complex requirements of their embedding application, leading to usability problems [2].

Related work on form design includes established best practices documented in books [1,3] and articles [4]. Research recognizes the need to make forms more dynamic and application-like; this applies to every aspect of form design as classified in [4]: (a) form content: e.g., assistive form elements [5], (b) form layout: combined form fields [6], (c) input types: free-text and multimodal data entry [7,8], (d) error handling, e.g., with multimodal form filling [8], and (e) form submission: e.g., versioned submissions in co-operative form filling [9,10].

But in addition, a deeper theoretical understanding and a unified concept for practical improvements are needed to adapt forms for use in complex applications. I hypothesize that form-filling can be improved in usability and user experience if forms more fully satisfy the entailments of the 'form' UI metaphor and put to use more of the interactive possibilities offered by digital media.

A. Holzinger et al. (Eds.): SouthCHI 2013, LNCS 7946, pp. 819–822, 2013.

Real-World Example and Scenario. In a form-based, medical documentation software named "Wound Healing Analysis Tool" [11], users were observed shouting across rooms to find out who else was documenting at the same time [1]. The forms did not update in real-time and did not provide enough awareness about concurrent usage. Moreover, data entry was complicated because the length of most forms required a lot of scrolling. This scenario demonstrates the practical need for better, more interactive forms.

2 Forms as User Interface Metaphors

Understanding forms as UI metaphor provides a deeper understanding of how forms are used in software, helps comparing forms with other UI metaphors [12], and allows to identify relevant research goals, as shown in this work. Metaphors declare two different concepts or things to be identical in order to assert their similarity [13]. UI metaphors likewise assert similarity, which helps to explain the functionality of a UI. Derived from [13], the 'form' UI metaphor can be defined as: *The 'form' UI metaphor is a device for explaining the functionality of a UI by asserting its similarity to conventional (e.g., paper) forms.* Consequently electronic forms are a deliberate choice [12] for designing a UI in a way that metaphorically reminds of conventional (e.g., paper) forms. This perspective allows for a systematical identification of improvements in form design, see Fig. 1: Firstly, not all metaphorical entailments are fulfilled by electronic forms. E.g., in contrast to paper forms, electronic forms typically cannot be freely annotated. Secondly, the 'form' metaphor does not yet fully make use of the interactive possibilities offered by digital media. E.g., attention-reactive UIs can dynamically adapt to the user's focus of attention [14], but forms are usually very static.

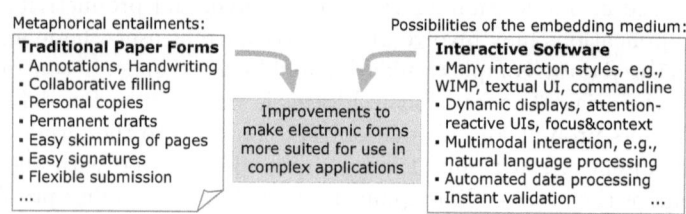

Fig. 1. To identify improvements in form design, this work considers unfulfilled entailments of the 'form' UI-metaphor and interactive possibilities offered by digital media

This approach leads to relevant improvements because firstly – referring to unfulfilled metaphorical entailments – paper is still the preferred medium of many users [15]; and porting paper abilities into the software medium will benefit domains where paper forms have traditionally been used. Secondly – referring to unused possibilities of the embedding medium – electronic forms could employ more interactive techniques to improve efficiency and user experience.

---

[1] Unpublished field study at Krankenhaus Göttlicher Heiland, www.khgh.at, 2010.

3   Research Goals and Methods

Relevant goals for form-filling interfaces that reflect the semiotics of historical (paper) forms and that more fully use the interactive possibilities of digital media are shown in Fig. 1. Methodologically, I propose to treat each goal using an iterative UI design process and subsequent empirical evaluation in the context of a specific domain, application and user group. The design process should include sketches, prototypes, and usability tests. The short length of this paper only permits a very brief overview on four particularly relevant goals:

Focus-and-Context Navigation. Long forms require a lot of scrolling, or else they are split into multiple pages or tabs. Both options lead to a loss of context for the user. This work proposes to apply the focus-and-context principle [16] and attention-reactive UIs [14] to form design: Only those parts of the form with the user's focus shall be fully shown; the rest is shown in a compact and aggregated way, see Fig. 2ab. I will research navigation patterns in other application fields (e.g., master/detail view, drill-down) and evaluate different granularities (i.e., single fields or whole fieldsets may toggle between full and compact views).

Collaborative Form Filling. Support for co-operative form filling would benefit applications where multiple users work on shared artifacts, e.g., as demonstrated in co-operative web browsing [9] and in a customer support system [10]. I propose design and evaluation of a prototype for real-time collaborative form filling in the medical platform [11] described in the example scenario.

Combined Input Fields. Forms tend to be split into many small fields to simplify automated data processing, but this can lead to inefficient data entry. A related paper proposes to combine complex search fields into one smart field [6]. This can be generalized for arbitrary forms: Combined input fields match the users input to the underlying form schema, see Fig. 2c. A usability evaluation shall quantify the improvement in form filling performance. Biggest benefits are expected in scenarios with repetitive data entry in sparsely filled forms.

A unified concept. The proposed improvements can and should work together, creating a unified concept for form-based interactions. For this purpose, a JavaScript framework could provide modules to enhance web forms with dynamic behavior (e.g., real-time collaboration, focus-and-context navigation). The modules could be loaded individually as required for a specific application.

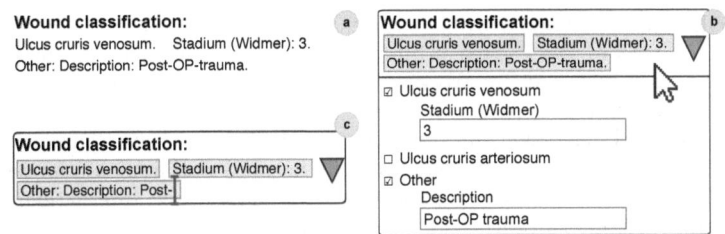

Fig. 2. Smart input fields: (a) Out-of-focus state, (b) Focussed state, with dropdown menu revealing the underlying structure, (c) Combined field with a textual editing UI

4   Discussion and Future Work

The contribution of this paper is to explain forms as UI metaphors, allowing to systematically identify relevant usability improvements, which are presented in this paper as goals for future research (Fig. 1). The author's future research can only cover select goals, starting with focus-and-context navigation in long forms, as described in this paper. Other researchers are encouraged to likewise discuss the future of interactive forms. These efforts shall lead to a unified concept that evolves the 'form' metaphor towards more interactiviy and better usability.

References

1. Wroblewski, L.: Web Form Design. Filling the Blanks. Louis Rosenfeld (2008)
2. Nielsen, J.: Forms vs. Applications (2005),
   http://www.nngroup.com/articles/forms-vs-applications/
3. Jarrett, C., Gaffney, G.: Forms that work. Morgan Kaufmann (2008)
4. Bargas-Avila, J., Brenzikofer, O., Roth, S., Tuch, A., Orsini, S., Opwis, K.: Simple but crucial user interfaces in the world wide web: Introducing 20 guidelines for usable web form design. In: Matrai, R. (ed.) User Interfaces, ch.1. InTech (2010)
5. Frohlich, D., Crossfield, Gilbert: Requirements for an intelligent form-filling interface. In: People and Computers: Designing the Interface, pp. 102–116 (1985)
6. Tjin-Kam-Jet, K., Trieschnigg, D., Hiemstra, D.: Free-text search over complex Web Forms. In: Hanbury, A., Rauber, A., de Vries, A.P. (eds.) IRFC 2011. LNCS, vol. 6653, pp. 94–107. Springer, Heidelberg (2011)
7. Tange, H.J., Hasman, A., de Vries Robbé, P.F., Schouten, H.C.: Medical Narratives in Electronic Medical Records. Int. J. Med. Inform. 46, 7–29 (1997)
8. Sturm, J., Boves, L.: Effective error recovery strategies for multimodal form-filling applications. Speech Communication 45(3), 289–303 (2005)
9. Jacobs, S., Gebhardt, M., Kethers, S., Rzasa, W.: Filling HTML forms simultaneously: CoWeb architecture and functionality. In: Computer Networks and ISDN Systems, vol. 28(7-11), pp. 1385–1395. Elsevier (1996)
10. Amrhein, D., Ivory, A.: Enable a Collaborative Experience for Html Forms. IBM (2010), http://ibm.com/developerworks/web/library/wa-twowayforms/
11. Strobl, S., Bernhart, M., Grechenig, T.: An Experience Report on the Incremental Adoption and Evolution of an SPL in eHealth. In: Proc. 2010 ICSE Workshop on Product Line Approaches in Software Engineering, pp. 16–23. ACM (2010)
12. Alty, J., Knott, R., Anderson, B., Smyth, M.: A framework for engineering metaphor at the user interface. In: Interacting with Computers, vol. 13(2), pp. 301–322 (2000)
13. Barr, P., Biddle, R., Noble, J.: A Semiotic Model of User-Interface Metaphor. In: Virtual, Distributed and Flexible Organisations, pp. 189–215. Springer (2005)
14. Card, S., Nation, D.: Degree-of-Interest Trees: A Component of an Attention-Reactive User Interface. In: Working Conference on Advanced Visual Interfaces, AVI 2002, pp. 231–245. ACM, New York (2002)
15. Holzinger, A., Baernthaler, M., Pammer, W., Katz, H., Bjelic-Radisic, V., Ziefle, M.: Investigating paper vs. screen in real-life hospital workflows: Performance contradicts perceived superiority of paper in the user experience. International Journal of Human-Computer Studies 69(9), 563–570 (2011)
16. Card, S., Mackinlay, J., Shneiderman, B.: Readings in Information Visualization: Using Vision to Think. Morgan Kaufmann (1999)

Intentions: A Confident-Based Interaction Design for Smart Spaces

Mario Vega-Barbas and Miguel A. Valero

T>SIC group, Universidad Politécnica de Madrid, Spain
{mvega,mavalero}@diatel.upm.es

Abstract. The paradigm of ubiquitous computing has become a reference for the design of Smart Spaces. Current trends in Ambient Intelligence are increasingly related to the scope of Internet of Things. This paradigm has the potential to support cost-effective solutions in the fields of telecare, e-health and Ambient Assisted Living. Nevertheless, ubiquitous computing does not provide end users with a role for proactive interactions with the environment. Thus, the deployment of smart health care services at a private space like the home is still unsolved. This PhD dissertation aims to define a person-environment interaction model to foster acceptability and users confidence in private spaces by applying the concept of user-centred security and the human performance model of seven stages of action.

Keywords: Person-Smart Space Interaction, Confident, Ubiquitous Computing.

1 Research Situation

The presented work is framed into the context of TALISEC+ project[1] and supported up to 2015 by a PhD scholarship (FPI) granted by the Spanish Ministry of Economy and Competitiveness. Currently I have completed my training period (MSc) that led to the beginning of the research stage of my thesis. Also this thesis is going to be support by a double doctorate cooperation agreement between the Royal Institute of Technology (KTH) from Sweden and Universidad Politécnica de Madrid from Spain.

Along the training period of my PhD studies I was able to specify the problem domain of my research as well as the expected results of my thesis work. Besides, a brief stay in the Smart Environment Research Group at the University of Ulster allowed me the validation of the objectives detailed below. However, expert researchers about Human-Computer Interaction (HCI) can contribute in an effective way to enhance the validity and feasibility of this work. This is my motivation to attend to the Doctoral Consortium of SouthCHI 2013.

---

[1] http://www.morelab.deusto.es/talisman/index_en.html

A. Holzinger et al. (Eds.): SouthCHI 2013, LNCS 7946, pp. 823–826, 2013.
© Springer-Verlag Berlin Heidelberg 2013

2   Background and Motivation

Current HCI models aim to look at the person as the center of all interaction activities [1]. Ubiquitous computing (ubicomp), smart spaces and the applications and services envisaged for these domains need to define new users' roles [2]. It is complex to include human beings in the traditional computational loop of these scenarios without degrading their capabilities [2][3].

Some studies analyze the implications of the inclusion of ubicomp into living spaces such as the home [4]. The majority of papers do focus on improving other required aspects like interoperability, devices self-discovery or the capability to program smart spaces in the Future Internet [5][6]. Thus, the field of ubicomp interaction has been dealt in an isolated way from a viewpoint of services and applications which does not include the end user [3][7]. Therefore, a new global approach needs to be defined in order to situate the user in the requested place.

Usage of ubicomp and proactivity in daily routine at health care area is still a challenge [4][7]. Telecare and e-health services could be enhanced by ubicomp if and only if users accept this emerging interaction way.

The aim of this PhD work is the creation of a new Person-Smart Space interaction model that maximizes users´ acceptance and confidentiality of pervasive healthcare and e-health services. This research addresses to identify those factors that should guide a new model and its application in the paradigm of ubiquitous computing, enhancing other acceptance model such as Pervasive Technology Acceptance Model (PTAM) [8] and Technology Acceptance Model 3 (TAM) [9].

3   Statement of Thesis

This thesis tries to solve the intrinsic problem that arises from the inclusion of ubiquitous and proactive technology in homes or private environments where personal information is managed. Consequently, the following problems are stated:

1. Identification of indicators that specify the level of confidence and acceptance of a person in relation with the application of pervasive technology at home.
2. Specification of suitable interaction models to support users at ubiquitous computing home based scenarios that manage confidential data such us e-health, telecare and Ambient Assisted Living.
3. The definition and implementation of hardware and software modules requested by a smart home e-health or telecare service to provide the expected confidence.
4. Finally, verification and validation of the interaction model developed. This process will be done using three methods of evaluation tools: interviews and group dynamics, validation through use cases and scenarios and prototyping into real deployments at several research projects.

4   Research Goals and Methods

The presented PhD dissertation would pursues the following goals:

— **Goal 1.** To define a measurable set of indicators capable of describing the willingness and barriers of a person, related to confidence, in order to accept a ubiquitous computing service at a smart home environment. The level of achievement of this goal will be validated in telecare and e-health domains.

Previous experiences will be reviewed to extract an initial set of indicators about users' attitudes towards confidentiality and privacy in ubicomp scenarios. Then, guided interviews with end users of telecare and e-health services will be carried out in order to fine-tune these indicators and validate its application.

— **Goal 2.** To set out a scalable interaction model in private ubicomp scenarios that integrates users' roles and attitudes. This model should enhance the acceptability and confidence of users by providing an accessible way to understand and verify the behavior of his surrounding environment.

Published results from related field works as well as the set of indicators defined in Goal 1 will be the basis to design the interaction model. Next, a validation home telecare or e-health service will be deployed including the requested interaction facilities, software and hardware, that provides end users with expected confidence. In this way, its verification and validation will be done through a proof of concept to be deployed and evaluated with end users into real scenarios such as their own homes and the Accessible Digital Home sited at Technical University of Madrid[2]. Moreover, the model developed will be use in order to supply prototypes for several e-health research projects at KTH, Sweden. Those prototypes and group dynamics and interviews help me to refine and validate the proposal.

The presented work should furnish guides or interaction models to guarantee an optimal level of user understanding of what happens in a smart environment. The result should contribute with a new approach to defining user roles in ubiquitous computing and should also lead to new ways of designing and developing smart environments designed for the people.

5   Dissertation Status

To date there have been two interviews to a set of users to determine which technologies should be used to make the process of interaction within homes and a survey about the confidence on smart spaces. Additionally, we have finished a complete study about confidence into smart environments with 200 people. With this information I have could define and enhance a user model for the specific case of telecare in the home with four different types of players (inhabitants, technology

---

[2] http://hogardigitalaccesible.euitt.upm.es/

integrators, services providers and other caregivers as family). Furthermore, I have designed software and hardware architecture to support this future interaction model based on actions and intentions, following the schema shown in the Fig. 1.

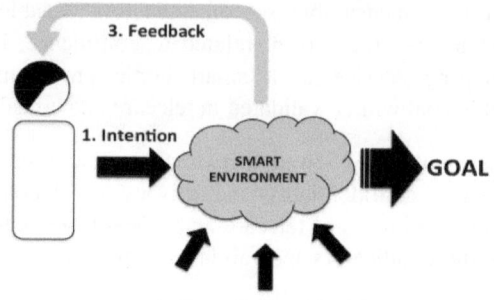

Fig. 1. Intention-based Interaction Model

This base work has been contrasted by a number of congress contributions. Additionally, through a research brief stay in the SERG group at the University of Ulster, has been able to verify the feasibility and validity of the aforementioned architecture design. Besides, the Suggestive Autonomy[3] research project that the author was co-director put into practice the basic ideas of this doctorate.

References

1. Sharp, H., Rogers, Y., Preece, J.: Interaction Design: Beyond Human-Computer Interaction, 3rd edn. Wiley Publishing (2012)
2. Tennenhouse, D.: Proactive computing. Commun. ACM 43(5), 43–50 (2000)
3. Poslad, S.: Ubiquitous Computing: Smart Devices, Environments and Interactions. Wiley Publishing (2009)
4. Bohn, J., Coroama, V., Langheinrich, M., Mattern, F., Rohs, M.: Social, Economic, and Ethical Implications of Ambient Intelligence and Ubiquitous Computing. Journal of Human and Ecological Risk Assessment 10(5), 763–786 (2004)
5. King, J., Bose, R., Yang, H., Pickles, S., Helal, A.: Atlas – A Service-Oriented Sensor Platform. In: Proceedings of the First IEEE International Workshop on Practical Issues in Building Sensor Network Applications (SenseApp 2006) (2006)
6. Kuniavsky, M.: Smart Things: Ubiquitous Computing User Experience Design. MK Publishers (2010)
7. Aarts, E., Ruyter, B.: New Research Perspectives on Ambient Intelligence. Journal of Ambient Intelligence and Smart Environments 1(1), 5–14 (2009)
8. Connelly, K.: On Developing a Technology Acceptance Modelfor Pervasive Computing. In: Proceedings of Ubiquitous System Evaluation (USE) at the Ninth International Conference on Ubiquitous Computing (UBICOMP) (2007)
9. Venkatesh, V., Bala, H.: TAM 3: Advancing the Technology Acceptance Model with a Focus on Interventions. Manuscript in-preparation

---

[3] http://www.autonomiasugestiva.es

Combining Spatial and Temporal Information of Eye Movements in Goal-Oriented Tasks

Monchu Chen, Nelson Alves, and Ricardo Sol

Madeira Interactive Technologies Institute, Funchal, Portugal
monchu@m-iti.org, {jose.nelson.afonseca,ricardosolj}@gmail.com

Abstract. Eye tracker is a tool commonly used to analyze and study cognition and usability of interfaces. Heat-maps and scan-paths are two well known visualizations to analyze eye tracker data. This work presents a new technique by combining both methods to visualize eye movements when conducting a goal-oriented task.

Keywords: Eye tracking, visualization, trajectory analysis.

1   Introduction

Gaze attention represents a rich and interesting source for generating novel and meaningful forms of visualizations. With a plethora of devices and apps / services competing for the average user's attention today, a better visual understanding of their gaze holds the promise to inform appropriate design decisions. Eye tracking is popular in evaluating web pages and advertisements and have helped designers and researchers analyze patterns of users' attention and consequently make content more accessible to them. Heat-maps and scan-paths are the most commonly used forms of visualizing eye tracking data. Although the individual forms of visualizations are well researched and heavily utilized, the combination of these visualizations presents itself as a unique opportunity for a better understanding of user goals in typical user studies.

2   Related Work

Heat-maps are visualizations where fixation time stands out and relative data distribution is displayed. Pomplun et al. conceived heat-maps in 1996 [1], but it only become popular after 2002 with Wooding's work [2]. Stellmach's work [3] in 2010 presented three visualizations: projected, object-based, and triangle-based. In 2012 Duchovsky et al. [4] presented an aggregate visualization with real-time heat-maps by implementing a popular heat-map rendering and making a qualitative argument for the use of a luminance-scale color gradients instead of a rainbow map.

Scan-paths are visualizations where the chronology of the fixations stands out. A string editing based scan-path comparison framework was introduced by Privitera and Stark [5] and further developed by Duchovski et al. [6]. Raschke et al. [7] presented

A. Holzinger et al. (Eds.): SouthCHI 2013, LNCS 7946, pp. 827–830, 2013.

Parallel Scan-Path Visualization that has three types of visualizations: gaze duration sequence diagram, a fixation point diagram, and a gaze duration distribution diagram.

At a broad level, there are several visualization techniques for describing data from an eye tracker. A dimensional framework is commonly used when classifying these visualizations techniques. The visualizations techniques could be divided in [8]: one-dimensional, (temporal), two-dimensional, three-dimensional, multi-dimensional.

One-dimensional category typically includes sequential organized textual information, e.g., log files. In this category, one may also vary parameters like for example: color, size, and thickness.

Temporal category refers to visualizations that are mapped against time, e.g., timelines. Keogh et al. [9] presented time boxes in order to deal with time series, filtering important data. Areas of Interest (AOIs) were a temporal visualization introduced by Lessing and Linge in 2002 [10] that gives goal, order, and duration to the user's actions.

The two-dimensional category, apart from scan-paths and heat-maps, also includes the following [8]: Fixation saccades graphs, Clustering fixations, Semitransparent fixations and Fixation maps. Fixation saccades graphs are scanpaths with some data clustering that aim at taking out the blur and show a more explicit visualization. Clustering fixations are important if the viewer only needs to see fixations. Semitransparent fixations are a representation of fixation that has a certain degree of image processing. Schiessl et al. presented EyeSquare [11] where the area surrounding the fixation is semitransparent. Fixation maps is a technique introduced by Wooding [2] wherein the majority of the image is not observable; however the areas next to the items that have more fixation time become transparent.

3   Heatmap of Scanpath

In this paper, we present a visualization technique that combines heat-maps and scan-paths into a single visualization. This technique enables researchers to observe the path users took to reach their target that is essentially an area of interest on the screen. This visualization applies to cases where users need to select from a series of options based on a specific goal (e.g., selecting a page from web search results).

To calculate the distance (our main metric), we first calculate a line from where the users started to look at, to where the user clicked on at the end. This line indicates the optimal path the user could take to reach his or her goal (Fig-1 Left). Then at any given time during the experiment, we calculate the distance between the eye focus and that line. This distance measures how much the user deviated away from his goal. Further on we plot this into a triangle and generate a heat-map.

4   Data Collection and Representation

11 users were asked to read a series of questions and select an answer from 4 available options for each one. At the end of each question, we asked the user about

their confidence level for the answer they selected. Eye movements were recorded. Selected answers and confidence levels were extracted and the data was analyzed for further analysis. Raw data as well as users' responses were exported to a MySQL database for easy access. We finally used a triangle-based visualization overlaid by a heat-map containing the distance path. This visualization meets the intention of being not just novel but also visually balanced in design.

We arrived at this after trying out various other forms of visualizations. The first one plotted where the user's eyes moved along the screen, while the second one included time dimension for the y-axis - so for the x-axis we used the horizontal distance from the current position to the final answer. Then we changed the horizontal distance to the distance between the line that intersects the question and the selected answer. Finally we adjusted the selection to the center, and scaled the plotting area to a triangle (Fig-1 Right).

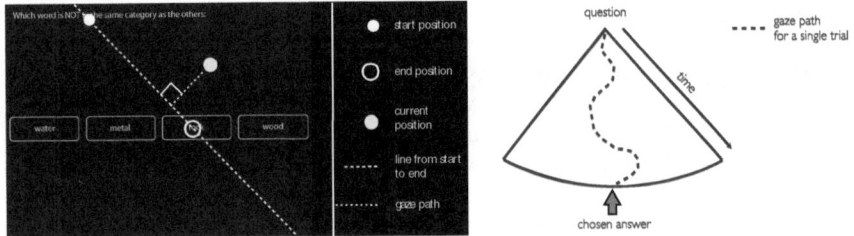

Fig. 1. Left: Screenshot of a single trail. Right: Transformation of Eye Gaze Scan-path.

5   Results

It is expected that the visualization will produce a bell shape that is short at the beginning, broad towards the middle and short at the end. The width of the bell shape would be inversely proportional to the confidence level, as a high confidence level would indicate the user spent little time selecting the answer. The images on figure-2 show the resulting visualization with the eye data broken down into different confidence levels. As expected, higher confidence levels produce a smaller heat-map, with less divergence from the center, as opposed to low confidence levels where there's a less concentrated heat-map.

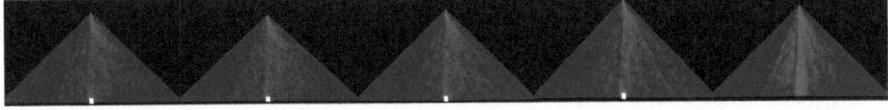

Fig. 2. Results of eye traces for all users by confidence levels (0%, 25%, 50%, 75%, 100%), where eye traces with higher confidence level seem to be more convergent comparing to trails with lower confidence levels. Each red dot represents transformed gaze point.

6   Conclusion

We introduced a novel way of looking at visual attention for users. The new visualization preserves both benefits of showing the temporal quality from a scanpath as well as the overall spatial quality of a heatmap. The results clearly show distinguishable tendency of both eye and mouse movements for different confidence level of their responses. The similarity between eye and mouse patterns may also signify the potential of eye-hand coordination in goal-oriented tasks with various confidence levels. We believe that the correlation between the pattern and the users' confidence level is interesting enough and deserves more attention and research.

Further work is needed, namely by expanding the research to include more subjects and refine the visual representation of the transformed scanpath. Additional efforts should also be devoted to investigate how the method can be applied to different tasks and domains.

References

1. Pomplun, M., Ritter, H., Velichkovsky, B.: Disambiguating Complex Visual Information: Towards Communication of Personal Views of a Scene. Perception 25(8), 931–948 (1996)
2. Wooding, D.S.: Fixation Maps: Quantifying Eye- Movement Traces. In: ETRA 2002: Proceedings of the 2002 Symposium on Eye Tracking Research & Applications, pp. 31–36. ACM, New York (2002)
3. Stellmach, S., Nacke, L., Dachselt, R.: 3D attentional maps: aggregated gaze visualizations in three- dimensional virtual environments. In: Proceedings of the International Conference on Advanced Visual Interfaces, AVI 2010, pp. 345–348. ACM, New York (2010)
4. Duchowski, A.T., et al.: Aggregate gaze visualization with real-time heatmaps. In: Proceedings of the Symposium on Eye Tracking Research and Applications. ACM (2012)
5. Privitera, C.M., Stark, L.W.: Algorithms for defining visual regions-of-interest: Comparison with eye fixations. IEEE Trans. Pattern Anal. Mach. Intell. 22, 970–982 (2000)
6. DuchowskI, A.T., Driver, J., Jolaoso, S., Tan, W., Ramey, B.N., Robbins, A.: Scanpath comparison revisited. In: Proceedings of the 2010 Symposium on Eye- Tracking Research and Applications (ETRA), pp. 219–226. ACM, New York (2010)
7. Raschke, M., Chen, X., Ertl, T.: Parallel scan-path visualization. In: Proceedings of the Symposium on Eye Tracking Research and Applications. ACM (2012)
8. Spakov, O.: iComponent—Device-Independent Platform for Analyzing Eye Movement Data and Developing Eye-Based Applications. PhD thesis, University of Tampere, Finland (2008)
9. Keogh, E.J., Hochheiser, H., Shneiderman, B.: An augmented visual query mechanism for finding patterns in time series data. In: Andreasen, T., Motro, A., Christiansen, H., Larsen, H.L. (eds.) FQAS 2002. LNCS (LNAI), vol. 2522, pp. 240–250. Springer, Heidelberg (2002)
10. Lessing, S., Linge, L.: IICap: A new environment for eye tracking data analysis. Master's thesis. University of Lund, Sweden (2002)
11. Schiessl, M., Duda, S., Thölke, A., Fischer, R.: Eye Tracking and Its Application in Usability and Media Research. MMI-Interaktiv Journal (6), 15–23 (2003)

Dyslexia Explorer: A Screening System for Learning Difficulties in the Arabic Language Using Eye Tracking

Arwa Al-Edaily[1], Areej Al-Wabil[2], and Yousef Al-Ohali[3]

[1] Information Technology Department, King Saud University, Saudi Arabia
aedaily@ksu.edu.sa
[2] Software Engineering Department, King Saud University, Saudi Arabia
aalwabil@ksu.edu.sa
[3] Computer Science Department, King Saud University, Saudi Arabia
yousef@ksu.edu.sa

Abstract. Dyslexia is a Specific Learning Difficulty (SpLD) that affects an individual's ability to process, store, and retrieve information. This consequently affects the educational development of children with dyslexia. Early diagnosis for people with dyslexia is important to assist them in the critical stages of learning. Research examining visual reading patterns in people with SpLDs has suggested that the readers' eye movements reflect the information processing difficulties that they experience. Visual reading patterns can be analyzed for screening purposes; eye tracking technology plays an essential role in this aspect. Research suggest that cognitive processing in reading Arabic demands stronger visual spatial processing abilities related to the nature of the Arabic language. This paper describes a screening system for people with dyslexia based on reading patterns of Arabic scripts using eye-tracking technology. The system records visual reading patterns in reading and provides objective measures of visual attention for SpLD specialists and practitioners to gain insights into the information processing difficulties and for them to design remedial plans for the individual.

Keywords: Dyslexia, Specific Learning Difficulty, Eye tracking, SpLD.

1 Introduction

Dyslexia is a persistent problem in reading and information processing. It affects an estimated 10% of the population (BDA, 2007). Researchers have found that the eye movement patterns and gaze intensity reflect the reading process of people with dyslexia [1]. Combining language-based screening with eye tracking methods provides practitioners with objective measures of visual attention in struggling readers which can consequently assist in detecting the specific difficulty in reading. Eye-gaze analysis in screening for SpLDs in Arabic have not been reported in the assistive technology research domain in reading Arabic text; this may be due to the complexity involved in the analysis of visual patterns exhibited in reading Arabic scripts such as the orthographic directionality of Arabic [2], cursive nature of this language, and the

A. Holzinger et al. (Eds.): SouthCHI 2013, LNCS 7946, pp. 831–834, 2013.

elaborate use of dots to differentiate between different graphemes[3].Variations in the Arabic language when compared to different orthographies may lead to different ma-nifestation of the SpLD in Arabic speaking readers [2][3]. In this paper, a screening system for dyslexia with Arabic texts using eye tracking technology is presented. The "Dyslexia Explorer" system is a screening program to help specialists analyze visual patterns of reading for people with SpLDs and explore individual and aggregate measures of eye gaze intensity and patterns that provide insights into understanding the differences between readers with and without dyslexia.

2   The Dyslexia Explorer System

"Dyslexia Explorer" is a screening program that uses eye-tracking technologies to decode visual patterns of reading in Arabic scripts in order to help SpLD specialists to identify reading problems in general and phonological difficulties in particular for the purpose of designing effective remedial programs for readers with dyslexia.

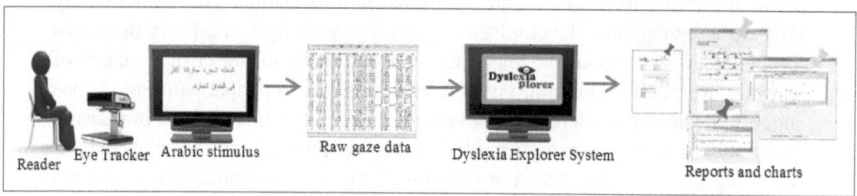

Fig. 1. The Conceptual Design of the Dyslexia Explorer System

The system is comprised of a configurable component for designing sessions with the stimuli and eye gaze analysis component as illustrated in Fig. 1.Dyslexia Explorer acquires the raw gaze data (x/y coordinates, timestamp for each gaze, and the validity code) by corneal reflection captured by a video-based eye tracking device while the individual is reading Arabic scripts. Following that, the system filters the gaze-readings to fixations and saccades using a *Fixation Filtering Algorithm*. Then, it ana-lyzes the fixations' duration and spatial distribution; measurements identified in study [4]. The measurements are: fixation duration in each/all Areas of Interest (AOI) – the areas around the words in the stimulus-, mean fixation duration in all/each AOI, total fixations' count for each/all AOI and backward saccades (regressive saccades). The backward saccade may pass on *one* word, *many* words or *cross* lines in the stimulus. The calculations of these measures and the fixations with saccades are displayed to the user. The reading analysis process is an essential step to explore and configure threshold values on these results (as described in the next section), and to generate understandable formatting reports for the SpLD specialists and practitioners.

2.1   Thresholds' Interactive Charts

Thresholds' interactive charts visualize the results in scattered plot diagrams depicting the results of gaze measures during readings (for individuals with and without dyslexia) with dynamic thresholds on the x and/or y axis (see Fig 2). The visualization provides insights into the type of problems individuals with dyslexia experience and facilitates exploratory analysis of aggregate data to determine normal and abnormal levels of eye gaze measures.

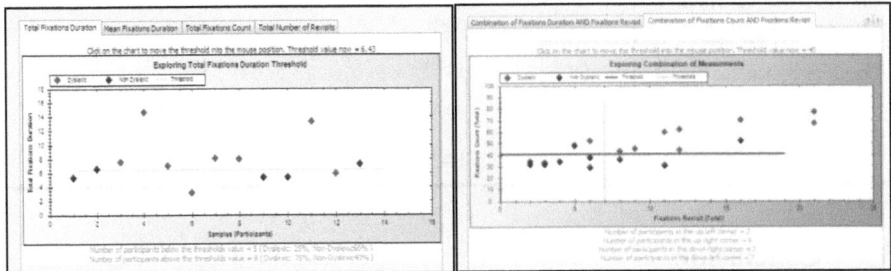

Fig. 2. Two types of interaction charts show reading analysis results for people with and without dyslexia. The second type (right) is a chart of combined measures for exploratory analysis.

2.2   Experiment and Results

Reading experiments with eye tracking were conducted to test the functionality of the screening system and to examine the efficiency of the measurements in differentiating between readers with and without dyslexia. The sample in this experiment was four-teen children (7 with dyslexia and 7 without dyslexia) with ages between 10 and 12 years. They were females in the fourth grade reading level. Six participants were asked to read Arabic text stimuli extracted from the third grade curriculum. The children's eye movements were captured using stand- alone X120 Tobii eye tracker with a sampling rate 120 Hz. The other eight participants were part of a previous study; recordings from the sample examined in an exploratory study described in [4] which involved the same reading task. In this experiment, the raw gaze data for all of the fourteen children was analyzed using the Dyslexia Explorer system.

The results of this experiment demonstrated that the system was effective in filtering and analyzing gaze points for readers efficiently. It reliably displays the fixations and saccades on each stimulus when compared to Tobii Studio visual analysis results. Moreover, the results of the fixation analysis for gaze duration and fixation counts were in agreement with manual review and comparison of these measures that were generated by both systems. The system was also examined for its ability to support SpLD specialists in examining thresholds for gaze measures to differentiate between readers with and without dyslexia on specific visual attention measures as shown in Table 1. For example, some visual attention measures such as fixation duration, mean fixation duration, fixations' count and three cases of backward saccade were able to segment the groups with accuracy levels of 70% and higher. In contrast, the measures backward saccade within a word (between letters) and backward after one fixation in another word were found to be less accurate as no threshold value could be found to separate the two groups with sufficient accuracy.

Table 1. Measurements of the efficiency in differentiating reader groups on a stimuli sample

Measurement	Threshold value	Percentage of readers with dyslexia above the threshold	Percentage of readers without dyslexia below the threshold
(1)Total Fixation Duration	5.8 s	77.98%	71.43%
(2)Mean Fixation Duration	0.19 s	85.71%	85.71%
(3)Total Fixation Count	24	100%	100%
(4)Backward after Multiple Fixations in Another Word	3	71.42%	100%
(5)Backward after Multiple Words	1	100%	71.42%
(6)Cross Line Backward	1	71.47%	100%

3   Conclusion

The "Dyslexia Explorer" system is designed to screen for dyslexia by examining visual attention in reading Arabic script. The system decodes visual patterns captured by eye tracking devices and analyzes the (x/y) coordinates of fixations to generate objective gaze measurements. The system also provides interactive charts with thresholds to explore the reading analysis' results. The system contributes in: screening readers who are at risk of having dyslexia before conducting extensive tests, discovering the strengths and weaknesses of the reader with dyslexia to inform the design of remedial plans and to explore visual attention measures exhibited on reading stimuli that can differentiate between readers with and without dyslexia. An exploratory experiment has shown that the system was able to acquire and analyze gaze data in readings efficiently and accurately. Also, it has found that the visual attention measures differ in their efficiency in distinguishing between readers with and without dyslexia.

Acknowledgements. The authors extend their appreciation to the Deanship of Scientific Research at King Saud University for funding the work through the research group project RGP-VPP-157.

References

1. Rayner, K.: Eye Movements in Reading and Information Processing: 20 Years of Research. Psychological Bulletin 124(3), 372–422 (1998)
2. Goulandris, N.: Dyslexia Diagnosis in Different Language. Whurr (1998)
3. Abu-Rabia, S.: Reading Arabic Texts: Effects of Text Type, Reader Type, and Vowelization. Reading and Writing: An Interdisciplinary Journal 10(2), 106–119 (1998)
4. Al-Wabil, A., Al-Sheaha, M.: Towards an Interactive Screening Program for Developmental Dyslexia: Eye Movement Analysis in Reading Arabic Texts. In: Miesenberger, K., Klaus, J., Zagler, W., Karshmer, A. (eds.) ICCHP 2010, Part II. LNCS, vol. 6180, pp. 25–32. Springer, Heidelberg (2010)

An Analysis of Social Interaction between Older and Children: Augmented Reality Integration in Table Game Design

Chan-Li Lin[1], Shih-Han Fei[2], and Shu-Wei Chang[2]

[1] Dept. of Cultural and Creative Industries Management, National Taipei University of Education, Taiwan
chanli@tea.ntue.edu.tw
[2] Dept. of Digital Multi-Media Design, China University of Technology, Taiwan
feishihhan@gmail.com, book@cute.edu.tw

Abstract. Digital information products are already a part of children's everyday lives, but the majority of older are unfamiliar with these products, widening the generational gap and divide between these groups. To resolve this problem, this study used augmented reality (AR) technology to construct a "barrier-free" digital environment for older. AR integrated game design was used to increase older' exposure to digital information and promote social interaction between children and older, thus reducing intergenerational separation. Consequently, it was possible to ascertain the usability of the table game design, as well as to pinpoint the subjective experiences and differences between the two groups.

Keywords: Augmented Reality, Table Game, Social Interaction.

1 Introduction

Considering the Historic Districts Conservation, Revitalization, and Value-Added Project of the Ministry of Education, the study researchers chose a well-known historical district of Taipei City, namely, Dihua Street of Dadaocheng, as the site for designing a table card game similar to Monopoly that combines 3D modeling and augmented reality (AR) technology in July 2011. The purposes of this game design were to preserve the cultural assets of the Dadaocheng area with digital archive technology and achieve dissemination and added value through digital media technology.

Taiwan has gradually become an aging society, and the digital divide phenomenon is continuously observed among seniors. The primary difference between seniors and schoolchildren is that seniors are less familiar with games and more apprehensive of complex game installation processes and content [1]. Therefore, how to construct a "barrier-free" digital environment for seniors and employing game designs using AR technology that enhance their experience of digital information and increase the interaction between seniors and schoolchildren to, thus, eliminate generation gaps have become crucial issues worthy of further exploration.

A. Holzinger et al. (Eds.): SouthCHI 2013, LNCS 7946, pp. 835–838, 2013.

2   Literature Review

2.1   Augmented Technology

AR technology combines 3D virtual modeling images with actual environments in real-time [2]. AR possesses the following three key features: (1) a combination of the virtual and real worlds; (2) instant interaction; and (3) 3D space [3]. AR technology integrates 3D virtual objects with actual environments in real-time, incorporating them into real-life scenarios. However, AR does not replace the real world; instead, it materializes real-life information. In addition, AR enables learners to immerse themselves in the learning content and, thus, can sustain children's focus for longer durations during the learning process [4].

2.2   Social Interaction

The population structure of Taiwan has significantly changed in recent years. The number of seniors over the age of 65 has increased progressively, accounting for 10.8% of the total population. Thus, Taiwan has gradually become an aging society. In addition to the emergence of senior population issues, the impact of this transformation into an aging society is reflected by the intergenerational estrangement that exists between seniors and younger generations because of a lack of interactions. Considered these issues from a psychological perspective and suggested that filial piety is no longer the primary reason for children to live in the same household as their parents; instead, multi-generational households are affected by various parent-child interactions, such as seniors caring for their grandchildren and family members caring for each other's daily lives.

The term "interaction" was coined by Isaac Taylor in 1832. He defined interaction as reciprocal action, that is, the effects or actions between people and objects [5]. Social interaction refers to a particular form of externalities, where the actions of a reference group affect an individual's preferences [6]. Interaction in social situations can be considered the dialogue between users and the by-products of civilization, or a certain level of interaction between integrated digitalized media and users [7].

2.3   Intergenerational Interactive Game Design

Appropriate opportunities for intergenerational communication and interaction can significantly improve positive relationships between generations. Therefore, various intergenerational programs have been developed [8] [9]. The UNESCO described intergenerational learning as an effective tool for resolving social problems. Intergenerational learning has the functions of (1) connecting estranged generations; (2) passing on cultural traditions; (3) encouraging cross-generational learning and living; (4) facilitating intergenerational resource sharing; (5) addressing the challenges presented by cross-generational social problems; and (6) assisting in lifelong learning [10].

3   Research Process

This study selected students from a class at Tucheng Elementary School, New Taipei City, as the sample for the intergenerational upbringing questionnaire. Overall, 30 questionnaires were distributed, and 29 questionnaires were returned. None of the returned questionnaires were incomplete; thus, all 29 questionnaires were valid. Subsequently, eight respondents who achieved a questionnaire score above 9 were selected to test the game. The selected participants, including seniors and schoolchildren, were all interested in promoting intergenerational relationships.

The research subjects comprised eight grandmothers, seven female schoolchildren, and one male schoolchild, for a total of 16 participants. To understand the subjects' pre-game conditions, 16 pretest questionnaires were distributed, and 16 posttest questionnaires and usability scales were distributed to assess the subjects' post-game changes and game performance.

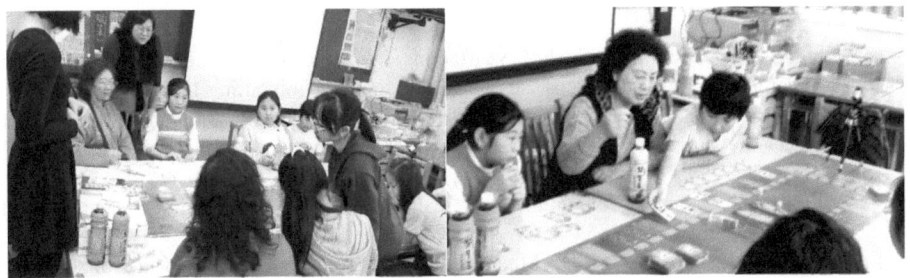

Fig. 1. The game play process

4   Discussion

This study developed an AR-integrated table card game that combines modern digital technology and traditional cultural assets. By video-recording the entire game play process, the study analyzed the social interaction between the subjects before, during, and after the game. The results show that two types of social behavior, that is, knowledge exchange behavior and function card social behavior involving functional cards, were observed. The function card social behavior was further classified as follows: (1) competitive behavior; (2) mutual-assistance behavior; and (3) opportunistic behavior. The results also indicate that the AR game design can promote intergenerational learning and interaction. The design of the function cards in the game encourages substantial intergenerational interaction, competition, and cooperation. The results of this study can provide a reference for game development in intergenerational programs.

In addition, the research results show that games designed with AR-integration and card game principles are widely accepted by seniors and schoolchildren, and successfully encourage both parties to play together. Unexpectedly, this study found that the opinions of seniors and schoolchildren regarding the AR 3D images differed. Generally, the seniors considered 3D images necessary because it increased their and the schoolchildren's interest in the game. By contrast, half the schoolchildren considered the 3D images unnecessary. Although the schoolchildren were initially attracted to the AR technology, they tended not to observe the 3D images displayed on the computer screen during the game; instead, they typically focused on the game behavior of the other players and how to win the game.

However, both the seniors and the schoolchildren agreed that they were attracted to play the game because of the AR technology. This suggests that the game content design successfully promoted intergenerational interaction and learning while providing a "barrier-free" digital environment to increase players' experience of digital information, reduce the digital wall phenomenon, and increase social interaction between players.

References

1. Mahmud, A.A., Mubin, O., Shahid, S., Martens, J.B.: Designing social games for children and older adults: Two related case studies. Entertainment Computing 1, 147–156 (2010)
2. Azuma, R., Baillot, Y., Behringer, R., Feiner, S., Julier, S., Macintyre, B.: Resent Advances in Augmented Reailty. IEEE Computer Graphics and Appilcations 21(6), 34–47 (2001)
3. Azuma, R.: A survey of augmented reality. Presence: Teleoperators and Virtual Environments 6(4), 355–385 (1997)
4. Kaufmann, H., Schmalstieg, D.: Mathematics and geometry education with collaborative augmented reality. Computers & Graphics 27, 339–345 (2003)
5. Keleti, P.: From action to interaction: Values, methods, and goals in philosophy, culture and education. Peter Lang, New York (1988)
6. Scheinkman, J.A.: Social interactions. In: Goulder, L.H., Pizer, W.A. (eds.) New Palgrave Dictionary of Economics, 2nd edn., Macmillan, New York (2004) (forthcoming)
7. Graham, L.: The principles of interactive design. Delmar, NY (1999)
8. Ohsako, T.: The role of intergenerational program in promoting lifelong learning for all ages (2002),
   http://www.unesco.org/education/uie/pdf/uiestud36.pdf (retrieved December 23, 2004)
9. Newman, S.: History and evolution of intergenerational program. In: Newman, S., Ward, C.R., Smith, T.B., Wilson, J.O., McCrea, J.M. (eds.) Intergenerational Program: Past, Present and Future, pp. 55–78. Taylor & Francis, Washington, DC (1997)
10. Bostrum, A.K., Hatton-Yeo, A., Ohsaka, T., Sawano, Y.: A general assessment of IP initiatives in the countries involved. In: Hatton-Yeo, A., Ohsako, T. (eds.) Intergenerational Programmes: Public Policy and Research Implications an International Perspective, pp. 3–8 (2000),
    http://www.unesco.org/education/uie/pdf/intergen.pdf (retrived November 20, 2004)

Justification of User Profiles Based
on the Mental Models' Competency

Ieva Bolakova, Svetlana Ignatjeva, and Nellija Bogdanova

Department of Computer Science, Daugavpils University, Latvia
{ieva.bolakova,svetlana.ignatjeva,nellija.bogdanova}@du.lv

Abstract. Information technologies (IT) environment of a researcher can include a large amount of computer tools. To raise the efficiency of research
process, one needs to identify the groups of users and clarify the functionality
of the IT environment for every individual user by considering the peculiarities
of the individual's work. The analysis of the structure of a researcher's competence model helped the authors to describe the content and structure of the researcher's as a user's mental model.

Keywords: users' mental model, competence, research work, user profile.

1 Introduction

The quality management and enhancing of the efficiency of research work imply
selection of optimal computer tools. Careful selecting of those tools is the task for
both the user-researcher, and the designer of the proper information and research environment.

The understanding of this proper information and research environment, its functionality, research methodology, and ways of interacting with software comprises the
essence of the user's mental model or concept model [3], which is characterized by
the following features: (i) obscurity – user's understanding of a system is ill defined
by the user himself/herself [3]; (ii) adaptivity and the dynamics – models change due
to one's experience with the system, communication with other users, information
from other sources and even on the basis of interaction with other systems [7];
(iii) selectivity – user excludes those elements that do not agree with his/her mental
model and adds other elements that strengthen the existing model, gives more or less
intensive meaning to the external elements depending on whether they keep to the
current model or not [5]; (iv) inertia – user can expect the system behavior to be similar to the already familiar model [4]; (v) subjectivity – user plans his/her actions in
line with his/her personal mental models, which may differ from the existing
models [6].

Competencies are behaviors that encompass knowledge, skills, and attributes required for a successful performance. Competency modeling is the activity of determining specific competencies that are characteristic of high performance and success
in a given job [1]. The user's requirements regarding skills, knowledge and attributes

A. Holzinger et al. (Eds.): SouthCHI 2013, LNCS 7946, pp. 839–842, 2013.

of work with computer tools may be determined via the competence model of the researcher.

For practical purposes, it is important to identify qualitatively the content of mental models (constructing personas [3], ethnographic interviews [3]), and to quantify the extent to which the mental model user interface [2].

The aim of the research: to make up a set of computer tools for user profiles appropriate to their competence model.

2   Research Procedure and Findings

64 respondents – doctoral students and candidates for the scientific degree in such study programmes as Economics, Biology, Pedagogy and Psychology at Daugavpils University – took part in the research. They filled in questionnaires, answered questions about their real and desired level of research competencies, their research strategies, and evaluated their level of knowledge and skills concerning the IT and the use of computer tools.

The competence model comprises 38 indicators that reflect methodological, practical, organizational and communication aspects of research activity. The analysis of a researcher's competence model allowed formulating a set of IT competencies necessary for conducting an efficient scientific work.

The program package SPSS (Statistical Package for the Social Sciences, 19.0 version for Windows) was used for statistical analysis of the data and for presenting the research findings.

In order to analyze the structure of respondents' computer competency, the authors used exploratory factor analysis that was carried out according to the following scheme: Extraction Method: Principal Component Analysis. Rotation Method: Varimax with Kaiser Normalization.

Kaiser-Meyer-Olkin Measure of Sampling Adequacy (KMO) equals to 0,847, for the factor analysis based on the evaluation of real skills and knowledge, and exceeds 0,800 in all other situations, which demonstrates the expediency of this procedure in dealing with the current issue. The structure of factors obtained by means of the evaluation of those skills necessary for successful research work is represented by three factors that may be interpreted as

- Basic IT competency;
- Quantitative analysis of data;
- Modeling and Data Mining.

The structure of factors does not change during the factor analysis in various situations.

Table 1 illustrates the structure of factors necessary for the researchers' computer competency as Factor Matrix, and Factor Loadings of several indicators.

The table provides information on the percentage of summary variance that explains every separate factor.

The value of Cronbach'sAlfa criteria, according to the table, is in range of 0,950 - 0,974. This indicates the high coherence of separate points in the questionnaire. Factor Scores may be obtained by both in the result of exploratory factor analysis and as the result of summing up the respective indicators. In the second case, to gain better understanding and further interpretation, standardization of factor evaluation should take place.

Table 1. Factor Matrix

Factors	Alpha	% of variance	IT- competences	Factor Loadings	User Profile
Basic computer competencies	0,953	30,60%	Internet usage as scientific communication tool	0,920	MS Power Point
			Graphs and diagrams construction	0,919	MS Excel
			Presentation preparation	0,893	MS Word
			Data processing and visualization	0,870	Adobe Acrobat
			Obtaining necessary quantitative information with Internet	0,833	
			Data export to PDF format. PDF document editing	0,872	
			Document structuring and layout designing with use of styles	0,771	
			Presentation of research findings via Internet	0,742	
			Working in Adobe Acrobat	0,744	
			Effective participation in work of professional Internet associations	0,517	
Quantitative analysis of data	0,950	16,65%	Confirmatory factor analysis	0,415	SPSS Statistics
			Exploratory factor analysis	0,581	
			Receiving and analysis of descriptive statistics' results	0,488	
			Application of checking criteria of statistical hypotheses	0,528	
			Data classification and cluster analysis	0,758	
			Working with data in SPSS	0,735	
			Multidimensional data analysis	0,727	
			Correlation, dispersive, regression analysis of data	0,704	
Modeling and Data Mining	0,974	34,76%	Object-oriented analysis and modeling	0,914	SPSS Clementine AMOS MS Visio Bpwin
			Methodology of functional modeling SADT	0,898	
			Data Mining methods usage for data analysis	0,876	
			Modeling by the linear structural equations	0,872	
			Data Mining components usage	0,865	
			Semantic and graphical description of models with UML	0,863	
			Modeling and analysis in AMOS	0,856	
			Working with data and models construction	0,844	
			Decomposition and structuring of the studied phenomena	0,628	

Cluster Analysis of factors concerning the respondents' computer competency allowed forming of two homogenous clusters. Besides, the most considerable differentiation abilities were demonstrated by such factors as Quantitative analysis of data and Modeling and Data Mining. Only 30% of the respondents did not consider those important for successful research work. In addition, the level of the basic IT competencies for those clusters singled out by the respondents do not differ to a great statistical extent *(Mean(1) = 3,56*; *Mean(2) = 3,81*; *t-test for Equality of Means, Sig. (2-tailed) = 0,267)*.

3   Conclusions

The competency mental model of a researcher's information system has three functional parts: (i) basic competencies, (ii) quantitative analysis of data, (iii) modeling and data mining. Users' profile is a combination of these functional parts, the compulsory one being basic competencies.

The content of a user's profile to a lesser degree depends on the object area, in which the researcher works, but to a higher degree – on his/her research strategy (qualitative or quantitative approach).

The user's profile of a researcher should be created in accordance with the level necessary for successful research work and in line with the skills and knowledge of computer tools. The user's profile based on the real level of computer capabilities does not meet the competence model of a successful researcher.

Acknowledgements. This work has been supported by ERAF within the project "Daugavpils University Technology Transfer Bureau", agreement Nr.L-TPK-08-0004, ID Nr. TPK/2.1.2.1.2/08/01/009.

References

1. Bogzda, I., Olehnovic, E., Ignatjeva, S.: Doctoral Students' Competence for Reseach Activities in Internet Resources Implementation. In: Partycky, S. (ed.) The Network Society, vol. 2, pp. 182–187. WydawnistwoKul, Lublin (2011)
2. Calero Valdez, A., Ziefle, M., Alagöz, F., Holzinger, A.: Mental Models of Menu Structures in Diabetes Assistants. In: Miesenberger, K., Klaus, J., Zagler, W., Karshmer, A. (eds.) ICCHP 2010, Part II. LNCS, vol. 6180, pp. 584–591. Springer, Heidelberg (2010)
3. Cooper, A., Reimann, R., Cronin, D.: About Face 3: The Essentials of Interaction Design. Wiley (2007)
4. Korchanov, S.: Menta Models, = Корчанов, С. Ментальные модели,
   http://marketing.ru/page.php?ss=201&tp=P
5. Mandel, T.: The Elements of User Interface Design, 2nd edn. John Wiley & Sons (2007)
6. Raskin, J.: The Humane Interface: New Directions for Designing Interactive Systems. Addison-Wesley Professional (2000)
7. Torres, R.J.: Practitioner's Handbook for User Interface Design and Development. Prentice Hall (2001)

Author Index